MW01098544

Psychosocial Care of End-Stage Organ Disease and Transplant Patients

Yelizaveta Sher · José R. Maldonado
Editors

Psychosocial Care of End-Stage Organ Disease and Transplant Patients

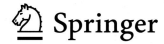

Editors
Yelizaveta Sher
Stanford University School of Medicine
Stanford, CA
USA

José R. Maldonado
Stanford University School of Medicine
Stanford, CA
USA

ISBN 978-3-319-94913-0   ISBN 978-3-319-94914-7   (eBook)
https://doi.org/10.1007/978-3-319-94914-7

Library of Congress Control Number: 2018958603

This Springer imprint is published by the registered company Springer Nature Switzerland AG
The registered company address is: Gewerbestrasse 11, 6330 Cham, Switzerland

Contents

Part I   Introduction

1   Introduction...   3
     Yelizaveta Sher and José R. Maldonado

2   Overview of Solid Organ Transplantation and the
     United States National Organ Transplant Act (NOTA).....................   9
     Oscar Salvatierra and José R. Maldonado

**Part II   Pre-transplant Psychosocial Evaluation
         of Prospective Recipients and Donors**

3   The Psychosocial Evaluation of Transplant Candidates....................   17
     José R. Maldonado

4   The Psychosocial Evaluation of Live Donors............................   49
     Akhil Shenoy

Part III   Renal Patient

5   Chronic and End-Stage Renal Disease and Indications
     for Renal Transplantation   63
     Adetokunbo Taiwo

6   Mental Health in Chronic and End-Stage Renal Disease   73
     Paula C. Zimbrean, Jennifer Braverman, and Marta Novak

7   Dialysis: Medical and Psychological Considerations......................   91
     Filza Hussain and Paula C. Zimbrean

8   History of Renal Transplantation 103
     John D. Scandling

9   Medical Course and Complications After Renal Transplantation............ 111
     Aleah Brubaker, Dan Stoltz, and Amy Gallo

10   Post-transplant Psychosocial and Mental Health Care of the Renal Recipient..... 119
     Mary Amanda Dew, Larissa Myaskovsky, Jennifer L. Steel, and Andrea F.
     DiMartini

Part IV   Liver Patient

11   End-Stage Liver Disease and Indications for Liver Transplantation.......... 139
     Aparna Goel, Osama Siddique, and Aijaz Ahmed

12   Mental Health in Chronic and End-Stage Liver Disease 147
     Rebekah Nash, Eric Golden, Mary Amanda Dew, and Andrea F. DiMartini

13 History of Liver Transplantation 159
Adam X. Sang and Carlos O. Esquivel

14 Medical Course and Complications After Liver Transplantation 169
Rajanshu Verma and Sanjaya K. Satapathy

**15 Post-transplant Psychosocial and Mental Health Care
of the Liver Recipient** 181
Andrea F. DiMartini, Eric Golden, Andrew Matz, Mary Amanda Dew, and
Catherine Crone

Part V   Cardiac Patient

16 End-Stage Heart Disease and Indications for Heart Transplantation 195
June Rhee and Randall Vagelos

17 Mental Health in Chronic and End-Stage Heart Disease 205
Yelizaveta Sher

18 ICDs, VADs, and Total Artificial Heart Implantation 215
Jared J. Herr

19 History of Heart Transplantation 225
Sharon A. Hunt

20 Medical Course and Complications After Heart Transplantation 227
Ranjan Ray and Michael Pham

**21 Post-transplant Psychosocial and Mental Health Care
of the Cardiac Recipient** 237
Peter A. Shapiro, Luis F. Pereira, Katherine E. Taylor, and Ilona Wiener

Part VI   Lung Patient

22 End-Stage Lung Disease and Indications for Lung Transplantation 247
Joshua J. Lee and Laveena Chhatwani

23 Mental Health in Chronic and End-Stage Lung Disease 255
Yelizaveta Sher

**24 Extracorporeal Membrane Oxygenation: Medical and Psychological
Considerations** 267
Joshua J. Lee and Joshua J. Mooney

25 History of Lung Transplantation 273
Kapil Patel and David Weill

26 Medical Course and Complications After Lung Transplantation 279
Guillermo Garrido and Gundeep S. Dhillon

**27 Post-transplant Psychosocial and Mental Health Care
of the Lung Recipient** 289
Yelizaveta Sher

Part VII   Visceral Transplantation

28 Intestinal Failure and Indications for Visceral Transplantation 301
Yelizaveta Sher

29   History of Visceral Transplantation 307
Sherif Armanyous, Mohammed Osman, Neha Parekh, Masato Fujiki,
Raffaele Girlanda, Guilherme Costa, and Kareem M. Abu-Elmagd

**30   Mental Health in Patients Requiring Pancreas
and Visceral Transplantation**.. 321
Catherine Crone and Jacqueline Posada

**31   Enteral and Parenteral Nutrition: Considerations for Visceral
Transplant Patients**.. 329
Neha D. Shah and Michelle Stroebe

32   Medical Course and Complications After Visceral Transplantation 337
Waldo Concepcion and Lung-Yi Lee

**33   Post-transplant Psychosocial and Mental Health Care
of Pancreas and Visceral Transplant Recipients** 343
Jaqueline Posada and Catherine Crone

Part VIII   Vascularized Composite Allotransplantation (VCA)

34   Psychological and Psychosocial Aspects of Face Transplantation 353
Kathy L. Coffman

35   Psychological and Psychosocial Aspects of Limb Transplantation............ 365
Martin Kumnig and Sheila G. Jowsey-Gregoire

**36   Psychological and Psychosocial Aspects of Uterine
and Penile Transplantation** 377
Andrea Ament and Sheila G. Jowsey-Gregoire

Part IX   Hematopoietic Cell Transplantation

**37   Bone Marrow Malignancies and Indications for Hematopoietic Cell
Transplantation**... 387
Laura Johnston

38   Mental Health Prior to Hematopoietic Cell Transplantation................ 401
Sheila Lahijani

39   History of Hematopoietic Cell Transplantation.......................... 413
Jaroslava Salman, Kimberly Shapiro, and Stephen J. Forman

**40   Medical Course and Complications After Hematopoietic
Cell Transplantation**.. 417
Janice (Wes) Brown and Judith A. Shizuru

**41   Post-transplant Psychosocial and Mental Health Care
of Hematopoietic Cell Transplant Recipients**........................... 439
Renee Garcia

Part X   General Considerations in the Treatment of Transplant Patients

42   Psychopharmacology in Transplant Patients............................ 453
Martha C. Gamboa and Stephen J. Ferrando

43   Psychotherapy in Transplant Patients 471
Mariana Schmajuk, Earl DeGuzman, and Nicole Allen

**44 Social Work Interventions in End-Stage Organ Disease
     and Transplant Patients** **483**
     Caitlin J. West and Kelsey Winnike

Part XI Other Considerations

45 Substance Use Disorders in Transplant Patients **493**
     Marian Fireman

46 Special Considerations in Pediatric Transplant Patients **505**
     Lauren M. Schneider, Catherine Naclerio, and Carol Conrad

47 Palliative Care in Transplant Patients **517**
     Anna Piotrowski and Susan Imamura

48 Ethical Considerations in Transplant Patients. **527**
     Nuriel Moghavem and David Magnus

49 Cultural Aspects of Transplantation **539**
     Sheila Lahijani and Renee Garcia

50 Patient Perspectives **547**
     Eirik Gumeny, Gerardine Hernandez, Tyson Hughes, and Yelizaveta Sher

Index **553**

Contributors

Kareem M. Abu-Elmagd, MD, PhD, FACS Center for Gut Rehabilitation and Transplantation, Department of Surgery, Digestive Disease and Surgery Institute, Cleveland Clinic, Cleveland, OH, USA

Aijaz Ahmed, MD Division of Gastroenterology and Hepatology, Department of Medicine, Stanford University School of Medicine, Stanford, CA, USA

Nicole Allen, MD Department of Psychiatry, Lenox Hill Hospital/Northwell Health, New York, NY, USA

Department of Psychiatry, Donald and Barbara Zucker School of Medicine at Hofstra/Northwell, Hempstead, NY, USA

Department of Psychiatry, SUNY Downstate School of Medicine, Brooklyn, NY, USA

Andrea Ament, MD Department of Psychiatry and Behavioral Sciences, Stanford University School of Medicine, Stanford, CA, USA

Sherif Armanyous, MD Center for Gut Rehabilitation and Transplantation, Department of Surgery, Digestive Disease and Surgery Institute, Cleveland Clinic, Cleveland, OH, USA

Jennifer Braverman, MD Department of Psychiatry, University of Toronto, Toronto, ON, Canada

Centre For Mental Health, University Health Network-Toronto General Hospital, Toronto, ON, Canada

Janice (Wes) Brown, MD Division of Blood and Marrow Transplantation, Department of Medicine, Stanford University School of Medicine, Stanford, CA, USA

Aleah Brubaker, MD, PhD Department of General Surgery, Stanford University School of Medicine, Stanford, CA, USA

Laveena Chhatwani, MD Division of Pulmonary and Critical Care, Department of Medicine, Stanford University School of Medicine, Stanford, CA, USA

Kathy L. Coffman, MD, FACLP Department of Psychiatry and Psychology, Cleveland Clinic, Cleveland, OH, USA

Waldo Concepcion, MD Division of Abdominal Transplantation, Departments of Surgery and Pediatrics, Stanford University School of Medicine, Stanford, CA, USA

Carol Conrad, MD Pediatric Lung and Heart-Lung Transplant Program, Division of Pulmonary Pediatrics, Department of Pediatrics, Stanford University School of Medicine, Stanford, CA, USA

Guilherme Costa, MD Center for Gut Rehabilitation and Transplantation, Department of Surgery, Digestive Disease and Surgery Institute, Cleveland Clinic, Cleveland, OH, USA

Catherine Crone, MD, FACLP Department of Psychiatry, Inova Fairfax Hospital, Falls Church, VA, USA

Department of Psychiatry, Virginia Commonwealth University School of Medicine, Richmond, VA, USA

Department of Psychiatry, George Washington University School of Medicine, Washington, DC, USA

Earl DeGuzman, MD Traditions Behavioral Health, Napa, CA, USA

Mary Amanda Dew, Phd Departments of Psychiatry, Psychology, Epidemiology, Biostatistics and the Clinical and Translational Science Institute, University of Pittsburgh, Pittsburgh, PA, USA

Gundeep S. Dhillon, MD Division of Pulmonary and Critical Care, Department of Medicine, Stanford University School of Medicine, Stanford, CA, USA

Andrea F. DiMartini, MD, FACLP Departments of Psychiatry and Surgery and the Clinical and Translational Science Institute, University of Pittsburgh, Pittsburgh, PA, USA

Carlos O. Esquivel, MD, PhD Division of Abdominal Transplantation, Department of Surgery, Stanford University School of Medicine, Stanford, CA, USA

Stephen J. Ferrando, MD Department of Psychiatry and Behavioral Sciences, New York Medical College, Valhalla, NY, USA

Marian Fireman, MD Department of Psychiatry, Oregon Health and Science University, Portland, OR, USA

Stephen J. Forman, MD Department of Hematology and Hematopoietic Cell Transplantation, City of Hope, Duarte, CA, USA

Masato Fujiki, MD Center for Gut Rehabilitation and Transplantation, Department of Surgery, Digestive Disease and Surgery Institute, Cleveland Clinic, Cleveland, OH, USA

Amy Gallo, MD Division of Abdominal Transplantation, Department of General Surgery, Stanford University School of Medicine, Stanford, CA, USA

Martha C. Gamboa, MD Department of Psychiatry and Behavioral Sciences, New York Medical College, Valhalla, NY, USA

Renee Garcia, MD Department of Psychiatry and Behavioral Sciences, Stanford University School of Medicine, Stanford, CA, USA

Hoag Presbyterian Memorial Hospital, Newport Beach, Stanford, CA, USA

Guillermo Garrido, MD Division of Pulmonary and Critical Care, Department of Medicine, Stanford University School of Medicine, Stanford, CA, USA

Raffaele Girlanda, MD Center for Gut Rehabilitation and Transplantation, Department of Surgery, Digestive Disease and Surgery Institute, Cleveland Clinic, Cleveland, OH, USA

Aparna Goel, MD Division of Gastroenterology and Hepatology, Department of Medicine, Stanford University School of Medicine, Stanford, CA, USA

Eric Golden, MD Department of Psychiatry, University of Pittsburgh, Pittsburgh, PA, USA

Eirik Gumeny, BA Stanford University Medical Center, Stanford, CA, USA

Gerardine Hernandez, BS Stanford University Medical Center, Stanford, CA, USA

Jared J. Herr, MD Sutter Health Center for Advanced Heart Failure Therapies, California Pacific Medical Center, San Francisco, CA, USA

Tyson Hughes, AA Stanford University Medical Center, Stanford, CA, USA

Sharon A. Hunt, MD Division of Cardiovascular Medicine, Department of Medicine, Stanford University, Stanford, CA, USA

Filza Hussain, MD Department of Psychiatry and Behavioral Sciences, Stanford University School of Medicine, Stanford, CA, USA

Susan Imamura, MD Department of Psychiatry, Kaiser Permanente, San Jose, CA, USA

Laura Johnston, MD Division of Blood and Marrow Transplantation, Department of Medicine, Stanford University School of Medicine, Stanford, CA, USA

Sheila G. Jowsey-Gregoire, MD Department of Psychiatry and Psychology and Department of Surgery, Mayo Graduate School of Medicine, Mayo Clinic Rochester, Rochester, MN, USA

Martin Kumnig Department of Medical Psychology, Center for Advanced Psychology in Plastic and Transplant Surgery, Innsbruck Medical University, Innsbruck, Austria

Sheila Lahijani, MD Department of Psychiatry and Behavioral Sciences, Stanford University School of Medicine, Stanford, CA, USA

Joshua J. Lee, MD Division of Pulmonary and Critical Care, Department of Medicine, Stanford University School of Medicine, Stanford, CA, USA

Lung-Yi Lee, MD Division of Abdominal Transplantation, Department of Surgery, Stanford University School of Medicine, Stanford, CA, USA

David Magnus, PhD Center of Biomedical Ethics, Stanford University School of Medicine, Stanford, CA, USA

José R. Maldonado, MD, FACLP, FACFE Department of Psychiatry & Behavioral Sciences, Stanford University School of Medicine, Stanford, CA, USA

Andrew Matz, MD Department of Psychiatry at Inova Fairfax Hospital and George Washington University Medical Center, Inova Fairfax Hospital, Church, VA, USA

Nuriel Moghavem, MD Department of Neurology and Neurological Sciences, Stanford University School of Medicine, Stanford, CA, USA

Joshua J. Mooney, MD Division of Pulmonary and Critical Care, Department of Medicine, Stanford University School of Medicine, Stanford, CA, USA

Larissa Myaskovsky, Phd Department of Internal Medicine, Nephrology Division and the Center for Healthcare Equity in Kidney Disease, University of New Mexico School of Medicine, Albuquerque, NM, USA

Catherine Naclerio, PsyD PGSP-Stanford Psy.D. Consortium, Palo Alto, CA, USA

Department of Psychology, Holtz Children's Hospital, Jackson Health System, Miami, FL, USA

Rebekah Nash, MD Department of Psychiatry, University of North Carolina Hospitals, Chapel Hill, NC, USA

Marta Novak, MD, PhD Department of Psychiatry, University of Toronto, Toronto, ON, Canada

Centre For Mental Health, University Health Network-Toronto General Hospital, Toronto, ON, Canada

Mohammed Osman, MD Center for Gut Rehabilitation and Transplantation, Department of Surgery, Digestive Disease and Surgery Institute, Cleveland Clinic, Cleveland, OH, USA

Neha Parekh, RD Center for Gut Rehabilitation and Transplantation, Department of Surgery, Digestive Disease and Surgery Institute, Cleveland Clinic, Cleveland, OH, USA

Kapil Patel, MD Center for Advanced Lung Disease, Division of Pulmonary and Critical Care Medicine, Morsani College of Medicine, University of South Florida, Tampa, FL, USA

Luis F. Pereira, MD Department of Psychiatry, Columbia University Irving Medical Center, New York, NY, USA

Michael Pham, MD Center for Advanced Heart Failure Therapies, Palo Alto Foundation Medical Group, San Francisco, CA, USA

Anna Piotrowski, MD Department of Psychiatry, Kaiser Permanente, San Jose, CA, USA

Jacqueline Posada, MD Department of Psychiatry, George Washington University School of Medicine, Washington, DC, USA

Ranjan Ray, MD Center for Advanced Heart Failure Therapies, Palo Alto Foundation Medical Group, San Francisco, CA, USA

June Rhee, MD Division of Cardiovascular Medicine, Department of Medicine, Stanford University School of Medicine, Stanford, CA, USA

Jaroslava Salman, MD Department of Psychiatry and Psychology, City of Hope, Duarte, CA, USA

Oscar Salvatierra, MD Stanford University School of Medicine, Stanford, CA, USA

Adam X. Sang, MD Department of Surgery, Stanford University School of Medicine, Stanford, CA, USA

Sanjaya K. Satapathy, MBBS, MD, DM, FACG, FASGE, AGAF Division of Transplantation, Methodist University Hospital Transplant Institute/University of Tennessee Health Sciences Center, Memphis, TN, USA

John D. Scandling, MD Division of Nephrology, Department of Medicine, Stanford University School of Medicine, Stanford, CA, USA

Mariana Schmajuk, MD Department of Psychiatry and Behavioral Sciences, Stanford University School of Medicine, Stanford, CA, USA

Lauren M. Schneider, PsyD Division of Child and Adolescent Psychiatry, Department of Psychiatry and Behavioral Sciences, Stanford University School of Medicine, Stanford, CA, USA

Neha D. Shah, MPH, RD, CNSC Intestinal and Transplant Program, Digestive Health Center, Stanford Health Care, Palo Alto, CA, USA

Kimberly Shapiro, MD Department of Psychiatry and Psychology, City of Hope, Duarte, CA, USA

Peter A. Shapiro, MD Department of Psychiatry, Columbia University Irving Medical Center, New York, NY, USA

Akhil Shenoy, MD, MPH Department of Psychiatry, Columbia University Medical Center, New York, NY, USA

Yelizaveta Sher, MD Department of Psychiatry and Behavioral Sciences, Stanford University School of Medicine, Stanford, CA, USA

Judith A. Shizuru, MD, PhD Division of Blood and Marrow Transplantation, Department of Medicine, Stanford University School of Medicine, Stanford, CA, USA

Osama Siddique, MD Department of Medicine, Memorial Hospital of Rhode Island/Alpert Medical School of Brown University, Providence, RI, USA

Jennifer L. Steel, PhD Departments of Surgery, Psychiatry, and Psychology, University of Pittsburgh, Pittsburgh, PA, USA

Dan Stoltz, BS Stanford University School of Medicine, Stanford, CA, USA

Michelle Stroebe, MS, RD Center for Advanced Lung Disease, Stanford Health Care, Palo Alto, CA, USA

Adetokunbo Taiwo, MD Division of Nephrology, Kidney Pancreas Transplant Program, Department of Medicine, Stanford University School of Medicine, Palo Alto, CA, USA

Katherine E. Taylor, MD Department of Psychiatry, Columbia University Irving Medical Center, New York, NY, USA

Department of Psychiatry, New York University Medical Center, New York, NY, USA

Randall H. Vagelos, MD Division of Cardiovascular Medicine, Department of Medicine, Stanford University School of Medicine, Stanford, CA, USA

Rajanshu Verma, MD Division of Transplantation, Methodist University Hospital Transplant Institute/University of Tennessee Health Sciences Center, Memphis, TN, USA

David Weill, MD Weill Consulting Group, New Orleans, LA, USA

Caitlin J. West, LCSW Department of Social Work, University of Colorado Hospital, Aurora, CO, USA

Ilona Wiener, MD Department of Psychiatry, Columbia University Irving Medical Center, New York, NY, USA

Kelsey Winnike, MSW, LCSW, CCTSW Department of Social Work and Case Management, Stanford Health Care, Stanford, CA, USA

Paula C. Zimbrean, MD, FAPA, FACLP Transplant Psychiatry Services at Yale New Haven Hospital, Departments of Psychiatry and Surgery, New Haven, CT, USA

Part I
Introduction

Introduction

Yelizaveta Sher and José R. Maldonado

Organ transplantation aims to extend lives, improve quality of life, and deliver hope to many patients and their families. However, the path to transplantation is fraught with angst and challenges. Failing health is usually associated with changes in social (e.g., loss of work, loss of status), interpersonal (e.g., change in relationships, loss of activities), and psychological (e.g., anxiety, depression, panic attacks) struggles.

There are numerous emotional, behavioral, and psychological aspects to organ transplantation, and psychiatric consultants have been involved with the transplantation process since its inception. In fact, Richard Herrick, the first successful kidney recipient, experienced an episode of delirium just before his transplant surgery, causing concern to his providers and complicating his care. Dr. Joseph Murray, the pioneer plastic surgeon turned transplant surgeon, described this dramatic episode in his autobiography *Surgery of the Soul* [1]. Richard Herrick was admitted to the Peter Bent Brigham Hospital on October 26, 1954, with chronic nephritis. Dr. Murray described the clinical challenges the patient and his medical team experienced due to "Richard's difficult behavior as a result of his illness." He borrows the following excerpts from Richard's medical record [1]:

> Since admission patient has been extremely uncooperative. Has knocked over infusions, has been restrained, has been moved to side room because of loud outbursts. Restless, cursing all members of the House Staff…
> Rather a difficult p.m. … Is extremely uncooperative. Behavior erratic and unpredictable. Bit nurse on hand while bed linen being changed…

The consulting psychiatrist who evaluated and treated the patient subsequently reported [1]:

> …[Prior] to dialysis, patient showed a varying disorientation as to time, place, and person… During his excited stages he would pull out his indwelling urethral catheter and would struggle against doctors and nurses, accusing them of attacking him sexually. Impression: toxic psychosis reaction superimposed on a paranoid personality. Offhand, I feel the patient will recover from his psychosis with the use of medications and removal of toxic agents by dialysis…

The behavioral and cognitive changes experienced by this famous patient are very familiar to the mental health professionals of today, who consult and assist transplant teams in the care of patients during the peri-transplant process. Today, we know that cognitive dysfunction and delirium pre- and post-transplantation are not only common but can adversely affect post-transplant clinical outcomes. Several studies have been done on liver and lung transplant patients demonstrating that pre-transplant cognitive impairment is associated with worse post-transplant cognitive status and survival, while post-transplant delirium is associated with longer ventilation times, hospital stays, and potentially increased mortality [2–7].

In Dr. Murray's account, the psychiatric consultant also played a pivotal role in conducting the first live donor psychosocial evaluation, highlighting the ethical considerations as to whether the team should proceed with surgery in a healthy individual to remove a kidney to assist his ailing brother [1].

Emotional challenges and setbacks have influenced and determined the pre- and post-transplant course of many end-stage organ failure patients. Studies have found a high prevalence of pre-transplant anxiety and depression among these patients [8–14]. Significant correlations between preoperative psychiatric diagnoses and poor medical adherence [15, 16] as well as between the presence of various psychosocial factors and postoperative coping and social support [17] have been demonstrated. Over a quarter of solid organ transplant recipients experience depression and/or anxiety after transplant, and the occurrence of depression and anxiety affects post-transplant medical outcomes [18–32]. Indeed, studies have demonstrated that many pre-transplant

Y. Sher (✉) · J. R. Maldonado
Department of Psychiatry & Behavioral Sciences,
Stanford University School of Medicine, Stanford, CA, USA
e-mail: ysher@stanford.edu; jrm@stanford.edu

© Springer International Publishing AG, part of Springer Nature 2019
Y. Sher, J. R. Maldonado (eds.), *Psychosocial Care of End-Stage Organ Disease and Transplant Patients*,
https://doi.org/10.1007/978-3-319-94914-7_1

psychosocial problems continued after transplantation and that psychiatric challenges after transplantation led to a higher risk of infections, hospital readmissions, and higher medical costs [30]. Moreover, specific psychosocial variables are significantly associated with shortened post-transplant survival [18, 33, 34]. Finally, substance use disorders may profoundly affect both the pre- and post-transplant outcomes [16, 35–41]. Psychosocial consultants may thus assist not just in the assessment but in developing a treatment plan and process to help patients achieve the utmost success.

In some cases, the psychological influences affect patients just as much as physical complications do. In her book *I'll Take Tomorrow,* Mary Gohlke, the courageous woman to undergo the first successful heart-lung transplant at Stanford, frankly described and shared her illness and emotional journey and the post-transplant challenges [42]. In her book, Mrs. Gohlke takes the readers through the whole array of the tumultuous psychological and psychiatric experiences associated with the pre- and post-transplant course. She shared the incredible aloneness she felt while sick and dying before the transplant, deteriorating due to advancing pulmonary hypertension. She described the courage and determination she had to master in order to keep fighting and taking a chance with an experimental endeavor, a lung-heart transplantation, to go on living. During the post-transplant period, she had to struggle with postoperative delirium likely due to steroid-induced psychosis, the burden of multiple immunosuppressant agents, the surgery itself, and renal insufficiency. She described feeling confused, irritable, and paranoid during her delirious state, which affected not only her but her primary social support, her husband. She experienced demoralization for not getting stronger fast enough; frustration for being stuck in the hospital; and exasperation at the daunting task of getting better [42].

After she left Stanford hospital, she experienced a whole host of emotional disturbances, including panic attacks and a debilitating anxiety. For a period of time, she became paralyzed with anxiety, terrified to leave her newly established safety net. Life was different, she was different, and she had to find her new balance and confidence. She acknowledges the invaluable assistance she received from the transplant team's consulting psychiatrist. Later after returning home to Arizona, she developed depression: not only did she not enjoy many activities and lacked concentration and motivation, but she could not gain much needed weight due to her lack of appetite. Again receiving psychological help was paramount to her ability to gain weight and continue with success. Although Mary Gohlke frequently bemused in her honest and straightforward memoir of why people reached out to her commending her courage to undergo this experimental at that time surgery, her courage indeed must be commended: not only for undergoing the surgery, surviving, and sharing her story with the world, but also for such honesty sharing her emotional experience.

Transplantation has revolutionized what patients with end-stage organ disease can imagine for themselves. The transplantation field has had many firsts and will undoubtedly continue to develop. It has been built by many talented, courageous, brilliant, and determined people: scientists, immunologists, pathologists, surgeons, physicians, mental health professionals, and, of course, the brave individuals and their families who have donated organs for those in need.

As described above, the first successful renal transplant occurred in 1954 in Boston, USA [1, 43]. The first successful liver transplant took place in 1967 in Denver, USA [43]. The first successful heart transplant took place in 1967 in Cape Town, South Africa [43]. The field was revolutionized by the discovery of cyclosporine, an immunosuppressant, in the 1970s in Switzerland [43]. The first successful heart-lung transplant took place in 1981 at Stanford, USA, as narrated by Mary Gohlke in her book [42, 44]. The first successful long-term single-lung and then double-lung transplant occurred in Toronto, Canada, in 1983 and 1986, respectively [44]. The year 2005 saw the first successful partial face transplant in France [45], and 2011 welcomed the first double-leg transplant in Spain [46].

These firsts have allowed thousands of people to live longer lives, have better quality of life, and discover new hope. However, with these growing opportunities, increasing demands follow. In the United States, every 10 minutes, someone is added to the national transplant waiting list [47]. As of April 15, 2018, 114,807 patients with end-stage organ failure are on the national waiting list in need of a life-saving transplant [48]. The demand much outweighs the supply of donated organs, and on average 22 people die each day waiting for the organs [48]. The psychosocial strain and distress that all of these patients experience throughout their transplant and life journeys are significant.

This is where psychosocial consultants (i.e., transplant mental health clinicians, social workers, psychologists, and psychiatrists) can make a difference. The psychosocial team can enhance the candidate selection process by fine-tuning the assessment of patients being considered for transplantation. They play an important role in the overall transplant theater: improving outcomes, survival, and the quality of life of transplant patients and their families. They play an integral part assisting the rest of the transplant team in caring for the inevitable cognitive and behavioral complications of organ dysfunction, both before and after the transplant surgery. And they have an indispensable role addressing the psychological and emotional reactions when life expectancy is threatened, when hope is taken away. These are the times psychosocial consultants are most needed, and their participation can make a unique difference, helping teams to take care of the whole person and assisting patients to make sense of their experiences and find meaning in their lives. Patients, as all of us, crave witnesses to their lives. We can be that witness.

We are profoundly grateful to many who taught us, mentored us, and served as pioneers and role models in transplantation psychiatry. Multiple articles have been written and quoted throughout this book. Several books have been published regarding the psychosocial aspects of transplantation. For instance, Drs. Paula T. Trzepacz and Andrea F. Dimartini edited an excellent textbook covering the biological, psychological, and ethical considerations in organ transplantation in 2000 [49]. Their work and that of the mental health professionals who tirelessly strive every day to improve the life of transplant patients has served as an inspiration to this volume.

What we envisioned in this textbook is an up-to-date, comprehensive, evidence-based guide to our transplant colleagues for the multidisciplinary psychosocial care of end-stage organ disease and transplant patients. To assist in the process of caring for our transplant patients in the most knowledgeable, collaborative, and compassionate way, we need to understand the underlying end-stage organ disease process; the details of transplantation; the prognosis and possible complications after surgery; the neuropsychiatric complications of organ failure; and the complex immunosuppressive medication regimen, associated neuropsychiatric effects, and interactions with other medications. We need to be aware of the expectations of our patients, their families, and the rest of the medical team. We need to understand the complex psychological reactions experienced by patients who face extraordinary medical challenges. Of course, above all, we need to understand our patients as people with their unique life experiences, goals, and values.

Our hope is that this book will offer a comprehensive starting point for mental health professionals working with this complex patient population through their incredible medical journeys. This book is also intended to assist medical professionals working with end-stage organ disease and transplant patients, by providing a wider glance into their patient's psychological world, and thus offering an opportunity to appreciate the implications of mental health for their overall wellbeing.

This book is organized into several parts. Several sections are based on organ systems (i.e., kidney, liver, heart, lung, visceral, and hematopoietic cell transplant) and include chapters on pre-transplant medical indications, pre-transplant psychosocial and psychiatric concerns, history of respective transplantation field, post-transplant medical course and complications, post-transplant psychosocial and psychiatric care considerations, and some special subjects (e.g., dialysis in renal patients, extracorporeal membrane oxygenation (ECMO) in lung patients). Other chapters are dedicated to topics such as vascularized composite transplantation, pediatric populations, substance use disorders, psychopharmacology, psychotherapy, palliative care, ethics, and cultural factors.

This book contains contributions from specialists that span the entire spectrum of transplant care (e.g., psychiatrists, psychologists, medical subspecialists, surgeons, dieticians, social workers, and ethicists). The voices reflect their specific expertise and experiences, but as they do every day in clinics and hospitals, across the globe, these experts have come together in this book to share their expertise and wisdom. However, in this book, the most treasured voice is that of those who themselves have gone through the transplant process, our patients. These writers have generously shared their very personal journeys with us, reflecting on their unique emotional experiences. They are our best teachers.

It has been an honor to put this book together, and we hope that it will continue to advance the care of end-stage organ disease and transplant patients.

References

1. Murray JE. Surgery of the soul: reflections on a curious career. 2nd ed. Cape Cod: Science History Publications; 2012.
2. Smith PJ, Rivelli SK, Waters AM, Hoyle A, Durheim MT, Reynolds JM, et al. Delirium affects length of hospital stay after lung transplantation. J Crit Care. 2015;30(1):126–9.
3. Sher Y, Mooney J, Dhillon G, Lee R, Maldonado JR. Delirium after lung transplantation: association with recipient characteristics, hospital resource utilization, and mortality. Clin Transpl. 2017;17.
4. Lescot T, Karvellas CJ, Chaudhury P, Tchervenkov J, Paraskevas S, Barkun J, et al. Postoperative delirium in the intensive care unit predicts worse outcomes in liver transplant recipients. Can J Gastroenterol. [Research Support, Non-U.S. Gov't]. 2013;27(4):207–12.
5. Wang SH, Wang JY, Lin PY, Lin KH, Ko CJ, Hsieh CE, et al. Predisposing risk factors for delirium in living donor liver transplantation patients in intensive care units. PLoS One. 2014;9(5):e96676.
6. Lee H, Oh SY, Yu JH, Kim J, Yoon S, Ryu HG. Risk factors of postoperative delirium in the intensive care unit after liver transplantation. World J Surg. 2018;6.
7. Anderson BJ, Chesley CF, Theodore M, Christie C, Tino R, Wysoczanski A, et al. Incidence, risk factors, and clinical implications of post-operative delirium in lung transplant recipients. J Heart Lung Transplant. 2018;2.
8. Mai FM, McKenzie FN, Kostuk WJ. Psychiatric aspects of heart transplantation: preoperative evaluation and postoperative sequelae. Br Med J (Clin Res Ed). 1986;292(6516):311–3.

9. Surman OS, Dienstag JL, Cosimi AB, Chauncey S, Russell PS. Psychosomatic aspects of liver transplantation. Psychother Psychosom. 1987;48(1–4):26–31.

10. Kuhn WF, Myers B, Brennan AF, Davis MH, Lippmann SB, Gray LA, Pool GE. Psychopathology in heart transplant candidates. J Heart Transplant. 1988;7(3):223–6.

11. Maricle RA, Hosenpud JD, Norman DJ, Woodbury A, Pantley GA, Cobanoglu AM, Starr A. Depression in patients being evaluated for heart transplantation. Gen Hosp Psychiatry. 1989;11(6):418–24.

12. Chacko RC, Harper RG, Kunik M, Young J. Relationship of psychiatric morbidity and psychosocial factors in organ transplant candidates. Psychosomatics. 1996;37(2):100–7.

13. Soyseth TS, Lund MB, Bjortuft O, Heldal A, Soyseth V, Dew MA, et al. Psychiatric disorders and psychological distress in patients undergoing evaluation for lung transplantation: a national cohort study. Gen Hosp Psychiatry. 2016;42:67–73.

14. Schneekloth TD, Jowsey SG, Biernacka JM, Burton MC, Vasquez AR, Bergquist T, et al. Pretransplant psychiatric and substance use comorbidity in patients with cholangiocarcinoma who received a liver transplant. Psychosomatics. 2012;53(2):116–22.

15. Mai FM, McKenzie FN, Kostuk WJ. Psychosocial adjustment and quality of life following heart transplantation. Can J Psychiatr. 1990;35(3):223–7.

16. Shapiro PA, Williams DL, Foray AT, Gelman IS, Wukich N, Sciacca R. Psychosocial evaluation and prediction of compliance problems and morbidity after heart transplantation. Transplantation. 1995;60(12):1462–6.

17. Chacko RC, Harper RG, Gotto J, Young J. Psychiatric interview and psychometric predictors of cardiac transplant survival. Am J Psychiatry. 1996;153(12):1607–12.

18. Dew MA, Rosenberger EM, Myaskovsky L, DiMartini AF, DeVito Dabbs AJ, Posluszny DM, et al. Depression and anxiety as risk factors for morbidity and mortality after organ transplantation: a systematic review and meta-analysis. Transplantation. 2015;100(5):988–1003.

19. Dew MA, Kormos RL, DiMartini AF, Switzer GE, Schulberg HC, Roth LH, et al. Prevalence and risk of depression and anxiety-related disorders during the first three years after heart transplantation. Psychosomatics. 2001;42(4):300–13.

20. Dew MA, DiMartini AF, DeVito Dabbs AJ, Fox KR, Myaskovsky L, Posluszny DM, et al. Onset and risk factors for anxiety and depression during the first 2 years after lung transplantation. Gen Hosp Psychiatry. 2012;34(2):127–38.

21. Jones BM, Chang VP, Esmore D, Spratt P, Shanahan MX, Farnsworth AE, et al. Psychological adjustment after cardiac transplantation. Med J Aust. 1988;149(3):118–22.

22. Rosenberger EM, DiMartini AF, DeVito Dabbs AJ, Bermudez CA, Pilewski JM, Toyoda Y, et al. Psychiatric predictors of long-term transplant-related outcomes in lung transplant recipients. Transplantation. [Research Support, N.I.H., Extramural]. 2016;100(1):239–47.

23. Favaro A, Gerosa G, Caforio AL, Volpe B, Rupolo G, Zarneri D, et al. Posttraumatic stress disorder and depression in heart transplantation recipients: the relationship with outcome and adherence to medical treatment. Gen Hosp Psychiatry. 2011;33(1):1–7.

24. Havik OE, Sivertsen B, Relbo A, Hellesvik M, Grov I, Geiran O, et al. Depressive symptoms and all-cause mortality after heart transplantation. Transplantation. 2007;84(1):97–103.

25. Dew MA, Kormos RL, Roth LH, Murali S, DiMartini A, Griffith BP. Early post-transplant medical compliance and mental health predict physical morbidity and mortality one to three years after heart transplantation. J Heart Lung Transplant. 1999;18(6):549–62.

26. DiMartini A, Dew MA, Chaiffetz D, Fitzgerald MG, Devera ME, Fontes P. Early trajectories of depressive symptoms after liver

transplantation for alcoholic liver disease predicts long-term survival. Am J Transplant. 2011;11(6):1287–95.

27. Zipfel S, Schneider A, Wild B, Lowe B, Junger J, Haass M, et al. Effect of depressive symptoms on survival after heart transplantation. Psychosom Med. 2002;64(5):740–7.

28. DiMatteo MR, Lepper HS, Croghan TW. Depression is a risk factor for noncompliance with medical treatment: meta-analysis of the effects of anxiety and depression on patient adherence. Arch Intern Med. 2000;160(14):2101–7.

29. Woodman CL, Geist LJ, Vance S, Laxson C, Jones K, Kline JN. Psychiatric disorders and survival after lung transplantation. Psychosomatics. 1999;40(4):293–7.

30. Paris W, Muchmore J, Pribil A, Zuhdi N, Cooper DK. Study of the relative incidences of psychosocial factors before and after heart transplantation and the influence of posttransplantation psychosocial factors on heart transplantation outcome. J Heart Lung Transplant. 1994;13(3):424–30. discussion 31–2.

31. Annema C, Drent G, Roodbol PF, Stewart RE, Metselaar HJ, van Hoek B, et al. Trajectories of anxiety and depression after liver transplantation as related to outcomes during 2-year follow-up: a prospective cohort study. Psychosom Med. 2018;80(2):174–83.

32. Palmer S, Vecchio M, Craig JC, Tonelli M, Johnson DW, Nicolucci A, et al. Prevalence of depression in chronic kidney disease: systematic review and meta-analysis of observational studies. Kidney Int. [Meta-Analysis Research Support, Non-U.S. Gov't Review]. 2013;84(1):179–91.

33. Owen JE, Bonds CL, Wellisch DK. Psychiatric evaluations of heart transplant candidates: predicting post-transplant hospitalizations, rejection episodes, and survival. Psychosomatics. 2006;47(3):213–22.

34. Maldonado JR, Sher Y, Lolak S, Swendsen H, Skibola D, Neri E, et al. The Stanford integrated psychosocial assessment for transplantation: a prospective study of medical and psychosocial outcomes. Psychosom Med. 2015;77(9):1018–30.

35. Karman JF, Sileri P, Kamuda D, Cicalese L, Rastellini C, Wiley TE, et al. Risk factors for failure to meet listing requirements in liver transplant candidates with alcoholic cirrhosis. Transplantation. 2001;71(9):1210–3.

36. Hanrahan JS, Eberly C, Mohanty PK. Substance abuse in heart transplant recipients: a 10-year follow-up study. Prog Transplant. 2001;11(4):285–90.

37. Dew MA, DiMartini AF, De Vito DA, Myaskovsky L, Steel J, Unruh M, et al. Rates and risk factors for nonadherence to the medical regimen after adult solid organ transplantation. Transplantation. [Research Support, N.I.H., Extramural Research Support, Non-U.S. Gov't]. 2007;83(7):858–73.

38. Pfitzmann R, Schwenzer J, Rayes N, Seehofer D, Neuhaus R, Nussler NC. Long-term survival and predictors of relapse after orthotopic liver transplantation for alcoholic liver disease. Liver Transpl. 2007;13(2):197–205.

39. Faure S, Herrero A, Jung B, Duny Y, Daures JP, Mura T, et al. Excessive alcohol consumption after liver transplantation impacts on long-term survival, whatever the primary indication. J Hepatol. 2012;57(2):306–12.

40. Iruzubieta P, Crespo J, Fabrega E. Long-term survival after liver transplantation for alcoholic liver disease. World J Gastroenterol. 2013;19(48):9198–208.

41. Nagele H, Kalmar P, Rodiger W, Stubbe HM. Smoking after heart transplantation: an underestimated hazard? Eur J Cardiothorac Surg. 1997;12(1):70–4.

42. Gohlke M, Jennings M. I'll take tomorrow. New York: M. Evans and Compnay, Inc.; 1985.

43. Linden PK. History of solid organ transplantation and organ donation. Crit Care Clin. [Historical Article]. 2009;25(1):165–84, ix.

44. Venuta F, Van Raemdonck D. History of lung transplantation. J Thorac Dis. [Review]. 2017;9(12):5458–71.

45. Devauchelle B, Badet L, Lengele B, Morelon E, Testelin S, Michallet M, et al. First human face allograft: early report. Lancet. 2006;368(9531):203–9.

46. de Lago M. World's first double leg transplantation is carried out in Spain. BMJ. [Case Reports News]. 2011;343:d4541.

47. OPTN. Organ Procurement and Transplantation Network. Organ Procurement and Transplantation Network; 2016 [4/16/2018]. Available from: https://optn.transplant.hrsa.gov/.

48. UNOS. National data: transplants by organ type United Network for Organ Sharing; 2018 [cited 2018 4/16/2018]. Available from: https://unos.org/data/.

49. Trzepacz PT, DiMartini AF. The transplant patient: biological, psychiatric and ethical issues in organ transplantation. Cambridge: Cambridge University Press; 2000.

Overview of Solid Organ Transplantation and the United States National Organ Transplant Act (NOTA)

2

Oscar Salvatierra and José R. Maldonado

Introduction

Psychosocial consultants have been an important, necessary, and integral part of solid organ transplantation due to the wide spectrum of challenging psychiatric and social issues encountered by this complex therapy.

Transplantation is a field that has required much more in its development than to just continue with the traditional methodologies that have provided for the successful clinical practice of medicine. Hospitals are generally autonomous in their operation and reign supreme. In contrast, organ transplantation has been an emerging medical specialty that has involved the retrieval of multiple organs from multiple hospitals with essentially no organizational infrastructure. There has thus been a great need to provide cooperation from a disparate group of practitioners and hospitals to better assure successful transplantation of all available donated organs. These organs are a precious public commodity for which transplant programs and practitioners assume fiduciary responsibility – the organs belong to the public, which has graciously donated them to save the lives of their fellow citizens with end-stage organ failure.

Early History

Since the first successful organ transplant performed in 1954 by Dr. Joseph Murray at the Peter Bent Brigham Hospital, now the Brigham and Women's Hospital in Boston, many firsts have taken place in the field of transplantation between 1950s and 1960s, as detailed in Chap. 1.

However, the early evolvement of organ transplantation had been challenging, primarily because of problems incurred

Table 2.1 1- and 3-year deceased donor graft and patient survival rates

	1 year	3 year
	% graft/patient	% graft/patient
Kidney	94.5/96.7	87.9/92
Liver	89.1/90.9	79.7/82.1
Heart	90.4/90.7	84.8/85.2

Note: Outcomes are currently similar for kidney, liver, and heart transplants as depicted in the following survival rates reported by the Scientific Registry of Transplant Recipients (SRTR) shown for a higher-risk older patient cohort (aged 50–64) [1]

with complications from the immunosuppression required to control the immune response in genetically dissimilar donor-recipient pairs, present for almost all kidney, liver, and heart transplants, except for the rare identical twin donor-recipient pairs. Because of some technical difficulties with the surgical procedures, the few liver and heart transplant centers that then existed entered into self-imposed moratoriums in 1970, in order to carefully evaluate outcomes so as to obtain future improvement in graft and patient survival rates.

Since then, all organ transplant results have substantially improved, and at present most solid organs (i.e., kidney, liver, and heart) essentially achieve similar graft and patient survival rates as reported by the Scientific Registry of Transplant Recipients (SRTR) for a higher-risk older patient cohort (aged 50–64) (see Table 2.1) [1].

Challenges Leading to Drafting of the National Organ Transplant Act (NOTA)

The development of organ transplantation is one of the outstanding medical achievements of this century [2]. When congressional hearings on transplantation were held by Congressmen Gore and Waxman in the autumn of 1983, the full implications were not obvious to many who testified, including Oscar Salvatierra, Norman Shumway, and Thomas E. Starzl [3].

O. Salvatierra ·J. R. Maldonado (✉)
Department of Psychiatry and Behavioral Sciences,
Stanford University School of Medicine, Stanford, CA, USA
e-mail: jrm@stanford.edu

© Springer International Publishing AG, part of Springer Nature 2019
Y. Sher, J. R. Maldonado (eds.), *Psychosocial Care of End-Stage Organ Disease and Transplant Patients*,
https://doi.org/10.1007/978-3-319-94914-7_2

9

Key to the marked improvement in transplant outcomes was the passage by the US Congress of the National Organ Transplant Act (NOTA) on October 19, 1984 [4–6], which facilitated and brought together all participants in organ transplantation. This was a monumental and strikingly pivotal achievement opening the door for the unimpeded, yet carefully monitored, clinical and scientific advancement of organ transplantation in the United States. The NOTA was critically important to patients with end-stage organ failure, as many were dying awaiting transplantation [6]. It not only established the framework for the US organ transplant system but has served as a model for development of other transplant networks worldwide [7].

There were several significant infrastructural challenges preceding and precipitating the creation and passage of NOTA. First of all, transplant programs lacked a much-needed infrastructure to unify transplant programs in their fiduciary responsibility to protect every organ removed for transplantation and to assure the appropriate most efficient life-saving use of this precious public commodity. For this infrastructure to develop, transplant programs and their hospitals had to abandon what appeared to be an unintended operational independence that for more than a century had been the hallmark of medical practice in the United States. The organ transplant centers required a more efficient and cooperative team environment at both regional and national levels to best protect and assure that every donated organ met its intended use. Organ transplantation is multifaceted and quite complex, involving multiple organs, multiple disciplines, and multiple locations and thus requiring a well-organized and functional infrastructure, not present before the passage of NOTA.

Second, heart and liver transplantation were still considered experimental in the early 1980s, so the third-party payers refused to provide reimbursement. This resulted in only a very few active centers where liver and heart transplantation were available. In addition, the general public's acceptance of transplantation was primarily focused on kidney transplantation with little awareness of heart and liver transplantation.

In addition, there was evidence of kidney wastage with some transplant programs where several organs removed for transplantation were discarded or allocated out of country. For example, if a transplant center procured kidneys that could not be used with one of their patients, it was not uncommon to send the organs to another country instead of another center at a closer distance in its own geographic region.

Despite these challenges, it was apparent that organ transplantation was outstripping its roots in its favorable evolvement and growth and with time was exceeding expectations in its clinical success. With the remarkable improvement in graft and patient survival that occurred with the then new immunosuppressive agent cyclosporine in clinical trials,

it was anticipated that there would be continued further meaningful future advancement of the field. Thus, faced with significant clinical promise of the field on one hand and considerable challenges on the other, there was an urgent necessity to (1) develop a well-functioning national infrastructure that would assure maximum utilization and equitable distribution of organs, (2) promote organ donation to help meet the expected increasing need for more organs, and (3) recognize life-saving nonrenal transplants as non-experimental. It was against this background that the drafting and passage of NOTA was achieved despite strong opposition by many powerful professional organizations, such as the American Medical Association (AMA), the American College of Surgeons (ACS), and even the Reagan Administration who believed the bill represented an incursion into the private practice of medicine and the imposition of controls that inevitably would permeate other aspects of medical care [3, 5].

The NOTA provided a single piece of legislation to best address the problems faced by the organ transplantation community, especially with a progressively increasing large numbers of patients desiring an organ transplant. No longer could 244 transplant programs operate independently, but instead, an organizational structure was required to bring transplant surgeons, physicians, immunologists, psychiatrists, and other research and technical personnel together to optimize the procurement, preservation, and distribution of organs to provide the best possible transplant outcomes.

NOTA Provisions

The objectives were clear: (1) to increase the supply of organs with a small grants program that could strengthen procurement agencies already in existence or stimulate the development of new programs in underserved areas, including the establishment of a national network for organ distribution; (2) to pay for novel and expensive immunosuppressant medicines, which were predicted to be too costly for many patients to afford; and (3) to prohibit the purchase and sale of organs [3].

The implementation of NOTA authorized (1) an Organ Procurement and Transplantation Network (OPTN), (2) the development of regional organ procurement organizations (OPOs), and (3) the establishment of a compulsory national scientific registry for all organs. Through the establishment of a national OPTN, the law directed that organ allocation would be managed on a national basis and be developed through a unique public-private partnership. Since the initial network contract was finalized in 1986, the United Network for Organ Sharing (UNOS) has served as the OPTN under contract with the US Department of Health and Human Services [7]. "The primary purposes of the OPTN are to operate and monitor an equitable system for allocating organs donated for transplantation; maintain a waiting list of potential recipients; match potential recipients with organ donors according to established medical criteria for allocation of organs and, to the extent feasible, for listing and delisting transplant patients; facilitate the efficient, effective placement of organs for transplantation; and increase organ donation" [6].

These three provisions of NOTA provided an immediate course correction for organ transplantation in the United States. Most importantly, NOTA provided for a highly functional three-tier infrastructure (Fig. 2.1) to sustain and support transplantation with equal consideration given to enhancing the success of all transplantable organs [8]. Additional major NOTA provisions included (4) establishment of a task force on organ transplantation, (5) prohibition of organ purchases, and (6) a bone marrow registry, demonstration, and study. NOTA represented the first and only time that Congress has provided for the infrastructure of a major medical specialty.

The bill mandated the Health Care Financing Administration (HCFA) to establish a national organ procurement and distribution network, which was granted to the UNOS, a previously private and nonprofit organization. The OPTN is a unique public-private partnership that links all professionals involved in the US donation and transplantation system [9].

The OPTN is operated under contract with the U.S. Dept. of Health and Human Services by the United Network for Organ Sharing (UNOS). As such, the OPTN has provided transplantation with an operational system and structure that has been inclusive of all aspects of organ procurement and distribution of organs [9]. A major area of debate in the drafting of the legislation was whether the effort to develop a

national operational system for organ transplantation should be managed privately, publicly, or as a private/public entity, the latter being the ultimate outcome. This is well described by the *New England Journal of Medicine* (NEJM) which highlights and encapsulates the debate [5].

At this time in the early 1980s, the discovery of new immunosuppressant agent cyclosporine led to new excitement in the field, as it heralded the improved results in graft and patient survival. This served as a major stimulus to request that the passage of NOTA legislation included assistance with the costs of outpatient cyclosporine therapy.

However, several senators and congressmen expressed reluctance to proceed with this authorization and instead called for a Task Force to "conduct comprehensive examinations of the medical, legal, ethical, economic and social issues presented by human organ procurement and transplantation," as well as "an analysis of the safety, effectiveness, and costs (including cost savings from improved success rates of transplantation) of different modalities of treatment" [6].

The NEJM reported on the sharply contrasting testimonies at a congressional hearing between the proponents for voluntary private management of organ transplantation in the United States versus those advocating a private/public system [5]. This article indicated that "with a few exceptions, no other issue confronting the Public Health Service at this time [was] as emotionally charged as this one" [5]. The AMA was also vehemently opposed to the legislation. The AMA's principal witness, Dr. James Davis, vice-speaker of the House of Delegates, testified that the legislation "would authorize the cookbook approach to medical practice, with chapter and verse written by the secretary of HHS [the Department of Health and Human Services]." Dr. Norman Shumway (Chair of the Department of Cardiovascular Surgery at Stanford University), Dr. Tom Starzl (Director of Transplantation at the University of Pittsburg), and Dr. Oscar Salvatierra (President of the American Society of Transplant Surgeons) proved to be the important congressional testimony in the effort to obtain the passage of NOTA [3, 5]. They argued that transplantation of all organs (kidney, heart, lung, liver, and pancreas) with their dramatically improving success rates under cyclosporine should be available to all patients with an equitable distribution of organs regardless of patients' financial status, race, or ethnicity. Their testimony on behalf of patients awaiting transplantation was very well received and eventually resulted in an almost unanimous vote for passage of NOTA by both the Senate and House of Representatives.

An extremely important part of NOTA was the establishment of organ procurement organizations [9] which brought together all transplant programs in a region for a cooperative and more efficient and effective management of organ donation, procurement, and the distribution. "All organs" were no longer just kidney organs, but included the heart, lung, liver,

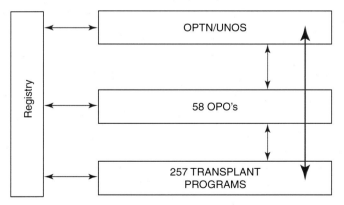

Fig. 2.1 NOTA established a highly functional 3-tier infrastructure designed to sustain and support transplantation of all organs with equal consideration given to enhancing the success of all transplantable organs. NOTA = the National Organ Transplant Act (NOTA) enacted by the US Congress on October 19, 1984; OPTN = Organ Procurement and Transplantation Network; UNOS = United Network for Organ Sharing; OPO's = organ procurement organizations

and pancreas. NOTA specifically stated that "[the] term 'organ' means the human kidney, liver, heart, lung, pancreas…" [6]. It also stated that an OPO "has procedures to obtain payment for non-renal organs provided to transplant centers" [6]. Thus, without directly saying so, the "experimental" label that nonrenal organs had carried for more than 15 years was now forever removed and third-party payers could no longer use "experimental" as a reason to decline reimbursement for nonrenal transplants.

Currently, there are 58 regional OPOs in operation in the United States under the OPTN/UNOS umbrella [4].

Scientific Registry

A reliable Scientific Registry was essential to a vibrant, successful and forward-looking national system in organ transplantation. The Scientific Registry authorized by NOTA is particularly effective because it is a compulsory registry where information on every patient must be provided by a transplant center in order for it to continue its existence. It thus provides reliable data to make policy decisions and to identify areas to be targeted for future investigation and research. In addition, organ specific data on every center is now available to the public in yearly reports from what is now called the Scientific Registry of Transplant Recipients (SRTR). See Fig. 2.2 for an overview of the organizational structure established by NOTA, including SRTR [10]. Founded in 1987, the SRTR is a national database of all transplant statistics. SRTR analyzes data from multiple sources and draws conclusions regarding allocation of organs, organ transplant waiting lists, and transplant patients' mortality, morbidity, quality of life, and other post-transplant outcomes [1].

Outcomes

NOTA and subsequent federal regulations call on the OPTN to emphasize fair and equitable patient access to transplantation, as well as reliance on objective medical evidence and adaptability to rapid evolution in clinical treatment and scientific understanding [7]. The results reported by UNOS and the SRTR [4], after passage of NOTA, show a favorable increase in yearly number of transplants performed from <6,500 in 1983 to a current >34,000 per year in 2017, which has been due to an increase in organ donation.

The success of transplantation in the United States currently depends upon a system of altruistic organ donation from living or cadaveric (deceased) donors [11]. Congress then made it "unlawful for any person to knowingly acquire, receive, or otherwise transfer any human organ for valuable consideration in human transplantation use if the transfer affects interstate commerce" [11]. Congress also imposed penalty for persons who engage in the exchange of human organs for valuable consideration with the maximum fine of $50,000 and/or a maximum 5-year imprisonment [6].

Despite advances in medicine and technology as well as an increased awareness of organ donation and transplantation, there has been a widening gap between organ donation and transplantation of patients on the waiting list. The marked improved success of organ transplantation is reflected in increased numbers of patients with end-stage organ failure now desiring this life-saving therapy. Yet, while a sizeable number of individuals receive organ transplants each year (i.e., 34,768 in 2017), the demand for available organs exceeds the supply [12], with currently with more than 118,000 people awaiting organ transplantation in the United States [13].

In 2004, Congress passed the Organ Donation and Recovery Improvement Act [14] to address the considerable concern over the growing organ transplant waiting list by implementing measures necessary to improve the existing altruism-based organ procurement and transplantation system. The 2004 Act sought to respond to the growing problem by authorizing the DHHS to provide funding for public awareness efforts addressing the need for organ donation, awarding grants to organ procurement organizations and hospitals to better coordinate and increase the rate of organ donation, and funding studies to "improve the recovery, preservation, and transportation of organs" [15]. It also

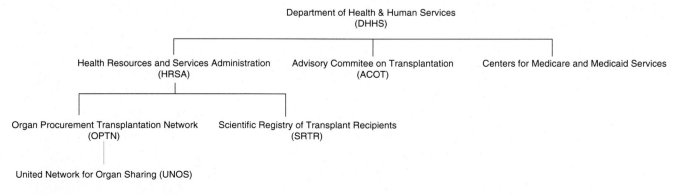

Fig. 2.2 Relationship between UNOS, OPTN, SRTR, and the Federal Government. (Source: [10])

authorized the DHHS to award grants to states, transplant centers, qualified organ procurement organizations, or other public or private entities for providing reimbursement for travel and subsistence expenses incurred by individuals making a living organ donation [14, 15].

The 2004 Act reflected a preference to improve and maintain the solely altruistic scheme of organ donation [14], but missed a unique opportunity to adopt provisions that would have permitted financial incentives that would encourage cadaveric organ donation, a potentially effective policy-alternative response to the organ shortage [15]. Congress considered, but ultimately rejected, an amendment to allow for the implementation of indirect financial incentives in cadaveric organ donation in the form of a fixed financial remuneration that could be used by the family "to help pay for funeral or hospital costs, as a donation to the deceased's favorite charity, or could simply remain the deceased donor's estate upon the family's decision to 'give the gift of life'" [15].

Conclusions

NOTA has unquestionably provided by statue the framework for structure, organization, discipline, future direction, and cooperation between the OPTN, SRTR, OPOs, HRSA, and transplant professionals. This remarkable private/public partnership has proven to be absolutely necessary and essential for organ transplantation in the United States to continue to improve with future increasing maximum benefit to patients with end-stage organ failure. The ultimate objective is a successful transplant for all patients requiring an organ transplant.

Organ transplantation from its very beginning has been blessed with many dedicated, skilled, and selfless professionals, which have included scientists, transplant surgeons, other transplant physicians, psychiatrists, social workers, nurses, coordinators, and technicians working with the various facets of organ transplantation. They have all worked tirelessly through the years since the first successful transplant and have been inseparably united in doing everything possible to give patients a second chance at life with a new organ. Most notable has been the ever presence and involvement of psychiatrists and other psychosocial specialists without whose very meaningful and compassionate support the complex field of organ transplantation would not exist as it does today. The extraordinary humanitarianism of organ donors, whether living or deceased, has been nothing short of exceptional and deserving of our greatest grati-

tude. These donated organs represent a precious public commodity in needs of utmost respect, careful protection, and equitable distribution to provide good-quality life to as many patients as possible. That was what NOTA has been all about and we hope that it will continue to foster patient-driven advancements in this spectacular field of solid organ transplantation. To fulfill the ultimate goals of NOTA, we must continue to ensure that the national transplant network allocates organs efficiently and fairly. We must also build public knowledge and trust in organ donation to help increase transplant opportunities for everyone in need [7].

References

1. SRTS. Scientific Registry of Transplant Recipients: US Department of Health & Human Services. Available from: https://srtr.transplant.hrsa.gov/default.aspx.
2. Salvatierra O Jr. Renal transplantation – the Starzl influence. Transplant Proc. 1988;20(1 Suppl 1):343–9.
3. Starzl TE, Shapiro R, Teperman L. The point system for organ distribution. Transplant Proc. 1989;21(3):3432–6. discussion 40–4.
4. Salvatierra O, Jr. Optimal use of organs for transplantation. N Engl J Med. 1988;318(20):1329–31. DHHS. Organ Donation and Transplantation Statistics: Graph Data. 2018; https://www.organdonor.gov/statistics-stories/statistics/data.html. Accessed September 30, 2018.
5. Iglehart JK. The politics of transplantation. N Engl J Med. 1984;310(13):864–8.
6. National Organ Transplant Act, Congress of the United States, 98th Congress Sess. (1984).
7. UNOS. National Organ Transplant Act enacted 30 years ago UNOS Website 2014 Available from: https://unos.org/national-organ-transplant-act-enacted-30-years-ago/.
8. Salvatierra O Jr. The status of the American Society of Transplant Surgeons on its tenth anniversary. Presidential address. Transplantation. 1984;38(6):727–30.
9. Organ procurement and transplantation network, US Congress, 101th Congress Sess. (1990).
10. 101 LD. Public Policy Organizations – Who are they and what do they do? Living Donor 101 Website 2018. Available from: http://www.livingdonor101.com/public_policy_organizations.shtml.
11. Sanford J, Rocchiccioli J. Cash for kidneys: the use financial incentives for organ donation. Policy Polit Nurs Pract. 2003;4(4):275–6.
12. UNOS. National Data: Transplants by Organ Type United Network for Organ Sharing; 2018. Available from: https://unos.org/data/.
13. OPTN. Organ Procurement and Transplantation Network OPTN website: U.S. Department of Health & Human Services; 2018 [4/21/2018]. Available from: https://optn.transplant.hrsa.gov/.
14. Organ Donation and Recovery Improvement Act, Congress of the United States, 108th Congress Sess. (2004).
15. Carlson PD. The 2004 organ donation recovery and improvement act: how congress missed an opportunity to say "yes" to financial incentives for organ donation. J Contemp Health Law Policy. 2006;23(1):136–66.

The Psychosocial Evaluation of Transplant Candidates

3

José R. Maldonado

Because donated organs are a severely limited resource, the best potential recipients should be identified. The probability of a good outcome must be highly emphasized to achieve the maximum benefit for all transplants.
(From: OPTN/UNOS Ethics Committee General Considerations in Assessment for Transplant Candidacy White Paper–2010) [1, 2]

Introduction

The number of transplant surgeries has risen steadily in the last 30 years in the USA (see Table 3.1; Fig. 3.1). For example, in 1991, a total of 15,756 transplants were performed in the USA, while the number of patients on the waiting list hovered around 23,198 (all organs). At present, nearly 100 transplants are performed each day in the USA [7]. Thus, by April 2018 (the last set of statistics available at time of publication), a total of 730,013 transplants had been performed in the USA, since 1988 (Table 3.2) [3].

Unfortunately, the availability of donated organs has not kept pace with the clinical demands. In fact, the number of available organs has remained relatively flat (see Fig. 3.1) [7]. According to the Organ Procurement and Transplantation Network (OPTN), every 10 minutes someone is added to the national transplant waiting list [7]. This has translated into a staggering statistic: on average, 20 patients die each day (which translates into 7300 candidates a year) while waiting for a transplant [3]. On average, 10–20% of all heart, liver, and lung transplant candidates die before an organ becomes available [4]. Transplant teams thus have become stewards of a very precious and limited resource.

Benefits of Using Objective Psychosocial Assessment Tools

Despite the exponential growth in the need for organs, the method by which the medical community selects transplant recipients has seen little in terms of definitive change or the establishment of recipient selection standards. When evaluating a patient's candidacy as a potential transplant recipient, we must consider not only medical listing criteria, but also the patient's psychosocial makeup.

Medical listing criteria have been relatively well established and specifically defined for each end-organ system by the United Network for Organ Sharing (UNOS) (see Table 3.3) (e.g., for liver transplant recipients, the Model for End-Stage Liver Disease (MELD) system [16]; for lung transplant, the Lung Allocation System (LAS) [23]).

On the other hand, psychosocial listing criteria are less standardized, both regarding tools and techniques used. Unfortunately, OPTN/UNOS guidelines regarding the psychosocial evaluation process are too broad and provide little direction: "All transplant programs should identify appropriately trained individuals who are designated members of the transplant team and have primary responsibility for coordinating the psychosocial needs of transplant candidates, recipients, living donors and families (OPTN Evaluation Plan, page IV-6)" [29]. In fact, the OPTN/UNOS Ethics Committee recognized that "the concept of non-medical transplant candidate criteria is an area of great concern. Most transplant programs in the United States use some type of non-medical evaluation of patients for transplantation... There is general agreement that non-medical transplant candidate criteria need to be evaluated. The legitimate substance of such an evaluation could cover a very wide range of topics" [2].

Over the years, studies have demonstrated a strong association between pre-transplant psychosocial vulnerability factors and a number of negative outcomes. These include negative medical outcomes, such as higher infection rates, treatment adherence, increased rejection episodes, acute late rejection, hospital readmissions, increased cost of care, post-transplant malignancies, graft loss, and decreased transplant survival. In addition, there are a number of adverse

J. R. Maldonado
Department of Psychiatry and Behavioral Sciences, Stanford University School of Medicine, Stanford, CA, USA
e-mail: jrm@stanford.edu

© Springer International Publishing AG, part of Springer Nature 2019
Y. Sher, J. R. Maldonado (eds.), *Psychosocial Care of End-Stage Organ Disease and Transplant Patients*,
https://doi.org/10.1007/978-3-319-94914-7_3

Table 3.1 US transplantation data: all organs

Year	Patients on the waiting list	Transplants performed	Donors recovered (both deceased and living donors)
2018 (January to March)	114,921	8509	4110
2017	127,374	34,768	16,476
2016	124,723	33,611	15,943
2015	122,071	30,975	15,071
2014	123,851	29,540	14,416
2013	121,272	28,954	14,256
2012	117,040	28,053	14,010
2011	112,766	28,540	14,149
2010	110,375	28,662	14,504
2009	105,567	28,459	14,632
2008	100,775	27,964	14,207
2007	97,670	28,366	14,400
2006	94,441	28,940	14,750
2005	90,526	28,118	14,497
2004	87,146	27,040	14,154
2003	83,731	25,473	13,285
2002	80,790	24,910	12,821
2001	79,524	24,239	12,702
2000	74,078	24,239	11,934
1999	67,224	22,026	10,869
1998	60,381	21,523	10,362
1997	53,167	20,314	9545
1996	46,961	19,765	9222
1995	41,203	19,396	8859
1994	35,271	18,298	8203
1993	31,355	17,631	7766
1992	27,563	16,134	7091
1991	23,198	15,756	6953

Ref. [3–5]

psychosocial outcomes, including the development of depression, anxiety, and other psychiatric conditions and need for psychiatric admissions, relapse to substance use, as well as social complications (e.g., loss of social support, financial stress). The occurrence of these medical and psychosocial outcomes has been linked to the ultimate transplant success or failure [26, 30–54].

Yet, despite the fact that every organization regulating transplantation procedures recommends or requires a psychosocial evaluation as a prerequisite for transplantation, psychosocial evaluations have remained less standardized, regarding both the assessment tools used and the listing criteria considered. A literature review demonstrates that there is a relative absence of evidence-based guidelines for pre-transplant psychosocial and behavioral screening [36, 39] and that transplant programs and psychosocial expert consultants utilize different techniques and psychosocial eligibility criteria to

evaluate prospective transplant candidates [46, 55]. In fact, data suggests that psychosocial assessments differ in content and application to candidate selection depending on the transplant program [46, 55, 56]. A survey of transplant psychosocial experts provided evidence for the need of expanding routine screening and support services to candidates for and recipients of transplants [57].

Until recently, the only national survey demonstrated a wide variability in the psychosocial listing criteria used by transplant programs. Even though there are no national standards or psychosocial minimal listing criteria, the survey found for example that there were certain conditions (i.e., current addictive drug use, active schizophrenia, current heavy alcohol use, history of multiple suicide attempts, current suicide ideation, dementia) which were endorsed as "absolute contraindications to transplantation" by 70% of responders [46].

More recently, a Stanford research group conducted an online survey through Qualtrics of all 650 adult and pediatric heart, kidney, liver, and lung programs in the USA, as identified by the OPTN [58]. A total of 343 programs submitted complete responses, representing 234 adult programs and 101 pediatric programs (response rate = 52.8%). The survey listed 38 psychosocial pertinent characteristics, and participants were asked to determine to which degree these were relevant in their listing deliberation consideration (i.e., irrelevant (IR), an absolute (AC), or a relative contraindication (RC) to listing). The survey found that although programs reached consensus during listing deliberations on all characteristics, 6–40% of programs had no formal guidelines for these. Among the findings, we discovered that programs differed regarding the active use of cigarettes (AC heart 75.6%, kidney 22.0%, liver 17.6%, lung 93.3%, $p < 0.001$), recreational marijuana (AC heart 56.4%, kidney 23.6%, liver 23.5%, lung 71.1%, $p < 0.001$), and alcohol (AC heart 75.6%, kidney 58.3%, liver 56.5%, lung 88.9%, $p < 0.001$) (see Fig. 3.2) and lacked consensus regarding undocumented status (AC 24.8%, IR 21.2%, $p < 0.001$). Adult programs are more likely to consider psychiatric factors to listing (AC dementia, adult 47.9%, pediatric 26.8%; current suicidal ideation, adult 82.9%, pediatric 57.4%; unstable schizophrenia, adult 87.6%, pediatric 61.4%; unstable affective disorder, adult 66.7%, pediatric 39.6%; unstable personality disorder, adult 60.3%, pediatric 36.6%). We found that programs today are more stringent compared to those surveyed in 1993 [46] with regard to cigarette use (current AC 17.6%~93.3% vs Levenson AC 1.3%~43.6%), current incarceration (current AC 41.2%~61.4% vs Levenson AC 20.6%~46.2%), and lack of social support (current AC 37.2%~64.4% vs Levenson AC 2.6%~9.0%) but less stringent with regard to use of recreational drugs

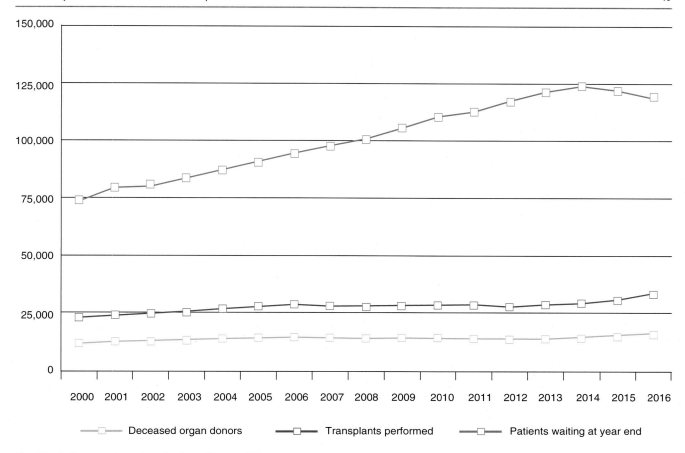

Fig. 3.1 Solid organ transplant shortage. (Source: [6])

Table 3.2 Transplants performed in the USA by organ type: January 1, 1988 to March 31, 2018. Based on OPTN data as of April 26, 2018

Organ	Transplants performed (*January 1, 1988 to April 28, 2018*)
Kidney	430,054
Liver	157,902
Pancreas	8609
Kidney/pancreas	23,104
Heart	69,711
Lung	36,426
Heart/lung	1237
Intestine	2941
Abdominal wall	1
Head and neck: craniofacial	5
Head and neck: scalp	1
GU: penile	2
GU: uterus	10
Upper limb: bilateral	6
Upper limb: unilateral	4
Total	**730,013**

Ref. [3]

other than marijuana (current AC 60.0%~88.9% vs Levenson AC 69.5%~92.3%) [58]. These results demonstrate that there continues to be a high degree of variability among transplant programs across the USA today.

Despite the lack of standardization, psychosocial consultants can enhance the candidate selection process by fine-tuning the assessment of patients being considered for transplantation [30, 39, 44, 46, 49]. This can most effectively be done by focusing on risk factors that are associated with poor adherence/compliance and ultimate medical and psychosocial transplant success [34, 45, 59–63].

Data suggest that there is not only a strong association between pre-transplant psychosocial vulnerability markers and post-transplant psychosocial outcomes [41], but also between specific psychosocial factors and ultimate transplant success or failure [31, 33, 34, 38, 42, 43, 45–47, 49–52, 54, 56, 64–66]. In fact, studies have demonstrated that many pre-transplant psychosocial problems continued after transplantation and that psychiatric problems after transplantation led to a higher risk of infection, hospital readmissions, and

Table 3.3 Medical listing criteria per end-organ system

End organ	1st Txp	Medical criteria	Developing entity	Reference
Kidney	1954 (first successful kidney transplant, Boston)	Kidney allocation score (KAS)	UNOS	De Meester et al. (1998) [8] Fuggle et al. (1998) [9] Nyberg et al. (2001) [10] Baskin-Bey et al. (2007) [11] UNOS (2009) [12] Desschans et al. (2008) [13]
Pancreas	1966 (first simultaneous kidney/pancreas transplant, Minnesota) 1968 (first successful isolated pancreas transplant)	Pancreas allocation score (PAS)	OPTN/UNOS pancreas transplantation committee	UNOS 2007 Desschans et al. (2008) [13] Revised (2009) [14]
Heart	1967 (S. Africa) 1968 (first successful heart transplant, Stanford, CA)	New York heart association (NYHA) functional classification	NYHA	NYHA (1994) [15]
Liver	1967 (first successful liver transplant, Denver) 1988 (first split-liver transplant) 1989 (first successful living donor liver transplant) 1998 (first successful adult-to-adult living donor liver transplant)	Model for end-stage liver disease (MELD)	Mayo Clinic	Kamath et al. (2001) [16] Wiesner et al. (2003) [17] Horslen (2004) [18] Kamath and Kim (2007) [19] Desschans et al. (2008) [13] Freeman (2008) [20] Singal and Kamath (2013) [21]
Lung	1981 (first successful heart-lung transplant) 1983 (first successful single-lung transplant, Toronto) 1986 (first successful double-lung transplant) 1990 (first successful living donor lung transplant)	Lung allocation score (LAS)	OPTN/UNOS	De Meester et al. (2001) [22] UNOS (2005) [23] OPTN (2015) [24] Smits et al. (2018) [25]
Intestine	1987 (first successful intestinal transplant)	Intestine allocation score (IAS)	OPTN/UNOS Liver and intestinal organ transplantation committee	UNOS (2015) Desschans et al. (2008) [13] Revised (2011)

Source: [26–28]

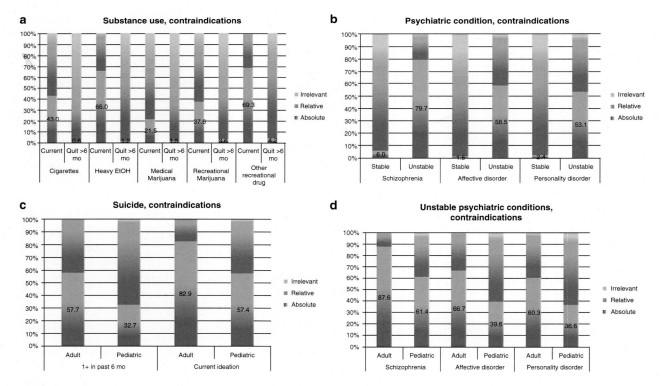

Fig. 3.2 Stanford 2018 online survey of transplant program psychosocial listing criteria. (Source: [58])

higher medical costs [67]. While some researchers demonstrated that the global psychosocial risk was associated with the number of rejection episodes and medication adherence after transplantation [68], others found that increasing psychiatric risk classification (i.e., high risk versus acceptable versus good candidates) was associated with a greater hazard of post-transplant mortality [63]. Four psychosocial variables (i.e., previous suicide attempts, poor adherence to medical recommendations, past history of substance abuse, and depression) were significantly associated with shortened post-transplant survival and/or greater risk for post-transplant infection [63]. In fact, differences among risk groups emerged early in the post-transplant process, with patients in the high-risk group experiencing greater mortality shortly after transplant, compared with the acceptable and good groups. More recently, a prospective study demonstrated that selected pre-transplant psychosocial factors predicted both post-transplant nonadherence to treatment and poor clinical outcome (i.e., nonadherence to immunosuppressant medications, late acute rejection, graft loss, and resource utilization), after controlling for medical predictors of poor outcome [60].

We thus suggest that the transplant recipient selection process should follow a continuum from (1) the determination that a patient suffers from end-stage organ disease to (2) an assessment for indications for transplantation, (3) a parallel screening for both medical and psychosocial fitness and/or contraindications to transplantation, (4) being wait-listed for the specific organ transplant, and (5) transplantation (see Fig. 3.3).

At the end, the goals of a psychosocial pre-transplant evaluation should include the following:

- To identify patient's level of neuropsychiatric and cognitive functioning in order to address current psychiatric issues and help minimize preventable challenges.
- To identify patient's social support network, thus allowing the identification of candidates with suboptimal social support systems, allowing for strengthening of existing systems, and providing the needed resources to develop a robust support system.
- To promote fairness and equal access to care.
- To maximize optimal outcomes and the wise use of scarce resources.
- To ensure that the potential for benefits outweighs surgical and medical risks to the patient by identifying potential risk factors (i.e., substance abuse, adherence issues, or serious psychopathological conditions) that may result in increased risk of postoperative nonadherence and morbidity.
- To provide clinicians the information required to develop and implement treatment plans addressing psychosocial vulnerabilities for individuals at high risk, in order to

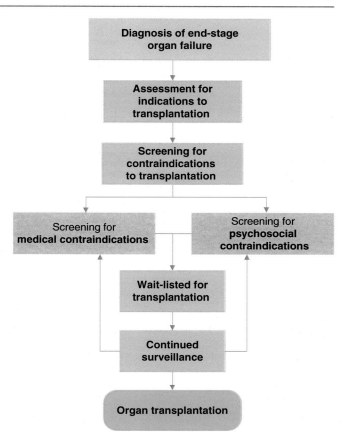

Fig. 3.3 Road to transplantation. (Source: [26])

reduce harm, mitigate risk, and optimize graft survival and patient's level of functioning and overall quality of life [47].

Psychosocial Assessment Tools

Over the years, a number of psychosocial assessment tools have been developed. Table 3.4 summarizes all transplant psychosocial assessment tools published to date. Each tool has its own characteristics and psychometric properties.

The Psychosocial Assessment of Candidates for Transplantation (PACT) consists of eight items, each rated on a 5-point scale, plus the rater's overall impressions [69]. The Psychosocial Levels System (PLS) assesses patients on three gradations of intensity, taking into account seven psychosocial variables, suggesting it was "the first stage in developing a system to reliably identify high-risk Bone Marrow Transplant (BMT) patients at the onset of medical treatment" [70]. The Transplant Evaluation Rating Scale (TERS), a revision of the PLS, consists of 10 items rated on a 3-point scale. The tool provides a single summary score that indicates a patient's current level of functioning as well

Table 3.4 Psychosocial pre-transplant assessment tools

1989	PACT PACT: Psychosocial Assessment of Transplant Candidates [69]	Eight items rated on a five-point scale plus the rater's overall impressions: a "final rating" that can overrule the total score
1991	PLS PLS: Psychosocial Levels System [70]	Three gradations of intensity, accounting for seven psychosocial variables Developed for BMT patients
1993	TERS: Transplant Evaluation Rating Scale [71]	Revision of the PLS Ten items rated on a three-point scale Single summary score to indicate functioning, plus weighted score for each variable
2012	SIPAT Stanford Integrated Psychosocial Assessment for Transplantation [26]	Determined 18 risk factors in 4 domains: Patient readiness Social support Psychological stability Substance abuse Certain items more heavily weighted based on evidence that they are more predictive of nonadherence and clinical outcomes
2014	mPACT Modified PACT [72]	Revision of PACT for VAD patients
2018	*SIPAT-MCS*: [†] Stanford Integrated Psychosocial Assessment for Transplantation – *Cardiac Mechanical Circulatory Support (MCS) Version*	Adaptation of the SIPAT tool for the assessment of candidates for cardiac mechanical circulatory support (MCS)

Sources: [26, 48, 69–73]
† = Tool already developed; currently is being tested and validated

as a weighted score for each variable, suggesting it "can become a valuable instrument enabling consultants to organ transplant programs to predict patients' psychosocial adjustment" [71].

Each scale has different interpretative characteristics. After the original 1991 paper, no further manuscripts have been published using the PLS, which seems to have been replaced by the TERS. One study compared the PACT to TERS on candidates for BMT and found comparable inter-rater reliability, although the authors suggested that "the 5-point scaling of PACT items allows more leeway in making ratings" [74]. In addition, the PACT allows for a clinician's subjective experience (via the "final rating") to overcome the total items score thus defeating the attempt at objectivity [74]. A more recent study explored the association of the PACT subscales and the final rating with 16 post-transplant medical outcomes and found significant relationships ($P \leq 0.05$) between PACT subscales and several medical outcomes, yet the final rating score and medical outcomes were not significantly correlated [75].

A study of lung transplant patients ($n = 110$) divided recipients into high and low psychosocial risk cohorts using a PACT score cutoff of 2 (i.e., recipients with an initial PACT score < 2 deemed as poor or borderline candidates and scores ≥2 deemed as acceptable, good, or great candidates). The authors found that an initial PACT score of <2 was modestly associated with higher mortality (adjusted hazard ratio = 2.73, $p = 0.04$) [76].

Similarly, a prospective study of patients undergoing hematopoietic cell transplantation (HCT) ($n = 366$) assessed the relationship between the TERS scores and objective outcome measures (e.g., length of hospitalization stay [LOS] and survival) [77]. For purposes of the study, patients were stratified into two groups (low/moderate risk vs high risk), based on their predicted psychosocial risk for problems pre-transplant (i.e., TERS scores). There was a significant difference in the median length of hospitalization between patients who scored low/moderate (LOS = 10 days) and those who scored high (LOS = 21.5 days) on the TERS. Furthermore, 2-year overall survival was significantly improved in allogeneic transplant patients who scored low/moderate versus those who scored high on the TERS (72% vs 46%; $p < =0.02$). These findings suggest a strong correlation between pre-transplant psychosocial risk factors, resource utilization, and patient outcomes in HCT [77].

There is no data regarding how widespread the use of PACT or TERS is.

The Stanford Integrated Psychosocial Assessment for Transplantation (SIPAT)

In an attempt to eliminate selection bias and standardize the psychosocial evaluation process for solid organ transplant candidates, the Psychosocial Medicine Team at Stanford studied the available literature on transplantation and the psychosocial factors contributing to the graft success or failure. The aims of the study were to (1) to develop an objective tool to assess the psychosocial factors that better predict patients' adherence and graft survival and (2) to develop a set of psychosocial listing criteria to help guide transplant program's selection process [26]. The team conducted a comprehensive review of the literature on the psychosocial factors that influence transplant clinical outcomes and reviewed all available published data regarding currently utilized psychosocial criteria for candidate selection. The result of this process was the development of a comprehensive pre-transplant candidate evaluation tool: the Stanford Integrated Psychosocial Assessment for Transplantation (SIPAT). The scale addresses only psychosocial variables that are supported by evidence-based data for treatment adherence, quality of life, and graft survival [73]. According to our review of the literature, the psychosocial factors that appear to better

Fig. 3.4 Stanford Integrated Psychosocial Assessment for Transplantation (SIPAT). (Refs: [26, 48])

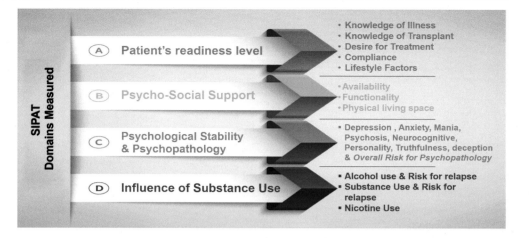

predict patient's adherence and graft survival fall in the following four domains (which include a total of 18 identified risk factors) (see Fig. 3.4):

- Patient's readiness level and illness management (5 items).
- Social support system's level of readiness (3 items).
- Psychological stability and psychopathology (5 items).
- Substance use disorders (5 items).

Based on the assessment of these factors, the SIPAT provides an overall risk severity score for psychosocial variables important in predicting post-transplant behavior, psychosocial support viability and effectiveness, treatment adherence, substance abuse and recidivism, and mental health. Studies have shown that the psychosocial and behavioral characteristics were comparable among solid organ, pre-transplant candidates [26]. Thus instead of performing the pre-transplant psychosocial screening in an organ-specific fashion, we designed and recommend a more general screening protocol.

Our review of the evidence suggested that some of the measured factors are more predictive of treatment nonadherence and clinical outcomes than others. Therefore, the SIPAT items scoring system is weighted more heavily to compensate for this reality. When administering the SIPAT or conducing a psychosocial transplant evaluation in general, it is important that, whenever possible, psychosocial consultants utilize as many sources of collateral information as possible (e.g., review of medical and psychiatric records, prior pre-transplant evaluation records, interview of family members and medical/psychosocial providers) in order to establish and verify the facts provided. This is particularly important in patients suffering from end-stage organ failure or encephalopathy, even more so in the case of candidates presenting in fulminant organ failure. Developing good collaborative relationships with the patient's medical providers and family members can provide a wealth of useful and corroborating

(or conflicting) information, which may be beneficial for the evaluation process.

SIPAT: Rationale for the Inclusion of Specific Psychosocial Variables

For organ transplantation to be an effective treatment, many factors must work in concert: the quality of the donated organ and degree of match between the donor and recipient, the surgical skill, ischemic time, the right postsurgical immunosuppressant therapy regimen, and the active cooperation of the patient with the therapeutic plan. Similarly, the presence of psychosocial factors appears to be a major contributor to poor post-transplant adherence, reduced quality of life [26, 48, 56, 78–82], and increased physical morbidity in the years after transplantation.

Treatment adherence (i.e., the active cooperation of patients with their healthcare professionals regarding attendance to clinics and laboratory appointments, following a specified medication schedule without deviations, following a diet and/or exercise/rehabilitation plan, and the notification of problems to the treatment team) significantly affects the life span and quality of life of recipients. Conversely, nonadherence is a major risk factor for graft rejection episodes and is responsible for up to 25% of deaths after the initial recovery period in all organ transplants [83]. Overall, it has been estimated that post-transplantation nonadherence rates range between 20% and 50% [67, 84–88].

Thus, it is fair to say that the main purpose of pre-transplant psychosocial evaluations is to "assess for the presence of psychosocial vulnerabilities that may contribute to treatment nonadherence and diminish post-transplant quality of life and use objective screening tools to identify patients in need of help with psychosocial problems in order to increase the odds of maximizing good outcomes after transplantation" [26, 47]. Indeed, others have demonstrated that perioperative psychosocial characteristics are strong and significant predictors of post-transplant nonadherence [87].

A study of alcoholic liver disease patients (ALD) ($n = 99$), evaluated for potential liver transplantation (LT), demonstrated that the presence of a number of psychosocial factors (i.e., history of suicidal ideation, $p = 0.03$; living alone, $p = 0.006$; history of alcohol-related hospitalization, $p = 0.01$; lack of alcohol rehabilitation, $p = 0.001$; failure to accept further rehabilitation before transplantation, $p = 0.01$) were associated with a failure to comply with transplant listing requirements, leading to patients never being listed or being removed from the transplant list due to nonadherence [45].

Among heart transplant (HT) recipients ($n = 125$), post-transplant nonadherence was associated with substance abuse history ($p = 0.0007$), personality disorder ($p = 0.007$), living arrangements (e.g., with family vs alone) ($p = 0.02$), and global psychosocial risk ($p = 0.001$) (see Fig. 3.5) [68]. Two factors contributed to the overall variance in compliance: substance abuse (odds ratio (OR) of nonadherence 3.69 [95% confidence intervals (CI) 1.07–12.71, Pearson's chi-squared test (X^2) =4.28, $P = 0.039$]) and global psychosocial risk (OR of nonadherence 3.76 [95% CI 1.18–11.97, $X^2 = 5.03$, $P = 0.025$]). In addition, the number of rejection episodes was associated with global psychosocial risk ($P = 0.029$), and trends were observed for rejection episodes and personality disorder ($r = 0.22$, $P = 0.06$) and support group attendance ($r = 0.16$, $P = 0.08$). Another preliminary finding of the study was the inverse relationship between development of transplant coronary artery disease (CAD) and education ($P = 0.01$). These results suggest that pre-transplant evaluations of psychosocial risk factors can identify patients with an increased risk of post-transplant nonadherence and increased morbidity [68].

A prospective analysis of HT recipients ($n = 145$) indicated that specific areas of medical nonadherence and specific types of psychiatric problems occurring during the first year post-transplant were robustly related to acute graft rejection, incident CAD, and mortality from 1 to 3 years post-transplant [83]. Figure 3.6 shows that recipients who missed medications during the first year post-transplant were 4.17 times more likely to experience acute rejection episodes during the follow-up period, and the experience of acute rejection led to a 6.88 times greater risk of mortality [83]. Similarly, recipients with persistently elevated levels of depressive symptoms and/or anger/hostility symptoms were over four to eight times more likely to develop CAD. In fact, patients who met criteria for transplant-related post-traumatic stress disorder (PTSD-T) during the year after the transplant were over 13 times more likely to have died by 3 years post-transplant (Fig. 3.6) [83].

Among HT recipients ($n = 191$), a multivariate analysis demonstrated a strong "dose-response effect" of the presence of the number of psychosocial risk factors (i.e., pre-transplant psychiatric history, female gender, longer hospitalization, more impaired physical functional status, and lower social supports from caregiver and family in the perioperative period) to post-transplant nonadherence (see Fig. 3.7) [89]. Risk factors' effects were additive; the presence of an increasing number of risk factors bore a dose-response relationship to cumulative risk of developing psychiatric disorders post-transplant. For example, among HT recipients by 3 years post-transplant, if one or no psychosocial risk factor was present, the probability of post-transplant psychiatric disorder was <20%; the probability rose to 50%, if two to three factors were present; but prevalence of a psychiatric dis was as high as 70% if ≥4 psychosocial factors were present ($p < 0.0001$) [89].

Finally, among HT recipients, a number of psychosocial variables (i.e., previous suicide attempts, poor adherence to medical recommendations, previous drug or alcohol rehabilitation, depression) significantly predicted attenuated survival times ($p = 0.004$) (see Fig. 3.8) [90]. In this cohort, a history of suicide attempt(s) was also strongly associated with time to infection and/or rejection episode ($p < 0.001$).

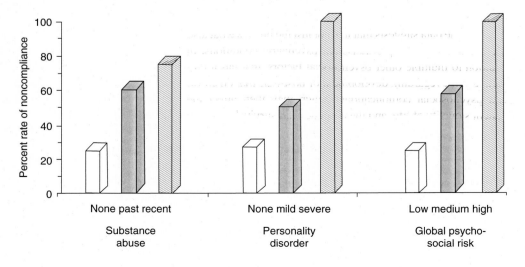

Fig. 3.5 Rates on nonadherence for various psychosocial factors among heart transplant recipients. (Source: [68])

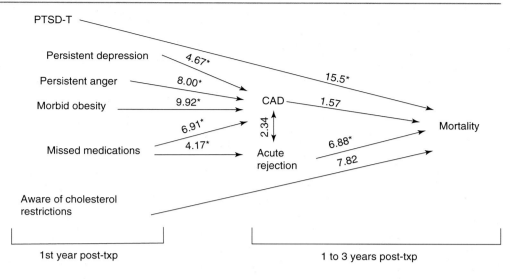

Fig. 3.6 Process by which medical adherence and mental health affect risk for morbidity and mortality post-transplant (Coefficients are odds ratios from logistic regression analyses) *p* < 0.05. (Source: [83]) CAD = coronary artery disease; PTSD-T = post-traumatic stress disorder related to PTSD; post-txp = post-heart transplant

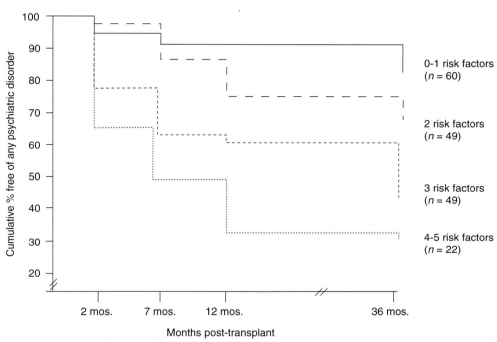

Fig. 3.7 Effect of total number of risk factors on time to onset of any psychiatric disorder post-transplant (Test of overall differences between survival curves, D(3) = 27.31, P < 0.0001). (Source: [89])

Thus, the data suggests that it is not just the presence but also the additive effect of pre-transplant psychiatric conditions, in addition to multiple other psychosocial factors, that has a predictive value regarding development of post-transplant medical and psychosocial complications, which may then affect the patient's quality of life, and the ultimate graft survival.

A prospective, cross-sectional study of HT patients ($n = 147$) demonstrated that 24.5% of post-transplant patients experienced some symptoms of depression. It further demonstrated that the survival outcome was significantly different among the three depression subgroups (log-rank X^2: 9.48, $P = 0.01$). Thus, higher level of depressive symptoms was associated with an almost threefold increase in the risk of mortality (see Fig. 3.9) [62].

Similarly, researchers studied patients who received LT for the treatment of ALD ($n = 167$) and found three trajectories of depressive symptoms evolving within the first post-LT year: a group with consistently *low* depression levels at all timepoints, a group with initially low depression levels that rose over time (i.e., *increasing*), and a group with consistently *high* depression levels [91]. After controlling for medical factors associated with poorer survival, compared to *low* depression patients, the *increasing* and *high* depression groups were more than twice as likely to die (all-cause mortality) over the subsequent year (hazard ratio [HR] 2.25, CI 1.2–4.3, and HR 2.38, CI 1.2–4.7, respectively) (see Fig. 3.10). The *increasing* and *high* depression groups had significantly poorer survival beyond the first post-LT year ($\chi2 = 34$, $p = 0.000$) compared to those

Fig. 3.8 Survival as a
function of psychiatric risk
classification. (Source: [63])

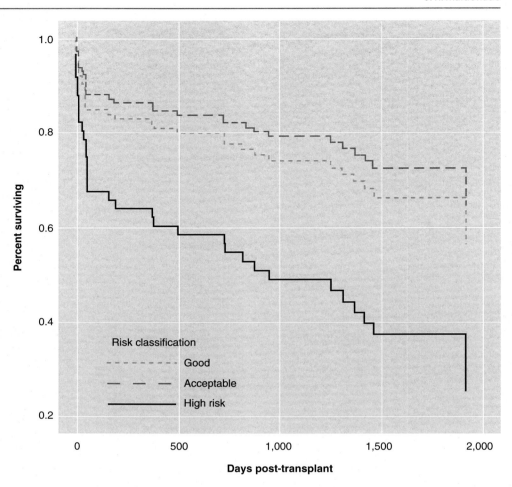

in the *low* depression group. At 10 years post-LT, the survival rate was 66% for the *low* depression group, but only 46% and 43%, respectively, for the *increasing* depression and *high* depression groups [91].

SIPAT: Domains Measured

Domain A: Patient's Level of Readiness

(Item 1) Knowledge and Understanding of Medical Illness Process (that Caused Specific Organ Failure), (Item 2) Knowledge and Understanding of the Process of Transplantation, (Item 3) Willingness and Desire for Transplantation, (Item 4) Treatment Adherence, and (Item 5) Lifestyle Factors Influencing the Medical Process.

The effectiveness of any treatment does not only depend on the right choice of therapy but largely also on the active cooperation of the patient in the therapeutic regimen (i.e., adherence). Lack of cooperation on the part of the patient often means that therapy fails [31].

Studies have demonstrated the link between a patient's understanding of their diagnosed illness and treatment adher-

ence. In fact, studies have found that cause and understanding of patient's illness affect patient's engagement in their treatment regimen and that lack of understanding can lead to frustration and ambivalence, leading to nonadherence [92]. It is not only important for patients to understand just what to do with their medications and how to do it, but for them to understand their disease and how medication compliance greatly impacts their well-being, as well as the adverse consequences of immunosuppressive nonadherence [93].

Others have demonstrated that improved health knowledge was associated with a strengthened sense of control in patients, which resulted in high levels of patient satisfaction. The authors concluded that with improved understanding of their illness, patients were better able to predict disease outcomes, which led to a perceived enhanced sense of control over their lives and a better understanding of how they were able to live with their disease [94]. Studies have found that inaccurate self-report or low awareness of chronic disease may be associated with increased risk of death by as much as 46% for coronary intervention, 34% for ischemic heart disease, and 40% for chronic obstructive pulmonary disease [95].

A number of studies link understanding of transplant process to post-transplant adherence. A study on the effects of a

Fig. 3.9 Kaplan-Meier survival curves according to level of depressive symptoms assessed by the Beck Depression Inventory (BDI). (Source: [62])

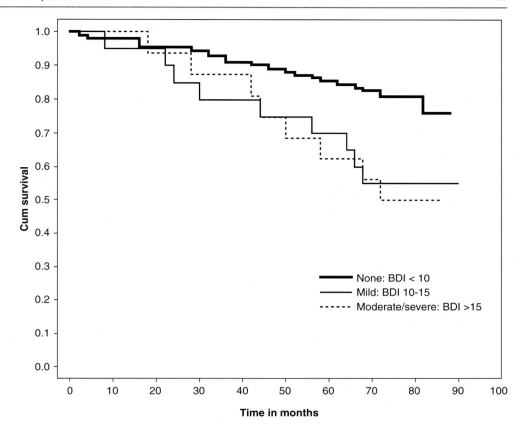

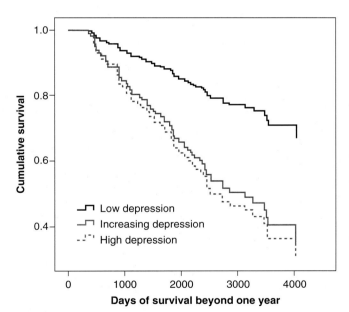

Fig. 3.10 Survival for three groups of liver transplant recipients based on the presence of depressive symptoms post-transplantation. (Source: [91])

pre-transplant interdisciplinary orientation among LT patients demonstrated that group interventions can enhance a patient's understanding regarding the process of transplantation, what to expect during the peri-transplant period, the use and impor-

tance of immunosuppressive drugs, and general and specific transplant requirements, thus enhancing patients' role in their own care [96]. Others have found that enhanced understanding can improve the patient's adherence to medications and minimize the nonadherence (from 43% to 19%) [97].

Inadequate knowledge by patients of their condition and treatment is a predictor of nonadherence after LT. In fact, many patients desire a comprehensive understanding of the medical regimen with an appropriate rationale for each aspect of the regimen, along with information about expected health outcomes, suggesting that patients are more likely to adhere to the post-transplant medical regimen when they fully understand its rationale [98]. Adherence with post-transplant recommendations requires patients to better understand the following elements: the anticipated wait for a deceased donor, the surgical procedure, the immediate postoperative management, and the long-term reality of transplantation [99].

While transplantation is a life-saving procedure for patients with end-stage organ failure, it remains an elective procedure, despite the reality of a poor prognosis should a patient choose not to undergo this complex procedure and associated lifelong management. Thus, it is not just important to assess the candidate's understanding of their illness and transplant procedure, but also important to ascertain their grasp of the lifelong commitment involved in transplantation. Patients must be able to comprehend the risks and benefits of the surgery and the importance of adherence to a medical regimen (i.e., informed consent). The literature suggests that a patient's wishes and degree of motivation for transplantation should be included in the psychosocial assessment [44, 99].

Many providers have met patients who are not fully motivated to proceed with transplantation because they "feel too well" or have not developed enough of the end-stage organ failure symptoms that interfere with their quality of life, despite the objective clinical data presented by their physician. Studies have demonstrated that denial of illness severity may be a potential contraindication to HT [31]. Others have found that recipients who had had positive expectations regarding the transplantation process were significantly more compliant in all areas post-transplantation [100]. Similarly, a survey of transplant clinician's perceptions of compliance found that 53% of clinicians identified lack of knowledge about the post-transplant regimen as a major determinant of nonadherence [101].

Poor preoperative adherence with medical treatment and/or restrictions (e.g., not keeping clinic appointments, refusal to pursue investigations of medical issues with no particular grounds, and self-medication or willfully switching medication doses) seems to persist postoperatively and is the major determinant of postoperative nonadherence [31, 39, 66].

Available data suggests that, among those with chronic illnesses, a history of nonadherence with medical treatment predicts future treatment nonadherence [60]. In fact, a prospective study of transplant patients ($N = 141$; lung 52, heart 28, liver 61) demonstrated that self-reported pre-transplant medication nonadherence was an independent predictor of post-transplant nonadherence (OR = 7.9) and of late acute rejection (OR = 4.4), and it predicted a trend towards greater number of hospitalization days after transplantation [60].

Similarly, a retrospective chart review of 126 kidney transplant (KT) recipients over a 3-year period demonstrated that pre-transplant nonadherence predicted post-transplant nonadherence and graft loss or death [102]. Others have demonstrated that nonadherence with immunosuppression therapy after HT was associated with a significant increase in transplant coronary artery disease (TxCAD) ($p = 0.025$) and was associated with significantly shorter clinical-event–free time compared with compliers (mean, 1318 vs 1612 days; p = 0.043) [103]. In addition, nonadherent patients experienced a greater rate of late acute rejection (11.8% vs 2.4%) and re-transplantation (13.3% vs 2.5%), although these differences were not statistically significant [103].

Some data have suggested that younger age and low socioeconomic status were predictive of nonadherence in prospective studies of KT recipients [51], having devastating effects in the post-transplant period. In fact, in this study, 91% of recipients who were nonadherent with taking medication and follow-up care experienced graft loss or death.

In addition, recipients who reported higher stress and more depression, who coped with stress by using avoidant coping strategies, and who believed that health outcomes are beyond their control were less compliant with both medications and follow-up (all p's < 0.05). Regression analyses revealed that stress was the strongest predictor of nonadherence for medications and follow-up care [104].

Many have already demonstrated that medication nonadherence is a contributing factor to acute organ rejection episodes, thus leading to premature death [66, 67, 81, 82, 85, 105–107]. A prospective study of HT patients demonstrated that poor medication adherence during the first year post-transplant increased risk for acute rejection by over fourfold (see Fig. 3.6) [83]. Furthermore, studies have demonstrated that adherence to various medical (i.e., medication taking, monitoring blood pressure, completing blood work, clinic follow-up visits) and lifestyle (i.e., diet, exercise, alcohol consumption, smoking) restrictions worsened significantly ($p < 0.05$) over time, after transplantation [87].

Poor adherence with other lifestyle factors (e.g., diet, exercise, and weight control) has been hypothesized to contribute to the development and progression of CAD in HT recipients [67, 83, 108–110]. Behavioral interventions should be introduced at the time of the pre-transplant evaluation, given the impact of health behaviors on survival, comorbidities, and quality of life [111].

Domain B: Social Support System

(Item 6) Social Support Availability, (Item 7) Functionality of the Social Support System, and (Item 8) Appropriateness of Physical Living Space and Environment

There are an abundance of studies in the scientific literature that validate the essential role of social support and its link to treatment adherence, quality of life, and graft survival in transplant patients [32, 37, 44, 57, 87, 112]. There is no doubt that the family and psychosocial support network play an important role with respect to survival and morbidity [52, 65, 113–116]. In fact, in some studies the support from a spouse was one of the most important factors in predicting the success of the transplant [117, 118]. A study of LT candidates demonstrated that the absence of a psychosocial support network was a significant risk factor predicting failure to meet listing requirements among end-stage liver disease patients ($p = 0.006$) [45]. See Table 3.5 for a description of the factors to consider when assessing the availability of a candidate's psychosocial support system.

A prospective study of transplant patients (i.e., heart, liver, and lung) also confirmed that the presence of low social support prior to transplant was an independent predictor of post-transplant nonadherence (OR = 0.9) [50]. In addition, among transplant patients, living in an unstable relationship predicted post-transplant graft loss (OR = 4.9) [60].

Others have demonstrated that marital status and living with another person increase adherence modestly, suggesting that the functioning of the social support network may be equally, if not more, influential [119].

Not only is the presence of a social support system imperative for transplant success, but also the functionality of this support network exerts significant influence. In considering the support system's functionality, we must understand that sheer numbers are not enough. Significant quality and functionality, versus a large quantity, are imperative when considering the complex medical regimen and care of the transplant patient in both the pre- and post-transplant phases [120, 121]. The literature regarding the emotional, physical, and financial toll on caregivers who have provided care for their loved ones suffering from chronic illness is well established [122]. A study of patients with end-stage heart disease found that spousal behavioral disengagement (i.e., giving up or withdrawing effort from attempting to reach the goal that is blocked by the stressor) during the pre-transplant evaluation was significantly associated with HT candidates' depression [123].

A meta-analysis of studies over a 50-year period demonstrated that practical support had the highest correlation with adherence to medical treatments [119]. In fact, adherence was 1.74 times higher in patients from cohesive families, but 1.53 times lower in patients from families in conflict [119]. Similarly, among lung transplant patients, the absence of an adequate caregiver support system was associated with the development of major depressive disorder (MDD) after transplantation [124]. See Table 3.6 for a description of the factors to consider when assessing the functionality of a candidate's psychosocial support system.

Finally, data suggest that social and environmental variables, such as poor financial status and living at increased distance from the transplant center, both play a significant role in inhibiting adherence. Living arrangements, specifically in terms of distance to transplant center and appropriateness of facilities, were found to be a significant risk factor for trans-

plant failure [46, 86]. The World Health Organization (WHO) 2003 report found that nonadherence to medication regimen was associated with socioeconomic factors (e.g., demographics, social support) among chronically ill patients [125].

Domain C: Psychological Stability and Psychopathology

(Item 9) Presence of Psychopathology, (Item 10) Organic Psychopathology or Neurocognitive Impairment, (Item 11) Influence of Personality Traits or Disorder, (Item 12) Truthfulness or Deceptive Behavior, (Item 13) Overall Risk for Psychopathology

Multiple studies have demonstrated a correlation between the presence of pre-transplant psychopathology and poor medical and psychosocial outcomes after transplantation. For example, high levels of psychiatric distress often affect the adherence behaviors that lead to negative medical outcomes [26, 67, 87].

Available data and clinical experience suggest that psychiatric problems before transplantation are consistently reported to persist after transplantation, which are highly associated with nonadherence (see Table 3.7) [45, 50, 67, 83, 86, 126–132]. Many have described a strong influence of psychiatric illness (i.e., depression, anxiety, and personality disorders) on post-transplant morbidity and mortality [83, 133].

A study of pre-transplant candidates across organ systems (i.e., heart, kidney, lung, and liver transplant candidates; $n = 311$) found that over 60% of candidates met criteria for a major psychiatric disorder and that 32% meet criteria for personality disorders [33]. As expected, the presence of an active (current) major psychiatric disorder was associated with a past history of psychiatric disorders ($X^2 = 32.36$, df = I, $P = 0.0000$), and family history of psychiatric illness ($X^2 = 6.27$, df = I, $P = 0.0 I$), which was also associated with

Table 3.5 Factors to consider when assessing the availability of a patient's psychosocial support system

Who is/are the patient's support person(s)
How long has patient known the support person(s)
What is the nature of the relationship of the support to the patient
What seems to be the motivating factors for the support in making the commitment to provide help
How easy or difficult would it be for the support person(s) to take the necessary time off from their lives and/or employment in order to fulfill the commitment of providing support
Is the support person(s) willing to relocate, if needed, in order to participate in the transplant education process and/or participate in the pre- and post-transplant care

Table 3.6 Factors to consider when assessing the functionality of a patient's psychosocial support system

Their historical facts that would predict failure or success in this relationship
How well does the patient and support person(s) know each other
What is the nature of their current relationship
Does the support person(s) display a healthy emotional investment in the patient and their recovery
Is there evidence of tension, resentment, reluctance – including the fact the identified support person(s) was chosen because "there is no one else"
How stable is the identified support person's health (i.e., is there a history of physical or mental illness, which may interfere with the support persons' ability to provide the needed help)
Are there any substance use issues in the support team, which may interfere with their ability to assist or adversely influence the status of the recipients

current personality disorder ($X^2 = 5.61$, df = I, $P = 0.018$) [33]. Pre-transplant coping was related to the presence of any major psychiatric ($X^2 = 52.52$, df = 2, $P = 0.0000$) and personality disorders ($X^2 = 49.20$, df = 2, $P = 0.0000$); and both major psychiatric diagnoses and personality disorders were significantly associated with ratings of marital disharmony and inadequacy of social support. Similarly, the presence of a major psychiatric disorder was associated with increasingly poorer psychosocial adjustment and health status after transplantation, while the presence of a personality disorder was significantly associated with global medical nonadherence ($X^2 = 26.69$, df = 2, $P = 0.0000$), including drug misuse ($X^2 = 6.63$, df = I, $P = 0.01$) [33]. Further examination of the HT recipient's sample ($n = 94$) examined before surgery and followed up to 56 months after transplantation revealed that the presence of a psychiatric disorder pre-transplant was specifically related to post-transplant hospital utilization ($p = 0.01$), while personality disorders were related to post-transplant health behaviors/coping style and social support problems ($p = 0.004$) [32]. The authors then divided the sample into low and high psychosocial risk based on a composite score of psychometric indexes of health behavior/coping style and social support measures, which was highly correlated with post-transplant survival ($p < 0.009$) (see Fig. 3.11) [134].

In a study of HT patients ($n = 152$), the authors found that baseline depression and anxiety levels were higher in ischemic cardiomyopathy patients (ICMP) as compared with those with dilated cardiomyopathy (DCMP). The authors divided the sample into low and high anxiety and depression, based on standardized scores. The dichotomized pre-HT anxiety scores were not a predictive factor in postoperative outcome. On the other hand, among those with ICMP, patients in the high depression group preoperatively experienced significantly higher mortality rates after HT compared with those in the low preoperative depression group (RR 5.06; 95% CI, 1.07–23.89; $p < 0.05$) (see Fig. 3.12) [134].

Similarly, Dew et al. [133] confirmed that a history of pre-transplant psychiatric problems, poor social supports, the use of avoidant coping strategies, and low self-esteem were associated with increased major psychiatric disorders post-transplant [133]. Furthermore, data suggest that transplant candidates and recipients exhibiting high levels of psycho-

Table 3.7 Psychological variables associated with nonadherence after transplantation

Depressive disorders
Anxiety disorders
Anger/hostility
Denial
Personality disorders
Psychosis
Suicidality

logical distress in formal testing seem to experience greater mortality rates [135].

In a cohort of HT recipients, those with persistently elevated levels of depressive symptoms and/or anger/hostility symptoms were over four to eight times more likely to develop CAD during the period 1–3 years post-transplant [83].

Among thoracic transplant recipients (i.e., heart and lung; $n = 304$), pre-transplant symptoms of depression and anxiety were associated with an increased risk of post-transplant panic disorder (HR 9; 95% CI, 2.71–30.30; $p < 0.001$), increased MDD (HR 2.5; 95% CI, 1.43–4.39; $p < 0.01$), and increased PTSD-T (HR 2.6; 95% CI, 1.21–5.68; $p < 0.05$) [124]. In fact, the risk for each of these psychiatric disorders was increased over twofold to ninefold by a pre-transplant history of mood or anxiety disorder [124].

A study of LT candidates found that a history of suicide ideation was significant risk factor predicting failure to meet listing requirements among end-stage liver disease patients ($p = 0.03$) [45].

Similarly, the presence of psychopathology after transplantation has been associated with medical comorbidities. For example, among HT recipients, those who developed PTSD-T experienced significantly increased mortality (RR 13.74) [83]. Prospective studies have demonstrated that the presence of depression and persistent anger-hostility significantly increased the risk of incident CAD in HT recipients [83].

A study of bone marrow transplant (BMT) patients found that 9% of recipients developed MDD and that this was associated with a significantly increased mortality at 1 year (HR 2.59; 95% CI, 1.21–5.53; $P = 0.014$) and 3 years (HR 2.04; 95% CI, 1.03–4.02; $P = 0.041$) [136].

Many have described a relationship between personality traits or disorders and negative sequelae after organ transplan-

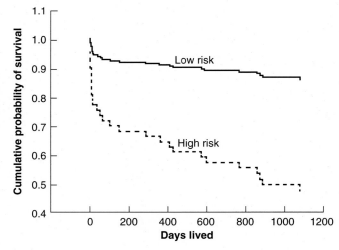

Fig. 3.11 Survival function for additive psychosocial risk factors by days lived at completion of the study for 94 heart transplant patients. (Source: [33])

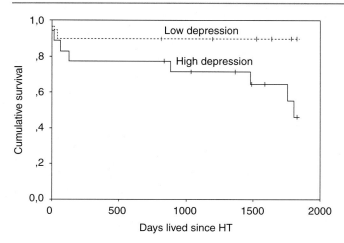

Fig. 3.12 Comparison of post-transplant survival between subgroups of ICMP patients with high and low preoperative depression scores (log rank: $x^2 = 5.18$, $p = 0.023$). (Source: [134])

tation. Personality disorders impair adherence and relationships with treatment team and caregivers. The data suggest that, among transplant patients, more refractory personality disorders may be associated with adherence-adjustment difficulties and appear to be a risk factor for poor outcomes after organ transplantation [105, 106, 135, 137–144].

In fact, a dose-dependent relationship between personality disorders and nonadherence has been described in HT recipients ($p = 0.007$) (see Fig. 3.5) [68]. Similarly, among HT patients, the presence of a personality disorder was significantly associated with global nonadherence ($P = 0.0000$) and specific nonadherence to diet ($P = 0.05$), smoking cessation ($P = 0.001$), keeping appointments ($P = 0.03$), not following medication regimen ($p = 0.006$), and misusing other drugs ($p = 0.0009$) [33]. In another study of HT recipients, those with mild personality disorder were 1.85 times more likely to be nonadherent, and those in the most severe personality disorder group were 3.7 times more likely (in which 100% of the patients were rated nonadherent), compared to recipients with no personality disorder [68]. In addition, personality disorder patients were viewed by the transplant team personnel as having more behavioral problems [32].

Finally, the presence of a personality disorder independently predicted recidivism among patients with a history of alcohol use disorder who underwent LT (relative hazard ratio 6.0 (95% CI, 1.9–18.7; $P = 0.002$) [145].

Given that many psychiatric disorders are characterized by a relapsing-remitting nature, the presence of presurgical psychiatric disorders should be considered as increasing the risk of post-transplant psychiatric complications, thus allowing an opportunity for early identification and intervention.

It is also important to consider the effects of organic psychopathology, including hepatic encephalopathy (HE). Hepatic encephalopathy (HE) is usually interpreted as a sign

of liver failure, but the prognosis of patients with HE is not uniform [146]. Advanced HE is a marker of the severity of liver function and of the presence of intracranial hypertension. Severe HE (grades 3–4) upon admission and during hospitalization is a significant determinant of poor outcome [147]. A study of patients with cirrhosis ($n = 226$) demonstrated that there are residual effects on cognitive function, especially executive functions, which result in learning impairment and working memory problems in patients with overt HE, even after adequate therapy and the attainment of clinical "normal mental status" [148]. Furthermore, the available data has shown that the psychometric performance deterioration continues and expands to the more basic cognitive domains of psychomotor speed, set shifting, and divided attention with increasing numbers of episodes and hospitalizations for overt HE [148].

Despite previous thoughts that HE is a neuropsychiatric syndrome fully reversible by LT, an increasing body of data has demonstrated that is not the case. Studies that have assessed neuropsychological function following LT found a heterogeneous outcomes with persistent cognitive deficits [149–152]. Some have found that patients with a history of HE are at higher risk of developing neurological complications following LT [153], while others have found evidence for "dementia-like" deficits that may not completely recover following LT [154].

The irreversibility of minimal HE (i.e., cognitive deficits) may reflect the neurological sequelae of underlying brain pathology, which is supported by studies demonstrating brain imaging abnormalities, presumed to be secondary to brain edema and gross atrophy in cirrhotic patients, reflecting permanent central nervous system disturbance [151, 154]. Others have found that brain volume after transplantation was smaller in patients with prior HE [155]. Similarly, they found that global cognitive function after LT was poorer in patients with a lower educational level, alcohol etiology, diabetes mellitus, or a history of HE prior to LT and that recipients with prior HE had persistent impaired cognitive and motor function after LT [148, 155]. In general, overall cognitive function may be impaired after LT in the absence of major neurological complications related to the surgical procedure or the postoperative management, due to evidence of central nervous system damage [154, 155].

There is a 25–35% risk of cerebral edema in patients with grade 3 HE. That risk increases to more than 75% of the patients with hepatic coma (grade 4 HE) [156, 157]. A study of LT in patients with hepatic coma demonstrated a significant difference in outcomes, both neurological recovery and overall survival, when comparing early transplantation [ELT] (i.e., within 48 hours of onset of coma) versus late transplantation [LLT] (i.e., after 48 hours of onset of coma). All patients with ELT experienced a complete neurological recovery, while only 50% of LLT recovered. The 3-year survival for ELT was 85% as compared to 50% for LLT (see Fig. 3.13) [158].

There is also data to indicate that patients suffering from HE at the time of LT may be more vulnerable to the metabolic stresses of surgery and the neurotoxicity of the drugs used and were at highest risk for such complications [159]. In fact, in a study of perioperative neurological complications after LT, 90% of HE recipients experienced neurological complications, compared with 6.5% of recipients without HE prior to LT [159]. In this study, logistic regression identified active preoperative HE as the strongest predictor of postoperative morbidity (OR 10.7; 95%, CI 3.8–29.9) [159].

Finally, resting-state functional magnetic resonance imaging (fMRI) data from cirrhotic patients with HE and without HE (noHE) was collected pre- and post-LT ($n = 63$) [160]. Long- and short-range functional connectivity strength (FCS) analysis indicated that before transplantation, both noHE and HE groups showed diffuse FCS abnormalities relative to healthy controls. For the noHE group, the abnormal FCS found before LT largely returned to normal levels after LT, except for in the cerebellum, precuneus, and orbital middle frontal gyrus. However, the FCS abnormalities prior to LT were largely preserved in the HE group after LT, including high-level cognition-related areas (frontal and parietal lobes) and vision-related areas (occipital lobe, cuneus, and precuneus). In addition, comparisons between HE and noHE groups revealed that weaker FCS in default mode network (DMN) in HE group persisted from pre- to post-LT. Correlation analysis showed that changes in FCS in the left postcentral and right middle frontal gyrus correlated with alterations in neuropsychological performance. These findings may suggest a mechanism to explain how pre-LT-related HE may prevent post-LT brain function recovery and

reveal that the DMN may be the most affected brain region by HE, which may not be reversed by LT [160].

The above studies strongly suggest that HE is not a purely metabolic syndrome that will completely reverse with LT. All these findings regarding HE have serious implications as pre-LT HE predicts post-LT neurocognitive deficits that must be considered during the pre-LT evaluation process, as these may affect post-LT functional daily activities, social interactions and the need for ongoing care, and quality of life. This further stresses the importance of cognitive evaluation pre-transplant, adapting the education level to the cognitive status of the patient if possible, maximum mobilization of the support system, and setting of appropriate expectations for the patient, family, and transplant teams.

Domain D: Effects of Substance Use

(Items 14 and 15) Alcohol Use Disorder and Risk for Relapse, (Items 16 and 17) Other Substance Use Disorder and Risk for Relapse [Including Prescribed and Illicit Substances], and (Item 18) Nicotine Use Disorder

A history of substance use disorder has been found to be both highly predictive of post-transplant substance use and of post-transplant treatment nonadherence [161]. Issues to explore include extent of use, time and conditions to substance use cessation, and risk of recidivism [47]. Some have found that, compared with patients with no history of substance use disorder, those with a history of substance use disorder were 2.4-fold more likely, and those with a recent history were three times more likely, to be nonadherent with medical treatment after transplantation [68]. Among HT patients, a history of substance use disorder was the most

Fig. 3.13 Overall survival of acute liver failure patients with hepatic coma after liver transplantation. (Source: [158]). *ELT* early liver transplantation, *LLT* late liver transplantation)

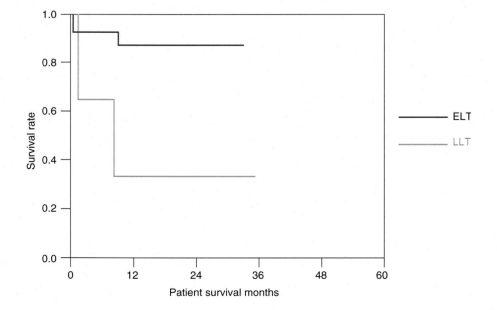

powerful predictor of treatment nonadherence [68]. In fact, a meta-analysis of 147 studies demonstrated that pre-transplant substance abuse predicts post-transplant substance use, and in turn, post-transplant substance abuse correlates with post-transplant nonadherence and decreased overall survival [34].

Preoperative alcohol and substance use disorders have repeatedly been shown to be important predictors for postoperative adherence difficulties [34, 50, 86, 108, 161, 162]. Some have considered the following patient groups to be most at risk for poor post-transplant treatment adherence with sobriety [86]:

- Patients whose substance abuse has not been in longstanding remission.
- Patients whose substance abuse continues after the development of end-stage organ damage and symptoms.
- Patients who ceased substance use only in the face of acute illness.

Specifically among patients undergoing LT for ALD, the cumulative experience has demonstrated that the 1-year actuarial survival after LT for patients with ALD (66–93%) is equal, if not slightly better, to that of patients transplanted for nonalcoholic liver disease (56–87%), as long as they do not resume alcohol use [163]. Unfortunately, multiple studies have found that the alcoholic relapse rate after LT varies from 10% to 50% [145, 164–170] and that alcohol use relapse is associated with a reduced long-term post-transplant survival [170–172].

A study of LT candidates found that a history of previous alcohol-related hospitalization ($p = 0.01$), lack of previous alcoholic rehabilitation before transplant evaluation ($p = 0.001$), and a failure to accept further alcoholic rehabilitation before LT ($p = 0.01$) were all significant risk factors predicting failure to meet listing requirements among end-stage liver disease patients [45]. Similarly, among pre-transplant candidates across organ systems (i.e., heart, kidney, lung, and liver transplant candidates; $n = 311$), a past or current (at time of psychosocial evaluation) history of substance abuse and drinking was significantly associated with nonadherence after transplantation ($P = 0.0000$) [34].

A randomized prospective study of sociological and/or alcohol-related behavioral factors predictive of relapse after LT for ALD patients demonstrated a rate of alcohol use relapse of 11% 1 year after transplantation and 30% after 2 years [173]. In this study, the only variable leading to a significantly lower rate of relapse was abstinence for ≥6 months before LT (23% vs 79%, $P = 0.0003$) (see Fig. 3.14) [173].

Abstinence for >6 months before transplant has been shown to significantly lower the rate of relapse (23% versus

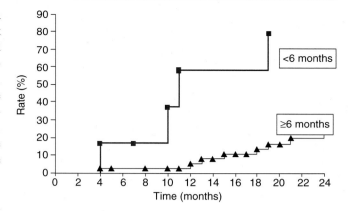

Fig. 3.14 Abstinence as predictive factor of alcohol relapse after OLT for ALD. (Source: [173])

79%, $p = 0.0003$) [174]. In general, while longer abstinence period has been shown to be predictive of ongoing sobriety, the "6-month rule" per se has not been validated. Similarly, among patients with ALD undergoing LT, patients who received substance abuse treatment both before and after transplantation had significantly lower rates of alcohol relapse (16%) than patients who received no substance abuse treatment (41%) or substance abuse treatment only before LT (45%, $p = 0.03$) [175].

Another study assessing the relevance of sobriety for outcome after LT for ALD followed 300 recipients for up to 89 months after orthotopic liver transplantation (OLT) and found that drinking of various degrees was observed in 19% of recipients [167]. Factors associated with an increased risk of recidivism to alcohol consumption included pre-transplant sobriety of less than 6 months, absence of companion in life or lack of adequate social support, presence of young children, and a predicted poor psychosocial prognosis. Pre-transplant sobriety had a significant impact on the recurrence of alcohol consumption after OLT: the longer pre-OLT sobriety, the later time to recidivism. In particular, recurrent alcohol consumption was observed among patients with <6 months of abstinence before transplantation. In this sample, a significantly better survival was observed among patients who remained abstinent compared to those who resumed drinking. In contrast to the uniformly excellent survival rates of patients undergoing OLT for ALD who remained sober (in this sample, 81.5% at 10 years), patients who resumed occasional drinking experienced a 69.1% 10-year survival, and those who resumed abusive drinking demonstrated a 20.1% 10-year survival (see Fig. 3.15) [167].

Researchers studied the potential factors associated with alcohol consumption relapse (recidivism) in a large cohort of patients undergoing LT for alcoholic cirrhosis ($n = 387$) [176]. They found that the overall relapse rate of

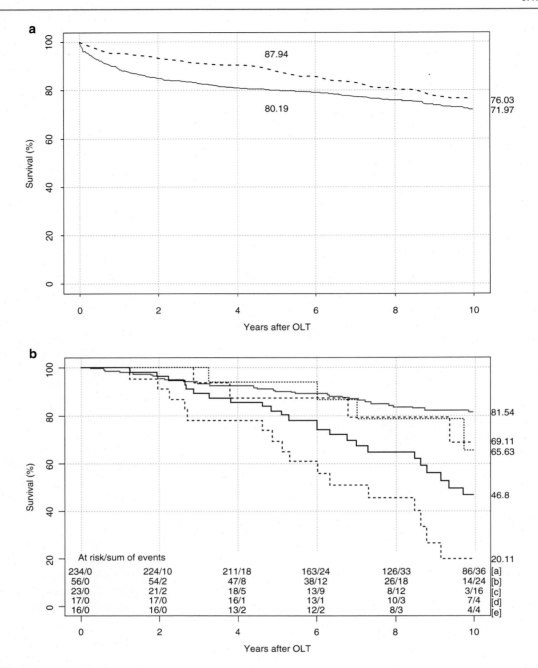

Fig. 3.15 Survival rates of OLT for ALD patients based on recidivism rate and pattern of alcohol use after transplantation. (Source: [167]). Note: Survival rates of patients who remained abstinent after OLT for ALD (n = 234, gray solid line; at risk/sum of events [a]) and patients who resumed drinking after OLT for ALD (n = 56, black solid line; at risk/sum of events [b]). Patients who resumed drinking were divided into three groups according to the severity of alcohol consumption: 23 (41%) patients resumed abusive drinking (dashed line; at risk/sum of events [c]), 17 (30%) patients slipped (dotted line; at risk/sum of events [d]), and in 16 (29%) patients the severity of alcohol consumption remained unknown (dash-dot line; at risk/sum of events [e]))

harmful alcohol consumption after LT was 11.9%. In univariate analysis, alcohol relapse was significantly associated with age greater than 50 years ($p = 0.04$), year of LT 1995 or earlier ($p < 0.05$), duration of abstinence less than 6 months ($p = 0.02$), presence of psychiatric comorbidities ($p < 0.001$), absence of a life partner (i.e., psychosocial support) ($p < 0.05$), and a high score on the High-Risk Alcoholism Relapse (HRAR) ($p < 0.001$). Multivariate logistic regression revealed the following independent factors of relapse: duration of abstinence of less than 6 months (OR 3.3; 95% CI, 1.2–9.3) ($p = 0.02$), presence of psychiatric comorbidities (OR, 7.8; 95% CI, 3.1–20.0)

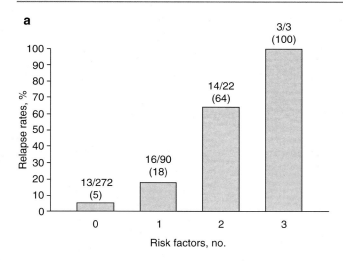
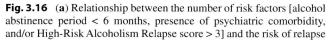

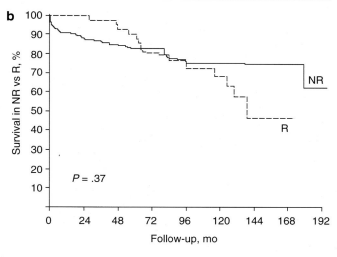

Fig. 3.16 (**a**) Relationship between the number of risk factors [alcohol abstinence period < 6 months, presence of psychiatric comorbidity, and/or High-Risk Alcoholism Relapse score > 3] and the risk of relapse to heavy drinking after liver transplantation. (**b**) Survival curve according to alcohol relapse after liver transplantation; R indicates relapse; NR, no relapse. (Source: {De Gottardi et al. [176])

($p < 0.001$), and HRAR score > 3 (OR, 10.7; 95% CI, 3.8–30.0) ($p = 0.001$). In contrast, in patients with none of these factors, alcohol relapse was only 5%. On the other hand, the presence of 1, 2, or 3 factors was associated with relapse rates of 18%, 64%, and 100% of the patients, respectively (see Fig. 3.16) [176].

In addition, in a prospective cohort of 441 patients who underwent LT, 281 of whom admitted to a history of excessive alcohol consumption prior to LT, alcohol consumption was reported by 32.3% of the study population after transplantation, including 43.7% of ALD patients and 24.3% of non-ALD patients [170]. A multivariable analysis indicated that resumption of alcohol use had a negative impact on long-term survival after transplantation ($p = 0.006$; HR = 2.08 [1.23–3.52]). Although the 5-year survival probability was similar between those who resumed alcohol use after transplantation (82% for relapse patients vs 86% for patients without relapse), the survival gap progressively spread thereafter, with a 10-year survival of 49% among patients with excessive alcohol relapse and 75% among non-relapsers (see Fig. 3.17) [170].

Finally, a meta-analysis including 54 studies ($n = 3263$) revealed that the 5-year survival rate was similar between relapsers and non-relapsers (92.9% vs 92.4%, respectively), but after 10 years, the survival rate decreased significantly in the relapse patients (45.1% vs 85.5%), with malignant tumors and cardiovascular events the main cause of death in these patients (Fig. 3.18) [171].

Regarding alcohol use disorder risk factors associated with graft failure include the following [45]:

- A history of previous alcohol-related hospitalization.
- Lack of or ineffective alcohol rehabilitation.

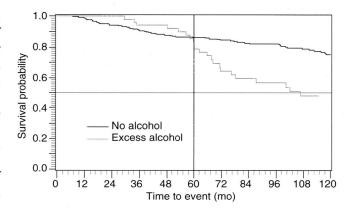

Fig. 3.17 Comparison of Kaplan-Meier survival curves between excessive alcohol relapsers and other patients. Black line: abstinent patients, occasional relapsers, slip relapsers. Gray line: excessive relapsers. (Source: [170])

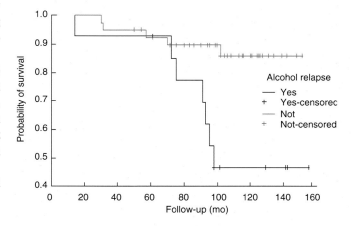

Fig. 3.18 Kaplan-Meier survival curves from patients with alcoholic liver diseases, with or without alcohol recidivism. (Source: [171])

- Failure to accept further alcohol rehabilitation before transplantation.
- Shorter abstinence time prior to transplant.

The attitude toward LT for ALD changed in 1988, when Starzl et al. published data demonstrating that the survival of patients receiving a transplant for alcoholic cirrhosis was not different from the survival of other transplant recipients. Since that report, ALD has become the most common indication for LT [177].

A review of 96 published studies regarding LT for ALD revealed that future abstinence (post-transplant) was associated with social stability, the absence of close relatives with alcohol problems, older age (>40), absence of repeated alcohol treatment failures, good adherence with medical care, no current polysubstance misuse, and an absence of coexisting severe mental disorder [178]. A more recent and simplified criteria are the "A to D transplantation selection criteria," wherein "A" refers to *demonstrated abstention* from alcohol for *over 6 months*, "B" *biology* (a negative family history for alcoholism), "C" *coinhabitants* not consuming alcohol, and "D" no concurrent *drug use disorder* [179].

Finally, we must consider the relationship between alcohol use and an increased incidence of cancer after organ transplantation [180–184]. Although the specific mechanisms of alcohol-mediated oncogenesis are poorly understood, the carcinogenic properties of acetaldehyde and/or the inhibition of DNA methylation via the alteration of retinoid processing have been proposed as potential mechanisms [185, 186]. It is also important to note that alcohol use disorder is associated with an increased risk for malignancies, even in non-immunosuppressed individuals [187–191]. In fact, some have found that excessive alcohol consumption has a negative impact on long-term survival after liver transplant, irrespective of the primary indication, with death being mainly due to liver disease and non-hepatic cancer [170]. Many have demonstrated that excessive drinkers have an increased risk for cancer of the mouth, pharynx, larynx, esophagus, liver, pancreas, stomach, and colon [192–194]. Others have found that both light drinking as well as moderate to heavy alcohol consumption significantly increased the risks of gastrointestinal cancers [187, 195, 196]. There are many mechanisms by which alcohol use may lead to an increased cancer risk, including intestinal stem cells dysregulation, the induction of cytochrome P-4502E1 (which is associated with an enhanced production of free radicals and enhanced activation of various procarcinogens present in alcoholic beverages), alterations in cell cycle behavior, the induction of microsomal enzymes which convert procarcinogens to carcinogens, and the generation of acetaldehyde, the major metabolite of ethanol and a proven carcinogenic and mutagenic agent [193, 197–202]. Considering the increased cancer risk for post-transplant recipient and that carcinogenesis can be enhanced even by relatively low daily doses of ethanol, everything possible should be done to decrease the risk of alcohol use after organ transplantation [199].

Tobacco use is the leading preventable cause of mortality in the general population of the USA [203]. According to the CDC, an estimated 15.5% of the population still smokes tobacco (that's about 37 million people), of which 76% do so on a daily basis [204]. In 2004, the US Surgeon General released a report on tobacco effects, "The Health Consequences of Smoking on the Human Body," detailing the specific end-organ problems caused by tobacco per each organ system (also see Fig. 3.19) [205].

Thus, it is important to understand the relationship between tobacco use and other substances, as well as the effects of tobacco on morbidity and mortality of transplant patients. For example, nearly 90% of alcohol use disorder patients smoke [206]. In a recent meta-analysis, active smoking was revealed as one of the major risk cofactors, independent of alcoholic relapse, of long-term morbidity and mortality in transplant recipients, either from cardiovascular complications or from de novo neoplasms [162]. These findings have been confirmed by numerous studies [207–218]. In fact, researchers observed that patients with a smoking history who continued smoking after the LT presented a hazard ratio of approximately 20 for the development of neoplasms associated with tobacco (head and neck, lung, esophagus, kidney, and urinary tract carcinomas) [219].

While data is not available for all transplant types, a recent online survey of abdominal transplant programs reported that tobacco smoking was an absolute contraindication to transplantation at 38% of kidney, 15% of liver, and 50% of pancreas programs [220].

Studies have found that nearly 40% of ALD recipients resume smoking and resume it early post-LT, increase their consumption over time, and quickly become tobacco dependent [209]. Similarly, some studies have found that in general 14% of KT recipients admit to tobacco use after transplantation [221]. Another study reported continued smoking in 90% of patients who smoked at the time of pre-transplant evaluation [111], while, among HT patients, studies have estimated a 32.6% tobacco relapse rate after transplantation [222].

Nicotine use dramatically potentiates morbidity and mortality after transplantation. When analyzing survival, patients who were smokers preoperatively had a significantly worse prognosis than nonsmokers. In fact, smoking after transplantation (all transplants) in combination with immunosuppressive treatment is associated with perioperative morbidity (e.g., malignancy and end-stage renal failure) and mortality, usually associated with cardiovascular events (e.g., myocardial infarction and cerebrovascular accident). Decreased survival associated with nicotine use has been confirmed in heart [223], lung [224], kidney [225], and liver [217] transplant recipients, with an associated increased length of hospital stay and cost of care, specifically in smokers who received LT [226].

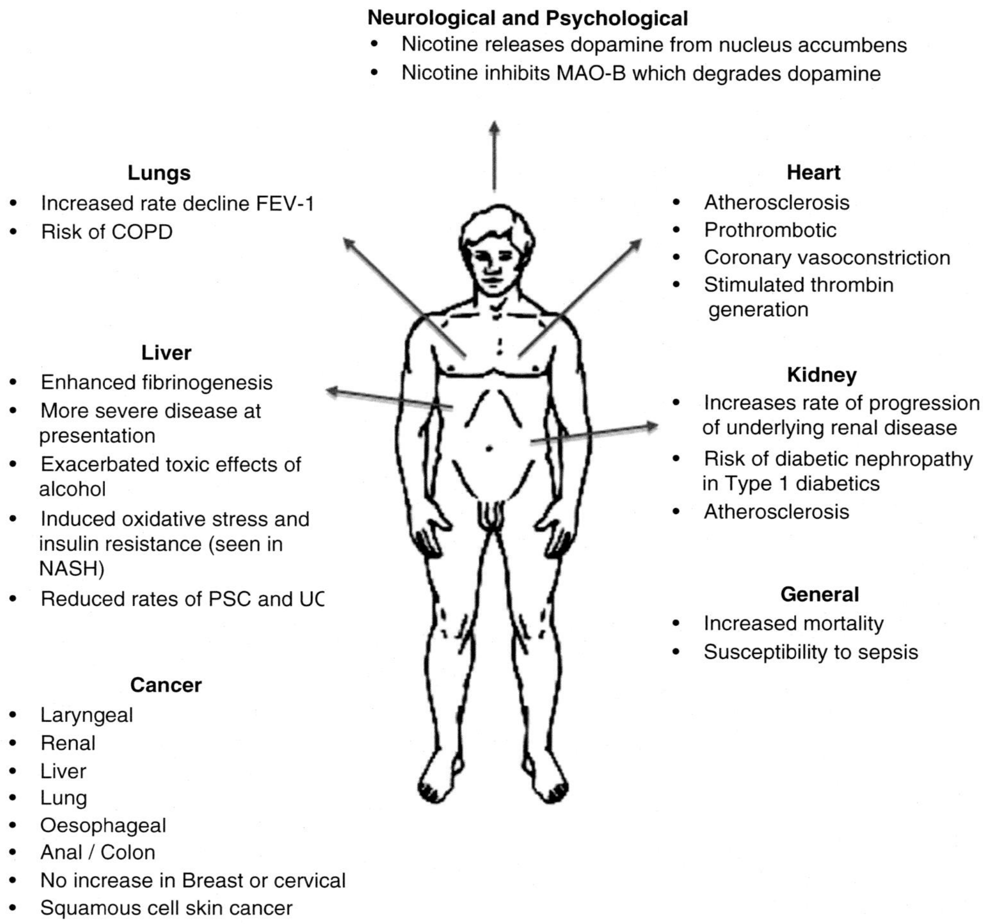

Fig. 3.19 Physiological and psychological effects of smoking on humans. (Source: Corbett et al. [203]). Notes: MAO-B monoamine oxidase B, FEV-1 forced expiratory volume in one second, COPD chronic obstructive pulmonary disease, NASH nonalcoholic steatohepatitis, PSC primary sclerosing cholangitis, UC ulcerative colitis

Neurological and Psychological
- Nicotine releases dopamine from nucleus accumbens
- Nicotine inhibits MAO-B which degrades dopamine

Lungs
- Increased rate decline FEV-1
- Risk of COPD

Liver
- Enhanced fibrinogenesis
- More severe disease at presentation
- Exacerbated toxic effects of alcohol
- Induced oxidative stress and insulin resistance (seen in NASH)
- Reduced rates of PSC and UC

Cancer
- Laryngeal
- Renal
- Liver
- Lung
- Oesophageal
- Anal / Colon
- No increase in Breast or cervical
- Squamous cell skin cancer

Heart
- Atherosclerosis
- Prothrombotic
- Coronary vasoconstriction
- Stimulated thrombin generation

Kidney
- Increases rate of progression of underlying renal disease
- Risk of diabetic nephropathy in Type 1 diabetics
- Atherosclerosis

General
- Increased mortality
- Susceptibility to sepsis

Studies among HT recipients ($n = 84$) found a high rate of patients who smoked after transplantation (26%) [223], which was associated with a 5- and 10-year survival that was significantly reduced in smokers vs nonsmokers (37 vs 80% and 10 vs 74%, respectively; $P < 0.0001$). They also found that smokers had a higher prevalence of transplant vasculopathy as revealed by coronary angiography and/or autopsy ($P < 0.00001$) and a higher rate of malignancies ($P = 0.0001$) [223]. In fact, they found that in patients with a carboxyhemoglobin (CO-Hb) level $\geq 2.5\%$, no patient survived after 4 years (mortality, 100%), and 51% of the patients with lower values were still alive and well after 10 years (see Fig. 3.20) [223].

Tobacco smoke exposure in either donors or recipients results in heightened systemic inflammation and increased oxidative stress, accelerates cardiac allograft rejection (reducing post-transplantation cardiac allograft survival by 33–57%), and increases intra-graft inflammation (tumor necrosis factor-α, interferon-γ, interleukin-6) and alloimmune activation (CD3, interleukin-1 receptor 2, programmed cell death-1, and stromal cell-derived factor-1) with consequent myocardial and vascular destruction [227].

Similarly, tobacco smoking has been found to be an independent risk factor for the development of infectious pulmonary complications in a dose-dependent manner after allogeneic hematopoietic cell transplantation (allo-HCT) [228].

In most cases, participation in a substance use disorder treatment program, ongoing toxicology monitoring, prolonged abstinence for several months, and efforts to improve associated psychosocial aspects are usually necessary to enhance the likelihood of continued sobriety, to improve adherence, and to ensure a good transplant outcome.

As the use of marijuana is increasingly legalized in the USA, questions arise frequently about whether organ transplant recipients who are using marijuana should be assessed or listed. There are some important facts to consider, such as the potency of tetrahydrocannabinol (THC), one of the main psychoactive ingredients in marijuana has been steadily increasing over the years and along with it, the number of Emergency Department visits due to its effects (see Fig. 3.21a, b) [229, 230]. Even when considering the use of other substances (i.e., cocaine and heroin), only marijuana, used either in combination with other drugs or alone, was associated with significant increases in the number of visits

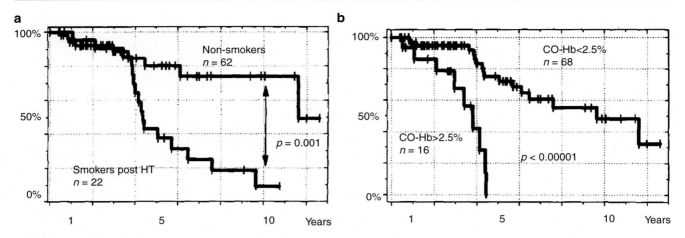

Fig. 3.20 Kaplan-Meier analysis of > 6 month survivors after heart transplantation: (**a**) survival of smokers vs nonsmokers; (**b**) survival of smokers based on HbCO level. (Source: [223]) HT = heart transplant

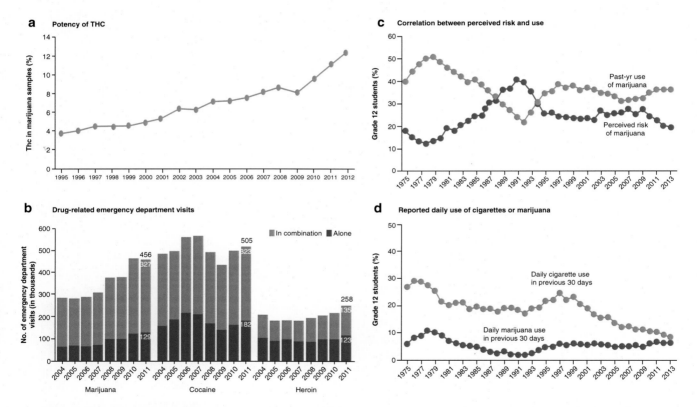

Fig. 3.21 Potency of THC in marijuana, number of ED visits, and perceived marijuana risk over time. (Source: [229]). Panel A shows the increasing potency of marijuana (i.e., the percentage of THC) in samples seized by the Drug Enforcement Administration (DEA) between 1995 and 2012. Panel B provides estimates of the number of emergency department visits involving the use of selected illicit drugs (marijuana, cocaine, and heroin) either singly or in combination with other drugs between 2004 and 2011. Among these three drugs, only marijuana, used either in combination with other drugs or alone, was associated with significant increases in the number of visits during this period (a 62% increase when used in combination with other drugs and a 100% increase when used alone, $P < 0.05$ for the two comparisons). Panel C shows the inverse correlation between the perception of the risk associated with marijuana use and actual use. Perceived risk corresponds to the percentage of teenagers who reported that the use of marijuana is dangerous. Panel D shows the percentage of students who reported daily use of tobacco cigarettes or marijuana in the previous 30 days)

during this period (a 62% increase when used in combination with other drugs and a 100% increase when used alone, $p < 0.05$ for the two comparisons) [231]. At the same time, there is an inverse correlation between the perception (i.e., the percentage of teenagers who reported that the use of marijuana is dangerous) of the risk associated with marijuana use and actual use among adolescents [232]. Of interest, as the daily use of cigarette smoking (a perceived dangerous product) goes down, the daily use of marijuana is on the rise (see Fig. 3.21c, d) [232].

Analysis of the smoke contents of marijuana and tobacco reveals much the same gas-phase constituents, including chemicals known to be toxic to respiratory tissue, including hydrocyanic acid, acetaldehyde, and acrolein [233–236]. In fact, cannabis smoke contains many of the same carcinogens as does tobacco smoke, with some in higher concentrations [237]. It is also mutagenic and carcinogenic in the mouse skin test, and chronic cannabis smokers show pathological changes in lung cells that precede the development of lung cancer in tobacco smokers [238–240]. For comparison, one marijuana joint was equivalent in effect to between 2.5 and 6 tobacco cigarettes, in measures of airflow obstruction [241]. Thus the concerns about its carcinogenic effects and other detrimental effects are the same as for tobacco. In fact, studies have found that the risk of lung cancer increased 8% (95% CI, 2–15%) for each joint-year of cannabis smoking, after adjustment for confounding variables including cigarette smoking, and 7% (95% CI, 5–9%) for each pack-year of cigarette smoking, after adjustment for confounding variables including cannabis smoking [242].

There have been several outbreaks of Mycobacterium tuberculosis due to marijuana use [243]. It appears that tobacco and marijuana may be subject to fungal and *Actinomycetes* contamination, including *Aspergillus*, *A. flavus*, *A. Niger*, *Mucor*, and *Penicillium* [244, 245]. There have been several cases of transplant patients and other immunosuppressed patients contracting infections from marijuana use, including a rare fungal infection with *Ochroconis gallopavum* [246], *Aspergillus* infection in solid organ transplant recipients [247], and lipid pneumonia associated with smoking weed oil [248]. Cases of fatal pulmonary aspergillosis in a bone marrow recipient have been associated with smoking marijuana for several weeks prior to the transplant, with positive cultures of *Aspergillus fumigatus* obtained from the marijuana being smoked [249].

There is also the issue of marijuana's psychoactive effects. A nationally representative sample of US adults, followed over 36 months, found that cannabis use was significantly associated with substance use disorders (any substance use disorder (OR 6.2; 95% CI, 4.1–9.4), any alcohol use disorder (OR 2.7; 95% CI, 1.9–3.8), any cannabis use disorder (OR 9.5; 95% CI, 6.4–14.1), any other drug use disorder (OR 2.6; 95% CI, 1.6–4.4), and nicotine dependence (OR 1.7; 95% CI, 1.2–2.4)) [250]. Similarly, there are a number of negative psychosocial effects of short- and long-term marijuana use that must be taken into consideration (see Table 3.8a) [229]. There is moderate to high level of confidence regarding the evidence for these negative effects (see Table 3.8b) [229].

Finally, consider the pharmacokinetic changes associated with marijuana use. Exogenous cannabinoids (either smoked or edibles) are a group of chemicals that both inhibit cytochrome P450 enzymes 3A4 and 3A5 (the metabolic pathway for the calcineurin inhibitor substances, like tacrolimus and cyclosporine) and inhibit the function of the P-glycoprotein transporter, which has a major role in tacrolimus absorption from the gut and distribution to other tissues, with both mechanisms affecting the bioavailability of immunosuppressant agents, thus potentially contributing to adverse drug-drug interactions and potential toxicity [251–253].

Several states (i.e., AZ, CA, DE, IL, MN, NH, WA) prohibit discrimination against medical cannabis patients in the organ transplant process. As in all cases, it is important to evaluate the patient's specific circumstances and determine whether, from a medical perspective as in the examples above, the use of cannabis is clinically contraindicated. In that situation, the same restrictions would apply to cannabis use as they do for any other legal and prescribed substance use in potential transplant patients. This discussion is neither an endorsement of nor an argument against MJ use per se. Rather, a note of caution given our previous similar experience with tobacco, a once considered a substance that was once considered to have medicinal benefits and is now well known for its adverse medical and carcinogenic effects. It would be a shame to find ourselves in a similar position, 20 years from now, "discovering" that marijuana was harmful to organ transplant patients. Certainly, more safety studies are required before an endorsement is guaranteed. Many programs across the USA prohibit the use of many other potentially harmful substances, despite their legal status.

There are a number of prescribed substances, whose abuse may pose a problem and, although legal, transplant programs may request prospective recipients to decrease or discontinue their use prior to listing (e.g., benzodiazepines, barbiturates, opioids). Depending on their pattern of use, a predetermined period of sobriety, formal drug abuse treatment, and drug surveillance tests may also be required. The question of other substances use by transplant patients is less controversial, as most transplant programs recognize their physiological and psychosocial detrimental effects. Same criteria should apply to marijuana use in transplant candidates. For further discussion, please refer to Chap. 45.

Table 3.8 (**a**) Adverse effects of marijuana; (**b**) Level of confidence in the evidence for adverse effects

a

Adverse Effects of Short-Term Use and Long-Term or Heavy
Use of Marijuana.

Effects of short-term use
Impaired short-term memory, making it difficult to learn and to retain information
Impaired motor coordination, interfering with driving skills and increasing the risk of injuries
Altered judgment, increasing the risk of sexual behaviors that facilitate the transmission of sexually transmitted diseases
In high doses, paranoia and psychosis
Effects of long-term or heavy use
Addiction (in about 9% of users overall, 17% of those who begin use in adolescence, and 25 to 50% of those who are daily users)*
Altered brain development*
Poor educational outcome, with increased likelihood of dropping out of school*
Cognitive impairment, with lower IQ among those who were frequent users during adolescence*
Diminished life satisfaction and achievement (determined on the basis of subjective and objective measures as compared with such ratings in the general population)*
Symptoms of chronic bronchitis
Increased risk of chronic psychosis disorders (including schizophrenia) in persons with a predisposition to such disorders

*The effect is strongly associated with initial marijuana use early in adolescence.

b

Level of Confidence in the Evidence for Adverse Effects of
Marijuana on Health and Well-Being.

Effect	Overall Level of Confidence*
Addiction to marijuana and other substances	High
Abnormal brain development	Medium
Progression to use of other drugs	Medium
Schizophrenia	Medium
Depression or anxiety	Medium
Diminished lifetime achievement	High
Motor vehicle accidents	High
Symptoms of chronic bronchitis	High
Lung cancer	Low

*The indicated overall level of confidence in the association between marijuana use and the listed effects represents an attempt to rank the strength of the current evidence, especially with regard to heavy or long-term use and use that starts in adolescence.

Source: [229]

SIPAT Psychometric Qualities

The SIPAT is a comprehensive screening tool designed to enhance the psychosocial assessment of organ transplant candidates. Its strengths include the standardization of the evaluation process and its ability to identify subjects who are at risk for negative outcomes after the transplant, in order to allow for the development of interventions directed at improving the patient's candidacy. In a study of 102 patients, SIPAT has demonstrated excellent inter-rater reliability, even among novice raters ($P < 0.001$) [26]. Another study of 217 transplant recipients demonstrated that a higher SIPAT score was significantly correlated with the probability of poor medical and psychosocial outcomes [48]. The SIPAT scores were associated with various post-transplant medical complications, such as organ rejection episodes ($p = 0.02$), medical hospitalizations ($p < 0.0001$), and infection rates ($p = 0.02$) within 1 year post transplantation. SIPAT scores also predicted the occurrence of various post-transplant psychosocial complications, such as psychiatric decompensation ($p < 0.005$), presence of nonadherence ($p = 0.09$), and failure of support system ($p = 0.02$). Logistic regression analysis on pooled outcomes data confirmed that higher SIPAT scores increased the probability of an occurrence of undesirable medical outcomes ($p = 0.04$) and negative psychosocial outcomes ($p = 0.03$) (see Fig. 3.22) [48].

At the end, SIPAT was not developed to just have a cutoff at which patients are "declined," but rather it is a standardized, objective, and evidence-based system to evaluate a patient's psychosocial candidacy, in order to determine his/her strengths, identify areas of weakness needing attention or referral (e.g., to social work, psychiatry, addiction services), and allow for timely intervention, so that we can optimize

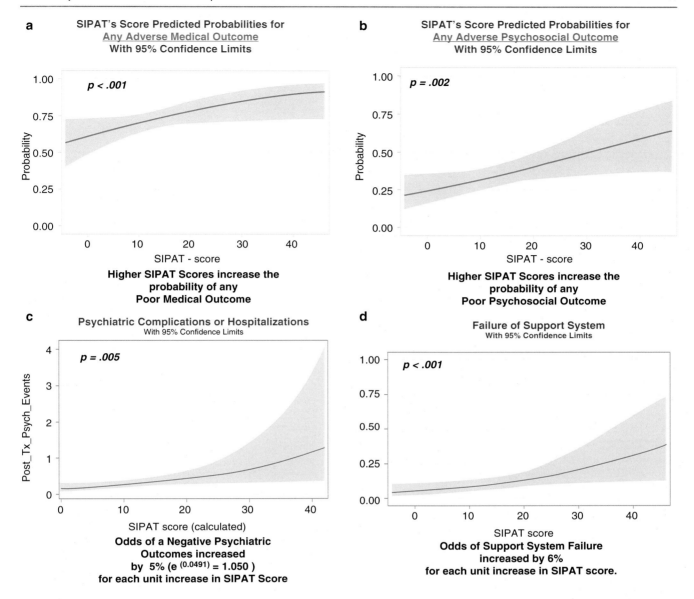

Fig. 3.22 SIPAT score prediction of any negative (**a**) medical and (**b**) psychosocial outcomes, within the psychosocial predictors; SIPAT scores predicted both (**c**) psychiatric complications and (**d**) failures of the psychosocial support system

patient's candidacy and improve their chance of successful transplantation and outcomes.

One of the strengths of the SIPAT is that it standardizes the psychosocial assessment evaluation process, so all transplant candidates undergo the same rigorous psychosocial scrutiny helping identify areas of strengths that can be built upon and areas of weaknesses needing assistance or further consultation and treatment.

The use of SIPAT may not only help to improve the selection process of transplant candidates, but it may also serve to identify a patient's level of social, neuropsychiatric, and cognitive functioning. Clinicians may use the SIPAT to complement and standardize the psychosocial evaluation process,

although it should not be used as the sole determinant of eligibility for transplantation. Instead, the content items of the SIPAT may enhance the selection process by identifying risk factors that may be amenable to clinical intervention before the transplant or that may require extra attention after transplantation.

The function of psychosocial consultants should not be to make a determination regarding "the patient's worthiness as a candidate" but to assist the transplant selection committee in making the best clinical decisions based on the current available data and to provide transplant candidates and teams with the best psychosocial recommendations and treatments to strengthen patients' candidacy, improve quality of life pre- and post-transplant, and increase the chance of post-transplant success. Our hope is that a universal agreed-upon use of a structured standardized tool, such as the SIPAT, in addition to a set of agreed upon minimal psychosocial listing criteria and organ-specific medical listing criteria, would allow for the establishment of a standardized process and criteria for the selection of solid organ transplant recipients in a way that promotes fairness, allows for the identification and timely management of potential problems, and maximizes graft survival and quality of life.

Conclusions

The assessment of transplant candidates is challenging and includes potential clinical, ethical, and social factors. The data available to date confirms that in addition to typical medical factors, psychosocial and behavioral issues may affect the ultimate success of the transplantation process. There is data to suggest that pre-transplant psychiatric history can predict psychological outcomes after transplant and that post-transplant psychosocial outcomes may predict physical morbidity and mortality. Accordingly, most guidelines suggest that the pre-transplant screening process must include both a comprehensive medical evaluation and a thorough psychological assessment.

Thus, psychosocial consultants should find data regarding those risk factors for which there is evidence supporting predictive value: the patient's readiness level to serve as a partner in the management of end-stage organ failure and post-transplant period, patient's understanding of their medical illness and the transplant process and expectations, the status and functionality of their social support network, history of transplant candidate's adherence to medical treatment and recommendations from medical teams, the candidate's psychological stability, and the candidate's extent of substance use, sobriety, and conditions under which it was achieved. These appear to be the most significant factors relating to the success of a transplant. Whenever possible, we should use sources of collateral information (e.g., family, healthcare providers, and medical records) to build on and verify the facts provided, particularly in patients with end-stage organ disease or fulminant failure. In addition, developing a good collaborative relationship with the social workers and nurse coordinators for the transplant teams will be rewarding, because they usually are the best at knowing the patient and can provide a wealth of useful and corroborating (or conflicting) information that may be helpful in making decisions regarding the patient's truthfulness with the process. The use of objective psychosocial assessment tools, such as the SIPAT, can assist transplant teams not only in eliminating the emotional factor from the assessment but also in presenting the facts of the case as they are. The role of psychosocial consultants should not be to make a determination regarding the patient's worthiness as a candidate but to assist the transplant selection committee in making the best clinical decision based on current available data.

References

1. OPTN. OPTN/UNOS Ethics Committee: ethical principles to be considered in the allocation of human organs: HRSA. 2010. [Updated June 22, 2010. Available from: http://optn.transplant.hrsa.gov/resources/bioethics.asp?index=5.
2. OPTN/UNOS. OPTN/UNOS Ethics Committee General considerations in assessment for transplant candidacy: HRSA. 2010. [Available from: http://optn.transplant.hrsa.gov/resources/bioethics.asp?index=5.
3. UNOS. National Data: transplants by organ type united network for organ sharing. 2018. [Available from: https://unos.org/data/.
4. OPTN. https://onlinelibrary.wiley.com/toc/16006143/18/S1. Am J Transplant. 2018;18(S1):1–503.
5. DHS. Organ donation and transplantation statistics: graph data: U.S. Department of Health & Human Services. 2018. Available from: https://www.organdonor.gov/statistics-stories/statistics/data.html.
6. OPTN. Need continues to grow: organ procurement and transplantation network. 2018. [cited 2018. Available from: https://optn.transplant.hrsa.gov/need-continues-to-grow/.
7. OPTN. Organ Procurement and Transplantation Network: Organ Procurement and Transplantation Network. 2016. [Available from: https://optn.transplant.hrsa.gov/.
8. De Meester J, Persijn GG, Wujciak T, Opelz G, Vanrenterghem Y. The new eurotransplant kidney allocation system: report one year after implementation. Eurotransplant International Foundation. Transplantation. 1998;66(9):1154–9.
9. Fuggle SV, Belger MA, Johnson RJ, Ray TC, Morris PJ. A new national allocation scheme for adult kidneys in the United Kingdom. United Kingdom Transplant Support Service Authority (UKTSSA) Users' Kidney Advisory Group and its task forces. Clin Transpl. 1998:107–13.
10. Nyberg SL, Matas AJ, Rogers M, Harmsen WS, Velosa JA, Larson TS, et al. Donor scoring system for cadaveric renal transplantation. Am J Transplant. 2001;1(2):162–70.
11. Baskin-Bey ES, Kremers W, Nyberg SL. A recipient risk score for deceased donor renal allocation. Am J Kidney Dis. 2007;49(2):284–93.
12. UNOS. "Kidney Allocation Policy Development." 2009. [Updated June 22, 2010. Available from: http://www.unos.org/kars.asp.
13. Desschans B, Van Gelder F, Van Hees D, de Rocy J, Monbaliu D, Aerts R, et al. Evolution in allocation rules for renal, hepatic, pancreatic and intestinal grafts. Acta Chir Belg. 2008;108(1):31–4.
14. UNOS. Standardizing the process: a look at the OPTN/UNOS pancreas transplantation committee. 2009. [Available from: http://www.unos.org/ContentDocuments/Committees_May_June09.pdf.
15. NYHA. Nomenclature and criteria for diagnosis of diseases of the heart and great vessels. Boston, Mass: Little, Brown & Co; 1994.
16. Kamath PS, Wiesner RH, Malinchoc M, Kremers W, Therneau TM, Kosberg CL, et al. A model to predict survival in patients with end-stage liver disease. Hepatology. 2001;33(2):464–70.
17. Wiesner R, Edwards E, Freeman R, Harper A, Kim R, Kamath P, et al. Model for end-stage liver disease (MELD) and allocation of donor livers. Gastroenterology. 2003;124(1):91–6.

18. Horslen S. Organ allocation for liver-intestine candidates. Liver Transpl. 2004;10(10 Suppl 2):S86–9.

19. Kamath PS, Kim WR. Advanced Liver Disease Study G. The model for end-stage liver disease (MELD). Hepatology. 2007;45(3):797–805.

20. Freeman RB Jr. Model for end-stage liver disease (MELD) for liver allocation: a 5-year score card. Hepatology. 2008;47(3):1052–7.

21. Singal AK, Kamath PS. Model for End-stage Liver Disease. J Clin Exp Hepatol. 2013;3(1):50–60.

22. De Meester J, Smits JM, Persijn GG, Haverich A. Listing for lung transplantation: life expectancy and transplant effect, stratified by type of end-stage lung disease, the Eurotransplant experience. J Heart Lung Transplant. 2001;20(5):518–24.

23. UNOS. The Lung Allocation Score (LAS) System. 2005. [Available from: http://www.unos.org/resources/frm_LAS_Calculator.asp?index=96.

24. OPTN. Lung allocation system: U.S. Department of Health & Human Services. 2015. [cited 2018 2018]. Available from: https://optn.transplant.hrsa.gov/learn/professional-education/lung-allocation-system/.

25. Smits JM, Nossent G, Evrard P, Lang G, Knoop C, Kwakkel-van Erp JM, et al. Lung Allocation Score - The Eurotransplant Model vs. the revised U.S. model. Transpl Int. 2018.

26. Maldonado JR, Dubois HC, David EE, Sher Y, Lolak S, Dyal J, et al. The Stanford Integrated Psychosocial Assessment for Transplantation (SIPAT): a new tool for the psychosocial evaluation of pre-transplant candidates. Psychosomatics. 2012;53(2):123–32.

27. OPTN. Organ Procurement and Transplantation Network (OPTN) Policies. OPTN Webite. 2018.

28. UNOS. History of Transplantation UNOS Website: United Network for Organ Sharing (UNOS). 2018. [cited 2018 4/21/2018]. Available from: https://unos.org/transplantation/history/?gclid=EAIaIQobChMI8fHeq73M2gIVkNdkCh2Nsgn_EAAYAiAAEgIW-fD_BwE.

29. OPTN. OPTN Evaluation Plan. 2010. [Updated 12/31/2010. Available from: http://optn.transplant.hrsa.gov/SharedContentDocuments/Evaluation_Plan_508_123110.pdf.

30. Barbour KA, Blumenthal JA, Palmer SM. Psychosocial issues in the assessment and management of patients undergoing lung transplantation. Chest. 2006;129(5):1367–74.

31. Bunzel B, Laederach-Hofmann K. Solid organ transplantation: are there predictors for posttransplant noncompliance? A literature overview. Transplantation. 2000;70(5):711–6.

32. Chacko RC, Harper RG, Gotto J, Young J. Psychiatric interview and psychometric predictors of cardiac transplant survival. Am J Psychiatry. 1996;153(12):1607–12.

33. Chacko RC, Harper RG, Kunik M, Young J. Relationship of psychiatric morbidity and psychosocial factors in organ transplant candidates. Psychosomatics. 1996;37(2):100–7.

34. Dew MA, DiMartini AF, De Vito DA, Myaskovsky L, Steel J, Unruh M, et al. Rates and risk factors for nonadherence to the medical regimen after adult solid organ transplantation. Transplantation. 2007;83(7):858–73.

35. Dew MA, DiMartini AF, Switzer GE, Kormos RL, Schulberg HC, Roth LH, et al. Patterns and predictors of risk for depressive and anxiety-related disorders during the first three years after heart transplantation. Psychosomatics. 2000;41(2):191–2.

36. Dobbels F, De Geest S, Cleemput I, Fischler B, Kesteloot K, Vanhaecke J, et al. Psychosocial and behavioral selection criteria for solid organ transplantation. Prog Transplant. 2001;11(2):121–30. quiz 31-2

37. Dobbels F, Vanhaecke J, Desmyttere A, Dupont L, Nevens F, De Geest S. Prevalence and correlates of self-reported pretransplant nonadherence with medication in heart, liver, and lung transplant candidates. Transplantation. 2005;79(11):1588–95.

38. Dobbels F, Vanhaecke J, Nevens F, Dupont L, Verleden G, Van Hees D, et al. Liver versus cardiothoracic transplant candidates and their pretransplant psychosocial and behavioral risk profiles: good neighbors or complete strangers? Transpl Int. 2007;20(12):1020–30.

39. Dobbels F, Verleden G, Dupont L, Vanhaecke J, De Geest S. To transplant or not? The importance of psychosocial and behavioural factors before lung transplantation. Chron Respir Dis. 2006;3(1):39–47.

40. Goetzmann L, Klaghofer R, Wagner-Huber R, Halter J, Boehler A, Muellhaupt B, et al. Psychosocial vulnerability predicts psychosocial outcome after an organ transplant: results of a prospective study with lung, liver, and bone-marrow patients. J Psychosom Res. 2007;62(1):93–100.

41. Goetzmann L, Ruegg L, Stamm M, Ambuhl P, Boehler A, Halter J, et al. Psychosocial profiles after transplantation: a 24-month follow-up of heart, lung, liver, kidney and allogeneic bone-marrow patients. Transplantation. 2008;86(5):662–8.

42. Hoodin F, Weber S. A systematic review of psychosocial factors affecting survival after bone marrow transplantation. Psychosomatics. 2003;44(3):181–95.

43. Huffman JC, Popkin MK, Stern TA. Psychiatric considerations in the patient receiving organ transplantation: a clinical case conference. Gen Hosp Psychiatry. 2003;25(6):484–91.

44. Jowsey SG, Taylor ML, Schneekloth TD, Clark MM. Psychosocial challenges in transplantation. J Psychiatr Pract. 2001;7(6):404–14.

45. Karman JF, Sileri P, Kamuda D, Cicalese L, Rastellini C, Wiley TE, et al. Risk factors for failure to meet listing requirements in liver transplant candidates with alcoholic cirrhosis. Transplantation. 2001;71(9):1210–3.

46. Levenson JL, Olbrisch ME. Psychosocial evaluation of organ transplant candidates. A comparative survey of process, criteria, and outcomes in heart, liver, and kidney transplantation. Psychosomatics. 1993;34(4):314–23.

47. Maldonado J. I have been asked to work up a patient who requires a liver transplant; how should I proceed? Focus. 2009;7(3):332–5.

48. Maldonado JR, Sher Y, Lolak S, Swendsen H, Skibola D, Neri E, et al. The Stanford Integrated Psychosocial Assessment for Transplantation: a prospective study of medical and psychosocial outcomes. Psychosom Med. 2015;77(9):1018–30.

49. Olbrisch ME, Benedict SM, Ashe K, Levenson JL. Psychological assessment and care of organ transplant patients. J Consult Clin Psychol. 2002;70(3):771–83.

50. Rivard AL, Hellmich C, Sampson B, Bianco RW, Crow SJ, Miller LW. Preoperative predictors for postoperative problems in heart transplantation: psychiatric and psychosocial considerations. Prog Transplant. 2005;15(3):276–82.

51. Schweizer RT, Rovelli M, Palmeri D, Vossler E, Hull D, Bartus S. Noncompliance in organ transplant recipients. Transplantation. 1990;49(2):374–7.

52. Teichman BJ, Burker EJ, Weiner M, Egan TM. Factors associated with adherence to treatment regimens after lung transplantation. Prog Transplant. 2000;10(2):113–21.

53. Jowsey SG, Schneekloth TD. Psychosocial factors in living organ donation: clinical and ethical challenges. Transplant Rev (Orlando). 2008;22(3):192–5.

54. Rudis R, Rudis E, Lupo Y, Safady R, Bonne O. Psychosocial model for evaluation and intervention with candidates for organ transplantation. Transplant Proc. 2000;32(4):761–2.

55. Withers N, Hilsabeck R, Maldonado J. Ethical and psychosocial challenges in liver transplantation. J Psychosom Res. 2003;55:116.

56. Dew MA, Switzer GE, DiMartini AF, Matukaitis J, Fitzgerald MG, Kormos RL. Psychosocial assessments and outcomes in organ transplantation. Prog Transplant. 2000;10(4):239–59. quiz 60-1

57. Skotzko CE, Stowe JA, Wright C, Kendall K, Dew MA. Approaching a consensus: psychosocial support services for solid organ transplantation programs. Prog Transplant. 2001;11(3):163–8.

58. Gun Ho Lee BA, David Magnus PD, Maldonado JR. Psychosocial contraindications to transplant listing decisions: a national survey of adult and pediatric heart, kidney, liver, and lung programs. Academy of psychosomatic medicine. Palm Springs, CA: Not yet published; 2017.

59. Denhaerynck K, Dobbels F, Cleemput I, Desmyttere A, Schafer-Keller P, Schaub S, et al. Prevalence, consequences, and determinants of nonadherence in adult renal transplant patients: a literature review. Transpl Int. 2005;18(10):1121–33.

60. Dobbels F, Vanhaecke J, Dupont L, Nevens F, Verleden G, Pirenne J, et al. Pretransplant predictors of posttransplant adherence and clinical outcome: an evidence base for pretransplant psychosocial screening. Transplantation. 2009;87(10):1497–504.

61. Drent G, Haagsma EB, SDvdB G, Aad P, Ten Vergert EM, van den Bosch HJ, MJH S, et al. Prevalence of prednisolone (non) compliance in adult liver transplant recipients. Transpl Int. 2005;18(8):960–6.

62. Havik OE, Sivertsen B, Relbo A, Hellesvik M, Grov I, Geiran O, et al. Depressive symptoms and all-cause mortality after heart transplantation. Transplantation. 2007;84(1):97–103.

63. Owen JE, Bonds CL, Wellisch DK. Psychiatric evaluations of heart transplant candidates: predicting post-transplant hospitalizations, rejection episodes, and survival. Psychosomatics. 2006;47(3):213–22.

64. Messias E, Skotzko CE. Psychiatric assessment in transplantation. Revista de saude publica. 2000;34(4):415–20.

65. Molassiotis A, van den Akker OB, Boughton BJ. Perceived social support, family environment and psychosocial recovery in bone marrow transplant long-term survivors. Social Sci & Med (1982). 1997;44(3):317–25.

66. Rodriguez A, Diaz M, Colon A, Santiago-Delpin EA. Psychosocial profile of noncompliant transplant patients. Transplant Proc. 1991;23(2):1807–9.

67. Paris W, Muchmore J, Pribil A, Zuhdi N, Cooper DK. Study of the relative incidences of psychosocial factors before and after heart transplantation and the influence of posttransplantation psychosocial factors on heart transplantation outcome. J Heart Lung Transplant. 1994;13(3):424–30. discussion 31–2

68. Shapiro PA, Williams DL, Foray AT, Gelman IS, Wukich N, Sciacca R. Psychosocial evaluation and prediction of compliance problems and morbidity after heart transplantation. Transplantation. 1995;60(12):1462–6.

69. Olbrisch M, Levenson J, Hamer R. The PACT: a rating scale for the study of clinical decision making in psychosocial screening of organ transplant candidates. Clin Transpl. 1989;3:164–9.

70. Futterman AD, Wellisch DK, Bond G, Carr CR. The psychosocial levels system. A new rating scale to identify and assess emotional difficulties during bone marrow transplantation. Psychosomatics. 1991;32(2):177–86.

71. Twillman RK, Manetto C, Wellisch DK, Wolcott DL. The transplant evaluation rating Scale. A revision of the psychosocial levels system for evaluating organ transplant candidates. Psychosomatics. 1993;34(2):144–53.

72. Maltby MC, Flattery MP, Burns B, Salyer J, Weinland S, Shah KB. Psychosocial assessment of candidates and risk classification of patients considered for durable mechanical circulatory support. J Heart Lung Transplant. 2014;33(8):836–41.

73. Maldonado J, David E, Plante R, Dubois H, Dyal J. "The Stanford Integrated Psychosocial Assessment for Transplant (SIPAT): a new tool for the psychosocial evaluation of solid organ pre-transplantat candidates." 55th Annual Meeting of the Academy of Psychosomatic Medicine; November 2008; Miami, FL: APPI, 2008.

74. Presberg BA, Levenson JL, Olbrisch ME, Best AM. Rating scales for the psychosocial evaluation of organ transplant candidates. Comparison of the PACT and TERS with bone marrow transplant patients. Psychosomatics. 1995;36(5):458–61.

75. Foster LW, McLellan L, Rybicki L, Dabney J, Visnosky M, Bolwell B. Utility of the psychosocial assessment of candidates for transplantation (PACT) scale in allogeneic BMT. Bone Marrow Transplant. 2009;44(6):375–80.

76. Hitschfeld MJ, Schneekloth TD, Kennedy CC, Rummans TA, Niazi SK, Vasquez AR, et al. The psychosocial assessment of candidates for transplantation: a cohort study of its association with survival among lung transplant recipients. Psychosomatics. 2016;57(5):489–97.

77. Speckhart DS, Solomon SR. Psychosocial factors as measured by the transplant evaluation rating scale (TERS) predict length of hospitalization and transplant outcomes following hematopoietic stem cell transplantation. Blood. 2006;108(11):75.

78. Crone CC, Wise TN. Psychiatric aspects of transplantation, III: Postoperative issues. Crit Care Nurse. 1999;19(4):28–38.

79. Dew MA, Switzer GE, Goycoolea JM, Allen AS, DiMartini A, Kormos RL, et al. Does transplantation produce quality of life benefits? A quantitative analysis of the literature. Transplantation. 1997;64(9):1261–73.

80. Mai FM, McKenzie FN, Kostuk WJ. Psychosocial adjustment and quality of life following heart transplantation. Can J Psychiatr. 1990;35(3):223–7.

81. Surman OS. Psychiatric aspects of liver transplantation. Psychosomatics. 1994;35(3):297–307.

82. Surman OS, Cosimi AB, DiMartini A. Psychiatric care of patients undergoing organ transplantation. Transplantation. 2009;87(12):1753–61.

83. Dew MA, Kormos RL, Roth LH, Murali S, DiMartini A, Griffith BP. Early post-transplant medical compliance and mental health predict physical morbidity and mortality one to three years after heart transplantation. J Heart Lung Transplant. 1999;18(6):549–62.

84. De Geest S, Abraham I, Moons P, Vandeputte M, Van Cleemput J, Evers G, et al. Late acute rejection and subclinical noncompliance with cyclosporine therapy in heart transplant recipients. J Heart Lung Transplant. 1998;17(9):854–63.

85. De Geest S, Borgermans L, Gemoets H, Abraham I, Vlaminck H, Evers G, et al. Incidence, determinants, and consequences of subclinical noncompliance with immunosuppressive therapy in renal transplant recipients. Transplantation. 1995;59(3):340–7.

86. Shapiro PA, Williams D, Gelman I, Foray AT, Wukich N. Compliance complications in cardiac patients. Am J Psychiatry. 1997;154(11):1627–8.

87. Dew MA, Roth LH, Thompson ME, Kormos RL, Griffith BP. Medical compliance and its predictors in the first year after heart transplantation. J Heart Lung Transplant. 1996;15(6):631–45.

88. Grady KL, Russell KM, Srinivasan S, Costanzo MR, Pifarre R. Patient compliance with annual diagnostic testing after heart transplantation. Transplant Proc. 1993;25(5):2978–80.

89. Dew MA, Kormos RL, DiMartini AF, Switzer GE, Schulberg HC, Roth LH, et al. Prevalence and risk of depression and anxiety-related disorders during the first three years after heart transplantation. Psychosomatics. 2001;42(4):300–13.

90. Owens B. Breastfeeding an infant after heart transplant surgery. J Hum Lact. 2002;18(1):53–5.

91. DiMartini A, Dew MA, Chaiffetz D, Fitzgerald MG, Devera ME, Fontes P. Early trajectories of depressive symptoms after liver transplantation for alcoholic liver disease predicts long-term survival. Am J Transplant. 2011;11(6):1287–95.

92. Anderson K, Devitt J, Cunningham J, Preece C, Cass A. "All they said was my kidneys were dead": Indigenous Australian patients' understanding of their chronic kidney disease. Med J Aust. 2008;189(9):499–503.

93. Chisholm MA, Mulloy LL, Jagadeesan M, DiPiro JT. Impact of clinical pharmacy services on renal transplant patients' compliance with immunosuppressive medications. Clin Transpl. 2001;15(5):330–6.
94. Meyer C, Muhlfeld A, Drexhage C, Floege J, Goepel E, Schauerte P, et al. Clinical research for patient empowerment--a qualitative approach on the improvement of heart health promotion in chronic illness. Med Sci Monit. 2008;14(7):CR358–65.
95. Cavanaugh KLM, Merkin SS, Plantinga LC, Fink NE, Sadler JH, Powe NR. Accuracy of patients' reports of comorbid disease and their association with mortality in ESRD. Am J Kidney Dis. 2008;52(1):118–27.
96. Guimaro MS, Lacerda SS, Bacoccina TD, Karam CH, de Sa JR, Ferraz-Neto BH, et al. Evaluation of efficacy in a liver pre-transplantation orientation group. Transplant Proc. 2007;39(8):2522–4.
97. Beck DE, Fennell RS, Yost RL, Robinson JD, Geary D, Richards GA. Evaluation of an educational program on compliance with medication regimens in pediatric patients with renal transplants. J Pediatr. 1980;96(6):1094–7.
98. Lisson GL, Rodrigue JR, Reed AI, Nelson DR. A brief psychological intervention to improve adherence following transplantation. Ann Transplant. 2005;10(1):52–7.
99. Steinman TI, Becker BN, Frost AE, Olthoff KM, Smart FW, Suki WN, et al. Guidelines for the referral and management of patients eligible for solid organ transplantation. Transplantation. 2001;71(9):1189–204.
100. Leedham B, Meyerowitz BE, Muirhead J, Frist WH. Positive expectations predict health after heart transplantation. Health Psychol. 1995;14(1):74–9.
101. Hathaway DK, Combs C, De Geest S, Stergachis A, Moore LW. Patient compliance in transplantation: a report on the perceptions of transplant clinicians. Transplant Proc. 1999;31(4A):10S–3S.
102. Douglas S, Blixen C, Bartucci MR. Relationship between pre-transplant noncompliance and posttransplant outcomes in renal transplant recipients. J Transpl Coord. 1996;6(2):53–8.
103. Dobbels F, De Geest S, van Cleemput J, Droogne W, Vanhaecke J. Effect of late medication non-compliance on outcome after heart transplantation: a 5-year follow-up. J Heart Lung Transplant. 2004;23(11):1245–51.
104. Frazier PA, Davis-Ali SH, Dahl KE. Correlates of noncompliance among renal transplant recipients. Clin Transpl. 1994;8(6):550–7.
105. Freeman AM 3rd, Folks DG, Sokol RS, Fahs JJ. Cardiac transplantation: clinical correlates of psychiatric outcome. Psychosomatics. 1988;29(1):47–54.
106. Brennan AF, Davis MH, Buchholz DJ, Kuhn WF, Gray LA Jr. Predictors of quality of life following cardiac transplantation. Psychosomatics. 1987;28(11):566–71.
107. Wolcott DL. Organ transplantation psychiatry. Psychosomatics. 1993;34(2):112–3.
108. Berlakovich GA. Wasting your organ with your lifestyle and receiving a new one? Ann Transplant. 2005;10(1):38–43.
109. Colonna P, Sorino M, D'Agostino C, Bovenzi F, De Luca L, Arrigo F, et al. Nonpharmacologic care of heart failure: counseling, dietary restriction, rehabilitation, treatment of sleep apnea, and ultrafiltration. Am J Cardiol. 2003;91(9A):41F–50F.
110. Stilley CS, DiMartini AF, de Vera ME, Flynn WB, King J, Sereika S, et al. Individual and environmental correlates and predictors of early adherence and outcomes after liver transplantation. Prog Transplant. 2010;20(1):58–66. quiz 7
111. Ehlers SL. Ethical analysis and consideration of health behaviors in organ allocation: focus on tobacco use. Transplant Rev (Orlando). 2008;22(3):171–7.
112. Lopez Sanchez J, Fernandez Lucas M, Miranda B, et al. editors. Adhesion to the treatment in renal transplant recipients: a Spanish multicentric trial. The first European symposium on non-compliance in transplantation. 1999.
113. Christensen AJ, Turner CW, Slaughter JR, Holman JM Jr. Perceived family support as a moderator psychological well-being in end-stage renal disease. J Behav Med. 1989;12(3):249–65.
114. Debray Q, Plaisant O. Pulmonary transplantation. Psychological aspects. The medical context and indications. Ann Med Psychol. 1990;148(1):105–7. discussion 8–9
115. Feinstein S, Keich R, Becker-Cohen R, Rinat C, Schwartz SB, Frishberg Y. Is noncompliance among adolescent renal transplant recipients inevitable? Pediatrics. 2005;115(4):969–73.
116. Schlebusch L, Pillay BJ, Louw J. Depression and self-report disclosure after live related donor and cadaver renal transplants. South African Medical Journal = Suid-Afrikaanse tydskrif vir geneeskunde. 1989;75(10):490–3.
117. Dew MA, Goycoolea JM, Stukas AA, Switzer GE, Simmons RG, Roth LH, et al. Temporal profiles of physical health in family members of heart transplant recipients: predictors of health change during caregiving. Health Psychol. 1998;17(2):138–51.
118. Jalowiec A, Grady KL, White-Williams C. Predictors of perceived coping effectiveness in patients awaiting a heart transplant. Nurs Res. 2007;56(4):260–8.
119. DiMatteo MR. Social support and patient adherence to medical treatment: a meta-analysis. Health Psychol. 2004;23(2):207–18.
120. Bolkhir A, Loiselle MM, Evon DM, Hayashi PH. Depression in primary caregivers of patients listed for liver or kidney transplantation. Prog Transplant. 2007;17(3):193–8.
121. Cohen M, Katz D, Baruch Y. Stress among the family caregivers of liver transplant recipients. Prog Transplant. 2007;17(1):48–53.
122. Brodaty H, Donkin M. Family caregivers of people with dementia. Dialogues Clin Neurosci. 2009;11(2):217–28.
123. Burker EJ, Evon DM, Ascari JC, Loiselle MM, Finkel JB, Mill MR. Relationship between coping and depression in heart transplant candidates and their spouses. Prog Transplant. 2006;16(3):215–21.
124. Dew MA, DiMartini AF, DeVito Dabbs AJ, Fox KR, Myaskovsky L, Posluszny DM, et al. Onset and risk factors for anxiety and depression during the first 2 years after lung transplantation. Gen Hosp Psychiatry. 2012;34(2):127–38.
125. Burkhart PV, Sabate E. Adherence to long-term therapies: evidence for action. J Nurs Scholarsh. 2003;35(3):207.
126. Achille MA, Ouellette A, Fournier S, Vachon M, Hebert MJ. Impact of stress, distress and feelings of indebtedness on adherence to immunosuppressants following kidney transplantation. Clin Transpl. 2006;20(3):301–6.
127. Cohen L, Littlefield C, Kelly P, Maurer J, Abbey S. Predictors of quality of life and adjustment after lung transplantation. Chest. 1998;113(3):633–44.
128. Grulke N, Larbig W, Kachele H, Bailer H. Pre-transplant depression as risk factor for survival of patients undergoing allogeneic haematopoietic stem cell transplantation. Psychooncology. 2008;17(5):480–7.
129. Kiley DJ, Lam CS, Pollak R. A study of treatment compliance following kidney transplantation. Transplantation. 1993;55(1):51–6.
130. Kuhn WF, Brennan AF, Lacefield PK, Brohm J, Skelton VD, Gray LA. Psychiatric distress during stages of the heart transplant protocol. J Heart Transplant. 1990;9(1):25–9.
131. Smith C, Chakraburtty A, Nelson D, Paradis I, Kesinger S, Bak K, et al. Interventions in a heart transplant recipient with a histrionic personality disorder. J Transpl Coord. 1999;9(2):109–13.
132. Phipps L. Psychiatric evaluation and outcomes in candidates for heart transplantation. Clin Invest Med. 1997;20(6):388–95.
133. Dew MA, Roth LH, Schulberg HC, Simmons RG, Kormos RL, Trzepacz PT, et al. Prevalence and predictors of depression and anxiety-related disorders during the year after heart transplantation. Gen Hosp Psychiatry. 1996;18(6 Suppl):48S–61S.
134. Zipfel S, Schneider A, Wild B, Lowe B, Junger J, Haass M, et al. Effect of depressive symptoms on survival after heart transplantation. Psychosom Med. 2002;64(5):740–7.

135. Brandwin M, Trask PC, Schwartz SM, Clifford M. Personality predictors of mortality in cardiac transplant candidates and recipients. J Psychosom Res. 2000;49(2):141–7.

136. Prieto JM, Atala J, Blanch J, Carreras E, Rovira M, Cirera E, et al. Role of depression as a predictor of mortality among cancer patients after stem-cell transplantation. J Clin Oncol. 2005;23(25):6063–71.

137. Frierson RL, Lippmann SB. Heart transplant candidates rejected on psychiatric indications. Psychosomatics. 1987;28(7):347–55.

138. Kuhn WFM, Myers B, Brennan AF, Davis MH, Lippmann SB, Gray LA, Pool GE. Psychopathology in heart transplant candidates. J Heart Transplant. 1988;7(3):223–6.

139. Phipps L. Psychiatric aspects of heart transplantation. Can J Psychiatr. 1991;36(8):563–8.

140. Denollet J, Holmes RV, Vrints CJ, Conraads VM. Unfavorable outcome of heart transplantation in recipients with type D personality. J Heart Lung Transplant. 2007;26(2):152–8.

141. Dobbels F, Put C, Vanhaecke J. Personality disorders: a challenge for transplantation. Prog Transplant. 2000;10(4):226–32.

142. Gorevski E, Succop P, Sachdeva J, Cavanaugh TM, Volek P, Heaton P, et al. Is there an association between immunosuppressant therapy medication adherence and depression, quality of life, and personality traits in the kidney and liver transplant population? Patient Prefer Adherence. 2013;7:301–7.

143. Telles-Correia D, Barbosa A, Mega I. Personality and transplantation. Acta Medica Port. 2010;23(4):655–62.

144. Weitzner MA, Lehninger F, Sullivan D, Fields KK. Borderline personality disorder and bone marrow transplantation: ethical considerations and review. Psychooncology. 1999;8(1):46–54.

145. Gish RG, Lee A, Brooks L, Leung J, Lau JY, Moore DH 2nd. Long-term follow-up of patients diagnosed with alcohol dependence or alcohol abuse who were evaluated for liver transplantation. Liver Transpl. 2001;7(7):581–7.

146. Garcia-Martinez R, Simon-Talero M, Cordoba J. Prognostic assessment in patients with hepatic encephalopathy. Dis Markers. 2011;31(3):171–9.

147. Ichai P, Samuel D. Etiology and prognosis of fulminant hepatitis in adults. Liver Transpl. 2008;14(Suppl 2):S67–79.

148. Bajaj JS, Schubert CM, Heuman DM, Wade JB, Gibson DP, Topaz A, et al. Persistence of cognitive impairment after resolution of overt hepatic encephalopathy. Gastroenterology. 2010;138(7):2332–40.

149. Sotil EU, Gottstein J, Ayala E, Randolph C, Blei AT. Impact of preoperative overt hepatic encephalopathy on neurocognitive function after liver transplantation. Liver Transpl. 2009;15(2):184–92.

150. Mechtcheriakov S, Graziadei IW, Mattedi M, Bodner T, Kugener A, Hinterhuber HH, et al. Incomplete improvement of visuo-motor deficits in patients with minimal hepatic encephalopathy after liver transplantation. Liver Transpl. 2004;10(1):77–83.

151. Tarter RE, Switala JA, Arria A, Plail J, Van Thiel DH. Subclinical hepatic encephalopathy. Comparison before and after orthotopic liver transplantation. Transplantation. 1990;50(4):632–7.

152. Lewis MB, Howdle PD. Cognitive dysfunction and health-related quality of life in long-term liver transplant survivors. Liver Transpl. 2003;9(11):1145–8.

153. Pujol A, Graus F, Rimola A, Beltran J, Garcia-Valdecasas JC, Navasa M, et al. Predictive factors of in-hospital CNS complications following liver transplantation. Neurology. 1994;44(7):1226–30.

154. Rose C, Jalan R. Is minimal hepatic encephalopathy completely reversible following liver transplantation? Liver Transpl. 2004;10(1):84–7.

155. Garcia-Martinez R, Rovira A, Alonso J, Jacas C, Simon-Talero M, Chavarria L, et al. Hepatic encephalopathy is associated with posttransplant cognitive function and brain volume. Liver Transpl. 2011;17(1):38–46.

156. Stravitz RT, Kramer AH, Davern T, Shaikh AO, Caldwell SH, Mehta RL, et al. Intensive care of patients with acute liver failure: recommendations of the U.S. Acute Liver Failure Study Group. Crit Care Med. 2007;35(11):2498–508.

157. Munoz SJ. Difficult management problems in fulminant hepatic failure. Semin Liver Dis. 1993;13(4):395–413.

158. Yang HR, Thorat A, Jeng LB, Hsu SC, Li PC, Yeh CC, et al. Living donor liver transplantation in acute liver failure patients with grade IV encephalopathy: is deep hepatic coma still an absolute contraindication? a successful single-center experience. Ann Transplant. 2018;23:176–81.

159. Dhar R, Young GB, Marotta P. Perioperative neurological complications after liver transplantation are best predicted by pre-transplant hepatic encephalopathy. Neurocrit Care. 2008;8(2):253–8.

160. Cheng Y, Zhang G, Shen W, Huang LX, Zhang L, Xie SS, et al. Impact of previous episodes of hepatic encephalopathy on short-term brain function recovery after liver transplantation: a functional connectivity strength study. Metab Brain Dis. 2018;33(1):237–49.

161. Hanrahan JS, Eberly C, Mohanty PK. Substance abuse in heart transplant recipients: a 10-year follow-up study. Prog Transplant. 2001;11(4):285–90.

162. Kotlyar DS, Burke A, Campbell MS, Weinrieb RM. A critical review of candidacy for orthotopic liver transplantation in alcoholic liver disease. Am J Gastroenterol. 2008;103(3):734–43. quiz 44

163. Maldonado JR, Keeffe EB. Liver transplantation for alcoholic liver disease: selection and outcome. Clin Liver Dis. 1997;1(2):305–21.

164. Donnadieu-Rigole H, Perney P, Pageaux GP. Alcohol consumption after liver transplantation in patients transplanted for alcoholic cirrhosis. Presse Med. 2015;44(5):481–5.

165. Jauhar S, Talwalkar JA, Schneekloth T, Jowsey S, Wiesner RH, Menon KV. Analysis of factors that predict alcohol relapse following liver transplantation. Liver Transpl. 2004;10(3):408–11.

166. Coffman KL, Hoffman A, Sher L, Rojter S, Vierling J, Makowka L. Treatment of the postoperative alcoholic liver transplant recipient with other addictions. Liver Transpl Surg. 1997;3(3):322–7.

167. Pfitzmann R, Schwenzer J, Rayes N, Seehofer D, Neuhaus R, Nussler NC. Long-term survival and predictors of relapse after orthotopic liver transplantation for alcoholic liver disease. Liver Transpl. 2007;13(2):197–205.

168. Mackie J, Groves K, Hoyle A, Garcia C, Garcia R, Gunson B, et al. Orthotopic liver transplantation for alcoholic liver disease: a retrospective analysis of survival, recidivism, and risk factors predisposing to recidivism. Liver Transpl. 2001;7(5):418–27.

169. Pereira SP, Howard LM, Muiesan P, Rela M, Heaton N, Williams R. Quality of life after liver transplantation for alcoholic liver disease. Liver Transpl. 2000;6(6):762–8.

170. Faure S, Herrero A, Jung B, Duny Y, Daures JP, Mura T, et al. Excessive alcohol consumption after liver transplantation impacts on long-term survival, whatever the primary indication. J Hepatol. 2012;57(2):306–12.

171. Iruzubieta P, Crespo J, Fabrega E. Long-term survival after liver transplantation for alcoholic liver disease. World J Gastroenterol. 2013;19(48):9198–208.

172. Rice JP, Eickhoff J, Agni R, Ghufran A, Brahmbhatt R, Lucey MR. Abusive drinking after liver transplantation is associated with allograft loss and advanced allograft fibrosis. Liver Transpl. 2013;19(12):1377–86.

173. Miguet M, Monnet E, Vanlemmens C, Gache P, Messner M, Hruskovsky S, et al. Predictive factors of alcohol relapse after orthotopic liver transplantation for alcoholic liver disease. Gastroenterol Clin Biol. 2004;28(10 Pt 1):845–51.

174. Mehra MR, Kobashigawa J, Starling R, Russell S, Uber PA, Parameshwar J, et al. Listing criteria for heart transplantation: International Society for Heart and Lung Transplantation guidelines for the care of cardiac transplant candidates--2006. J Heart Lung Transplant. 2006;25(9):1024–42.

175. Rodrigue JR, Hanto DW, Curry MP. Substance abuse treatment and its association with relapse to alcohol use after liver transplantation. Liver Transpl. 2013;19(12):1387–95.

176. De Gottardi A, Spahr L, Gelez P, Morard I, Mentha G, Guillaud O, et al. A simple score for predicting alcohol relapse after liver transplantation: results from 387 patients over 15 years. Arch Intern Med. 2007;167(11):1183–8.

177. Maldonado J. Liver Transplantation in alcoholic liver disease: selection and outcome. J Psychosom Res. 2003;55:115–6.

178. McCallum S, Masterton G. Liver transplantation for alcoholic liver disease: a systematic review of psychosocial selection criteria. Alcohol Alcoholism (Oxford, Oxfordshire). 2006;41(4):358–63.

179. Gong A, Minuk GY. Predictors of alcohol relapse following liver transplantation for alcohol-induced liver failure. consideration of "A-D" selection criteria. Ann Transplant. 2018;23:129–35.

180. Duvoux C, Delacroix I, Richardet JP, Roudot-Thoraval F, Metreau JM, Fagniez PL, et al. Increased incidence of oropharyngeal squamous cell carcinomas after liver transplantation for alcoholic cirrhosis. Transplantation. 1999;67(3):418–21.

181. Watt KD, Pedersen RA, Kremers WK, Heimbach JK, Sanchez W, Gores GJ. Long-term probability of and mortality from de novo malignancy after liver transplantation. Gastroenterology. 2009;137(6):2010–7.

182. Jain A, DiMartini A, Kashyap R, Youk A, Rohal S, Fung J. Long-term follow-up after liver transplantation for alcoholic liver disease under tacrolimus. Transplantation. 2000;70(9):1335–42.

183. Saigal S, Norris S, Muiesan P, Rela M, Heaton N, O'Grady J. Evidence of differential risk for posttransplantation malignancy based on pretransplantation cause in patients undergoing liver transplantation. Liver Transpl. 2002;8(5):482–7.

184. Zanus G, Carraro A, Vitale A, Gringeri E, D'Amico F, Valmasoni M, et al. Alcohol abuse and de novo tumors in liver transplantation. Transplant Proc. 2009;41(4):1310–2.

185. Nakajima T, Kamijo Y, Tanaka N, Sugiyama E, Tanaka E, Kiyosawa K, et al. Peroxisome proliferator-activated receptor alpha protects against alcohol-induced liver damage. Hepatology. 2004;40(4):972–80.

186. Seitz HK, Stickel F. Molecular mechanisms of alcohol-mediated carcinogenesis. Nat Rev Cancer. 2007;7(8):599–612.

187. Mufti SI, Darban HR, Watson RR. Alcohol, cancer, and immunomodulation. Crit Rev Oncol Hematol. 1989;9(3):243–61.

188. Chirigos MA, Schultz RM. Animal models in cancer research which could be useful in studies of the effect of alcohol on cellular immunity. Cancer Res. 1979;39(7 Pt 2):2894–8.

189. Ratna A, Mandrekar P. Alcohol and Cancer: Mechanisms and Therapies. Biomolecules. 2017;7(3)

190. Schottenfeld D. Alcohol as a co-factor in the etiology of cancer. Cancer. 1979;43(5 Suppl):1962–6.

191. Su LJ, Arab L. Alcohol consumption and risk of colon cancer: evidence from the national health and nutrition examination survey I epidemiologic follow-up study. Nutr Cancer. 2004;50(2):111–9.

192. Haas SL, Ye W, Lohr JM. Alcohol consumption and digestive tract cancer. Curr Opin Clin Nutr Metab Care. 2012;15(5):457–67.

193. Seitz HK, Maurer B, Stickel F. Alcohol consumption and cancer of the gastrointestinal tract. Dig Dis. 2005;23(3-4):297–303.

194. Salaspuro MP. Alcohol consumption and cancer of the gastrointestinal tract. Best Pract Res Clin Gastroenterol. 2003;17(4):679–94.

195. Choi YJ, Lee DH, Han KD, Kim HS, Yoon H, Shin CM, et al. The relationship between drinking alcohol and esophageal, gastric or colorectal cancer: A nationwide population-based cohort study of South Korea. PLoS One. 2017;12(10):e0185778.

196. Testino G, Borro P. Alcohol and gastrointestinal oncology. World J Gastrointest Oncol. 2010;2(8):322–5.

197. Lu R, Voigt RM, Zhang Y, Kato I, Xia Y, Forsyth CB, et al. Alcohol Injury Damages Intestinal Stem Cells. Alcohol Clin Exp Res. 2017;41(4):727–34.

198. Taylor B, Rehm J. Moderate alcohol consumption and diseases of the gastrointestinal system: a review of pathophysiological processes. Dig Dis. 2005;23(3-4):177–80.

199. Poschl G, Seitz HK. Alcohol and cancer. Alcohol and alcoholism (Oxford, Oxfordshire). 2004;39(3):155–65.

200. Badger TM, Ronis MJ, Seitz HK, Albano E, Ingelman-Sundberg M, Lieber CS. Alcohol metabolism: role in toxicity and carcinogenesis. Alcohol Clin Exp Res. 2003;27(2):336–47.

201. Mufti SI. Alcohol-stimulated promotion of tumors in the gastrointestinal tract. Cancer Detect Prev. 1998;22(3):195–203.

202. Lieber CS, Seitz HK, Garro AJ, Worner TM. Alcohol-related diseases and carcinogenesis. Cancer Res. 1979;39(7 Pt 2):2863–86.

203. CDC. Burden of Tobacco Use in the U.S. 2018; https://www.cdc.gov/tobacco/campaign/tips/resources/data/cigarette-smoking-in-united-states.html, 2018.

204. Jamal A, King BA, Neff LJ, Whitmill J, Babb SD, Graffunder CM. Current Cigarette Smoking Among Adults - United States, 2005-2015. MMWR Morb Mortal Wkly Rep. 2016;65(44):1205–11.

205. The 2004 United States Surgeon General's Report: The Health Consequences of Smoking. NSW Public Health Bull. 2004;15(5–6):107.

206. Burling TA, Ziff DC. Tobacco smoking: a comparison between alcohol and drug abuse inpatients. Addict Behav. 1988;13(2):185–90.

207. Cuadrado A, Fabrega E, Casafont F, Pons-Romero F. Alcohol recidivism impairs long-term patient survival after orthotopic liver transplantation for alcoholic liver disease. Liver Transpl. 2005;11(4):420–6.

208. Herrero JI, Lorenzo M, Quiroga J, Sangro B, Pardo F, Rotellar F, et al. De Novo neoplasia after liver transplantation: an analysis of risk factors and influence on survival. Liver Transpl. 2005;11(1):89–97.

209. DiMartini A, Javed L, Russell S, Dew MA, Fitzgerald MG, Jain A, et al. Tobacco use following liver transplantation for alcoholic liver disease: an underestimated problem. Liver Transpl. 2005;11(6):679–83.

210. Rubio E, Moreno JM, Turrion VS, Jimenez M, Lucena JL, Cuervas-Mons V. De novo malignancies and liver transplantation. Transplant Proc. 2003;35(5):1896–7.

211. Scheifele C, Reichart PA, Hippler-Benscheidt M, Neuhaus P, Neuhaus R. Incidence of oral, pharyngeal, and laryngeal squamous cell carcinomas among 1515 patients after liver transplantation. Oral Oncol. 2005;41(7):670–6.

212. Jimenez C, Manrique A, Marques E, Ortega P, Loinaz C, Gomez R, et al. Incidence and risk factors for the development of lung tumors after liver transplantation. Transpl Int. 2007;20(1):57–63.

213. Dumortier J, Guillaud O, Adham M, Boucaud C, Delafosse B, Bouffard Y, et al. Negative impact of de novo malignancies rather than alcohol relapse on survival after liver transplantation for alcoholic cirrhosis: a retrospective analysis of 305 patients in a single center. Am J Gastroenterol. 2007;102(5):1032–41.

214. Chak E, Saab S. Risk factors and incidence of de novo malignancy in liver transplant recipients: a systematic review. Liver Int. 2010;30(9):1247–58.

215. van der Heide F, Dijkstra G, Porte RJ, Kleibeuker JH, Haagsma EB. Smoking behavior in liver transplant recipients. Liver Transpl. 2009;15(6):648–55.

216. Corbett C, Armstrong MJ, Neuberger J. Tobacco smoking and solid organ transplantation. Transplantation. 2012;94(10):979–87.

217. Borg MA, van der Wouden EJ, Sluiter WJ, Slooff MJ, Haagsma EB, van den Berg AP. Vascular events after liver transplantation: a long-term follow-up study. Transpl Int. 2008;21(1):74–80.

218. Pungpapong S, Manzarbeitia C, Ortiz J, Reich DJ, Araya V, Rothstein KD, et al. Cigarette smoking is associated with an increased incidence of vascular complications after liver transplantation. Liver Transpl. 2002;8(7):582–7.

219. Herrero JI, Pardo F, D'Avola D, Alegre F, Rotellar F, Inarrairaegui M, et al. Risk factors of lung, head and neck, esophageal, and kidney and urinary tract carcinomas after liver transplantation: the effect of smoking withdrawal. Liver Transpl. 2011;17(4):402–8.

220. Cote DR, Chirichella TJ, Noon KA, Shafran DM, Augustine JJ, Schulak JA, et al. Abdominal organ transplant center tobacco use policies vary by organ program type. Transplant Proc. 2016;48(6):1920–6.

221. Sung RS, Althoen M, Howell TA, Ojo AO, Merion RM. Excess risk of renal allograft loss associated with cigarette smoking. Transplantation. 2001;71(12):1752–7.

222. Mehra MR, Uber PA, Prasad A, Scott RL, Park MH. Recrudescent tobacco exposure following heart transplantation: clinical profiles and relationship with athero-thrombosis risk markers. Am J Transplant. 2005;5(5):1137–40.

223. Nagele H, Kalmar P, Rodiger W, Stubbe HM. Smoking after heart transplantation: an underestimated hazard? Eur J Cardiothorac Surg. 1997;12(1):70–4.

224. Okayasu H, Ozeki Y, Chida M, Miyoshi S, Shimoda K. Lung transplantation in a Japanese patient with schizophrenia from brain-dead donor. Gen Hosp Psychiatry. 2013;35(1):102 e11–3.

225. Cosio FG, Falkenhain ME, Pesavento TE, Yim S, Alamir A, Henry ML, et al. Patient survival after renal transplantation: II. The impact of smoking. Clin Transpl. 1999;13(4):336–41.

226. McConathy K, Turner V, Johnston T, Jeon H, Bouneva I, Koch A, et al. Analysis of smoking in patients referred for liver transplantation and its adverse impact of short-term outcomes. J Ky Med Assoc. 2007;105(6):261–6.

227. Khanna AK, Xu J, Uber PA, Burke AP, Baquet C, Mehra MR. Tobacco smoke exposure in either the donor or recipient before transplantation accelerates cardiac allograft rejection, vascular inflammation, and graft loss. Circulation. 2009;120(18):1814–21.

228. Hanajiri R, Kakihana K, Kobayashi T, Doki N, Sakamaki H, Ohashi K. Tobacco smoking is associated with infectious pulmonary complications after allogeneic hematopoietic stem cell transplantation. Bone Marrow Transplant. 2015;50(8):1141–3.

229. Volkow ND, Baler RD, Compton WM, Weiss SR. Adverse health effects of marijuana use. N Engl J Med. 2014;370(23):2219–27.

230. ElSohly M. Potency Monitoring Program quarterly report no 123 — reporting period: 09/16/2013-12/15/2013.: University of Mississippi, National Center for Natural Products Research. 2014.

231. SAMHSA. Drug abuse warning network, 2011: national estimates of drug-related emergency department visits. Rockville: MD; 2011.

232. Johnston LD, O'Malley PM, Miech RA, et al Monitoring the Future: national survey results on drug use, 1975–2013 — overview, key findings on adolescent drug use. Ann Arbor, MI; 2014.

233. Hoffmann D, Brunneman D, Gori G, Wynder E. On the carcinogenicity of marijuana smoke. Recent Adv Phytochem. 1975;9:63–81.

234. Novotny M, Lee ML, Bartle KD. A possible chemical basis for the higher mutagenicity of marijuana smoke as compared to tobacco smoke. Experientia. 1976;32(3):280–2.

235. Novotny M, Lee ML, Low CE, Maskarinec MP. High-resolution gas chromatography/mass spectrometric analysis of tobacco and marijuana sterols. Steroids. 1976;27(5):665–73.

236. Novotny M, Lee ML, Low CE, Raymond A. Analysis of marijuana samples from different origins by high-resolution gas-liquid chromatography for forensic application. Anal Chem. 1976;48(1):24–9.

237. Moir D, Rickert WS, Levasseur G, Larose Y, Maertens R, White P, et al. A comparison of mainstream and sidestream marijuana and tobacco cigarette smoke produced under two machine smoking conditions. Chem Res Toxicol. 2008;21(2):494–502.

238. Tashkin DP. Effects of marijuana smoking on the lung. Ann Am Thorac Soc. 2013;10(3):239–47.

239. Tashkin DP. Effects of marijuana on the lung and its defenses against infections and cancer. Sch Psychol Int [Internet]. 1999:pp. 20–3.

240. Tashkin DP, Baldwin GC, Sarafian T, Dubinett S, Roth MD. Respiratory and immunologic consequences of marijuana smoking. J Clin Pharmacol. 2002;42(11 Suppl):71S–81S.

241. Aldington S, Williams M, Nowitz M, Weatherall M, Pritchard A, McNaughton A, et al. Effects of cannabis on pulmonary structure, function and symptoms. Thorax. 2007;62(12):1058–63.

242. Aldington S, Harwood M, Cox B, Weatherall M, Beckert L, Hansell A, et al. Cannabis use and risk of lung cancer: a case-control study. Eur Respir J. 2008;31(2):280–6.

243. Coffman KL. The debate about marijuana usage in transplant candidates: recent medical evidence on marijuana health effects. Curr Opin Organ Transplant. 2008;13(2):189–95.

244. Verweij PE, Kerremans JJ, Voss A, Meis JF. Fungal contamination of tobacco and marijuana. JAMA. 2000;284(22):2875.

245. Kagen SL, Kurup VP, Sohnle PG, Fink JN. Marijuana smoking and fungal sensitization. J Allergy Clin Immunol. 1983;71(4):389–93.

246. Boggild AK, Poutanen SM, Mohan S, Ostrowski MA. Disseminated phaeohyphomycosis due to Ochroconis gallopavum in the setting of advanced HIV infection. Med Mycol. 2006;44(8):777–82.

247. Marks WH, Florence L, Lieberman J, Chapman P, Howard D, Roberts P, et al. Successfully treated invasive pulmonary aspergillosis associated with smoking marijuana in a renal transplant recipient. Transplantation. 1996;61(12):1771–4.

248. Vethanayagam D, Pugsley S, Dunn EJ, Russell D, Kay JM, Allen C. Exogenous lipid pneumonia related to smoking weed oil following cadaveric renal transplantation. Can Respir J. 2000;7(4):338–42.

249. Hamadeh R, Ardehali A, Locksley RM, York MK. Fatal aspergillosis associated with smoking contaminated marijuana, in a marrow transplant recipient. Chest. 1988;94(2):432–3.

250. Blanco C, Hasin DS, Wall MM, Florez-Salamanca L, Hoertel N, Wang S, et al. Cannabis Use and Risk of Psychiatric Disorders: Prospective Evidence From a US National Longitudinal Study. JAMA Psychiatry. 2016;73(4):388–95.

251. Vanhove T, Annaert P, Kuypers DR. Clinical determinants of calcineurin inhibitor disposition: a mechanistic review. Drug Metab Rev. 2016;48(1):88–112.

252. Zhu HJ, Wang JS, Markowitz JS, Donovan JL, Gibson BB, Gefroh HA, et al. Characterization of P-glycoprotein inhibition by major cannabinoids from marijuana. J Pharmacol Exp Ther. 2006;317(2):850–7.

253. Hauser N, Sahai T, Richards R, Roberts T. High on Cannabis and Calcineurin Inhibitors: A Word of Warning in an Era of Legalized Marijuana. Case Rep Transplant. 2016;2016:4028492.

The Psychosocial Evaluation of Live Donors

4

Akhil Shenoy

Background

Solid organ transplantation as a treatment for end-stage organ failure has allowed patients to live longer and have greater quality of life. While the number of patients waiting for a transplant significantly exceeds available deceased donors, the living organ donors come forward to transplant centers with the expressed interest to help another person despite risk and cost. Live donation helps ease burden on the deceased donor supply, prevents delay in transplant, minimizes cold ischemic time, and allows control over scheduling. There is no medical benefit for the donor, although the donor may benefit psychologically (e.g., increased self-esteem).

Living donation traces its history back to the first successful solid organ transplantation. In 1954 at the Peter Bent Brigham Hospital in Boston, Ronald Herrick willingly gave one of his kidneys to his identical twin brother Richard who had chronic nephritis, in a pioneering surgery by Dr. Joseph Murray. Richard Herrick did not require immunosuppression and lived for 8 years with his brother's kidney, while Ronald, the donor, died in 2010 at the age of 79, after several years of maintenance dialysis. Since then, living donor kidney transplantation (LDKT) has been performed for over 50 years, and many studies have shown that the surgery is safe and most donors lead normal lives with a solitary kidney. Without the need for perfect human leukocyte antigen (HLA) matching, genetically unrelated persons have increasingly been able to be donors.

The liver has long been known to regenerate to its original size and function. Living donor liver transplantation (LDLT) began in 1989 with the first in the United States at the University of Chicago of a 29-year-old teacher from Texas donating her left liver lobe to her 21-month-old daughter with biliary atresia. Both the donor and recipient continued to be healthy with the recipient successfully discontinuing immunosuppression [1]. With cautious optimism for donor safety, LDLT for children grew in places such as Japan, where there is less opportunity for deceased donor transplants. Since 1998, adult-to-adult LDLT, which usually involves the right liver lobe, had been increasing in the United States to over 500 LDLT surgeries per year until a donor death in 2002. While liver donation, especially of the right lobe, has higher postsurgical risks than kidney donation, it is believed to be safe enough to perform at experienced centers.

Lung, intestine, and pancreas donations have been performed; however, they are rare today given the risks along with slightly more favorable demand versus deceased donor ratio. Uterine transplant has almost exclusively used live donors but is still quite rare. Live kidney and liver donors continue to meet a great need, especially in places where the waitlist for organ far exceeds the number of deceased donors available. Worldwide, these two most commonly donated organs supply one-third of all kidney and liver transplants [2]. Living kidney donors meet this demand through traditional direct donation or through networks of paired exchange donation. In the United States, both kidney and liver donation had been increasing and reaching a plateau in recent years (Fig. 4.1).

Today live donation is a subspecialty of transplantation, and the successful management of a live donor requires a multidisciplinary team approach to their care before, during, and after transplant [3]. Guidelines on the psychosocial assessment and follow-up of living donors from Australia, the United Kingdom, the United States, Continental Europe, and Canada have been reviewed showing similar areas of concern with few offering specific psychosocial recommendations [4]. The Organ Procurement and Transplantation Network/United Network for Organ Sharing (OPTN/UNOS) implemented policy requirements for all living liver and kidney donors in the United States to foster consistency with informed consent, as well as medical and psychosocial evaluation. Similarly, the European Society for Organ

A. Shenoy
Department of Psychiatry, Columbia University Medical Center, New York, NY, USA
e-mail: as5549@cumc.columbia.edu

© Springer International Publishing AG, part of Springer Nature 2019
Y. Sher, J. R. Maldonado (eds.), *Psychosocial Care of End-Stage Organ Disease and Transplant Patients*,
https://doi.org/10.1007/978-3-319-94914-7_4

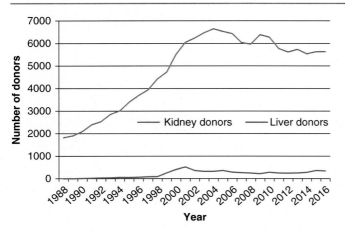

Fig. 4.1 Live kidney and liver donors in the United States

Table 4.1 Live donor psychosocial evaluation goals

1. Identify and appraise any potential risks for poor psychosocial outcomes
2. Ensure that the prospective donor comprehends the risks, benefits, and potential outcome of the donation for herself or himself and the recipient
3. Assess the donor's capacity to make the decision to donate and ability to cope with a major surgery and related stress
4. Assess the donor's motives and the degree to which the donation decision was made free of guilt, undue pressure, enticements, or impulsive response
5. Review lifestyle circumstances (e.g., employment, relationships) that might be affected by donation
6. Determine that a support system is in place and ensure a realistic plan for donation and recovery
7. Identify any factors that warrant educational or therapeutic intervention before donation can proceed

Reprinted with permission from LaPointe Rudow et al. [5], adapted from the CMS survey and Certification letter: Organ transplant interpretive guidelines, 2014

Transplantation (ESOT) has deemed that a psychosocial team is integral to the mission of live organ donation. UNOS has laid out broad goals for the psychosocial evaluation and these have been adapted to practice [5] (Table 4.1). The live donor psychosocial team must maintain a balance between overall encouragement of living donation and advocacy for the individual donor's autonomy and safety.

The Psychosocial Evaluation of the Live Donor

The live donor is assigned an evaluation team separate from the recipient team, consisting of a live donor transplant coordinator, medical specialist, donor surgeon, and an often-called "psychosocial team." The composition of the psychosocial team varies greatly among transplant centers, but it most frequently consists of a mental health professional (e.g., psychiatrist or psychologist) and a licensed social

worker. The live donor transplant coordinator provides education to the donor and families and makes an early assessment of the donor's ability to comprehend risk and desire to proceed with donation. Advanced practice nurses coordinate multidisciplinary care around the time of surgery and postdonation. UNOS has mandated that a member of the living donor team serves as an independent living donor advocate (ILDA). Often the social worker serves in dual roles as a psychosocial evaluator and ILDA. The ILDA helps facilitate the donor's independent decision-making given the variety of internal and external pressures they can face.

The OPTN offers some guidance regarding absolute and relative contraindications to live donation but leaves it to individual centers to practice discretion [6]. There is some agreement that the psychosocial evaluation should take place in two phases: an initial psychosocial screen along with medical prescreening, followed by a more extensive evaluation [7]. The initial screening often happens on the phone or in an online questionnaire with the goal to provide basic information to the donor, probe for the donor's motivations, and assess risk factors [8]. There is no clear guidance on which donor candidates should require a more extensive evaluation. After a liver donor death in 2002, the New York State Department of Health formalized rules requiring an evaluation by a "donor advocate team" including an independent medical specialist and social worker, who are not part of the recipient team, and a transplant psychiatrist. A sample process is outlined in Table 4.2. In most centers the in-person psychosocial evaluation proceeds in tandem with the medical evaluation after some early education and screening.

The Medical and Surgical Evaluation

The goals of the medical evaluation are to ensure the immunological compatibility between the donor and the recipient, analyze the general health and surgical risk for the donor, rule out diseases in the donor that could be transmitted to the recipient, and assess the anatomy and function of the organ to be donated. The transplant team usually conducts this evaluation along with consultation from cardiology, radiology, and nutrition. If needed, other specialists are invited to evaluate donors whenever the initial work-up reveals medical diagnoses that are uncommon or have unclear impact on donation. The donor may need to be reevaluated or their information and laboratory analyses updated if a significant time has passed after the evaluation.

The surgeon reviews the recipient and donor body magnetic resonance imaging (MRI) and makes a determination of surgical approach. In the case of LDKT, the team usually chooses the kidney safest for removal and optimal for donation with the caveat that the kidney with the better function should stay with the donor. Laparoscopy with minimal

Table 4.2 Live donor evaluation process

Prescreen	Online/phone or in-person
	    Medical questionnaire by the registered nurse (RN)
	    Social work (SW) for mini-assessment for active psychosocial issues
	    SW for distant donors

Length of evaluation	Liver, 2 days Kidney, 1–2 days Transplant Coordinator, Medical Evaluation, Cardiology, Dietician
SW/ILDA	Scheduled after RN education and MD evaluation, 60–90-minute interview

Psychiatry referral	Liver donors:
	    All are pre-scheduled
	Kidney donors:
	    Pre-scheduled with additional referral when indicated for:
	    Altruistic, non-directed donors or social media donors
	    Suspicion of secondary gain or questionable relationship
	    Neurocognitive problems or symptoms
	    Ambivalence
	    Current psychiatric symptoms
	    History of significant psychiatric disorder or substance abuse
	    Paired exchange or chained donors

Committee review	Donor advocate team (medical and psychosocial) discuss clearance of donor Surgeon and radiology review anatomy and potential for surgery
Cooling-off period	2 weeks; expectation of donor to contact the center with decision to move forward

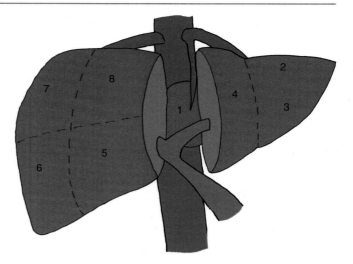

Fig. 4.2 Liver donor anatomy

Table 4.3 Potential risk factors for adverse psychosocial outcomes

Pre-donation
Financial motivations [9]
Feeling morally obligated to donate [10]
Concerns about post-donation health effects [11]
High ambivalence [12]
Lack of partner [13]
Psychiatric disorder [14]
Post-donation
Longer recovery time [10, 11]
Fatigue [15]
Pain [16]
Recipient graft failure [17–22]
Financial stress [10, 11]

scarring is available to kidney donors. In the case of LDLT, the surgical approach requires a transverse incision and a possible additional incision. Left lobe donation (segments 2, 3, and 4) is generally safer than right lobe donation (segments 5, 6, 7, and 8). In donation to a child, often only the smaller left lateral lobe, roughly 15% of the total volume (segments 2 and 3) is needed. Right liver lobe donation (sometimes 60% of the total volume) is often required for an adult recipient (Fig. 4.2).

Psychosocial Factors

The goals of the live donor psychosocial evaluation are to ensure that donors who move forward are highly motivated, capable of informed consent, have not been coerced to donate, and are not receiving payment for their donation. In addition, any ambivalence and sense of expectations for their own recovery and their recipient's recovery should be explored. Particular attention is paid to donor candidates' coping, psychological stability, emotional support, recovery support, and financial stability. The evaluator reviews the donor's psychiatric and substance abuse history and assesses for the presence of any signs of current psychopathology. A meeting report from the American Society of Transplantation directs the components of a psychosocial evaluation of living-unrelated kidney donors where there is heightened concern regarding motivation and informed consent. As the donor is accepting a surgery that they themselves do not need, the ethical dictum "do no harm" remains a guiding principle in the evaluation of the live donor. Regret for going through donation is one unfortunate donor outcome, and there is growing evidence that some pre-donation factors predict poor psychosocial outcomes (Table 4.3).

Psychosocial risk and protective factors can include individual features and interpersonal relations, along with their social and environmental milieu. Psychological vulnerability, such as poor coping, should be identified and addressed accordingly. A psychiatric interview can uncover subtle coercive factors contributing to the donor's decision. Psychiatric and substance use disorders have long been considered risk factors and concerns for donor screening. Potential donors with psychiatric disorders should be afforded the same access to candidacy as others but may need further evaluation by a mental health professional. The psychiatrist or psychologist working with a living donor program should serve the best interests of the individual donor.

Little is known about the psychosocial outcomes of donors who are psychosocially excluded from donation.

Part of ESOT, a European platform on ethical, legal, and psychosocial aspects of organ transplantation (ELPAT), conducted a recent review of all available literature describing the psychosocial screening of living kidney and liver donor candidates. Most guidelines, consensus statements, and protocols recommend a standardized structured interview (36%) or a semi-structured interview (57%) [7]. The psychosocial domains and factors that have been consistently recommended for inclusion are described in this section.

Motivation

The evaluator must empathetically query all the motivators or reasons for the donor's presentation. More than any other psychosocial factor, donor motivation is considered an essential area to explore [7]. The donor should narrate the story of how their interest grew, including the relationship with the recipient, their learning about the process, their knowledge of risks, and any periods of ambivalence. While most directed donors describe an immediate positive response and agreement to the opportunity, not all donors maintain this enthusiasm [23]. Internal pressure or a sense of obligation may be in the realm of acceptable reasons, while signs of coercion from the recipient or external pressure to move forward should be met with concern for the donor's independence in making a decision.

In directed donations, the motivation of a parent to help their young child is often easily understood. Similarly an adult donor to their elderly parent may seem obvious, but additional secondary motivations should be reviewed such as the desire to relieve caregiver burden or return to work. Wishing to relieve guilt or repair a troubled relationship may be problematic. Clarifying the donor's experience with the recipient and their expectations for the future relationship is a critical feature of fully exploring the donor's motivations. One qualitative study of kidney donors has identified multiple reasons for wanting to donate. These include compelled altruism, inherent responsibility, accepting risks, family expectation, personal benefit, and spiritual confirmation [24].

Non-directed donors (NDD), also known as altruistic or "Good Samaritan" donors, should be expected to provide a more detailed explanation of their personal motivations for donation. These explanations usually fit a pattern of "compelled altruism" related to a deep sense of purpose related to a past history of good deeds. The interviewer can explore past altruistic behavior or core values and beliefs. If the primary goal is to improve their own self-esteem or their standing within their family or work, extreme care must be taken to describe these expectations. Some NDDs are also solicited from their religious community [25] or social media [26] without findings of coercion. NDDs should be discouraged to donate if it appears that there is a strong desire for recognition or an attempt to curry favor with a recipient. NDDs are commonly viewed with some skepticism and are evaluated with greater caution than related donors.

Organ sale is illegal in most of the world. In Iran where an organ market is legal, motivation for financial reward has been found to leave donors regretful [9]. When donors are paid, the emphasis on the commercial transaction may dampen the sense of altruistic intention. In the United States, the donor surgery and aftercare is paid by the recipient's insurance, but extraneous costs and lost wages have been found to be a deterrent for donation [27]. Securing grants, stipends, and even private funds to recover some of these costs are ethically justified and encouraged by the transplant team, but possibility for additional payment must be queried. This should be a consideration whenever the donor is impoverished or in a subordinate relationship with the recipient.

Relationship with Recipient

In the cases of directed donation, a full history of the relationship between live donor and recipient helps appreciate the motivations and the expectations placed on the recipient after donation. First degree relative donors may experience better outcomes than unrelated donors [28]. Nonetheless, directed donation from unrelated and non-spousal donors has increased. The initially identified NDD may grow close to the recipient through the clearance process. In the case of NDD, the expectation for the future relationship should still be explored. Given the sacrifice and investment, will the donor respect the recipient's autonomy after donation? If the recipient's lifestyle is not guided toward protection of the new graft, will this affect their relationship with the donor? A lack of stability in the relationship may prompt further exploration of the expectations for the relationship after donation. Due to the additional risks of liver donation, UNOS guidelines recommend a strong emotional bond in LDLT. In the cases of unrelated and non-spousal friends, the closeness of relationship should meet the standard of a "strong emotional bond." When adhering to this guideline, the psychosocial evaluator should try to ensure that the donor is truly "like a brother" to the recipient in length and depth of the relationship.

Informed Consent

For an adequate informed consent process to occur, the donor's wishes to proceed with surgery must be voluntary, and they must have the relevant information and the capacity for decision-making. Although donors often commit to donation before knowing all the risks [23], informed consent is developed after weeks of conversations with various team members and a 2-week cooling-off period ending ultimately in a situation-dependent decision to move forward on the day of surgery. The specific knowledge about their organ donation and recovery process is essential for the donor's decision-making. Living donors should be aware of the various risks of short-term morbidity and mortality, as well as long-term risks discussed below. Adapted education should be provided to potential donors. Throughout the evaluation process, the risks are discussed and re-discussed in person by multiple team members with a final surgical consent completed just prior to surgery.

The psychosocial evaluation is completed along the medical assessment, and psychosocial evaluators should be aware that the donor's knowledge of the material may still be nascent. Donors should demonstrate early knowledge level and capacity to learn new information. General competency referring to global decision-making ability and capability to comprehend information should also be assessed. Donors tend to interpret new information in a selective fashion in support of their initial choice [29]. Hence they may minimize risks or be passive about seeking information that could help them more effectively prepare for donation. One of the major goals of the psychosocial evaluation is to allow the potential donor to feel comfortable to openly share their concerns and to encourage this type of openness throughout the process.

Expectations After Donation

Donors may have unrealistic expectations about the donation experience and recipient outcomes. Some donors and patients have the erroneous expectations that transplantation will result in a cure for end-organ damage, with a return to premorbid health. Donors with unrealistic expectations and anxious avoidance of problem confrontation had more problematic postoperative courses [30]. Donors' baseline understanding must be assessed and corrected early in the evaluation process. Papachristou and colleagues completed a qualitative analysis of 28 donor interviews and describe four different attitudes donors displayed in dealing with the risks (Table 4.4) [23]. The donor's attitude toward outcomes for themselves and the recipient should be individually considered. Donors may retain hope and trust in the medical system to minimize risks, but concerns about outcomes for the recipient may remain.

Ambivalence

Ambivalence about donation is not uncommon and has been found to predict poor post-donation psychosocial outcomes

Table 4.4 Donor attitudes toward risks

Heroic/ optimistic	These donors present with an overly optimistic or fatalistic attitude	"I know anything can happen… it's ok if I die… we are putting our faith in God's hands"
Optimistic/ apprehensive	These donors were less positive and took in less knowledge about risks	"I don't want to think too much about it, but I'm sure it will be ok"
Informed/ balanced	These donors carefully weighed the pros and cons and made a deliberate decision	"We have considered all those possibilities and we are comfortable with risks"
Uncertain/ anxious	These donors fearfully avoid the risks and feel they cannot manage	"I'm not sure I know all the risks yet, I have to think about it more"

Adapted from Ref. [23]. Used with permission

[12]. Ambivalence may play a central role in the motivation to donate and the donor's relationship with the recipient. Ambivalence has been the only psychosocial factor studied and targeted for intervention in a randomized controlled trial. Kidney and liver living donors were provided with motivational interviewing to target donor's residual ambivalence and found that the reduction in ambivalence in their intervention group was also predictive of improved medical and psychosocial outcomes for the donors [12]. Interestingly, in the Adult-to-Adult Living Donor Liver Transplantation Cohort Study (A2ALL), some pre-donation ambivalence along with motivation and purpose was associated with donors' perceptions of being better people and experiencing psychological growth following donation [28]. Liver donors may be more ambivalent about donation than kidney donors [31]. This may stem from the higher risks involved. The degree of ambivalence may be increased by anxiety, depression, physical symptoms, as well as low social support [32]. Ambivalence is not an uncommon internal struggle but may be salient in potential donors who may be exploited or coerced to donate, and thus should be always further explored and understood.

Social Support and Stability in Life

A functional social support network is usually reviewed in both recipient and donor evaluations. Family support may predict a donor's stability and sense of coherence [33]. Low social support may influence other factors such as donor ambivalence. In one cross-sectional study of liver donor candidates with a high incidence of ambivalence, higher social support was able to mitigate other psychosocial factors' impact on ambivalence [34]. A lack of a partner may impact post-donation well-being and increase in psychological symptoms [13]. The evaluator should also query the donor for possible disapproval from family and friends. It is not uncommon for potential donors to not speak with their social support prior to evaluation; this can be problematic especially when the donor needs to ensure social support and help. Financial instability along with other stressors such as divorce, unstable work, and children's illness should also be queried. Some of the social concerns may be mitigated through grants from private foundations and patient advocacy groups. For example, the National Kidney Foundation (NKF) can help offset the costs of travel.

Psychiatric Disorders, Unhealthy Coping, and Substance Use Disorders

Candidates with severe psychiatric conditions, especially with suicidal behavior, require a thorough evaluation with a psychiatrist or psychologist. Psychiatric disorders may be minimized prior to donation, being prevalent after donation and associated with worse quality of life post-donation [14]. Personality disorders and/or personality traits should be addressed, especially if it is believed that severe, unmanaged disorders may be contributing to the wish to donate. The candidate with motivation for donation stemming from a latent wish to be psychologically stable cannot be accepted. Similarly, those with ongoing suicidality and severe untreated mental illness should be discouraged to donate. In 1 study of 205 sequential liver donor candidates, with 66 going on to donate, 11 were rejected for psychiatric conditions and substance abuse [35]. It may be prudent for the transplant psychiatrist to meet these declined candidates in person and conduct a risk assessment prior to referring them for ongoing psychiatric care.

For those not declined, mental health professionals can further evaluate severe anxiety or impulsivity that may be barriers to successful donation. This may be especially pertinent in donors going into a chain or paired exchange to prevent discontinuation to the organ chain due to ambivalence. Published data suggest that accepted donors tend to be more resilient than the general population [36]. Pre-donation resilience predicted higher quality of life 3 months post-donation [37]. Potential donors with a history of trauma, substance use disorders, or personality disorders may sense their own vulnerability and not move forward early in the evaluation process.

Excessive alcohol use may both impact the donated liver, as well as be a great risk for complicating hepatic regeneration in the donor. Some have called for the same cessation requirements for donors as for liver recipients [38] and donors should be carefully monitored for any alcohol use disorder behaviors prior to and after donation [28]. Active opioid use disorder or regular opioid use for chronic pain should also be ruled out. Tobacco use in kidney donors is associated with negative renal function in both the recipient and donor post-donation with smoking cessation possibly improving this outcome [39].

Obstacles to the Psychosocial Evaluation

Naturally, potential donors will often highlight their strengths and minimize areas of concern. This type of impression management can at times come across as "too good to be true." Rigid denial of all symptoms or minimizing minor or remote history of substance use should alert the evaluator to potential problems with truthfulness. Deceptive behavior can be often uncovered by a thorough assessment of all the key psychosocial domains. The evaluator should attempt to question any areas of deception in the most nonjudgmental and professional manner. Cultural differences and language translation can further complicate the full evaluation and may require extra time and additional meetings.

Psychosocial Assessment Tools

Psychometric tools can be helpful to standardize the psychosocial assessment given the subjective reporting of many variables. Standardization can be a boon to improving communication between team members, creating efficiencies in workflow, educating new team members, and encouraging research endeavors.

Self-assessment questionnaires using Likert scales can be mailed to potential donors prior to presenting to the center. The Living Donation Expectancies Questionnaire (LDEQ) focuses on the potential donor expectations for personal well-being after donation [40]. In a wish to also include donor expectations for the recipient's well-being, the Donation Cognition Instrument (DCI) was developed to assess a fuller range of motivations, expectations, and worries surrounding donation [41]. While these tools have not been tested for post-donation outcomes, they may be helpful with aiding in donor decision-making and to intervene if expectations are problematic. Another set of self-assessment scales developed for kidney donors by Roberta Simmons was used to test ambivalence through a motivational interviewing intervention [12]. Two tests of knowledge about kidney and liver donation have been developed: the Rotterdam Renal Replacement Knowledge-Test (R3K-T) for kidney donors [42] and the Evaluation of Donor Informed Consent Tool (EDICT) for liver donors [43].

Two comprehensive evaluation tools have been developed for use with all solid organ living donor candidates, the living organ donor Psychosocial Assessment Tool (EPAT) and Live Donor Assessment Tool (LDAT). Both tools require a semi-structured interview and offer concrete guidance for psychosocial screening of live organ donors. The EPAT was developed by members of the European Society for Organ Transplantation (ESOT) and consists of a selection of 28 validated questionnaires, 43 interview questions, and a 14-point red flag checklist [44]. The LDAT was designed at New York's Mount Sinai Hospital to encompass the various

Table 4.5 Live Donor Assessment Tool (LDAT)

1. Motivation (internal/external motivation, types of motives, relationship)
2. Feelings (coercion, anxiety, indecision, impulsivity, ambivalence)
3. Knowledge (health literacy, knowledge of process, recipient's diagnosis)
4. Expectations (post-donation recovery, recipient outcomes, change in relationship)
5. Social support (functional status, relationships, support's attitude toward donation)
6. Stability in life (early life, employment, financial, stressors, coping, sleep)
7. Psychiatric issues (symptoms, personality traits, truthfulness)
8. Substance abuse (alcohol, substances, marijuana, nicotine)

psychosocial areas of concern and should be used by a member of the psychosocial team familiar with living donation. Modeled in part on the Stanford Integrated Psychosocial Assessment for Transplantation (SIPAT) [45], the current LDAT consists of 33 items across 8 major domains. The LDAT has good inter-rater reliability between psychiatrists and social workers, as well as construct validity for the usual risk stratification of donors and has been shown to predict post-donation adherence problems [46]. The LDAT was easily integrated into different centers' psychosocial evaluation process and a multi-center prospective study across four varied US transplant centers.

The components of the LDAT are demonstrated in Table 4.5.

Independent Living Donor Advocate (ILDA)

Consensus recommendations have suggested that all potential live donors meet with an independent living donor advocate (ILDA) who is not a member of the recipient transplant team in order to minimize potential conflicts of interest. The role of the ILDA has been evolving since 2007. At present, the ILDA responsibilities include many of the components of a general psychosocial evaluation with a focus on independently evaluating the potential donor's willingness and competence to donate. The ILDA also ensures that the donor understands their rights to withdraw at any time and the concept of the opt-out or so-called medical out.

In order to protect the donor's right to self-determination, they are repeatedly reminded of their *option to opt out*. A common script instructs "As a potential donor, you have the right to decline to donate at any time. Additionally, you may discontinue the donor consent or evaluation process if you wish; you may do so in a way that is protected and confidential." This remains a difficult option for close relatives who wish to maintain an ongoing trusting relationship with their relative. The donor should feel comfortable to share these concerns and manage their wish to secure "permission" to back out from their relative [47]. Strong feelings of guilt for

backing out can be overwhelming to potential donors and should be processed by the ILDA, along with other members of the psychosocial team.

Live Donor Outcomes

Living donors can improve outcomes for organ recipients by improving survival rates and optimizing the timing of transplant. Kidney recipients wish to time the surgery for when they are most prepared and to avoid dialysis. For donors themselves, a well-deserved "halo" effect may enhance the sense of well-being that donors enjoy but can quickly give way to loss of attention when the focus turns to the recipient. Donors often directly benefit by increased satisfaction and meaning in their life, but there are psychosocial risks beyond the surgery.

Clinicians have an ethical duty to the donor to ensure that the known risks of donation are understood. While the actual outcomes of kidney and liver donation may be better than the perceived risks [48] in one study, while donors felt well-informed of perioperative donor risks (94%) and their short-term complications (85.3%) as well as recipient risks (97%) and hazards of graft dysfunction (88%), only 53% of donors felt well-informed of the donor long-term complications, with 47% stating that they had little or no information on this topic [49].

Donor Surgery, Acute Recovery Period, and Long-Term Medical Outcomes

The live organ donor must manage a variety of short-term physical, emotional, and social challenges. Kidney donor surgery has evolved from open laparotomy to a laparoscopic procedure with on average a 2-day hospital stay and a 2-week recuperation. Kidney donors should expect to miss 4–6 weeks of work, if their jobs require heavy lifting, but can expect to return to a desk job after 2 weeks. Donor nephrectomy through laparoscopy causes less pain, shorter hospital stays, quicker recovery times, and better cosmetic results. Fatigue [15] and pain [16] remain concerning patient-reported outcomes that can impact psychosocial well-being. While the short-term risks of kidney donation are lower than with liver donation, the long-term risk of end-stage renal disease (ESRD) is increased relative to other healthy controls with a low absolute risk (incidence rate 0.5 event per 1000 person-years). The same meta-analysis observed a higher rate of preeclampsia (incidence rate 5.9 events per 100 pregnancies) [50]. Studies of long-term outcomes of kidney donors are based on younger, non-obese donors. Removing risk factors such as high blood pressure, weight, glycemic control, and tobacco use may reduce the risk of long-term ESRD in the donor.

Hepatectomy is more surgically complex and invasive than nephrectomy. Often, these donors suffer more short-term complications than their kidney donor counterparts. In most adult-to-adult liver donation, the larger right lobe is removed, with an estimated mortality rate around 0.4–0.5% 60–90 days after partial hepatectomy. When the recipient is a child or a smaller recipient, the left lobe is donated. In these cases, the risk of death may be much lower, at around 0.09%. During the initial hospitalization, the most common complications are ileus (27%) and atelectasis (26%). The mostly minor perioperative morbidity of around 25% lends support to the current donor selection process [51].

In 2016, there were 354 LDLTs performed with a 10-year recipient graft and patient survival of 65% and 80%, respectively. The improved survival over deceased donor transplant is one of the reasons to justify the potential risks of directed liver donation. Post-donation, the liver donor must routinely manage discomfort, fatigue, and pain. In the A2ALL group at 3 months post-transplantation, nearly 80% of complications have resolved, with a 95% resolution after 12 months [52]. Similarly, even though donors have reported decreased sexual function at 3 months, most reported complete return to normal activities after 1 year [53]. Another study of long-term follow-up suggests that over half of liver donors experience persistent intolerance to fatty food and one-third had gastrointestinal reflux and nausea [17]. Decreased platelet counts have been a consistent finding with 19% average lower count at 3 years post-donation [54].

Long-Term Psychosocial Outcomes

In addition to medical outcomes, centers are studying post-donation quality of life, psychiatric disorders, resilience, substance abuse, relationships, and financial impact [10, 55]. Concerns of securing future insurance due to a preexisting condition continue to loom.

Kidney
In an effort to realize long-term psychosocial outcomes of kidney donors, the Renal and Lung Living Donors Evaluation (RELIVE) study completed a cross-sectional survey of 2455 kidney donors across 3 transplant centers. The majority of kidney donors reported high satisfaction with their lives [56] and had a rate of post-donation depression of 8% comparable to the general population. Those with poor psychosocial outcomes felt morally obligated to donate, had increased recovery time, and revealed financial stress [10]. Recipient graft failure was also an independent risk factor for low donor satisfaction [18]. While many kidney donors report an increase in self-esteem, those with recipients who died had less optimal psychosocial outcomes [19]. Two recent prospective studies of psychological health also exposed mild donor vul-

nerability around setbacks in recipient's health but overall return to baseline psychosocial health [20, 21].

Liver
Three to 10 years after live liver donation, 95% of donors reported that they would donate again [52]. Other studies have shown similar findings. In one group of donors, 47% suggested ways to improve the donation process such as providing more detail in the informed consent, but still 94% of liver donors were willing to donate again [17]. Half of donors reported improved relationships with their recipients with one-third reporting better relationships with their own families, while 44% of donors found their out-of-pocket expenses burdensome [57]. It is likely that the close relationship with their recipients helped engender the wish to donate, despite the costs. Positive medical and psychosocial outcomes aside, other concerns still exist. Quality of life decreased for liver donors whose recipient died in the first 2 years [22]. Higher than normal levels of anxiety in females and alcohol use disorder in males were observed in follow-up [11]. Two patients committed suicide as a late complication of donation among the 390 donors in the A2ALL series, and 11 patients (2.8%) experienced severe psychiatric complications [58].

The Ethics of Live Donation

Transplant professionals must balance the ethical principles of preserving the donor's autonomy and protecting them from risk. Short- and long-term risks should be explained, minimized as much as possible, and clarified for the donor's understanding to facilitate an autonomous and informed process. Autonomy should be curtailed when donors are requesting to act in clinically hopeless situations. Autonomy may also be called into question in cases where unnecessary risks are present, there is evidence of coercion, or motivations are not consistent with maintaining good donor outcomes. A significant number of living kidney and liver donors feel their own lives have been enhanced by the process of donation, reporting a heightened sense of satisfaction, self-esteem, and psychological growth [19, 56, 59]. These findings raise an interesting question about the balance of beneficence and non-malfeasance for donors, independent of the benefits experienced by recipients. In this line of thinking, the transplant community could be encouraging more non-directed donation where the outcome for the specific recipient is less important to the donor.

Allowing donors with their own increased medical and/or psychosocial risk is also an ethical question. The consensus has been for non-directed kidney donors to meet the same degree of medical suitability of related donors, but heightened concerns about informed consent and true autonomy for decision-making remain [8]. Current practices allow the psychosocial team to decline donors with inappropriate relationships or strong unconscious or latent motivations that may not be resolved through the donation process. The team's suspicions that these donors may be regretful after donation may compete with the donor's autonomy. The act of declining these candidates can cause its own interpersonal conflict and may raise questions as to how well the psychosocial team can predict poor outcomes. The overall struggle to ensure good outcomes for the program, in the face of individual autonomy, is a regular theme.

Ensuring donor's privacy and the freedom to opt out at any time during the evaluation process is the current doctrine. The "medical out" or so-called alibi helps preserve donor autonomy, but it raises questions about the "invention" of a medical illness as cause for disqualifying a prospective donor. It is common practice for the specific reasons for excluding a donor not be disclosed to the recipient. Coercion may also occur at the institutional level when donors joining a kidney exchange or chain enter a commitment to donate especially when several people are depending on that individual.

Future of Live Donation and Conclusions

Live donation will continue to grow before synthetic organs or xenotransplantation are clinical feasible. The transplant community has documented clear success in LKLT and LDLT through the high-quality care and outcomes. Kidney recipients, in particular, have improved outcomes, and the health system can save approximately $20 million for every 100 kidneys transplanted, averting dialysis over a 5-year period [60]. Transplant professionals and government agencies must continue to study outcomes, barriers to access, and ways to improve donor recruitment.

OPTN/UNOS has mandated a 2-year follow-up of all organ donors. Future studies should try to include donors who are older, overweight, and members of racial and ethnic minorities to best represent the demographics of future donors.

Paired and chained donation are transforming live kidney donation. The National Kidney Registry (NKR) has used matching algorithms to large sets of potential donors and their intended recipients to allow large chains expanding the donor pool. The recent findings that show good recipient outcomes with HLA incompatible pairs will help the many live donors who wish to directly donate to their loved one [61].

After a peak of donors in 2004, the number of annual live kidney donors has leveled, while the proportion of NDD has increased. Four main barriers to living kidney donation were identified: lack of education of patients and families, lack of public awareness about living donor kidney transplantation, financial costs incurred by donors, and healthcare system-level inefficiencies [60]. Proposed strategies to expand the live donor pool include allowing more medically complex and older donors, improving outreach to potential family donors, increasing encouragement of altruistic or NDD, participating in paired and pooled exchange programs, and offering subsidies to offset cost to the donor [5].

Live organ donation is an essential and thriving part of organ transplantation. Research into the medical and psychosocial outcomes will continue to help educate future donors to come forward. Care must be taken to ensure that donors are not coerced or complicit with exploitative financial transactions. There is a strong role for the psychosocial team to ensure that a careful selection of organ donors ensures ongoing and perhaps improved donor outcomes.

References

1. University of Chicago Medicine [Internet]. Archive of press releases 2010. Available from: http://www.uchospitals.edu/news/2010/20100507-smith.html
2. World Health Organization (WHO) Global Knowledge Base on Transplantation [Internet]. Available from: http://www.who.int/transplantation/gkt/statistics/en/
3. LaPointe Rudow D. Experiences of the live organ donor: lessons learned pave the future. Narrat Inq Bioeth. 2012;12(1):45–54.
4. Tong A, Chapman JR, Wong G, de Bruijn J, Craig JC. Screening and follow-up of living kidney donors: a systematic review of clinical practice guidelines. Transplantation. 2011;92(9):962–72.
5. LaPointe RD, Hays R, Baliga P, Cohen DJ, Cooper M, Danovitch GM, et al. Consensus conference on best practices in live kidney donation: recommendations to optimize education, access, and care. Am J Transplant. 2015;15(4):914–22.
6. Organ Procurement and Transplantation Network (OPTN). Policies on live donation. Available from: https://optn.transplant.hrsa.gov/media/1200/optn_policies.pdf
7. Duerinckx N, Timmerman L, Van Gogh J, van Busschbach J, Ismail SY, Massey EK, Dobbels F. ELPAT psychological care for living donors and recipients working group. Predonation psychosocial evaluation of living kidney and liver donor candidates: a systematic literature review. Transpl Int. 2014;27(1):2–18.
8. Adams PL, Cohen DJ, Danovitch GM, Edington RM, Gaston RS, Jacobs CL, et al. The nondirected live-kidney donor: ethical considerations and practice guidelines: a National Conference Report. Transplantation. 2002;74(4):582–9.
9. Zargooshi J. Iranian kidney donors: motivations and relations with recipients. J Urol. 2001;165(2):386–92.
10. Jowsey SG, Jacobs C, Gross CR, Hong BA, Messersmith EE, Gillespie BW, RELIVE Study Group, et al. Emotional well-being of living kidney donors: findings from the RELIVE study. Am J Transplant. 2014;14(11):2535–44.
11. Dew MA, Butt Z, Liu Q, Simpson MA, Zee J, Ladner DP, et al. Prevalence and predictors of patient-reported long-term mental and physical health after donation in the adult-to-adult living-donor liver transplantation cohort study. Transplantation. 2018;102(1):105–18.
12. Dew MA, DiMartini AF, DeVito Dabbs AJ, Zuckoff A, Tan HP, McNulty ML, et al. Preventive intervention for living donor psychosocial outcomes: feasibility and efficacy in a randomized controlled trial. Am J Transplant. 2013;13(10):2672–84.

13. Timmerman L, Timman R, Laging M, Zuidema WC, Beck DK, IJzermans JN, et al. Predicting mental health after living kidney donation: the importance of psychological factors. Br J Health Psychol. 2016;21(3):533–54.

14. Smith GC, Trauer T, Kerr PG, Chadban SJ. Prospective psychosocial monitoring of living kidney donors using the short Form-36 health survey: results at 12 months. Transplantation. 2004;78(9):1384–9.

15. Meyer K, Wahl AK, Bjørk IT, Wisløff T, Hartmann A, Andersen MH. Long-term, self-reported health outcomes in kidney donors. BMC Nephrol. 2016;17:8.

16. Rodrigue JR, Vishnevsky T, Fleishman A, Brann T, Evenson AR, Pavlakis M, Mandelbrot DA. Patient-reported outcomes following living kidney donation: a single center experience. J Clin Psychol Med Settings. 2015;22(2–3):160–8.

17. Sotiropoulos GC, Radtke A, Molmenti EP, Schroeder T, Baba HA, Frilling A, et al. Long-term follow-up after right hepatectomy for adult living donation and attitudes toward the procedure. Ann Surg. 2011;254(5):694–700.

18. Jacobs CL, Gross CR, Messersmith EE, Hong BA, Gillespie BW, Hill-Callahan P, RELIVE Study Group, et al. Emotional and financial experiences of kidney donors over the past 50 years: the RELIVE study. Clin J Am Soc Nephrol. 2015;10(12):2221–31.

19. Clemens KK, Thiessen-Philbrook H, Parikh CR, Yang RC, Karley ML, Boudville N, et al. DONOR nephrectomy outcomes research (DONOR) network. Psychosocial health of living kidney donors: a systematic review. Am J Transplant. 2006;6(12):2965–77.

20. Timmerman L, Laging M, Timman R, Zuidema WC, Beck DK, IJzermans JN, et al. The impact of the donors' and recipients' medical complications on living kidney donors' mental health. Transpl Int. 2016;29(5):589–602.

21. Maple H, Chilcot J, Weinman J, Mamode N. Psychosocial wellbeing after living kidney donation – a longitudinal, prospective study. Transpl Int. 2017;30(10):987–1001.

22. Ladner DP, Dew MA, Forney S, Gillespie BW, Brown RS Jr, Merion RM, et al. Long-term quality of life after liver donation in the adult to adult living donor liver transplantation cohort study (A2ALL). J Hepatol. 2015;62(2):346–53.

23. Papachristou C, Walter M, Frommer J, Klapp BF. Decision-making and risk-assessment in living liver donation: how informed is the informed consent of donors? A qualitative study. Psychosomatics. 2010;51(4):312–9.

24. Tong A, Chapman JR, Wong G, Kanellis J, McCarthy G, Craig JC. The motivations and experiences of living kidney donors: a thematic synthesis. Am J Kidney Dis. 2012;60(1):15–26.

25. Serur D, Bretzlaff G, Christos P, Desrosiers F, Charlton M. Solicited kidney donors: are they coerced? Nephrology (Carlton). 2015;20(12):952–5.

26. Chang A, Anderson EE, Turner HT, Shoham D, Hou SH, Grams M. Identifying potential kidney donors using social networking web sites. Clin Transpl. 2013;27(3):E320–6.

27. Thiessen C, Jaji Z, Joyce M, Zimbrean P, Reese P, Gordon EJ, Kulkarni S. Opting out: a single-centre pilot study assessing the reasons for and the psychosocial impact of withdrawing from living kidney donor evaluation. J Med Ethics. 2017;43(11):756–61.

28. Butt Z, Dew MA, Liu Q, Simpson MA, Smith AR, Zee J, et al. Psychological outcomes of living liver donors from a multicenter prospective study: results from the adult-to-adult living donor liver transplantation cohort Study2 (A2ALL-2). Am J Transplant. 2017;17(5):1267–77.

29. Surman OS, Fukunishi I, Allen T, Hertl M. Live organ donation: social context, clinical encounter, and psychology of communication. Psychosomatics. 2005;46:1.

30. Schweitzer J, Seidel-Wiesel M, Verres R, et al. Psychological consultation before living kidney donation: finding out and handling problem cases. Transplantation. 2003;76:1464–70.

31. Shenoy A, Iacoviello B, Klipstein K, Filipovic Z, LaPointe Rudow D. Formative evaluation of the Living Donor Assessment Tool (LDAT): a review of cases histories, poster session, Academy of Psychosomatic Medicine, Fort Lauderdale, November 13th, 2014.

32. Weng LC, Huang HL, Tsai HH, Lee WC. Predictors of decision ambivalence and the differences between actual living liver donors and potential living liver donors. PLoS One. 2017;12(5):e0175672.

33. Erim Y, Beckmann M, Kroencke S, Schulz KH, Tagay S, Valentin-Gamazo C, et al. Sense of coherence and social support predict living liver donors' emotional stress prior to living-donor liver transplantation. Clin Transpl. 2008;22(3):273–80.

34. Lai YC, Lee WC, Juang YY, Yen LL, Weng LC, Chou HF. Effect of social support and donation-related concerns on ambivalence of living liver donor candidates. Liver Transpl. 2014;20(11):1365–71.

35. Erim Y, Beckmann M, Valentin-Gamazo C, Malago M, Frilling A, Schlaak J, et al. Selection of donors for adult living-donor liver donation: results of the assessment of the first 205 donor candidates. Psychosomatics. 2008;49(2):143–51.

36. LaPointe RD, Iacoviello BM, Charney D. Resilience and personality traits among living liver and kidney donors. Prog Transplant. 2014;24(1):82–90.

37. Erim Y, Kahraman Y, Vitinius F, Beckmann M, Kröncke S, Witzke O. Resilience and quality of life in 161 living kidney donors before nephrectomy and in the aftermath of donation: a naturalistic single center study. BMC Nephrol. 2015;16:164.

38. Bramstedt KA. Alcohol abstinence criteria for living liver donors and their organ recipients. Curr Opin Organ Transplant. 2008;13(2):207–10.

39. Heldt J, Torrey R, Han D, Baron P, Tenggardjaja C, McLarty J, et al. Donor smoking negatively affects donor and recipient renal function following living donor nephrectomy. Adv Urol. 2011;2011:929263.

40. Rodrigue JR, Guenther R, Kaplan B, Mandelbrot DA, Pavlakis M, Howard RJ. Measuring the expectations of kidney donors: initial psychometric properties of the living donation expectancies questionnaire. Transplantation. 2008;85(9):1230–4.

41. Wirken L, van Middendorp H, Hooghof CW, Sanders JF, Dam RE, van der Pant KAMI, et al. Pre-donation cognitions of potential living organ donors: the development of the donation cognition instrument in potential kidney donors. Nephrol Dial Transplant. 2017;32(3):573–80.

42. Ismail SY, Timmerman L, Timman R, Luchtenburg AE, Smak Gregoor PJ, Nette RW, et al. A psychometric analysis of the Rotterdam renal replacement knowledge-test (R3K-T) using item response theory. Transpl Int. 2013;26(12):1164–72.

43. Gordon EJ, Mullee J, Butt Z, Kang J, Baker T. Optimizing informed consent in living liver donors: evaluation of a comprehension assessment tool. Liver Transpl. 2015;21(10):1270–9.

44. Massey EK, Timmerman L, Ismail SY, Duerinckx N, Lopes A, Maple H, et al. ELPAT psychosocial care for living donors and recipients working group. The ELPAT living organ donor psychosocial assessment tool (EPAT): from 'what' to 'how' of psychosocial screening – a pilot study. Transpl Int. 2018;31(1):56–70.

45. Maldonado JR, Dubois HC, David EE, Sher Y, Lolak S, Dyal J, Witten D. The Stanford integrated psychosocial assessment for transplantation (SIPAT): a new tool for the psychosocial evaluation of pre-transplant candidates. Psychosomatics. 2012;53(2):123–32.

46. Iacoviello BM, Shenoy A, Hunt J, Filipovic-Jewell Z, Haydel B, LaPointe Rudow D. A prospective study of the reliability and validity of the live donor assessment tool. Psychosomatics. 2017;58(5):519–26.

47. Lapointe Rudow D, Swartz K, Phillips, et al. The psychosocial and independent living donor advocate evaluation and post-surgery care of living donors. J Clin Psychol Med Settings. 2015;22:136–49.

48. LaPointe RD, Charlton M, Sanchez C, et al. Kidney and liver living donors: a comparison of experiences. Prog Transplant. 2005;15(2):185–91.

49. Castedal M, Andersson M, Polanska-Tamborek D, Friman S, Olausson M, Fehrman-Ekholm I. Long-term follow-up of living liver donors. Transplant Proc. 2010;42(10):4449–54.

50. O'Keeffe LM, Ramond A, Oliver-Williams C, Willeit P, Paige E, Trotter P, et al. Mid- and long-term health risks in living kidney donors: a systematic review and meta-analysis. Ann Intern Med. 2018. doi:https://doi.org/10.7326/M17-1235. [Epub ahead of print].

51. Hall EC, Boyarsky BJ, Deshpande NA, Garonzik-Wang JM, Berger JC, Dagher NN, Segev DL. Perioperative complications after live-donor hepatectomy. JAMA Surg. 2014;149(3):288–91.

52. Abecassis MM, Fisher RA, Olthoff KM, et al. Complications of living donor hepatic lobectomy—a comprehensive report. Am J Transplant. 2012;12(5):1208–17.

53. DiMartini AF, Dew MA, Butt Z, Simpson MA, Ladner DP, Smith AR, Hill-Callahan P, Gillespie BW. Patterns and predictors of sexual function after liver donation: the adult-to-adult living donor liver transplantation cohort study. Liver Transpl. 2015;21(5):670–82.

54. Trotter JF, Gillespie BW, Terrault NA, Abecassis MM, Merion RM, Brown RS Jr, et al. Adult-to-adult living donor liver transplantation cohort study group. Laboratory test results after living liver donation in the adult-to-adult living donor liver transplantation cohort study. Liver Transpl. 2011;17(4):409–17.

55. Dew MA, Butt Z, Humar A, DiMartini AF. Long-term medical and psychosocial outomes in living liver donors. Am J Transplant. 2017;17:880–92.

56. Messersmith EE, Gross CR, Beil CA, Gillespie BW, Jacobs C, Taler SJ, RELIVE Study Group, et al. Satisfaction with life among living kidney donors: a RELIVE study of long-term donor outcomes. Transplantation. 2014;98(12):1294–300.

57. DiMartini A, Dew MA, Liu Q, Simpson MA, Ladner DP, Smith AR, et al. Social and financial outcomes of living liver donation: a prospective investigation within the adult-to-adult living donor liver transplantation Cohort Study 2 (A2ALL-2). Am J Transplant. 2017;17(4):1081–96.

58. Trotter JF, Hill-Callahan MM, Gillespie BW, Nielsen CA, Saab S, Shrestha R, et al. A2ALL study group. Severe psychiatric problems in right hepatic lobe donors for living donor liver transplantation. Transplantation. 2007;83(11):1506–8.

59. Dew MA, DiMartini AF, Ladner DP, Simpson MA, Pomfret EA, Gillespie BW, et al. Psychosocial outcomes 3 to 10 years after donation in the adult to adult living donor liver transplantation cohort study. Transplantation. 2016;100(6):1257–69.

60. Getchell LE, McKenzi SQ, Sontrop JM, Hayward JS, McCallum MK, Garg AX. Increasing the rate of living donor kidney transplantation in Ontario: donor- and recipient-identified barriers and solutions. Can J Kidney Health Dis. 2017;4:1–8.

61. Orandi BJ, Luo X, Massie AB, Garonzik-Wang JM, Lonze BE, Ahmed R, et al. Survival benefit with kidney transplants from HLA-incompatible live donors. N Engl J Med. 2016;374(10):940–50.

Part III

Renal Patient

Chronic and End-Stage Renal Disease and Indications for Renal Transplantation

5

Adetokunbo Taiwo

Introduction

Chronic kidney disease (CKD) is the ninth leading cause of mortality in the United States (USA) [1]. CKD is defined by changes in kidney structure or function, as evidenced by imaging abnormalities, albuminuria ($\geq$30 mg/g), and/or a reduced estimated glomerular filtration rate (eGFR) of less than 60 ml/minute/1.73 m^2 for 3 months or more [2, 3]. The Kidney Disease Improving Global Outcomes (KDIGO) group classifies CKD by stage according to eGFR and albuminuria (see Table 5.1) [3]. Of note, end-stage renal disease (ESRD) is an administrative term in the United States, based on the conditions for payment for healthcare by the Medicare ESRD Program, specifically the level of eGFR and the occurrence of signs and symptoms of kidney failure necessitating initiation of treatment by replacement therapy. ESRD includes patients treated by dialysis or transplantation, irrespective of the level of GFR.

The progression between CKD stages is variable, however it generally takes years for one to reach stages 4 and 5. Rapid onset and progression is possible, such as with rapidly progressive glomeruloneprhitis and in cases where there is additional kidney injury, such as medication nephrotoxicity or sepsis. After reaching stages 5 with uremic symptoms or in cases of severe acute kidney injury, renal replacement therapy (RRT) is usually recommended. RRT includes continuous and intermittent dialysis modalities (i.e hemodialysis and peritoneal dialysis) and kidney transplantation. Continuous RRT can be done via continuous hemodialysis, hemofiltration, or hemodiafiltration; these interventions are done in acute situations, typically during treatment in intensive care unit. Many patients with CKD eventually require intermittent dialysis (often referred to as "dialysis"), which can be performed at a qualified center or at home (see Chap. 7 for further discussion of dialysis).

Albuminuria alone is an independent risk factor for CKD progression and is associated with increased mortality from cardiovascular disease [4–8]. Increasing stages of CKD carry an incremental risk of mortality [3]. Cardiovascular disease is the leading cause of death in CKD and remains so in patients who receive kidney transplants [9].

Patients with CKD, particularly those who have advanced to ESRD, utilize a disproportionate amount of healthcare resources. According to the United States Renal Data System (USRDS), Medicare expenditure for CKD approached $100 billion in 2015 and $34 billion of that amount was spent on care for patients with ESRD [10, 11]. Despite this, the awareness of CKD remains quite low among individuals who have the disease and the general population [10, 12]. Nearly half of patients with advanced stages of kidney disease are unaware of having CKD [12]. Patients may be aware of having diabetes or hypertension, and though they may have concurrent albuminuria and/or reduced eGFR, they often do not make the association that they have CKD. Many patients who present for transplantation report being unaware of having chronic kidney disease until they were near or had reached ESRD. Early referral from primary care providers to nephrology helps to bridge this gap and allows for patient education and dialysis planning. The general consensus is to refer patients with stage 3 CKD to nephrology. Early referral to nephrology allows for early referral to a kidney transplant center, which helps facilitate preemptive (i.e., transplant prior to needing dialysis) kidney transplantation. Transplanting patients just before they require dialysis is associated with better allograft and patient survival outcomes [13–15]. Given the extensive workup needed for kidney transplant (discussed later), early referral also allows patients time to complete required studies prior to transplantation.

A. Taiwo
Division of Nephrology, Kidney Pancreas Transplant Program, Department of Medicine, Stanford University School of Medicine, Palo Alto, CA, USA
e-mail: ataiwo@stanford.edu

© Springer International Publishing AG, part of Springer Nature 2019
Y. Sher, J. R. Maldonado (eds.), *Psychosocial Care of End-Stage Organ Disease and Transplant Patients*,
https://doi.org/10.1007/978-3-319-94914-7_5

Table 5.1 Classification and prognosis of chronic kidney disease by GFR and albuminuria categories [3]

eGFR categories (ml/min/1.73m²)			Albuminuria categories (mg/g)		
			A1 Normal to Midly increased	A2 Moderately increased	A3 Severely increased
			< 30 mg/g	30-300 mg/g	> 300 mg/g
G1	Normal or high	≥ 90			
G2	Mildly decreased	60-89			
G3a	Mildly to moderately decreased	45-59			
G3b	Moderately to severely decreased	30-44			
G4	Severly decreased	15-29			
G5	Kidney failure	<15			

Green, low risk (if no other markers of kidney disease, no CKD); yellow, moderately increased risk; orange, high risk; red, very high risk
2012 KDIGO guidelines incorporate prognosis as predicted by accompanying albuminuria. Abbreviations: *eGFR* estimated glomerular filtration rate. Source: Adapted from: http://kdigo.org/home/guidelines/ckd-evaluation-management/

Epidemiology

According to the USRDS, the prevalence of CKD was 14.8% between 2011 and 2014 [10]. This number has been relatively stable over the past 2 decades and translates to approximately 30 million Americans with CKD. In 2015, the adjusted prevalence of patients on dialysis was 2128 persons per million/year, and there were 124,114 new ESRD cases with an adjusted incidence rate of 357 persons per million/year. Prevalent ESRD cases continue to rise due an aging population and increased patient survival on dialysis. In the United States, the vast majority of patients requiring renal replacement therapies are on hemodialysis compared to peritoneal dialysis and kidney transplantation. In 2015, among prevalent ESRD patients, 63.2% were on hemodialysis, 7.0% were on peritoneal dialysis, and 29.6% had received kidney transplants [10].

There are racial and ethnic differences in the prevalence and incidence of CKD. In 2015, the adjusted incidence rate ratio for ESRD compared to Caucasians was 3.0 for African Americans, 1.2 for American Indians/Alaska Natives, and 1.0 for Asians [10]. All groups experienced a decline in incidence rate over a 15-year period. The incidence rate ratio in Native Hawaiians/Pacific Islanders was 8.4; however, due to the significant discrepancy in this race designation in the US Census data versus USRDS, this data is inconclusive. In African Americans, the excess risk of ESRD is attributed to inheritance of apolipoprotein L1 (APO-L1) gene variants. Carrying two risk alleles confers a tenfold higher risk of ESRD from

hypertension and a 17-fold higher risk from focal segmental glomerulosclerosis (FSGS) [16]. The APO-L1 risk alleles are found predominantly in people with West African Ancestry. Having one risk allele is reported to protect against *African Trypanosomiasis* similar to protection from Malaria seen in heterozygote carriers of the sickle cell gene [17].

Mortality among patients on dialysis decreased by 28% between 2001 and 2015. Adjusted mortality rates were 136, 166, and 29 per 1000 patient-years in ESRD, dialysis, and transplant patients, respectively [10]. In Medicare patients, the mortality rate among CKD patients is more than twice higher than that of patients without CKD at 109.8 per 1000 patient-years. CKD patients also experience higher rates of re-hospitalization compared to patients without CKD [10].

Etiologies of CKD

Diabetes and hypertension are the two leading causes of CKD in the United States and other developed countries [10]. The etiology of ESRD from diabetes and hypertension is often presumptive as it is not typical to obtain biopsies in these patients. Nonetheless, 40% of patients with CKD have diabetes and 32% have hypertension [10]. Advancing age is the largest predictor of low eGFR, while hypertension is the largest predictor of albuminuria [10]. Figure 5.1 shows the etiologies of incident ESRD based on data from USRDS [10].

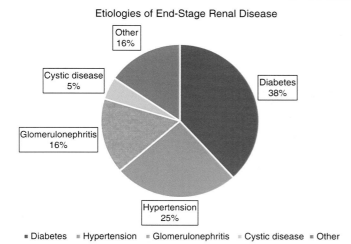

Etiologies of End-Stage Renal Disease

■ Diabetes ■ Hypertension ■ Glomerulonephritis ■ Cystic disease ■ Other

Fig. 5.1 Etiologies of incident ESRD according to 2015 USRDS data [10]

Table 5.2 Recurrence rates of kidney disease after transplant

Disease	Risk of recurrence	Risk of graft loss at 5–10 years
Primary FSGS	20–40%	20–30%
Membranoproliferative glomerulonephritis (MPGN) type I (monoclonal and polyclonal IgG)	20–60%	10–50%
MPGN type II (C3 glomerulopathy and dense deposit disease)	50–90%	10–50%
Membranous nephropathy	10–55%	20–50%
IgA nephropathy	50–60%	2–20%
Lupus nephritis	2–40%	15%
Anti-GBM disease	<5–50%	5%
Atypical hemolytic uremic syndrome	30–50%	>50%
Amyloidosis	25%	Rare
Primary hyperoxaluria	100%	80%

Glomerulonephritis or glomerular disease is the third leading cause of ESRD in the United States [10]. A study looking at the temporal and geographic trends in 21,374 biopsy-proven cases between 1986 and 2001 found that focal segmental glomerular sclerosis accounted for 25%; membranous nephropathy, 13%; lupus nephritis, 12.5%; IgA nephropathy, 10%; pauci-immune glomerulonephritis, 8%; minimal change disease, 5%; and membranoproliferative glomerulonephritis, 3% of cases of glomerular disease [18]. Glomerulopathies recur at variable time periods posttransplant and are an important cause of allograft loss/failure, particularly in living donor recipients [19].

It is important to know the cause of kidney disease due to the risk of disease recurrence in the transplanted kidney (see Table 5.2) [19–21]. This allows the transplant provider to counsel patients about their disease-specific risks. Some kidney diseases (e.g., primary FSGS and C3 glomerulopathies) can recur aggressively early and lead to allograft loss. The rates of disease recurrence and risk of graft loss reported in the litterature is variable based on different study design used

and ascertainment and followup timeframes. This information is particularly important for patients with living donors.

Complications of Advanced Kidney Disease

Anemia

In advanced stages of kidney disease, anemia is caused by reduced erythropoietin production and shortened lifespan of red blood cells [22, 23]. The use of erythropoietin stimulating agents has greatly reduced the need for blood transfusions in the dialysis population [24]. Limiting sensitizing events is paramount in patients who are likely to need a kidney transplant. Sensitizing events (e.g., transfusions, pregnancies, prior transplants) increase the chance of developing panel reactive antibodies (PRA) to the general population. Patients with greater sensitization have smaller pools of available donors. Patients with PRA greater than 20% are considered sensitized, and those with PRA greater than 80% are considered highly sensitized. Previously patients who were considered highly sensitized had disproportionately long waitlist times. In December 2014, the US organ allocation rules changed to allow a sliding scale of points based on PRA. In addition, patients who are hypersensitized with PRA of 99 and 100 gained access to regional and national organ sharing, respectively.

Acid-base Imbalances

Patients with advanced stages of kidney disease tend to develop a chronic metabolic acidosis. Treatment of chronic metabolic acidosis with bicarbonate supplementation may mitigate uremic bone disease, malnutrition, and muscle wasting and may help slow the progression of kidney disease [3, 25–27]; however, the level at which supplementation should be initiated and whether to target a normal serum bicarbonate level is somewhat controversial in the nephrology community. The KDIGO group recommends treating chronic metabolic acidosis with bicarbonate supplementation to achieve serum bicarbonate levels above 22 mmol/L [3].

Electrolyte Imbalances

Hyperkalemia is the more common and feared electrolyte abnormality in patients with CKD as it may lead to fatal cardiac arrhythmias [28]. Chronic exposure to a high-potassium milieu raises the threshold at which cardiac arrhythmias occur, such that many dialysis patients adapt to serum potassium of greater than 6.0 mmol/l without the clinical consequences, levels that could pose a significant risk if acutely developed. As kidney disease progresses, patients are prone to hyperkalemia due to oliguria, high-potassium diet, and/or the use of medications that induce a hypoaldosterone state (e.g., renin-angiotensin system blockers) [29].

Hyperkalemia is treated by adhering to a low-potassium diet, the use of potassium-binding resins (e.g., Kayexalate and Patiromer), discontinuing renin-angiotensin-aldosterone-system-blocking medications, and dialysis.

Hyponatremia is another common electrolyte abnormality in advanced CKD, and it is often caused by impaired free water excretion as eGFR declines. Hyponatremia may be confounded by a concurrent syndrome of inappropriate antidiuretic hormone secretion (SIADH) and/or hypervolemic states. It is important to decipher the exact etiology of hyponatremia and chronicity to determine appropriate treatment.

Mineral Bone Disease

Mineral bone disease (MBD) occurs from derangements in the phosphorus-calcium-parathyroid hormone axis that occur in advanced kidney disease [30]. Manifestations of MBD include osteitis fibrosa, osteomalacia, and adynamic bone disease. As kidney function declines, serum phosphorus rises and calcium decreases (due to decreased production of activated vitamin D by the kidney). The rise in phosphorus is initially mitigated by an elevated fibroblast growth factor (FGF)-23 level and then rising parathyroid hormone (PTH), both of which are phosphatonins [31]. The rise in PTH helps to normalize both phosphorus and calcium. This process leads to a development of secondary hyperparathyroidism. Treatment includes adhering to a low-phosphorous diet, taking phosphate binders with meals, and using active vitamin D analogs (e.g., calcitriol) and calcimimetics (e.g., Sensipar) [32, 33]. A selected number of patients with secondary hyperparathyroidism go on to develop tertiary hyperparathyroidism requiring parathyroidectomy. Some transplant centers require patients with uncontrolled hyperparathyroidism undergo parathyroidectomy prior to kidney transplantation. However, kidney transplantation alone may restore the calcium-phosphorous-PTH axis and lead to resolution of secondary hyperparathyroidism within several months. Patients with persistent hyperparathyroidism after kidney transplantation may then be referred for parathyroidectomy.

Hypertension and Volume Overload

Patients with advanced CKD are less adapt to changes in sodium and volume expansion. With development of oliguria or anuria, management of volume overload is quite challenging and may require near daily dialysis in some patients. Fluid restriction is paramount for reduction of intradialytic weight gains but is challenging for many patients. In these more challenging cases, longer (4 hours or more) and/or frequent (4 days a week or more) dialysis may be needed for volume management. To enable more aggressive ultrafiltration (fluid removal on dialysis), nocturnal dialysis or home hemodialysis modalities can accommodate longer or more frequent dialysis sessions in patients who can manage the timing, training, and equipment. Other treatment options include sodium restriction (< 2 grams per day), fluid restriction, and diuretics in patients who are not auric [3, 34].

Malnutrition

Malnutrition is a common consequence of advanced CKD [35]. Patients with CKD have diminished appetite and anorexia which is confounded by many dietary restrictions (e.g., sodium, potassium, phosphorus), and they lose amino acids in dialysate fluids. Renal dieticians are available in many kidney clinics and the US dialysis centers to help with frequent education and recommendations about diet.

Kidney Transplant Evaluation

Indications

Kidney transplant is an elective procedure and it is not without risks; nonetheless, it is the treatment of choice for stage 5 CKD/ESRD [20, 36]. Compared to dialysis, kidney transplantation improves quantity and quality of life. Unlike other solid organ transplants where the sickest patients get transplanted first, priority for kidney transplants is largely based on the waiting time and sensitization status.

Patients can receive transplants from a living donor or a deceased donor. The average waiting time for deceased donor kidney transplantation in the United States depends on geography, blood type, and sensitization status and ranges from 3 to 10 years, thus transplantation from an eligible living donor represents a much faster path [37]. Given the impact of dialysis vintage (i.e., length of time on dialysis) on outcomes, this is an important consideration. In December 2014, the United Network for Organ Sharing (UNOS) implemented a new kidney allocation system to improve equity and fairness for disadvantaged groups: highly sensitized patients, ethnic minorities, blood group B patients, and patients who experience late referral [38].

Timing of Referral

Patients with CKD are eligible for kidney transplant listing if they are on dialysis or if their eGFR is 20 ml/min/1.73 m² or less [38]. At this eGFR, patients are generally asymptomatic, and many do not develop symptoms that would require dialysis until eGFR falls below 12–15 mL/min/1.73m². The optimum timing for kidney transplant in patients who are not yet in ESRD is not defined. The goal is to wait for as long as possible such that the timing occurs right before uremic symptoms and complications develop. There is no survival (patient or graft) benefit to transplantation well in advance of the need for dialysis. The new kidney allocation system allows for backdating wait time to the dialysis start date [38]. This mitigates the disadvantage to patients who qualified for kidney transplantation but were referred late. A patient who had been on dialysis for 5 years at the time of referral would automatically get 5 years of waiting time.

Medical Evaluation

A comprehensive medical history, physical examination, laboratory and diagnostic studies (see Table 5.3), and psychosocial assessment are crucial in evaluating patients for kidney transplantation [39, 40]. The goal of the evaluation process is to detect conditions or disease that would make patients ineligible for transplantation. There are few absolute contraindications to kidney transplantation and these are represented in Table 5.4. In areas of the country where the waiting time is long, it is reasonable to undergo a limited workup to see if patients can be listed in their current state and defer the more extensive workup until the patient is closer to transplantation. In areas of the country with long waiting times, yearly updates and follow-up clinic visits closer to the time of transplant is often needed to ensure patients remain medically and psychosocially suitable for transplantation.

Table 5.3 Comprehensive workup for kidney transplantation. Limited life expectancy minimizes the potential benefit of transplantation

Blood type, complete blood count, comprehensive metabolic panel, coagulation studies
Infectious serologies: HIV, RPR, hepatitis B and C, varicella, EBV, CMV, gold quantiferon, and endemic fungi (e.g coccidioidomycosis, cryptococcus, and histoplasmosis) in applicable regions
Anti-A isoagglutinin titers should be measured in blood type B candidates who are willing to accept a kidney from an A2 or A2B donor
Chest X-ray
Cardiac screening with EKG, stress testing (pharmacologic echocardiography), myocardium perfusion scan or coronary angiogram as determined based on age and comorbid conditions
Age appropriate cancer screening as recommended by the USPSTF and cancer societies for the general population
Other testing determined based on clinical history, e.g., random drug screen in patients with a history of substance abuse

Table 5.4 Absolute contraindications to kidney transplantation

Active ischemic heart disease or severe cardiomyopathy
Severe peripheral vascular disease involving iliofemoral vessels
Active infection
Recent history of cancer other than non-melanoma skin cancers and carcinoma in-situ
Cirrhosis or advanced liver fibrosis (unless liver transplant candidate)
Primary oxalosis (unless liver transplant candidate)
Active psychosis
Active substance abuse or dependence
Incorrigible noncompliance
Body mass index (BMI) > 40
Lack of adequate social/caregiver support

Factors to Consider During the Evaluation Process

Age

There is no age limit for kidney transplantation; however, in general, patients over the age of 65–70 should be "well otherwise" (i.e., wow), with well-managed comorbidities. The benefits of transplantation should outweigh the risk of surgery, anesthesia, and chronic immunosuppression. With appropriate patient selection, those over the age of 70 do well with good long-term graft outcomes. Older patients or those with an expected post-transplant survival of around 5 years or more can be good candidates for deceased donor kidneys with a kidney donor profile index (KDPI) of 85% or higher, which can achieve satisfactory graft outcomes [41]. The KDPI is composed of ten donor factors (age, diabetes, hypertension, race/ethnicity, height, weight, creatinine, cause of death, donation after cardiac death (DCD) status, and hepatitis C status) and is a marker of organ quality. A KDPI of 85% percent has 85% higher expected risk of allograft failure compared to all kidney donors from the prior year. The estimated post-transplant survival is a score composed of four factors (diabetes, hypertension, prior transplant, dialysis vintage). Lower estimated post-transplant survival (EPTS) scores translate to higher post-transplant survival. Patients with scores of 20% or less primarily receive offers from KDPI kidneys of 20% or less. The KDPI and EPTS scores are used in the organ allocation system to help improve longevity matching, i.e., kidneys with the longest chance of survival go to the patient with the longest life expectancy [38].

Considering expected post-transplant survival in the evaluation process helps with counseling patients regarding staying on dialysis versus moving toward transplantation. Patients should be expected to survive longer than the half-life of a transplanted kidney. For older patients, it is also important to consider that the risk of death rises in the immediate postoperative period and is higher than in patients who are waitlisted for transplant. It takes about 3.5 years for the mortality rate to drop below that of patients who remain on the waiting list [42]. Older patients may have acceptable quality of life on dialysis and may not experience a survival benefit with transplantation [43].

Cardiovascular Disease

The burden of cardiovascular disease is high in CKD patients [44, 45]. Noninvasive cardiac testing has limited utility in patients with CKD who have diabetes. Noninvasive testing (e.g., stress echocardiogram) is permissible in asymptomatic low-risk patients; however, higher-risk patients (i.e., those with diabetic nephropathy or long-standing diabetes, over the age of 50, with risk factors for coronary artery disease such as smoking, hypertension, hyperlipidemia, family history, or heart failure with reduced ejection fraction) should undergo coronary angiogram [46–48].

Cerebrovascular Disease

There is an increased risk of ischemic stroke in CKD after kidney transplantation [49]. Patients with history of ischemic stroke should undergo screening for carotid stenosis and repair. Patients with risk factors for stroke (e.g., hypertension, smoking, hyperlipidemia, transient ischemic attacks) or carotid artery bruits on physical examination should be evaluated. Patients with autosomal dominant polycystic kidney disease who have a family history of strokes, cerebral aneurysms, or chronic headaches should undergo screening to assess for cerebral aneurysms, and those who meet the size criteria should be repaired prior to kidney transplantation [50].

Peripheral Vascular Disease

The vascular physical examination is a crucial part of the kidney transplant evaluation. Kidney transplantation can be technically impossible in patients with severe vascular calcifications involving the iliofemoral system. Bilateral femoral and pedal pulses should be palpated. Patients with reduced or non-palpable pulses should have imaging to assess their vasculature (e.g., Doppler studies or non-contrast computed tomography (CT) of the abdomen/pelvis). Patients with severe distal stenosis are at risk for steal syndrome (i.e., shunting of blood flow leading to reduced distal perfusion) with a transplant and can risk limb loss, ulcer development, and/or poor wound healing. Patients with claudication symptoms should undergo evaluation and repair of flow-limiting stenosis.

Malignancy

All patients should undergo age-appropriate cancer screening as recommended by the United States Preventative Services Task Force (USPSTF) and professional cancer societies. Immunosuppression increases the risk for cancers in

Table 5.5 Cancer waiting period

Renal cell cancer	
Symptomatic < 5 cm	2 years
≥ 5 cm or invasive	5 years
Incidental (< 5 cm)	None
Wilms' tumor	2 years
Bladder	
In situ or noninvasive papillomas	None
Invasive	Inadequate evidence
Cervix	
In situ	None
Invasive	2–5 years
Uterus	2 years
Testis	2 years
Thyroid	2 years
Kaposi's and other sarcomas	2 years
Breast	2–5 years
Colorectal	2–5 years
Prostate	2 years
Liver	Contraindicated
Myeloma	Contraindicated
Lymphoma	2 years
Leukemia	2 years
Melanoma	5 years
In situ	2 years
Non-melanoma skin cancer	None
Lung	5 years

Adapted from Kasiske et al. [40] and Pham et al [36]

kidney transplant patients. Patients who have been treated for certain malignancies and remain disease-free for 2–5 years (depending on the type of cancer) may proceed to kidney transplantation (see Table 5.5) [51, 52].

Hematologic Disease

Patients with a history of recurrent miscarriage, arterial/venous thrombosis, hemodialysis graft or fistula thrombosis, lupus, or a prior history of unexplained kidney allograft thrombosis should undergo a hypercoagulable workup [20, 37]. Hematology referral may be needed to assess thrombosis risk prior to transplantation. In addition, patients with monoclonal gammopathies or history of paraproteinemias may require hematology evaluation and recommendations regarding risk.

Obesity

Centers vary on their body mass index (BMI) cutoff point at which patients are required to lose weight prior to transplantation. Many centers consider a BMI over 35 kg/m^2 as an absolute contraindication to transplantation [20]. Obese patients are at increased risk for delayed graft function (defined as the need for dialysis in the first week of transplant), poor wound healing, and infections. Obesity is not associated with kidney transplant rejection, graft loss, or death.

Gastrointestinal Disease

Having recent gastrointestinal malignancy or cirrhosis that is not eligible for liver transplant are absolute contraindications to kidney transplant. Patients with evidence of advanced liver disease or cirrhosis should be referred to hepatology for liver transplant evaluation. For advanced stages of liver disease, combined liver-kidney transplant may be an option. Gastrointestinal ulcers should be under control as they may worsen with induction therapy and high-dose corticosteroids. Perforated visicus is a rare but feared complication of ulcers. Patients with chronic nausea and vomiting should be evaluated as these symptoms can worsen and cause patients to be unable to comply with transplant medications which could lead to rejection and allograft loss. In patients with chronic diarrhea and ESRD, hyperoxaluria (excess loss of oxalate in the urine that leads to calcium oxalate stones and crystal deposits) should be considered as a cause for ESRD and ruled out. If this diagnosis is missed, it can lead to rapid loss of a kidney transplant [20, 36]. Primary oxalosis is treated with combined liver and kidney transplantation.

Infection

Patients undergoing kidney transplant should be free of active infection before transplantation [20]. Patients with chronic viral infections like human immunodeficiency virus (HIV) may be transplanted if their disease is under good control. Transplants in patients with HIV should be done at centers with experience managing these patients. The new antiviral mediations for hepatitis C treatment yield excellent sustained viral clearance, making transplantation in this group permissible. This also opens up a pool of hepatitis C donors for hepatitis C positive recipients. Patients with latent tuberculosis should receive an adequate course of treatment (e.g., 9 months of isoniazid) before or after transplantation. For patients who did not complete their course prior to transplant, it is permissible to proceed and complete the course after transplant. Patients with poor dentition should see a dentist for deep cleaning and extractions as indicated prior to transplantation. Oral surgery in the early months post-transplant while immunosuppression is still intense is generally not advised. Although response to vaccination is poor in ESRD patients, live vaccines should be offered when indicated at this time, as they are contraindicated after transplantation.

Frailty

The prevalence of frailty rises with increasing stages of CKD [53–55]. Frailty is associated with increased length of stay, delayed graft function, higher risk of readmission, and mortality in kidney transplant patients [56–58]. Centers use various batteries to assess for frailty (e.g., sit-stand test, walking speed, test, grip strength, Fried criteria, short physical performance battery). Frail patients can undergo pre-transplant rehabilitation to improve outcomes post-transplant. Studies are being done to assess the impact of rehabilitation in kidney transplant recipients on their post-transplant outcomes and survival.

Psychosocial Evaluation

Potential kidney transplant recipients must be motivated to have a transplant. They should be able to understand the risks and benefits of the transplantation and chronic immunosuppression and be able to make an informed decision. Mental health professionals (i.e., social workers, psychiatrists, psychologists) play a crucial role in the evaluation of potential kidney transplant recipients. The goals of the psychosocial evaluation are to determine behavioral, social, and financial barriers to transplantation. This assessment elicits behaviors that may be risk factors for medical nonadherence after transplant. Social workers contact dialysis units to determine patients' adherence with their dialysis appointments and treatments. Many centers insist on absolute adherence with outpatient dialysis regimens in order to consider patients for transplantation. Patient's psychiatric or cognitive disease may require neuropsychiatric assessment and a referral to transplant psychiatry.

Patients who have low literacy concerns or difficulty understanding their medications are referred to pre-transplant education. Transplant centers require that one or two able adults serve as a caregiver(s) in the post-transplant phase. Caregivers help with medication reminders, transportation to appointments, and supervising the patient at home. Patients cannot name their proposed living donor (e.g., a spouse, child, or parent) as a caregiver.

Patients with alcohol or substance abuse may be required to undergo treatment rehabilitation and pass random alcohol and drug screening. Patients with diabetes, peripheral vascular disease, or other risk factors for cardiovascular disease are required to stop smoking to be eligible for transplantation.

Patients require adequate insurance for transplantation. ESRD patients qualify for Medicare based on the disease alone; however, coverage for prescriptions expires 3 years after transplant if the patient does not qualify for Medicare by age. Three years represents a crucial time in the field of kidney transplantation as patients who lose prescription coverage risk rejection and subsequent allograft loss. Many patients with ESRD are on disability. Kidney transplantation should improve quality of life to an extent of enabling patients to return to the workforce, if the patient desires. Patients who return to the workforce may gain insurance coverage with their employer.

Surgical Evaluation

As patients get closer to the top of the list, they may be seen by surgeons to ensure the transplant is technically feasible. Concerning factors from the initial evaluation include known peripheral vascular disease, symptoms of claudication, history of amputation, and abnormal femoral and distal extremity pulses. These should prompt imaging of the iliofemoral system with a non-contrast CT scan evaluating for vascular calcification or ultrasound imaging evaluating for flow-limiting stenosis. Severe calcification of the iliofemoral system could make surgery technically infeasible.

Living Donation

About one third of kidney transplants in the United States come from living donors [59, 60]. The living donation rate has declined in recent years. Patients who receive living donors generally have immediate allograft function and a longer median survival of approximately 15 years compared to 10 years with deceased donors [59, 60]. Living donors must have a completely separate living donor advocate. Living donors should also undergo extensive medical, surgical, and psychosocial evaluation prior to living kidney donation [59, 60] (see Chap. 4 for more details).

Conclusions

CKD is an important cause of morbidity and the ninth leading cause of mortality in the United States. Diabetes and hypertension remain the most common causes of CKD in developed countries. Complications of advanced stages of CKD include anemia, chronic metabolic acidosis, electrolyte imbalances, volume overload, hypertension, and mineral bone disease. Kidney transplantation is the treatment of choice for patients with Stage 5 CKD and ESRD and leads to better health and cost-effective outcomes compared to dialysis. Nonetheless, kidney transplantation is an elective procedure with both short- and long-term risks and complications. The evaluation process requires the efforts of a multidisciplinary team to ensure appropriate candidate selection.

References

1. Heron M. Deaths: leading causes for 2015. National vital statistics reports: from the Centers for Disease Control and Prevention, National Center for Health Statistics. Natl Vital Stat Rep. 2017;66(5):1–76.
2. National Kidney Foundation. K/DOQI clinical practice guidelines for chronic kidney disease: evaluation, classification and stratification. Am J Kidney Dis. 2002;39(suppl 1):S1–S266.
3. Kidney Disease: Improving Global Outcomes (KDIGO) CKD Work Group. KDIGO 2012 clinical practice guideline for the evaluation and management of chronic kidney disease. Kidney Int. 2013;3(Suppl):1–150.
4. Gerstein HC, Mann JF, Yi Q, Zinman B, Dinneen SF, Hoogwerf B, et al. Albuminuria and risk of cardiovascular events, death, and heart failure in diabetic and nondiabetic individuals. JAMA. 2001;286(4):421–6.
5. Hong JW, Ku CR, Noh JH, Ko KS, Rhee BD, Kim DJ. Association between low-grade albuminuria and cardiovascular risk in Korean adults: the 2011–2012 Korea National Health and nutrition examination survey. PLoS One. 2015;10(3):e0118866.
6. Skaaby T, Husemoen LL, Ahluwalia TS, Rossing P, Jorgensen T, Thuesen BH, et al. Cause-specific mortality according to urine albumin creatinine ratio in the general population. PLoS One. 2014;9(3):e93212.
7. Toyama T, Furuichi K, Ninomiya T, Shimizu M, Hara A, Iwata Y, et al. The impacts of albuminuria and low eGFR on the risk of cardiovascular death, all-cause mortality, and renal events in diabetic patients: meta-analysis. PLoS One. 2013;8(8):e71810.
8. Matsushita K, van der Velde M, Astor BC, Woodward M, Levey AS, de Jong PE, et al. Association of estimated glomerular filtration rate and albuminuria with all-cause and cardiovascular mortality in general population cohorts: a collaborative meta-analysis. Lancet (London, England). 2010;375(9731):2073–81.
9. Go AS, Chertow GM, Fan D, McCulloch CE, Hsu CY. Chronic kidney disease and the risks of death, cardiovascular events, and hospitalization. N Engl J Med. 2004;351(13):1296–305.
10. United States Renal Data System. 2017 USRDS annual data report: Epidemiology of kidney disease in the United States. National Institutes of Health, National Institute of Diabetes and Digestive and Kidney Diseases, Bethesda, MD, 2017.
11. Saran R, Robinson B, Abbott KC, et al. US renal data system 2017 annual data report: epidemiology of kidney disease in the United States. Am J Kidney Dis. 2018;71(3, suppl 1):Svii,S1–S672.
12. Centers for Disease Control and Prevention. Chronic kidney disease surveillance system website. http://www.cdc.gov/ckd. Accessed 3 May 2018.
13. Kallab S, Bassil N, Esposito L, Cardeau-Desangles I, Rostaing L, Kamar N. Indications for and barriers to preemptive kidney transplantation: a review. Transplant Proc. 2010;42(3):782–4.
14. Perez-Flores I, Sanchez-Fructuoso A, Calvo N, Marques M, Anaya S, Ridao N, et al. Preemptive kidney transplant from deceased donors: an advantage in relation to reduced waiting list. Transplant Proc. 2007;39(7):2123–4.
15. Ishani A, Ibrahim HN, Gilbertson D, Collins AJ. The impact of residual renal function on graft and patient survival rates in recipients of preemptive renal transplants. Am J Kidney Dis. 2003;42(6):1275–82.
16. Friedman DJ, Kozlitina J, Genovese G, Jog P, Pollak MR. Population-based risk assessment of APOL1 on renal disease. J Am Soc Nephrol. 2011;22(11):2098–105.
17. Genovese G, Friedman DJ, Ross MD, Lecordier L, Uzureau P, Freedman BI, et al. Association of trypanolytic ApoL1 variants with kidney disease in African Americans. Science (New York, NY). 2010;329(5993):841–5.
18. O'Shaughnessy MM, Hogan SL, Poulton CJ, Falk RJ, Singh HK, Nickeleit V, et al. Temporal and demographic trends in glomerular disease epidemiology in the southeastern United States, 1986–2015. Clin J Am Soc Nephrol. 2017;12(4):614–23.
19. Blosser CD, Bloom RD. Recurrent glomerular disease after kidney transplantation. Curr Opin Nephrol Hypertens. 2017;26:501–8.
20. Scandling JD. Kidney transplant candidate evaluation. Semin Dial. 2005;18(6):487–94.
21. Yamamoto I, Yamakawa T, Katsuma A, et al. Recurrence of native kidney disease after kidney transplantation. Nephrology (Carlton, Vic). 2018;23(Suppl 2):27–30.
22. Astor BC, Muntner P, Levin A, Eustace JA, Coresh J. Association of kidney function with anemia: the third National Health and Nutrition Examination Survey (1988–1994). Arch Intern Med. 2002;162(12):1401–8.
23. Hsu CY, McCulloch CE, Curhan GC. Epidemiology of anemia associated with chronic renal insufficiency among adults in the United States: results from the third National Health and

Nutrition Examination Survey. Clin J Am Soc Nephrol. 2002 Feb;13(2):504–10.

24. Kliger AS, Foley RN, Goldfarb DS, Goldstein SL, Johansen K, Singh A, et al. KDOQI US commentary on the 2012 KDIGO clinical practice guideline for Anemia in CKD. Am J Kidney Dis. 2013;62(5):849–59.

25. Green J, Kleeman CR. Role of bone in regulation of systemic acid-base balance. Kidney Int. 1991;39(1):9–26.

26. Krieger NS, Frick KK, Bushinsky DA. Mechanism of acid-induced bone resorption. Curr Opin Nephrol Hypertens. 2004;13(4):423–36.

27. de Brito-Ashurst I, Varagunam M, Raftery MJ, Yaqoob MM. Bicarbonate supplementation slows progression of CKD and improves nutritional status. Clin J Am Soc Nephrol. 2009;20(9):2075–84.

28. Allon M. Hyperkalemia in end-stage renal disease: mechanisms and management. Clin J Am Soc Nephrol. 1995;6(4):1134–42.

29. Hsu CY, Chertow GM. Elevations of serum phosphorus and potassium in mild to moderate chronic renal insufficiency. Nephrol Dial Transplant. 2002;17(8):1419–25.

30. Hruska KA, Teitelbaum SL. Renal osteodystrophy. N Engl J Med. 1995;333(3):166–74.

31. Cunningham J, Locatelli F, Rodriguez M. Secondary hyperparathyroidism: pathogenesis, disease progression, and therapeutic options. Clin J Am Soc Nephrol. 2011;6(4):913–21.

32. Ketteler M, Block GA, Evenepoel P, Fukagawa M, Herzog CA, McCann L, et al. Executive summary of the 2017 KDIGO chronic kidney disease-mineral and bone disorder (CKD-MBD) guideline update: what's changed and why it matters. Kidney Int. 2017;92(1):26–36.

33. Isakova T, Nickolas TL, Denburg M, Yarlagadda S, Weiner DE, Gutierrez OM, et al. KDOQI US commentary on the 2017 KDIGO clinical practice guideline update for the diagnosis, evaluation, prevention, and treatment of chronic kidney disease-mineral and bone disorder (CKD-MBD). Am J Kidney Dis. 2017;70(6):737–51.

34. Shrout T, Rudy DW, Piascik MT. Hypertension update, JNC8 and beyond. Curr Opin Pharmacol. 2017;33:41–6.

35. Kopple JD, Greene T, Chumlea WC, Hollinger D, Maroni BJ, Merrill D, et al. Relationship between nutritional status and the glomerular filtration rate: results from the MDRD study. Kidney Int. 2000;57(4):1688–703.

36. Pham PT, Pham PA, Pham PC, Parikh S, Danovitch G. Evaluation of adult kidney transplant candidates. Semin Dial. 2010;23(6):595–605.

37. Hart A, Smith JM, Skeans MA, Gustafson SK, Wilk AR, Robinson A, et al. OPTN/SRTR 2016 annual data report: kidney. Am J Transplant. 2018;18(Suppl 1):18–113.

38. Stewart DE, Klassen DK. Early experience with the new kidney allocation system: a perspective from UNOS. Clin J Am Soc Nephrol. 2017;12(12):2063–5.

39. Knoll G, Cockfield S, Blydt-Hansen T, Baran D, Kiberd B, Landsberg D, et al. Canadian Society of Transplantation consensus guidelines on eligibility for kidney transplantation. CMAJ. 2005;173(10):1181–4.

40. Kasiske BL, Cangro CB, Hariharan S, Hricik DE, Kerman RH, Roth D, et al. The evaluation of renal transplantation candidates: clinical practice guidelines. Am J Transplant. 2001;1(Suppl 2):3–95.

41. Jay CL, Washburn K, Dean PG, Helmick RA, Pugh JA, Stegall MD. Survival benefit in older patients associated with earlier transplant with high KDPI kidneys. Transplantation. 2017;101(4):867–72.

42. Wolfe RA, Ashby VB, Milford EL, Ojo AO, Ettenger RE, Agodoa LY, et al. Comparison of mortality in all patients on dialysis, patients on dialysis awaiting transplantation, and recipients of a first cadaveric transplant. N Engl J Med. 1999;341(23):1725–30.

43. Schold JD, Meier-Kriesche HU. Which renal transplant candidates should accept marginal kidneys in exchange for a shorter waiting time on dialysis? Clin J Am Soc Nephrol. 2006;1(3):532–8.

44. Hart A, Weir MR, Kasiske BL. Cardiovascular risk assessment in kidney transplantation. Kidney Int. 2015;87(3):527–34.

45. Kahn MR, Fallahi A, Kim MC, Esquitin R, Robbins MJ. Coronary artery disease in a large renal transplant population: implications for management. Am J Transplant. 2011;11(12):2665–74.

46. De Lima JJ, Sabbaga E, Vieira ML, de Paula FJ, Ianhez LE, Krieger EM, et al. Coronary angiography is the best predictor of events in renal transplant candidates compared with noninvasive testing. Hypertension (Dallas, Tex : 1979). 2003;42(3):263–8.

47. Holley JL, Fenton RA, Arthur RS. Thallium stress testing does not predict cardiovascular risk in diabetic patients with end-stage renal disease undergoing cadaveric renal transplantation. Am J Med. 1991;90(5):563–70.

48. Pilmore H. Cardiac assessment for renal transplantation. Am J Transplant. 2006;6(4):659–65.

49. Masson P, Webster AC, Hong M, Turner R, Lindley RI, Craig JC. Chronic kidney disease and the risk of stroke: a systematic review and meta-analysis. Nephrol Dial Transplant. 2015;30(7):1162–9.

50. Niemczyk M, Gradzik M, Fliszkiewicz M, Kulesza A, Golebiowski M, Paczek L. Natural history of intracranial aneurysms in autosomal dominant polycystic kidney disease. Neurol Neurochir Pol. 2017;51(6):476–80.

51. Engels EA, Pfeiffer RM, Fraumeni JF Jr, Kasiske BL, Israni AK, Snyder JJ, et al. Spectrum of cancer risk among US solid organ transplant recipients. JAMA. 2011;306(17):1891–901.

52. Moosa MR. Racial and ethnic variations in incidence and pattern of malignancies after kidney transplantation. Medicine. 2005;84(1):12–22.

53. Reese PP, Cappola AR, Shults J, Townsend RR, Gadegbeku CA, Anderson C, et al. Physical performance and frailty in chronic kidney disease. Am J Nephrol. 2013;38(4):307–15.

54. Wilhelm-Leen ER, Hall YN, KT M, Chertow GM. Frailty and chronic kidney disease: the third National Health and Nutrition Evaluation Survey. Am J Med. 2009;122(7):664–71.e2.

55. Kutner NG, Zhang R, Bowles T, Painter P. Pretransplant physical functioning and kidney patients' risk for posttransplantation hospitalization/death: evidence from a national cohort. Clin J Am Soc Nephrol. 2006;1(4):837–43.

56. McAdams-DeMarco MA, King EA, Luo X, Haugen C, DiBrito S, Shaffer A, et al. Frailty, length of stay, and mortality in kidney transplant recipients: a national registry and prospective cohort study. Ann Surg. 2017;266(6):1084–90.

57. Garonzik-Wang JM, Govindan P, Grinnan JW, Liu M, Ali HM, Chakraborty A, et al. Frailty and delayed graft function in kidney transplant recipients. Arch Surg (Chicago, Ill : 1960). 2012;147(2):190–3.

58. McAdams-DeMarco MA, Law A, Salter ML, Chow E, Grams M, Walston J, et al. Frailty and early hospital readmission after kidney transplantation. Am J Transplant. 2013;13(8):2091–5.

59. Lentine KL, Kasiske BL, Levey AS, Adams PL, Alberu J, Bakr MA, et al. Summary of kidney disease: improving global outcomes (KDIGO) clinical practice guideline on the evaluation and care of living kidney donors. Transplantation. 2017;101(8):1783–92.

60. Lentine KL, Patel A. Risks and outcomes of living donation. Adv Chronic Kidney Dis. 2012;19(4):220–8.

Mental Health in Chronic and End-Stage Renal Disease

6

Paula C. Zimbrean, Jennifer Braverman, and Marta Novak

Abbreviations

AIS	Acceptance of Illness Scale
BDI	Beck Depression Inventory
BFI	Big Five Inventory
CAPD	Continuous automated peritoneal dialysis
CKD	Patients with chronic kidney disease not on HD or PD
COPE	Coping strategies with stress
CS	Cross-sectional study
DSI	Dialysis Symptom Index
DSM V	Diagnostic and Statistical Manual of Mental Disorders, Fifth Edition
DT	Distress Thermometer
ESRD	End-stage renal disease
ESS-r	Somatic Symptom Scale revised
FSFI	Female Sexual Function Index
GDS-4	Geriatric Depression Scale
HADS	Hospital Anxiety and Depression Scale
HARS	Hamilton Anxiety Rating Scale
HD	Patients on hemodialysis
HDRS	Hamilton Depression Rating Scale
HPS	Health perceptions questionnaire
IDDM	Insulin-dependent diabetes mellitus
IEFF	Erectile Function International Evaluation Form
KDQoL	Kidney Disease Quality of Life
MHLC	Multidimensional Health Locus of Control scale
MINI	Mini-International Neuropsychiatric Interview
MMSE	Mini Mental Status Examination
MOODS-SR	Self-report questionnaire to assess mood
MOS	Medical Outcomes Study
MR	Medical records
MSAS-SF	Renal Memorial Symptom Assessment Scale
MSPSS	Multidimensional Scale of Perceived Social Support
OL-HDF	Online hemodiafiltration
P	Prospective study
PAS-SR	Self-report questionnaire to assess panic and agoraphobia
PD	Patients on peritoneal dialysis
SCID-D	Structured Clinical Interview for Depression
SCLE 90	Symptom Checklist 90
SF-36	Short Form Health Survey
SOS	Significant Others Scale
TAS	Toronto Alexithymia Scale
TDQ	Taiwan Depression Questionnaire
THS	Trait Hope Scale
WHODAS 2	WHO Disability Assessment Schedule 2.0
WHOQOL-BREF	World Health Organization Quality of Life instrument
3MS	Modified Mini-Mental State Examination

P. C. Zimbrean (✉)
Departments of Psychiatry and Surgery, Yale University School of Medicine, New Haven, CT, USA
e-mail: Paula.zimbrean@yale.edu

J. Braverman · M. Novak
Department of Psychiatry, University of Toronto, Toronto, ON, Canada

Centre For Mental Health, University Health Network-Toronto General Hospital, Toronto, ON, Canada

Introduction

Psychiatrists are often asked to evaluate and treat psychiatric presentations during the course of chronic kidney disease (CKD). Due to a significant overlap between CKD and psychiatric presentations and between renal diseases in general and psychiatry, a new subspecialty has emerged over the past

© Springer International Publishing AG, part of Springer Nature 2019
Y. Sher, J. R. Maldonado (eds.), *Psychosocial Care of End-Stage Organ Disease and Transplant Patients*,
https://doi.org/10.1007/978-3-319-94914-7_6

decade. *Psychonephrology* is the field of psychosomatic medicine with focus on the psychiatric and psychological problems of patients with CKD, including patients on renal replacement therapy (RRT) [1, 2].

This chapter summarizes current knowledge related to the diagnosis, epidemiology, etiology, and management of psychiatric illness in patients with CKD prior to transplantation, as resulting from systematic reviews, pivotal trials, and pharmacological databases.

Disease Mechanisms in Psychonephrology

The association between CKD and psychiatric presentations can occur in different sequences: patients with chronic psychiatric illness can develop CKD or a patient with CKD may present with new onset psychiatric symptoms.

Patients with chronic psychiatric illnesses are at higher risk of developing CKD; for instance, patients with schizophrenia have a 25% increase in the risk of developing CKD compared to controls [3]. Several factors associated with chronic mental illness may mediate this risk, including direct toxicity of ingested substances (psychiatric medications, substances of abuse, misuse of medications such as Nonsteroidal anti-inflammatory drugs (NSAIDs)), and uncontrolled psychiatric illness leading to nonadherence with medical treatment for diabetes or hypertension and, indirectly, to CKD.

Psychiatric Medications and Nephrotoxicity

Among psychotropic medications, lithium is the most known agent linked to significant risk of developing kidney damage. A recent systematic review and meta-analysis of the lithium toxicity profile suggests that the risk of lithium-induced renal failure is small (0.5% of patients received RRT) [4]. A recent report of 630 patients who received lithium for more than 10 years showed that 32% of the patients had an estimated glomerular filtration rate (eGFR) below 60 mL/min per 1.73 m^2 and 5% of the patients developed stage 4 or 5 CKD [5]. Serum lithium level is routinely monitored in psychiatric treatment due to the medication narrow therapeutic index; however, some studies have questioned the importance of the serum lithium level in developing CKD [6]. Nephrogenic diabetes insipidus is present in 12% of lithium-treated patients [7]. Discontinuing lithium can lead to normalization of GFR, but kidney damage is irreversible in some patients.

Association Between Drugs of Abuse and Chronic Kidney Disease

A histological kidney analysis from 153 cases of deaths due to drug toxicology showed that glomerular pathology was associated with a history of alcohol abuse, while use of benzodiazepines was associated with vascular changes in the kidneys. Acetaminophen and cannabis use were associated with tubular damage, raising concerns for long-term use of these substances for pain [8]. Another postmortem analysis of over 5000 deaths in patients with history of drug use showed that severe intravenous drug use (IVDU) was associated with interstitial inflammation and renal calcification, whereas cocaine abuse was associated with hypertensive and ischemic damage. Cocaine is a well-known offender, contributing to kidney disease via hypertension; its use is detrimental in hepatitis C co-infected patients, leading to rapid onset of chronic renal impairment [9, 10]. Synthetic cannabinoids were also associated with acute kidney injury in case series [11]. Kidney disease can be the direct effect of drug use, such as opioids [12]. An analysis of renal biopsy results of 19 heroin users positive with hepatitis C showed 13 (68.4%) had membranoproliferative glomerulonephritis (MPGN), 2 had chronic interstitial nephritis, 2 had acute glomerulonephritis (GN), 1 had amyloidosis, and 1 had a combination of nephritis with GN [13]. Acute kidney injury has also been described in relation with energy drinks [14].

Neuropsychiatric Presentations in Patients with CKD

Causes for new onset neuropsychiatric presentations in patients with CKD include metabolic abnormalities, immune response, and vascular changes. Metabolic changes contributing to psychiatric presentations in CKD include hyponatremia [15], uremia [16], and higher homocysteine levels [17]. A study comparing cerebral glucose metabolism in patients with CKD pre-dialysis with healthy controls (21 each group) showed that pre-dialytic patients with CKD had decreased cerebral glucose metabolism in several areas, including decreased glucose metabolism in the orbitofrontal complex, which correlated with higher depression measured by Hamilton Depression Scale [18]. In vitro studies of asymmetric dimethylarginine (ADMA) and brain-derived neurotropic factor (BDNF) in CKD demonstrated that an increase of ADMA and decrease of BDNF correlated with depressive behavior [19]. Vascular alterations are considered to contribute to posterior reversible encephalopathy [20]. The role of the immune system in mental health presentations in CKD is also being investigated; however, the association between depression and interleukin (IL) levels in CKD is still uncertain [21].

Psychosocial Factors

As many kidney diseases are chronic conditions, patients often have to cope with the associated psychosocial stressors such as insurance eligibility in the United States [22] or lack of dialysis availability [23]. These factors can lead to significant psychological distress, impaired quality of life (QOL), impaired relationships, and adjustment disorders.

Epidemiology of Mental Health Problems in Chronic Kidney Disease

A significant body of evidence suggests a high prevalence of psychiatric concerns in patients with CKD. Table 6.1 Summarizes the most important studies investigating the prevalence of anxiety, depression, substance abuse, sleep disorders, and sexual dysfunctions. This literature consists mostly of cross-sectional studies without a control group, with most of the subjects belonging to the convenience samples, not always clearly representative of the population studied. The measures used have not always been validated in this population and do not always equal a diagnosis of psychiatric illness. In addition, many of the quality of life studies measure complaints or symptoms as opposed to psychiatric disorders. Studies rarely control for other medical conditions which are themselves associated with an increased risk of psychiatric comorbidities; therefore, it cannot be ascertained if the psychiatric symptoms are driven by the kidney disease or by its frequent medical comorbidities, such as diabetes and coronary artery disease.

Depression

Screening and Evaluation
Over the past 30 years, tens of studies have described and/or measured depression in patients with CKD. The definitions and measurements of depression have significantly varied in this context: from psychological distress measures reported on QOL scales, to qualitative measures of depression without a threshold for clinical significance. Even when structured instruments are used, only a few have been validated in this population (Table 6.2).

Prevalence of Depression in CKD
Depression is the most common psychiatric disorder among patients with CKD [29]. The prevalence of depressive disorders varies between 6.8% [30] and 47.1% [31]. When the *Diagnostic and Statistical Manual of Mental Disorders*, 4th Edition (DSM IV) criteria were applied, 40% of hemodialysis (HD) patients met criteria for a depressive disorder at some point in their life: MDD, 19.6%; dysthymic disorder, 9.8%; and depressive disorder not otherwise specified (NOS), 2.8% [28]. A study of CKD patients that used Structured Clinical Interview for DSM

Disorders (SCID) for evaluation showed a prevalence of MDD of 27.9%, similar in men and women [32]. Eighty-five percent of patients who initially screened positive for depression were eventually diagnosed with a depressive disorder after the clinical evaluation [33].

Suicide is significantly elevated in dialysis patients and is discussed in detail in Chap. 7.

Risk Factors for Depression in CKD
Multiple studies have analyzed the risk factors contributing to the emergence of depression in patients with CKD. With very few longitudinal studies available, these risk factors are mostly associations found in cross-sectional studies.

Demographic factors such as female gender or being older are considered to increase the risk to develop depression [34]. Not all studies confirmed the role of these demographic factors; one cross-sectional study of 140 patients with CKD in various stages showed that age, gender, income, employment status, and education were not associated with depression [32]. Early studies showed significant variation in the prevalence of depression in CKD by geographic region, with a 2% prevalence in Japan and 21.7% in the United States [35]. It was considered that these differences were mostly due to a variation in how depression was diagnosed or screened and they have not been yet replicated.

Among the potential biological risk factors, lower albumin and lower indoxyl sulfate [36], lower phosphorus, and high levels of CRP [37] have been associated with increased prevalence of depressive symptoms in this population.

The number of comorbid medical conditions [38] and especially the presence of diabetes mellitus (DM) increase the risk of depression in patients with CKD [37]. Although the risk of depression is not always linked with the general severity of somatic illness in CKD [39], recent findings suggest that patients with CKD stage 3 and above are more likely to develop depression [40].

Several studies have supported the notion that compared with pre-dialysis CKD patients, patients on HD have a higher risk for depression, since their kidney disease is more advanced and they have to face the psychosocial hurdles of their treatments [41–43].

Psychological factors linked to increased risk of depression in CKD include less religiosity [44], lower level of hope [45], and external locus of control [46, 47]. HADS-total score is associated with the use of denial as a psychological defense mechanism, and positively correlated with difficulties in identifying and expressing emotions, and with the intensity of subjective somatic complaints [39]. Additional risk factors for depression in CKD include the presence of pain [48], decreased sexual functioning [49], and lack of aerobic activity [50].

Table 6.1 Prevalence of psychiatric disorders in chronic kidney disease

Author	Year	Type of study	Population	N	Control (N)	Instruments	Findings (prevalence)	Findings (risk factors)
Adamczak et al.	2012	CS	CKD HD	697		BDI	Depression 38.6%	Age (older), central catheter, higher serum CPR, coronary artery disease, history of myocardial infarction, stroke, or COPD
Al Zaben et al.	2014	CS	HD	310		SCID-D HDRS	Depressive disorders 6.8%, major depression 3.2%, minor depression 3.6%, significant depressive symptoms 24.2%	Saudi nationality, marital status, stressful life events, poor physical functioning, cognitive impairment, overall severity of medical illness, and history of family psychiatric problems
Al Zaben et al.	2015	P	HD	39		SCID-D HDRS	20/39 patients with major or minor depressive disorder	Eight (40%) fully remitted by 6 weeks and an additional three patients remitted over the next 6 weeks, leaving 45% with significant depressive symptoms persisting beyond 12 weeks
Aribi et al.	2015	CS	HD	50		HADS KDQoL	86.48% sexual dysfunction, 26% sexually inactive, 62% had decrease of sexual activity	Positively correlated with age > 55 years, personal medical history, some nephropathy data, HD period greater than or equal to 1 year, depression, anxiety, and impaired quality of life
Azegbeobor et al.	2015	CS	CKD	160	160 general medical clinic	MINI WHODAS 2	Depression prevalence 17.5% (4.4% in control groups)	Depression was a predictor for disability
Baykan et al.	2012	CS	CAPD and HD	41 CAPD, 42 HD		SCID I HADS SF-36 COPE	Psychiatric disorder: 59.5% in HD group, 53.7% in CAPD group, 26.8% among controls	In all three groups, the most common psychiatric disorder was depressive disorder
Billington et al.	2008	CS	HD	193		THS SOS MHLC HADS	Anxiety 39 (38%), depression 40 (39%)	Hope emerged as an independent significant predictor in five of the multiple regressions: anxiety, depression, effects and symptoms of kidney disease, and mental health quality of life
Cantekin et al.	2014	CS	pre-HD	120		HADS	Depression 35%, anxiety 53.4%	
Chen et al.	2010	CS	HD	200		MINI HADS CFS	Depression 70 (35.0%); 43 (21.5%) had had suicidal ideation in the previous month	Low body mass index (BMI), number of comorbid physical illnesses, greater levels of fatigue and anxiety, more common suicidal ideation, poorer quality of life
Chiang et al.	2013	CS	CKD	270		TDQ	Depression 22.6%	Sleep disturbances, lack of religious beliefs, no regular exercise regimen, CKD stage 3 or above
Cukor et al.	2008	CS	HD	70		HADS SCID I	Any axis I diagnosis 71%, anxiety disorder 45.7%, mood disorder 40%	Anxiety disorder associated with worsened QOL
de Barros et al.	2011	CS	PKD and GN	52 GN, 38 PKD		STAI BDI SF-36	Depression 34.6% of familial GN, depression 60.5% of PKD	
De Vecchi et al.	2000	CS	PD and HD	84 PD, 87 HD		Self-administered questionnaire	Problems sleeping: 49% of PD and 65% of HD	
Donia et al.	2015	CS	HD	76		BDI II, SF-36	Depression 76.3%, 32.9% of total-severe depression	

Table 6.1 (continued)

Author	Year	Type of study	Population	N	Control (N)	Instruments	Findings (prevalence)	Findings (risk factors)
Esen et al.	2015	Cs	Pre-HD	53		FSFI IEFF SF-36 BDI	Sexual dysfunction: Male 46%, Females 51%	No gender differences
Feng et al.	2013	P	CKD 3 and 4	362		GDS SF-12	Depression 13% at baseline	Baseline cognitive impairment, functional disability, and other chronic illnesses were significantly associated with both increasing GDS scores and depressive symptoms
Ferreira et al.	2016	CS	OL-HDF	114		GDS	Depression 28.9%	Depression associated with low social support and decreased muscular mass and creatinine serum levels
Garcia et al.	2010	CS	HD male	47		HADRS	Depression 68.1%	List of symptoms and problems (rs = −0.399; p = 0.005), quality of social interaction (rs = −0.433; p = 0.002), and quality of sleep (rs = −0.585; p < 0.001)
Gonzalez-De-Jesus	2011	CS	CKD	75		HADS SCLE 90	Depressive symptoms 25.3%, anxiety symptoms 30.7%	
Knowles et al.	2014	CS	CKD	80		HADS COPE HPS	Moderate or severe anxiety 16.3%, moderate depression 7.5%	Perception of an illness rather than the actual symptoms themselves best account for adaption to CKD
Kokoszka et al.	2016	CS	HD	107		M.I.N.I. BDI AIS	Depressive disorders 78.5%, MDD 29%, dysthymia 28%, an episode of depression with melancholic features 21.5%. Patients met no criteria for a mental disorder 21.5%	
Lee J. et al.	2013	CS	CKD	280		HADS, WHOQOL-BREF	Depression 47.1%, anxiety 27.6%	Prevalence of depression/anxiety did not differ across CKD stages; depression correlated positively with age, employment, income, education, comorbidity index, hemoglobin level, albumin concentration, and anxiety score and negatively with all WHOQOL-BREF domain scores; Anxiety correlated significantly with QOL, but not with socioeconomic factors
Li et al.	2014	CS	CAPD	42		PSQI Restless legs syndrome criteria HADRS	Sleep disorders 47.6%	Lower albumin, depression
Mauri et al.	2016	CS	ESRD or severe IDDM (awaiting kidney/ pancreas txp)	227	IDDM	SCID I and II MOODS-SR PAS-SR	Current axis I disorders 13.2%, agoraphobia 4.8%, major depressive episode 4.0%	No difference in the distribution of axis I disorders between the two groups (ESRD and IDDM)

(continued)

Table 6.1 (continued)

Author	Year	Type of study	Population	N	Control (N)	Instruments	Findings (prevalence)	Findings (risk factors)
McKercher et al.	2013	P	CKD	49		PHQ 9 BAI MSPSS 3MS	MDD 10%, anxiety 9%	
Novick et al.	2016	P	CKD	2286		Interview	15% opioid use, 22% cocaine use	
Peng et al.	2013	CS	CKD	57		SF-36 HARS HADRS	Depression 38.6%, anxiety 54.4%	
Perales et al.	2016	CS	HD	52		SF-36 HADS ESS-r	Anxiety 36.5%, depression 27%	
Saeed et al.	2012	CS	HD	180		BDI	Depression 75%	Married, unemployed
Saglimbene et al.	2016	CS	HD	659		FSFI	Either no sexual activity or high sexual dysfunction in all measured domains (orgasm 75.1%, arousal 64.0%, lubrication 63.3%, pain 60.7%, satisfaction 60.1%, sexual desire 58.0%)	Age, depression, previous cardiac event higher scores; being on transplant-protective
Sanchez-Roman et al.	2011	CS	CKD	120	41	HADS NEUROPSI Attention and Memory	Cognitive impairment 23%	Anemia a risk factor Stage 5 the worse
Silva et al.	2014	CS	CKD on transplant wait-list	50		BAI Lipp Stress Symptoms for Adults Inventory	Anxiety 56%	Stress associated with longer wait time and less education
Simms et al.	2016	CS	PKD not on HD or transplant	349		KDQoL PHQ9 MSPSS	Depression 22%	Female gender was associated with overall poorer psychosocial well-being, whereas increasing age, lower kidney function, larger kidneys, and loss of a first-degree relative from ADPKD were additional risk factors for QOL, depression or psychosocial risk
Spoto et al.	2015	CS	HD and PD	128 HD, 27 PD		BDI, HADS	HD group: depression 22.5% on BDI, 9.3% on HADS; anxiety 25.7% on BDI, 14% on HADS for PD, depression 29.6% BDI, 14.8% HADS; anxiety 11.1% BDI, no anxiety on HADS	No differences in anxiety/depression between PD and HD
Sumanathissa et al.	2011	CS	CKD	140		SCID	MDD 27.9%: Males 27% (95% CI 17.6–36.3), Females 29.4% (95% CI 16.5–42.4)	Age, gender, income, employment status, and education were not associated with depression. The only significant variable associated with depression was patient's understanding of prognosis
Van Zwieten et al.	2016	CS	HD; median age 70	538		DSM V criteria	Major neurocognitive disorder 52.4%, minor neurocognitive disorder 17.3%	

Table 6.1 (continued)

Author	Year	Type of study	Population	N	Control (N)	Instruments	Findings (prevalence)	Findings (risk factors)
Vazquez-Martinez et al.	2016	CS	HD	40	40	HADS	Depression 27.7%	Risk factors: literate, being a housewife, big family, HD more than 5 years but not statistically significant
Vikhram et al.	2012	CS	HD	130		MINI	40% had a psych disease, moderate depressive episode 13.1%, hx of alcohol use disorder 31.5%	
Zaben et al.	2014	CS	HD	310		SCID-D, HDRS	Depressive disorder 6.8%, MDD 3.2%, minor depression 3.6%, significant depressive symptoms 24.2%	Saudi nationality, marital status, stressful life events, poor physical functioning, cognitive impairment, overall severity of medical illness, and history of family psychiatric problems
Wuerth et al.	2005	CS	PD	380		BDI	Depression 45%	Out of positive screen, 85% were clinically diagnosed with MDD

Table 6.2 Validated measures for depression and anxiety in patients with CKD

Scale	Cutoff	Validity	Author
Beck Depression Inventory (BDI)	11	Sensitivity 89% Specificity 88%	[24]
	16	Sensitivity 91% Specificity 59% Positive predictive value (PPV) 59% Negative predictive value (NPV) 71%	[25]
16-item Quick Inventory of Depressive Symptomatology-Self Report	10	Sensitivity 91% Specificity 88%	[24]
	8	Sensitivity 96% Specificity 79%	[26]
Center for Epidemiologic Studies Depression Scale (CES-D)	18	Sensitivity 69% Specificity 83% PPV 60% NPV 88%	[27]
Patient Health Questionnaire 9 (PHQ 9)	10	Sensitivity 92% Specificity 92% PPV 71% NPV 98%	[25]
Hospital Anxiety and Depression Scale (HADS)	N/A	The anxiety score did not correlate with presence of anxiety disorder on SCID	[28]

Anxiety Disorders

Prevalence of Anxiety Disorders in CKD

The prevalence of anxiety in patients with CKD is reported to range between 16.3% [51] and 54.4% [52], higher than in general population [53] (Table 6.1). As with depression, most of the measures used to assess anxiety have not been validated for CKD population (such as Beck Anxiety Inventory (BAI) or State Trait Anxiety Inventory (STAI)) or have been shown to have poor validity. For instance, compared to SCID, HADS was found to be a poor predictor for an anxiety disorder in HD patients [28], although sensitivity might be better with a lower cutoff of 6 for HADS as compared to 8 or 11 [54]. Most of patients with CKD report some degree of anxiety associated with the illness, starting dialysis, or the dialysis treatments themselves. A recent study of patients with ESRD awaiting kidney transplant that used SCID I and II found that agoraphobia was the most common axis I diagnosis (4.8%) [55].

Risk Factors for Anxiety in CKD

Anxiety is more likely to occur in patients with chronic pain [48, 56]), decreased sexual functioning [49], lower level of hope [45], and higher level of IL-6 production [57].

Cognitive Impairment

The presence of cognitive impairment in patients with CKD has been documented in multiple studies. It is worth noting that many of these studies do not address significant confounders such as cardiovascular risk factors or mood disorders [58].

Screening and Assessment

Montreal Cognitive Assessment (MOCA) and Mini-Mental State Examination (MMSE) are widely used screening tests of cognition. In clinical practice, results on these screening tests in association with the clinical evaluation typically lead to the diagnosis of a cognitive disorder. More detailed neuropsychological testing is done when there are discrepancies between the subjective and objective findings, or to plan additional services (e.g., supportive services, surrogate decision maker, or neuropsychological rehabilitation). Some of the most used instruments to assess cognition in CKD include: California Verbal Learning Test–Second Edition (CVLTII), Delis-Kaplan Executive Function System (D-KEFS) [59], Consortium to establish a registry for Altzheimer's Disease Neuropsychological Assessment Battery, lexical fluency, digit span test, 64 card Wisconsin Cared Sorting Test [60], NEUROPSY Attention and Memory [61], Rey Auditory–Verbal Learning Test, and Trail making Test [62].

Prevalence of Cognitive Impairment in CKD

In one study, 23% of CKD patients had cognitive impairment when measured with the NEUROPSI Attention and Memory battery [61]. Women with moderate CKD had worse delayed recall and backward digit span [62]. The INVADE study (Project on Cerbrovascular Diseases and Dementia) showed that 10.8% of patients with CKD had cognitive impairment; in addition, 6.2% developed new onset cognitive impairment in 2 years [63]. The BRINK study (Brain in Kidney disease) showed that patients with CKD had worse cognitive function than controls on MMSE, Hopkins Verbal Learning Test-Revised, Digit Span and Symbol-Digit-Modality Test [64].

Risk factors for cognitive impairment in CKD include high serum creatinine [62], anemia, hypertension, diabetes, somnolence, cardiovascular risk factors [61], HD treatment (versus peritoneal dialysis (PD)), 24-hour urine volume, systolic blood pressure, GFR, weight, time in dialysis [61], winter time [65], moderate to severe CKD [60], frailty [66], albumin and prealbumin levels [67], and comorbid obstructive sleep apnea (OSA) [68].

Sleep Disorders

The sleep architecture is significantly altered in patients with CKD and sleep disorders are common. Stages 1 and 2 non-rapid eye movement (REM) sleep are increased, while REM sleep [69] and sleep efficiency are decreased [70]. Even in early CKD, general sleep disturbance is estimated to be present in 84.6% of patients [71].

Screening and Assessment

Several sleep disorder screening questionnaires have been used in studies of CKD populations (e.g., Pittsburgh Sleep Quality Index, Epworth Sleepiness Scale, etc.), while the electroencephalography-based monitoring tests such as actigraphy (ambulatory monitoring) or polysomnography remain the gold standard for certain sleep disorder diagnoses. It is important to notice that sleep disorders have been found in CKD patients with no subjective complaints. A cost-effectiveness study done in Japan argues that even screening with a simple self-administered scale such as Epworth Sleepiness Scale is cost effective for patients with CKD [72].

Prevalence of Sleep Disorders in Patients with CKD

Breathing-related sleep disorder, such as OSA, is estimated to be present in 54% of CKD patients not receiving dialysis [73] and in 20–54% of HD patients [74].

Dyssomnias such as restless legs syndrome (RLS) or periodic limb movement syndrome (PLMS) have long been considered an expected finding in CKD. RLS was present in 3.5% of patients with CKD versus 1.5% of controls [75]. More recent studies demonstrated RLS in 17.5% of patients with CKD [76].

Risk Factors for Sleep Disorders in CKD

There is contradictory information about whether sleep disorders correlate with the stages of CKD or dialysis status. Some authors argue that sleep disorders tend to improve over time [77]. Other authors found that more advanced CKD correlates with more sleep disturbances: stage 4 CKD was associated with higher odds ratio for RLS in older hospital patients [78]. Severity of sleep apnea correlated with a lower GFR [79]. In one study, PLMS prevalence increased with CKD stages, but this relationship was unclear for RLS [76]. Other risk factors for sleep disorders in CKD are low albumin [80], low ferritin [78], depression, anxiety, male gender, and duration of CKD [81].

Other Mental Health Presentations in CKD

Fatigue

Often mistaken for depression, fatigue is a common finding in patients with CKD. A recent systematic review and meta-analysis found the prevalence of fatigue in CKD between 42% and 89% [82]. Several structured measures are available to document fatigue: Functional Assessment of Chronic

Illness Therapy-Fatigue (FACIT-F), Piper Fatigue Scale (PFS), or Fatigue Severity Scale (FSS).

Fatigue was associated with elevated phosphate serum levels, creatinine, advanced age, albumin (nutritional status), post-dialysis serum urea level, anemia [83], higher BMI, poor sleep quality, and mood disturbance [84]. In patients with pronounced fatigue, serum IL-6 levels were significantly higher, while albumin and creatinine levels were significantly lower [85]. Presence of cardiovascular disease, low serum albumin, depression, anxiety, unemployment, poor subjective sleep quality, excessive daytime sleepiness, and RLS were associated with greater fatigue [82, 83, 86, 87].

Chronic Psychotic Disorders

Prevalence of chronic psychotic disorders in CKD population is estimated at 10.2% [28]. For comparison, median lifetime prevalence of schizophrenia in the general population is estimated at 0.4% [88]. This difference in reported prevalence may be due to variation of measurements (some studies measured chronic psychotic disorders, while others focused on schizophrenia only). In addition, patients with chronic psychosis have a high incidence of diabetes [89], which leads to CKD and may contribute to the finding of higher prevalence of psychosis in this group. Patients with schizophrenia and ESRD received suboptimal pre-dialysis care and had a higher risk for mortality than general ESRD patients [90]. Another cohort study showed that patients with serious and persistent mental illness (SPMI) and CKD are more likely to be re-hospitalized than CKD patients without SPMI [91].

Substance Use Disorders

Substance use disorders have an estimated prevalence of 18% in patients with CKD [28]. In an Iranian sample of patients with CKD, 35.9% of patients used tobacco, 14.1% used opium, and 3.1% used alcohol [92]. A cross-sectional study of 2286 US patients with CKD showed a 15% prevalence of opioid use (with "use" defined as > = 5 times lifetime uses) and 22%-cocaine [93]. There is extensive evidence to support the deleterious effects of nicotine upon kidney function [94, 95], although prevalence studies about nicotine dependence in CKD are lacking.

Psychological Adjustments in CKD

Similar to other chronic medical illnesses, living with CKD requires significant adjustments in order to cope with physical limitations, loss of independence, often loss of income and social status, and significant alterations in relationships. In addition, the logistics of dialysis treatments lead to significant life changes. It is not uncommon that the initial diagnosis of CKD or the recommendation for dialysis is met with denial, demoralization, anger, or displacement which, if not resolved, can lead to poor adherence with treatment and significant medical complications.

Emotional defensiveness as a main coping skill tends to negatively affect the mental component of QOL in these patients [96]. Use of denial initially appears to be protective against depression and anxiety, however, may impact the medication adherence [39]. Blame as a defense mechanism was associated with worse adjustment [97], while hope was considered an independent predictor of better QOL [45]. Greater use of reappraisal was associated with lower levels of anxiety, while suppression was associated with greater depression [98]. Hemodialysis systematically affected personality in patients with CKD, with both neuroticism and psychoticism decreasing after initiation of HD [99].

Impact of Mental Health Problems in CKD

There is overwhelming evidence that mental health problems impact QOL of patients with CKD. A systematic review of 38 studies demonstrated a negative impact of depression, anxiety, and perceived stress upon health-related QOL [100]. Levels of depression and anxiety correlated with lower QOL in patients with CKD in multiple studies [28, 31, 52, 101–104]. A meta-analysis of 81 studies including 13,240 patients showed a medium effect size for impact of affect, cognition, and stress level upon QOL in patients with ESRD [105]. In a linear regression analysis, depression and anxiety independently correlated with QOL after adjustments for age, alcohol use, employment, income, education, hemoglobin level, and albumin concentration [31].

Mental health problems have been associated with worse medical outcomes ranging from medical complications to increased health care utilization measures. Major depressive episodes were independent risk factor for negative events (defined as death, hospitalizations, or dialysis initiation) in patients with CKD not on HD [106]. Depression in PD was associated with higher incidence of peritonitis [107]. Periodic limb movement disorder was associated with increased cardiovascular and cerebrovascular risk in CKD patients [108]. Central sleep apnea has been found to be a risk factor for mortality in non-dialyzed CKD patients compared to those without CKD, while mixed sleep apnea was related to rapid decline of renal function in non-dialyzed subjects [109]. Poor sleep quality was shown to be an independent risk factor for cardiovascular damage in CKD [110]. Depression in early CKD was a predictive factor for initiation of HD [40] and was associated with more days spent in the hospital [111, 112].

Studies investigating the impact of depression upon the mortality of patients with CKD have shown contradictory results. MDD measured by PHQ was associated with 2.95-fold greater risk of death in patients with diabetes mellitus on HD [113]. Depression was associated with increased mortality in geriatric patients with stage 2–3 CKD [114]. A meta-analysis of 22 studies (83,381 participants) comprising 12,063 cases of depression with a follow-up of 3 months to 6.5 years concluded that depression consistently increased the risk of death from any cause but had less certain effects on cardiovascular mortality [115]. In at least two studies, however, depression did not predict mortality in kidney disease [116, 117].

The studies investigating the psychological adaptation to CKD are illustrative of some aspects that can improve the QOL and overall outcomes. Surprisingly, high level of social support had no influence on the adherence of patients with high conscientiousness, while it actually decreased the adherence of patients with low conscientiousness levels [118]. Extraversion and neuroticism were found to be associated with a higher health-related QOL [119]. Acceptance level correlated with higher QOL in patients with CKD [120]. Social adaptability index has been associated with increased survival [121].

Treatment of Mental Health Conditions in Chronic Kidney Disease

Pharmacological Interventions

It is important to remember that renal impairment affects the hepatic metabolism of medications, by inducing or suppressing liver enzymes or by affecting the availability of protein binding [122]. Furthermore, intestinal and hepatic transporters are altered in patients with CKD, on or off dialysis [123]. Authors have suggested that drug development should include information on pharmacokinetics in patients with CKD, on PD and HD, even for nonrenally cleared medications [123]; however, that is not yet the case in the United States. In general, patients with CKD are excluded from psychopharmacological trials due to safety concerns, so information about the safety, tolerability, and efficacy of psychotropics in patients with CKD is limited. For most psychotropics, dose adjustment is recommended once the creatinine clearance decreases, but medications can be continued. Special attention needs to be given to psychotropic agents with nephrotoxic potential (e.g., lithium and topiramate) and to those excreted primarily through the kidney (e.g., gabapentin and baclofen). Detailed information about the dose adjustments necessary in CKD and about possible drug to drug interactions during CKD can be found elsewhere [124]. In addition, Chap. 7 further discusses use of psychotropic medications in patients on dialysis.

Depression

There is poor evidence about the efficacy and safety of antidepressant treatment in patients with CKD [125, 126]. While several open trials suggested the benefit of antidepressants, two randomized controlled trials (RCTs) of antidepressants (fluoxetine and escitalopram) showed no differences in efficacy [126]. In an open randomized study, citalopram was reported to be efficacious in improving symptoms of anxiety and depression in HD patients, but interestingly these improvements were similar to psychological training, consisting of stress management training and education about kidney disease [127]. The Chronic Kidney Disease Antidepressant Sertraline Trial (CAST) study, a double-blind placebo-controlled study examining efficacy and safety of sertraline in patients with CKD and not dialysis-dependent, did not show any difference between sertraline and placebo upon depressive symptoms [128].

Fatigue

Epoetin is reported to help fatigue in CKD [129]. To our knowledge, there is no information about the efficacy of modafinil or methylphenidate in CKD. Recent in vivo findings suggest a potential for nephrotoxicity for methylphenidate; therefore, it should be used cautiously [130].

Cognitive Impairment

The initiation of HD significantly improved cognitive status in patients with ESRD. There is only anecdotal evidence about the use of acetylcholinesterase inhibitors in patients with dementia and CKD [131]. Interestingly, a population study of 11,943 patients with CKD in Taiwan demonstrated that receiving the flu vaccine was protective against developing dementia, regardless of other risk factors [132].

Sleep Disorders

Dopamine agonists, such as ropinirole and rotigotine, have been found helpful for RLS in patients with CKD [133, 134]. In vitro studies showed that melatonin may have protective effects against oxidative stress and inflammation in renal disorders [135], but clinical trials are lacking at this time. Treatment of sleep apnea with continuous positive airway pressure has been shown to reveal increased symptoms of PLMS [136].

Pharmacokinetics in CKD

CKD can modify the psychopharmacology of psychotropic agents even for medications not primarily excreted by the kidneys. Chronic kidney disease can induce changes in distribution, protein binding, metabolism, and excretion. Obviously when the medication is primarily metabolized and excreted in the kidneys (e.g., gabapentin or topiramate), the dose will need to be decreased if the patient develops CKD. The use of psychotropic medications in patients with CKD can be limited due to comorbid illness, such as impaired hepatic function, electrolyte disturbances, cardiac arrhythmias, or QTC prolongation. For further detailed information, the reader is referred to additional materials [137].

Other Use of Psychotropics in CKD

An interesting topic is represented by the use of psychotropic medications for nonpsychiatric conditions. Sertraline was shown to be effective for pruritus in ESRD patients [138].

Non-Pharmacological Treatments for Mental Health Symptoms in Patients with Chronic Kidney Disease

Psychotherapeutic Interventions

In nonmedically ill patients, it has been shown that psychological interventions have important advantages in comparison to pharmacological treatment. Psychotherapy allows one to avoid the risk of medication side effects and low adherence with drug therapy. In addition, for many patients, psychotherapy may be easier to accept [139]. Research also indicates that psychotherapy may be more effective in reducing the risk of depression relapse compared to pharmacological therapy [140]. Although there is an increased interest in psychological interventions for patients with CKD, the research, while expanding, is still limited.

A systematic review and meta-analysis of 8 RCTs aimed to evaluate effects of psychological interventions on depression, sleep quality, QOL, and fluid intake restriction adherence, demonstrated that the psychological interventions significantly reduced the Beck Depression Inventory scores and inter-dialysis weight gain [141]. The most widely used psychological intervention was cognitive behavioral therapy (CBT). Another systematic review and meta-analysis concluded that psychosocial interventions were associated with a medium effect size for reduction in depressive symptoms and a small effect size for improved QOL in patients with CKD/ESRD and their caregivers and some evidence suggested also a reduction in anxiety [142].

CBT is an especially helpful modality for depression, anxiety, insomnia, and adherence. It can also teach patients skills to facilitate communication with care providers, problem-solve when necessary, reduce arousal, and correct misconceptions and distortions [143, 144]. A RCT conducted in Brazil compared the effectiveness of 12 weekly sessions of group CBT in chronic hemodialysis patients diagnosed with MDD ($N = 41$) compared to usual care con-

sisting of education and emotional support offered in the dialysis unit ($N = 44$) [144]. The intervention group demonstrated significant improvements compared to the control in average BDI scores, Mini-International Neuropsychiatric Interview (MINI) score, and Kidney Quality of Life dimensions.

Another randomized crossover trial in HD patients with 48.5% meeting criteria for MDD administered chairside CBT during dialysis treatments for 3 months. The study demonstrated that the treatment-first group achieved significantly larger reductions in BDI-II and HAM-D scores, as compared to the wait-list control. Mean scores for the treatment-first group did not change significantly at the 3-month follow-up, indicating persistence of a treatment effect beyond the end of the treatment period [145]. The treatment-first group experienced greater improvements in QOL and inter-dialytic weight gain than the wait-list group, although no effect on adherence was evident.

Another RCT found that group-based CBT was effective in improving adherence to fluid restrictions in patients undergoing hemodialysis [146]. Yet, a more recent RCT of PD patients evaluating the effectiveness of a CBT group approach to improve patient adherence demonstrated a statistically significant difference in edematous status at 6-week follow-up, potentially indicative of fluid restriction adherence [147].

A randomized active-controlled, open-label trial is currently being carried out to test whether a mindfulness-based stress reduction (MBSR) program delivered in a novel workshop-teleconference format would reduce symptoms and improve health-related quality of life (HRQOL) in patients awaiting kidney transplantation. Telephone-adapted MBSR (tMBSR) significantly improved mental HRQOL at follow-up, with over 90% of tMBSR participants reporting practicing mindfulness and finding it helpful for stress management [148].

A group therapy intervention in 48 HD patients significantly reduced depression and improved self-care, self-efficacy, and QOL in this patient population [149].

Case studies and some controlled studies suggest that relaxation and imagery techniques can be successfully used with hemodialysis patients to improve their adjustment. However, a RCT on a specific visual imagery technique in a sample of HD patients did not demonstrate an effect of this intervention on emotional adjustment or QOL, although the rate of patient compliance with the intervention was moderately high and patients reported their satisfaction with the intervention procedures [150].

Tsay and Hung [151] examined the effects of an empowerment intervention program in HD patients in a RCT in Taiwan. The results indicated that scores of the empowerment, self-care, self-efficacy, and depression in the intervention group had a significantly greater improvement compared to controls [151].

Exercise

Aerobic exercises have been shown to improve not only physical functioning but also nutritional status, hematological indices, inflammatory cytokines, depression, and HRQOL in ESRD patients [152]. There have been a few RCTs examining the effects of exercise on depression in hemodialysis patients. In one such study on the effect of exercise training on heart rate variability and depression in HD patients, BDI scores decreased by 34.5% in HD patients randomized to a 1-year intradialytic exercise training program [153]. In another RCT in patients with reduced aerobic capacity, patients randomized to a 10-month intradialytic exercise training program demonstrated a 21% increase in maximal oxygen uptake (VO_2 max) in the exercise group and a 39% reduction in BDI scores, while control groups had no such changes [154].

Alternative Therapies

Music therapy has been investigated in ESRD. Thirty-six hemodialysis patients in Seoul, Korea, treated with music therapy reported lower scores in both depression and anxiety levels compared to the control group with no therapy [155].

Authors of another study observed that patients who listened to music during the dialysis sessions exhibited significant reductions in perceived stressors and adverse reactions, a fact that led the authors to conclude that music could be beneficial for promoting well-being in hemodialysis patients [156].

Self-Management

Self-management is another approach to target mental health symptoms in patients with kidney disease. Self-management in CKD involves developing knowledge, skills, and behaviors necessary to manage illness and treatments, as well as developing collaborative relationships with healthcare team providers. Self-management in dialysis necessitates that patients and families develop specific skills related to managing the dialysis treatment itself ranging from organizational tasks, such as coordinating transportation, to more active participation in the dialysis treatment, such as preparation for cannulation. Developing strategies to manage the psychosocial consequences of CKD and its treatment is an important part of self-management. Activities such as evaluating one's condition, negotiating treatment plans with care providers, and voicing one's preference for treatment reflect the cognitive dimensions of self-management in this population [157].

Psychoeducation

Pre-dialysis psychoeducational interventions present information about normal function of the kidneys, diseases of the kidneys, nutrition, medications, alternative modes of RRT, and lifestyle.

An important goal of pre-dialysis psychoeducational interventions is to socialize patients into a collaborative role in relating to service providers. Pre-dialysis psychoeducational intervention helps patients learn about CKD and its medical management and supports long-term knowledge retention [158]. Pre-dialysis psychoeducational intervention facilitates vocational rehabilitation and promotes QOL. Devins et al. have shown that pre-dialysis psychoeducational interventions extended time to dialysis therapy [159] and survival [160].

Conclusions

Patients with CKD have a high prevalence of psychiatric symptoms due to biological risk factors and psychosocial burdens of a chronic medical illness requiring significant time and resources for treatment. The most common mental health conditions encountered are depression, anxiety, and cognitive impairments, which in turn worsen adherence with medical treatments. The literature supports screening for depression and cognitive impairment in patients with CKD. Treatment of the psychiatric comorbidities in CKD leads to improvements in QOL and outcomes and increase in survival. The safety and efficacy data on psychopharmacological agents in patients with ESRD are lacking. At the same time, non-pharmacological methods, including psychotherapies, lifestyle and behavioral interventions, as well as complementary therapies, are becoming increasingly utilized in patients with CKD.

References

1. Novak M. Psychonephrology: an emerging field. Prim Psychiatry. 2008;15(1):43–4.
2. Levy NB. What is psychonephrology? J Nephrol. 2008;21(SUPPL. 13):S51–S3.
3. Tzeng NS, Hsu YH, Ho SY, Kuo YC, Lee HC, Yin YJ, et al. Is schizophrenia associated with an increased risk of chronic kidney disease? A nationwide matched-cohort study. BMJ Open. 2015;5(1):e006777.
4. McKnight RF, Adida M, Budge K, Stockton S, Goodwin GM, Geddes JR. Lithium toxicity profile: a systematic review and meta-analysis. Lancet. 2012;379(9817):721–8.
5. Aiff H, Attman PO, Aurell M, Bendz H, Ramsauer B, Schon S, et al. Effects of 10 to 30 years of lithium treatment on kidney function. J Psychopharmacol. 2015;29(5):608–14.
6. Bendz H, Schon S, Attman PO, Aurell M. Renal failure occurs in chronic lithium treatment but is uncommon. Kidney Int. 2010;77(3):219–24.

7. Aiff H, Attman PO, Aurell M, Bendz H, Schon S, Svedlund J. End-stage renal disease associated with prophylactic lithium treatment. Eur Neuropsychopharmacol. 2014;24(4):540–4.

8. Blessing M, Reichard RR, Maleszewski JJ, Dierkhising R, Langman L, Alexander MP. Nephropathy in the setting of substance abuse: an analysis of 153 medicolegal deaths. Lab Investig. 2015;95:405A–6A.

9. Buettner M, Toennes SW, Buettner S, Bickel M, Allwinn R, Geiger H, et al. Nephropathy in illicit drug abusers: a postmortem analysis. Am J Kidney Dis. 2014;63(6):945–53.

10. Rossi C, Cox J, Cooper C, Martel-Laferriere V, Walmsley S, Gill J, et al. Frequent injection cocaine use increases the risk of renal impairment among hepatitis C and HIV coinfected patients. AIDS. 2016;30(9):1403–11.

11. Buser GL, Gerona RR, Horowitz BZ, Vian KP, Troxell ML, Hendrickson RG, et al. Acute kidney injury associated with smoking synthetic cannabinoid. Clin Toxicol. 2014;52(7):664–73.

12. Ambruzs JM, Serrell PB, Rahim N, Larsen CP. Thrombotic microangiopathy and acute kidney injury associated with intravenous abuse of an oral extended-release formulation of oxymorphone hydrochloride: kidney biopsy findings and report of 3 cases. Am J Kidney Dis. 2014;63(6):1022–6.

13. do Sameiro Faria M, Sampaio S, Faria V, Carvalho E. Nephropathy associated with heroin abuse in Caucasian patients. Nephrol Dial Transplant. 2003;18(11):2308–13.

14. Greene E, Oman K, Lefler M. Energy drink-induced acute kidney injury. Ann Pharmacother. 2014;48(10):1366–70.

15. Baar JM. Organic mood disorder, manic type, associated with hyponatremia: a case report. Int J Psychiatry Med. 1994;24(3):223–8.

16. Thomas CS, Neale T. Organic manic syndrome associated with advanced uraemia due to polycystic kidney disease. Br J Psychiatry. 1991;158:119–21.

17. Yeh YC, Kuo MC, Hwang SJ, Hsioa SM, Tsai JC, Huang MF, et al. Homocysteine and cognitive impairment in chronic kidney disease. European Psychiatry Conference: 21st European Congress of Psychiatry, EPA. 2013;28 (no pagination).

18. Song SH, Kim IJ, Kim SJ, Kwak IS, Kim YK. Cerebral glucose metabolism abnormalities in patients with major depressive symptoms in pre-dialytic chronic kidney disease: statistical parametric mapping analysis of F-18-FDG PET, a preliminary study. Psychiatry Clin Neurosci. 2008;62(5):554–61.

19. Suntharalingam M, Kielstein H, Rong S, Perthel R, Bode-Boger SM, Kielstein JT. Role of the endogenous nitric oxide inhibitor ADMA and BDNF in depression and behavioral changes-clinical and preclinical data in chronic kidney disease. Nephrol Dial Transplant. 2015;30:iii161.

20. Dhooria GS, Bains HS, Pooni PA, Bhat D. Posterior reversible encephalopathy syndrome in children with nephrotic syndrome: a report of 2 cases. Arch Dis Child. 2014;99:A152.

21. Taraz M, Taraz S, Dashti-Khavidaki S. Association between depression and inflammatory/anti-inflammatory cytokines in chronic kidney disease and end-stage renal disease patients: a review of literature. Hemodial. 2015;19(1):11–22.

22. Golin CO, Johnson AM, Fick G, Gabow PA. Insurance for autosomal dominant polycystic kidney disease patients prior to end-stage renal disease. Am J Kidney Dis. 1996;27(2):220–3.

23. Isreb M, Al Kukhun H, Al-Adwan SAS, Kass-Hout TA, Murad L, Rifai AO, et al. Psychosocial impact of war on Syrian refugees with ESRD. Am J Kidney Dis. 2016;67(5):A56.

24. Hedayati SS, Minhajuddin AT, Toto RD, Morris DW, Rush AJ. Validation of depression screening scales in patients with CKD. Am J Kidney Dis. 2009;54(3):433–9.

25. Watnick S, Wang PL, Demadura T, Ganzini L. Validation of 2 depression screening tools in dialysis patients. Am J Kidney Dis. 2005;46(5):919–24.

26. Jain N, Carmody T, Minhajuddin AT, Toups M, Trivedi MH, Rush AJ, et al. Prognostic utility of a self-reported depression questionnaire versus clinician-based assessment on renal outcomes. Am J Nephrol. 2016;44(3):234–44.

27. Hedayati SS, Bosworth HB, Kuchibhatla M, Kimmel PL, Szczech LA. The predictive value of self-report scales compared with physician diagnosis of depression in hemodialysis patients. Kidney Int. 2006;69(9):1662–8.

28. Cukor D, Coplan J, Brown C, Friedman S, Newville H, Safier M, et al. Anxiety disorders in adults treated by hemodialysis: a single-center study. Am J Kidney Dis. 2008;52(1):128–36.

29. Baykan H, Yargic I. Depression, anxiety disorders, quality of life and stress coping strategies in hemodialysis and continuous ambulatory peritoneal dialysis patients. Klinik Psikofarmakoloji Bulteni. 2012;22(2):167–76.

30. Al Zaben F, Khalifa DA, Sehlo MG, Al Shohaib S, Shaheen F, Alhozali H, et al. Depression in patients with chronic kidney disease on dialysis in Saudi Arabia. Int Urol Nephrol. 2014;46(12):2393–402.

31. Lee YJ, Kim MS, Cho S, Kim SR. Association of depression and anxiety with reduced quality of life in patients with predialysis chronic kidney disease. Int J Clin Pract. 2013;67(4):363–8.

32. Sumanathissa M, De Silva VA, Hanwella R. Prevalence of major depressive episode among patients with pre-dialysis chronic kidney disease. Int J Psychiatry Med. 2011;41(1):47–56.

33. Wuerth D, Finkelstein SH, Finkelstein FO. The identification and treatment of depression in patients maintained on dialysis. Semin Dial. 2005;18(2):142–6.

34. Simms RJ, Thong KM, Dworschak GC, Ong ACM. Increased psychosocial risk, depression and reduced quality of life living with autosomal dominant polycystic kidney disease. Nephrol Dial Transplant. 2016;31(7):1130–40.

35. Lopes AA, Albert JM, Young EW, Satayathum S, Pisoni RL, Andreucci VE, et al. Screening for depression in hemodialysis patients: associations with diagnosis, treatment, and outcomes in the DOPPS. Kidney Int. 2004;66(5):2047–53.

36. Hsu HJ, Yen CH, Chen CK, Wu IW, Lee CC, Sun CY, et al. Erratum to "Association between uremic toxins and depression in patients with chronic kidney disease undergoing maintenance hemodialysis". Gen Hosp Psychiatry. 2013;35(4):450.

37. Su SF, Ng HY, Huang TL, Chi PJ, Lee YT, Lai CR, et al. Survey of depression by Beck depression inventory in uremic patients undergoing hemodialysis and hemodiafiltration. Ther Apher Dial. 2012;16(6):573–9.

38. Chen CK, Tsai YC, Hsu HJ, Wu IW, Sun CY, Chou CC, et al. Depression and suicide risk in hemodialysis patients with chronic renal failure. Psychosomatics. 2010;51(6):528–.e6.

39. Jadoulle V, Hoyois P, Jadoul M. Anxiety and depression in chronic hemodialysis: some somatopsychic determinants. Clin Nephrol. 2005;63(2):113–8.

40. Chiang HH, Guo HR, Livneh H, Lu MC, Yen ML, Tsai TY. Increased risk of progression to dialysis or death in CKD patients with depressive symptoms: a prospective 3-year follow-up cohort study. J Psychosom Res. 2015;79(3):228–32.

41. Alston H, Vickerstaff V, Low J, Beaty C, Da Silva GM, Burns A. Haemodialysis patients experience higher levels of psychosocial distress than equivalent CKD patients. Nephrol Dial Transplant. 2015;30:iii614–ii5.

42. Ch'ng AS, Chen LL, Lim SK, Poi PJ. Haemodialysis versus non-dialysis therapy among older adults with stage 5 chronic kidney

disease: a comparison of health-related quality of life. Value Health. 2015;18(7):A745.

43. Chen SF, Wang IJ, Lang HC. Risk of major depression in patients with chronic renal failure on different treatment modalities: a matched-cohort and population-based study in Taiwan. Hemodial. 2016;20(1):98–105.

44. Chiang HH, Livneh H, Yen ML, Li TC, Tsai TY. Prevalence and correlates of depression among chronic kidney disease patients in Taiwan. BMC Nephrol. 2013;14:78.

45. Billington E, Simpson J, Unwin J, Bray D, Giles D. Does hope predict adjustment to end-stage renal failure and consequent dialysis? Br J Health Psychol. 2008;13(Pt 4):683–99.

46. Christensen AJ, Turner CW, Smith TW, Holman JM Jr, Gregory MC. Health locus of control and depression in end-stage renal disease. J Consult Clin Psychol. 1991;59(3):419–24.

47. Karamanidou C, Theofilou P, Ginieri-Coccossis M, Synodinou C, Papadimitriou G. Anxiety, depression and health beliefs in end stage renal disease (ESRD) patients. Eur Psychiatry. 2009;24:S651.

48. Santoro D, Satta E, Messina S, Costantino G, Savica V, Bellinghieri G. Pain in end-stage renal disease: a frequent and neglected clinical problem. Clin Nephrol. 2013;79(Suppl 1):S2–11.

49. Theofilou PA. Sexual functioning in chronic kidney disease: the association with depression and anxiety. Hemodial. 2012;16(1):76–81.

50. Lopes AA, Lantz B, Morgenstern H, Wang M, Bieber BA, Gillespie BW, et al. Associations of self-reported physical activity types and levels with quality of life, depression symptoms, and mortality in hemodialysis patients: the DOPPS. Clin J Am Soc Nephrol. 2014;9(10):1702–12.

51. Knowles S, Swan L, Salzberg M, Castle D, Langham R. Exploring the relationships between health status, illness perceptions, coping strategies and psychological morbidity in a chronic kidney disease cohort. Am J Med Sci. 2014;348(4):271–6.

52. Peng T, Hu Z, Guo L, Xia Q, Li D, Yang X. Relationship between psychiatric disorders and quality of life in nondialysis patients with chronic kidney disease. Am J Med Sci. 2013;345(3):218–21.

53. Gonzalez-De-Jesus LN, Sanchez-Roman S, Morales-Buenrostro LE, Ostrosky-Solis F, Alberu J, Garcia-Ramos G, et al. Assessment of emotional distress in chronic kidney disease patients and kidney transplant recipients. Rev Investig Clin. 2011;63(6):558–63.

54. Preljevic VT, Osthus TB, Sandvik L, Opjordsmoen S, Nordhus IH, Os I, et al. Screening for anxiety and depression in dialysis patients: comparison of the hospital anxiety and depression scale and the Beck depression inventory. J Psychosom Res. 2012;73(2):139–44.

55. Mauri M, Calderone A, Calabro PF, Augusto S, Ceccarini G, Piaggi P, et al. Quality of life and psychopathology of patients awaiting kidney/pancreas transplants. J Psychopathol. 2016;22(2):118–26.

56. Gamondi C, Galli N, Schonholzer C, Marone C, Zwahlen H, Gabutti L, et al. Frequency and severity of pain and symptom distress among patients with chronic kidney disease receiving dialysis. Swiss Med Wkly. 2013;143:w13750.

57. Montinaro V, Iaffaldano GP, Granata S, Porcelli P, Todarello O, Schena FP, et al. Emotional symptoms, quality of life and cytokine profile in hemodialysis patients. Clin Nephrol. 2010;73(1):36–43.

58. Todica O, Schwanitz A, Dalis M, Wolters N, Volsek M, Kribben A, et al. Cognitive disturbances in chronic kidney disease: cardiovascular risk factors and mood disorders as underestimated confounders. Eur J Neurol. 2010;17:212.

59. Gelb S, Shapiro RJ, Hill A, Thornton WL. Cognitive outcome following kidney transplantation. Nephrol Dial Transplant. 2008;23(3):1032–8.

60. Lee JJ, Chin HJ, Byun MS, Choe JY, Park JH, Lee SB, et al. Impaired frontal executive function and predialytic chronic kidney disease. J Am Geriatr Soc. 2011;59(9):1628–35.

61. Sanchez-Roman S, Ostrosky-Solis F, Morales-Buenrostro LE, Nogues-Vizcaino MG, Alberu J, McClintock SM. Neurocognitive profile of an adult sample with chronic kidney disease. J Int Neuropsychol Soc. 2011;17(1):80–90.

62. Tsai CF, Wang SJ, Fuh JL. Moderate chronic kidney disease is associated with reduced cognitive performance in midlife women. Kidney Int. 2010;78(6):605–10.

63. Etgen T, Sander D, Chonchol M, Briesenick C, Poppert H, Forstl H, et al. Chronic kidney disease is associated with incident cognitive impairment in the elderly: the INVADE study. Nephrol Dial Transplant. 2009;24(10):3144–50.

64. Murray AM, Knopman DS, Rossom RC, Heubner B, Tupper D, Amiot E. Cognitive impairment in moderate chronic kidney disease: the brain in kidney disease (BRINK) study. Alzheimers Dement. 2014;10:P499–500.

65. Afsar B, Kirkpantur A. Are there any seasonal changes of cognitive impairment, depression, sleep disorders and quality of life in hemodialysis patients? Gen Hosp Psychiatry. 2013;35(1):28–32.

66. McAdams-Demarco MA, Tan J, Salter ML, Gross A, Meoni LA, Jaar BG, et al. Frailty and cognitive function in incident hemodialysis patients. Clin J Am Soc Nephrol. 2015;10(12):2181–9.

67. Fidan C, Tutal E, Bal Z, Sezer S. Musclewasting is associated with depression and altered mental stage in dialysis patients. Nephrol Dial Transplant. 2016;31:i538.

68. Kang EW, Abdel-Kader K, Yabes J, Glover K, Unruh M. Association of sleep-disordered breathing with cognitive dysfunction in CKD stages 4-5. Am J Kidney Dis. 2012;60(6):949–58.

69. Unruh M, Tamura MK. Introduction: sleep and neurologic disorders in chronic kidney disease. Semin Nephrol. 2015;35(4):303.

70. Pierratos A, Hanly PJ. Sleep disorders over the full range of chronic kidney disease. Blood Purif. 2011;31(1–3):146–50.

71. De Santo RM, Bartiromo M, Cesare MC, Di Iorio BR. Sleeping disorders in early chronic kidney disease. Semin Nephrol. 2006;26(1):64–7.

72. Okubo R, Kondo M, Hoshi SL, Yamagata K. Cost-effectiveness of obstructive sleep apnea screening for patients with diabetes or chronic kidney disease. Sleep Breath. 2015;19(3):1081–92.

73. Markou N, Kanakaki M, Myrianthefs P, Hadjiyanakos D, Vlassopoulos D, Damianos A, et al. Sleep-disordered breathing in nondialyzed patients with chronic renal failure. Lung. 2006;184(1):43–9.

74. Molnar MZ, Novak M, Mucsi I. Management of restless legs syndrome in patients on dialysis. Drugs. 2006;66(5):607–24.

75. Aritake-Okada S, Nakao T, Komada Y, Asaoka S, Sakuta K, Esaki S, et al. Prevalence and clinical characteristics of restless legs syndrome in chronic kidney disease patients. Sleep Med. 2011;12(10):1031–3.

76. Ogna A, Forni Ogna V, Haba Rubio J, Tobback N, Andries D, Preisig M, et al. Sleep characteristics in early stages of chronic kidney disease in the HypnoLaus cohort. Sleep. 2016;39(4):945–53.

77. De Santo RM, Bilancio G, Santoro D, Vecchi ML, Perna A, De Santo NG, et al. A longitudinal study of sleep disorders in early-stage chronic kidney disease. J Ren Nutr. 2010;20(5 Suppl):S59–63.

78. Quinn C, Uzbeck M, Saleem I, Cotter P, Ali J, O'Malley G, et al. Iron status and chronic kidney disease predict restless legs syndrome in an older hospital population. Sleep Med. 2011;12(3):295–301.

79. Sakaguchi Y, Shoji T, Kawabata H, Niihata K, Suzuki A, Kaneko T, et al. High prevalence of obstructive sleep apnea and its association with renal function among nondialysis chronic kidney disease patients in Japan: a cross-sectional study. Clin J Am Soc Nephrol. 2011;6(5):995–1000.

80. Li H, Li XB, Feng SJ, Zhang GZ, Wang W, Wang SX. Sleep disorders and its related risk factors in patients undergoing chronic peritoneal dialysis. Chin Med J. 2014;127(7):1289–93.

81. Ceyhun HA, Kirpinar I, Yazici E, Ozan E. A comparative study on subjective sleep quality and predictive factors in renal transplant and dialysis patients. J Psychosom Res. 2010;68(6):614.

82. Artom M, Moss-Morris R, Caskey F, Chilcot J. Fatigue in advanced kidney disease. Kidney Int. 2014;86(3):497–505.

83. Karakan S, Sezer S, Ozdemir FN. Factors related to fatigue and subgroups of fatigue in patients with end-stage renal disease. Clin Nephrol. 2011;76(5):358–64.

84. Rodrigue JR, Mandelbrot DA, Hanto DW, Johnson SR, Karp SJ, Pavlakis M. A cross-sectional study of fatigue and sleep quality before and after kidney transplantation. Clin Transpl. 2011;25(1):E13–21.

85. Bossola M, Pepe G, Vulpio C. Fatigue in kidney transplant recipients. Clin Transpl. 2016;30(11):1387–93.

86. Jhamb M, Liang K, Yabes J, Steel JL, Dew MA, Shah N, et al. Prevalence and correlates of fatigue in chronic kidney disease and end-stage renal disease: are sleep disorders a key to understanding fatigue? Am J Nephrol. 2014;38(6):489–95.

87. Williams AG, Crane PB, Kring D. Fatigue in African American women on hemodialysis. Nephrol Nurs J. 2007;34(6):610–7, 44; quiz 8.

88. McGrath J, Saha S, Chant D, Welham J. Schizophrenia: a concise overview of incidence, prevalence, and mortality. Epidemiol Rev. 2008;30:67–76.

89. Annamalai A, Kosir U, Tek C. Prevalence of obesity and diabetes in patients with schizophrenia. World J Diabetes. 2017;8(8):390–6.

90. Hsu YH, Cheng JS, Ouyang WC, Lin CL, Huang CT, Hsu CC. Lower incidence of end-stage renal disease but suboptimal pre-dialysis renal care in schizophrenia: a 14-year nationwide cohort study. PLoS One. 2015;10(10):e0140510.

91. McPherson S, Barbosa-Leiker C, Daratha K, Short R, McDonell MG, Alicic R, et al. Association of co-occurring serious mental illness with emergency hospitalization in people with chronic kidney disease. Am J Nephrol. 2014;39(3):260–7.

92. Ahmadi J, Benrazavi L. Substance use among Iranian nephrologic patients. Am J Nephrol. 2002;22(1):11–3.

93. Novick T, Liu Y, Alvanzo A, Zonderman AB, Evans MK, Crews DC. Lifetime cocaine and opiate use and chronic kidney disease. Am J Nephrol. 2016;44:447–53.

94. Orth SR, Viedt C, Ritz E. Adverse effects of smoking in the renal patient. Tohoku J Exp Med. 2001;194(1):1–15.

95. Molander L, Hansson A, Lunell E, Alainentalo L, Hoffmann M, Larsson R. Pharmacokinetics of nicotine in kidney failure. Clin Pharmacol Ther. 2000;68(3):250–60.

96. Kaltsouda A, Skapinakis P, Damigos D, Ikonomou M, Kalaitzidis R, Mavreas V, et al. Defensive coping and health-related quality of life in chronic kidney disease: a cross-sectional study. BMC Nephrol. 2011;12:28.

97. Rich MR, Smith TW, Christensen AJ. Attributions and adjustment in end-stage renal disease. Cogn Ther Res. 1999;23(2):143–58.

98. Gillanders S, Wild M, Deighan C, Gillanders D. Emotion regulation, affect, psychosocial functioning, and well-being in hemodialysis patients. Am J Kidney Dis. 2008;51(4):651–62.

99. Koutsopoulou V, Theodosopoulou E, Vantsi E, Kotrosiou E, Kostandinou V, Dounousi E. Personality dimensions of haemodialysis patients related to initial renal disease. EDTNA-ERCA J. 2002;28(1):21–4.

100. Garcia-Llana H, Remor E, Del Peso G, Selgas R. The role of depression, anxiety, stress and adherence to treatment in dialysis patients health-related quality of life: a systematic review of the literature. Nefrologia. 2014;34(5):637–57.

101. Varela L, Vazquez MI, Bolanos L, Alonso R. Psychological predictors for health-related quality of life in patients on peritoneal dialysis. Nefrologia. 2011;31(1):97–106.

102. Abuyassin B, Sharma K, Ayas NT, Laher I. Obstructive sleep apnea and kidney disease: a potential bidirectional relationship? J Clin Sleep Med. 2015;11(8):915–24.

103. Lee J, Nicholl DD, Ahmed SB, Loewen AH, Hemmelgarn BR, Beecroft JM, et al. The prevalence of restless legs syndrome across the full spectrum of kidney disease. J Clin Sleep Med. 2013;9(5):455–9.

104. Rhee C, Chen A, You A, Jing J, Nakata T, Kovesdy C, et al. Relationship between depression and health-related quality of life in a prospective hemodialysis cohort. Am J Kidney Dis. 2016;67(5):A90.

105. Chan R, Brooks R, Steel Z, Heung T, Erlich J, Chow J, et al. The psychosocial correlates of quality of life in the dialysis population: a systematic review and meta-regression analysis. Qual Life Res. 2012;21(4):563–80.

106. Hedayati SS, Minhajuddin AT, Afshar M, Toto RD, Trivedi MH, Rush AJ. Association between major depressive episodes in patients with chronic kidney disease and initiation of dialysis, hospitalization, or death. JAMA. 2010;303(19):1946–53.

107. Troidle L, Watnick S, Wuerth DB, Gorban-Brennan N, Kliger AS, Finkelstein FO. Depression and its association with peritonitis in long-term peritoneal dialysis patients. Am J Kidney Dis. 2003;42(2):350–4.

108. Lindner AV, Novak M, Bohra M, Mucsi I. Insomnia in patients with chronic kidney disease. Semin Nephrol. 2015;35(4):359–72.

109. Xu J, Yoon IY, Chin HJ. The effect of sleep apnea on all-cause mortality in nondialyzed chronic kidney disease patients. Sleep Med. 2016;27-28:32–8.

110. Zhang J, Wang C, Gong W, Peng H, Tang Y, Li CC, et al. Association between sleep quality and cardiovascular damage in pre-dialysis patients with chronic kidney disease. BMC Nephrol. 2014;15:131.

111. Hedayati SS, Finkelstein FO. Epidemiology, diagnosis, and management of depression in patients with CKD. Am J Kidney Dis. 2009;54(4):741–52.

112. Adamczak M, Wiecek A, Nowak L. High prevalence of depression in haemodialysed patients. Nephrol Dial Transplant. 2012;27:ii511.

113. Young BA, Von Korff M, Heckbert SR, Ludman EJ, Rutter C, Lin EH, et al. Association of major depression and mortality in stage 5 diabetic chronic kidney disease. Gen Hosp Psychiatry. 2010;32(2):119–24.

114. Feng L, Bee Yap K, Pin NT. Depressive symptoms in older adults with chronic kidney disease: mortality, quality of life outcomes, and correlates. Am J Geriatr Psychiatr. 2013;21(6):570–9.

115. Palmer SC, Vecchio M, Craig JC, Tonelli M, Johnson DW, Nicolucci A, et al. Association between depression and death in people with CKD: a meta-analysis of cohort studies. Am J Kidney Dis. 2013;62(3):493–505.

116. Tsai YC, Chiu YW, Hung CC, Hwang SJ, Tsai JC, Wang SL, et al. Association of symptoms of depression with progression of CKD. Am J Kidney Dis. 2012;60(1):54–61.

117. Assari S. Renal disease mortality in the U.S. general population; demographic, socioeconomic, behavioral, and medical risk factors. Nephrourol Mon. 2017;9 (1):e42357 (no pagination).

118. Moran PJ, Christensen AJ, Lawton WJ. Social support and conscientiousness in hemodialysis adherence. Ann Behav Med. 1997;19(4):333–8.
119. Ibrahim N, Teo SS, Che Din N, Abdul Gafor AH, Ismail R. The role of personality and social support in health-related quality of life in chronic kidney disease patients. PLoS One. 2015;10(7):e0129015.
120. Poppe C, Crombez G, Hanoulle I, Vogelaers D, Petrovic M. Improving quality of life in patients with chronic kidney disease: influence of acceptance and personality. Nephrol Dial Transplant. 2013;28(1):116–21.
121. Goldfarb-Rumyantzev AS, Rout P, Sandhu GS, Khattak M, Garg J, DeSilva R, et al. Social adaptability index predicts survival in chronic disease (CKD) patients. Am J Kidney Dis. 2011;57(4):A42.
122. Rowland Yeo K, Aarabi M, Jamei M, Rostami-Hodjegan A. Modeling and predicting drug pharmacokinetics in patients with renal impairment. Expert Rev Clin Pharmacol. 2011;4(2):261–74.
123. Thomson BK, Nolin TD, Velenosi TJ, Feere DA, Knauer MJ, Asher LJ, et al. Effect of CKD and dialysis modality on exposure to drugs cleared by nonrenal mechanisms. Am J Kidney Dis. 2015;65(4):574–82.
124. Levenson JL. Renal and urological disorders. In: Levenson J, Ferrando SJ, editors. Clinical manual of psychopharmacology in the medically ill. Arlington: American Psychiatric Association Publishing; 2016. p. 195–214.
125. Hedayati SS, Yalamanchili V, Finkelstein FO. A practical approach to the treatment of depression in patients with chronic kidney disease and end-stage renal disease. Kidney Int. 2012;81(3):247–55.
126. Nagler EV, Webster AC, Vanholder R, Zoccali C. Antidepressants for depression in stage 3–5 chronic kidney disease: a systematic review of pharmacokinetics, efficacy and safety with recommendations by European Renal Best Practice (ERBP). Nephrol Dial Transplant. 2012;27(10):3736–45.
127. Hosseini SH, Espahbodi F, Mirzadeh Goudarzi SM. Citalopram versus psychological training for depression and anxiety symptoms in hemodialysis patients. Iran J Kidney Dis. 2012;6(6):446–51.
128. Hedayati SS, Gregg LP, Carmody T, Jain N, Toups M, Rush AJ, et al. Effect of sertraline on depressive symptoms in patients with chronic kidney disease without dialysis dependence: the CAST randomized clinical trial. JAMA. 2017;318(19):1876–90.
129. Johansen KL, Finkelstein FO, Revicki DA, Evans C, Wan S, Gitlin M, et al. Systematic review of the impact of erythropoiesis-stimulating agents on fatigue in dialysis patients. Nephrol Dial Transplant. 2012;27(6):2418–25.
130. Salviano LH, Linhares MI, de Lima KA, de Souza AG, Lima DB, Jorge AR, et al. Study of the safety of methylphenidate: focus on nephrotoxicity aspects. Life Sci. 2015;141:137–42.
131. Suwata J, Kamata K, Nishijima T, Yoshikawa T, Sano M. New acetylcholinesterase inhibitor (donepezil) treatment for Alzheimer's disease in a chronic dialysis patient. Nephron. 2002;91(2):330–2.
132. Liu JC, Hsu YP, Kao PF, Hao WR, Liu SH, Lin CF, et al. Influenza vaccination reduces dementia risk in chronic kidney disease patients: a population-based cohort study. Medicine (United States). 2016;95 (9):e2868 (no pagination).
133. Gopaluni S, Sherif M, Ahmadouk NA. Interventions for chronic kidney disease-associated restless legs syndrome. Cochrane Database Syst Rev. 2016;11:CD010690.
134. Dauvilliers Y, Benes H, Partinen M, Rauta V, Rifkin D, Dohin E, et al. Rotigotine in hemodialysis-associated restless legs syndrome: a randomized controlled trial. Am J Kidney Dis. 2016;68(3):434–43.
135. Russcher M, Koch B, Nagtegaal E, van der Putten K, ter Wee P, Gaillard C. The role of melatonin treatment in chronic kidney disease. Front Biosci (Landmark Ed). 2012;17:2644–56.
136. Benz RL, Pressman MR, Wu X. Periodic limb movements in sleep revealed by treatment of sleep apnea with continuous positive airway pressure in the advanced chronic kidney disease population. Clin Nephrol. 2011;76(6):470–4.
137. Levenson JL, Ferrando SJ. Chapter 5- Renal and urological disorders. In: Clinical manual of psychopharmacology in the medically ill. 2nd ed. Arlington: American Psychiatric Publishing; 2016.
138. Shakiba M, Sanadgol H, Azmoude HR, Mashhadi MA, Sharifi H. Effect of sertraline on uremic pruritus improvement in ESRD patients. Int J Nephrol. 2012;2012:363901.
139. ten Doesschate MC, Bockting CLH, Schene AH. Adherence to continuation and maintenance antidepressant use in recurrent depression. J Affect Disord. 115(1):167–70.
140. Guidi J, Fava GA, Fava M, Papakostas GI. Efficacy of the sequential integration of psychotherapy and pharmacotherapy in major depressive disorder: a preliminary meta-analysis. Psychol Med. 2011;41(2):321–31.
141. Xing L, Chen R, Diao Y, Qian J, You C, Jiang X. Do psychological interventions reduce depression in hemodialysis patients?: a meta-analysis of randomized controlled trials following PRISMA. Medicine (Baltimore). 2016;95(34):e4675.
142. Pascoe MC, Thompson DR, Castle DJ, McEvedy SM, Ski CF. Psychosocial interventions for depressive and anxiety symptoms in individuals with chronic kidney disease: systematic review and meta-analysis. Front Psychol. 2017;8:992.
143. Wright JH, Sudak DM, Turkington D, Thase ME. High-yield cognitive-behavior therapy for brief sessions: an illustrated guide. Washington, DC: American Psychiatric Publishing; 2010.
144. Duarte PS, Miyazaki MC, Blay SL, Sesso R. Cognitive-behavioral group therapy is an effective treatment for major depression in hemodialysis patients. Kidney Int. 2009;76(4):414–21.
145. Cukor D, Ver Halen N, Asher DR, Coplan JD, Weedon J, Wyka KE, et al. Psychosocial intervention improves depression, quality of life, and fluid adherence in hemodialysis. J Am Soc Nephrol. 2014;25(1):196–206.
146. Sharp J, Wild MR, Gumley AI, Deighan CJ. A cognitive behavioral group approach to enhance adherence to hemodialysis fluid restrictions: a randomized controlled trial. Am J Kidney Dis. 2005;45(6):1046–57.
147. Hare J, Clark-Carter D, Forshaw M. A randomized controlled trial to evaluate the effectiveness of a cognitive behavioural group approach to improve patient adherence to peritoneal dialysis fluid restrictions: a pilot study. Nephrol Dial Transplant. 2014;29(3):555–64.
148. Gross CR, Reilly-Spong M, Park T, Zhao R, Gurvich OV, Ibrahim HN. Telephone-adapted mindfulness-based stress reduction (tMBSR) for patients awaiting kidney transplantation. Contemp Clin Trials. 2017;57:37–43.
149. Lii YC, Tsay SL, Wang TJ. Group intervention to improve quality of life in haemodialysis patients. J Clin Nurs. 2007;16(11C):268–75.
150. Krespi MR, Oakley D, Bone M, Ahmad R, Salmon P. The effects of visual imagery on adjustment and quality in life of hemodialysis patients. Turk Psikiyatri Derg. 2009;20(3):255–68.
151. Tsay SL, Hung LO. Empowerment of patients with end-stage renal disease--a randomized controlled trial. Int J Nurs Stud. 2004;41(1):59–65.
152. Mitrou GI, Grigoriou SS, Konstantopoulou E, Theofilou P, Giannaki CD, Stefanidis I, et al. Exercise training and depression in ESRD: a review. Semin Dial. 2013;26(5):604–13.
153. Kouidi E, Karagiannis V, Grekas D, Iakovides A, Kaprinis G, Tourkantonis A, et al. Depression, heart rate variability, and exercise training in dialysis patients. Eur J Cardiovasc Prev Rehabil. 2010;17(2):160–7.

154. Ouzouni S, Kouidi E, Sioulis A, Grekas D, Deligiannis A. Effects of intradialytic exercise training on health-related quality of life indices in haemodialysis patients. Clin Rehabil. 2009;23(1):53–63.

155. Kim Y, Evangelista LS, Park YG. Anxiolytic effects of music interventions in patients receiving Incenter hemodialysis: a systematic review and meta-analysis. Nephrol Nurs J. 2015;42(4):339–47. quiz 48

156. Lin YJ, Lu KC, Chen CM, Chang CC. The effects of music as therapy on the overall well-being of elderly patients on maintenance hemodialysis. Biol Res Nurs. 2012;14(3):277–85.

157. Novak M, Costantini L, Schneider S, Beanlands H. Approaches to self-management in chronic illness. Semin Dial. 2013;26(2):188–94.

158. Devins GM, Hollomby DJ, Barre PE, Mandin H, Taub K, Paul LC, et al. Long-term knowledge retention following predialysis psychoeducational intervention. Nephron. 2000;86(2):129–34.

159. Devins GM, Mendelssohn DC, Barre PE, Binik YM. Predialysis psychoeducational intervention and coping styles influence time to dialysis in chronic kidney disease. Am J Kidney Dis. 2003;42(4):693–703.

160. Devins GM, Mendelssohn DC, Barre PE, Taub K, Binik YM. Predialysis psychoeducational intervention extends survival in CKD: a 20-year follow-up. Am J Kidney Dis. 2005;46(6):1088–98.

Dialysis: Medical and Psychological Considerations

7

Filza Hussain and Paula C. Zimbrean

Introduction

After reaching chronic kidney disease (CKD) stages 4 or 5, renal replacement therapy (RRT) is usually recommended. RRT encompasses continuous and intermittent modalities as well as kidney transplantation. Continuous RRT can be done via continuous dialysis, hemofiltration, hemodiafiltration, or high-flux dialysis; these interventions are done in acute situations, typically during treatment in intensive care unit. Many patients with CKD eventually require intermittent dialysis (often referred to as "dialysis"), which can be performed at a qualified center or at home. Intermittent dialysis can be hemodialysis (HD) (uses an arteriovenous fistula which connects to the dialysis machine) or peritoneal dialysis (PD) (uses catheters from the peritoneal cavity connecting to exchange bags or pumps). Although traditionally HD has been done in HD centers, 3 times a week, there is increased interest in performing HD at home. PD can be machine-free (done by patient 4–5 times a day) or automated (APD) done by machine typically at night when the patient is asleep. All RRT have advantages and disadvantages, but they all require significant lifestyle adjustments.

Since the year 2000, the use of hemodialysis has been increasing [1]. In 2015, 63% of all incident end-stage renal disease (ESRD) patients were receiving hemodialysis, 7% were treated with peritoneal dialysis, and the remainder received a kidney transplant [1]. Four decades ago in 1977, continuous renal replacement therapy (CRRT) was introduced as a treatment for critically ill patients with acute renal failure. Prior to CRRT, treatment of these patients led to significant hypotension as a side effect of intermittent

Table 7.1 Summary of renal replacement modalities [2]

Renal replacement modality	Clinical situation used in	Other considerations
Hemodialysis	End-stage renal disease	Usually 3–6 h 3 days a week Other prescriptions of length and frequency exist
Peritoneal dialysis	End-stage renal disease	Patients not bound to a machine, have more flexibility and autonomy
1. Continuous ambulatory peritoneal dialysis (CAPD)	Manual exchanges performed can be done several times a day	
2. Automated peritoneal dialysis (APD or CCPD)	Machine performs exchanges overnight	
Intermittent hemodialysis	Acute renal failure	3–6 h per treatment More cost effective Slower rates can improve risk for hypotension
Continuous renal replacement	Acute renal failure in critically ill patients	Continuous over 24 h Better control of hypotension, better solute removal Better management of intravascular volume
1. Continuous venovenous hemofiltration (CVVH)	CVVH better at removing middle and larger weight substances	
2. Continuous venovenous hemodialysis (CVVHD)	CVVHD better at removing small molecular weight substances (e.g., urea, creatinine, potassium)	
3. Continuous venovenous hemodiafiltration (CVVHDF)	CVVHDF combines diffusion and convective clearance to remove small to large weight substances	

hemodialysis. Table 7.1 summarizes the different renal replacement modalities currently in clinical use. The focus of this chapter will be on hemodialysis (HD) and peritoneal dialysis (PD) in patients with ESRD.

F. Hussain (✉)
Department of Psychiatry and Behavioral Sciences, Stanford University School of Medicine, Stanford, CA, USA
e-mail: hussainf@stanford.edu

P. C. Zimbrean
Transplant Psychiatry Services at Yale New Haven Hospital, Departments of Psychiatry and Surgery, New Haven, CT, USA

© Springer International Publishing AG, part of Springer Nature 2019
Y. Sher, J. R. Maldonado (eds.), *Psychosocial Care of End-Stage Organ Disease and Transplant Patients*,
https://doi.org/10.1007/978-3-319-94914-7_7

Choosing the Right Modality for a Patient

Investigation of various dialysis modalities (e.g., PD versus HD, continuous ambulatory versus automated PD) did not demonstrate superiority of one method over the other [3, 4]. Conservative non-dialysis care may be the appropriate decision for older patients with multiple comorbidities [5], while transplantation might be more suitable for others. All treatment modalities add a burden to the already encumbered patients and their families; hence early conversations between medical teams and patients and their caregivers are important.

In a review of 18 qualitative studies on the experience of 375 patients and 87 caregivers, Morton et al. [6] identified 4 major themes central to treatment choices: (1) *confronting mortality* (choosing life or death, being a burden, living in limbo), (2) *lack of choice* (medical decision, lack of information, constraints on resources), (3) *gaining knowledge about options* (peer influence, timing of information), and (4) *weighing alternatives* (maintaining lifestyle, family influence, maintaining status quo). For these decisions to be made in an informed manner, adequate time for education and assimilation of the information provided is necessary.

When to Start Dialysis

The Kidney Disease Outcomes Quality Initiative (KDOQI) workgroup in its most recent guidelines [7] recommends an individualized approach to initiating hemodialysis. Focusing only on the appearance of uremic symptoms (Table 7.2) [8] or basing the decision on estimated glomerular filtration rate (GFR) may be fraught with challenges and does not lead to improved clinical outcomes. Patients may have other reversible causes associated with uremia, and serum creatinine levels may appear spuriously decreased secondary to low muscle mass [7]. Conversely, patients may have a high GFR but have refractory hypervolemia or hyperkalemia that warrants initiating HD. To assist the decision-making process, in selected cases, direct measurement of GFR, measurement of filtration markers in the urine, and measures of

Table 7.2 Common symptoms of uremia [8]

Neurological	Endocrine and metabolic
Anergia	Amenorrhea and sexual dysfunction
Confusion	Insulin resistance
Anorexia	Increased protein muscle catabolism
Gustatory and olfactory alterations	Pruritus
Sleep disturbances	
Neuropathy	

serum cystatin C and other serum biomarkers of kidney function not dependent on muscle mass may yield more precise estimates in people with advanced kidney disease [9, 10].

The Initiating Dialysis Early and Late (IDEAL) study conducted in 32 centers in Australia and New Zealand randomized patients to begin dialysis early at creatinine clearance of 10–14 mL/min/1.73m^2 versus later at creatinine clearance of 5–7 mL/min/1.73m^2. The results did not show a difference between two groups for cost, time to death, cardiovascular outcomes, infectious events, or complications of dialysis [11, 12]. Limitations of this study included a narrow difference in actual creatinine clearance between the two groups (average of 12.0 and 9.8 mL/min/1.73m^2 in the early and late groups, respectively) which may account for a clear lack of difference between the two groups.

Although the KDOQI does not describe a certain creatinine clearance limit to initiate HD [7], the recommendations are quite clear about educating patients early about their disease course and treatment options, including different HD modalities as well as the option for transplant or conservative care without dialysis.

Frequency of Dialysis

Conventional HD remains the most common treatment for ESRD worldwide and is usually performed for 3–5 hours (h), 3 days per week [1, 7]. Some dialysis programs now offer intensive HD regimens, characterized by either longer duration, increased frequency, or both. There are no randomized controlled studies investigating intensive HD, but Kraus and colleagues in a narrative review note intensive HD can address important clinical problems such as left ventricular hypertrophy, hypertension, hyperphosphatemia, low quality of life, and poor tolerability of conventional HD [13]. Intensive HD may, however, increase the risks of infections, complications of frequent vascular access, and burden to the patient and caregivers. It may also lead to an accelerated decline in residual kidney function [7, 13].

Quality of Life

Quality of life (QOL) is an important measure of treatment efficacy and improves communication and understanding between patients and physicians. The health-related quality of life (HRQOL) in dialysis patients is lower compared to that of age-matched subjects in the general population [14, 15] due to loss of vocational capacity; effects of a chronic, physically demanding frequent therapy; decline in functional capacity; medication side effects; loss of social support; and impact of a multitude of physical and emotional symptoms [16].

There has been a debate about which dialysis modality (HD vs. PD) has better HRQOL measures.

Systematic reviews [15, 17] have not found significant differences in outcomes of physical function, recreation, freedom, or ability to work between PD and HD.

Each modality has its advantages and disadvantages. HD affords patients less responsibility for the procedure and allows for the development of community and socialization with other HD patients as well as HD center staff [18]. On the other hand, patients on HD have access complications, the risk of infections, and a higher mortality just before and 12 h after dialysis due to electrolyte fluctuations. In a systematic review of 24 studies including 221 patients on home HD [19], 5 themes of psychological adaptation were identified: (1) *vulnerability of dialyzing independently* (fear of self-needling, feeling unqualified, and anticipating catastrophic complications), (2) *fear of being alone* (social isolation and medical disconnection), (3) *concern of family burden* (emotional demands on caregivers, imposing responsibility), (4) *opportunity to thrive* (reestablishing a healthy self-identity, gaining control and freedom, strengthening relationships), and (5) *appreciating medical responsiveness* (attentive monitoring and communication and clinician validation).

PD is not only lower in cost but also allows patients to have more autonomy, schedule flexibility, better maintenance of residual renal function, and greater satisfaction with medical care team despite less frequent contact than the HD cohort. The one-on-one relationship with the PD nurse fosters patient confidence and support in a way that leads to more satisfaction than that experienced by in-center HD patients. PD patients also have an improved survival over those on HD in the first 1–2 years after initiation of treatment. The risk of death in PD patients becomes equivalent or greater than HD patients after the initial 1.5–2 years depending on patient age and medical comorbidities such as diabetes. Patients on PD do experience more technique failure, weight gain, and caregiver burnout [18].

Much like the earlier reviews [15, 17], a recent meta-analysis [20] that included seven studies comparing HD and PD across different measures on the Kidney Disease Quality of Life (KDQOL) Short Form version 1.3 (KDQOL-SF 1.3) and KDQOL-SF 36 was inconclusive. The quantitative analysis, however, showed that the only statistically significant difference between the QOL of patients on hemodialysis and those on PD concerned the KDQOL-SF 1.3 domain on effects of kidney disease (question 15 a-h). This domain evaluates the impact of kidney disease on fluid and dietary restrictions, ability to complete chores, travel, dependence on medical professionals, level of worries and stress, and changes to personal appearance and sex life. Patients undergoing PD scored better on this domain (P = 0.032). Improving social support and reducing role limitations in patients using either modality improved emotional well-being, quality of sleep, and symptom management by patients.

Ultimately, the choice of dialysis modality needs to be individualized [17]. Modality selection should in most cases be patient/family directed, with primary considerations focused on lifestyle and social issues such as patient autonomy, geographic location (as it affects transportation to and from the dialysis center) living situation, patient motivation, and patient and family employment [18].

Psychiatric Disorders in Dialysis Patients

Depression

In the international Dialysis Outcomes and Practice Patterns Study (DOPPS) [21], 21.5% of dialysis patients self-reported depression, while 17.7% of patients on chronic dialysis had depression diagnosed by a physician. This is significantly higher than the estimated prevalence (10%) of depression in the general population [22]. In a study that measured depressive symptoms monthly via Patient Health Questionnaire 9 (PHQ-9) in 280 patients on chronic dialysis, Weisbord et al. identified moderate to severe depressive symptoms on 18% of the assessments [23]. A recent meta-analysis showed the prevalence of depression in dialysis population varied from 22.8% using interview-based diagnosis to 39.3% using self- or clinician-administered rating scales [24].

Depression in this population is associated with lower QOL, sexual dysfunction, and nonadherence to medical treatment [25]. Studies comparing the prevalence of depression in patients undergoing various types of dialysis treatment (e.g., HD versus PD) have been contradictory [26–28]. Increased risk for MDD has been reported with standard HD versus those receiving hemodiafiltration [29]. Levels of depression were equivalent in assisted PD and self-care PD [30]. Increased risk for depression in HD patients has also been linked to generalized weakness and loss of strength as measured by a lower body mass index (BMI) [31], muscle wasting as measured by 10-meter walking test [32], and hand grip strength [33]. On the other hand, HD parameters (uremic toxin removal indices) or nutrition indices do not appear to influence the level of depression [34].

Depressed patients on hemodialysis have a higher risk of death and hospitalizations compared with those without depressive symptoms [35]. A recent meta-analysis of 31 observational studies, although limited by the heterogeneity of studies and depression assessment methods, showed a significant association between mortality and depression in patients on both PD and HD [36]. Higher levels of inflammatory cytokines and stress hormones, increased platelet aggregation, reduced adherence to dietary and fluid restrictions, and medications in depressed patients contribute to increased incidence of hospitalizations, worse cardiovascular outcomes, and increased mortality [25, 37]. Weisbord et al. noted an independent association between depression and missed or abbreviated dialysis sessions in 65 patients with depression [23].

In addition to etiologic factors of depression present in the general population such as genetic predisposition and neurotransmitter dysregulation, patients with ESRD have an increased level of cytokines, difficulties with sleep, and social risk factors of role disruptions, financial implications of illness, and a perception of lack of control contributing to the development of depression [38]. Greater symptom burden and a lower QOL experienced by depressed individuals lead to social withdrawal and low family support [39], resulting in a vicious cycle. Despite growing evidence of the importance of early detection, depression remains underdiagnosed and undertreated in dialysis patients [40, 41].

The Beck Depression Inventory (BDI) is a self-report questionnaire that has been validated and widely used to assess depressive symptoms in dialysis patients [42]. Screening for depression in this population is complex due to an overlap with symptoms of uremia. The Cognitive Depression Index (CDI), a truncated version of the BDI with somatic symptoms omitted, may also be used to avoid confounding between symptoms from the medical illness and depression. In a study comparing the BDI, Hospital Anxiety and Depression Scale (HADS), and CDI, Preljevic et al. found the BDI and HADS to be acceptable screening tools in this population [43]. The authors recommend using a cutoff of 17 or higher for depression on the BDI, higher than the previously recommended 13 or 16 [44]. CDI was found to be only slightly more specific than the BDI [43].

Suicide in Dialysis Patients

Traditionally, patients with CKD, specifically those on dialysis, have been considered at higher risk for suicide. Some early studies reported a suicide risk up to 400 times higher than in general population [45]. It is important to note that most of the initial studies considered stopping dialysis treatment as a form of suicide. With time, clinicians and researchers started differentiating cessation of RRT from suicidal behavior. Studies focused on cessation of RRT show that more than half of these cases occur in patients with cognitive impairment and multiple medical complications and that in the majority of these cases, the proposal to discontinue treatment had been originated by the medical providers [46]. Even when cessation of RRT is not considered suicidal behavior, the suicide rate in patients with CKD is 84% higher compared with the general US population [47].

Comorbid anxiety, fatigue, reduced QOL, alcohol or drug use disorder, and an inability to cope with the stressors of illness contribute to this risk [31]. Additional risk factors for suicidal ideations or behavior in these patients are low BMI [48], male gender, age over 75 years, white or Asian race, depression, substance use disorders, medical comorbidities such as cancer or COPD, serum albumin less than 3.5 g/dl, and hospitalization within the past 12 months [47].

A recent retrospective study of 65,000 patients in Taiwan found suicide risk to be 140% in patients on dialysis when compared to the general population. The study population displayed a risk of suicide by cutting, 20 times higher than that of the general population [49]. Other means of suicide in dialysis patients may involve nonadherence to dietary and fluid restrictions, manipulating the graft leading to massive hemorrhage, and firearms [50]. On the other hand, a recent cross-sectional study in Brazil concluded that spiritual and religious beliefs were protective, leading to better mental health and lower suicide risk [51].

Comprehensive care of patients on dialysis should include screening for depression and inquiries by nephrology/dialysis staff about thoughts of suicide so a risk assessment can be undertaken and a prevention plan is generated [52]. Close collaboration with mental health clinicians and collaborative care models will be helpful.

Treatment Options and Challenges

There is a paucity of data on pharmacological and non-pharmacological treatments of depression in dialysis patients. Patients on dialysis who have screened positive for depression have shown disinterest in modifying or initiating treatment for depression. For example, Pena-Polanco and colleagues assessed depression monthly in participants of a clinical trial for symptom management during dialysis from 2009 to 2011 and found that these patients were frequently not interested in modifying or initiating treatment for depression. They also found renal providers to be unwilling to modify or initiate antidepressants [53].

Studies investigating the efficacy of antidepressant medications in dialysis-dependent patients have been limited due to small sample size, lack of randomization, short treatment durations, low adherence, high dropout rates, and nonstandard criteria for diagnosing depression [54].

A systematic review and meta-analysis found 4 studies of 170 participants assessing the efficacy of antidepressants for depression in patients on dialysis and reported that evidence for antidepressant use in the dialysis population is sparse and inconclusive [55]. In a randomized controlled feasibility trial comparing sertraline to placebo, 709 patients were screened, and only 30 made the inclusion criteria with 21 completing the trial. Although no benefit of sertraline was observed, the study highlighted recruitment issues in this population [56].

This dearth of data limits careful use of antidepressants in a population with cardiovascular risk factors. In a small, single-center study of patients on chronic peritoneal dialysis, Wuerth and colleagues faced similar challenges with patients resistant to start medications. However, they found that the small subgroup of patients treated with antidepressants had improvement in their BDI scores following 12 weeks of therapy, suggesting clinical depression can be treatable by antidepressants in this patient population [57].

Other studies have found paroxetine and fluoxetine to be tolerated in dialysis populations [58, 59]. CBT and mindfulness training are two psychotherapeutic approaches which have been found to be helpful for depression in dialysis patients [60, 61]. They are discussed in more detail in Chap. 6.

In summary, depression in dialysis patients is an important comorbidity with multiple risk factors and subsequent important downstream consequences, including increased suicide risk and worsening HRQOL outcomes. The evidence establishing safety and efficacy of treatment of depression in this population remains scant, and further research is warranted.

Anxiety in Dialysis Patients

The exact prevalence of anxiety disorders in the dialysis population remains unclear, as there are no large nationally representative studies. With SCID remaining the gold standard instrument for a psychiatric diagnosis, a study of 70 patients on HD showed that 45.7% meet criteria for anxiety disorders: 26.6% had specific phobias, 21% panic disorder, 4.2% post-traumatic stress disorder (PTSD), and 4.3% social phobia [62]. Levels of anxiety were equivalent in assisted PD and self-care PD [30].

Smaller studies using a variety of diagnostic tools and self-report measures report a broad range of anxiety prevalence in these patients, from 12% to 52% [63]. Similar to the depression literature, this represents the heterogeneity in diagnostic tools and thresholds of diagnoses. Compared to patients with depression, patients with anxiety have reported better QOL; however, when these same patients are compared to those dialysis patients with no psychiatric illness, they score lower on the QOL scales [64]. In a recent cross-sectional study of 414 patients from 24 different dialysis centers in Greece, Gerogianni and colleagues found female gender, lack of a secondary education, being a pensioner, having more financial difficulties, comorbid illness, and not being a transplant candidate to be associated with higher levels of anxiety in dialysis patients [65].

For a patient reporting symptoms of a panic attack during a dialysis treatment (e.g., shortness of breath, lightheadedness, palpitations), it takes a very detailed assessment to diagnose anxiety and differentiate it from physical symptoms caused by the treatment or by medical comorbidities. Very few studies measuring anxiety take this into consideration, in order to accurately diagnose anxiety disorders.

The Hospital Anxiety and Depression Scale (HADS), a self-report screening measure, has been reported to perform well in assessments of both the diagnosis and symptom severity of anxiety and depression. The HADS-A is acceptable for screening anxiety in this population; however, lower cutoff scores (6 versus 8 or 11) than other populations may be needed for improved sensitivity and specificity [43].

In a cross-sectional study of 170 patients on maintenance dialysis for 6 months or more, 155 HD and 15 on PD, Feroze and colleagues [66] found that 53% of patients experienced some anxiety when coming for a dialysis treatment, especially if there were changes in routine, such as a different dialysis technician. Alarm bells on the machine and presence of paramedics in the dialysis unit were also found to be anxiety-provoking for patients. Despite having been in dialysis for 6 months or more, patients found the experience of dialysis and common occurrences happening within each treatment anxiety-provoking.

Anxiety is often comorbid with depression and increases the risk for substance use disorders as well. Cohen and colleagues recommend screening for anxiety before the initiation of dialysis and during annual mental health assessments. A change in patient behavior from their norm, including disruption on the HD unit, new onset nonadherence, and avoidance behaviors, should also trigger screening for anxiety and depression [67].

Treatment

There have been limited studies for the treatment of anxiety in the dialysis populations. SSRIs are considered first-line treatment for anxiety disorders in adults [68]. Benzodiazepines have also been used for short-term relief of anxiety [69], but risk of dependence and cognitive challenges make their longer-term use less desirable. Other medications, such as quetiapine, gabapentin, and buspirone, have also been used in the treatment of anxiety disorders [69], but safety data for patients on dialysis is limited.

Sleep Disorders

Dialysis patients frequently experience sleep difficulties with a reported prevalence of sleep disorders ranging from 20 to 70% [70]. Insomnia, restless legs syndrome (RLS), and sleep-disordered breathing are the most common disorders. Sleep disorders have been found in 47.6% of patients on continuous PD [71]. The prevalence of insomnia in HD patients varies from 15% [72] to 69% [73]. RLS prevalence in patients on dialysis ranges from 12 to 25% [73, 74], while the prevalence of periodic limb movement disorder (PLMD) was reported at 42% in HD patients [75]. RLS has been associated with prematurely stopping dialysis and decreased

QOL [74]. These patients also experience more anxiety, daytime sleepiness, and sexual dysfunction [76].

The severity of sleep disorders progresses with worsening kidney function; however, this is not linearly related to uremia [40]. Short sleep, in turn, is associated with decreased kidney function [77] and a 50% increase in mortality rate compared to those without sleep difficulties [78]. The Pittsburgh Sleep Quality Index (PSQI) and Epworth Sleepiness Scale (ESS) have not been validated in this population but can be used as screening instruments. Instruments screening for sleep apnea commonly focus on hypertension, snoring, and body habitus. These have not proven to be sensitive enough to be used in the ESRD population [79]. Comorbidity with depression in ESRD also impacts sleep and leads to downstream cognitive challenges discussed later in this chapter.

Treatment of Sleep Disorders in Dialysis Patients

There are few trials on treatment of sleep disorders in dialysis patients. General initial recommendations include the use of non-pharmacological interventions and reversal of any potential causes of sleep disruption. Treatment should begin with reviewing basic sleep hygiene. If these conservative measures do not improve the underlying sleep problems, cognitive behavioral therapy for insomnia (CBT-I) can be helpful. A trial of 98 maintenance HD patients randomized to CBT-I versus controls who received no CBT showed improvement in depression, anxiety, and sleep quality in the CBT-I treatment group [80]. The Following Rehabilitation, Economics and Everyday-Dialysis Outcome Measurements (FREEDOM) Study [81] and Frequent Hemodialysis Network (FHN) [82] trials both found short daily HD (6 times per week) to cause improvement in sleep quality as compared to matched conventional HD, although this improvement was not sustained beyond a year.

In a meta-analysis of 9 studies and 220 patients on HD, ropinirole proved to have a modest effect for RLS in CKD [83]. Rotigotine has also been reported helpful for RLS in patients with CKD on dialysis in one randomized study [84]. Other than low-dose dopaminergic medications, gabapentin or pregabalin is helpful for control of RLS symptoms, although no large randomized controlled studies exist [70]. Caution should be used when using gabapentin given its renal excretion. Dosages of 100–300 mg given right after dialysis have been efficacious but require close monitoring for adverse effects [70]. Intradialytic aerobic exercise and shorter daily HD can also decrease the severity of RLS symptoms as reported by a few small studies [70].

Non-benzodiazepine medications, such as eszopiclone, zaleplon, and zopiclone, do not require dose reduction in reduced renal clearance and can be used to treat insomnia in this patient population for short periods of time, starting at low doses and titrating slowly [70]. Small randomized studies have found zaleplon [85] and melatonin [86] to be helpful for short periods of time without significant adverse effects.

Unlike the general population, patients on dialysis differ in characteristics pertaining to sleep-disordered breathing (SDB). There is no gender difference in this group, and neck circumference (>40 cm) rather than BMI is recognized as a better marker for SDB risk [87]. An increased neck circumference resulting from fluid overload can cause narrowing of airways and hence more symptoms. Small studies [87, 88] have shown improvement in symptoms subsequent to fluid removal.

Cognitive Dysfunction

Patients on dialysis are at an increased risk of developing cognitive impairment [89]. This, in turn, is associated with increased mortality, hospitalization rate, and cerebrovascular events, as well as decreased QOL [90, 91]. A recent cross-sectional study using SCID and DSM V criteria showed that 52.4% of HD patients met criteria for a major neurocognitive disorder and 17.3% for a minor neurodegenerative disorder [92].

Hypertension, diabetes, and hyperlipidemia, frequently associated with and leading to CKD, compromise the brain substrate. Subsequent exposures to fluctuating levels of uremic toxins, hypoxemia, changing fluid and electrolyte levels during dialysis, hospitalizations, and alterations in drug metabolism further increase the risk of cognitive dysfunction, especially delirium [91, 93]. In addition, depression and sleep disorders worsen performance on measures of cognition. The absence of residual renal function, malnutrition, and low hemoglobin concentration have also been found in the DOPPS to be independently associated with diagnosed dementia [94]. Diagnosed dementia was associated with an increased risk of death and dialysis withdrawal, independent of a number of confounding factors.

A retrospective cohort study of nearly 122,000 patients comparing the incidence of dementia in patients on HD versus PD found the annual incidence in the total cohort to be 2.3% compared with 1% in a non-dialysis matched cohort. When compared to patients on HD, persons on PD were found to have a 25% lower risk of being diagnosed with dementia. This lower risk persisted after adjusting for the younger age and ethnicities of patients on PD. Patients on PD do not experience the hypotension and large volume shifts associated with HD and potentially leading to cerebral injury. There may also be a selection bias where cognitively more intact patients are referred for PD rather than HD. The difference in cognitive effects of the two modalities needs to be investigated further [95].

There are no screening cognitive tests developed specifically for the CKD population [96]. Compared to the Mini-Mental Status Examination (MMSE), the Montreal Cognitive Assessment (MoCA) has good sensitivity and specificity to discriminate the cognitively impaired from the non-impaired dialysis patients [97].

A study of 26 patients on hemodialysis found that cognitive scores vary depending on the timing and setting of the cognitive test. Hypotension and fatigue during dialysis compromise test scores. Authors recommended testing patients before dialysis in a room different from where dialysis occurs [98].

Treatment of Cognitive Dysfunction

Management of cognitive impairment in this population mostly relies on identification, reversal of possible etiologies, and non-pharmacological interventions. For those with delirium, addressing the underlying uremia, anemia, and fluid and electrolyte shifts can help. Caregivers should accompany patients to their treatments and appointments which may decrease anxiety for the patient and ensure adequate adherence to treatment and dietary restrictions. Pharmacologically, there has been no published data on cholinesterase inhibitors (e.g., donepezil) or N-methyl-D-aspartate (NMDA) antagonists (e.g., memantine) in this patient population [90].

Sexual Dysfunction

Sexual dysfunction is reported in up to 86% of patients on dialysis [99]. The prevalence of erectile dysfunction in dialysis patients increases with age, and up to 55% of female dialysis patients report difficulty with sexual arousal, impaired vaginal lubrication, dyspareunia, and anorgasmia [99]. Sexual dysfunction in this population is correlated with depression and anxiety [100].

Psychopharmacology in Dialysis

When choosing and dosing a psychotropic medication in patients on dialysis, clinicians should consider certain pharmacokinetic variables given changes in fluid volumes, muscle wasting, and body habitus due to ESRD [7]. Specific considerations for dialysis patients include protein binding (e.g., fluoxetine and its metabolite norfluoxetine are not removed by dialysis given its protein binging), fat solubility, and volume of distribution [101]. Most psychotropics are large fat-soluble molecules that are highly protein bound (e.g., haloperidol and sertraline) and hence not effectively reduced by dialysis. Lithium which is completely dialyzed needs a post-dialysis dose to maintain steady state. In addi-

tion, the percentage of drug renally cleared should be considered: if the medication is less than 30% renally cleared, then dose adjustments post dialysis are not necessary. Medications such as gabapentin and amantadine that are excreted unchanged as well as drugs with active metabolites (e.g., bupropion) that are renally cleared can accumulate in ESRD and should be avoided or used in smaller quantities.

Lithium is water soluble and completely dialyzable. Despite its deleterious renal effects, in carefully selected patients, lithium has been used for the treatment of bipolar disorder in patients receiving hemodialysis with specific monitoring of the blood levels [102, 103].

The important pharmacokinetic considerations for commonly used psychotropics are presented in Table 7.3. Also refer to the reviews by Baghdady et al. [104] and Eyler [101] for further details.

Declining Dialysis

Initiation and withdrawal of dialysis are both important decisions requiring careful considerations of prognostic outcomes, the burden of treatment, and burden of managing illness without dialysis. Withdrawal of dialysis is a separate entity from suicide and euthanasia and is better characterized as a complex end-of-life decision [105] influenced by the quality of life, frailty, and medical futility. Crude mortality rates related to withdrawal of dialysis have increased over time across the United States from 3 per 1000 person-years in 1966 to 48.6 per 1000 person-years in 2010. In the United States, crude mortality rates preceded by dialysis withdrawal are higher in the older population and have increased over time in the age group of 65 and above. In this age group, the crude mortality rate from dialysis withdrawal was 89.4 per 1000 person-years compared with 26.1 per 1000 person-years in the 50–64-year-old age group (2008–2010) [106].

Shared decision-making is an important construct allowing patients to promote their values and balance ethical principles of autonomy, beneficence, and non-maleficence.

Nephrologists are developing clinical protocols to address the cessation of RRT, which take into considerations the type of treatment, medical complications, psychiatric comorbidities, QOL, and family preferences [107]. The Renal Physicians Association and the American Society of Nephrology released a revised second edition of the guidelines for dialysis withdrawal [108]. It emphasizes relying on shared decision-making between the patient, family, and physicians, obtaining informed consent, estimating the prognosis on dialysis, adopting a systematic approach for conflict resolution of disagreements, honoring advance directives, and ensuring the provision of palliative care. Most importantly, the guidelines note that the patient with decision-making capacity has the right to refuse dialysis, even if the

Table 7.3 Commonly used psychotropic medications and their pharmacokinetic considerations in dialysis [104]

Medications	Renal clearance	Effects of dialysis	Dose changes required	Other considerations	Side effects
Selective serotonin reuptake inhibitors Fluoxetine Citalopram Paroxetine	Elimination half-life of citalopram increases by 35% and clearance decreases by 40%. Paroxetine drug exposure increased at lower creatinine clearance.	Highly protein bound. Not removed by dialysis.	No dose change for fluoxetine. Use caution for citalopram. Paroxetine: start. low go slow.	Fluoxetine efficacious and well tolerated. QT prolongation by citalopram.	Nausea, headache, may be confounded by uremia Bleeding issues Sexual dysfunction
Serotonin Norepinephrine Reuptake Inhibitors Venlafaxine Desvenlafaxine Duloxetine	Venlafaxine and desvenlafaxine renally cleared and elimination half-life increased. Duloxetine is also renally cleared.	Not removed by dialysis, dose supplementation not needed.	Decrease dose to half for venlafaxine per manufacturer. Desvenlafaxine not to exceed 50 mg every other day. Duloxetine dosing information advises against use in patients with CrCl less than 30.	Useful in chronic pain, such as diabetic neuropathy. Less muscarinic and histaminic compared to tricyclic antidepressants. Avoid abrupt discontinuation.	Can increase blood pressure due to noradrenergic effects.
Trazodone Vilazodone	No studies	No studies	US dosing information indicates no changes needed.		Hypotension
Tricyclic Antidepressants Amitriptyline Nortriptyline Desipramine	Metabolites can accumulate	Conjugated metabolites are removed. Nortriptyline, a metabolite of amitriptyline, is not removed.	Start low and monitor levels	Used for pruritus, insomnia, and depression. Not first line for treatment.	Dry mouth, weight gain, excessive sedation, hypotension, cardiac side effects
Bupropion	Metabolites threohydrobupropion and hydroxybupropion can accumulate	Some clearance of bupropion and threohydrobupropion; none for hydroxybupropion	Decrease dose because of active metabolites	Most appropriate dose unknown but usually lower than that for healthy adults	Decreases seizure threshold
Mirtazapine	50% reduction in clearance in ESRD	85% protein bound. Minimally removed by dialysis.	Yes, lower dosages given reduction in clearance	Has been used to treat uremic pruritus	Weight gain, sedation
Benzodiazepines	Active metabolites are renally cleared	Highly protein bound. Not removed by dialysis.	50% lower dose for chlordiazepoxide. Free drug concentration may be increased in dialysis patients.	Used to treat RLS and other sleep disorders. Caution with p450 3A4 inhibitors.	Cognitive and sexual side effects
Buspirone	Increased serum levels of active drug and metabolites in CKD patients	Metabolites are removed but unpredictably	Use lower dosages	Can be used for anxiolysis	
Atypical antipsychotics	Risperidone and active metabolite both with reduced clearance in CKD	Not removed by HD	Dose reduction needed for risperidone	Other atypicals have limited information but no change in pharmacokinetics noted	Careful dose titration and monitoring for side effects
First-generation antipsychotics	Not enough data, fewer concerns about accumulation	Highly protein bound	No dose reduction needed	Phenothiazine can promote hypotension	Careful dosing in patients taking other QT-prolonging agents
Lithium	Renal clearance declines proportionally to a threshold of 30 ml/min	Completely removed in dialysis	Dose reduction to avoid toxicity	Single post-dialysis dose to maintain steady state	Cardiovascular side effects, anemia, mineral bone disease

Table 7.3 (continued)

Medications	Renal clearance	Effects of dialysis	Dose changes required	Other considerations	Side effects
Antiepileptic Carbamazepine Oxcarbazepine Valproic acid Gabapentin	Carbamazepine: metabolites renally cleared. Oxcarbazepine: renally excreted. Minimal renal excretion for valproic acid. Gabapentin renally cleared with dose-dependent toxicity.	20–50% carbamazepine removed by dialysis but post-dialysis dose not needed	None needed for carbamazepine. Oxcarbazepine requires a 50% dose reduction.	Monitor sodium levels on carbamazepine. Oxcarbazepine can cause hyponatremia.	
		20% valproic acid removed by dialysis	Gabapentin 200 to 300 mg single dose after dialysis		
		Gabapentin extracted 35%			
NMDA antagonists* Amantadine Memantine	Amantadine and memantine excreted renally, unchanged	Amantadine is highly protein bound and not dialyzed	Dose reduction for amantadine per package insert, contraindicated if CrCl less than 15. Package insert for memantine suggests dose halved for CrCl of 5–29 mL/min.		Myoclonus
Acetylcholinesterase inhibitors* Rivastigmine Donepezil	Rivastigmine 97% renally excreted. Donepezil 57% renally excreted, 17% unchanged.	Rivastigmine 40% protein bound, not dialyzable. Donepezil 96% protein bound, dialyzability unknown.	Per package insert for GFR less than 50, use lower dosages of rivastigmine.		
Stimulants* Modafinil Methylphenidate Dextroamphetamine	Methylphenidate 78–97% renally excreted. Renal excretion for dextroamphetamine dependent on pH.	Methylphenidate 10–33% protein bound. Dialyzability not established.	No dose adjustment needed		
Antihistamines* Hydroxyzine	Only 0.8% of the dose is renally excreted	Metabolite cetirizine not dialyzed	Reduce dose to avoid metabolite accumulation		Anticholinergic side effects QT prolongation

Medications with * information from package inserts

team disagrees with the patient. On the other hand, if the patient or family demands dialysis in a situation where it is deemed not beneficial or may bring forth more harm, the physicians can refuse to initiate or to maintain dialysis [109].

Patients who wish to withdraw from dialysis must be evaluated for decision-making capacity as well as depression in order to understand motivations behind the decision to withdraw. The request to discontinue dialysis may come from a patient, the family, or both. Important considerations include the motivations and level of support of family members [110].

Conclusions

The number of people worldwide on renal replacement therapy as well as their length of survival with this therapy are increasing. However, patients on dialysis face unique challenges of being dependent on a machine and experiencing loss of flexibility of schedule and societal roles. These patients face fatigue, depression, and anxiety at rates higher than the general population. Sleep and cognitive disorders are frequent. Unfortunately, mental health issues in this population are underrecognized and undertreated, leading to poorer quality of life and hence outcomes. Once a diagnosis of a mental health condition has been made, treatment poses unique challenges given the change in the pharmacokinetics of renally cleared drugs as well as removal in dialysis. Suicide and its risk factors need to be addressed, while withdrawal of dialysis understood as a complex end-of-life decision, rather than an act of suicide. Joint decision-making between physicians and patients can help with decisions to commence or withdraw dialysis to preserve patient autonomy, support their values, improve QOL, and achieve best possible outcomes.

References

1. Saran R, Robinson B, et al. US renal data system 2016 annual data report: epidemiology of kidney disease in the United States. Am J Kidney Dis. 2017;69(3 Suppl 1):A7–8.

2. Pannu N, Gibney RN. Renal replacement therapy in the intensive care unit. Ther Clin Risk Manag. 2005;1:141–50.

3. Bieber SD, Burkart J, Golper TA, Teitelbaum I, Mehrotra R. Comparative outcomes between continuous ambulatory and automated peritoneal dialysis: a narrative review. Am J Kidney Dis. 2014;63:1027–37.

4. Chiu Y-W, Jiwakanon S, Lukowsky L, Duong U, Kalantar-Zadeh K, Mehrotra R. An update on the comparisons of mortality outcomes of hemodialysis and peritoneal dialysis patients. Semin Nephrol. 2011;31:152–8.

5. Davison SN. End-of-life care preferences and needs: perceptions of patients with chronic kidney disease. Clin J Am Soc Nephrol. 2010;5:195–204.

6. Morton RL, Tong A, Howard K, Snelling P, Webster AC. The views of patients and carers in treatment decision making for chronic kidney disease: systematic review and thematic synthesis of qualitative studies. BMJ. 2010;340:c112–c112.

7. By National Kidney Foundation, Transl. DD Ivanov. KDOQI clinical practice guideline for hemodialysis adequacy: 2015 update. Kidney. 2016;53–6.

8. Meyer TW, Hostetter TH. Approaches to uremia. J Am Soc Nephrol. 2014;25:2151–8.

9. Levey AS, Inker LA, Coresh J. GFR estimation: from physiology to public health. Am J Kidney Dis. 2014;63:820–34.

10. Delanaye P, Mariat C. The applicability of eGFR equations to different populations. Nat Rev Nephrol. 2013;9:513–22.

11. Johnson DW, Wong MG, Cooper BA, et al. Effect of timing of dialysis commencement on clinical outcomes of patients with planned initiation of peritoneal Dialysis in the Ideal trial. Perit Dial Int. 2012;32:595–604.

12. Harris A, Cooper BA, Li JJ, et al. Cost-effectiveness of initiating dialysis early: a randomized controlled trial. Am J Kidney Dis. 2011;57:707–15.

13. Kraus MA, Kansal S, Copland M, Komenda P, Weinhandl ED, Bakris GL, Chan CT, Fluck RJ, Burkart JM. Intensive hemodialysis and potential risks with increasing treatment. Am J Kidney Dis. 2016;68(5S1):S51–8.

14. Kim J-Y, Kim B, Park K-S, Choi J-Y, Seo J-J, Park S-H, Kim C-D, Kim Y-L. Health-related quality of life with KDQOL-36 and its association with self-efficacy and treatment satisfaction in Korean dialysis patients. Qual Life Res. 2012;22:753–8.

15. Boateng EA, East L. The impact of dialysis modality on quality of life: a systematic review. J Ren Care. 2011;37:190–200.

16. Weisbord SD. Patient-centered dialysis care: depression, pain, and quality of life. Semin Dial. 2016;29:158–64.

17. Purnell TS, Auguste P, Crews DC, et al. Comparison of life participation activities among adults treated by hemodialysis, peritoneal dialysis, and kidney transplantation: a systematic review. Am J Kidney Dis. 2013;62:953–73.

18. Sinnakirouchenan R, Holley JL. Peritoneal dialysis versus hemodialysis: risks, benefits, and access issues. Adv Chronic Kidney Dis. 2011;18(6):428–32.

19. Walker RC, Morton RL, Tong A, Marshall MR, Palmer S, Howard K. Patient and caregiver preferences for home dialysis--the home first study: a protocol for qualitative interviews and discrete choice experiments. BMJ Open. 2015;5(4):e007405.

20. Zazzeroni L, Pasquinelli G, Nanni E, Cremonini V, Rubbi I. Comparison of quality of life in patients undergoing hemodialysis and peritoneal dialysis: a systematic review and meta-analysis. Kidney Blood Press Res. 2017;42:717–27.

21. Lopes AA, Bragg J, Young E, Goodkin D, Mapes D, Combe C, et al. Depression as a predictor of mortality and hospitalization among hemodialysis patients in the United States and Europe. Kidney Int. 2002;62(1):199–207.

22. Major depression [Internet]. NIMH. [cited 2018 Feb 12]. Available from: www.nimh.nih.gov/health/statistics/major-depression.

23. Weisbord SD, Mor MK, Sevick MA, Shields AM, Rollman BL, Palevsky PM, Arnold RM, Green JA, Fine MJ. Associations of depressive symptoms and pain with dialysis adherence, health resource utilization, and mortality in patients receiving chronic hemodialysis. Clin J Am Soc Nephrol. 2014;9:1594–602.

24. Palmer S, Vecchio M, Craig JC, et al. Prevalence of depression in chronic kidney disease: systematic review and meta-analysis of observational studies. Kidney Int. 2013;84:179–91.

25. Vecchio M, Palmer SC, Tonelli M, Johnson DW, Strippoli GFM. Depression and sexual dysfunction in chronic kidney disease: a narrative review of the evidence in areas of significant unmet need. Nephrol Dial Transplant. 2012;27:3420–8.

26. Ch'ng AS, Chen LL, Lim SK, Poi PJ. Haemodialysis versus non-dialysis therapy among older adults with stage 5 chronic kidney disease: a comparison of health-related quality of life. Value Health. 2015;18(7):A745.

27. Chen SF, Wang IJ, Lang HC. Risk of major depression in patients with chronic renal failure on different treatment modalities: a matched-cohort and population-based study in Taiwan. Hemodial Int. 2016;20(1):98–105.

28. Ginieri-Coccossis M, Theofilou P, Synodinou C, Tomaras V, Soldatos C. Quality of life, mental health and health beliefs in haemodialysis and peritoneal dialysis patients: investigating differences in early and later years of current treatment. BMC Nephrol. 2008;9:14.

29. Su SF, Ng HY, Huang TL, Chi PJ, Lee YT, Lai CR, et al. Survey of depression by Beck Depression Inventory in uremic patients undergoing hemodialysis and hemodiafiltration. Ther Apher Dial. 2012;16(6):573–9.

30. Augustine KWC, Li YZ, Juan NH, Foo M, Mooppil N, Griva K. QOL and emotional adjustment in peritoneal dialysis vs. hemodialysis: the paradox of higher care satisfaction in peritoneal dialysis patients despite higher depression and poorer physical health. Perit Dial Int. 2010;30:S159.

31. Saeed Z, Ahmad AM, Shakoor A, Ghafoor F, Kanwal S. Depression in patients on hemodialysis and their caregivers. Saudi J Kidney Dis Transpl. 2012 Sep;23(5):946–52.

32. Simms RJ, Thong KM, Dworschak GC, Ong ACM. Increased psychosocial risk, depression and reduced quality of life living with autosomal dominant polycystic kidney disease. Nephrol Dial Transplant. 2016;31(7):1130–40.

33. Adamczak M, Wiecek A, Nowak L. High prevalence of depression in haemodialysed patients. Nephrol Dial Transplant. 2012;27:ii511.

34. Lopes AA, Lantz B, Morgenstern H, Wang M, Bieber BA, Gillespie BW, et al. Associations of self-reported physical activity types and levels with quality of life, depression symptoms, and mortality in hemodialysis patients: the DOPPS. Clin J Am Soc Nephrol. 2014;9(10):1702–12.

35. Hedayati SS, Grambow SC, Szczech LA, Stechuchak KM, Allen AS, Bosworth HB. Physician-diagnosed depression as a correlate of hospitalizations in patients receiving long-term hemodialysis. Am J Kidney Dis. 2005;46(4):642–9.

36. Farrokhi F, Abedi N, Beyene J, Kurdyak P, Jassal SV. Association between depression and mortality in patients receiving long-term dialysis: a systematic review and meta-analysis. Am J Kidney Dis. 2014;63:623–35.

37. Cukor D, Rosenthal DS, Jindal RM, Brown CD, Kimmel PL. Depression is an important contributor to low medication

adherence in hemodialyzed patients and transplant recipients. Kidney Int. 2009;75:1223–9.

38. Kimmel PL. Depression in patients with chronic renal disease: what we know and what we need to know. Journal of Psychosomatic Research. 2002;53(4):951–6.

39. Bohlke M, Nunes DL, Marini SS, Kitamura C, Andrade M, Von-Gysel MPO. Predictors of quality of life among patients on dialysis in southern Brazil. Sao Paulo Med J. 2008;126:252–6.

40. Claxton RCAN, Blackhall L, Weisbord SD, Holley JL. Undertreatment of symptoms in patients on maintenance hemodialysis. J Pain Symptom Manag. 2010;39:211–8.

41. Weisbord SD, Fried LF, Mor MK, et al. Renal provider recognition of symptoms in patients on maintenance hemodialysis. Clin J Am Soc Nephrol. 2007;2:960–7.

42. Hedayati S, Bosworth H, Kuchibhatla M, Kimmel P, Szczech L. The predictive value of self-report scales compared with physician diagnosis of depression in hemodialysis patients. Kidney Int. 2006;69:1662–88.

43. Preljevic VT, Østhus TBH, Sandvik L, Opjordsmoen S, Nordhus IH, Os I, Dammen T. Screening for anxiety and depression in dialysis patients: comparison of the Hospital Anxiety and Depression Scale and the Beck Depression Inventory. J Psychosom Res. 2012;73:139–44.

44. Loosman WL, Siegert CEH, Korzec A, Honig A. Validity of the Hospital Anxiety and Depression Scale and the Beck Depression Inventory for use in end-stage renal disease patients. Br J Clin Psychol. 2010;49:507–16.

45. Abram HS, Moore GL, Westervelt FB Jr. Suicidal behavior in chronic dialysis patients. Am J Psychiatry. 1971;127(9):1199–204.

46. Catalano C, Goodship TH, Graham KA, Marino C, Brown AL, Tapson JS, et al. Withdrawal of renal replacement therapy in Newcastle upon Tyne: 1964-1993. Nephrol Dial Transplant. 1996;11(1):133–9.

47. Kurella M, Kimmel PL, Young BS, Chertow GM. Suicide in the United States end-stage renal disease program. J Am Soc Nephrol. 2005;16(3):774–81.

48. Chen CK, Tsai YC, Hsu HJ, Wu IW, Sun CY, Chou CC, et al. Depression and suicide risk in hemodialysis patients with chronic renal failure. Psychosomatics. 2010;51(6):528–528.e6.

49. Chen I-M, Lin P-H, Wu V-C, Wu C-S, Shan J-C, Chang S-S, et al. Suicide deaths among patients with end-stage renal disease receiving dialysis: a population-based retrospective cohort study of 64,000 patients in Taiwan. J Affect Disord. 2018;227:7–10.

50. Pompili M, Venturini P, Montebovi F, Forte A, Palermo M, Lamis DA, Serafini G, Amore M, Girardi P. Suicide risk in Dialysis: review of current literature. Int J Psychiatry Med. 2013;46:85–108.

51. Loureiro ACT, Coelho MCDR, Coutinho FB, Borges LH, Lucchetti G. The influence of spirituality and religiousness on suicide risk and mental health of patients undergoing hemodialysis. Compr Psychiatry. 2018;80:39–45.

52. Keskin GCBC, Engin E. The evaluation of depression, suicidal ideation and coping strategies in haemodialysis patients with renal failure. J Clin Nurs. 2011;20(19–20):2721–32.

53. Pena-Polanco JE, Mor MK, Tohme FA, Fine MJ, Palevsky PM, Weisbord SD. Acceptance of antidepressant treatment by patients on hemodialysis and their renal providers. Clin J Am Soc Nephrol. 2017;12:298–303.

54. Hedayati SS, Gregg LP, Carmody T, Jain N, Toups M, Rush AJ, Toto RD, Trivedi MH. Effect of sertraline on depressive symptoms in patients with chronic kidney disease without dialysis dependence. JAMA. 2017;318:1876.

55. Palmer SC, Natale P, Ruospo M, Saglimbene VM, Rabindranath KS, Craig JC, Strippoli GF. Antidepressants for treating depression in adults with end-stage kidney disease treated with dialysis. Cochrane Database Syst Rev. 2016; https://doi.org/10.1002/14651858.cd004541.pub3.

56. Friedli K, Guirguis A, Almond M, et al. Sertraline versus placebo in patients with major depressive disorder undergoing hemodialysis: a randomized, controlled feasibility trial. Clin J Am Soc Nephrol. 2017;12:280–6.

57. Wuerth D, Finkelstein SH, Kliger AS, Finkelstein FO. RENAL RESEARCH INSTITUTE SYMPOSIUM: chronic peritoneal dialysis patients diagnosed with clinical depression: results of pharmacologic therapy. Semin Dial. 2003;16:424–7.

58. Koo J-R, Yoon J-Y, Joo M-H, et al. Treatment of depression and effect of antidepression treatment on nutritional status in chronic hemodialysis patients. Am J Med Sci. 2005;329:1–5.

59. Blumenfield M, Levy NB, Spinowitz B, Charytan C, Beasley CM, Dubey AK, Solomon RJ, Todd R, Goodman A, Bergstrom RF. Fluoxetine in depressed patients on Dialysis. Int J Psychiatry Med. 1997;27:71–80.

60. Cukor D, Halen NV, Asher DR, Coplan JD, Weedon J, Wyka KE, Saggi SJ, Kimmel PL. Psychosocial intervention improves depression, quality of life, and fluid adherence in hemodialysis. J Am Soc Nephrol. 2013;25:196–206.

61. Thomas ZCAB, Novak M, Platas SGT, et al. Brief mindfulness meditation for depression and anxiety symptoms in patients undergoing hemodialysis. Clin J Am Soc Nephrol. 2017;12:2008–15.

62. Cukor D, Coplan J, Brown C, Friedman S, Newville H, Safier M, et al. Anxiety disorders in adults treated by hemodialysis: a single-center study. Am J Kidney Dis. 2008;52(1):128–36.

63. Murtagh FE, Addington-Hall J, Higginson IJ. The prevalence of symptoms in end-stage renal disease: a systematic review. Adv Chronic Kidney Dis. 2007;14:82–99.

64. Cukor D, Coplan J, Brown C, Peterson RA, Kimmel PL. Course of depression and anxiety diagnosis in patients treated with hemodialysis: a 16-month follow-up. Clin J Am Soc Nephrol. 2008;3:1752–8.

65. Gerogianni G, Lianos E, Kouzoupis A, Polikandrioti M, Grapsa E. The role of socio-demographic factors in depression and anxiety of patients on hemodialysis: an observational cross-sectional study. Int Urol Nephrol. 2017; https://doi.org/10.1007/s11255-017-1738-0.

66. Feroze U, Martin D, Kalantar-Zadeh K, Kim JC, Reina-Patton A, Kopple JD. Anxiety and depression in maintenance dialysis patients: preliminary data of a cross-sectional study and brief literature review. J Ren Nutr. 2012;22:207–10.

67. Cohen SD, Cukor D, Kimmel PL. Anxiety in patients treated with hemodialysis. Clin J Am Soc Nephrol. 2016;11:2250–5.

68. Reinhold JA, Rickels K. Pharmacological treatment for generalized anxiety disorder in adults: an update. Expert Opin Pharmacother. 2015;16:1669–81.

69. Stein MB, Sareen J. Generalized anxiety disorder. N Engl J Med. 2015;373:2059–68.

70. Scherer JS, Combs SA, Brennan F. Sleep disorders, restless legs syndrome, and uremic pruritus: diagnosis and treatment of common symptoms in dialysis patients. Am J Kidney Dis. 2017;69:117–28.

71. Pierratos A, Hanly PJ. Sleep disorders over the full range of chronic kidney disease. Blood Purif. 2011;31(1–3):146–50.

72. De Santo RM, Bartiromo M, Cesare MC, Di Iorio BR. Sleeping disorders in early chronic kidney disease. Semin Nephrol. 2006;26(1):64–7.

73. Okubo R, Kondo M, Hoshi SL, Yamagata K. Cost-effectiveness of obstructive sleep apnea screening for patients with diabetes or chronic kidney disease. Sleep Breath. 2015;19(3):1081–92.

74. Novak M, Shapiro CM, Mendelssohn D, Mucsi I. Diagnosis and management of insomnia in dialysis patients. Semin Dial. 2006;19(1):25–31.

75. Markou N, Kanakaki M, Myrianthefs P, Hadjiyanakos D, Vlassopoulos D, Damianos A, et al. Sleep-disordered breath-

ing in nondialyzed patients with chronic renal failure. Lung. 2006;184(1):43–9.

76. Dikici S, Bahadir A, Baltaci D, Ankarali H, Eroglu M, Ercan N, et al. Association of anxiety, sleepiness, and sexual dysfunction with restless legs syndrome in hemodialysis patients. Hemodial Int. 2014;18(4):809–18.

77. Mcmullan CJ, Curhan GC, Forman JP. Association of short sleep duration and rapid decline in renal function. Kidney Int. 2016;89:1324–30.

78. Benz RL, Pressman MR, Hovick ET, Peterson DD. Potential novel predictors of mortality in end-stage renal disease patients with sleep disorders. Am J Kidney Dis. 2000;35:1052–60.

79. Chu G, Choi P, Mcdonald VM. Sleep disturbance and sleep-disordered breathing in hemodialysis patients. Semin Dial. 2017;31:48–58.

80. Hou Y, Hu P, Liang Y, Mo Z. Effects of cognitive behavioral therapy on insomnia of maintenance hemodialysis patients. Cell Biochem Biophys. 2014;69:531–7.

81. Jaber BL, Schiller B, Burkart JM, Daoui R, Kraus MA, Lee Y, Miller BW, Teitelbaum I, Williams AW, Finkelstein FO. Impact of short daily hemodialysis on restless legs symptoms and sleep disturbances. Clin J Am Soc Nephrol. 2011;6:1049–56.

82. Unruh ML, Larive B, Eggers PW, Garg AX, Gassman JJ, Finkelstein FO, Kimmel PL, Chertow GM. The effect of frequent hemodialysis on self-reported sleep quality: frequent hemodialysis network trials. Nephrol Dial Transplant. 2016;31:984–91.

83. Gopaluni S, Sherif M, Ahmadouk NA. Interventions for chronic kidney disease-associated restless legs syndrome. Cochrane Database Syst Rev. 2016;11:CD010690.

84. Dauvilliers Y, Benes H, Partinen M, Rauta V, Rifkin D, Dohin E, et al. Rotigotine in hemodialysis-associated restless legs syndrome: a randomized controlled trial. Am J Kidney Dis. 2016;68(3):434–43.

85. Sabbatini M, Crispo A, Pisani A, Ragosta A, Cesaro A, Mirenghi F, Cianciaruso B, Federico S. Zaleplon improves sleep quality in maintenance hemodialysis patients. Nephron Clin Pract. 2004;94:c99–c103.

86. Russcher M, Koch B, Nagtegaal E, van der Putten K, ter Wee P, Gaillard C. The role of melatonin treatment in chronic kidney disease. Front Biosci (Landmark Ed). 2012;17:2644–56.

87. Ogna A, Ogna VF, Mihalache A, et al. Obstructive sleep apnea severity and overnight body fluid shift before and after hemodialysis. Clin J Am Soc Nephrol. 2015;10:1002–10.

88. Lyons OD, Chan CT, Yadollahi A, Bradley TD. Effect of ultrafiltration on sleep apnea and sleep structure in patients with end-stage renal disease. Am J Respir Crit Care Med. 2015;191:1287–94.

89. Weiner DE, Seliger SL. Cognitive and physical function in chronic kidney disease. Curr Opin Nephrol Hypertens. 2014;23:291–7.

90. Tamura MK, Yaffe K. Dementia and cognitive impairment in ESRD: diagnostic and therapeutic strategies. Kidney Int. 2011;79:14–22.

91. Mcquillan R, Jassal SV. Neuropsychiatric complications of chronic kidney disease. Nat Rev Nephrol. 2010;6:471–9.

92. Todica O, Schwanitz A, Dalis M, Wolters N, Volsek M, Kribben A, et al. Cognitive disturbances in chronic kidney disease: cardiovascular risk factors and mood disorders as underestimated confounders. Eur J Neurol. 2010;17:212.

93. Helmer C, Stengel B, Metzger M, Froissart M, Massy Z-A, Tzourio C, Berr C, Dartigues J-F. Chronic kidney disease, cognitive decline, and incident dementia: the 3C study. Neurology. 2011;77:2043–51.

94. Kurella M, Mapes DL, Port FK, Chertow GM. Correlates and outcomes of dementia among dialysis patients: the dialysis outcomes and practice patterns study. Nephrol Dial Transplant. 2006;21:2543–8.

95. Wolfgram DF, Szabo A, Murray AM, Whittle J. Risk of Dementia in Peritoneal Dialysis Patients Compared with Hemodialysis Patients. *Peritoneal Dialysis International*. 2015;35(2):189–98. https://doi.org/10.3747/pdi.2014.00213.

96. Schneider SM, Kielstein JT, Braverman J, Novak M. Cognitive function in patients with chronic kidney disease: challenges in neuropsychological assessments. Semin Nephrol. 2015;35:304–10.

97. Tiffin-Richards FE, Costa AS, Holschbach B, et al. The montreal cognitive assessment (MoCA) – a sensitive screening instrument for detecting cognitive impairment in chronic hemodialysis patients. PLoS One. 2014; https://doi.org/10.1371/journal.pone.0106700.

98. Tholen S, Schmaderer C, Kusmenkov E, Chmielewski S, Förstl H, Kehl V, et al. Variability of cognitive performance during hemodialysis: standardization of cognitive assessment. Dement Geriatr Cogn Disord. 2014;38(1–2):31–8.

99. Vecchio M, Navaneethan SD, Johnson DW, Lucisano G, Graziano G, Querques M, et al. Treatment options for sexual dysfunction in patients with chronic kidney disease: a systematic review of randomized controlled trials. Clin J Am Soc Nephrol. 2010;5(6):985–95.

100. Varela L, Vazquez MI, Bolanos L, Alonso R. Psychological predictors for health-related quality of life in patients on peritoneal dialysis. Nefrologia. 2011;31(1):97–106.

101. Eyler RF, Unruh ML, Quinn DK, Vilay AM. Psychotherapeutic agents in end-stage renal disease. Semin Dial. 2015;28(4):417–26.

102. Knebel RJ, Rosenlicht N, Colllins L. Lithium carbonate maintenance therapy in a hemodialysis patient with end-stage renal disease. Am J Psychiatry. 2010;167(11):1409–10.

103. Bjarnason NH, Munkner R, Kampmann JP, Tornoe CW, Ladefoged S, Dalhoff K. Optimizing lithium dosing in hemodialysis. Ther Drug Monit. 2006;28(2):262–6.

104. Baghdady NT, Banik S, Swartz SA, Mcintyre RS. Psychotropic drugs and renal failure: translating the evidence for clinical practice. Adv Ther. 2009;26:404–24.

105. Bostwick JM, Cohen LM. Differentiating suicide from life-ending acts and end-of-life decisions: a model based on chronic kidney disease and Dialysis. Psychosomatics. 2009;50:1–7.

106. Murphy E, Germain MJ, Cairns H, Higginson IJ, Murtagh FE. International variation in classification of dialysis withdrawal: a systematic review. Nephrol Dial Transplant. 2013;29:625–35.

107. Maurizi Balzan J, Cartier JC, Calvino-Gunther S, Carron PL, Baro P, Palacin P, et al. Dialysis withdrawal: impact and evaluation of a multidisciplinary deliberation within an ethics committee as a shared-decision-making model. Ther Apher Dial. 2015;19(4):385–92.

108. Renal Physicians Association [Internet]. Renal Physicians Association. [cited 2018 Feb 12]. Available from: http://www.renalmd.org/.

109. Moss AH. Revised dialysis clinical practice guideline promotes more informed decision-making. Clin J Am Soc Nephrol. 2010;5:2380–3.

110. Schmidt RJ, Moss AH. Dying on dialysis: the case for a dignified withdrawal. Clin J Am Soc Nephrol. 2013;9:174–80.

History of Renal Transplantation

John D. Scandling

Introduction

Transplantation has held human imagination for millennia. Twins Cosmas and Damian, patron saints of medicine and transplantation, were early Christians who practiced medicine, and refused payment, in the Roman province of Syria. Around the turn of the fourth century, they were martyred, along with their three brothers, under the persecution of the Roman emperor Diocletian. In the early sixth century, Pope Felix IV dedicated the Basilica of Saints Cosmas and Damian, located on the Roman Forum in what was the Temple and Library of Peace, where the physician Galen lectured during the second century. In the mid-fifteenth century, the miraculous transplantation of a deacon, Justinian, was depicted by Fra Angelico in a small painting in the predella of the altarpiece in the Convent San Marco, Florence (Fig. 8.1). The saints are shown transplanting a donor leg from a deceased black man, replacing the diseased leg of Justinian, a white man.

Transplantation has long been a prominent interface of medicine and ethics. The miracle of the saints illustrates one of the first ethical inquiries at that interface, the use of a body part from one to save another.

Early Twentieth Century

Experimental transplantation dates to the turn of the twentieth century and was centered in Europe. The work of Alexis Carrel, a future Nobel Prize winner (1912), in technique of vascular anastomosis, made transplantation technically possible [1]. In 1902, experimental kidney transplantation was first attempted by Emerich Ullmann in Vienna, including autotransplantation (i.e., donor is the recipient) and allotrans-

plantation (i.e., donor is genetically dissimilar to the recipient but of the same species) in the dog and xenotransplantation (i.e., donor is of a different animal species) in a dog from a goat [2]. That year Ullmann also attempted xenotransplantation in a human, using the kidney of a pig, but failed due to technical difficulty and the anesthetic death of the donor animal [3]. In 1906, experimental kidney transplantation was done in humans, using xenografts (from pig and goat), in Lyon by Mathieu Jaboulay, one of Carrel's teachers [4]. In 1933, the first human kidney transplant using an allograft from a non-heart beating deceased donor was performed by Yurii Voronoy in Ukraine [5]. He went on to perform another five deceased donor kidney transplantations. Voronoy was the first to place the transplant kidney in the thigh with anastomoses to the femoral vessels, but this was not known to the world until some years later. During the 1930s, attention also turned to organ preservation, as Charles Lindbergh, the famed aviator, and Carrel collaborated to design a pulsatile pump to sustain organs for transplantation in vitro with perfusion fluid designed by Carrel [6].

The first "successful" human kidney transplant using a non-heart-beating deceased donor allograft occurred in Boston in 1945, performed by Ernest Landsteiner and Charles Hufnagel [7]. The transplant kidney was extracorporeal and anastomosed to the brachial vessels. The transplant was successful in that the recipient, a young woman, survived, as urine output of the native kidneys resumed within hours of the transplantation. However, the transplant kidney excreted little urine and was removed after 48 hours.

Postwar Revival

Following World War II (WWII), experimental work in clinical transplantation took hold on both sides of the Atlantic as treatment for both acute kidney injury and presumed end-stage kidney disease. Dialysis as treatment for kidney failure was in its infancy, so there was no alternative for kidney

J. D. Scandling
Division of Nephrology, Department of Medicine,
Stanford University School of Medicine, Stanford, CA, USA
e-mail: jscand@stanford.edu

© Springer International Publishing AG, part of Springer Nature 2019
Y. Sher, J. R. Maldonado (eds.), *Psychosocial Care of End-Stage Organ Disease and Transplant Patients*,
https://doi.org/10.1007/978-3-319-94914-7_8

Fig. 8.1 Healing of Deacon Justinian, 1438–1443, Fra Angelico

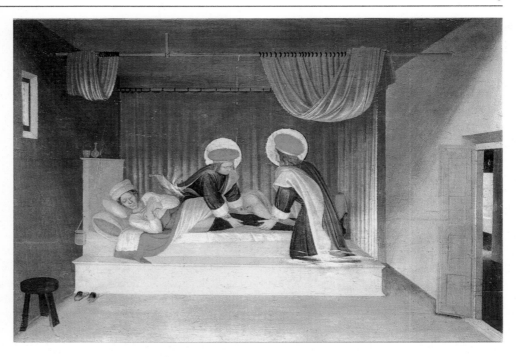

replacement therapy. There was a series of kidney transplants using deceased donor allografts performed in both Europe and North America in the early 1950s, without immunosuppression and with survival of only days to perhaps a few weeks, when the allografts succumbed to rejection. The extraperitoneal, pelvic placement of the transplant kidney originated during this time, an approach advanced by Rene Kuss in France [8]. Kuss eventually concluded that given the experience of these early attempts and the emerging understanding of immune response, "the only rational basis for kidney replacement would be between monozygotic twins."

The first live donor transplant, from a mother to son, was done in late December 1952, at the Necker Hospital in Paris by a team led by Jean Hamburger (who is thought to have coined the term nephrology) [9]. The kidney functioned initially, before its loss to rejection at 3 weeks.

The first truly successful kidney transplant was performed in late December 1954 at Peter Bent Brigham Hospital in Boston, between identical twins (Fig. 8.2) [10]. This transplantation illustrated that a donor organ could function normally in the recipient. The Brigham team was led by John Merrill, who is considered a father of American nephrology. (Nephrology was not a developed subspecialty of internal medicine at the time.) The donor surgeon was a urologist, J. Hartwell Harrison. The recipient surgeon, a plastic surgeon, Joseph Murray, was awarded the Nobel Prize in 1990 (he was the sole survivor of the original team; Nobel Prizes are not awarded posthumously). The transplantation was between 23-year-old identical twins, Ronald (donor) and Richard (recipient) Herrick. Richard died of a myocardial infarction complicating apparently recurrent kidney disease 8 years later. Ronald died in 2010, at age 79, after years of

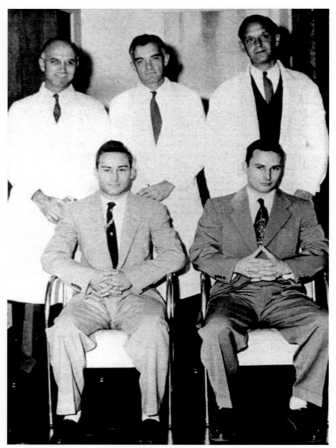

Drs. Joseph Murray (1919–2012), John P. Merrill (1917–1984) and J. Hartwell Harrison (1909–1984) Richard Herrick (recipient, 1931–1963) and Ronald Herrick (donor, 1931–2010)

Fig. 8.2 The participants in the world's first successful kidney transplantation, performed in December 1954

dialysis. Successful transplants performed through the remainder of the 1950s were between identical twins.

Paralleling the clinical experiment in kidney transplantation were advances in understanding human immunology. WWII had prompted investigation in skin grafting to treat burns. (Indeed, this was Murray's initial interest in transplantation.) The humoral mechanism of rejection of skin grafts, which had been hypothesized for some time, was furthered by the work of Thomas Gibson and Peter Medawar [11]. Ray Owen's discovery of red blood cell chimerism and immune tolerance in fraternal twin cattle [12], the theory of acquired immune tolerance of F.M. Burnet [13], and the experimental work of Rupert Billingham, Leslie Brent, and Medawar in acquired tolerance in chimeric neonatal mice [14, 15] provided the foundation of investigation in organ transplant tolerance, the "Holy Grail" of transplantation. Burnet and Medawar were awarded the Nobel Prize in 1960.

The roots of matching donor and recipient by tissue type date to 1958, when human leukocyte antigens (HLAs) were identified by Jean Dausset, another future Nobel Prize winner (1980), of the Paris team [16]. An underappreciated investigator in early HLA identification and its immunologic importance was Rose Payne of Stanford [17]. The early understanding of HLA underpinned progress in transplantation in France, as the Necker Hospital team focused on tissue typing as the key to successful transplantation.

Nonidentical Twin Transplantation

Since the early years of the twentieth century it was known that radiation had immunosuppressive properties, and in the 1950s radiation was being used for treatment of hematologic malignancy. In 1958, total body irradiation to prevent rejection was introduced in nonidentical twin transplantation, first in Boston and then in Paris [18–20]. This success with an immunosuppressive treatment opened the door to transplantation beyond identical twins. Rapid development and prompt use of immunosuppressive drugs soon followed, with cyclophosphamide and 6-mercaptopurine (6-MP) in the United Kingdom and corticosteroid in the United States. Azathioprine, the prodrug of 6-MP, was first used in Boston in 1962 by Murray and Roy Calne, who conducted the preclinical work in a dog in the United Kingdom. This resulted in the first successful deceased donor kidney transplantation, defined by recipient survival exceeding a year [21]. In 1963, Thomas Starzl, the first to perform clinical liver transplantation, introduced the use of combined therapy with azathioprine and corticosteroid to kidney transplantation [22]. The success of this combined regimen encouraged the development of transplant programs across the United States [23], and the regimen became the standard for the next two decades. During this time there was also a short revival of xenotransplantation, with a nonhuman primate as the donor.

Keith Reemtsma and colleagues achieved some short-term success in this endeavor, with recipient survival of days and up to 9 months in one case [24]. Given the limited supply of human organs for transplantation, xenotransplantation is considered by many to be the future of transplantation despite its immunologic challenge, risk of transmission of zoonoses, and potential ethical concerns.

Clinical Application

Due to the development of clinically applicable immunosuppression, the 1960s brought rapid expansion of kidney transplantation to medical centers across the United States. Chronic dialysis was in its infancy and not readily available due its technical demand and expense. It was a harrowing time. Transplantation was the only viable treatment for end-stage kidney disease, causing all effort directed to success of the transplant. Unfortunately, patients would commonly succumb to kidney failure as a consequence of rejection or infection as a consequence of immunosuppression. Nonetheless, some met with success, and some have lived decades thereafter with functioning transplant kidneys.

The 1960s brought greater understanding of transplant rejection and its mechanisms. Hyperacute rejection, wherein the transplant kidney is rejected immediately as a consequence of pre-existing antibody in the recipient, often during the transplant surgery, came to be recognized and was well described in 1968 [25]. This observation was corroborated by the work of Paul Terasaki in 1969, instituting crossmatch testing between potential donor and intended recipient as essential to transplantation [26]. Terasaki had earlier devised a microdroplet lymphocytotoxicity test, which was quickly adopted as the international standard for tissue typing [27].

The Cyclosporine Era

The 1970s saw continuation of the rapid development of immunosuppressive drugs that began a decade earlier. The most notable drug developed was cyclosporine, a calcineurin inhibitor, which would revolutionize the field and truly open the door to transplantation of organs other than the kidney. Cyclosporine was isolated from a soil fungus in 1970. Within 2 years its immunosuppressive properties were appreciated. By 1978 clinical trials of cyclosporine in transplant centers in the United States and Europe were begun. It was released for use in the United States in late 1983.

Cyclosporine is a drug with a narrow therapeutic window, frequently resulting in over- and under-immunosuppression. Indeed, there was no improvement in transplant kidney survival in the United States in the first 2 years after its release, due to the challenge of its use. Later in the decade, "triple immunosuppression," consisting of cyclosporine, azathioprine, and corticosteroid, and resulting in improved efficacy and safety, became the standard maintenance immunosuppression regimen.

Muromonab-CD3, the first monoclonal antibody, was created in 1976 and released in the United States in 1986 after its clinical utility was first reported in 1981. It would supplant antilymphocyte antibody preparations, a number of which had been developed in the 1960–1970s, and was the cornerstone of induction therapy for the next decade. (Induction therapy is given during the first days to week after transplantation, particularly to those recipients at increased risk for acute rejection.)

Understanding and knowledge of transplant immunology continued to grow. The "transfusion effect" was first described in 1973 [28], and "donor-specific" transfusion effect in living donor transplantation was described in 1980 [29]. This led to the purposeful blood transfusion of both deceased donor and living donor transplant candidates, as those who received transfusions were found to have greater acceptance of the transplant kidney. Early on after the introduction of cyclosporine, it was found that there was no transfusion effect with its use. Consequently, intentional transfusion of transplant candidates ceased and is now avoided, to reduce risk of HLA sensitization, a barrier to transplantation. (HLA sensitization limits access to transplantation by reducing the pool of potential donors for a transplant candidate. HLA sensitization occurs through blood transfusion, pregnancy, and transplantation.) The advent of epoetin in 1989 for treatment of the secondary anemia of end-stage kidney disease greatly enabled the restriction of blood transfusion in transplant candidates.

Knowledge of histocompatibility continued to advance during the 1970s, such that the overall structure of the HLA system was identified. Matching for HLA-DR loci, which are present on B cells but not T cells, was introduced to clinical transplantation in 1978. Matching for DR improved transplant kidney survival [30].

The 1970s brought the institution of chronic dialysis as a viable treatment for end-stage kidney disease in the United States. In 1972 Congress, following years of advocacy by the National Kidney Foundation, an organization with roots to 1950, passed legislation that began Medicare funding for the treatment of end-stage kidney disease. No longer did a patient have no alternatives other than transplantation or death. With the available backup of dialysis, no longer did the transplant kidney have to be saved at all costs.

Further national interest and support of transplantation followed. In 1980, brain death was established as an alternative definition of biological death (the commonly accepted definition being total failure of the cardiorespiratory system), by the Uniform Determination of Death Act drafted by the National Conference of Commissioners on Uniform State Laws [31]. The Act was approved by both the American

Medical Association (1980) and the American Bar Association (1981) and subsequently codified by all US states and the District of Columbia. Adoption of this Act across the country enabled the coming growth of deceased donor kidney transplantation, and the establishment of heart and liver transplantation, allowed by the new immunosuppressive drug, cyclosporine.

In 1984, the US Congress passed the National Organ Transplant Act, which outlawed payment for human organs for transplantation [32] (See Chap. 2 for further details). Additionally, the Act charged the Secretary of Health and Human Services with the creation of a Task Force on Organ Procurement and Transplantation to oversee transplantation. The Act also established the Organ Procurement and Transplantation Network to unite the nation's organ procurement organizations and transplant centers in their work in deceased donor organ retrieval and allocation. Since its inception, management of the OPTN has been contracted to the United Network for Organ Sharing (UNOS), based in Richmond, Virginia, and the successor to the South-Eastern Organ Procurement Foundation founded in 1975. This legislation also resulted in the creation of the Scientific Registry of Transplant Recipients, a publicly available guide to all US organ procurement organizations and organ transplant centers (www.srtr.org).

An Expanding Pharmacopeia (and the Age of Generics)

Tacrolimus, the second calcineurin inhibitor, was approved in the United States for liver transplantation in 1994 and for kidney transplantation in 1997. Within a decade it had supplanted cyclosporine as the cornerstone immunosuppressant in kidney transplantation. This occurred despite the release of modified cyclosporine in 1995, which greatly improved cyclosporine's bioavailability and thus reliability. Mycophenolate mofetil, a more specific antimetabolite, was also released in the United States in 1995 and over a number of years came to replace azathioprine. In 1998, two anti-CD25 monoclonal antibodies that inhibit interleukin-2, the humanized daclizumab and the chimeric basiliximab, were released. Within a year muromonab-CD3 as induction therapy was replaced by these two new drugs, due to their efficacy and greater safety and tolerability. However, daclizumab is no longer available, and in the United States, the use of basiliximab for induction therapy has now largely given way to rabbit antithymocyte globulin. The year of 1999 saw the release of a drug with a new mechanism of immunosuppressive action, inhibition of the mammalian target of rapamycin (mTOR). This drug is sirolimus, also known as rapamycin. Sirolimus holds appeal because it is not nephrotoxic and consequently has been studied repeatedly as an alternative to the calcineurin inhibitors. However, its efficacy and safety profiles have limited its use. A second mTOR inhibitor, everolimus, is available, but it is not in common use.

The Achilles heel of the calcineurin inhibitors is their nephrotoxicity, albeit seemingly a greater risk with cyclosporine than with tacrolimus. Given the pace of new drug development in transplantation during the 1990s, the anticipation was that a newer, safer drug would be developed with time, but this has not happened. Two drugs with new mechanisms of action and early promise, fingolimod (now used in treatment of multiple sclerosis) and tofacitinib (now used in treatment of rheumatoid arthritis), were not advanced for use in transplantation, the former due to safety concerns and the latter due to a business decision of the pharmaceutical company. Akin to sirolimus in that it is not nephrotoxic, belatacept, released in 2011 and a blocker of T-cell costimulation, is in use in maintenance immunosuppressive regimens designed to minimize and replace the calcineurin inhibitors. However, again akin to sirolimus, its efficacy and safety profiles, as well as the logistics of its parenteral administration, have limited its use.

The drugs now in common use for maintenance immunosuppression are now available in generic formulation. Generic cyclosporine was approved in 2000, and generic tacrolimus and mycophenolate mofetil were approved in 2009. Thus, the three primary drugs, tacrolimus, mycophenolate mofetil, and prednisone, are all now available as generics. With 1-year transplant kidney survival rates in the United States now at 95%, the bar to clear for entry of a new drug into the field is set very high. Future immunosuppressive drug development in transplantation is seemingly a victim of success.

These drugs have relatively narrow therapeutic windows. Thus, their use is challenging. There is no substitute for clinical experience in transplant medicine, as much of their use in practice remains art not science.

The Current State and Challenges in Kidney Transplantation

It was not until 1999 that kidney transplantation was definitely shown to be superior to dialysis as kidney replacement therapy (Fig. 8.3). Risk of death with transplantation was shown to be up to threefold greater in the first 100 days following transplant surgery but then fell to less than that in the comparator group, transplant candidates who did not undergo transplantation. Consequently, transplantation on average doubles life expectancy when compared to maintenance dialysis. This survival advantage has been shown to hold true in higher-risk transplant subgroups, including African Americans, older recipients (transplant recipients in the United States are on average almost two decades younger than dialysis patients), and those who receive organs from

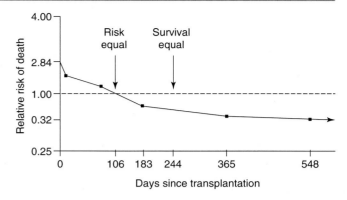

Fig. 8.3 Relative risk of death following first deceased donor kidney transplant, United States, 1991–1996. (From Wolfe et al. [34])

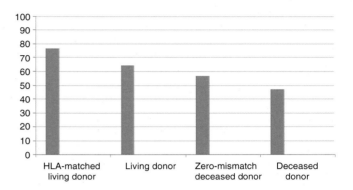

Fig. 8.4 Actuarial 10-year transplant kidney survival in US recipients transplanted during years 2005–2007. An HLA-matched living donor can only be a sibling. A zero-mismatch deceased donor does not have an HLA epitope against which the recipient has a preformed antibody. Based on OPTN data as of January 26, 2018. This work was supported in part by the Health Resources and Services Administration contract 234-2005-37011C. The content is the responsibility of the author alone and does not necessarily reflect the views or policies of the Department of Health and Human Services, nor does mention of trade names, commercial products, or organizations imply endorsement by the US Government.

less than optimal donors (recipients of organs from "expanded criteria" donors).

The success of transplantation has continued to advance over the last two decades, such that there are now over 200,000 recipients alive with functioning transplant kidneys in the United States. One-year transplant kidney survival is 95%. Ten-year transplant kidney survival is 50% for deceased donor recipients and over 60% for living donor recipients (and 75% for HLA-matched living donor recipients) (Fig. 8.4). The primary cause for the loss of a transplant kidney in the long term is death, an undesired cause as it reflects the lesser life expectancy of patients with end-stage kidney disease, but a desired cause for many patients because they do not want to return to life on maintenance dialysis.

The present-day success of transplantation is a reflection of improvements in organ retrieval, preservation, and sharing, in transplant surgical technique, in histocompatibility (a field of rapid evolution), and in immunosuppressive drugs. Transplant success also requires attentive surveillance; virtually all transplant centers now have specialized teams dedicated to the management and coordination of the multiple steps involved.

Since its description over two decades ago, the minimally invasive (laparoscopic) approach has become the standard living donor surgery. Without question, this has greatly improved donor recovery and perhaps fueled an increase in donation, but growth in living donor transplantation has stagnated over the last decade. There are now 5000-6000 living donor transplants annually in the United States. Smaller families, the aging population, and the all-important responsibility to donor safety are likely factors contributing to the plateau. Immediate family members were the traditional donors, but nowadays as many as half of living donors are not blood relatives.

So, it is a good time to be transplanted. But there are challenges. Demand far outstrips organ supply, resulting in the United States in an average waiting time of 4 years for deceased donor transplantation. The deceased donor pool has been relatively static for over a decade. Adopting "presumed consent" for deceased donation, which has resulted in an increase in donation in other countries, is unlikely in the United States. The living donor pool has also been static over the last decade, despite the growth of donor exchange. Expansion of the human organ donor pool has limits and would still not meet demand, fueling continued experimentation in xenotransplantation, which many consider the future of transplantation, and now organogenesis.

While most kidney transplant recipients enjoy excellent short- and intermediate- term success, improving long-term transplant kidney survival has proven stubborn. There are a number of threats. The primary threat is death as a consequence of extrarenal cause, whether a consequence of immunosuppression, the immunosuppressive drugs, or otherwise (chronic kidney disease carries and contributes to comorbidities already present at transplantation). A second threat is the toll of histoincompatibility over time, resulting in transplant organ loss to chronic rejection. A third threat is the contradictory use of a class of nephrotoxic drugs, the calcineurin inhibitors, as the primary immunosuppressants. A threat in the longer term is recurrent disease, usually a glomerulonephritis but also diabetic nephropathy. Recurrent glomerulonephritis is particularly vexing. De novo diabetic nephropathy is becoming more prevalent, due to post-transplant diabetes mellitus. A final category of threat to long-term success is socioeconomic. This is most evident in younger transplant recipients given the greater risk of nonadherence in the second (teenage) and third (twenty-something) decades. The immunosuppressive drugs are expensive; inadequate medical insurance can lead to medication nonadherence at any age. Complete rehabilitation following transplantation, with

return to full engagement in work and personal life, can be a challenge. For some, moving from the medically insured and social safety net of the dialysis unit to the relative freedom of transplantation is difficult.

Federal regulatory oversight came to transplantation in the United States in the 1980s and has increased over the ensuing decades. Regulation initially pertained to deceased donor transplantation, directed at systematic organization of organ retrieval, and justice and utility in organ allocation. It has been an evolutionary process, responding to both public and professional input, and now encompassing living donor transplantation as well. The regulatory environment has arguably resulted in transplantation being the most transparent of medical disciplines. All US transplant centers are required to submit data on all transplantations to the federal agency with oversight responsibility. The data are collated, analyzed, and reported on a semiannual basis in transplant program-specific reports (www.srtr.org). While most would agree that this transparency has been for the good, some argue that it has resulted in risk aversion, manifest as reduced use of higher-risk donor organs and reduced access for high-risk transplant candidates, and is a threat to innovation.

Short of solving the overarching challenge of organ shortage, there is opportunity in the nearer term for improvement that may extend transplant life. Areas of focus include ischemia-reperfusion injury, immune monitoring, and immune tolerance. Ischemic-reperfusion injury is a stubborn problem, resulting in delayed function of the transplant kidney in approximately 25% of deceased donor transplants, measured as need for supportive dialysis during the first week following transplantation. This injury compromises both function and survival of the transplant kidney over time. Immune monitoring holds great appeal to transplant recipients and physicians alike, as reliable biomarkers could theoretically allow true tailoring of the immunosuppressive drugs to avoid over- and under-immunosuppression, an attractive goal in this nascent era of precision medicine. Immune tolerance, wherein transplantation is successful without need for long-term maintenance immunosuppression, is becoming reality in a small number of clinical trials. Advances in all these areas should extend transplant life, perhaps even achieving the laudable goal of "one transplant for life" [33].

References

1. Carrel A. La technique operatoire des anastomoses vasculaires et la transplantation des visceres. Lyon Med. 1902;98:859.
2. Ullman E. Experimentelle nierentransplantation. Wien Klin Wochenschr. 1902;11:281–5.
3. Ullman E. Tissue and organ transplantation. Ann Surg. 1914;60:195–219.
4. Jaboulay M. Greffe de reins au pli de coude par soudures artérielles et veineuses. Lyon Med. 1906;107:575–7.

5. Voronoy Y. Sobre el bloqueo del aparato reticuloendotelial del hombre en algunas formas de intoxicacion por el sublimado y sobre la transplantacion del rinon cadaverico como metodo de tratamiento de la anuria consecutive a aquella intoxicacion. Siglo Med. 1936;97:296–7.
6. Redman E. To save his dying sister-in-law, Charles Lindbergh invented a medical device. Smithsonian.com. September 9, 2015.
7. Hume DM, Merrill JP, Miller BF, Thorn GW. Experiences with renal homotransplantations in the human: report of nine cases. J Clin Invest. 1955;34:327–82.
8. Kuss R, Teinturier J, Milliez P. Quelques essais de greffe de rein chez l'homme. Mem Acad de Chir. 1951;77:755–64.
9. Michon L, Hamburger J, Oeconomos N, Delinotte P, Richet G, Vaysse J, Antoine B. Un etentative de transplantation renale chez l'homme: aspects medicaux et biologique. Presse Med. 1953;61:1419–23.
10. Merrill JP, Murray JE, Harrison JH, Guild WR. Successful homotransplantation of the human kidney between identical twins. JAMA. 1956;160:277–82.
11. Gibson T, Medawar PB. The fate of skin homografts in man. J Anat. 1943;77:299–310.
12. Owen RD. Immunogenetic consequences of vascular anastomoses between bovine twins. Science. 1945;102:400–1.
13. Burnet FM, Fenner F. The production of antibodies. Melbourne: Macmillan; 1949.
14. Billingham RE, Brent L, Medawar PB. 'Actively acquired tolerance' of foreign cells. Nature. 1953;172:603–6.
15. Billingham RE, Brent L, Medawar PB. Quantitative studies on tissue transplantation immunity. III Actively acquired tolerance. Phil Trans R Soc Lond B. 1956;239:357–414.
16. Dausset J. Iso-leuco-anticorps. Acta Haematol. 1958;20:156–66.
17. Payne R. Leukocyte agglutinins in human sera: correlation between blood transfusions and their development. AMA Arch Intern Med. 1957;99:587–606.
18. Murray JE, Merrill JP, Dammin GJ, Dealy JB Jr, Alexandre GW, Harrison JH. Kidney transplantation in modified recipients. Ann Surg. 1962;156:337–55.
19. Hamburger J, Vaysse J, Crosnier J, Auvert J, Lalanne CM, Hopper J Jr. Renal homotransplantation in man after radiation of the recipient: experience with six patients since 1959. Am J Med. 1962;32:854–71.
20. Kuss R, Legrain M, Mathe G, Nedey R, Camey M. Homologous human kidney transplantation: experience with six patients. Postgrad Med J. 1962;38:528–31.
21. Murray JE, Merrill JP, Harrison JH, Wilson RE, Dammin GJ. Prolonged survival of human-kidney homografts by immunosuppressive drug therapy. N Engl J Med. 1963;268:1315–23.
22. Starzl TE, Marchioro TL, Waddell WR. The reversal of rejection in human renal homografts with subsequent development of homograft tolerance. Surg Gynecol Obstet. 1963;117:385–95.
23. Barker CF, Markmann JF. Historical overview of transplantation. Cold Spring Harb Perspect Med. 2013;3:a014977.
24. Reemtsma K, McCracken BH, Schlegel JU, Pearl MA, Pearce CW, DeWitt CW, Smith PE, Hewitt RL, Flinner RL, Creech O Jr. Renal heterotransplantation in man. Ann Surg. 1964;160:384–410.
25. Williams GM, Hume DM, Hudson RP Jr, Morris PJ. Hyperacute renal-homograft rejection in man. N Engl J Med. 1968;279:611–8.
26. Patel R, Terasaki PI. Significance of the positive crossmatch test in kidney transplantation. N Engl J Med. 1969;280:735–9.
27. Terasaki PI, McClelland JD. Microdroplet assay of human serum cytotoxins. Nature. 1964;204:998–1000.
28. Opelz G, Sengar DP, Mickey MR, Terasaki PI. Effect of blood transfusions on subsequent kidney transplants. Transplant Proc. 1973;5:253–9.
29. Salvatierra O Jr, Vincenti F, Amend W, Potter D, Iwaki Y, Opelz G, Terasaki P, Duca R, Cochrum K, Hanes D, Stoney RJ, Feduska NJ. Deliberate donor-specific blood transfusions prior to living related renal transplantation. A new approach. Ann Surg. 1980;192:543–52.
30. Ting A, Morris P. Matching for B-cell antigens of the HLA-DR series in cadaver renal transplantation. Lancet. 1978;311:575–7.
31. Delmonico FL. The concept of death and deceased organ donation. Int J Organ Transplant Med. 2010;1:15–20.
32. United States. National Organ Transplant Act: Public Law 98-507. US Statut Large. 1984;98:2339–48.
33. Montgomery RA. One kidney for life. Am J Transplant. 2014;14:1473–4.
34. Wolfe RA, Ashby VB, Milford EL, Ojo AO, Ettenger RE, Agodoa LY, Held PJ, Port FK. Comparison of mortality in all patients on dialysis, patients on dialysis awaiting transplantation, and recipients of a first cadaveric transplant. N Engl J Med. 1999;341:1725–30.

Medical Course and Complications After Renal Transplantation

Aleah Brubaker, Dan Stoltz, and Amy Gallo

Introduction

Kidney transplantation can be life changing for many patients. As medical and surgical care has evolved, the pre-operative, perioperative, and postoperative course can be fairly predictable and standardized for most patients. However, complexities remain as multifactorial details determine outcomes in each particular case. Varying donor and recipient factors influence a patient's course tremendously. Serious complications are rare but can be devastating when they occur, both medically and psychologically. Successful transplantation requires frequent evaluation and meticulous attention to details, often making patients feel that they have traded one disease for another. This chapter outlines the fundamentals of kidney transplantation including pre-transplant factors that play a role in the postoperative management, specifics of the transplant hospital course, and a typical outpatient medical regimen.

The Kidney Transplant

Scheduling the Transplant

In the majority of kidney transplants, the medical course begins without warning when a suitable deceased donor organ becomes available. Frequently the potential recipient receives a phone call in the middle of the night after waiting 8 or more years, with less than three total appointments with the transplant center, and is told to pack their belongings to

relocate for months. Once admitted, if a donor organ does not meet the expectations extrapolated from the donor history or provided by the donor surgeon, the transplant team will ask the candidate to return home until another more suitable offer becomes available.

Living donor kidney recipients have more preparation time but can also be plagued by false starts depending on lab variations or common colds that increase operative risk factors and subsequently require rescheduling. Ideally a transplant center optimized both the donor and recipient for the elective surgery. If a recipient has a living donor that is incompatible, the pair may enter a national kidney swap where a recipient can acquire another living donor kidney in exchange for their incompatible living donor kidney. In reality, this is often a chain of transplants traveling throughout the United States. If a single recipient or donor within the chain has a complication halting the transplant, all transplants are often canceled.

This process can be psychologically difficult and tiring for patients. Long wait times, repeated phone calls to check-in for a potential donor, and the hope that a chain donation will come to fruition can all lead to mental exhaustion for patients that are very hopeful for transplantation to be their answer to daily dialysis.

Donor Quality

On average, a deceased donor kidney has a half-life of 12 years [1], but each individual deceased donor kidney may have a different expected survival based on donor characteristics. The Kidney Donor Profile Index (KDPI) is a value assigned to a deceased donor kidney to summarize its quality compared to other offered grafts. The KDPI is based on the Kidney Donor Risk Index (KDRI), ten characteristics that help to predict the risk of graft failure (Table 9.1). KPDI scores range from 1% to 100%, with higher scores indicating greater graft failure risk and decreased graft longevity. A kidney with a score of 99% has a graft failure risk greater than 99% of all kidney donors recovered the year prior and a

A. Brubaker · D. Stoltz
Department of General Surgery, Stanford University School of Medicine, Stanford, CA, USA
e-mail: abrubake@stanford.edu; djstoltz@stanford.edu

A. Gallo (✉)
Division of Abdominal Transplantation, Department of General Surgery, Stanford University School of Medicine, Stanford, CA, USA
e-mail: agallo@stanford.edu

© Springer International Publishing AG, part of Springer Nature 2019
Y. Sher, J. R. Maldonado (eds.), *Psychosocial Care of End-Stage Organ Disease and Transplant Patients*,
https://doi.org/10.1007/978-3-319-94914-7_9

25.9% 8-year survival rate. Comparatively, a score of 1% has a graft failure risk greater than only 1% of recovered kidneys and with a 72.2% 8-year survival. While the KDPI is a helpful tool to access organs, other donor details, anatomic variations, and organ visualization provide additional valuable information about a particular kidney.

Surgery

A kidney transplant is a major operation, lasting approximately 3 hours. From initiation of general anesthesia, placement of adequate intravenous access, and a Foley catheter into the bladder, the total operative time is about 5 hours. The

Table 9.1 Donor characteristics that are used to calculate KDRI

Age
Height
Weight
Ethnicity
History of hypertension
History of diabetes
Cause of death
Serum creatinine
Hepatitis C virus status
Donation after circulatory death (DCD) status

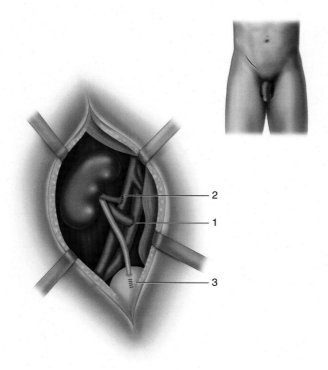

Fig. 9.1 An illustration of a kidney transplant incision, the three typical surgical anastomoses and the order in which they are performed: (**1**) the donor renal vein to the recipient external iliac vein, (**2**) the donor renal artery to the recipient external iliac artery, (**3**) the donor ureter to the recipient bladder

donor kidney has three major connections to the recipient, the artery, vein, and ureter (Fig. 9.1). In adult transplant recipients, the vascular connection is commonly to the external iliac artery and vein. A sutured anastomosis connects the donor ureter to the recipient bladder for drainage.

Ceasing Dialysis

Patients routinely have the expectation that they will cease dialysis post-transplantation. However, 57% of deceased donor kidney transplants result in delayed graft function (DGF) [2]. The definition of DGF is the requirement of dialysis during the first week following transplant. The majority of transplant recipients with DGF will require dialysis for weeks to months but will eventually cease dialysis. However, approximately 10% will remain with primary graft nonfunction (PNF). Organ cold times, or the time the organ is on ice, donor quality, and recipient factors are the most common explanations for DGF or PNF. Patients with PNF out to three months' post-transplant can reclaim their accumulated pre-transplant waiting times for re-listing, but they must remain on immunosuppression, unless they undergo a transplant nephrectomy.

Postoperative Course

Immunosuppression

Details of immunosuppression regimens are often center-specific, but the majority of patients undergo induction immunosuppression followed by maintenance immunosuppression. Immunosuppression regimens are also tailored based on each patient's risk stratification. High-risk patients, including those with multiple human leukocyte antigen (HLA) mismatches, high panel reactive antibody (PRA), positive donor-specific antibodies (DSA), prolonged cold ischemia time, African-American ethnicity, young recipients of older donor organs, and blood group incompatibility, may undergo more intensive induction and/or maintenance regimens [3]. Induction immunosuppression acts to depress the immune system more dramatically, is started during or immediately following transplant to prevent early acute rejection, and allows for reduction in maintenance medications. Common induction agents include antithymocyte globulin (ATG), rituximab, intravenous immunoglobulin (IVIG), basiliximab, and high-dose glucocorticoids.

Maintenance immunosuppression is generally long-term immunotherapy to minimize graft rejection and prevent allograft loss. This must be delicately balanced with toxicity, infection, and malignancy that can occur if dosing is supratherapeutic or overall immunosuppression burden is too high. Typical regimens include a calcineurin inhibitor (i.e., cyclosporine, tacrolimus), an antimetabolite (i.e., mycophenolate mofetil, azathioprine), glucocorticoids (e.g., prednisone), and mammalian target of rapamycin (mTOR) inhibitors (i.e., sirolimus, everolimus). Calcineurin inhibitors (CNIs) can be nephrotoxic at high doses. Additional side effects include headache, altered mental status, insomnia, tremor, diabetes, diarrhea, emesis, alopecia, and hypertension. Antimetabolites cause dose-related bone marrow suppression, persistent diarrhea, abdominal cramping, nausea, and hepatitis. Glucocorticoids are known to cause a variety of side effects when used for an extended duration, such as osteoporosis, hypertension, cardiac remodeling, hyperlipidemia, and diabetes. Some centers attempt to use reduced doses or wean completely off glucocorticoids to minimize these effects. mTOR inhibitors are less common as first-line agents in maintenance immunosuppression regimens as they interfere with wound healing, but are often used for patients that develop CNI toxicity or intolerance.

Particularity important for non-transplant providers caring for transplant recipients is understanding medication interactions. For neurologists and psychiatrists, anticonvulsants including barbiturates, carbamazepine, and phenytoin induce hepatic clearance and reduce CNI levels. mTOR inhibitors may mildly affect aripiprazole and clozapine. St. John's wort can decrease everolimus concentrations, and concomitant use is not recommended. These interactions are further discussed in Chap. 42.

Immediate Postoperative Complications

Bleeding and Hemorrhage

As with all operations, bleeding and hemorrhage can occur after renal transplantation. Inadequate hemostasis in the setting of uremia can cause ongoing bleeding. A less common etiology for postoperative bleeding is fracture of the allograft parenchyma. This can occur due to allograft swelling secondary to acute rejection. As the transplanted kidney is usually placed in the retroperitoneum, bleeding is usually limited by the size of the retroperitoneal space. Patients will complain of flank pain and may have a brisk hematocrit drop. If there is significant compression of the kidney, they may present with normotension or hypertension, rather than the expected hypotension. Evacuation of the hematoma is necessary if there is significant graft compression, evidence of graft compromise, or infection [4, 5].

Vascular Complications

Arterial or venous thrombosis is much less common, but can cause serious graft compromise in the early postoperative period. The most common cause of inflow or outflow obstruction is kinking of the vascular pedicle due to graft position. Technical anastomotic errors and clamping can also cause

intraluminal narrowing or thrombosis. Arterial thrombosis may also be secondary to acute rejection. A brisk decline in urine output in a patient that was previously diuresing well should be an early clue to an inflow or outflow problem. Patients may also develop hematuria, graft pain, and increasing serum creatinine. Duplex ultrasound can help in diagnosis. Rapid surgical correction is usually required to preserve the graft [4]. Occasionally, patients may develop iliofemoral thrombosis without extension into the renal vein. This can be treated as a standard deep venous thrombosis with anticoagulation.

Urologic Complications

Following renal transplant, 2–9% of patients may develop urinary obstruction and 1–5% may develop a urine leak [4]. Urinary obstruction is most often related to poor vascular supply at the ureteroneocystostomy, eventually leading to stricture and discussed in more detail below. Obstruction may also be related to kinking from graft position or compression from a perinephric fluid collection, requiring either surgical repositioning, surgical drainage, or radiologic drainage. Patients with a urine leak will often present with swelling and pain within the first week following transplant. Urine leak in the early postoperative period is related to a technical failure at the ureteroneocystostomy. Diagnosis is made by sampling the surgical drain fluid and testing fluid creatinine. Fluid creatinine higher than serum creatinine is diagnostic. If the surgical drain was not placed or has been removed, image-guided fluid sampling by interventional radiology can be performed.

Lymphocele

Division of the recipient's lymphatics overlying the iliac vessel occurs routinely during renal transplant. Lymphatic leaks leading to a lymphocele can occur in upward of 18% of transplant recipients [4] and only require intervention if they are symptomatic (e.g., compression, pain). Simple aspiration is associated with high rates of recurrence. Definitive management requires drainage in conjunction with sclerotherapy or surgical marsupialization. Sclerotherapy uses chemical irritation, often ethanol, to collapse or scar the lymphatics. Marsupialization is the more commonly used approach, where the lymphocele is laparoscopically located from the abdominal cavity, and the peritoneum is fenestrated to allow for intraperitoneal drainage.

Wound Infection

Wound infection remains a common problem following transplant, with 1–10% of patients developing a postoperative wound infection [6]. Preoperative antibiotics are administered to minimize this risk. Transplant patients are at heightened risk given the high levels of immunosuppression and steroid use in the perioperative window. Diabetes and obesity further elevate a patient's risk.

Typical Hospital Course and Discharge

Depending on the graft and recipient, some patients make urine almost immediately. Others demonstrate delayed graft function and may require some duration of dialysis. For our purposes here, we will focus on the hospital course for patients with immediate graft function and cessation of dialysis.

Following renal transplant, the patient will leave the operating room with a Foley catheter and surgical drain in place. The patient is typically started on a clear liquid diet on the night of postoperative day 0 but maintained on intravenous fluids. Urine output is monitored closely. Replacement fluids with bicarbonate are started if the patient is making more than 200 mL of urine per hour. If urine output is marginal, patency of the Foley is ensured, and the patient's volume status is assessed to decide additional clinical management.

Timing and administration of induction immunosuppression is dependent of the degree of sensitization and can affect the duration of hospital stay. Patients with a PRA less than 25% or a haplotype match living-related transplant are at low immunologic risk, do not necessitate induction therapy, and are started on maintenance immunosuppression on postoperative day 0. Highly sensitized patients (>25% PRA) undergo thymoglobulin induction for approximately 3–5 days. Induction therapy may be started as early as postoperative day 0. Patients on an immunosuppression regimen including steroids either undergo a rapid taper with intravenous solumedrol or a standard taper with 3 days of intravenous solumedrol followed by a slow outpatient taper of oral prednisone.

On postoperative day 1, a renal ultrasound may be ordered based on surgeon preference or if there is concern for delayed graft function. Generally, the patient is advanced to a regular diet and started on oral pain medications. Antibiotics and intravenous fluids are generally continued until postoperative day 2. The Foley catheter is removed on postoperative day 2 or 3. The surgical drain is removed after the Foley catheter is discontinued to ensure that once the bladder is no longer decompressed, a urinoma does not develop. The majority of patients are able to be discharged home between postoperative days 3–5, once their pain is adequately controlled with oral medications, they are tolerating a regular diet, and are voiding independently without the Foley catheter. Some patients may require a longer hospital course for their immunosuppression induction.

Post-transplant Course

Frequency of Office Visits and Blood Draws

Following kidney transplantation, patients are followed by a transplant specialist to monitor allograft function and minimize immunosuppression side effects such as infection, malignancy, diabetes, and cardiovascular disease. A typical schedule involves clinic visits twice weekly for the first month post-transplant, weekly for the second month, every 2 weeks for the third month, and every 2 months for the remainder of the first-year post-transplant. The type and frequency of laboratory testing also varies among transplant centers. A typical monitoring scheme is shown in Table 9.2.

Complications

Rejection and Graft Loss

Acute rejection is a major cause of allograft dysfunction and is generally associated with a reduction in long-term allograft survival. Acute rejection can be broadly classified into T-cell-mediated (cellular) rejection (TCMR) and antibody-mediated rejection (ABMR). Both may coexist simultaneously. Allogeneic risk factors for acute rejection include the presence of DSAs or a high PRA, a higher degree of HLA

Table 9.2 A representative medical schedule of a kidney transplant recipient

	Month 1	Month 2	Months 3–4	Months 4–6	Months 6–12	>1 year
Labs	2×/week	Weekly	Every 2 weeks	Every 2 weeks	Monthly	Every 1–2 months
Clinic	2×/week	Weekly	Every 2 weeks	Months 4 and 6	Months 8, 10, and 12	Months 18 and 24 and then yearly
Driving	2 weeks or off pain meds					
Travel			Local		Out of state <2 weeks	Out of country >2 weeks
Return to work		X				
Eye exam				X		
Dental exam				X		
Flu shot						Yearly
Pneumovax						Every 2–3 years

mismatches, and blood group incompatibility [7, 8]. Patients with a previous episode of rejection, history of a previous transplant, or issues with medication nonadherence are also at increased risk. Nonadherence aside, the majority of acute rejection episodes occur within the first 6 months. The majority of patients are asymptomatic, other than an acute rise in serum creatinine, which tends to occur relatively late in the course of a rejection episode. When symptoms are present, they may include fever, malaise, oliguria, and graft discomfort. Hypertension, pyuria or proteinuria may also be present. The standard for the diagnosis of rejection is a renal allograft biopsy. Treatment depends on the type and severity of the acute rejection episode. Generally, TCMR is treated with pulse high-dose intravenous glucocorticoids followed by an oral glucocorticoid taper, augmentation of maintenance immunosuppression, and rabbit antithymocyte globulin if necessary. ABMR is typically treated with a combination of pulse high-dose intravenous glucocorticoids followed by an oral glucocorticoid taper, plasmapheresis, IVIG, augmentation of maintenance immunosuppression, and rituximab as needed.

While short-term allograft loss has significantly improved in recent decades, long-term allograft loss remains a significant issue in kidney transplantation. In 2005, 10-year graft failure for deceased donor transplants was 52.8%, while 10-year graft failure for living donor transplants was 37.3%. Etiologies of graft loss change with the time of presentation after kidney transplantation. Surgical complications are more commonly seen in the immediate post-transplant period, while graft loss secondary to infection or recurrent disease tends to present later. Some causes, such as rejection, can occur at any time after transplant. Numerous risk prediction models have identified many risk factors for long-term graft loss, including graft cold ischemia time, cadaveric donor, delayed graft function, a higher degree of HLA mismatching, preformed or de novo DSAs, nonadherence, cytomegalovirus (CMV) seropositivity, acute rejection, and recurrent glomerular disease [9].

Urinary Tract Infections

Urinary tract infection (UTI) is the most common infectious complication after kidney transplant, with reported rates as high as 80% [10]. Risk factors include receiving a cadaveric allograft, female sex, diabetes mellitus, and ureteral stent placement [11]. Uncomplicated UTIs typically present with local urinary symptoms (dysuria, frequency, urgency), while complicated UTIs can present with fever, chills, malaise, and allograft pain. Urinalysis is often positive for leukocyte esterase and nitrites, while urine microscopy can show pyuria. A positive urine culture establishes the diagnosis. The majority of UTIs are caused by gram-negative uropathogens. Though antibacterial prophylaxis has decreased the incidence of UTIs, it has also led to increased rates of resistant organisms. Timely diagnosis and treatment is crucial, as UTIs are associated with acute cellular rejection, impaired allograft function, allograft loss, and death [12].

Ureteric Strictures

Ureteric strictures are a common urological complication following renal transplant, with an incidence of 1–3% [13, 14]. The majority of strictures occur within the first several months after transplantation and are most frequently located near the distal portion of the ureter. Common etiologies include technical issues related to the ureter implantation, ischemia of the ureter secondary to disruption of its blood supply, allograft rejection, and infection [15]. Patients may be asymptomatic with normal serum creatinine levels and adequate urine output until the stricture progresses to an advanced stage. Proximal dilation of the urinary collection system may be appreciated on imaging studies. Significant ureteral strictures are initially treated with minimally invasive percutaneous or endoscopic stenting before attempting open surgical reconstruction. Prompt and effective treatment is critical to prevent negative impact on graft survival.

BK Virus

BK virus is a human polyomavirus named after the initials of the index patient diagnosed with the virus. Most BK primary infections are asymptomatic, though the virus establishes latency in the kidney and urinary tract of healthy individuals and can manifest as BK viremia or BK virus nephropathy months to years after kidney transplant [16]. The incidence of BK virus nephropathy ranges from 1% to 10% [17]. The strongest risk factor for progression is the cumulative immunosuppression burden. A majority of transplant centers focus on polymerase chain reaction (PCR)-based screening techniques, though timing and testing methodologies are not standardized. Diagnosis requires renal transplant biopsy. Currently, there is no effective pharmacologic prophylaxis or treatment for BK viremia or BK virus nephropathy. Reduction of immunosuppression is typically initiated upon a diagnosis of BK nephropathy [16], though this can result in rejection or formation of DSAs, both of which can threaten long-term allograft survival. The mean incidence of allograft loss secondary to BK virus nephropathy is approximately 45% [17] but can vary widely depending on the center-specific screening and intervention protocols.

Cytomegalovirus

CMV is the most prevalent opportunistic infection after kidney transplant. Approximately 60% of patients will have an active CMV infection and 20% will develop symptomatic disease [18, 19]. Infection occurs by endogenous reactivation in the recipient, transmission via the donor allograft or by acquiring a new infection from the general population. The incidence of CMV infection and associated complications is highly contingent upon the serostatus of the donor-recipient pair, with CMV-seronegative recipients who receive a kidney from a CMV-seropositive donor having the highest risk [20]. Clinically, CMV infection can present as three entities: asymptomatic viremia, CMV viral syndrome (i.e., fever, malaise, arthralgia, and leukopenia), and CMV tissue-invasive disease (i.e., CMV present on tissue biopsy specimen accompanied by end-organ damage such as nephritis, colitis, hepatitis, pneumonitis, or retinitis). In all cases, laboratory confirmation, typically via PCR, is required for a diagnosis. The two principal strategies to prevent CMV disease are preemptive therapy based on routine CMV PCR monitoring and general antiviral prophylaxis following transplant. Both are equally effective, though prophylaxis is recommended in CMV-seropositive donors/CMV-seronegative recipient pairs. Active CMV disease treatment requires reduction of immunosuppression and/or initiation of an antiviral agent.

EBV/PTLD

Epstein-Barr virus (EBV) is a γ-herpesvirus transmitted via direct person-to-person contact, primarily through saliva. Most immunocompetent individuals do not demonstrate EBV-associated disease after primary infection, though in kidney transplant recipients, EBV is associated with post-transplantation lymphoproliferative disorder (PTLD) [21]. The cumulative incidence of PTLD in kidney transplant recipients ranges from 1% to 5%. Risk factors include cumulative immunosuppression burden (principally T-cell suppression) and EBV-seronegative recipients who receive a kidney from an EBV-seropositive donor [22]. Routine EBV monitoring is recommended for these patients. Patients with PTLD have highly variable clinical presentations. Constitutional symptoms such as fatigue, fever, and weight loss are typical. Other symptoms may be related to dysfunction of involved organs including the gastrointestinal tract, lungs, liver, central nervous system, skin, and the kidney allograft. Diagnosis relies on tissue biopsy and imaging studies for localization and staging. Management depends on the type of lymphoproliferative disease but commonly involves immunosuppression reduction and rituximab. Chemotherapy, radiation therapy or surgery may also be offered if necessary. Prognosis depends on the type and stage of the malignancy.

Skin Cancer

Morbidity and mortality secondary to skin cancer are dramatically increased in kidney transplant recipients. Chronic immunosuppression regimens can have direct carcinogenic effects and promote proliferation of oncogenic viruses. Risk factors include the intensity and duration of immunosuppression, sun exposure, and a past history of skin cancer. Squamous cell carcinoma (SCC) and basal cell carcinoma (BCC) account for the majority of skin cancers in kidney transplant recipients [23]. Contrary to the general population, SCC is more common in immunosuppressed transplant recipients that BCC. The natural course of SCC in kidney transplant recipients is often aggressive with local invasion, early recurrence following treatment, higher rates of metastases, and increased mortality [24]. Though rare, melanoma, cutaneous lymphoma, and Kaposi sarcoma are also found at higher rates compared to the general population [25]. Skin biopsy is a crucial component in establishing a diagnosis and prognosis.

Nonadherence

Nonadherence by kidney transplant recipients manifests as a range of behaviors, such as not completing laboratory work, missing scheduled outpatient appointments, and not taking prescribed medications. Nonadherent patients are seven times more likely to suffer graft failure when compared to patients who are adherent [26]. The etiology of nonadherence is multifactorial, though the strongest risk factor is prior nonadherence. Sociodemographic factors (e.g., minority ethnicity, low socioeconomic status) and patient-related psychosocial factors (e.g., low health literacy, poor social support) also play an important role [27]. Treatment-related factors (e.g., multiple medications, side effects) and health system factors (e.g., access to care, insurance status, poor reinforcement by healthcare providers) can also negatively impact adherence [27].

Disease Recurrence

Recurrence of primary renal disease is a significant cause of allograft dysfunction and loss after kidney transplantation. Primary glomerular renal diseases such as membranoproliferative glomerulonephritis (MPGN), focal segmental glomerulosclerosis (FSGS), primary membranous nephropathy, and hemolytic uremic syndrome have the highest propensity to recur and induce allograft loss [28] (Also see Chap. 5 for more details). Late recurrence can be seen with many systemic diseases, including diabetic nephropathy. In all cases of suspected recurrence, renal transplant biopsy is required for diagnosis. Individuals seeking a re-transplant account for 12.5% of patients on the adult kidney waitlist in the United States [29]. Allograft survival in kidney re-transplant recipients is inferior to first-time kidney transplant recipients when controlling donor factors [30].

Conclusions

Kidney transplant not only extends life expectancy compared to dialysis, but it can also significantly improve quality of life. These benefits will only be appreciated if patients have a successful operative and postoperative course. Acknowledging and understanding potential pitfalls help to ensure successful outcomes.

References

1. Matas AJ, Kandaswamy R, Dunn TB, Payne WD, Sutherland DER, Humar A. NIH public access. Transplantation. 2009;49(18):1841–50. https://doi.org/10.1016/j.jacc.2007.01.076.White.

2. Taber DJ, DuBay D, McGillicuddy JW, et al. Impact of the new kidney allocation system on perioperative outcomes and costs in kidney transplantation. J Am Coll Surg. 2017;224(4):585–92. https://doi.org/10.1016/j.jamcollsurg.2016.12.009.

3. Kasiske BL, Zeier MG, Craig JC, et al. Kidney Disease: Improving Global Outcomes (KDIGO) Transplant Work Group. Journal A. Special issue: KDIGO clinical practice guideline for the care of kidney transplant recipients. Am J Transplant 2009;9(Suppl 3):S1–155. https://doi.org/10.1111/j.1600-6143.2009.02834.x.

4. Hedegard W, Saad WEA, Davies MG. Management of vascular and nonvascular complications after renal transplantation. Tech Vasc Interv Radiol. 2009;12(4):240–62. https://doi.org/10.1053/j.tvir.2009.09.006.

5. Richard HM. Perirenal transplant fluid collections. Semin Intervent Radiol. 2004;21(4):235–7. https://doi.org/10.1055/s-2004-861557.

6. Mehrabi A, Fonouni H, Wente M, et al. Wound complications following kidney and liver transplantation. Clin Transpl. 2006;20(s17):97–110. https://doi.org/10.1111/j.1399-0012.2006.00608.x.

7. Aubert O, Loupy A, Hidalgo L, et al. Antibody-mediated rejection due to preexisting versus De Novo donor-specific antibodies in kidney allograft recipients. J Am Soc Nephrol. 2017;28(6):1912–23. https://doi.org/10.1681/ASN.2016070797.

8. Higgins RM, Daga S, Mitchell DA. Antibody-incompatible kidney transplantation in 2015 and beyond. Nephrol Dial Transplant. 2015;30(12):1972–8. https://doi.org/10.1093/ndt/gfu375.

9. Kaboré R, Haller MC, Harambat J, Heinze G, Leffondré K. Risk prediction models for graft failure in kidney transplantation: a systematic review. Nephrol Dial Transplant. 2017;32:ii68–76. https://doi.org/10.1093/ndt/gfw405.

10. Hollyer I, Ison MG. The impact of urinary tract infections in renal transplant recipients. Transpl Infect Dis. 2018;78(8):719–21. https://doi.org/10.1038/ki.2010.219.

11. Lee JR, Bang H, Dadhania D, et al. Independent risk factors for urinary tract infection and for subsequent bacteremia or acute cellular rejection: a single-center report of 1166 kidney allograft recipients. Transplantation. 2013;96(8):732–8. https://doi.org/10.1097/TP.0b013e3182a04997.

12. Chuang P, Parikh CR, Langone A. Urinary tract infections after renal transplantation: a retrospective review at two US transplant centers. Clin Transpl. 2005;19(2):230–5. https://doi.org/10.1111/j.1399-0012.2005.00327.x.

13. Xie L, Lin T, Wazir R, Wang K, Lu Y. The management of urethral stricture after kidney transplantation. Int Urol Nephrol. 2014;46(11):2143–5. https://doi.org/10.1007/s11255-014-0798-7.

14. Shoskes DA, Hanbury D, Cranston D, Morris PJ. Urological complications in 1,000 consecutive renal transplant recipients. J Urol. 1995;153(1):18–21. https://doi.org/10.1097/00005392-199501000-00008.

15. Giessing M. Transplant ureter stricture following renal transplantation: surgical options. Transplant Proc. 2011;43(1):383–6. https://doi.org/10.1016/j.transproceed.2010.12.014.

16. Nickeleit V, Klimkait T, Binet IF, et al. Testing for polyomavirus type BK DNA in plasma to identify renal-allograft recipients with viral nephropathy. N Engl J Med. 2000;342(18):1309–15.

17. Hirsch HH, Brennan DC, Drachenberg CB, et al. Polyomavirus-associated nephropathy in renal transplantation: interdisciplinary analyses and recommendations. Transplantation. 2005;79(10):1277–86. https://doi.org/10.1097/01.TP.0000156165.83160.09.

18. Sagedal S, Nordal KP, Hartmann A, et al. A prospective study of the natural course of cytomegalovirus infection and disease in renal allograft recipients. Transplantation. 2000;70(8):1166–74.

19. Helanterä I, Schachtner T, Hinrichs C, et al. Current characteristics and outcome of cytomegalovirus infections after kidney transplantation. Transpl Infect Dis. 2014;16(4):568–77. https://doi.org/10.1111/tid.12247.

20. Hartmann A, Sagedal S, Hjelmesæth J. The natural course of cytomegalovirus infection and disease in renal transplant recipients. Transplantation. 2006;82(SUPPL. 2):15–7. https://doi.org/10.1097/01.tp.0000230460.42558.b0.

21. Kotton CN. Viral infection in the renal transplant recipient. J Am Soc Nephrol. 2005;16(6):1758–74. https://doi.org/10.1681/ASN.2004121113.

22. Caillard S, Dharnidharka V, Agodoa L, Bohen E, Abbott K. Posttransplant lymphoproliferative disorders after renal transplantation in the United States in era of modern immunosuppression. Transplantation. 2005;80(9):1233–43. https://doi.org/10.1097/01.tp.0000179639.98338.39.

23. Moloney FJ, Comber H, O'Lorcain P, O'Kelly P, Conlon PJ, Murphy GM. A population-based study of skin cancer incidence and prevalence in renal transplant recipients. Br J Dermatol. 2006;154(3):498–504. https://doi.org/10.1111/j.1365-2133.2005.07021.x.

24. Euvrardl S, Kanitakisl J, Touraind JL. Skin cancers in organ transplant recipients. Ann Transplant. 1997;2(4):28–32.

25. Sullivan AN, Bryant EA, Mark LA. Patients: a case report and review of the literature. CUTIS do not copy. CUTIS. 2012;89(March):133–6.

26. Dew MA, Switzer GE, DiMartini AF, Matukaitis J, Fitzgerald MG, Kormos RL. Psychosocial assessments and outcomes in organ transplantation. Prog Transplant. 2000;10(4):231–9.

27. Nevins TE, Nickerson PW, Dew MA. Understanding medication nonadherence after kidney transplant. J Am Soc Nephrol. 2017:2290–301. https://doi.org/10.1681/ASN.2017020216.

28. Blosser CD, Bloom RD. Recurrent glomerular disease after kidney transplantation. Curr Opin Nephrol Hypertens. 2017;26(6):501–8. https://doi.org/10.1097/MNH.0000000000000358.

29. Hart A, Smith JM, Skeans MA, et al. OPTN/SRTR 2016 annual data report: kidney. Am J Transplant. 2018;18(Suppl 1):18–113. https://doi.org/10.1111/ajt.14557.

30. Khalil AK, Slaven JE, Mujtaba MA, et al. Re-transplants compared to primary kidney transplants recipients: a mate kidney paired analysis of the OPTN/UNOS database. Clin Transpl. 2016;30(5):566–78. https://doi.org/10.1111/ctr.12722.

Post-transplant Psychosocial and Mental Health Care of the Renal Recipient

10

Mary Amanda Dew, Larissa Myaskovsky, Jennifer L. Steel, and Andrea F. DiMartini

Introduction

The psychosocial and mental health care needs of kidney transplant recipients assume increasing importance as the size of this population and duration of life expected post-transplant continue to grow. In the United States, over 19,000 individuals received kidney transplants in 2016; this represents a 40% increase over the number of kidney transplants in 2000 [1]. Kidney transplantation accounts for 80% of all organ transplants [1], and kidney transplant recipients enjoy higher survival rates than any other type of solid organ recipient. Patient survival rates are 97%, 93%, and 86% at 1, 3, and 5 years post-transplant, respectively, and graft survival is 95%, 88%, and 78% at these time points [1]. Graft survival exceeds 60% even at 10 years post-transplant [2], and 20 or more years of graft function is not uncommon [3]. Moreover, in the event of graft failure, kidney recipients have more treatment options than other types of organ recipients. In particular, patients may receive dialysis and/or be listed for

retransplantation. The retransplantation rate in kidney recipients (13% of all kidney transplants in 2016) is higher than the retransplantation rates for recipients of liver, heart, or lung transplantation (3–5% of transplants) [1]. Given high survival rates plus the possibility of retransplantation, the population of individuals living with a kidney transplant has more than doubled since 2000: as of June 2015, there were more than 200,000 recipients alive with a functioning graft in the United States [2].

Significant resources must be deployed to provide ongoing clinical care and monitoring of this sizable population. Such care necessarily focuses on graft functioning, common medical comorbidities, and complications of immunosuppression. However, the psychosocial and mental health needs of these recipients require consideration as well: it is well-known, for example, that psychosocial and behavioral factors encompassing adherence to the medical regimen, mental health, and substance use can affect clinical outcomes, including risks for both morbidity and mortality [4–10]. Thus, providing care to address emerging psychosocial issues can be essential for prolonging patients' duration and quality of life after kidney transplantation.

In this chapter, we describe the prevalence, risk factors, and interventions tested to prevent or treat three key psychosocial issues in kidney transplant recipients: adherence to the multifactorial medical regimen, mental health problems, and substance use. We consider the implications of this information for the care of kidney recipients and suggest work that is needed in the future in order to expand the set of evidence-based treatment strategies available to healthcare professionals who provide this care. Our review of the evidence and our clinical recommendations pertain to adult kidney recipients. The psychosocial issues of key importance in pediatric transplantation are very different than in adults, and a variety of reviews summarize evidence and care recommendations for pediatric kidney recipients [11–16].

M. A. Dew (✉)
Departments of Psychiatry, Psychology, Epidemiology, Biostatistics and the Clinical and Translational Science Institute, University of Pittsburgh, Pittsburgh, PA, USA
e-mail: dewma@upmc.edu

L. Myaskovsky
Nephrology Division and the Center for Healthcare Equity in Kidney Disease, Department of Internal Medicine, University of New Mexico School of Medicine, Albuquerque, NM, USA

J. L. Steel
Departments of Surgery, Psychiatry, and Psychology, University of Pittsburgh, Pittsburgh, PA, USA

A. F. DiMartini
Departments of Psychiatry and Surgery and the Clinical and Translational Science Institute, University of Pittsburgh, Pittsburgh, PA, USA

© Springer International Publishing AG, part of Springer Nature 2019
Y. Sher, J. R. Maldonado (eds.), *Psychosocial Care of End-Stage Organ Disease and Transplant Patients*,
https://doi.org/10.1007/978-3-319-94914-7_10

How Common Are Psychosocial Problems After Renal Transplantation?

Information on prevalence is important for estimating how likely any given kidney recipient is to have psychosocial difficulties. From a clinical standpoint, understanding which types of problems are most common is the first step toward identifying and prioritizing new educational and preventive efforts for this patient population. In addition, such information is relevant for deciding how to modify existing clinical care strategies.

Nonadherence to the Medical Regimen

The post-transplant medical regimen is multifaceted and must be followed by patients for the remainder of their lives with their transplanted kidney. Immunosuppressant medication-taking is a central element, but patients are also expected to adhere to other requirements: they must attend routine clinic appointments for health monitoring by the transplant program, complete required laboratory and other tests, engage in routine self-monitoring of vital signs (e.g., blood pressure, temperature), and engage in healthy lifestyle behaviors (e.g., routine exercise, following prescribed diets, avoiding prolonged sun exposure). Several systematic reviews have reported on the prevalence of medical regimen nonadherence after kidney transplantation [17–20]. Most focus on immunosuppressant medication adherence. In the only analysis to date to report on prevalence rates of nonadherence for each of the multiple areas of the post-transplant medical regimen, we found 147 studies of organ recipients, including 72 studies of kidney recipients [20]. The rates of nonadherence among kidney recipients are shown in Fig. 10.1. Immunosuppressant nonadherence was the most common problem across the various areas assessed: approximately 36 per 100 kidney recipients per year (i.e., 36% during any given year) were nonadherent to these medications. Rates of nonadherence to requirements for blood work and testing, as well as nonadher-

ence to lifestyle requirements including exercise and diet, also appear to be relatively common. However, kidney recipients had low rates of nonadherence to monitoring vital signs (e.g., blood pressure) and attending required clinic appointments. In additional analyses, we found that the immunosuppressant nonadherence rate was in fact significantly higher than the rates found in studies of other types of organ recipients, which ranged from 7% to 14% [20]. However, kidney recipients were indistinguishable from other types of recipients in terms of nonadherence rates for other areas of the regimen [20].

An important question concerns how the prevalence of nonadherence in any given area of the post-transplant medical regimen changes over time. Neither our meta-analysis nor other systematic reviews and meta-analyses have provided a detailed consideration of this issue in kidney or other organ transplantation. However, individual studies examining temporal patterns of change show that, even in such critical areas of the post-transplant regimen as taking immunosuppressants, nonadherence begins within months of the transplant surgery and grows more common over time [21–26]. These findings are consistent with evidence from the general chronic disease treatment literature which also shows increasing rates of nonadherence with time after treatment initiation [27, 28].

Mental Health Problems

There have been several recent reviews discussing the prevalence of psychiatric difficulties in kidney recipients [29–32]. Depressive and anxiety disorders, and elevated levels of depression and anxiety symptoms, are the most common mental health problems identified in organ transplant recipients [33, 34]. In kidney recipients, most studies have focused on depression. Point prevalence rates of clinically significant depressive symptom levels range widely from 4% to 49%, with most rates falling between 20% and 40%. A recent meta-analysis found that the pooled estimate (an

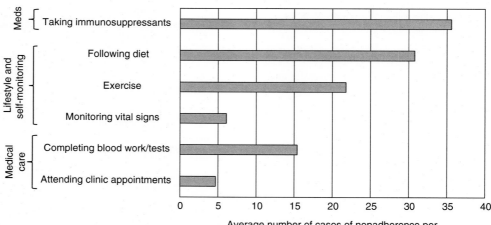

Fig. 10.1 Average rates of nonadherence to components of the medical regimen after kidney transplantation, meta-analysis results [20]

average across studies, weighted by sample size) was 27% [31]. The great heterogeneity in rates across studies likely reflects factors such as variability in measures used to assess depression, cut points chosen to indicate elevated distress, and whether the study sample was one of convenience rather than a sample constructed more systematically. Although the studies' samples also vary in time since transplant, this factor has not been found to be associated with point prevalence rates of depression or other mental health problems [32].

Only rarely have diagnosable depressive disorders been considered in kidney recipients. Vasquez et al. [35] reported a point prevalence rate of 12% for depressive disorders in a Central American sample, and Dobbels et al. [36], relying on Medicare claims data in a national sample in the United States, found that the cumulative annual incidence of depression was 5%, 7%, and 9% across the first 3 years after kidney transplantation.

Kidney recipients' risk for depression appears to be lower than that of end-stage renal disease patients, including candidates listed for transplant [31]. However, recipients' risk remains elevated above that of the general population [32]. Despite lack of evidence that the point prevalence rates of depression vary with time post-transplant, a better understanding of patients' typical trajectory of depression over time is needed. For example, duration of episodes and patients' risk for episode recurrence are unknown.

Anxiety-related conditions have received little attention in kidney recipients, despite the well-known high comorbidity between anxiety and depression. From 10% to 25% of kidney recipients have been found to have elevated anxiety symptom levels [37, 38]. Vasquez et al. [35] reported a 15% point prevalence rate of anxiety disorders in their cohort. Anxiety levels in kidney recipients appear higher than those found in healthy general community samples [39].

There is limited evidence on the prevalence of rare but severe psychiatric disorders, such as psychosis and bipolar disorder, after any type of organ transplantation. In a national renal transplant database in Ireland, less than 1% of kidney recipients had histories of schizophrenia or bipolar disorder. However, this report did not consider recurrence of symptoms after transplant [40]. In the largest study to date, Abbott et al. [41] examined administrative data from the United States Renal Data System and found that the incidence of hospitalized psychosis after kidney transplantation was 7.5 per 1000 person years (PY) of observation. This rate did not differ from that of the population of patients on dialysis (7.2/1000 PY). However, 94% of the transplant recipients were aged 65 or less. When the dialysis population was restricted to those aged 65 or less, the risk of hospitalized psychosis was lower in kidney recipients than the rate of 9.6/1000 PY in dialysis patients [41]. This report did not compare these rates to rates in the general population.

Substance Use

Transplant programs require abstinence from illicit drug use after kidney transplantation. Recipients should also refrain from tobacco use. Although recipients are not generally required to abstain from all alcohol consumption, alcohol use must be limited. Research has largely focused on tobacco smoking in kidney recipients, with less consideration of alcohol or other substance use [4, 7, 10, 20]. In our meta-analysis of adherence-related behaviors after organ transplantation [20], we found a rate of tobacco smoking of 3 per 100 kidney recipients seen in any given year (3% annually), while the rates of annual use of illicit drugs and annual use of alcohol above limits set by patients' transplant programs were each 1%. Consistent with these findings of particularly low rates of alcohol and illicit drug use, research since our analysis has concluded there is little evidence that alcohol abuse or dependence are prevalent problems in the kidney recipient population [42]. (This is unlikely to be due to selection of patients for transplantation; it more likely reflects relatively low rates of alcohol use in the population of patients needing kidney transplants, especially compared to other populations such as patients needing liver transplants [10].)

Whether substance use reflects a relapse to prior use or incident cases is an important issue. With respect to tobacco, a study examining Medicare claims data in the United States identified kidney recipients who had no history of tobacco smoking before transplantation but had claims on which post-transplant tobacco use was recorded [43]. The authors report that the incidence rate of smoking (i.e., new-onset smoking) was 4.6% (and this was apparently across a maximum of 5 years post-transplant). The time to smoking use onset (adjusted for censored observations due, for example, to patient death) was 1.3 years post-transplant.

We have not identified any studies of incident alcohol or illicit drug use in kidney recipients. However, there is a literature on rates of relapse to alcohol and illicit drug use in organ recipients with histories of substance abuse or dependence before transplantation, as summarized in a meta-analysis [44]. (Studies examining this subgroup of patients were excluded from our previous meta-analysis described above, which focused on general samples, and not samples selected on the basis of pre-transplant histories.) While there were no studies of relapse to alcohol use in kidney recipients with histories of abuse/dependence (all studies focused on liver recipients), we found that relapse to illicit drug use was 6% annually in kidney recipients, a rate equal to that in heart recipients but lower than the 2% annual rate found in liver recipients.

There has been little to no examination of the specific types of illicit drugs used by kidney recipients. One recent report examined recreational marijuana use in kidney recipients (in a state in the United States where use is not legal) and estimated 3% of patients were active users (by on either self-report or urine toxicology screen data) [45]. However, patients differed dramatically in time since transplant, and, given no adjustments for survival time, the 3% rate may underestimate the risk of marijuana use post-transplant.

The timing of substance use onset after kidney transplantation has received no consideration. However, as for other behavioral problems post-transplant such as medication nonadherence, it seems likely that substance use would begin in the early months post-transplant. This pattern has been documented in other types of transplant recipients (e.g., liver recipients [44]).

What Factors Increase Risk for Psychosocial Problems After Renal Transplantation?

Identification of key risk factors can be important for targeting patients who may need additional monitoring and early intervention, should they begin to show any signs of psychosocial problems.

Nonadherence to the Medical Regimen

In chronic disease populations in general, five categories of risk factors appear important for medical regimen adherence [46]. These are listed below, along with specific examples of factors found relevant for nonadherence risk in kidney transplant recipients [5, 9]:

- Sociodemographic characteristics (e.g., younger age, minority race/ethnicity, low socioeconomic status).
- Patient-related psychosocial factors (e.g., past nonadherence, low health literacy, low knowledge about one's illness and treatment options, psychological distress, low self-efficacy, poor social supports, forgetfulness/cognitive impairment, daily routine changes).
- Treatment-related factors (e.g., more frequent medication doses, greater total number of medications, side effects of medications or other treatments).
- Condition-related factors (e.g., longer time since transplant, transplant from a living donor, better perceived health, physical limitations).
- Healthcare system and provider-level factors (e.g., insurance status, access to care, provider-patient communication, transition from a pediatric to an adult transplant program).

In kidney transplantation, as in other areas of transplantation, the strongest and most consistent risk factor for post-transplant nonadherence, particularly with respect to immunosuppressant medications, is a history of nonadher-

ence before transplantation [8, 19, 20, 23, 47]. Similar to findings in other chronic disease groups [48], more complex regimens (involving multiple doses of one or more medications daily and a greater total number of medications) also increase risk for medication nonadherence in kidney recipients [17]. It is noteworthy, however, that the impact of each of the factors listed above may be modest [9, 20], and thus interventions would likely need to simultaneously address and ameliorate more than a single factor in order to be effective. Additionally, in some cases, the evidence for a given factor's importance is inconsistent. For example, minority race/ethnicity emerges as a risk factor for medication nonadherence after kidney transplantation in some studies [26, 49–52] but not others [53–56]. The inconsistency in findings may arise because race/ethnicity likely is a proxy for characteristics such as insurance status and access to care that are the true contributors to nonadherence risk.

There is also an informative qualitative literature describing kidney recipients' own views about factors that affect their self-management of health issues, including adherence to the post-transplant medical regimen. In a systematic review of this literature, Jamieson et al. [57] concluded that patients' comments about their self-management challenges reflected five themes: (a) empowerment (strategies used to gain personal control over the medical regimen); (b) fear of adverse health outcomes (e.g., graft loss); (c) managing medical regimen demands (e.g., attempts to adhere despite changes in daily routines); (d) feelings that life has become overmedicalized (e.g., feelings of burnout at having to manage the medical regimen); and (e) accountability to others (e.g., gratitude to the donor and the transplant program, motivation to care for the kidney).

Recipients' comments indicated recognition of the need to overcome many of the factors found in empirical studies to increase risk for nonadherence (e.g., by gaining a better understanding of the regimen and their responsibilities, by establishing daily routines, and by setting up reminders for various activities). Patients also introduced additional ideas about areas potentially relevant for nonadherence risk reduction, including the need to improve problem-solving skills and the opportunity to learn from peers about ways to remain adherent.

In a separate systematic review focused specifically on kidney recipients' medication-taking activities, Tong et al. [58] extracted themes that characterized recipients' beliefs, experiences, and perspectives on medication-taking. Thus, poor adherence was often described as the result of patient forgetfulness, intolerable side effects, inability to pay for medications, difficulty accessing a pharmacy to obtain the medications, and the occurrence of disrupting life events. In contrast, high degrees of vigilance and adherence to the medication regimen were described by patients who strongly endorsed a desire to protect their new chance at life, who felt powerful obligations to both donors and the transplant team, and who described the importance of taking personal responsibility for their health. Patients able to maintain a high level of medication adherence also felt that they were able to tolerate side effects and had developed strategies to keep from forgetting doses. Finally, patients who showed variable degrees of success at taking their medications felt that this arose because they were attempting to change drugs or dosing requirements in order to manage side effects. They also felt that they missed doses due to forgetfulness or took doses late due to changes in routines. Taken together, the findings from the qualitative literature indicate the importance of asking patients directly about the factors they consider to be the most important barriers and facilitators for achieving high levels of medication adherence.

Mental Health Problems

In all types of organ transplant recipients, the strongest risk factor for depression, anxiety, other psychiatric disorders, or elevated symptom levels is a pre-transplant history of distress in these areas [30, 33, 34]. The bulk of research in kidney recipients has focused on risk for depression, and several key risk factors have emerged. Principal among these are clinical factors: a longer duration of dialysis before transplantation [36, 59], poor graft function after transplantation [59–61], the occurrence of rejection episodes [62], and the presence of physical comorbidities, including obesity [36, 59–61, 63].

A range of psychosocial factors have also been examined. Demographic characteristics such as female sex and lower levels of education are well-known risk factors for depression in kidney recipients [29], just as they are in other transplant populations and in general community samples. In addition, in kidney recipients, among the psychosocial factors found to most consistently increase depression risk are post-transplant unemployment and personal financial difficulties [35, 59, 61, 64] and poor social support [35, 60–62, 64]. Both poor availability of support persons and poorer perceived quality of support appear important. Thus, unmarried individuals and individuals living alone are at higher risk than married individuals [38, 60–62, 64], and perceptions of low social supports, including tangible support and emotional support, also increase depression risk [35, 61].

There is less evidence on whether other aspects of recipients' psychosocial environments are associated with depression risk. Thus, factors related to coping styles and strategies may increase risk or in some cases may protect against depression. However, the findings are inconsistent to date. For example, Christensen et al. [65] found that a coping style characterized by information-seeking in order to manage health problems reduced kidney recipients' risk for enduring or increasing depression symptom levels after transplant. In contrast, Knowles et al. [37] found no large or statistically significant association between either "maladaptive" coping strategies (e.g., attempting to avoid thinking about problems) or "adaptive" strategies (e.g., active problem-solving efforts), and other studies have also failed to find that coping strategies are related to depression [38]. However, so few studies have evaluated coping styles and strategies that it is difficult to conclude whether they play an important role for depression or not.

Very little work has examined risk factors for anxiety or severe mental disorders such as psychosis. One report found that greater severity of self-reported transplant-related stressors (in areas such as perceived medication side effects, occurrence of problems such as graft rejection, and perceived physical limitations) was related to higher anxiety levels [66]. Interestingly, these authors did not find social supports to be correlated with anxiety levels. Knowles et al. [37] reported that illness perceptions (encompassing greater perceived impact of illness on daily life and feelings of little control over the illness) were associated with heightened anxiety symptoms. Similar to findings for depression, whether or not coping strategies affect risk for anxiety symptoms is unclear. Two recent studies suggest that maladaptive coping strategies, such as avoidance and denial, are associated with increased anxiety [37, 39]. With regard to psychosis, in the study described earlier on the occurrence of hospitalizations for psychosis after kidney transplantation [41], both delayed graft function after transplant and the occurrence of graft rejection episodes were risk factors for psychiatric hospitalizations. No demographic risk factors for hospitalization for psychosis were identified.

Unlike the literature on medical adherence, which includes rich quantitative as well as qualitative reports, studies identifying risk factors for poor mental health are empirical and have not routinely sought to include patient views on factors that affect their psychological status. One qualitative report notes that patients may feel that their expectations for life after the transplant are not met, which can lead to disappointment and disillusionment [67]. However, it is not clear that patients were specifically queried about any linked feelings of depression or anxiety. The qualitative literature on self-management of the medical regimen, however, notes that patients themselves feel that poor graft function and the risks of serious side effects (e.g., cancers from the immunosuppressants) lead to considerable anxiety [57]. The feelings of "burnout" at being a patient, feelings that their lives have become "overmedicalized", and patient descriptors of such experiences appear to include depressive elements [57]; it seems likely that patients with heightened feelings of burnout either are at risk for depression or are depressed [68].

Substance Use

Not surprisingly, a history of substance use is the most important risk factor for post-transplant substance use in organ recipients, including kidney recipients [7, 20, 44]. Organ transplant recipients who use one substance are likely to use others (e.g., smoking is correlated with alcohol and illicit drug use; alcohol and illicit drug use are correlated [7, 42, 43, 45]).

There has been relatively limited consideration of other risk factors. The bulk of work pertains to post-transplant tobacco smoking. Duerinckx et al. [7] provide a comprehensive examination of risk factors and correlates of smoking post-transplant, but they do not distinguish between types of organ received. Kidney transplant studies were, however, more numerous than studies of other types of recipients. They found that male sex, younger age, and higher body mass index (BMI) increased risk for smoking, while prevalent comorbidities including hypertension, diabetes, and cardiovascular disease were not reliable risk factors. They noted that many potential factors (e.g., psychiatric symptoms, coping styles) had been examined in very few studies, thus precluding firm conclusions about their possible roles. In particular, they found that duration of abstinence from smoking before transplantation has been examined in only a few studies, with conflicting results. Duerinckx et al. [7] focused largely on studies of recipients with histories of tobacco use before transplant. In a large US study of tobacco use incidence after kidney transplantation, Hurst et al. [43] found that new smokers were more likely than nonsmokers to be male, younger, and African American. They were also likely to have more medical comorbidities and to have histories of alcohol and/or drug dependence.

Few studies have considered risk factors for alcohol or drug use specifically in kidney recipients. Male sex appears to increase risk for post-transplant heavier alcohol use, while age is not a risk factor [42, 69]. Zelle et al. [42] found that kidney recipients who used alcohol had a shorter time on dialysis before transplant. However, post-transplant kidney function or ability to return to work was not associated with alcohol use risk. Similarly, Fierz et al. [69] found that clinical variables such as comorbidities and occurrence of graft rejection were not related to alcohol use, but they found that patients who returned to work were at higher risk for alcohol use. They speculated that kidney recipients who are employed may be those who perceive their health to be better. Fierz et al. [69] examined but found no evidence that level of education, depressive symptoms, coping styles or strategies, or clinical variables such as comorbidities and the occurrence of graft rejection were independent risk factors for alcohol use.

Finally, Greenan et al. [45] reported that kidney recipients who used marijuana recreationally were more likely to be unmarried, have less education, currently use alcohol and tobacco, and have histories of treated substance addiction. Interestingly, in contrast to the risk factors we have discussed for other substance use in kidney recipients, male sex was not associated with marijuana use.

What Interventions Have Been Tested to Address Psychosocial Problems After Renal Transplantation?

In order to provide evidence-based care to transplant recipients, clinicians must understand the range of treatment options that have been tested for efficacy specifically in kidney transplant recipients. Gaps in that evidence may be partially filled by considering intervention efficacy studies in other transplant or chronic disease populations, although whether or not the findings would generalize to kidney recipients is often unclear.

Nonadherence to the Medical Regimen

Among the psychosocial problems that we have addressed in this chapter, the greatest focus of intervention trials has been on immunosuppressant medication adherence after transplantation. Table 10.1 shows the interventions tested and key results in studies published since 2000 [70–86]. The majority of studies used multicomponent interventions focused on providing education about medication-taking, assessing barriers to adherence, providing feedback on adherence levels achieved (often using data from electronic medication monitoring devices in pill bottles given to patients), and encouraging problem-solving and goal setting. These interventions usually required multiple sessions with an interventionist over a period of months. Interventionists were often nurses but sometimes included pharmacists, psychologists, or multidisciplinary teams. Exceptions to these "coaching" interventions included an intervention that simply involved switching from twice-daily dosing of the key immunosuppressant to once-daily dosing [75] and an intervention that used electronic medication monitoring along with text messaging and feedback to clinicians on medication-taking patterns [84]. Studies varied in terms of whether medication adherence was assessed by electronic monitoring, patient self-report, blood levels of the immunosuppressant medication, or combinations of these assessments.

Across these 16 trials, 11 found that the intervention improved medication-taking. Interestingly, although most of the trials involved labor-intensive complex interventions, even some of those with simpler strategies (e.g., the modification in doses per day) found benefits in improved adherence. Important remaining issues concern the durability of intervention effects,

Table 10.1 Controlled trials testing interventions to improve immunosuppressant medication adherence in adult kidney recipients[a]

First author, year	Sample size and follow-up duration	Intervention	Impact on adherence
Chisholm, 2001 [70]	N = 24, end of intervention (first year post-transplant)	– Medication review, education – 12 monthly face-to-face or phone sessions with clinical pharmacist	Intervention group had significantly higher adherence (pharmacy refills) than usual care control group
Hardstaff, 2003 [71]	N = 48, up to 6 months post-intervention	– Feedback (appeared to focus on EM data) – 1 clinic visit with nurse practitioner	No differences noted between intervention and usual care control groups in adherence (based on EM)
De Geest, 2006 [72]	N = 18, 6 months post-intervention	– EM data feedback, education, goal setting, problem-solving, use of social supports – 1 home visit, 3 monthly phone calls with research nurse	Nonsignificant trend for intervention group to show greater initial adherence increase (based on EM) than enhanced usual care control group, but advantage not maintained
Russell, 2011 [73]	N = 15, end of intervention	– EM data feedback, planning and review of behavior change efforts – 1 home visit, 6 monthly phone calls with research clinical nurse specialist	Intervention group had significantly higher adherence (based on EM) during follow-up than health education control group, but no between-group differences by the end of trial
Chisholm-Burns, 2013 [74]	N = 150, 3 months post-intervention	– Behavioral contracting, education, adherence barrier identification, goal setting, problem-solving – 5 20–30 min face-to-face or phone sessions over 12 mos with clinical pharmacist	Intervention group had significantly higher adherence (pharmacy refills) than usual care group at each time point after baseline
Kuypers, 2013 [75]	N = 219, 6 months post-randomization	– Switch from twice- to once-daily tacrolimus	Intervention group had significantly higher adherence (based on EM) compared to usual dosing group
McGillicuddy 2013 [76]	N = 19; end of intervention	– EM medication box with alerts, BP monitoring, text message reminders, transplant team alerted to medication or BP monitoring nonadherence, physician given feedback on patient data – 3 mos of use of strategies	Intervention group had significantly higher medication adherence (based on EM) than usual care controls at each time point after baseline
Joost, 2014 [77]	N = 67, end of intervention (12 months after hospital discharge post-transplant)	– Medication-taking education, adherence barrier identification, goal setting, use of social support – 3 30-min sessions pre-discharge, outpatient sessions ≥ quarterly for 12 mos	Intervention group had significantly higher adherence (based on EM and pill count) than usual care group
Annunziato, 2015 [78]	N = 22, 1 year after transfer from pediatric to adult program	– Education on transfer process, patient self-management problem-solving – ≥ 2 meetings with patient/family by pediatric team social worker, social worker completion of transition checklist and discussion with adult team	No significant group differences between intervention and usual transfer control group; all patients showed adherence decline (blood levels) with trend toward less decline in intervention group
Garcia, 2015 [79]	N = 111, 3 months post-transplant	– Medication-taking education, goal setting, problem-solving – 10 weekly 30-min clinic sessions with nurse	Intervention group had significantly better adherence (self-report) than usual care control group
McQuillan, 2015 [80]	N = 32, 1 year after transfer to adult program	– 1 visit by patient/parent to new transfer clinic, patient and parent small groups to discuss transition and self-management, patient completion of online education, adult and pediatric team meeting	Intervention group had significantly less nonadherence (self-report) during follow-up and greater decline in nonadherence from pre- to post-intervention than usual transfer control group. No significant group differences on blood level data
Bessa, 2016 [81]	N = 126, end of intervention	– Medication-taking education – 9 sessions (duration not noted) in first 90 days post-transplant	No significant differences in adherence (blood levels, self-report) between intervention and usual care groups No significant differences between groups in rates of infections, acute graft rejection, graft function, death, graft loss, or hospital readmissions

(continued)

Table 10.1 (continued)

First author, year	Sample size and follow-up duration	Intervention	Impact on adherence
Breu-Dejean, 2016 [82]	N = 110, 3 months post-intervention	– Medication-taking education – 8 weekly 2-hr small group sessions with multidisciplinary team	Intervention group had significantly better adherence (self-report) than usual care group at end of intervention and end of follow-up
Cukor, 2017 [83]	N = 33, ~4 weeks post-intervention	– Cognitive behavioral therapy, motivational interviewing focused on barriers to and motivations for adherence – 2 2-hr small group sessions with psychologists over 1–2 week period	Intervention group had significantly higher adherence (self-report pill counts) at follow-up and more improvement in adherence pre- to post-intervention than usual care control No significant difference in blood level data from baseline but significant improvement in intervention group after intervention compared to control group
Reese, 2017 [84]	N = 117, last 90 days of intervention (EM data), 6 mos post-intervention (blood levels), end of intervention (self-report)	– EM monitor with alerts, used alone or with provider notification. Text and email reminders could be sent. Providers in one intervention arm called patients if adherence declined and informed clinical team – 6-mo use of monitor and other components	Reminders+provider notification group and reminder alone group had significantly better adherence (based on EM) than usual care control group; the former group was also marginally better than reminder alone group No group differences in blood levels or self-report
Schmid, 2017 [85]	N = 46, end of intervention (first year post-transplant)	– Telemonitoring, education, support and coaching provided on demand – Daily monitoring by nurse case manager (with physician support), case management	Intervention group had significantly better adherence (composite of clinician ratings, self-report, blood levels) at all assessments than usual care control group

Abbreviations: *BP* Blood Pressure, *EM* Electronic Monitoring

[a]All studies in the table were randomized controlled trials except for Joost et al. [77], Annunziato et al. [78], and McQuillan et al. (who compared the intervention cohort to historical or sequential controls) [80]. All samples varied in time since transplant except as noted. An additional report by Henriksson et al. [86] examined medication nonadherence in kidney recipients, but was excluded from this table because the authors did not distinguish adult recipients from pediatric recipients (many of whom were not responsible for their own adherence and would have required caregiver administration of medications)

whether the interventions benefit some patients more than others, and whether—as would be hoped—the interventions lead not only to improved medication-taking but to improved clinical outcomes. The follow-up periods in most of the trials were relatively brief: some studies followed patients only until the intervention ended; others continued to follow patients for a few months after the intervention. The studies did not identify subgroups of patients who appeared to show particular benefit from the interventions. However, the qualitative literature that we reviewed earlier suggests that medication adherence after kidney transplantation may be improved through explicit consideration of patients' perspectives and by tailoring a given intervention to address patients' perceived adherence barriers and facilitators [87].

Despite evidence that most of the interventions tested led to some improvement in immunosuppressant medication adherence, the studies' results concerning intervention impact on clinical outcomes have been disappointing. Several examined clinical outcomes, including rehospitalizations [74, 81, 85], emergency and outpatient visits [74, 85], infections [81], graft function [77–81], rejection episodes and graft loss [77, 78, 80, 81], and death [79, 81, 82]. Although rehospitalization risk was lowered by adherence interventions in two studies [74, 85], no other study in Table 10.1 observed any effects on clinical outcomes.

Another important consideration in future adherence-promoting trials in kidney transplantation would be to go beyond medication adherence to consider impact on other types of outcomes. Hsiao et al. [88] evaluated a support group-based intervention designed to increase feelings of self-care empowerment and found that participants improved in their overall self-reported ability to adhere to the medical regimen, relative to control participants receiving usual care. Some evidence in other areas of organ transplantation suggests that electronic health (e-health) interventions, including smartphone apps in particular, can lead to improved medical regimen adherence [5, 89].

A few studies have tested interventions in kidney recipients designed to improve lifestyle behaviors (e.g., weight control, exercise, diet [90, 91]). These interventions were modestly effective at changing patients' behaviors and improving related health parameters, at least in the short-term. Maintenance of these effects was not examined. In addition, large proportions of the patients in these studies dropped out. This suggests low intervention or research trial design acceptability.

Mental Health Problems

Mental health outcomes have been considered in only a very limited number of intervention trials in kidney recipients. Two investigative teams have examined nonmedication psychotherapeutic interventions. First, Baines et al. [92, 93] examined recipients randomized to receive 12 weeks of individual psychotherapy or 12 weeks of group sessions. A "control" group receiving usual care was also included (but this group was constructed separately and patients were not randomized into it). The psychotherapy sessions focused on adaptation to the transplant. Patients' depression symptom levels in both active psychotherapy conditions declined significantly from pre- to post-intervention, with sustained effects 12 months later. Individual psychotherapy appeared more effective than group therapy. Control group depression levels, in contrast, worsened over time.

Second, Gross and colleagues [94–96] conducted two studies examining an 8-week group-based Mindfulness-Based Stress Reduction (MBSR) intervention for reducing symptoms of depression, anxiety, and sleep disturbance in kidney, lung, or pancreas transplant recipients. In an initial study, Gross et al. [94] enrolled kidney, lung, or pancreas transplant recipients, and although they did not examine effects in kidney recipients alone, they found that across all types of recipients, both depression and sleep improved from baseline (pre-intervention) to immediately after the intervention ended. At 3-month follow-up [94] and at 6-month follow-up [96], sleep effects were maintained and anxiety was significantly lower than baseline. Depression symptom reductions were not maintained at either follow-up time point. A subsequent, larger study randomized kidney, kidney/pancreas, liver, heart, and lung recipients to receive the MBSR intervention or receive health education sessions [95]. The MBSR intervention showed significant and sustained anxiety and sleep disturbance reductions, relative to the control group, with effects sustained through 12 months post-intervention. Although depression levels also improved, they did not show as dramatic a change and were not distinguishable from control group depression levels.

Beyond kidney transplantation, other nonpharmacologic psychotherapeutic intervention trials in organ candidates and recipients suggest that telephone-based counseling using cognitive behavioral therapy principles and internet-based interventions involving problem-solving therapy can lead to reductions in depression and anxiety [95]. It seems likely that such interventions would be effective in kidney recipients. Additional strategies have been described for kidney recipients, but they have not been evaluated for efficacy. These include peer mentoring, internet-based education and support, and intensive support and education before discharge after the initial transplant surgery (see Dew and DiMartini [33] and DiMartini et al. [97], for reviews).

Psychopharmacologic strategies have not received study in controlled trials in kidney recipients. Randomized trials comparing the impact on depression of sertraline vs. placebo in chronic (nondialysis) kidney disease patients [98] and sertraline vs. cognitive behavioral therapy in dialysis patients [99] are completed or ongoing. In the former trial, sertraline was found to be no more effective than placebo at reducing depressive symptoms. It would be important to consider whether these findings would generalize to kidney transplant recipients.

Substance Use

Ten years ago, Tome et al. [100] noted that very little was known about addictions and their treatment in recipients of organs other than the liver and that this should be a research priority. However, there continues to be a dearth of intervention research. In kidney recipients, a recently published study protocol described a trial focused on smoking cessation using a nonpharmacologic intervention involving brief counseling plus feedback on patients' carbon monoxide oximetry [101]. No results have yet been reported and we could not identify any other completed studies focused on the efficacy of interventions for substance use in kidney recipients. Recent literature on liver recipients suggests that facilitating availability of alcohol addictions treatment specialists (by, e.g., embedding them within the transplant team) may reduce relapse rates post-transplant [102]. Whether this intervention would be feasible in kidney transplant programs—given that fewer kidney recipients have histories of alcohol abuse/dependence than do liver recipients—is not clear. A more feasible approach in kidney transplantation might employ a written "alcohol contract" (or contract for any other type of substance use), in which transplant candidates commit to abstinence after transplantation. However, Masson et al. [103] tested this approach in liver transplantation and found no effect on relapse rates among liver recipients with histories of alcoholic liver disease.

Clinical Strategies to Provide Psychosocial Care to Kidney Recipients After Transplantation: Recommendations

The evidence on prevalence, risk factors, and empirically evaluated interventions leads to two major types of recommendations regarding care for kidney recipients. First, such patients should be routinely screened for psychosocial problems in the areas of medical regimen adherence, mental health, and substance use. Recipients with strong risk factors for such problems may require more frequent or extensive screening. Second, when patients with psychosocial

Table 10.2 Strategies kidney transplant programs could use in order to improve psychosocial outcomes after kidney transplantation

Establish a foundation of trust to encourage patients to speak openly about psychosocial problems, including nonadherence to the medical regimen, mental health problems, and substance use.
Develop collaborative partnerships with patients' other healthcare providers.
Embed a focus on psychosocial outcomes into the transplant team's culture, including routine screening for and tracking of patient status on these outcomes.
Stratify patients by their needs and risk factors so that interventions can be appropriately deployed by the team or so that timely referrals can be made for care by specialists.
Employ multiple interventions; one size does not fit all.

Adapted from Oberlin et al. [104]

problems are identified, the choice of interventions to be offered should be guided by the evidence base on efficacious interventions in kidney recipients. In the absence of such evidence, the interventions should have been established as efficacious in other organ transplant and/or chronic and end-stage disease populations.

Although we focus below on these two major areas of recommendations, we note that additional factors will also likely need to be in place so that transplant programs can successfully screen for and intervene to treat psychosocial problems. Thus, a recent review focused on medication adherence intervention activities by kidney transplant programs concluded that transplant teams must change their "cultures" regarding their approach to addressing nonadherence in their patients [104]. We believe that a similar culture change may be needed to effectively address other psychosocial outcomes, including mental health and substance use problems. Therefore, we have adapted the elements that Oberlin and colleagues suggest are most important in order to encompass psychosocial outcomes in general, and our adaptation is shown in Table 10.2. As detailed in the table, screening and intervention are critical activities for improving psychosocial outcomes, but elements such as building collaborative relationships with kidney recipients' other healthcare providers and building a foundation of trust in order to encourage open conversation with patients may ultimately be equally important.

Screening for Psychosocial Problems

The importance of screening activities to identify psychosocial problems is well-recognized in clinical care guidelines for kidney recipients [105, 106]. Screening should be incorporated into every follow-up clinical visit after transplantation. We noted earlier that problems related to nonadherence, for example, can emerge very soon after transplantation. Fortunately, from a screening standpoint, kidney recipients return to their transplant centers relatively often during the first year after transplant. During routine follow-up clinic visits post-transplant, they typically see a nurse coordinator and a transplant team physician

(often a nephrologist), and it is likely that these professionals would have the greatest opportunity to perform routine psychosocial screening. Most teams providing post-transplant care do not include assessments by mental healthcare providers or other specialists in psychosocial issues, and the professionals who conduct the pre-transplant psychosocial evaluations of patients do not routinely follow patients post-transplant. Therefore, the nurse coordinator and team physician who are most likely to see patients during follow-up must be provided with psychosocial screening tools that are easy to use and provide clear indications of which patients are experiencing problems and may need referral to specialists within or beyond the team for intervention.

Beyond the first year post-transplant, patients are likely to return less frequently to the transplant program for care. In some cases, patients may only return if they develop problems related to the graft or to medical comorbidities linked to immunosuppression or other transplant-related medications. Thus, face-to-face screening may become less feasible. For patients with risk factors for psychosocial problems, programs could consider remote screening options including telephone screening. Recommending to recipients' local healthcare providers (e.g., primary care physicians or local nephrologists) that they should engage in screening may also be an option.

Nonadherence to the Medical Regimen As summarized in Table 10.3, several types of tools could be used to screen for adherence problems, including simple patient-report measures, biologic assays, and routine review of information in patients' electronic health records for trends and patterns on key parameters [107–147]. Historically, self-report screens for nonadherence, especially with regard to medication-taking, have been viewed as inferior to methods such as electronic medication monitoring. However, despite its use in research, electronic monitoring is generally not feasible in clinical practice [148]. Careful use of self-report measures can yield valid information on medication nonadherence [149]. A common clinical practice in transplant programs is to use open-ended questioning about medication-taking rather than any specific self-report questionnaire or checklist [150]. If such a strategy is adopted, clinicians should draw on lines of questioning recommended by experts [48], which focus on understanding the patient's perspective and building rapport. However, open-ended questions may not be asked in the same way across patients or across clinicians and thus may lead to varying degrees of success in identifying nonadherent patients. A stronger, more systematic alternative is to employ one of the several very brief, validated self-report measures of medication-taking recommended for clinical use with transplant patients [149, 151]. Prime examples are listed in Table 10.3. These measures focus on immunosuppressant nonadherence but may be adapted for other types of medication-taking. In fact, both the ITAS and the

Table 10.3 Approaches to screening for psychosocial problems after kidney transplantation

Psychosocial domain	Examples of screening approaches and tools for routine clinical use	Relevant references
Nonadherence to the medical regimen	*Medication-taking*	
	Patient self-report surveys	
	Immunosuppressant Therapy Adherence Scale (ITAS)	Chisholm et al., 2005; Wilks et al., 2010 [107, 108]
	Basel Assessment of Adherence to Immunosuppressive Medications Scale (BAASIS)	Shäfer-Keller et al., 2008 [109]
	Calculation of medication blood level variability	
	Medication Level Variability Index (MLVI)	Shemesh & Fine, 2010; Supelana et al., 2014 [110, 111]
	Coefficient of Variation (CV)	Maclean et al., 2011; Scheel et al., 2017 [112, 113]
	Clinic appointment attendance, completion of required blood work, and lifestyle issues	
	Review of patient medical record for repeated failure to complete clinic appointments and blood work	
	Review of medical record for elevated or rising BMI levels	
	Patient self-report of physical activity	
	International Physical Activity Questionnaire, Short Form "Past 7 days" (IPAQ-S7S)	Craig et al., 2003 [114]
	General Practice Physical Activity Questionnaire (GPPAQ)	Dept. of Health, UK, 2009 [115]
	Patient self-report of diet	
	Rapid Eating and Activity Assessment for Participants-Short Version (REAP-S)	Segal-Isaacson et al., 2004 [116]
Mental health problems	*Depression* (patient self-report surveys)	
	Patient Health Questionnaire-2 (PHQ-2)	Kroenke et al., 2003 [117]
	Patient Health Questionnaire-9 (PHQ-9)	Kroenke et al., 2001 [118]
	MOS-Depression Screener	Burnam et al., 1988 [119]
	Beck Depression Inventory-II (BDI-II)	Beck et al., 1996 [120]
	Beck Depression Inventory FastScreen for Medical Patients (BDI-FS)	Beck et al., 2000 [121]
	Center for Epidemiologic Studies-Depression Scale (CES-D)	Radloff et al., 1977 [122]
	CES-D Short Form (CES-D-SF)	Kohout et al., 1993 [123]
	Anxiety (patient self-report surveys)	
	Generalized Anxiety Disorder-2 (GAD-2)	Kroenke et al., 2007 [124]
	Generalized Anxiety Disorder-7 (GAD-7)	Spitzer et al., 2006 [125]
	Multiple areas of distress (patient self-report surveys)	
	Hospital Anxiety and Depression Scale (HADS)	Snaith, 2003 [126]
	Patient Health Questionnaire (PHQ)	Spitzer et al., 1994 [127]
	Hopkins Symptom Checklist and derivatives (e.g., Brief Symptom Inventory; Symptom Checklist-90-Revised)	Derogatis, 1974; 1993; 1994 [128–130]
	General Health Questionnaire (GHQ)	Goldberg & Williams, 1988 [131]
Substance use	*Tobacco use* (patient self-report surveys)	
	Fagerström Test for Nicotine Dependence (FTND)	Heatherton et al., 1991 [132]
	Fagerström Test for Nicotine Dependence-Smokeless Tobacco (FTND-ST)	Ebbert et al., 2006 [133]
	Alcohol use (patient self-report surveys)	
	CAGE Questionnaire	Mayfield et al., 1974 [134]
	Michigan Alcoholism Screening Test (MAST)	Selzer, 1971 [135]
	Short MAST (SMAST)	Selzer et al., 1975 [136]
	Brief MAST	Pokorny et al., 1972 [137]
	Alcohol Use Disorders Identification Test (AUDIT)	Saunders et al., 1993 [138]
	AUDIT-Alcohol consumption questions (AUDIT-C)	Bush et al., 1998 [139]
	Patient Health Questionnaire Alcohol items (PHQ-Alcohol items)	Spitzer et al., 1994 [127]
	Drug use and multiple areas of substance use (patient self-report surveys)	
	Single-Item Screen	Smith et al., 2010 [140]
	Drug Abuse Screening Test and its derivatives (DAST; DAST-20; DAST-10)	Skinner, 1982; Yudko et al., 2007 [141, 142]
	Alcohol, Smoking and Substance Involvement Screening Test (ASSIST)	WHO ASSIST Working Group, 2002 [143]
	CAGE Questionnaire Adapted to Include Drugs (CAGE-AID)	Brown & Rounds, 1995 [144]
	RAFFT Questionnaire (RAFFT)	Bastiaens et al., 2002 [145]
	Biologic measures of tobacco, alcohol, or other drug use	
	Blood, urine, hair, and saliva samples can be tested for tobacco, alcohol and other drug use	Richter & Johnson, 2001; Grigsby et al., 2017 [146, 147]

BAASIS originated from assessments of other types of medications.

Concerning use of biologic assays and other indicators of medication nonadherence, transplant programs have often relied on biopsy evidence of graft rejection or low blood levels of a given medication to infer nonadherence. However, the use of such data for this purpose should be avoided. Both biopsy results and blood levels may be influenced by factors other than nonadherence. For example, blood levels of immunosuppressants commonly fluctuate over time and can be affected by blood draw timing, other medications' impact on immunosuppressant metabolism, and dosing changes. To appropriately examine blood levels with respect to patient adherence, clinicians should employ one of the recently developed measures that determines whether blood level variability over time exceeds that expected due to biological factors or measurement error. Two examples of such measures are shown in Table 10.3. The calculations for these measures would not be difficult to perform routinely using the repeated laboratory testing results available in patients' medical records.

Both the self-report and blood level assessment strategies that we suggest focus on medication adherence. In some other areas of the regimen, nonadherence may relatively easily determined by periodic review of the patient's medical record. For example, repeated failure to attend clinic appointments or complete blood work and tests indicates nonadherence to these requirements. Similarly, elevated and/or rising BMI would suggest difficulties with lifestyle issues (e.g., diet and perhaps exercise). A variety of screening tools exist for physical activity and level of exercise, although these measures have not been evaluated in kidney recipients. Two such measures are shown in Table 10.3. The IPAQ-S7S appears particularly suitable for routine clinical use given its strong research base [152]. A second measure, the GPPAQ, has been recommended for use in primary care practice in the UK [153], and thus may be appropriate as well, although the evidence base for this measure's psychometric properties is incomplete [154]. A brief measure to evaluate diet and nutrition, the REAP-S, may also be useful as a screen for identifying eating habits that are problematic.

Mental Health Problems Similar to the common practice of asking a few open-ended questions to assess adherence issues in kidney recipients, transplant teams may not systematically screen for psychological distress aside from asking general, open-ended question about how patients are feeling or how their mood has been. There are, however, many self-report measures available that can be used to screen patients for the presence of the most common problems, depression

and anxiety. Prime examples are listed in Table 10.3. For depression, an ultra-brief screener, such as the PHQ-2, takes less than 1 minute to complete. Other measures such as the PHQ-9, the MOS-Depression Screener, the BDI-Primary Care, and the CES-D short form are also quite brief. Longer versions of these and other measures are also available, widely used, and have well-documented psychometric properties. The measures can be used as continuous scales to determine degree of distress. However, even more important from a screening standpoint, each has a cut point that can be used to identify patients with clinically significant distress warranting more extensive evaluation and, potentially, treatment.

Screeners such as the GAD-2 and GAD-7 are available to evaluate anxiety symptoms, and measures such as the HADS, the Patient Health Questionnaire, the Hopkins Symptom Checklist and its derivatives, and the General Health Questionnaire assess multiple areas of distress. Each of these measures has strong psychometric properties and, as for the depression scales, established thresholds to indicate clinically significant distress.

Substance Use Transplant teams do not routinely monitor kidney recipients for tobacco, alcohol, or other drug use unless patients were identified before transplant as having a substance use disorder. For patients with no history of diagnosable disorder (the majority of kidney recipients), resumption of substance use—particularly use at levels that exceed post-transplant care recommendations—may be discovered only if patients or families volunteer such information or if patients develop medical complications that lead to team suspicions and subsequent evaluation to determine whether patients are using proscribed substances. For patients at risk for substance use, transplant programs could consider employing self-report screens for areas of substance use that are of concern (see Table 10.3). There are many such screeners available, including those that are specific to one type of substance use and those that assess use of any of multiple substances.

There are also a variety of biological assessments available, as noted in Table 10.3. However, such assessments are more costly than self-report screeners, require the patient to be seen at the follow-up clinic or a laboratory and may not detect sporadic use. In general, their findings will depend on the timing of the sample relative to actual substance use. They should be reserved for situations in which substance use risk is high or when substance use is suspected to be occurring on a regular basis [146]. Careful clinical interviewing about possible substance use, conducted in conjunction with the use of self-report measures, may yield higher rates of substance use identification than a reliance on biological measures [155].

Clinical Intervention for Psychosocial Problems

The interventions tested in research summarized earlier should be considered for potential use with kidney recipients struggling with adherence or mental health problems. We noted earlier that there is a dearth of research evidence on substance use interventions in kidney recipients. It is noteworthy that, although the evidence base on adherence-related and mental health-related interventions appears to be growing within transplantation, there has been very little consideration of whether the interventions tested would be able to be translated into routine clinical use. Most of the successful adherence-focused interventions and psychotherapeutic interventions have involved multiple face-to-face sessions with patients. Perhaps the most important message from these studies is that one-on-one coaching of patients can indeed improve adherence, and that both individual and group-based nonpharmacologic psychotherapeutic strategies can be helpful for reducing patients' depressive and anxiety symptoms. However, these interventions are likely to be labor-intensive for most transplant teams, and teams may not have the expertise to mount some of the effective interventions. If patients have healthcare insurance coverage that allows for referral for counseling-based strategies for adherence problems (including interventions for "lifestyle" health-related issues such as diet, exercise, and obesity management) and/or for mental health services, such studies suggest that positive results could be obtained. Of note, the intervention tested by Reese and colleagues, involving text messaging and email reminders about medication-taking, was also quite effective and may be a more realistic option for transplant programs to adopt. However, it also required electronic medication monitoring which, as we noted above, is not generally feasible for routine use. Nevertheless, the study suggests that use of mobile or e-health intervention strategies may hold particular promise for kidney recipients, and this is supported by intervention research in other types of organ recipients, as we discussed earlier.

We also noted earlier that there have been few tests of pharmacologic strategies for mental health issues in kidney recipients. Clinicians, therefore, must draw on the evidence regarding the safety and efficacy of strategies tested in other populations. Concerns have been voiced that altered drug clearances, drug-drug interactions, and prevalent cardiovascular comorbidity may alter the risk/benefit profile of antidepressant and anxiolytic medications in patients with chronic kidney disease, even after kidney transplantation [31]. These concerns notwithstanding, there is a large practice-focused literature showing that psychopharmacologic options can be used safely and effectively with transplant recipients with stable organ function, including kidney recipients [34, 97, 156, 157]. DiMartini et al. [97] provide a detailed consideration of which psychotropic medications should be used as first-line strategies in organ recipients, who take a cocktail of immunosuppressants and other medications. In particular, many immunosuppressant agents are primarily metabolized by the cytochrome P450 (CYP 450) enzyme system. Thus, psychotropic medications that strongly inhibit CYP 450 3A4 should be avoided (e.g., fluvoxamine and nefazodone). The selective serotonin reuptake inhibitors escitalopram and citalopram are likely the best choices. They may also be the best choices for long-term treatment of anxiety in organ recipients [157]. Although sertraline may be considered, the recent trials that we reviewed earlier, which showed no benefit for the treatment of depression in patients with chronic kidney disease, suggest that sertraline may not be the best initial choice of antidepressant medication for kidney recipients if other options are available. Sertraline's efficacy for anxiety in kidney disease populations has not been examined.

With respect to substance use, little to no research has focused specifically on kidney recipients. However, Corbett et al. [4] summarized evidence on efficacy of tobacco smoking cessation therapies across multiple meta-analyses and systematic reviews in a variety of study populations, showing that all major nicotine replacement therapies were effective. In addition, nicotine replacement therapy in combination with smoking cessation counseling appeared to be particularly effective. The use of the medications bupropion and varenicline was also found to be effective. However, these medications require caution with transplant recipients [97]. Bupropion should not be used in patients with a seizure disorder history or with electrolytes disturbances that could contribute to a seizure. Varenicline is renally excreted and thus should be appropriately adjusted in kidney recipients, especially in the context of impaired graft function.

With respect to alcohol and other substance use, Parker et al. [10] provide an overview of counseling-based strategies of potential use in transplant recipients, including motivational interviewing and mutual self-help approaches (e.g., Alcoholics Anonymous and Narcotics Anonymous) that can be considered. Transplant programs would likely refer patients to such programs rather than attempt to offer them in-house. In transplant populations, care is needed in the use of pharmacotherapies for alcohol and other substance use [34, 97]. Medications to reduce cravings and relapse risk for alcohol (e.g., acamprosate, ondansetron, naltrexone) or opioids (naltrexone) have not been studied in kidney or other organ transplant patients. Acamprosate is renally excreted and, therefore, the dosage may require adjustment in kidney recipients with impaired renal function. Naltrexone has a small risk of hepatotoxicity and would not be recommended in kidney recipients with liver dysfunction. Disulfiram is not recommended in transplant recipients. Please refer to Chap. 42 for more details on psychopharmacology in transplant recipients.

Conclusions and Future Directions

Recent years have seen a great expansion in research examining psychosocial problems in the areas of medical regimen adherence, mental health, and substance use after kidney transplantation. The bulk of work has been descriptive and has focused on prevalence and risk factors for problems. Nevertheless, our understanding of true risk factors, as opposed to correlates of post-transplant psychosocial difficulties, has remained incomplete. The most potent risk factor for post-transplant psychosocial problems is a history of such problems before transplantation. This information, at the very least, is valuable because it allows transplant programs to identify kidney recipients who require more careful follow-up post-transplant regarding psychosocial outcomes. Future work to provide a more definitive risk factor profile, plus continued emphasis on exploring patients' own perceptions of the causes of nonadherence, mental health problems, and substance use problems, may allow (a) better identification of patients who may need close monitoring post-transplant and (b) tailoring of interventions to be more responsive to the specific issues of concern to patients.

The evidence base indicating what interventions are most effective for psychosocial problems is also relatively slim. The bulk of evidence focuses on interventions to reduce or avoid immunosuppressant medication nonadherence, with very limited work testing interventions for other areas of nonadherence or for mental health problems. Virtually no research has examined interventions for substance use in kidney recipients. Drawing on available evidence in kidney recipients, as well as intervention research findings from other transplant, chronic disease and/or community populations, several recommendations for the care of kidney recipients can reasonably be made. Thus, screening for psychosocial problems is critical, and many tools are available to accomplish such screening efficiently during routine follow-up care after kidney transplantation. In the case of nonadherence, transplant programs will likely need to develop and administer their own interventions to assist patients, ideally modeled after interventions already tested. While some research-based interventions may not be feasible for transplant programs to employ (e.g., because the interventions may be too labor-intensive given program resources), transplant programs may be able to employ elements of these interventions to assist their patients with adhering to the medical regimen. In the case of mental health and substance use interventions, it is likely that patients will need to be referred to specialists for care, unless transplant teams include mental health and addictions experts as team members. Future research with a focus on the dissemination and update of efficacious psychosocial interventions by kidney transplant programs is needed in order to provide teams with the best resources for aiding their patients with adherence-related, mental health, and substance use issues after transplantation.

Acknowledgement Preparation of this manuscript was supported in part by Grants R01 DK101715 and R01 DK110737 from the National Institute of Diabetes and Digestive and Kidney Diseases.

References

1. Organ Procurement and Transplantation Network. Data tables. https://optn.transplant.hrsa.gov/data/. Updated December 15, 2017.
2. Organ Procurement and Transplantation Network/Scientific Registry of Transplant Recipients (OPTN/SRTR). OPTN/SRTR Annual Data Report 2015. Am J Transplant. 2017;17(Suppl 1):1–564.
3. Matas AJ, Gillingham KJ, Humar A, Kandaswamy R, Sutherland DE, Payne WD, et al. 2202 kidney transplant recipients with 10 years of graft function: what happens next? Am J Transplant. 2008;8:2410–9. https://doi.org/10.1111/j.1600-6143.2008.02414.x.
4. Corbett C, Armstrong MJ, Neuberger J. Tobacco smoking and solid organ transplantation. Transplantation. 2012;94:979–87.
5. Dew MA, DeVito Dabbs AJ, Posluszny DM, DiMartini AF. Adherence and self-management in the context of chronic disease: transplantation. In: Howren MB, Christensen AJ, editors. Patient adherence to medical treatment regimens and health lifestyle behaviors: promoting evidence-based research and practice. New York: Springer Publishing. in press.
6. Dew MA, Rosenberger EM, Myaskovsky L, DiMartini AF, DeVito Dabbs AJ, Posluszny DM, et al. Depression and anxiety as risk factors for morbidity and mortality after organ transplantation: a systematic review and meta-analysis. Transplantation. 2015;100:988–1003. https://doi.org/10.1097/TP.0000000000000901.
7. Duerinckx N, Burkhalter H, Engberg SJ, Kirsch M, Klem ML, Sereika SM, et al. Correlates and outcomes of posttransplant smoking in solid organ transplant recipients: a systematic literature review and meta-analysis. Transplantation. 2016;100:2252–63.
8. Neuberger JM, Bechstein WO, Kuypers DR, Burra P, Citterio F, De Geest S, et al. Practical recommendations for long-term management of modifiable risks in kidney and liver transplant recipients: A Guidance Report and Clinical Checklist by the Consensus on Managing Modifiable Risk in Transplantation (COMMIT) Group. Transplantation. 2017;101(4S Suppl 2):S1–56. https://doi.org/10.1097/TP.0000000000001651.
9. Nevins TE, Nickerson PW, Dew MA. Understanding medication nonadherence after kidney transplant. J Am Soc Nephrol. 2017;28:2290–301.
10. Parker R, Armstrong MJ, Corbett C, Day EJ, Neuberger JM. Alcohol and substance abuse in solid-organ transplant recipients. Transplantation. 2013;96:1015–24.
11. Dew MA, DeVito Dabbs A, Myaskovsky L, Shyu S, Shellmer DA, DiMartini AF, et al. Meta-analysis of medical regimen adherence outcomes in pediatric solid organ transplantation. Transplantation. 2009;88:736–46.
12. Dobbels F, Ruppar T, De Geest S, Decorte A, Van Damme-Lombaerts R, Fine RN. Adherence to the immunosuppressive regimen in pediatric kidney transplant recipients: a systematic review. Pediatr Transplant. 2010;14:603–13.

13. Gerson AC. Psychosocial issues in children with chronic kidney disease. In: Geary D, Schaefer F, editors. Pediatric kidney disease. Berlin: Springer; 2016. p. 1603–24.

14. Stuber ML. Psychiatric issues in pediatric organ transplantation. Child Adolesc Psychiatr Clin N Am. 2010;19:285–300.

15. Tong A, Morton R, Howard K, Craig JC. Adolescent experiences following organ transplantation: a systematic review of qualitative studies. J Pediatr. 2008;155:542–9.

16. Yazigi NA. Adherence and the pediatric transplant patient. Semin Pediatr Surg. 2017;26:267–71.

17. Belaiche S, Décaudin B, Dharancy S, Noel C, Odou P, Hazzan M. Factors relevant to medication non-adherence in kidney transplant: a systematic review. Int J Clin Pharm. 2017;39:582–93.

18. Butler JA, Roderick P, Mullee M, Mason JC, Peveler RC. Frequency and impact of nonadherence to immunosuppressants after renal transplantation: a systematic review. Transplantation. 2004;77:769–76.

19. Denhaerynck K, Dobbels F, Cleemput I, Desmyttere A, Schäfer-Keller P, Schaub S, et al. Prevalence, consequences, and determinants of nonadherence in adult renal transplant patients: a literature review. Transpl Int. 2005;18:1121–33.

20. Dew MA, DiMartini AF, DeVito Dabbs A, Myaskovsky L, Steel J, Unruh M, et al. Rates and risk factors for nonadherence to the medical regimen after adult solid organ transplantation. Transplantation. 2007;83:858–73.

21. Chisholm MA, Vollenweider LJ, Mulloy LL, Jagadeesan M, Wynn JJ, Rogers HE, et al. Renal transplant patient compliance with free immunosuppressive medications. Transplantation. 2000;70:1240–4.

22. Couzi L, Moulin B, Morin MP, Albano L, Godin M, Barrou B, et al. Factors predictive of medication nonadherence after renal transplantation: a French observational study. Transplantation. 2013;95:326–32.

23. De Geest S, Burkhalter H, Bogert L, Berben L, Glass TR, Denhaerynck K, et al. Describing the evolution of medication nonadherence from pretransplant until 3 years post-transplant and determining pretransplant medication nonadherence as risk factor for post-transplant nonadherence to immunosuppressives: the Swiss Transplant Cohort Study. Transpl Int. 2014;27:657–66.

24. Nevins TE, Kruse L, Skeans MA, Thomas W. The natural history of azathioprine compliance after renal transplantation. Kidney Int. 2001;60:1565–70.

25. Nevins TE, Robiner WN, Thomas W. Predictive patterns of early medication adherence in renal transplantation. Transplantation. 2014;98:878–84.

26. Tsapepas D, Langone A, Chan L, Wiland A, McCague K, Chisholm-Burns M. A longitudinal assessment of adherence with immunosuppressive therapy following kidney transplantation from the Mycophenolic Acid Observational REnal Transplant (MORE) study. Ann Transplant. 2014;19:174–81.

27. Vrijens B, Vincze G, Kristanto P, Urquhart J, Burnier M. Adherence to prescribed antihypertensive drug treatments: longitudinal study of electronically compiled dosing histories. BMJ. 2008;17:1114–7.

28. Yeaw J, Benner JS, Walt JG, Sian S, Smith DB. Comparing adherence and persistence across 6 chronic medication classes. J Manag Care Pharm. 2009;15:728–40.

29. Chilcot J, Spencer BWJ, Maple H, Mamode N. Depression and kidney transplantation. Transplantation. 2014;97:717–21.

30. Corbett C, Armstrong MJ, Parker R, Webb K, Neuberger JM. Mental health disorders and solid-organ transplant recipients. Transplantation. 2013;96:593–600.

31. Palmer S, Vecchio M, Craig JC, Tonelli M, Johnson DW, Nicolucci A, et al. Prevalence of depression in chronic kidney disease: systematic review and meta-analysis of observational studies. Kidney Int. 2013;84:179–91.

32. Veater NL, East L. Exploring depression amongst kidney transplant recipients: a literature review. J Ren Care. 2016;42:172–84.

33. Dew MA, DiMartini AF. Transplantation. In: Friedman HS, editor. Oxford handbook of health psychology. New York: Oxford University Press; 2011. p. 522–59.

34. DiMartini AF, Shenoy A, Dew MA. Organ transplantation. In: Levenson JL, editor. The American Psychiatric Publishing textbook of psychosomatic medicine: psychiatric care of the medically ill. 3rd ed. Washington DC: American Psychiatric Publishing, Inc. in press.

35. Vasquez V, Novarro N, Valdes RA, Britton GB. Factors associated to depression in renal transplant recipients in Panama. Indian J Psychiatry. 2013;55:273–8.

36. Dobbels F, Skeans MA, Snyder JJ, Tuomari AV, Maclean JR, Kasiske BL. Depressive disorder in renal transplantation: an analysis of medicare claims. Am J Kidney Dis. 2008;51:819–28.

37. Knowles SR, Castle DJ, Biscan SM, Salzberg M, O'Flaherty EB, Langham R. Relationships between illness perceptions, coping and psychological morbidity in kidney transplant patients. Am J Med Sci. 2016;351:233–8.

38. Muller HH, Englbrecht M, Wiesener MS, Titze S, Heller K, Groemer TW, et al. Depression, anxiety, resilience and coping pre and post kidney transplantation - initial findings from the Psychiatric Impairments in Kidney Transplantation (PI-KT)-Study. PLoS One. 2015;10(11):e0140706. https://doi.org/10.1371/journal.pone.0140706.

39. Janiszewska J, Lichodziejewska-Niemierko M, Gołębiewska J, Majkowicz M, Rutkowski B. Determinants of anxiety in patients with advanced somatic disease: differences and similarities between patients undergoing renal replacement therapies and patients suffering from cancer. Int Urol Nephrol. 2013;45:1379–87.

40. Butler MI, McCartan D, Cooney A, Kelly PO, Ahmed I, Little D, et al. Outcomes of renal transplantation in patients with bipolar affective disorder and schizophrenia: a national retrospective cohort study. Psychosomatics. 2017;58:69–76.

41. Abbott KC, Agodoa LY, O'Malley PG. Hospitalized psychoses after renal transplantation in the United States: incidence, risk factors, and prognosis. J Am Soc Nephrol. 2003;14:1628–35.

42. Zelle DM, Agarwal PK, Ramirez JL, van der Heide JJ, Corpeleijn E, Gans RO, et al. Alcohol consumption, new onset of diabetes after transplantation, and all-cause mortality in renal transplant recipients. Transplantation. 2011;92:203–9.

43. Hurst FP, Altieri M, Patel PP, Jindal TR, Guy SR, Sidawy AN, et al. Effect of smoking on kidney transplant outcomes: analysis of the United States renal data system. Transplantation. 2011;92:1101–7.

44. Dew MA, DiMartini AF, Steel J, DeVito Dabbs A, Myaskovsky L, Unruh M, et al. Meta-analysis of risk for relapse to substance use after transplantation of the liver or other solid organs. Liver Transpl. 2008;14:159–72.

45. Greenan G, Ahmad SB, Anders MG, Leeser A, Bromberg JS, Niederhaus SV. Recreational marijuana use is not associated with worse outcomes after renal transplantation. Clin Transpl. 2016;30:1340–6. https://doi.org/10.1111/ctr.12828.

46. Sabaté E. Adherence to long-term therapies: evidence for action. Geneva: World Health Organization; 2003. http://apps.who.int/medicinedocs/pdf/s4883e/s4883e.pdf

47. Fine RN, Becker Y, De Geest S, Eisen H, Ettenger R, Evans R, et al. Nonadherence consensus conference summary report. Am J Transplant. 2009;9:35–41.

48. Osterberg L, Blaschke T. Adherence to medication. N Engl J Med. 2005;353:487–97.

49. Gaston RS, Hudson SL, Ward M, Jones P, Macon R. Late renal allograft loss: Noncompliance masquerading as chronic rejection. Transplant Proc. 1999;31(4, Suppl 1):21S–3S.

50. Gaynor JJ, Ciancio G, Guerra G, Sageshima J, Hanson L, Roth D, et al. Graft failure due to noncompliance among 628 kidney transplant recipients with long-term follow-up: a single-center observational study. Transplantation. 2014;97:925–33.

51. Israni AJ, Weng FL, Cen YY, Joffe M, Kamoun M, Feldman HI. Electronically-measured adherence to immunosuppressive medications and kidney function after deceased donor kidney transplantation. Clin Transpl. 2011;25:E124–31.

52. Taber DJ, Fleming JN, Fominaya CE, Gebregziabher M, Hunt KJ, Srinivas TR, et al. The impact of health care appointment non-adherence on graft outcomes in kidney transplantation. Am J Nephrol. 2017;45:91–8.

53. Chisholm-Burns MA, Kwong WJ, Mulloy LL, Spivey CA. Nonmodifiable characteristics associated with nonadherence to immunosuppressant therapy in renal transplant recipients. Am J Health Syst Pharm. 2008;65:1242–7.

54. Patzer RE, Serper M, Reese PP, Przytula K, Koval R, Ladner DP, et al. Medication understanding, non-adherence, and clinical outcomes among adult kidney transplant recipients. Clin Transpl. 2016;30:1294–305.

55. Weng FL, Israni AK, Joffe MM, Hoy T, Gaughan CA, Newman M, et al. Race and electronically measured adherence to immuno-suppressive medications after deceased donor renal transplantation. J Am Soc Nephrol. 2005;16:1839–48.

56. Weng FL, Chandwani S, Kurtyka KM, Zacker C, Chisholm-Burns MA, Demissie K. Prevalence and correlates of medication non-adherence among kidney transplant recipients more than 6 months post-transplant: a cross-sectional study. BMC Nephrol. 2013;14:261.

57. Jamieson NJ, Hanson CS, Josephson MA, Gordon EJ, Craig JC, Halleck F, et al. Motivations, challenges, and attitudes to self-management in kidney transplant recipients: a systematic review of qualitative studies. Am J Kidney Dis. 2016;67:461–78.

58. Tong A, Howell M, Wong G, Webster AC, Howard K, Craig J. The perspectives of kidney transplant recipients on medicine taking: a systematic review of qualitative studies. Nephrol Dial Transplant. 2011;26:344–54.

59. Zelle DM, Dorland HF, Rosmalen JG, Corpeleijn E, Gans RO, van der Heide JJ H, et al. Impact of depression on long-term outcome after renal transplantation: a prospective cohort study. Transplantation. 2012;94:1033–40.

60. Novak M, Molnar MZ, Szeifert L, Kovacs AZ, Vamos EP, Zoller R, et al. Depressive symptoms and mortality in patients after kidney transplantation: a prospective prevalent cohort study. Psychosom Med. 2010;72:527–34.

61. Szeifert L, Molnar MZ, Ambrus C, Koczy AB, Kovacs AZ, Vamos EP, et al. Symptoms of depression in kidney transplant recipients: a cross-sectional study. Am J Kidney Dis. 2010;55:132–40.

62. Tsunoda T, Yamashita R, Kojima Y, Takahara S. Risk factors for depression after kidney transplantation. Transplant Proc. 2010;42:1679–81.

63. Srifuengfung M, Noppakun K, Srisurapanont M. Depression in kidney transplant recipients: prevalence, risk factors, and association with functional disabilities. J Nerv Ment Dis. 2017;205:788–92.

64. Czira ME, Lindner AV, Szeifert L, Molnar MZ, Fornadi K, Kelemen A, et al. Association between the malnutrition-inflammation score and depressive symptoms in kidney transplanted patients. Gen Hosp Psychiatry. 2011;33:157–65.

65. Christensen AJ, Ehlers SL, Raichle KA, Bertolatus JA, Lawton WJ. Predicting change in depression following renal transplantation: effect of patient coping preferences. Health Psychol. 2000;19:348–53.

66. Pisanti R, Poli L, Lombardo C, Bennardi L, Giordanengo L, Berloco PB, et al. The role of transplant-related stressors and social support in the development of anxiety among renal trans-plant recipients: the direct and buffering effects. Psychol Health Med. 2014;19:650–5.

67. Schipper K, Abma TA, Koops C, Bakker I, Sanderman R, Schroevers MJ. Sweet and sour after renal transplantation: a quali-tative study about the positive and negative consequences of renal transplantation. Br J Health Psychol. 2014;19:580–91.

68. Bianchi R, Schonfeld IS, Laurent E. Burnout-depression overlap: a review. Clin Psychol Rev. 2015;36:28–41.

69. Fierz K, Steiger J, Denhaerynck K, Dobbels F, Bock A, De Geest S. Prevalence, severity and correlates of alcohol use in adult renal transplant recipients. Clin Transpl. 2006;20:171–8.

70. Chisholm MA, Mulloy LL, Jagadeesan M, DiPiro JT. Impact of clinical pharmacy services on renal transplant patients' com-pliance with immunosuppressive medications. Clin Transpl. 2001;15:330–6.

71. Hardstaff R, Green K, Talbot D. Measurement of compliance posttransplantation—the results of a 12-month study using elec-tronic monitoring. Transplant Proc. 2003;35:796–7.

72. De Geest S, Schäfer-Keller P, Denhaerynck K, Thannberger N, Köfer S, Bock A, et al. Supporting medication adherence in renal transplantation (SMART): a pilot RCT to improve adherence to immunosuppressive regimens. Clin Transpl. 2006;20:359–68.

73. Russell C, Conn V, Ashbaugh C, Madsen R, Wakefield M, Webb A, et al. Taking immunosuppressive medications effectively (TIMELink): a pilot randomized controlled trial in adult kidney transplant recipients. Clin Transpl. 2011;25:864–70.

74. Chisholm-Burns MA, Spivey CA, Graff Zivin J, Lee JK, Sredzinski E, Tolley EA. Improving outcomes of renal transplant recipients with behavioral adherence contracts: a randomized con-trolled trial. Am J Transplant. 2013;13:2364–73.

75. Kuypers DRJ, Peeters PC, Sennesael JJ, Kianda MN, Vrijens B, Kristanto P, et al. Improved adherence to tacrolimus once-daily formulation in renal recipients: a randomized controlled trial using electronic monitoring. Transplantation. 2013;95:333–40.

76. McGillicuddy JW, Gregoski MJ, Weiland AK, Rock RA, Brunner-Jackson BM, Patel SK, et al. Mobile health medication adher-ence and blood pressure control in renal transplant recipients: a proof-of-concept randomized controlled trial. JMIR Res Protoc. 2013;2:E32. https://doi.org/10.2196/resprot.2633.

77. Joost R, Dörje F, Schwitulla J, Eckardt KU, Hugo C. Intensified pharmaceutical care is improving immunosuppressive medica-tion adherence in kidney transplant recipients during the first post-transplant year: a quasi-experimental study. Nephrol Dial Transplant. 2014;29:1597–607.

78. Annunziato RA, Parbhakar M, Kapoor K, Matloff R, Casey N, Benchimol C, et al. Can transition to adult care for transplant recipients be improved by intensified services while patients are still in pediatrics? Prog Transplant. 2015;25:236–42.

79. Garcia MF, Bravin AM, Garcia PD, Contti MM, Nga HS, Takase HM, et al. Behavioral measures to reduce non-adherence in renal transplant recipients: a prospective randomized controlled trial. Int Urol Nephrol. 2015;47:1899–905.

80. McQuillan RF, Toulany A, Kaufman M, Schiff JR. Benefits of a transfer clinic in adolescent and young adult kidney transplant patients. Can J Kidney Health Dis. 2015;2:45.

81. Bessa AB, Felipe CR, Hannun P, Sayuri P, Felix MJ, Ruppel P, et al. Prospective randomized trial investigating the influ-ence of pharmaceutical care on the intra-individual variabil-ity of tacrolimus concentrations early after kidney transplant. Ther Drug Monit. 2016;38:447–55. https://doi.org/10.1097/FTD.0000000000000299.

82. Breu-Dejean N, Driot D, Dupouy J, Lapeyre-Mestre M, Rostaing L. Efficacy of psychoeducational intervention on allograft func-tion in kidney transplant patients: 10-year results of a prospective randomized study. Exp Clin Transplant. 2016;14:38–44.

83. Cukor D, Ver Halen N, Pencille M, Tedla F, Salifu M. A pilot randomized controlled trial to promote immunosuppressant adherence in adult kidney transplant recipients. Nephron. 2017;135:6–14.

84. Reese PP, Bloom RD, Trofe-Clark J, Mussell A, Leidy D, Levsky S, et al. Automated reminders and physician notification to promote immunosuppression adherence among kidney transplant recipients: a randomized trial. Am J Kidney Dis. 2017;69:400–9.

85. Schmid A, Hils S, Kramer-Zucker A, Bogatyreva L, Hauschke D, De Geest S, Pisarski P. Telemedically supported case management of living-donor renal transplant recipients to optimize routine evidence-based aftercare: a single-center randomized controlled trial. Am J Transplant. 2017;17:1594–605.

86. Henriksson J, Tydén G, Höijer J, Wadström J. A prospective randomized trial on the effect of using an electronic monitoring drug dispensing device to improve adherence and compliance. Transplantation. 2016;100:203–9.

87. Dew MA, DeVito Dabbs AJ. Harnessing the power of qualitative research in transplantation. Am J Kidney Dis. 2016;67:357–9.

88. Hsiao CY, Lin LW, Su YW, Yeh SH, Lee LN, Tsai FM. The effects of an empowerment intervention on renal transplant recipients: a randomized controlled trial. J Nurs Res. 2016;24:201–10.

89. Fleming JN, Taber DJ, McElligott J, McGillicuddy JW, Treiber F. Mobile health in solid organ transplant: the time is now. Am J Transplant. 2017;17:2263–76. https://doi.org/10.1111/ajt.14225.

90. Lorenz EC, Amer H, Dean PG, Stegall MD, Cosio FG, Cheville AL. Adherence to a pedometer-based physical activity intervention following kidney transplant and impact on metabolic parameters. Clin Transpl. 2015;29:560–8.

91. Tzvetanov I, West-Thielke P, D'Amico G, Johnsen M, Ladik A, Hachaj G, et al. A novel and personalized rehabilitation program for obese kidney transplant recipients. Transplant Proc. 2014;46:3431–7.

92. Baines LS, Joseph JT, Jindal RM. Emotional issues after kidney transplantation: a prospective psychotherapeutic study. Clin Transpl. 2002;16:455–60.

93. Baines LS, Joseph JT, Jindal RM. Prospective randomized study of individual and group psychotherapy versus controls in recipients of renal transplants. Kidney Int. 2004;65:1937–42.

94. Gross CR, Kreitzer MJ, Russas V, Treesak C, Frazier PA, Hertz MI. Mindfulness meditation to reduce symptoms after organ transplant: a pilot study. Altern Ther Health Med. 2004;10:58–66.

95. Gross CR, Kreitzer MJ, Thomas W, Reilly-Spong M, Cramer-Bornemann M, Nyman JA, et al. Mindfulness-based stress reduction for solid organ transplant recipients: a randomized controlled trial. Altern Ther Health Med. 2010;16:30–8.

96. Kreitzer MJ, Gross CR, Ye X, Russas V, Treesak C. Longitudinal impact of mindfulness meditation on illness burden in solid-organ transplant recipients. Prog Transplant. 2005;15:166–72.

97. DiMartini AF, Dew MA, Crone C. Organ transplantation. In: Sadock BJ, Sadock VA, Ruiz P, editors. Kaplan and Sadock's comprehensive textbook of psychiatry. 10th ed. Philadelphia: Wolters Kluwer; 2017. p. 2357–73.

98. Hedayati SS, Gregg LP, Carmody T, Jain N, Toups M, Rush AJ, et al. Effect of sertraline on depressive symptoms in patients with chronic kidney disease without dialysis dependence: the CAST randomized clinical trial. JAMA. 2017;318:1876–90.

99. Hedayati SS, Daniel DM, Cohen S, Comstock B, Cukor D, Diaz-Linhart Y, et al. Rationale and design of a trial of sertraline vs. cognitive behavioral therapy for end-stage renal disease patients with depression (ASCEND). Contemp Clin Trials. 2016;47:1–11.

100. Tome S, Said A, Lucey MR. Addictive behavior after solid organ transplantation: what do we know already and what do we need to know? Liver Transpl. 2008;14:127–9.

101. Pita-Fernández S, Seijo-Bestilleiro R, Pértega-Díaz S, Alonso-Hernández Á, Fernández-Rivera C, Cao-López M, et al. A randomized clinical trial to determine the effectiveness of CO-oximetry

and anti-smoking brief advice in a cohort of kidney transplant patients who smoke: study protocol for a randomized controlled trial. Trials. 2016;17:174.

102. Addolorato G, Mirijello A, Leggio L, Ferrulli A, D'Angelo C, Vassallo G, et al. Liver transplantation in alcoholic patients: impact of an alcohol addiction unit within a liver transplant center. Alcohol Clin Exp Res. 2013;37:1601–8.

103. Masson S, Marrow B, Kendrick S, Elsharkawy AM, Latimer S, Hudson M. An 'alcohol contract' has no significant effect on return to drinking after liver transplantation for alcoholic liver disease. Transpl Int. 2014;27:475–81.

104. Oberlin SR, Parente ST, Pruett TL. Improving medication adherence among kidney transplant recipients: findings from other industries, patient engagement, and behavioral economics-a scoping review. Sage Open Med. 2016;4:2050312115625026.

105. Bia M, Adey DB, Bloom RD, Chan L, Kulkarni S, Tomlanovich S. KDOQI US commentary on the 2009 KDIGO clinical practice guideline for the care of kidney transplant recipients. Am J Kidney Dis. 2010;56:189–218.

106. Kidney Disease: Improving Global Outcomes (KDIGO) Transplant Work Group. KDIGO clinical practice guideline for the care of kidney transplant recipients. Am J Transplant. 2009;9(Suppl 3):S1–157.

107. Chisholm MA, Lance CE, Williamson GM, Mulloy LL. Development and validation of the immunosuppressant therapy adherence instrument (ITAS). Patient Educ Couns. 2005;59:13–20.

108. Wilks SE, Spivey CA, Chisholm-Burns MA. Psychometric re-evaluation of the immunosuppressant therapy adherence scale among solid-organ transplant recipients. J Eval Clin Pract. 2010;16:64–8.

109. Shäfer-Keller P, Steiger J, Bock A, Denhaerynck K, De Geest S. Diagnostic accuracy of measurement methods to assess nonadherence to immunosuppressive drugs in kidney transplant recipients. Am J Transplant. 2008;8:616–26.

110. Shemesh E, Fine RN. Is calculating the standard deviation of tacrolimus blood levels the new gold standard for evaluating nonadherence to medications in transplant recipients? Pediatr Transplant. 2010;14:940–3.

111. Supelana C, Annunziato R, Schiano T, Anand R, Vaidya S, Chuang K, et al. The medication level variability index (MLVI) predicts rejection, possibly due to nonadherence, in adult liver transplant recipients. Liver Transpl. 2014;20:1168–77.

112. Maclean JR, Pfister M, Zhou Z, Roy A, Tuomari VA, Heifets M. Quantifying the impact of nonadherence patterns on exposure to oral immunosuppressants. Ther Clin Risk Manag. 2011;7:149–56. https://doi.org/10.2147/TCRM.S16870.

113. Scheel J, Reber S, Stoessel L, Waldmann E, Jank S, Eckardt KU, et al. Patient-reported non-adherence and immunosuppressant trough levels are associated with rejection after renal transplantation. BMC Nephrol. 2017;18:107.

114. Craig C, Marshall A, Sjostrom M, Bauman AE, Booth ML, Ainsworth BE, et al. International physical activity questionnaire: 12-country reliability and validity. Med Sci Sports Exerc. 2003;35:1381–95. https://doi.org/10.1249/01.MSS.0000078924.61453.FB.

115. Department of Health (UK). The general practice physical activity questionnaire: a screening tool to assess adult physical activity levels, within primary care. 2009 https://www.gov.uk/government/uploads/system/uploads/attachment_data/file/192453/GPPAQ_-_guidance.pdf.

116. Segal-Isaacson CJ, Wylie-Rosett J, Gans KM. Validation of a short dietary assessment questionnaire: the Rapid Eating and Activity Assessment for Participants short version (REAP-S). Diabetes Educ. 2004;30:774–10.

117. Kroenke K, Spitzer RL, Williams JBW. The Patient Health Questionnaire-2: validity of a two-item depression screener. Med Care. 2003;41:1284–92.

118. Kroenke K, Spitzer RL, Williams JBW. The PHQ-9: validity of a brief depression severity measure. J Gen Intern Med. 2001;16:606–13.

119. Burnam MA, Wells KB, Leake B, Landsverk J. Development of a brief screening instrument for detecting depressive disorders. Med Care. 1988;26:775–89.

120. Beck AT, Steer RA, Brown GK. Beck Depression Inventory: second edition manual. San Antonio: The Psychological Corporation; 1996.

121. Beck AT, Steer RA, Brown GK. BDI: FastScreen for Medical Patients manual. San Antonio: The Psychological Corporation; 2000.

122. Radloff LS. The CES-D scale: a self-report depression scale for research in the general population. Appl Psychol Meas. 1977;1:385–401.

123. Kohout FJ, Berman LF, Evans DA, Cornoni-Huntley J. Two shorter forms of the CES-D depression symptoms index. J Aging Health. 1993;5:179–93.

124. Kroenke K, Spitzer RL, Williams JBW, Monahan PO, Lowe B. Anxiety disorders in primary care: prevalence, impairment, comorbidity, and detection. Ann Intern Med. 2007;146:317–25.

125. Spitzer RL, Kroenke K, Williams JB, Löwe B. A brief measure for assessing generalized anxiety disorder: the GAD-7. Arch Intern Med. 2006;166:1092–7.

126. Snaith RP. The Hospital Anxiety and Depression Scale. Health Qual Life Outcomes. 2003;1:29.

127. Spitzer RL, Williams JBW, Kroenke K, Linzer M, de Gruy FV 3rd, Hahn SR, et al. Utility of a new procedure for diagnosing mental disorders in primary care: the PRIME-MD 1000 study. JAMA. 1994;272:1749–56.

128. Derogatis LR, Lipman RS, Rickels K, Uhlenhuth EH, Covi L. The Hopkins Symptom Checklist (HSCL): a self-report symptom inventory. Behav Sci. 1974;19:1–15.

129. Derogatis LR. BSI Brief Symptom Inventory: administration, scoring, and procedure manual. 4th ed. Minneapolis: Pearson Education, Inc.; 1993.

130. Derogatis LR. SCL-90-R administration, scoring and procedures manual. Minneapolis: Pearson Education, Inc.; 1994.

131. Goldberg D, Williams P. A user's guide to the General Health Questionnaire. Windsor: NFER-Nelson; 1988.

132. Heatherton TF, Kozlowski LT, Frecker RC, Fagerström KO. The Fagerström Test for Nicotine Dependence: a revision of the Fagerström Tolerance Questionnaire. Br J Addict. 1991;86:1119–27.

133. Ebbert JO, Patten CA, Schroeder DR. The Fagerström Test for Nicotine Dependence-Smokeless Tobacco (FTND-ST). Addict Behav. 2006;31:1716–21.

134. Mayfield D, McLeod G, Hall P. The CAGE questionnaire: validation of a new alcoholism screening instrument. Am J Psychiatry. 1974;131:1121–3.

135. Selzer ML. The Michigan Alcoholism Screening Test: the quest for a new diagnostic instrument. Am J Psychiatry. 1971;127:1653–8.

136. Selzer ML, Vinokur A, van Rooijan L. A self-administered short Michigan Alcoholism Screening Test (SMAST). J Stud Alcohol. 1975;36:117–26.

137. Pokorny AD, Miller BA, Kaplan HB. The brief MAST: a shortened version of the Michigan Alcoholism Screening Test. Am J Psychiatry. 1972;129:342–5.

138. Saunders JB, Aasland OG, Babor TF, de la Fuente JR, Grant M. Development of the Alcohol Use Disorders Identification Test (AUDIT): WHO collaborative project on early detection of persons with harmful alcohol consumption–II. Addiction. 1993;88:791–804.

139. Bush K, Kivlahan DR, McDonell MB, Fihn SD, Bradley KA. The AUDIT alcohol consumption questions (AUDIT-C): an effective brief screening test for problem drinking. Arch Intern Med. 1998;158:1789–95.

140. Smith PC, Schmidt SM, Allensworth-Davies D, Saitz R. A single-question screening test for drug use in primary care. Arch Intern Med. 2010;170:1155–60.

141. Skinner HA. The Drug Abuse Screening Test. Addict Behav. 1982;7:363–71.

142. Yudko E, Lozhkina O, Fouts A. A comprehensive review of the psychometric properties of the Drug Abuse Screening Test. J Subst Abuse Treat. 2007;32:189–98.

143. WHO ASSIST Working Group. The Alcohol, Smoking and Substance Involvement Screening Test (ASSIST): development, reliability and feasibility. Addiction. 2002;97:1183–94.

144. Brown RL, Rounds LA. Conjoint screening questionnaires for alcohol and other drug abuse: criterion validity in a primary care practice. Wis Med J. 1995;94:135–40.

145. Bastiaens L, Riccardi K, Sakhrani D. The RAFFT as a screening tool for adult substance use disorders. Am J Drug Alcohol Abuse. 2002;28:681–91.

146. Grigsby TJ, Sussman S, Chou CP, Ames SL. Assessment of substance misuse. In: VanGeest JB, Johnson TP, Alemagno SA, editors. Research methods in the study of substance abuse. Cham, Switzerland: Springer; 2017. p. 197–234.

147. Richter L, Johnson PB. Current methods of assessing substance use: a review of strengths, problems, and developments. J Drug Issues. 2001;31:809–32.

148. Park LG, Howie-Esquivel J, Dracup K. Electronic measurement of medication adherence. West J Nurs Res. 2015;37:28–49.

149. Stirratt MJ, Dunbar-Jacob J, Crane HM, Simoni JM, Czajkowski S, Hilliard ME, et al. Self-report measures of medication adherence behavior: recommendations on optimal use. Transl Behav Med. 2015;5:470–82. https://doi.org/10.1007/s13142-015-0315-2.

150. Berben L, Dobbels F, Kugler C, Russell CL, De Geest S. Interventions used by health care professionals to enhance medication adherence in transplant patients: a survey of current clinical practice. Prog Transplant. 2011;21:322–31.

151. Dobbels F, Berben L, De Geest S, Drent G, Lennerling A, Whittaker C, et al. The psychometric properties and practicability of self-report instruments to identify medication nonadherence in adult transplant patients: a systematic review. Transplantation. 2010;90:205–19.

152. Silsbury Z, Goldsmith R, Rushton A. Systematic review of the measurement properties of self-report physical activity questionnaires in healthy adult populations. BMJ Open. 2015;5:e008430.

153. National Institute for Health and Care Excellence (NICE). Physical activity: brief advice for adults in primary care. London: NICE Public Health Guidance; 2013. p. 44.

154. Smith TO, McKenna MC, Salter C, Hardeman W, Richardson K, Hillsdon M, et al. A systematic review of the physical activity assessment tools used in primary care. Fam Pract. 2017;34:384–91.

155. DiMartini A, Day N, Dew MA, Lane T, Fitzgerald MG, Magill J, et al. Alcohol use following liver transplantation: a comparison of follow-up methods. Psychosomatics. 2001;42:55–62.

156. Crone CC, Gabriel GM. Treatment of anxiety and depression in transplant patients: pharmacokinetic considerations. Clin Pharmacokinet. 2004;43(6):361–94.

157. Sher Y, Zimbrean P. Psychiatric aspects of organ transplantation in critical care: an update. Crit Care Clin. 2017;33:659–79.

End-Stage Liver Disease and Indications for Liver Transplantation

Aparna Goel, Osama Siddique, and Aijaz Ahmed

Epidemiology of Cirrhosis

End-stage liver disease or cirrhosis is the twelfth leading cause of death in the United States (USA), accounting for over 38,000, or 1.5%, of all deaths in 2014 [1]. Cirrhosis represents an irreversible outcome of progressive hepatic fibrosis, characterized by diffuse nodular regeneration surrounded by dense fibrotic septa with architectural distortion [2]. The marked distortion of the intrahepatic vasculature and hepatic parenchymal extinction result in increased portal pressures and hepatic synthetic dysfunction. In the early stages of fibrosis, treatment aimed at the underlying cause of liver disease may prevent progression of or even reverse hepatic fibrosis. However, without treatment, cirrhosis may result.

The most common etiologies of cirrhosis in the United States are chronic viral hepatitis, alcoholic liver disease (ALD), and nonalcoholic steatohepatitis (NASH).

The viral hepatitis infections that lead to chronic liver disease are hepatitis B and C. While the overall prevalence of chronic hepatitis B infection in the United States is low, there remains a disproportionately high rate of infection in persons emigrating from regions of high or intermediate endemicity. As these persons usually acquire hepatitis B via perinatal transmission, the rates of chronic infection are quite high. Treatment of hepatitis B virus certainly reduces the risk of hepatocellular cancer and cirrhosis, but these significant complications remain an important cause for liver transplantation. Exposure to hepatitis C virus results in chronic infection in 75–85% of persons [3]. The most significant risk factor for acquiring hepatitis C infection is a history of injection drug use. Unfortunately, nearly 75% of hepatitis C infections are undiagnosed in the United States, which is a significant public health concern [4]. There are large-scale screening efforts to diagnose hepatitis C in the community as the virus is readily treatable with new direct-acting antivirals [5, 6].

Alcohol use disorder is a major cause of morbidity and mortality in the United States and accounts for over 88,000 deaths annually [7]. Alcoholic liver disease encompasses a clinical and histologic spectrum of steatosis (fatty change in the liver), alcoholic hepatitis (inflammation, hepatocyte necrosis), and cirrhosis. There is a direct dose-dependent relationship between the amount of alcohol consumed and risk of liver disease; however, genetic factors likely contribute as well.

Nonalcoholic fatty liver disease (NAFLD) is rapidly rising in the United States and is prevalent in approximately 30% of the overall population [8]. It is considered the hepatic manifestation of metabolic syndrome and is seen most frequently in obese patients with diabetes, hypertriglyceridemia, and hypertension. Similar to ALD, NAFLD includes a spectrum of disease from simple steatosis to NASH to cirrhosis. It is unclear what percentage of patients with NAFLD will progress to NASH, but we believe that approximately 15% of patients with NASH will develop cirrhosis.

While chronic hepatitis C virus (HCV) infection is the leading indication for liver transplantation and accounts for approximately 25% of all transplants currently, this is expected to decrease with highly effective and curative treatment of HCV with direct-acting antivirals [9]. Recent trends on the liver transplant waiting list reveal that NASH will likely emerge as the leading indication for liver transplantation in the near future, as the rate of transplants for NASH has increased to over 20% in the past decade [10–12]. ALD remains an important cause of end-stage liver disease, accounting for nearly 20% of all liver transplants in the United States [13]. Of concern is the recent data from National Epidemiologic Survey on Alcohol indicating that the 12-month prevalence of alcohol use, high-risk drinking,

A. Goel · A. Ahmed (✉)
Division of Gastroenterology and Hepatology, Department of Medicine, Stanford University School of Medicine, Stanford, CA, USA
e-mail: aijazahmed@stanford.edu

O. Siddique
Department of Medicine, Memorial Hospital of Rhode Island/ Alpert Medical School of Brown University, Providence, RI, USA

© Springer International Publishing AG, part of Springer Nature 2019
Y. Sher, J. R. Maldonado (eds.), *Psychosocial Care of End-Stage Organ Disease and Transplant Patients*,
https://doi.org/10.1007/978-3-319-94914-7_11

and alcohol use disorder is on the rise across all sociodemographic groups in the United States [14]. Other causes of cirrhosis include, but are not limited to, cholestatic liver disease such as primary sclerosing cholangitis and primary biliary cholangitis, autoimmune hepatitis, alpha-1 antitrypsin deficiency, hemochromatosis, Wilson's disease, veno-occlusive disease such as Budd-Chiari, and drug-induced liver injury.

Natural History of Cirrhosis

The natural history of cirrhosis is characterized by an initial asymptomatic and often undiagnosed phase, termed compensated cirrhosis. Patients with compensated cirrhosis have normal liver synthetic function and a median survival greater than 12 years [15]. Regardless of the etiology, patients with cirrhosis are susceptible to developing a variety of complications of portal hypertension and liver dysfunction, classified as decompensated cirrhosis. The risk of developing complications of cirrhosis, and hence transitioning from compensated to decompensated cirrhosis, is approximately 5–7% per year [15]. Often, these complications are rapidly progressive, leading to a markedly reduced life expectancy, with a median survival of 1.6 years.

Complications of End-Stage Liver Disease

Portal Hypertension Complications

Many complications from end-stage liver disease are a result of portal hypertension, or increased pressures within the portal venous system. The structural distortion of hepatic parenchyma inherent to cirrhosis and increase in vasodilator production result in elevated resistance to portal blood flow and formation of collaterals [16]. Portal hypertension can lead to the development of ascites, varices, hepatic encephalopathy, hepatorenal syndrome, hepatopulmonary syndrome, and portopulmonary hypertension.

Ascites

Ascites is the pathologic accumulation of fluid within the peritoneal cavity and the most common complication of cirrhosis. Ascites develops as a consequence of sinusoidal fibrosis and systemic vasodilation. The dense fibrotic tissue and "capillarization" of hepatic sinusoids increase splanchnic capillary pressure and result in excess lymph formation that leaks into the peritoneal cavity from the hepatic surface [17]. Additionally, the profound systemic arterial vasodilation due to increased nitric oxide levels activates the renin-angiotensin-aldosterone system, resulting in water and sodium retention, expansion of plasma volume, and hence ascites [18].

All patients with new-onset ascites should have a diagnostic paracentesis performed to determine the serum-ascites albumin gradient (SAAG) and total cell count [19]. A SAAG >1.1 g/dL is consistent with ascites due to portal hypertension. A SAAG <1.1 g/dL warrants further investigation of the etiology of ascites, which may be from malignancy, tuberculosis, nephrotic syndrome, or another inflammatory condition. Ascites due to cirrhosis is initially treated with a combination of diuretics and salt restriction of 2000 mg per day. More stringent restriction in sodium intake is not recommended as it is poorly tolerated and likely to lead to malnutrition. Diuretic regimens usually include a combination of an aldosterone receptor antagonist, such as spironolactone, and a loop diuretic, such as furosemide [20]. Importantly, in patients with alcohol-induced liver injury, cessation of alcohol use is paramount in treating ascites [21]. In some patients with refractory ascites or significant hyponatremia limiting diuretic use, repeated therapeutic paracentesis or transjugular intrahepatic portosystemic shunt (TIPS) placement may be necessary. Hepatic encephalopathy is an unfortunate frequent complication of TIPS, occurring in 30–60% of patients within 1 year after the TIPS procedure [22]. A patent TIPS allows portal blood flow to bypass the liver, where toxic ammonia is converted to urea via the urea cycle. The accumulation of ammonia contributes to hepatic encephalopathy.

Cirrhotic patients with ascites are at risk of developing an infection in the peritoneal fluid, called spontaneous bacterial peritonitis (SBP). This infection occurs without evidence of an intra-abdominal secondary source and is characterized by an elevated ascites fluid absolute polymorphonuclear leukocyte count ≥ 250 cells/mm^3 or a positive bacterial culture [23]. In-hospital mortality after the first episode of SBP ranges from 10% to 50%, and among those who survive, 70% will have a recurrent episode within 1 year [24, 25]. Given the significant mortality associated with SBP, antimicrobial prophylaxis is recommended in patients at high risk of developing SBP or those with a prior episode of SBP [19, 26].

Hepatorenal Syndrome
Hepatorenal syndrome is the development of kidney failure in patients with advanced cirrhosis and marked portal hypertension. It is perhaps the most deleterious complication of refractory ascites and is associated with rapid deterioration and high mortality [27]. In hepatorenal syndrome, the kidneys are structurally normal, but the marked circulatory dysfunction in advanced cirrhosis results in renal failure. As liver disease progresses, increased nitric oxide production results in splanchnic arterial vasodilation and reduced systemic vascular resistance. When increases in cardiac output are unable to compensate for the reduced vascular resistance, arterial underfilling occurs. The underfilling of the renal arterioles results in sodium and water retention, leading to ascites and edema, and further activation of vasoconstrictor

systems. These compensatory mechanisms help maintain effective arterial blood volume but can ultimately lead to intrarenal vasoconstriction, hypoperfusion, and hence renal failure [27–29].

There are two types of hepatorenal syndrome, differing in the rapidity of decline in renal function. Type 1 is associated with a worse prognosis and is defined as a doubling of serum creatinine to greater than 2.5 mg/dL in less than 2 weeks. Type 2 hepatorenal syndrome is a slower, more progressive disease associated with a creatinine greater than 1.5 mg/dL or creatinine clearance less than 40 cc/min. Both are associated with refractory ascites. The median survival with type 1 hepatorenal syndrome is 1 month compared to 6 months with type 2 hepatorenal syndrome [30].

The diagnosis of hepatorenal syndrome is based upon clinical criteria including lack of improvement in renal function after withdrawal of diuretics and expansion of plasma volume, absence of shock, and lack of renal parenchymal disease. Treatment of hepatorenal syndrome includes volume expansion, midodrine for vasoconstriction to increase mean arterial pressure, and octreotide to decrease splanchnic vasodilation. The definitive cure for hepatorenal syndrome is liver transplantation. If liver transplant is not performed within 1 month of developing hepatorenal syndrome, the kidneys usually do not recover, and a combined liver and kidney transplantation may be necessary [30].

Variceal Bleeding

Varices develop due to the increased portal blood flow into a fibrotic liver with high intrahepatic resistance. This leads to the formation of portal-systemic collaterals, including the dilation of the coronary and gastric veins that then constitute gastroesophageal varices [31].

In patients with compensated cirrhosis, gastroesophageal varices are present in 30–40% of patients compared to 85% of patients with decompensated cirrhosis. Varices develop at a rate of approximately 7–8% per year in patients with compensated cirrhosis and progress from small to large varices at a rate of 10–20% per year [32]. Hence, screening for varices with esophagogastroduodenoscopy is recommended in all patients with cirrhosis to identify if varices are present and to stratify risk of bleeding. In patients with small varices at low risk of bleeding, nonselective beta-blockers, such as propranolol, nadolol, or carvedilol, may delay growth or prevent variceal hemorrhage. In patients with small varices with high risk of hemorrhage (stigmata of recent bleeding with red wale marks or varices in patients with decompensated cirrhosis), nonselective beta-blockers are recommended. Lastly, in patients with medium or large varices, either nonselective beta-blockers or serial endoscopic variceal ligation may be used to prevent bleeding [33].

Over 90% of variceal bleeding occurs from esophageal varices and only 10% due to gastric varices. Patients with variceal hemorrhage present with hematemesis and/or melena. Treatment of variceal hemorrhage requires a combination of vasoconstrictor (terlipressin, somatostatin, or analogues such as octreotide) and endoscopic therapy with possible band ligation or sclerotherapy [34]. In patients with bleeding due to gastric varices, the use of tissue adhesives such as N-butyl-2-cyanoacrylate is more effective than banding. Antibiotic prophylaxis with either norfloxacin or ceftriaxone is also important as infections, such as SBP, often precipitate variceal hemorrhage [35]. In approximately 10–20% of patients, this standard therapy fails and placement of a TIPS should be considered. The mortality after an episode of variceal hemorrhage ranges from 15 to 25% within 6 weeks. In the past two decades, this mortality has decreased, likely due to improved endoscopic and vasoactive therapies as well as management with antibiotics [31, 34].

Hepatic Encephalopathy

Hepatic encephalopathy describes the wide spectrum of neuropsychiatric complications seen in patients with cirrhosis. The pathogenesis of hepatic encephalopathy is incompletely understood but generally involves ammonia shunting into the systemic circulation. Hyperammonemia results in neuronal dysfunction and decreased excitatory neurotransmission [36]. The degree of serum ammonia elevation does not correlate with the severity of hepatic encephalopathy. The clinical features of hepatic encephalopathy can vary from reduced awareness and irritability to coma as noted in the West Haven Criteria (Table 11.1) [37].

The initial treatment for hepatic encephalopathy is to reduce ammonia absorption from the intestinal lumen with the use of lactulose. Lactulose alters the microbiome in the gut to favor non-urease-producing bacteria, thereby reducing intestinal ammonia production [36]. Rifaximin reduces serum ammonia levels in a similar manner [38, 39]. The nonabsorbable nature of lactulose also results in the production of ammonium from ammonia in the colon and creates a cathartic effect. In addition to these medications, L-ornithine-L-aspartate (LOLA) and probiotics may improve hepatic encephalopathy for some patients. Ornithine and aspartate

Table 11.1 West Haven criteria for hepatic encephalopathy

Stage	Consciousness	Intellect and behavior	Neurologic findings
0	Normal	Normal	Normal exam
1	Mild lack of awareness	Shortened attention span, impaired addition or subtraction	Mild asterixis or tremor
2	Lethargic	Disoriented, inappropriate behavior	Obvious asterixis, slurred speech
3	Somnolent but arousable	Gross disorientation, bizarre behavior	Muscular rigidity and clonus, hyperreflexia
4	Coma	Coma	Decerebrate posturing

are important substrates in the metabolic conversion of ammonia to urea and glutamine, respectively. LOLA thus provides substrates for both of these ammonia detoxification pathways. It is important to identify and address the triggers for hepatic encephalopathy, as infection, gastrointestinal bleeding, dehydration or electrolyte disturbances, and renal insufficiency may be contributing to encephalopathy as well.

Pulmonary Vascular Complications

Hepatopulmonary syndrome is characterized by arterial hypoxemia with a PaO2 of less than 70 mmHg and an arterial-alveolar gradient greater than 20 mmHg in patients with advanced liver disease. It affects anywhere from 10% to 30% of patients with cirrhosis. Hepatopulmonary syndrome develops due to excess nitric oxide and capillary vasodilation, which result in arteriovenous shunting or diffusion-perfusion defects [40]. Patients may have platypnea or orthodeoxia and may describe dyspnea. A transthoracic contrast echocardiogram may detect an intrapulmonary right-to-left shunt indicating intrapulmonary vascular dilations [41]. Rarely, a macroaggregated albumin scan is performed to confirm and quantify such a shunt.

Portopulmonary hypertension is the presence of pulmonary hypertension in patients with portal hypertension from chronic liver disease and occurs in approximately 2% of patients. The severity of liver disease does not correlate with the severity of portopulmonary hypertension. It is classified as group 1 in the current classification of pulmonary hypertension. Vasoactive substances that are usually metabolized by the liver reach the pulmonary circulation via portosystemic collaterals. The chronic exposure of the pulmonary vascular endothelium to these substances leads to smooth muscle endothelial proliferation, vasoconstriction, and obliteration of the vascular lumen. The diagnosis of pulmonary hypertension is by a right heart catheterization. For the diagnosis of pulmonary hypertension, the mean pulmonary pressure must be greater than 25 mmHg with a pulmonary capillary wedge pressure less than 15 mmHg [42].

Hepatocellular Carcinoma

In addition to the portal hypertensive complications noted above, patients with cirrhosis are at risk of developing hepatocellular carcinoma (HCC). Patients with chronic hepatitis B virus infection are also at risk of developing HCC in the absence of cirrhosis. The risk of developing HCC varies with the etiology of liver disease but, in general, ranges from 1% to 5% per year [43]. The incidence of HCC has been rapidly rising in the United States over the last 20 years and is expected to continue its upward trajectory until 2030, largely due to the hepatitis C virus epidemic [44]. Because HCC is asymptomatic in its early course, the diagnosis is often delayed. Hence,

screening at-risk patients for HCC with ultrasonography or cross-sectional imaging is recommended for early detection [45]. The diagnosis of HCC is suggested by elevated serum alpha-fetoprotein (AFP) or radiographic findings. The development of decompensation in a patient with previously compensated cirrhosis, abdominal pain, jaundice, and early satiety should all raise suspicion for HCC [46].

The only potentially curative treatment options for HCC are resection or liver transplantation. Treatment modality is dependent upon underlying liver function, degree of portal hypertension, and stage of the tumor. For patients unable to tolerate resection or awaiting liver transplantation, multiple therapeutic options exist including radiofrequency ablation, chemoembolization, radioembolization, and cryoablation [47]. These therapies are often not curative, but may control tumor growth for an interval of time. It is important to remember that a cirrhotic liver remains at risk of developing recurrent and de novo tumors.

Indications for Liver Transplantation and Evaluation

In general, the major indications for liver transplantation are irreversible hepatic failure or liver cancer as noted in Table 11.2. These indications are similar regardless of the etiology of liver disease. In the United States, there are approximately 14,000 candidates awaiting liver transplantation; yet only 7000 transplantations are performed annually [48]. Hence, the process of selecting appropriate candidates for liver transplantation is complicated by the realities of ration-

Table 11.2 Indications for liver transplantation

Fulminant hepatic failure
Complications of cirrhosis
Ascites
Hepatorenal syndrome
Spontaneous bacterial peritonitis
Hepatic encephalopathy
Variceal hemorrhage
Hepatopulmonary syndrome
Portopulmonary hypertension
Liver neoplasms
Hepatocellular carcinoma
Epithelioid hemangioendothelioma
Large hepatic adenomas
Liver-based metabolic conditions
Primary hyperoxaluria
Familial amyloidosis
Alpha-1 antitrypsin deficiency
Wilson's disease
Hemochromatosis
Acute intermittent porphyria
Glycogen storage diseases type I and IV
Tyrosinemia
Cystic fibrosis

ing a limited societal resource. To reduce the gap in available organs, transplant centers are now using organs previously considered unsuitable for transplantation, called extended criteria donor organs or living donors. The average 5-year survival following liver transplantation is more than 70%, owing to improved pre-transplant management, surgical techniques, organ preservation, and immunosuppression.

Timing of Liver Transplantation Referral

There are several predictive models to determine a patient's prognosis from end-stage liver disease. The two most common models are the Child-Pugh classification and Model for End-Stage Liver Disease (MELD) score. The Child-Pugh classification was originally developed to stratify the risk of portacaval shunt surgery in patients with cirrhosis but has since been shown to correlate with survival in patients not undergoing surgery. The variables included in this classification include serum albumin, bilirubin, prothrombin time, ascites, and encephalopathy, and scores range from 5 to 15. A score of 5 or 6 is indicative of Child-Pugh class A or well-compensated cirrhosis; a score of 7 to 9 is Child-Pugh class B cirrhosis or moderate hepatic impairment; and a score of 10–15 classifies as Child-Pugh class C or decompensated cirrhosis. The 1-year survival rates for patients with Child-Pugh class A, B, and C cirrhosis are approximately 100%, 80%, and 45%, respectively [49]. Due to subjectivity in categorizing ascites and encephalopathy in the Child-Pugh classification, the MELD score became more favorable. The MELD score is based entirely on laboratory data including serum bilirubin, creatinine, and international normalized ratio (INR). The MELD score was recently modified to incorporate serum sodium given its correlation with survival [50, 51]. As the MELD system offers objective data that is free of bias and directs donor organs to the sickest irrespective of waiting time, it is the current method of donor organ allocation.

A referral for liver transplantation is recommended in any patient that develops decompensated cirrhosis or has major complications of cirrhosis including cancer. The timely recognition of the need for transplant and referral to a transplant center are very important in this process. Patients with a MELD score ≥ 10 should be referred to a transplant center for evaluation. While transplantation is generally not considered beneficial until the MELD score is above 15, it is important to begin the evaluation process early and before a patient becomes significantly more ill [52].

Liver Transplant Evaluation Process

The evaluation to determine if a patient is a candidate for liver transplantation is relatively uniform across transplant centers and necessarily rigorous. The goal of the evaluation process is to determine (1) if transplantation is the best option for long-term survival, (2) if there are comorbid medical or psychosocial conditions that would outweigh the benefit of transplantation, and (3) the urgency of proceeding with transplantation.

The transplant evaluation process involves several sequential and simultaneous steps as outlined in Fig. 11.1. Ideally, this process can be completed within a few days, but it may be prolonged if additional subspecialty consultations are required. For example, patients with a substance use disorder or significant mental illness may require a referral to transplant and/or addiction psychiatry. Once a thorough medical and psychosocial evaluation of the transplant candidate has been performed, they are presented at a transplant selection meeting with attendees of disciplines from each step of the process above. Based on the discussion at this meeting, the candidate may be listed for transplant, deferred until additional evaluation is completed and/or suggested/required recommendations implemented or declined.

Each transplant center has its unique policies regarding absolute contraindications to transplant. These are listed in Table 11.3. In the past, most transplant centers adhered to a strict policy of requiring 6 months of sobriety prior to wait-listing patients with ALD for transplantation. However, more recent data suggest that the "6-month rule" may not be validated. Some patients with severe ALD

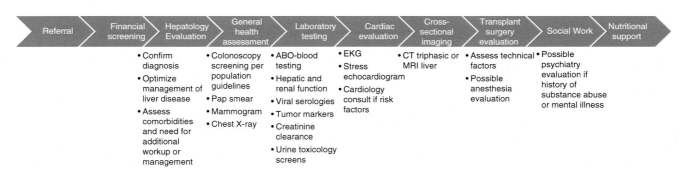

Fig. 11.1 Step-by-step process of evaluating candidacy for liver transplantation

Table 11.3 Contraindications to liver transplantation

Malignancy outside the liver (except non-melanoma skin cancer)
Hepatocellular cancer that has not been downsized to within UNOS criteria-tumor size guidelines, or with portal/hepatic vein invasion or extrahepatic spread
Extrahepatic cholangiocarcinoma > stage 2
Uncontrolled active bacterial infection outside the hepatobiliary system
Active or recent (less than 6 months) abuse of drugs including prescribed substances, failure to go for toxicology screen when requested
Active nicotine use
Advanced cardiopulmonary or other systemic disease
Inadequate social support system
Active opportunistic infection (including invasive fungal, mycobacterial or viral infection)
Active, uncontrolled psychiatric illness

might require longer time for sobriety and rehabilitation. On the other hand, patients with severe alcoholic hepatitis with 6-month survival of only 30% who fail to respond to medical therapy and are carefully selected might do well post-transplantation with less than 6-month sobriety [53]. Several transplant centers in the United States and Europe have developed protocols to consider liver transplantation in this group of patients [54, 55]. Importantly, the involvement of addiction psychiatrists is paramount in the adequate selection of candidates that have the highest predicted risk of relapse. Please see Chap. 45 on substance use disorders for further discussion.

Once a patient is deemed to be an acceptable transplant candidate, they are placed on the waiting list based on their MELD score and blood type. Donor organs are allocated first locally and then regionally. There are several possible exceptions or extra MELD points that candidates can receive for specific clinical conditions, including hepatocellular carcinoma, primary sclerosing cholangitis with biliary sepsis, and hepatopulmonary syndrome.

Conclusions

In summary, end-stage liver disease is a significant cause of morbidity and mortality in the United States. Once complications from cirrhosis arise, including hepatic encephalopathy, ascites, and esophageal variceal bleeding, a liver transplantation should be considered. Additionally, patients with fulminant hepatic failure, liver-based metabolic defect, hepatocellular carcinoma, or a systemic complication of liver disease should be referred for a transplant evaluation. The ensuing workup and decision regarding transplant candidacy is a process involving a multidisciplinary team at the transplant center.

References

1. Kochanek KD, Murphy SL, Xu J, Tejada-Vera B. National vital statisitcs reports. 65(4), (06/30/2016). 2014 [cited 2017 Sep 20]; Available from: https://www.cdc.gov/nchs/data/nvsr/nvsr65/nvsr65_04.pdf.
2. Rastogi A, Maiwall R, Bihari C, Ahuja A, Kumar A, Singh T, et al. Cirrhosis histology and Laennec staging system correlate with high portal pressure. Histopathology [Internet]. 2013 [cited 2017 Sep 20];62(5):731–41. Available from: http://doi.wiley.com/10.1111/his.12070.
3. Westbrook RH, Dusheiko G. Natural history of hepatitis C. J Hepatol [Internet]. 2014 [cited 2015 Apr 28];61(1 Suppl):S58–68. Available from: http://www.ncbi.nlm.nih.gov/pubmed/25443346.
4. Galbraith JW, Franco RA, Donnelly JP, Rodgers JB, Morgan JM, Viles AF, et al. Unrecognized chronic hepatitis C virus infection among baby boomers in the emergency department. Hepatology [Internet]. 2015 Mar 28 [cited 2015 Oct 5];61(3):776–82. Available from: http://www.ncbi.nlm.nih.gov/pubmed/25179527.
5. Goel A, Sanchez J, Paulino L, Feuille C, Arend J, Shah B, et al. A systematic model improves hepatitis C virus birth cohort screening in hospital-based primary care. J Viral Hepat [Internet]. 2016 [cited 2017 Mar 8]; Available from: http://doi.wiley.com/10.1111/jvh.12669.
6. Turner BJ, Taylor BS, Hanson JT, Perez ME, Hernandez L, Villarreal R, et al. Implementing hospital-based baby boomer hepatitis C virus screening and linkage to care: Strategies, results, and costs. J Hosp Med [Internet]. 2015 [cited 2016 Jan 21];10(8):510–6. Available from: http://www.ncbi.nlm.nih.gov/pubmed/26033458.
7. Alcohol-Attributable Deaths and Years of Potential Life Lost — 11 States, 2006–2010 [Internet]. [cited 2018 Feb 14]. Available from: https://www.cdc.gov/mmwr/preview/mmwrhtml/mm6310a2.htm.
8. Mittal S, Sada YH, El-Serag HB, Kanwal F, Duan Z, Temple S, et al. Temporal trends of nonalcoholic fatty liver disease–related hepatocellular carcinoma in the veteran affairs population. Clin Gastroenterol Hepatol [Internet]. 2015 [cited 2017 Apr 11];13(3):594–601.e1. Available from: http://www.ncbi.nlm.nih.gov/pubmed/25148760.
9. van der Meer AJ, Veldt BJ, Feld JJ, Wedemeyer H, Dufour J-F, Lammert F, et al. Association between sustained virological response and all-cause mortality among patients with chronic hepatitis C and advanced hepatic fibrosis. JAMA [Internet]. 2012 [cited 2017 Mar 8];308(24):2584–93. Available from: http://jama.jamanetwork.com/article.aspx?doi=10.1001/jama.2012.144878.
10. Goldberg D, Ditah IC, Saeian K, Lalehzari M, Aronsohn A, Gorospe EC, et al. Changes in the prevalence of hepatitis C virus infection, nonalcoholic steatohepatitis, and alcoholic liver disease among patients with cirrhosis or liver failure on the waitlist for liver transplantation. Gastroenterology [Internet]. 2017 [cited 2017 Apr 17];152(5):1090–1099.e1. Available from: http://www.ncbi.nlm.nih.gov/pubmed/28088461.
11. Kim WR, Lake JR, Smith JM, Skeans MA, Schladt DP, Edwards EB, et al. OPTN/SRTR 2015 Annual data report: liver. Am J Transplant [Internet]. 2017 [cited 2017 Apr 11];17(S1):174–251. Available from: http://doi.wiley.com/10.1111/ajt.14126.
12. Charlton MR, Burns JM, Pedersen RA, Watt KD, Heimbach JK, Dierkhising RA. Frequency and outcomes of liver transplantation for nonalcoholic steatohepatitis in the United States. Gastroenterology [Internet]. 2011 [cited 2017 Sep 20];141(4):1249–53. Available from: http://www.ncbi.nlm.nih.gov/pubmed/21726509.
13. Stepanova M, Wai H, Saab S, Mishra A, Venkatesan C, Younossi ZM. The portrait of an adult liver transplant recipient in the United States from 1987 to 2013. JAMA Intern Med [Internet]. 2014 [cited 2017 Oct 11];174(8):1407–9. Available from: http://archinte.jamanetwork.com/article.aspx?doi=10.1001/jamainternmed.2014.2903.

14. Grant BF, Chou SP, Saha TD, Pickering RP, Kerridge BT, Ruan WJ, et al. Prevalence of 12-month alcohol use, high-risk drinking, and *DSM-IV* alcohol use disorder in the United States, 2001–2002 to 2012–2013. JAMA Psychiatry [Internet]. 2017 [cited 2017 Oct 11];74(9):911. Available from: http://www.ncbi.nlm.nih.gov/pubmed/28793133.

15. D'Amico G, Garcia-Tsao G, Pagliaro L. Natural history and prognostic indicators of survival in cirrhosis: a systematic review of 118 studies. J Hepatol [Internet]. 2006 [cited 2017 Oct 11];44(1):217–31. Available from: http://linkinghub.elsevier.com/retrieve/pii/S0168827805006847.

16. García-Pagán J, Gracia-Sancho J, Bosch J. Functional aspects on the pathophysiology of portal hypertension in cirrhosis. J Hepatol [Internet]. 2012 [cited 2017 Oct 11];57(2):458–61. Available from: http://www.sciencedirect.com/science/article/pii/S0168827812002498?via%3Dihub.

17. Ginès P, Cárdenas A, Arroyo V, Rodés J. Management of cirrhosis and ascites. N Engl J Med [Internet]. 2004 [cited 2017 Oct 11];350(16):1646–54. Available from: http://www.nejm.org/doi/abs/10.1056/NEJMra035021.

18. Bosch J, Arroyo V, Betriu A, Mas A, Carrilho F, Rivera F, et al. Hepatic hemodynamics and the renin-angiotensin-aldosterone system in cirrhosis. Gastroenterology [Internet]. 1980 [cited 2017 Oct 11];78(1):92–9. Available from: http://www.ncbi.nlm.nih.gov/pubmed/7350041.

19. Runyon BA. Introduction to the revised American association for the study of liver diseases practice guideline management of adult patients with ascites due to cirrhosis 2012. Hepatology [Internet]. 2013;57(4):1651–3. Available from: https://www.aasld.org/sites/default/files/guideline_documents/adultascitesenhanced.pdf.

20. Runyon BA. Care of patients with ascites. N Engl J Med [Internet]. 1994 [cited 2017 Oct 11];330(5):337–42. Available from: http://www.nejm.org/doi/abs/10.1056/NEJM199402033300508.

21. Veldt BJ, Lainé F, Guillygomarc'h A, Lauvin L, Boudjema K, Messner M, et al. Indication of liver transplantation in severe alcoholic liver cirrhosis: quantitative evaluation and optimal timing. J Hepatol [Internet]. 2002 [cited 2017 Oct 11];36(1):93–8. Available from: http://www.ncbi.nlm.nih.gov/pubmed/11804670.

22. Casadaban LC, Parvinian A, Minocha J, Lakhoo J, Grant CW, Ray CE, et al. Clearing the confusion over hepatic encephalopathy after TIPS creation: incidence, prognostic factors, and clinical outcomes. Dig Dis Sci [Internet]. 2015 [cited 2018 Feb 14];60(4):1059–66. Available from: http://link.springer.com/10.1007/s10620-014-3391-0.

23. Wiest R, Krag A, Gerbes A. Spontaneous bacterial peritonitis: recent guidelines and beyond. Gut [Internet]. 2012;61(2):297–310. Available from: http://www.ncbi.nlm.nih.gov/pubmed/?term=Spontaneous+bacterial+peritonitis%3A+recent+guidelines+and+beyond.

24. Rimola A, García-Tsao G, Navasa M, Piddock LJV, Planas R, Bernard B, et al. Diagnosis, treatment and prophylaxis of spontaneous bacterial peritonitis: a consensus document. J Hepatol [Internet]. 2000 [cited 2014 Oct 28];32(1):142–53. Available from: http://www.journal-of-hepatology.eu/article/S0168827800802019/fulltext.

25. Thuluvath PJ, Morss S, Thompson R. Spontaneous bacterial peritonitis--in-hospital mortality, predictors of survival, and health care costs from 1988 to 1998. Am J Gastroenterol [Internet]. 2001 [cited 2015 May 14];96(4):1232–6. Available from: http://www.ncbi.nlm.nih.gov/pubmed/11316175.

26. EASL clinical practice guidelines on the management of ascites, spontaneous bacterial peritonitis, and hepatorenal syndrome in cirrhosis. J Hepatol [Internet]. 2010 [cited 2014 Oct 18];53(3):397–417. Available from: http://www.ncbi.nlm.nih.gov/pubmed/20633946.

27. Ginès P, Schrier RW. Renal failure in cirrhosis. N Engl J Med [Internet]. 2009 [cited 2017 Oct 16];361(13):1279–90. Available from: http://www.nejm.org/doi/abs/10.1056/NEJMra0809139.

28. Arroyo V, Ginès P, Gerbes AL, Dudley FJ, Gentilini P, Laffi G, et al. Definition and diagnostic criteria of refractory ascites and hepatorenal syndrome in cirrhosis. Hepatology [Internet]. 1996 [cited 2017 Oct 16];23(1):164–76. Available from: http://www.ncbi.nlm.nih.gov/pubmed/8550036.

29. Angeli P, Ginès P, Wong F, Bernardi M, Boyer TD, Gerbes A, et al. Diagnosis and management of acute kidney injury in patients with cirrhosis: revised consensus recommendations of the international club of ascites. J Hepatol [Internet]. 2015 [cited 2015 Apr 23];62(4):968–74. Available from: http://www.sciencedirect.com/science/article/pii/S0168827814009581.

30. Salerno F, Gerbes A, Gines P, Wong F, Arroyo V. Diagnosis, prevention and treatment of hepatorenal syndrome in cirrhosis. Postgrad Med J [Internet]. 2008 [cited 2017 Oct 16];84(998):662–70. Available from: http://www.ncbi.nlm.nih.gov/pubmed/17389705.

31. Garcia-Tsao G, Bosch J. Management of varices and variceal hemorrhage in cirrhosis. N Engl J Med [Internet]. 2010 [cited 2017 Oct 11];362(9):823–32. Available from: http://www.nejm.org/doi/abs/10.1056/NEJMra0901512.

32. Kovalak M, Lake J, Mattek N, Eisen G, Lieberman D, Zaman A. Endoscopic screening for varices in cirrhotic patients: data from a national endoscopic database. Gastrointest Endosc [Internet]. 2007 [cited 2017 Oct 11];65(1):82–8. Available from: http://linkinghub.elsevier.com/retrieve/pii/S0016510706027532.

33. Garcia-Tsao G, Abraldes JG, Berzigotti A, Bosch J. Portal hypertensive bleeding in cirrhosis: risk stratification, diagnosis, and management: 2016 practice guidance by the American association for the study of liver diseases. [cited 2017 Oct 11]; Available from: https://www.aasld.org/sites/default/files/Garcia-Tsao_et_al-2017-Hepatology.pdf.

34. Carbonell N, Pauwels A, Serfaty L, Fourdan O, Lévy VG, Poupon R. Improved survival after variceal bleeding in patients with cirrhosis over the past two decades. Hepatology [Internet]. 2004 [cited 2017 Oct 11];40(3):652–9. Available from: http://doi.wiley.com/10.1002/hep.20339.

35. Fernández J, Ruiz del Arbol L, Gómez C, Durandez R, Serradilla R, Guarner C, et al. Norfloxacin vs ceftriaxone in the prophylaxis of infections in patients with advanced cirrhosis and hemorrhage. Gastroenterology [Internet]. 2006 [cited 2017 Oct 11];131(4):1049–56; quiz 1285. Available from: http://linkinghub.elsevier.com/retrieve/pii/S0016508506015356.

36. Wijdicks EFM. Hepatic encephalopathy. Longo DL, editor. N Engl J Med [Internet]. 2016 [cited 2017 Oct 11];375(17):1660–70. Available from: http://www.nejm.org/doi/10.1056/NEJMra1600561.

37. Bajaj JS, Cordoba J, Mullen KD, Amodio P, Shawcross DL, Butterworth RF, et al. Review article: the design of clinical trials in hepatic encephalopathy--an International Society for Hepatic Encephalopathy and Nitrogen Metabolism (ISHEN) consensus statement. Aliment Pharmacol Ther [Internet]. 2011 [cited 2017 Oct 16];33(7):739–47. Available from: http://doi.wiley.com/10.1111/j.1365-2036.2011.04590.x.

38. Bajaj JS. Review article: potential mechanisms of action of rifaximin in the management of hepatic encephalopathy and other complications of cirrhosis. Aliment Pharmacol Ther [Internet]. 2016 [cited 2017 Apr 18];43:11–26. Available from: http://www.ncbi.nlm.nih.gov/pubmed/26618922.

39. Bass NM, Mullen KD, Sanyal A, Poordad F, Neff G, Leevy CB, et al. Rifaximin treatment in hepatic encephalopathy. N Engl J Med [Internet]. 2010 [cited 2017 Oct 16];362(12):1071–81. Available from: http://www.nejm.org/doi/abs/10.1056/NEJMoa0907893.

40. Tumgor G. Cirrhosis and hepatopulmonary syndrome. World J Gastroenterol [Internet]. 2014 [cited 2017 Oct 16];20(10):2586. Available from: http://www.ncbi.nlm.nih.gov/pubmed/24627594.

41. Aller R, Moya JL, Moreira V, Boixeda D, Cano A, Picher J, et al. Diagnosis of hepatopulmonary syndrome with contrast transesophageal echocardiography: advantages over contrast transthoracic echocardiography. Dig Dis Sci [Internet]. 1999 [cited 2017 Oct 16];44(6):1243–8. Available from: http://www.ncbi.nlm.nih.gov/pubmed/10389704.

42. Saleemi S. Portopulmonary hypertension. Ann Thorac Med [Internet]. 2010 [cited 2017 Oct 16];5(1):5–9. Available from: http://www.ncbi.nlm.nih.gov/pubmed/20351954.

43. Sherman M, Bruix J, Porayko M, Tran T. Screening for hepatocellular carcinoma: the rationale for the American association for the study of liver diseases recommendations. Hepatology [Internet]. 2012 [cited 2014 Feb 12];56(3):793–6. Available from: http://www.ncbi.nlm.nih.gov/pubmed/22689409.

44. Petrick JL, Kelly SP, Altekruse SF, McGlynn KA, Rosenberg PS. Future of hepatocellular carcinoma incidence in the United States forecast through 2030. J Clin Oncol [Internet]. 2016 [cited 2017 Oct 18];34(15):1787–94. Available from: http://www.ncbi.nlm.nih.gov/pubmed/27044939.

45. Heimbach J, Kulik LM, Finn R, Sirlin CB, Abecassis M, Roberts LR, et al. AASLD guidelines for the treatment of hepatocellular carcinoma. Hepatology. 2018 [cited 2017 Oct 18]; 67(1):358–380. Available from: https://www.aasld.org/sites/default/files/guideline_documents/Heimbach_et_al-2017-Hepatology.pdf.

46. Forner A, Llovet JM, Bruix J. Hepatocellular carcinoma. Lancet [Internet]. 2012 [cited 2017 Oct 18];379(9822):1245–55. Available from: http://www.ncbi.nlm.nih.gov/pubmed/22353262.

47. Graziadei IW, Sandmueller H, Waldenberger P, Koenigsrainer A, Nachbaur K, Jaschke W, et al. Chemoembolization followed by liver transplantation for hepatocellular carcinoma impedes tumor progression while on the waiting list and leads to excellent outcome. Liver Transpl [Internet]. 2003 [cited 2014 Feb 10];9(6):557–63. Available from: http://www.ncbi.nlm.nih.gov/pubmed/12783395.

48. Kim WR, Lake JR, Smith JM, Skeans MA, Schladt DP, Edwards EB, et al. OPTN/SRTR 2015 Annual data report: liver. Am J Transplant [Internet]. 2017 Jan [cited 2017 Jan 25];17(S1):174–251. Available from: http://doi.wiley.com/10.1111/ajt.14126.

49. Albers I, Hartmann H, Bircher J, Creutzfeldt W. Superiority of the child-pugh classification to quantitative liver function tests for assessing prognosis of liver cirrhosis. Scand J Gastroenterol [Internet]. 1989 [cited 2017 Oct 18];24(3):269–76. Available from: http://www.ncbi.nlm.nih.gov/pubmed/2734585.

50. Kim WR, Biggins SW, Kremers WK, Wiesner RH, Kamath PS, Benson JT, et al. Hyponatremia and mortality among patients on the liver-transplant waiting list. N Engl J Med [Internet]. 2008 [cited 2017 Oct 18];359(10):1018–26. Available from: http://www.ncbi.nlm.nih.gov/pubmed/18768945.

51. Bernardi M, Gitto S, Biselli M. The MELD score in patients awaiting liver transplant: strengths and weaknesses. J Hepatol [Internet]. 2011 [cited 2016 Apr 28];54(6):1297–306. Available from: http://www.ncbi.nlm.nih.gov/pubmed/21145851.

52. Merion RM, Schaubel DE, Dykstra DM, Freeman RB, Port FK, Wolfe RA. The survival benefit of liver transplantation. Am J Transplant [Internet]. 2005 [cited 2016 Apr 28];5(2):307–13. Available from: http://www.ncbi.nlm.nih.gov/pubmed/15643990.

53. Mathurin P, Moreno C, Samuel D, Dumortier J, Salleron J, Durand F, et al. Early liver transplantation for severe alcoholic hepatitis. N Engl J Med [Internet]. 2011 [cited 2017 Nov 12];365(19):1790–800. Available from: http://www.ncbi.nlm.nih.gov/pubmed/22070476.

54. Im GY, Kim-Schluger L, Shenoy A, Schubert E, Goel A, Friedman SL, et al. Early liver transplantation for severe alcoholic hepatitis in the United States--a single-center experience. Am J Transplant [Internet]. 2016 [cited 2017 Nov 12];16(3):841–9. Available from: http://doi.wiley.com/10.1111/ajt.13586.

55. Lee BP, Chen P-H, Haugen C, Hernaez R, Gurakar A, Philosophe B, et al. Three-year results of a pilot program in early liver transplantation for severe alcoholic hepatitis. Ann Surg [Internet]. 2017 [cited 2017 Nov 12];265(1):20–9. Available from: http://insights.ovid.com/crossref?an=00000658-201701000-00005.

Mental Health in Chronic and End-Stage Liver Disease

Rebekah Nash, Eric Golden, Mary Amanda Dew, and Andrea F. DiMartini

Introduction

Mental health care professionals caring for patients with liver disease require both an understanding of the inherent liver disease process and an awareness of mental health disorders that commonly co-occur with liver diseases. The main causes of cirrhosis worldwide, alcoholic liver disease (ALD) and some cases of viral hepatitis, develop due to substance use behaviors, and clinicians need to be aware of the evaluation and treatment of addiction disorders. In other liver diseases, the presenting symptoms can be psychiatric in nature, and patients may seek psychiatric care before the correct liver disease diagnosis is known. For all patients with liver disease, as sequelae of end-stage disease develop, associated physiological changes may affect cognition, physical functioning, and medication pharmacokinetics. In this chapter we review the symptoms, sequelae, and psychiatric conditions common to liver diseases. Although we will briefly review the basics of drug metabolism in end-stage liver disease, Chap. 42 Psychopharmacology in Transplant Patients provides a comprehensive overview of psychotropic medications following transplant. Additionally, while Chap. 3 covers the evaluation of transplant candidates in general, here we will briefly address psychotherapeutic issues more commonly encountered by mental health professionals evaluating end-stage liver disease patients undergoing transplant evaluation. The medical/surgical indications for liver transplantation (LT) are further reviewed in Chap. 11. Finally, we review the issues relevant to terminal care management, with consideration for palliative care consultation.

Specific Common Liver Diseases with Mental Health Disorder Implications

ALD, chronic hepatitis C, and nonalcoholic steatohepatitis are the most common causes of chronic liver disease (CLD) worldwide and the most common indications for LT in the USA [1–6].

Alcoholic Liver Disease

In addition to being a common liver disease and indication for LT, ALD accounts for 48% of all deaths from cirrhosis [7]. ALD represents a continuum of liver pathology caused by excessive alcohol consumption [8] that includes alcoholic steatosis, alcoholic hepatitis, and cirrhosis. Interestingly, a study examining the effects of alcohol on liver disease found that the total lifetime alcohol intake is similar in alcoholic patients who develop liver disease and those who do not develop liver disease [9]. However, among adult females who drink alcohol, an increased number of drinking days was associated with an increased risk of ALD. In addition, females with ALD had a lower overall lifetime alcohol intake than males with ALD, suggesting that females require lower overall alcohol exposure to progress to ALD than do males [9]. Nevertheless, while there is no specified amount of consumed alcohol that predictably results in ALD and while the diagnosis of ALD is not synonymous with a history of alcohol use disorder (AUD) [8, 10], heavy prolonged alcohol use (80 g/day in males or 20 g/d in females) is associated with

R. Nash
Department of Psychiatry, University of North Carolina Hospitals, Chapel Hill, NC, USA

E. Golden
Department of Psychiatry, University of Pittsburgh, Pittsburgh, PA, USA

M. A. Dew (✉)
Departments of Psychiatry, Psychology, Epidemiology, Biostatistics and the Clinical and Translational Science Institute, University of Pittsburgh, Pittsburgh, PA, USA
e-mail: dewma@upmc.edu

A. F. DiMartini
Departments of Psychiatry and Surgery and the Clinical and Translational Science Institute, University of Pittsburgh, Pittsburgh, PA, USA

© Springer International Publishing AG, part of Springer Nature 2019
Y. Sher, J. R. Maldonado (eds.), *Psychosocial Care of End-Stage Organ Disease and Transplant Patients*,
https://doi.org/10.1007/978-3-319-94914-7_12

Table 12.1 National Institute on Alcohol Abuse and Alcoholism definition of at-risk drinking levels for developing an AUD

	Men	Women
On any single day	>4 standard drinks[a] or >3–4 units[b]	>3 standard drinks or >2–3 units
Total drinks per week	>14 standard drinks or >21 units	>7 standard drinks or >14 units

Source: https://www.niaaa.nih.gov/alcohol-health/overview-alcohol-consumption/moderate-binge-drinking.

According to NIAAA, only 2 in 100 who drink below these limits have an AUD. However, low risk does not mean "no" risk especially for those with health problems.

[a]A US standard drink equals 0.6 fluid ounces or 14 g of pure alcohol (e.g., a 12 oz. 5% beer or 1.5 oz. of 80 proof liquor)

[b]In the UK, one unit of alcohol is defined as 10 mL (7.9 g of pure alcohol). In other European countries, units differ in size, ranging from 8 to 14 g of pure alcohol

ALD [8, 10, 11]. Indeed, 10–35% of heavy drinkers will develop alcoholic hepatitis, and 10% will go on to develop cirrhosis [12]. Of all patients diagnosed with ALD, 70–95% likely meet criteria for AUD [13–15] (see Table 12.1 for levels of at-risk drinking).

Clearly important to the diagnosis of ALD is the collection of an accurate, detailed alcohol consumption history. Mental health providers may be better suited to the task of asking such detailed questions in a nonjudgmental fashion, avoiding the constraints of patient denial, underreporting, or underestimation of alcohol-related problems by the clinician. Indirect phrasing using simple declarative sentences that invite the patient to agree or disagree can create a less confrontational interview and provide a context for more accurate disclosure [16]. While primary interventions for at-risk drinkers could prevent ALD, once developed, the definitive treatment is complete sustained abstinence, not reduced drinking. Clinicians should work diligently to get patients into addiction treatment (see section on AUDs below). Clinicians should additionally evaluate for and recommend treatment of other common comorbid psychiatric disorders. In a recent study, patients hospitalized for ALD had an increased prevalence of psychiatric diagnoses compared to patients hospitalized for non-ALD, with significantly higher rates of depression, anxiety disorders, adjustment disorders, post-traumatic stress disorder, and personality disorders [7].

Chronic Viral Hepatitis

Hepatitis C (HCV) is responsible for the vast majority of chronic viral hepatitis cases in the USA. The primary route of HCV transmission is intravenous (IV) drug use; once infected, 75–85% of individuals will develop a chronic HCV infection, and 60–70% will progress to CLD [17]. Early detection is key to preventing liver disease as newer extremely effective oral HCV treatments are resulting in

high cure rates with shorter treatment times. Ultimately treatment of the underlying drug addiction is needed as cured individuals can become reinfected. Hepatitis B (HBV) is implicated in a small percentage of CLD cases; its incidence decreased significantly following the introduction of the HBV vaccine [18, 19].

Chronic viral hepatitis B and C are associated with a lower health-related quality of life (QOL) as compared to the general population, including in domains of mental health and role limitation due to emotional problems [20, 21]. HCV is able to invade neuronal tissue, and HCV-positive patients have been shown to suffer from neurocognitive deficits, such as impaired concentration, working memory, and visuomotor processing [22, 23]. HCV is associated with an increased risk of psychiatric disorders [22–28], although there is significant variability in prevalence estimates between studies [21–29]. In addition, although many psychiatric diagnoses are associated with increased risk of HCV infection, it is often difficult to determine whether an individual's psychiatric disorder(s) antedated or developed after their HCV infection [27]. In contrast, rates of depression in patients with HBV (4–6.4%) [21, 26, 28] are similar to those of the general population but do tend to increase with disease severity [30, 31]. Individuals with HCV are also more likely to have a history of substance abuse, as compared to the general population and those with HBV. Studies have demonstrated that 51–88% of patients with HCV have a substance abuse history, compared with 10–20% of general population, and an estimated 16% of patients with HBV [11, 23, 32–34]. Similarly, 28–83% of patients with HCV have a history of IV drug use [11, 32, 34, 35], compared to 2.6% of the general population [36].

Nonalcoholic Steatohepatitis

Nonalcoholic fatty liver disease (NAFLD) is a growing cause of CLD and hepatocellular carcinoma [3, 4, 6, 37–39]. It encompasses a range of liver pathology, from incidental hepatic steatosis (also called nonalcoholic fatty liver, NAFL) to nonalcoholic steatohepatitis (NASH) [38, 39]. It is estimated that 27–55% of patients with NAFLD also hold a diagnosis of depression [28, 40], and a correlation between generalized anxiety disorder and major depressive disorder and severity of liver histological findings has been demonstrated [40]. Since obesity increases the risk for NAFLD, binge eating disorder and other overeating disorders are also overrepresented in the NAFLD population [41]. The connection between NAFLD and psychiatric disorders is multifactorial and bidirectional in nature. Common mediators of both include alterations in behavioral patterns (decreased activity), eating patterns, level of neuroinflammation and oxidative stress, and lack of access to health care [40, 41]. Many psychiatric disorders, including depression and psychotic disorders, are associated with poor adherence to medical interventions, and many psychotropic medications carry a risk of weight gain [40, 41]. Whether switching psychotropic medications could help weight reduction without destabilizing the underlying psychiatric disorder would need to be decided by the psychiatric provider.

Treatment guidelines for NAFLD recommend lifestyle changes prior to medication trials [42]. Behavioral therapies including cognitive behavioral therapy (CBT) can be effective in weight loss and improving markers of liver disease [41, 42]. Psychotherapeutic approaches combined with weight loss programs have also been studied, although patients often regain a portion of the weight lost during the intervention [41]. As obesity is a chronic health problem, some level of ongoing support is likely necessary to maintain long-term treatment effects [41]. However, such treatments are unlikely to be provided in the gastroenterologist's clinic. Mental health clinicians may be best suited to evaluating and arranging for such therapies. Collaborative care models are best suited to addressing the comorbid liver and mental health disorders in these complex cases [41]. If psychotropic medications are indicated, the potential risk of psychotropics that promote weight gain should be carefully considered.

Neurocognitive and Neuropsychiatric Manifestations of CLD

Hepatic Encephalopathy

Hepatic encephalopathy (HE) is a neuropsychiatric syndrome arising out of declining liver function and/or porto-systemic shunting [43]. Patients can present with alteration of consciousness (including stupor or coma), cognitive impairment, confusion/disorientation, affective/emotional dysregulation, psychosis, behavioral disturbances, and physical signs such as asterixis. HE can be episodic or persistent [44]. While overt HE is typically evident on clinical examination, subtle or subclinical HE may require neurocognitive testing to identify it [44] (see Vilstrup et al. [43] for review). While less obvious, subclinical HE can be deleterious to daily self-management tasks such as medication taking or complex tasks such as driving [45]. Mental health clinicians are more likely than other clinicians to use and be able to interpret basic neurocognitive testing. Commonly used HE screening instruments, such as the trail making tests, examine processing speed, concentration, and attention. To overcome time and provider barriers, a recent study piloted the use of neurocognitive testing through a self-scoring smart phone app using the Stroop test [46]. Eventually such apps may allow clinicians and patients to monitor minimal HE symptoms in real time, perhaps even remotely [46].

While high blood ammonia levels alone do not add any diagnostic, staging, or prognostic value in HE patients [43], they can aid in a questionable diagnosis, and if ammonia-lowering drugs are being used, repeated measurements of ammonia may be helpful to follow treatment efficacy [43]. Malnutrition is implicated in the development of HE, and the amelioration of nutritional status is an effective goal to decrease the prevalence of cognitive impairment in these patients [47]. As with other types of delirium, the use of antipsychotic medications may aid in severe symptom relief but not in treating the underlying disorder. Also see Chap. 11 for additional discussion of HE.

Alcohol Related Cognitive Impairment in CLD

Cognitive impairment in individuals with AUD and CLD is often multifactorial, reflecting a combination of alcohol neurotoxicity, nutritional derangements, and HE. In general, malnutrition is a common feature of CLD resulting from inadequate intake, impaired absorption, and altered metabolism that is often associated with neuropsychiatric complications as well as outcomes following LT [47]. Alcohol-related dementia encompasses clinical entities such as Wernicke-Korsakoff syndrome. Heavy alcohol use is associated with nutritional deficiencies including thiamine deficiency [48, 49]. Thiamine deficiency can result in Wernicke's encephalopathy, classically described as a triad of symptoms including oculomotor findings, cerebellar dysfunction, and altered mental status, but in reality presenting more subtly [50]. If untreated, Wernicke's encephalopathy can progress to Korsakoff's dementia, a syndrome of permanent cognitive impairment characterized by the inability to create new memories [49].

Wilson's Disease

Wilson's disease (WD) is an autosomal recessive disorder of copper transport resulting in the inappropriate deposition of copper in multiple organs, including the liver, eyes, and brain. Copper deposition in the liver parenchyma leads to an increased risk of HE. Copper deposition in the brain leads to direct damage to neuronal tissue and a broad variety of psychiatric and neurological symptoms. Neurological and psychiatric symptoms in WD typically begin in the second or third decade. Psychiatric symptoms include affective disorders, changes in personality/behavior, cognitive dysfunction, and psychotic symptoms [51–53]. Psychiatric or cognitive symptoms can antedate the diagnosis of WD, and almost half of patients will first present with neurological or psychiatric symptoms: 30–60% will have depressive symptoms, 18–30% will have bipolar illness, 46–71% will have personality changes, approximately 25% will have cognitive impairment, and 4–16% will engage in suicidal behaviors during the course of the disease [54, 55]. Patients can also present with extrapyramidal symptoms, as the caudate and putamen are the most common areas of the brain to be affected [52, 54]. Typically, the presence of the ocular findings of Kayser-Fleischer rings and serum ceruloplasmin <10 mg/dl are sufficient to establish the diagnosis [56]. In general, treatment options include the copper chelators, which must be taken lifelong. LT is a rare consideration in WD since the condition usually responds to medical therapy.

Porphyrias

Porphyrias are inherited or acquired disorders of heme production. Five of the eight classes of porphyrias result in the accumulation of heme precursors in the liver. Four of these five have prominent neuropsychiatric symptoms. Porphyrias present as discrete, acute "attacks" of psychiatric and physical symptoms. Common psychiatric symptoms include anxiety, depression, psychosis, delirium, and catatonia, and common physical symptoms include abdominal pain, constipation, vomiting, peripheral neuropathy, and bullous or erythematous rash. Of note, psychiatric symptoms can persist after the resolution of other symptoms associated with the acute episode [52, 57–59]. Porphyrias can be easily misdiagnosed as conversion disorders, primary psychotic disorders, personality disorders, primary mood disorders, and a chronic fatigue disorder [57]. Triggers for episodes can include stress, dieting/eating disorders, sun (if cutaneous), cocaine, certain alcoholic drinks (whisky and red wine), and a host of medications, many of which are psychotropics (http://www.drugs-porphyria.org/) [52, 57, 58]. Acute attacks of porphyria can be confirmed by demonstration of a markedly increased urinary porphobilinogen and aminolevulinic acid levels. If severe, LT can be pursued although this does not necessarily correct the underlying etiology [58].

Common Mental Health Disorders in Liver Disease

Depression

Depressive disorders are among the most prevalent mental health disorders in the general population, and depression can influence a patient's course and symptomatology in the presence of liver disease. While the WHO estimates 19% of US adults will experience depression in their lifetime [60], lifetime rates of depression were 35% in one study of patients with advanced liver disease, using a diagnostic structured lifetime interview [61]. The mechanisms underlying the association between liver disease and depression are not fully understood. A study found that after adjusting for confounding variables including age, sex, ethnicity, marital status, smoking status, and amount of alcohol consumed, patients with liver disease have a risk of developing depression that is 2.2 times that of individuals without liver disease [62]. There is some evidence to suggest that the etiology of the liver disease may explain the development of depressive symptoms. For example, in patients with HCV, the virus impacts dopaminergic and serotonergic neurotransmission [63]. There is also a psychological component to the etiology of depressive symptoms in HCV patients due to stigma associated with the diagnosis of a chronic infectious disease [25]. In addition to higher rates of depression diagnoses, liver disease is associated with a threefold increase in risk of a suicide attempt compared to those without liver disease [62]. As is seen in other chronic disease states, liver disease is associated with decreased overall health-related QOL [62]. HE is a relatively common finding in liver disease patients and can manifest as changes in mood, personality, cognition, and alertness as well as psychomotor changes. While there is overlap in the symptomatology of HE and major depressive disorder, these represent two distinct syndromes [63]. It is important to screen patients for depressive symptoms, as untreated depressive symptoms contribute to worse treatment outcomes throughout the course of CLD.

Alcohol and Substance Use Disorders in Liver Disease Patients

Alcohol As noted above, substance use disorders (SUDs) are commonly associated with alcoholic and viral liver disease. Perhaps due to the prevalence of ALD, the bulk of the literature addresses the co-occurrence of ALD and AUD. The definitive treatment for AUD and ALD is sustained abstinence—not reduced drinking—and this information should be made very clear so that patients do not "tailor" advice to suit their beliefs or denial [64]. Nevertheless, simply educating on the dangers of continued alcohol use, while necessary, is insufficient to produce sustained abstinence. Additionally, brief interventions in this population would likely not be effective. A meta-analysis of behavioral interventions in primary care settings found no evidence for the use of brief interventions for patients with AUD [65]. While ALD patients may seek treatment for their ALD symptoms, they often do not consider that they have any need for addiction counseling. In fact, study of ALD patients being evaluated for LT found these patients did not perceive themselves to have an addiction disorder, were more preoccupied with their medical treatments, and were reluctant or resistant to consider addiction counseling [66]. Motivational interviewing (MI) can be a helpful strategy to overcome ambivalence and resistance to seeking treatment [66, 67] and is described in more detail in Chap. 43. Clinicians should additionally evaluate carefully for comorbid psychiatric disorders as an estimated 36% of patients with AUD will also have a depressive disorder, 12% will have an anxiety disorder, and 25% will abuse substances other than alcohol [14].

Clinicians should work diligently to get patients into addiction treatment or dual diagnosis addiction treatment if indicated. Follow-up to ensure patients are participating in treatment may be necessary. Unfortunately, patients diagnosed with ALD often continue to consume alcohol and, even after a period of pre-transplant sobriety, can relapse following LT [12, 68–73]. The intensity of treatment will depend on the severity of the AUD, likelihood of requiring detoxification, and type and intensity of prior rehabilitation attempts. For patients with ALD, motivational enhancement therapy (MET), CBT, MI, supportive therapy, and psycho-education, either alone or in combination, have been used to reduce alcohol consumption [74, 75]. Weinrieb et al. [75] demonstrated a reduction in number of drinking days and total number of drinks for patients receiving MET, relative to a treatment as usual group who were referred to local resources. Other groups have achieved increased rates of abstinence and reduced rates of recidivism but have done so only when combining psychotherapy with medical treatment [74]. A multidisciplinary team approach in the gastroenterologist's office where ALD patients may initially seek care could be the most effective means to provide for the comprehensive care needs of ALD-AUD patients. In one center, embedding psychiatry and social work in a gastroenterology service resulted in a marked improvement in the accuracy of drinking histories obtained, ability to provide medical and psychiatric care at one appointment, and referral for addiction treatment and communication between patients, their families, and their clinicians [76]. Importantly, monitoring of alcohol abstinence by regular interviewing and random biological marker testing are necessary as both methods independently contribute to the identification of ongoing use [77].

Medications to reduce the positive effects of and cravings for alcohol and thereby reduce alcohol consumption can be used to augment psychotherapeutic treatments. Acamprosate may be a potential pharmacological treatment but is renally excreted, and the dose may require reduction if hepatorenal syndrome exists. While naltrexone could also be considered in stable cirrhosis, it is contraindicated in acute hepatitis or liver failure. In particular, naltrexone is not advised for patients with serum aminotransferase levels greater than 3–5 times the normal limit [78].

Tobacco Patients with AUD or ALD also have an increased prevalence of co-occurring tobacco use compared to others [7, 79]. Like alcohol use, tobacco use is also harmful to liver health. There is increasing evidence that cigarette smoking may negatively affect the incidence, severity, and clinical course of many types of CLDs, perhaps due in part to its promotion of fibrogenesis [80]. Cigarette smoking predicts reduced survival time in patients with hepatocellular carcinoma with concurrent HCV and HBV [81]. Thus, in addition to other potential health benefits, promoting and assisting patients in smoking cessation for liver health are strongly recommended. In addition to pharmacological therapies such as nicotine replacement therapy, varenicline or bupropion, there are a number of online self-help programs for smoking cessation (e.g., American Lung Association's Freedom From Smoking program, www.freedomfromsmoking.org).

Opioid Maintenance Therapy Opioid use disorders are common in patients with viral hepatitis/cirrhosis. Opioid maintenance therapy (OMT) (e.g., methadone or buprenorphine) can be an effective and long-term strategy for achieving stability for those with an opioid addiction. However, when stably abstinent methadone-maintained patients are tapered and discontinued from their methadone, relapse rates typically exceed 80% [67], and similar relapse rates exceeding 50% are seen in those who involuntarily discontinue buprenorphine [82]. Therefore, while dose adjustments may be required to accommodate deteriorating hepatic functioning and/or development of HE, the standard of care would be to continue OMT until the patient and treating addiction clinician determine the proper time to taper and discontinue treatment. A mandate to taper off OMT as prerequisite for LT or other medical treatments (e.g., HCV treatment) is not recommended and puts the patient at risk of relapse during a highly stressful time of medical illness. A 2000 survey of LT programs' approaches to OMT showed 56% of programs accepted patients on methadone maintenance, but 32% of programs required that patients discontinue methadone use [83]. Although attitudes may have since changed toward OMT LT candidates, mental health clinicians may need to educate the LT team about the appropriateness of continuing OMT.

Marijuana Aside from the health risks of smoked marijuana (e.g., respiratory inflammation and infection), there is equivocal evidence that cannabinoids directly affect the progression of liver disease. This is likely related to the fact that cannabinoid receptors produce complimentary effects on the liver, some exerting profibrogenic and pro-inflammatory effects, while others inhibit or even reverse liver fibrogenesis [84, 85]. Thus, while some studies of HCV and NAFLD patients demonstrate worsening of liver disease in those who used cannabis [86–88], others do not find such an association

[89, 90]. However, in healthy individuals, the use of exogenous cannabinoids is well known to impair cognition. In addition to these known effects, for those with liver disease, one subset of cannabinoid receptors may worsen symptoms of HE [91].

Although patients may assert a need to use cannabis for medicinal reasons, there is no medical indication for smoked marijuana, and no other medicine is smoked [92, 93]. Additionally, studies demonstrating the beneficial effects of cannabinoids for various medical illnesses and symptoms were conducted using pharmaceutical agents approved by the FDA (e.g., dronabinol and nabilone), not smoked or eaten cannabis [92, 93]. If use of marijuana is medically indicated, then rather than relying on medicinal marijuana which has no regulatory oversight for quality and purity [92, 93], using a prescribed pharmaceutical would be safer, especially in medically ill individuals. However, until the exact effects of cannabinoids on the progression of liver disease are fully understood, the use or prescription of any cannabinoid in patients with liver disease should be done with significant caution.

Pain in Cirrhosis

Pain is commonly reported in patients with cirrhosis, with recent studies suggesting upward of 80% of patients experiencing pain [94–96] and a similarly high percentage, 75% in one study, experiencing chronic pain-related disability [94]. Chronic pain in cirrhosis is associated with the disease stage and increases in prevalence as cirrhosis progresses [97, 98]. Disability related to pain is additionally associated with the severity of pain, psychiatric symptoms, prescription opioid use, and elevated inflammatory markers [94]. While patients with cirrhosis may experience non-liver-related pain, the high prevalence of abdominal pain is likely associated with liver disease-related factors including ascites, hepatic capsular distension, and splenomegaly [94, 99, 100]. Patients with ascites and abdominal pain require evaluation to rule out spontaneous bacterial peritonitis. HCV has been associated with irritable bowel symptoms and visceral hyperalgesia, which may further contribute to the prevalence of abdominal pain complaints in this population [101]. Furthermore, one of the key elements of cirrhosis pathophysiology is systemic inflammation with associated increased production of pro-inflammatory cytokines [102], the same cytokines associated with pain.

Despite the awareness of the opioid epidemic and increasingly strict regulations for the prescription of opioid analgesics, the use of prescribed opioids in this population is high. Prescription prevalence estimates of opioids are 24–54% for patients with cirrhosis [100]. Although the use of opioid analgesics is likely partly due to poor alternatives for the treatment of moderate to severe pain, cirrhosis is a risk factor for opioid-related complications (e.g., respiratory and central nervous system depression). Additionally, opioids can contribute to symptoms of HE and further slow intestinal motility, diminishing the efficacy of ammonia-reducing medications. Opioid use predicts hospital readmissions in cirrhosis [103] and, in a study of cirrhotic patients who underwent LT, the use of opioids before and after LT was associated with poor patient and graft survival [104]. Whether opioid use itself or comorbidities associated with opioid use are driving mortality requires further investigation. Additionally, only a minority of LT recipients who use opioids have been found able to taper and discontinue opioid analgesics following transplant, suggesting that perhaps a large proportion of patients had pain unrelated to liver disease [104].

While any cirrhotic patient must be carefully managed to assure they do not become addicted to opioids or develop complications, patients with prior opioid and other SUDs present an especially complicated pain treatment dilemma to clinicians. These patients can have legitimate pain but may find it difficult to obtain treatment in a pain clinic. Those in opioid agonist therapy programs may not be eligible for or may find it difficult to obtain additional pain medication. Patients with such complex needs may be best managed by pain specialists in chronic pain clinics where oversight and monitoring for abuse behaviors are provided. Liver disease specialists should be involved in collaborative care to provide advice on the severity of liver disease and potential issues with associated liver disease complications. The potentially negative effects of opioid use and the high prevalence of psychiatric symptoms and possible inflammation in cirrhosis suggest other pharmacological treatment targets for pain management in these patients. Pain clinics may be able to provide a range of therapies in addition to pharmacological management.

Pharmacotherapy in the Context of Liver Disease

As the liver plays a critical role in the metabolism and clearance of most medications, liver disease will impact most aspects of drug pharmacokinetics. Depending on the severity of liver disease and its associated sequela, pharmacokinetic processes from absorption to metabolism, protein binding, and volume of distribution can be altered. The loss of functional liver tissue with subsequent loss of hepatic enzymes (cytochrome P450 and conjugation/glucuronidation enzymes) will cause a reduction in intrinsic hepatic clearance and loss of biliary excretion. Loss of functional tissue can also reduce the production of binding proteins resulting in less drug binding and higher levels of free drug. Portal hypertension with portosystemic shunting of blood flow will reduce first pass metabolism, while vascular congestion can slow drug absorption. Development of ascites and peripheral edema can alter volume of drug distribution and, depending on whether a drug is less protein-bound or is water-soluble, can lower drug levels by increasing the volume of distribution. Finally, liver disease can be associated with renal insufficiency (e.g., hepatorenal syndrome), with associated reduced glomerular filtration and alteration in fluid status. However, while disease-related changes in metabolism and elimination can alter drug pharmacokinetics in complex and significant ways, compensatory mechanisms can offset clinically significant effects on free drug levels. For example, while the loss of hepatic enzymes reduces metabolism leading to higher drug levels, a reduction in binding proteins results in greater amount of free drug available for metabolism, thus lowering drug levels [105, 106].

Unlike the kidneys where a measure of elimination (creatinine clearance) can guide drug dosing, in liver disease, perhaps due to the multiplicity of the liver's contribution to overall pharmacokinetics, there is no precise measure of reduced intrinsic liver metabolism. Clinicians should consider the severity of the liver disease, the therapeutic drug level range, and potential for toxicity, as well as the presence of HE. A strategy of beginning with lower initial doses and possibly longer dosing intervals and then gradually titrating the dose may be the safest. As liver functioning deteriorates over time, drug doses and dosing schedules should be reevaluated. If HE is present, avoiding drugs that can worsen encephalopathy (i.e. sedatives, tranquilizers, anticholinergic medications) is recommended. Drugs metabolized into active metabolites (e.g., amitriptyline, venlafaxine), extended or slow release drug formulations, or those with long half-lives (e.g., fluoxetine) may be difficult to adjust or predict clinical response/toxicity and should be used with caution. Drugs distributed in total body water (e.g., lithium) can be difficult to manage with concurrent use of diuretics or therapeutic paracentesis that can dramatically alter the volume of distribution, potentially making previously therapeutic drug levels toxic. Serotonin reuptake inhibitors are the most commonly prescribed class of antidepressants for patients with liver disease [63]. However, concerns over increased risk for bleeding make them less desirable, especially if other antiplatelet medications or nonsteroidal anti-inflammatory drugs are concurrently prescribed [63]. Few psychotropic drugs are potentially toxic to the liver. While most of these reactions are idiosyncratic, there is some evidence that patients with existing liver disease are at heightened risk of developing toxicity (e.g., duloxetine) [107, 108]. Additionally, for patients with existing loss of hepatic function, additional tissue loss may not be well tolerated, and existing alterations in liver enzymes may mask a developing drug problem, making monitoring for toxicity difficult. Nevertheless, severe drug-induced liver injury is usually reversible and rarely results in fatality if the drug is discontinued.

Psychotherapeutic Issues in CLD

Patients with CLD face a slow decline in both physical and cognitive function, as their liver function slowly declines and ammonia levels rise [52, 109, 110]. For patients awaiting LT, this gradual decline is overlaid by the daily uncertainty of whether or not a matching organ is going to be found; this uncertainty is further compounded by the fear that the patient may become ineligible for an organ due to some unforeseen future illness or catastrophe [52, 109, 111, 112]. Patients are also not guaranteed resolution of symptoms following transplant and face an arduous postoperative course of immunosuppressive regimens and surveillance of transplant function [111]. These stressors are often magnified by comorbid psychiatric disorders including depression, anxiety, and substance use [109, 112–115].

Several groups have developed psychotherapeutic approaches to help patients with CLD improve their ability to effectively manage these challenges [109, 116–120]. As in the general population, therapies involving both pharmacological and psychotherapeutic approaches are likely most effective [115, 121]. However, for patients who are medically fragile, on an extensive number of medications, and who will hopefully be undergoing LT with immunosuppressive regimens, special care must be taken to avoid drug-drug interactions and drug-induced side effects that could further worsen the patient's liver function or symptoms [122]. As a result, psychotherapeutic approaches can be acceptable and safer alternatives to drug-based therapies [115, 123]. Approaches that have been tested specifically in CLD patients include CBT [118], bibliotherapy, scheduled telephone-based contacts with patients [109], mindfulness-based stress reduction (MBSR) [116], and multidisciplinary team approaches [119].

For example, Sharif et al. [120] demonstrated improvement in physical and psychological measures in patients with CLD after a series of four 90-minute sessions that combined education, relaxation training, and coping strategies, relative to care as usual. Evon et al. [117] described an integrated care approach for patients with chronic hepatitis C that combined counseling and case management and increased the patients' eligibility for interferon-based treatment relative to standard of care. Neri et al. [119] used multidisciplinary teams with psychotherapy to reduce the incidence of depression and the number of antidepressant and benzodiazepine prescriptions required for patients receiving interferon and ribavirin therapy, when compared to care as usual.

While many interventions resulted in improved patient outcomes over time or relative to care as usual, these gains were at times reduced when compared to an active comparator control group. For example, Bailey et al. [109] compared patients with CLD awaiting LT who either received a telephone-based psychotherapeutic intervention (CBT-based coping skills training and uncertainty in illness theory-based symptom management) or participated in an active control condition (telephone-based education regarding liver disease and symptoms management). Although neither group showed appreciable change in depression, anxiety, QOL, or illness uncertainty, both groups appeared to improve in perceived self-efficacy for managing liver disease symptoms, with no significance difference in degree of improvement.

Specific Coping Challenges During the Pre-transplant Period

Waiting Period

After acceptance onto the LT wait list, patients typically experience improved hopefulness and even elation. However, the realities of the wait for a scarce organ, the deteriorating health, and the need to be at the top of the list based on medical urgency in order to get the next available organ mean many LT candidates wait for years, and 10–15% each year do not survive to transplant. Many patients and families feel that the waiting period is the most psychologically stressful period of transplantation, and mental health providers should be aware of the stresses unique to this phase of the transplant process. In addition to the use of traditional psychotherapies to alleviate distress, therapeutic interventions based on transplant specific themes have been developed to help patients and families weather the uncertainty of the waiting period. In one example, a study of patients wait-listed for LT and their caregivers tested an intervention focused on uncertainty management, improvement in QOL, and caregiver support [109]. In this and other studies, the use of telephone-delivered therapy sessions aided in overcoming logistical issues for chronically ill patients and their caregivers (e.g., debility, transportation, time off work, traveling regularly to a clinic for therapy).

Maintaining Hope While Preparing for Eventualities

Patients and families often focus on the goal of obtaining a liver transplant, yet should consider preparation for the possibility that a donor organ will not come in time. As the patient's health deteriorates, they will become increasingly dependent on caregivers and may experience medical setbacks or hospitalizations. Patients may also develop complications making them ineligible for transplantation (e.g., stroke or metastasizing hepatocellular carcinoma), and both

patient and family should be made aware that their eligibility might change over time for many reasons. Discussions about end-of-life directives or palliative care consultation are not commonly undertaken for LT candidates [124, 125], yet the overlap in the intensity of the patient's medical care, the nature of the day-to-day clinical problems, and the intensity of the commitment to patients and their families makes consideration of engaging palliative care services a natural collaboration. Patients, families, and even the transplant team may be reluctant to consider such input, believing it is a sign of giving up hope or abandoning the goal of transplantation. However, palliative care input can assist in providing improvement in QOL in parallel with the intent to go forward with transplantation. Early engagement of palliative care services allows patients an opportunity to participate in treatment planning while they are still able. Two intervention studies using palliative care services for LT candidates demonstrated improved continuity of care and treatment planning, increased goals-of-care discussions, increased do-not-resuscitate status, reduced symptom burden, and improved depressive symptoms [126, 127]. Neither study found an increase in mortality rate compared to patients not in the interventions. Please see Chap. 47 for further discussion of palliative care in transplant patients.

Conclusions

Mental health-care professionals caring for patients with liver disease should be aware of the high prevalence of psychiatric disorders in this population, especially SUDs. For SUDs in particular, the complete abstinence from alcohol or drugs is the definitive strategy for the stabilization and ultimate treatment of the underlying liver disease. Mental health professionals serve a key role in identifying these disorders and arranging adequate addiction treatment.

For some types of liver diseases, the presenting symptoms may appear as primary psychiatric disorders, and patients may initially seek psychiatric help for their problems. Careful consideration of the differential diagnosis, with possible input from additional medical specialists, may be needed to identify the underlying liver disease.

Beyond traditional psychotherapies and addiction counseling, the psychiatric treatment of patients with liver disease may necessitate attention to disease-specific issues. Patients with CLD often need to adjust to being chronically ill, experiencing decrements in QOL, and enduring limitations in their daily functioning. For those facing LT, special challenges exist during the pre-transplant wait period, as health is typically deteriorating and the wait may be long. Strategies to address patients' and caregivers' particular needs during this period are required.

Pharmacotherapy is also complex in patients with liver disease. As the liver is responsible for the metabolism of most drugs, medication prescription requires careful consideration as liver disease progresses, with consideration of specific drug metabolism, severity of liver disease and potential for drug side effects. Additionally complex is the high prevalence of chronic pain disorders in this population. For patients with cirrhosis, strategies to minimize opioid analgesics would be best. The combination of potential ill effects of opioids coupled with the contributions to pain of psychiatric symptoms and possible systemic inflammation in cirrhosis suggest alternative treatment strategies targeting these issues may be beneficial. HE should also be considered with the use of drug therapies. Subclinical HE may not always be identifiable on clinical exam, and mental health clinicians may need to consider whether formal neurocognitive testing is required.

The traditional sub-specialization model of medicine lends to providers focusing on a patient's specific issues relative to their clinical expertise. In this model, each clinician may fashion a treatment plan in isolation of the patient's other comorbid yet interrelated disorders. However, many of these complex and comorbid disorders cannot be fully addressed in isolation. An interdisciplinary team approach for overall coordination of care would be the best strategy. As outlined above, depending on the specific needs of the individual patient, coordination of care may require simultaneous input from mental health providers, gastroenterologist/hepatologists, addiction and pain management specialists, and palliative care. In other comorbid chronic medical and mental health diseases, the use of a collaborative care team approach compared to usual care demonstrated overall better medical and mental health outcomes as well as greater patient satisfaction [128]. Additionally, as comorbid liver and psychiatric diseases are often chronic conditions, longitudinal care management will likely be required. By virtue of their comprehensive assessment of patient histories, mental health providers may be best suited to recognize the totality of the CLD patients' needs and recommend—if not facilitate—a more comprehensive approach to care.

References

1. Bell BP, Manos MM, Zaman A, Terrault N, Thomas A, Navarro VJ, et al. The epidemiology of newly diagnosed chronic liver disease in gastroenterology practices in the United States: results from population-based surveillance. Am J Gastroenterol. 2008;103(11):2727–36.
2. Davis GL, Albright JE, Cook SF, Rosenberg DM. Projecting future complications of chronic hepatitis C in the United States. Liver Transpl. 2003;9(4):331–8.
3. Goldberg D, Ditah IC, Saeian K, Lalehzari M, Aronsohn A, Gorospe EC, et al. Changes in the prevalence of hepatitis C virus infection, nonalcoholic steatohepatitis, and alcoholic liver disease among patients with cirrhosis or liver failure on the waitlist for liver transplantation. Gastroenterology. 2017;152(5):1090–9.
4. Younossi ZM, Otgonsuren M, Henry L, Venkatesan C, Mishra A, Erario M, et al. Association of nonalcoholic fatty liver disease (NAFLD) with hepatocellular carcinoma (HCC) in the United States from 2004 to 2009. Hepatology. 2015;62(6):1723–30. https://doi.org/10.1002/hep.28123.
5. National Institute of Diabetes and Digestive and Kidney Diseases (NIDDK). Monograph on cirrhosis. 2014. https://www.niddk.nih.gov/health-information/liver-disease/cirrhosis.
6. Organ Procurement and Transplantation Network. Data tables. Updated December 15, 2017. https://optn.transplant.hrsa.gov/data/.
7. Jinjuvadia R, Jinjuvadia C, Puangsricharoen P, Chalasani N, Crabb DW, Liangpunsakul S, et al. Concomitant psychiatric and nonalcohol-related substance use disorders among hospitalized patients with alcoholic liver disease in the United States. Alcohol Clin Exp Res. 2018;42(2):397–402.
8. Diehl AM. Alcoholic liver disease: natural history. Liver Transpl Surg. 1997;3(3):206–11.
9. Nielsen JK, Olafsson S, Bergmann OM, Runarsdottir V, Hansdottir I, Sigurdardottir R, et al. Lifetime drinking history in patients with alcoholic liver disease and patients with alcohol use disorder without liver disease. Scand J Gastroenterol. 2017;52(6–7):762–7.
10. DiMartini AF, Beresford TP. Alcoholism and liver transplantation. Curr Opin Organ Transplant. 1999;4(2):177–81.
11. DiMartini AF, Crone C, Dew MA. Alcohol and substance use in liver transplant patients. Clin Liver Dis. 2011;15(4):727–51.
12. Addolorato G, Mirijello A, Leggio L, Ferrulli A, Landolfi R. Management of alcohol dependence in patients with liver disease. CNS Drugs. 2013;27(4):287–99.
13. Beresford TP. Predictive factors for alcoholic relapse in the selection of alcohol-dependent persons for hepatic transplant. Liver Transpl Surg. 1997;3(3):280–91.
14. DiMartini AF, Dew MA, Javed L, Fitzgerald MG, Jain A, Day N. Pretransplant psychiatric and medical comorbidity of alcoholic liver disease patients who received liver transplant. Psychosomatics. 2004;45(6):517–23.
15. DiMartini A, Dew MA, Fitzgerald MG, Fontes P. Clusters of alcohol use disorders diagnostic criteria and predictors of alcohol use after liver transplantation for alcoholic liver disease. Psychosomatics. 2008;49(4):332–40.
16. Beresford TP, Wongngamnit N, Temple BA. Alcoholism: diagnosis and natural history in the context of medical disease. In: Neuberger J, DiMartini A, editors. Alcohol abuse and liver disease. Oxford: Wiley; 2015. p. 22–34.
17. Centers for Disease Control and Prevention. Hepatitis C FAQs for health professionals. 2018. https://www.cdc.gov/hepatitis/hcv/hcvfaq.htm#section1.
18. Centers for Disease Control and Prevention. Hepatitis B FAQs for health professionals. 2018. https://www.cdc.gov/hepatitis/hbv/hbvfaq.htm#overview.
19. Lok AS, McMahon BJ. Chronic hepatitis B. Hepatology. 2007;45(2):507–39.
20. Fontana RJ, Hussain KB, Schwartz SM, Moyer CA, Su GL, Lok AS. Emotional distress in chronic hepatitis C patients not receiving antiviral therapy. J Hepatol. 2002;36(3):401–7.
21. Karaivazoglou K, Iconomou G, Triantos C, Hyphantis T, Thomopoulos K, Lagadinou M, et al. Fatigue and depressive symptoms associated with chronic viral hepatitis patients. Health-related quality of life (HRQOL). Ann Hepatol. 2010;9(4):419–27.
22. Modabbernia A, Poustchi H, Malekzadeh R. Neuropsychiatric and psychosocial issues of patients with hepatitis C infection: a selective literature review. Hepat Mon. 2013;13(1):e8340.
23. Rifai MA, Gleason OC, Sabouni D. Psychiatric care of the patient with hepatitis C: a review of the literature. Prim Care Companion J Clin Psychiatry. 2010;12(6):PCC.09r00877. https://doi.org/10.4088/PCC.09r00877whi.

24. el-Serag HB, Kunik M, Richardson P, Rabeneck L. Psychiatric disorders among veterans with hepatitis C infection. Gastroenterology. 2002;123(2):476–82.

25. Golden J, O'Dwyer AM, Conroy RM. Depression and anxiety in patients with hepatitis C: prevalence, detection rates and risk factors. Gen Hosp Psychiatry. 2005;27(6):431–8.

26. Ozkan M, Corapcioglu A, Balcioglu I, Ertekin E, Khan S, Ozdemir S, et al. Psychiatric morbidity and its effect on the quality of life of patients with chronic hepatitis B and hepatitis C. Int J Psychiatry Med. 2006;36(3):283–97.

27. Quelhas R, Lopes A. Psychiatric problems in patients infected with hepatitis C before and during antiviral treatment with interferon-alpha: a review. J Psychiatr Pract. 2009;15(4):262–81.

28. Weinstein AA, Kallman Price J, Stepanova M, Poms LW, Fang Y, Moon J, et al. Depression in patients with nonalcoholic fatty liver disease and chronic viral hepatitis B and C. Psychosomatics. 2011;52(2):127–32.

29. Navines R, Castellvi P, Moreno-Espana J, Gimenez D, Udina M, Canizares S, et al. Depressive and anxiety disorders in chronic hepatitis C patients: reliability and validity of the Patient Health Questionnaire. J Affect Disord. 2012;138(3):343–51.

30. Altindag A, Cadirci D, Sirmatel F. Depression and health related quality of life in non-cirrhotic chronic hepatitis B patients and hepatitis B carriers. Neurosciences (Riyadh). 2009;14(1):56–9.

31. Modabbernia A, Ashrafi M, Malekzadeh R, Poustchi H. A review of psychosocial issues in patients with chronic hepatitis B. Arch Iran Med. 2013;16(2):114–22.

32. Ashrafi M, Modabbernia A, Dalir M, Taslimi S, Karami M, Ostovaneh MR, et al. Predictors of mental and physical health in non-cirrhotic patients with viral hepatitis: a case control study. J Psychosom Res. 2012;73(3):218–24.

33. Grant BF, Saha TD, Ruan WJ, Goldstein RB, Chou SP, Jung J, et al. Epidemiology of DSM-5 drug use disorder: results from the National Epidemiologic Survey on Alcohol and Related Conditions-III. JAMA Psychiat. 2016;73(1):39–47.

34. Yovtcheva SP, Rifai MA, Moles JK, Van der Linden BJ. Psychiatric comorbidity among hepatitis C-positive patients. Psychosomatics. 2001;42(5):411–5.

35. Cheung RC. Epidemiology of hepatitis C virus infection in American veterans. Am J Gastroenterol. 2000;95(3):740–7.

36. Lansky A, Finlayson T, Johnson C, Holtzman D, Wejnert C, Mitsch A, et al. Estimating the number of persons who inject drugs in the United States by meta-analysis to calculate national rates of HIV and hepatitis C virus infections. PLoS One. 2014;9(5):e97596.

37. Banini BA, Sanyal AJ. Nonalcoholic fatty liver disease: epidemiology, pathogenesis, natural history, diagnosis, and current treatment options. Clin Med Insights Ther. 2016;8:75–84.

38. Demir M, Lang S, Steffen HM. Nonalcoholic fatty liver disease—current status and future directions. J Dig Dis. 2015;16(10):541–57.

39. Noureddin M, Zhang A, Loomba R. Promising therapies for treatment of nonalcoholic steatohepatitis. Expert Opin Emerg Drugs. 2016;21(3):343–57.

40. Elwing JE, Lustman PJ, Wang HL, Clouse RE. Depression, anxiety, and nonalcoholic steatohepatitis. Psychosom Med. 2006;68(4):563–9.

41. Stewart KE, Levenson JL. Psychological and psychiatric aspects of treatment of obesity and nonalcoholic fatty liver disease. Clin Liver Dis. 2012;16(3):615–29.

42. Marchesini G, Suppini A, Forlani G. NAFLD treatment: cognitive-behavioral therapy has entered the arena. J Hepatol. 2005;43(6):926–8.

43. Vilstrup H, Amodio P, Bajaj J, Cordoba J, Ferenci P, Mullen KD, et al. Hepatic encephalopathy in chronic liver disease: 2014 Practice Guideline by the American Association for the Study of Liver Diseases and the European Association for the Study of the Liver. Hepatology. 2014;60(2):715–35.

44. Ferenci P, Lockwood A, Mullen K, Tarter R, Weissenborn K, Blei AT. Hepatic encephalopathy—definition, nomenclature, diagnosis, and quantification: final report of the working party at the 11th World Congresses of Gastroenterology, Vienna, 1998. Hepatology. 2002;35(3):716–21.

45. Bajaj JS, Saeian K, Schubert CM, Hafeezullah M, Franco J, Varma RR, et al. Minimal hepatic encephalopathy is associated with motor vehicle crashes: the reality beyond the driving test. Hepatology. 2009;50(4):1175–83.

46. Bajaj JS, Heuman DM, Sterling RK, Sanyal AJ, Siddiqui M, Matherly S, et al. Validation of EncephalApp, smartphone-based Stroop test, for the diagnosis of covert hepatic encephalopathy. Clin Gastroenterol Hepatol. 2015;13(10):1828–35.

47. Bémeur C, Butterworth RF. Nutrition in the management of cirrhosis and its neurological complications. J Clin Exp Hepatol. 2014;4(2):141–50.

48. Ridley NJ, Draper B, Withall A. Alcohol-related dementia: an update of the evidence. Alzheimers Res Ther. 2013;5(1):3.

49. Thomson AD, Guerrini I, Marshall EJ. The evolution and treatment of Korsakoff's syndrome: out of sight, out of mind? Neuropsychol Rev. 2012;22(2):81–92.

50. Galvin R, Bråthen G, Ivashynka A, Hillbom M, Tanasescu R, Leone MA. EFNS guidelines for diagnosis, therapy and prevention of Wernicke encephalopathy. Eur J Neurol. 2010;17(12):1408–18. https://doi.org/10.1111/j.1468-1331.2010.03153.x.

51. Dening TR, Berrios GE. Wilson's disease. Psychiatric symptoms in 195 cases. Arch Gen Psychiatry. 1989;46(12):1126–34.

52. Levenson JL, editor The American Psychiatric Publishing textbook of psychosomatic medicine: psychiatric care of the medically ill. 2nd ed. Washington, DC: American Psychiatric Publishing; 2011.

53. Srinivas K, Sinha S, Taly AB, Prashanth LK, Arunodaya GR, Janardhana Reddy YC, et al. Dominant psychiatric manifestations in Wilson's disease: a diagnostic and therapeutic challenge! J Neurol Sci. 2008;266(1–2):104–8. https://doi.org/10.1016/j.jns.2007.09.009.

54. Carta M, Mura G, Sorbello O, Farina G, Demelia L. Quality of life and psychiatric symptoms in Wilson's Disease: the relevance of bipolar disorders. Clin Pract Epidemiol Ment Health. 2012a;8:102–9.

55. Carta MG, Sorbello O, Moro MF, Bhat KM, Demelia E, Serra A, et al. Bipolar disorders and Wilson's disease. BMC Psychiatry. 2012b;12:52.

56. Bandmann O, Weiss KH, Kaler SG. Wilson's disease and other neurological copper disorders. Lancet Neurol. 2015;14(1):103–13.

57. Crimlisk HL. The little imitator—porphyria: a neuropsychiatric disorder. J Neurol Neurosurg Psychiatry. 1997;62(4):319–28.

58. National Institute of Diabetes and Digestive and Kidney Diseases (NIDDK). Porphyria. 2014. https://www.niddk.nih.gov/health-information/liver-disease/porphyria.

59. Tracy JA, Dyck PJ. Porphyria and its neurologic manifestations. Handb Clin Neurol. 2014;120:839–49.

60. Kessler RC, Bromet EJ. The epidemiology of depression across cultures. Annu Rev Public Health. 2013;34:119–38.

61. Ewusi-Mensah I, Saunders JB, Williams R. The clinical nature and detection of psychiatric disorders in patients with alcoholic liver disease. Alcohol Alcohol. 1984;19(4):297–302.

62. Le Strat Y, Le Foll B, Dubertret C. Major depression and suicide attempts in patients with liver disease in the United States. Liver Int. 2015;35(7):1910–6.

63. Mullish BH, Kabir MS, Thursz MR, Dhar A. Review article: depression and the use of antidepressants in patients with chronic liver disease or liver transplantation. Aliment Pharmacol Ther. 2014;40(8):880–92.

64. Blaxter M, Cyster R. Compliance and risk-taking: the case of alcoholic liver disease. Sociol Health Illn. 1984;6(3):290–310.

65. Jonas DE, Garbutt JC, Amick HR, Brown JM, Brownley KA, Council CL, et al. Behavioral counseling after screening for alcohol misuse in primary care: a systematic review and meta-analysis for the U.S. Preventive Services Task Force. Ann Intern Med. 2012;157(9):645–54.

66. Weinrieb RM, Van Horn DH, McLellan AT, Volpicelli JR, Calarco JS, Lucey MR. Drinking behavior and motivation for treatment among alcohol-dependent liver transplant candidates. J Addict Dis. 2001;20(2):105–19.

67. Weinrieb RM, Lucey MR. Treatment of addictive behaviors in liver transplant patients. Liver Transpl. 2007;13(11 Suppl 2):S79–82.

68. Bjornsson E, Olsson J, Rydell A, Fredriksson K, Eriksson C, Sjoberg C, et al. Long-term follow-up of patients with alcoholic liver disease after liver transplantation in Sweden: impact of structured management on recidivism. Scand J Gastroenterol. 2005;40(2):206–16.

69. Burra P, Lucey MR. Liver transplantation in alcoholic patients. Transpl Int. 2005;18(5):491–8.

70. Gedaly R, McHugh PP, Johnston TD, Jeon H, Koch A, Clifford TM, et al. Predictors of relapse to alcohol and illicit drugs after liver transplantation for alcoholic liver disease. Transplantation. 2008;86(8):1090–5.

71. Kodali S, Kaif M, Tariq R, Singal A. Alcohol relapse after liver transplantation for alcoholic cirrhosis—impact on liver graft and patient survival: a meta-analysis. Alcohol Alcohol. 2018;53(2):166-72. https://doi.org/10.1093/alcalc/agx098.

72. Pessione F, Ramond MJ, Peters L, Pham BN, Batel P, Rueff B, et al. Five-year survival predictive factors in patients with excessive alcohol intake and cirrhosis. Effect of alcoholic hepatitis, smoking and abstinence. Liver Int. 2003;23(1):45–53.

73. Yates WR, LaBrecque DR, Pfab D. Personality disorder as a contraindication for liver transplantation in alcoholic cirrhosis. Psychosomatics. 1998;39(6):501–11.

74. Khan A, Tansel A, White DL, Kayani WT, Bano S, Lindsay J, et al. Efficacy of psychosocial interventions in inducing and maintaining alcohol abstinence in patients with chronic liver disease: a systematic review. Clin Gastroenterol Hepatol. 2016;14(2):191–202.e1–4.

75. Weinrieb RM, Van Horn DH, Lynch KG, Lucey MR. A randomized, controlled study of treatment for alcohol dependence in patients awaiting liver transplantation. Liver Transpl. 2011;17(5):539–47.

76. Moriarty KJ, Platt H, Crompton S, Darling W, Blakemore M, Hutchinson S, et al. Collaborative care for alcohol-related liver disease. Clin Med (Lond). 2007;7(2):125–8.

77. DiMartini AF, Dew MA. Monitoring alcohol use on the liver transplant wait list: therapeutic and practical issues. Liver Transpl. 2012;18(11):1267–9.

78. Crowley P. Long-term drug treatment of patients with alcohol dependence. Aust Prescr. 2015;38(2):41–3.

79. Falk DE, Yi HY, Hiller-Sturmhofel S. An epidemiologic analysis of co-occurring alcohol and tobacco use and disorders: findings from the National Epidemiologic Survey on Alcohol and Related Conditions. Alcohol Res Health. 2006;29(3):162–71.

80. Bataller R. Time to ban smoking in patients with chronic liver diseases. Hepatology. 2006;44(6):1394–6.

81. Kolly P, Knopfli M, Dufour JF. Effect of smoking on survival of patients with hepatocellular carcinoma. Liver Int. 2017;37(11):1682–7.

82. Bentzley BS, Barth KS, Back SE, Book SW. Discontinuation of buprenorphine maintenance therapy: perspectives and outcomes. J Subst Abus Treat. 2015;52:48–57.

83. Koch M, Banys P. Liver transplantation and opioid dependence. JAMA. 2001;285(8):1056–8.

84. Parfieniuk A, Flisiak R. Role of cannabinoids in chronic liver diseases. World J Gastroenterol. 2008;14(40):6109–14.

85. Patsenker E, Stickel F. Cannabinoids in liver diseases. Clin Liver Dis. 2016;7(2):21–5.

86. Hézode C, Zafrani ES, Roudot-Thoraval F, Costentin C, Hessami A, Bouvier-Alias M, et al. Daily cannabis use: a novel risk factor of steatosis severity in patients with chronic hepatitis C. Gastroenterology. 2008;134(2):432–9.

87. Ishida JH, Peters MG, Jin C, Louie K, Tan V, Bacchetti P, et al. Influence of cannabis use on severity of hepatitis C disease. Clin Gastroenterol Hepatol. 2008;6(1):69–75.

88. Tam J, Liu J, Mukhopadhyay B, Cinar R, Godlewski G, Kunos G. Endocannabinoids in liver disease. Hepatology. 2011;53(1):346–55.

89. Adejumo AC, Alliu S, Ajayi TO, Adejumo KL, Adegbala OM, Onyeakusi NE, et al. Cannabis use is associated with reduced prevalence of non-alcoholic fatty liver disease: a cross-sectional study. PLoS One. 2017;12(4):e0176416.

90. Brunet L, Moodie EE, Rollet K, Cooper C, Walmsley S, Potter M, et al. Marijuana smoking does not accelerate progression of liver disease in HIV-hepatitis C coinfection: a longitudinal cohort analysis. Clin Infect Dis. 2013;57(5):663–70.

91. Magen I, Avraham Y, Berry E, Mechoulam R. Endocannabinoids in liver disease and hepatic encephalopathy. Curr Pharm Des. 2008;14(23):2362–9.

92. Schrot RJ, Hubbard JR. Cannabinoids: Medical implications. Ann Med. 2016;48(3):128–41.

93. Wilkinson ST, D'Souza DC. Problems with the medicalization of marijuana. JAMA. 2014;311(23):2377–8.

94. Rogal SS, Bielefeldt K, Wasan AD, Lotrich FE, Zickmund S, Szigethy E, et al. Inflammation, psychiatric symptoms, and opioid use are associated with pain and disability in patients with cirrhosis. Clin Gastroenterol Hepatol. 2015;13(5):1009–16.

95. Silberbogen AK, Janke EA, Hebenstreit C. A closer look at pain and hepatitis C: preliminary data from a veteran population. J Rehabil Res Dev. 2007;44(2):231–44.

96. Whitehead AJ, Dobscha SK, Morasco BJ, Ruimy S, Bussell C, Hauser P. Pain, substance use disorders and opioid analgesic prescription patterns in veterans with hepatitis C. J Pain Symptom Manag. 2008;36(1):39–45.

97. Imani F, Motavaf M, Safari S, Alavian SM. The therapeutic use of analgesics in patients with liver cirrhosis: a literature review and evidence-based recommendations. Hepat Mon. 2014;14(10):e23539.

98. Rogal SS, Bielefeldt K, Wasan AD, Szigethy E, Lotrich F, DiMartini AF. Fibromyalgia symptoms and cirrhosis. Dig Dis Sci. 2015b;60(5):1482–9.

99. Riley TR 3rd, Koch K. Characteristics of upper abdominal pain in those with chronic liver disease. Dig Dis Sci. 2003;48(10):1914–8.

100. Rogal SS, Winger D, Bielefeldt K, Szigethy E. Pain and opioid use in chronic liver disease. Dig Dis Sci. 2013;58(10):2976–85.

101. Fouad YM, Makhlouf MM, Khalaf H, Mostafa Z, Abdel Raheem E, Meneasi W. Is irritable bowel syndrome associated with chronic hepatitis C? J Gastroenterol Hepatol. 2010;25(7):1285–8.

102. Dirchwolf M, Ruf AE. Role of systemic inflammation in cirrhosis: from pathogenesis to prognosis. World J Hepatol. 2015;7(16):1974–81.

103. Acharya C, Betrapally NS, Gillevet PM, Sterling RK, Akbarali H, White MB, et al. Chronic opioid use is associated with altered gut microbiota and predicts readmissions in patients with cirrhosis. Aliment Pharmacol Ther. 2017;45(2):319–31.

104. Randall HB, Alhamad T, Schnitzler MA, Zhang Z, Ford-Glanton S, Axelrod DA, et al. Survival implications of opioid use before and after liver transplantation. Liver Transpl. 2017;23(3):305–14.

105. Adedoyin A, Branch RA. Pharmacokinetics. In: Zakim D, Boyer TD, editors. Hepatology: a textbook of liver disease. 3rd ed. Philadelphia: WB Saunders; 1996. p. 307–22.

106. Blaschke TF. Protein binding and kinetics of drugs in liver diseases. Clin Pharmacokinet. 1977;2(1):32–44.

107. DeSanty KP, Amabile CM. Antidepressant-induced liver injury. Ann Pharmacother. 2007;41(7):1201–11.

108. Russo MW, Watkins PB. Are patients with elevated liver tests at increased risk of drug-induced liver injury? Gastroenterology. 2004;126(5):1477–80.

109. Bailey DE Jr, Hendrix CC, Steinhauser KE, Stechuchak KM, Porter LS, Hudson J, et al. Randomized trial of an uncertainty self-management telephone intervention for patients awaiting liver transplant. Patient Educ Couns. 2017;100(3):509–17.

110. Singh N, Gayowski T, Wagener MM, Marino IR. Depression in patients with cirrhosis. Impact on outcome. Dig Dis Sci. 1997;42(7):1421–7.

111. Engle D. Psychosocial aspects of the organ transplant experience: what has been established and what we need for the future. J Clin Psychol. 2001;57(4):521–49.

112. Olbrisch ME, Benedict SM, Ashe K, Levenson JL. Psychological assessment and care of organ transplant patients. J Consult Clin Psychol. 2002;70(3):771–83.

113. Corbett C, Armstrong MJ, Parker R, Webb K, Neuberger JM. Mental health disorders and solid-organ transplant recipients. Transplantation. 2013;96(7):593–600.

114. Rogal SS, Dew MA, Fontes P, DiMartini AF. Early treatment of depressive symptoms and long-term survival after liver transplantation. Am J Transplant. 2013;13(4):928–35.

115. Stewart BJ, Turnbull D, Mikocka-Walus AA, Harley HA, Andrews JM. Acceptability of psychotherapy, pharmacotherapy, and self-directed therapies in Australians living with chronic hepatitis C. J Clin Psychol Med Settings. 2013;20(4):427–39.

116. Bajaj JS, Ellwood M, Ainger T, Burroughs T, Fagan A, Gavis EA, et al. Mindfulness-based stress reduction therapy improves patient and caregiver-reported outcomes in cirrhosis. Clin Transl Gastroenterol. 2017;8(7):e108.

117. Evon DM, Simpson K, Kixmiller S, Galanko J, Dougherty K, Golin C, et al. A randomized controlled trial of an integrated care intervention to increase eligibility for chronic hepatitis C treatment. Am J Gastroenterol. 2011;106(10):1777–86. https://doi.org/10.1038/ajg.2011.219.

118. Morana JG. Psychological evaluation and follow-up in liver transplantation. World J Gastroenterol. 2009;15(6):694–6.

119. Neri S, Bertino G, Petralia A, Giancarlo C, Rizzotto A, Calvagno GS, et al. A multidisciplinary therapeutic approach for reducing the risk of psychiatric side effects in patients with chronic hepatitis C treated with pegylated interferon alpha and ribavirin. J Clin Gastroenterol. 2010;44(9):e210–7. https://doi.org/10.1097/MCG.0b013e3181d88af5.

120. Sharif F, Mohebbi S, Tabatabaee HR, Saberi-Firoozi M, Gholamzadeh S. Effects of psycho-educational intervention on health-related quality of life (QOL) of patients with chronic liver disease referring to Shiraz University of Medical Sciences. Health Qual Life Outcomes. 2005;3:81.

121. Rizzo M, Creed F, Goldberg D, Meader N, Pilling S. A systematic review of non-pharmacological treatments for depression in people with chronic physical health problems. J Psychosom Res. 2011;71(1):18–27.

122. Grover S, Sarkar S. Liver transplant-psychiatric and psychosocial aspects. J Clin Exp Hepatol. 2012;2(4):382–92.

123. Gross CR, Kreitzer MJ, Thomas W, Reilly-Spong M, Cramer-Bornemann M, Nyman JA, et al. Mindfulness-based stress reduction for solid organ transplant recipients: a randomized controlled trial. Altern Ther Health Med. 2010;16(5):30–8.

124. Larson AM, Curtis JR. Integrating palliative care for liver transplant candidates: "too well for transplant, too sick for life". JAMA. 2006;295(18):2168–76.

125. Wright L, Pape D, Ross K, Campbell M, Bowman K. Approaching end-of-life care in organ transplantation: the impact of transplant patients' death and dying. Prog Transplant. 2007;17(1):57–61.

126. Baumann AJ, Wheeler DS, James M, Turner R, Siegel A, Navarro VJ. Benefit of early palliative care intervention in end-stage liver disease patients awaiting liver transplantation. J Pain Symptom Manag. 2015;50(6):882–6.

127. Lamba S, Murphy P, McVicker S, Harris Smith J, Mosenthal AC. Changing end-of-life care practice for liver transplant service patients: structured palliative care intervention in the surgical intensive care unit. J Pain Symptom Manag. 2012;44(4):508–19.

128. Katon WJ, Lin EH, Von Korff M, Ciechanowski P, Ludman EJ, Young B, et al. Collaborative care for patients with depression and chronic illnesses. N Engl J Med. 2010;363(27):2611–20.

History of Liver Transplantation

13

Adam X. Sang and Carlos O. Esquivel

"It was all nothing but a kind of a wild science fiction at the beginning, but as realistic as the dream of putting a man on the surface of the moon was at that time. They both did not sound like anything very rational, but they both turned out to work at around the same time."

Thomas Starzl, MD

Introduction

In the above quote from an interview at the 2014 International Small Bowel Transplant Symposium [1], Dr. Thomas Starzl compares the pioneering of liver transplantation to the Space Race. Starzl performed the first successful human liver transplantation in 1967. Two years later, the United States ended the Space Race by landing on the moon in 1969.

Beyond the contemporary nature of these two enormous achievements, however, are many deeper similarities. Both endeavors pushed what was once science fiction—the *Frankenstein* of Mary Shelley and *From the Earth to the Moon* of Jules Verne—into the forefront of reality. Both opened up entire frontiers of what was possible: replacing failing organs and traveling to another celestial body. Both were races against time, with human lives and national pride on the line. Most importantly, both stories are culminations of decades of perseverance through failures, setbacks, and surprises.

If there was ever a story that captured the elaborate dance between clinical medicine and scientific research, and how each propels the other to new heights, it would be the story of organ transplantation. The failure of the liver, an organ recognized since prehistoric times to be essential to life, had been universally fatal throughout mankind's history. We now have the ability to cure it. As you shall see, the journey was long and riddled with one obstacle after another, but they were overcome by scientists, physicians, surgeons, policymakers, and patients working toward a common goal. However, recording history is an imperfect art, and the story of liver transplantation continues to be revised and debated even today.

A lot has been accomplished in a relatively short timeframe, and today, liver transplantation is an established therapy that is safer than ever. In contrast, just 50 years ago, we simply could not treat patients with end-stage liver disease (ESLD). Thus, while caring for patients with ESLD today can be challenging and exhausting, we now have more surgical and medical options than ever before.

How Our Ancient Ancestors Viewed the Liver

Surgically replacing the liver is a very modern invention, but our ancestors knew a surprising amount about the liver, even if they could not manipulate it. Many scholars believe that the ancient Greek myth of Prometheus—a Titan who stole fire from Zeus and gifted it to man—was evidence that the Greeks knew about the incredible regenerative ability of the liver. As eternal punishment for his act, Prometheus was chained to a mountain in the Caucasus, and an eagle would peck out his liver every day, only for the liver to grow back, and the punishment repeated the next day.

Several prominent Greek physicians made particular observations of the liver. Herophilus and later Galen, for example, wrote about the lobar nature of liver anatomy [2], an observation that unlocked the secret of safe liver surgery two millennia later. Hippocrates and then Celsus also made mention of draining liver abscesses in their works [3].

Not surprisingly, liver medicine did not advance much during the Middle Ages. In the nineteenth century, there was anecdotal evidence depicting salvage liver resections in the setting of trauma [2]. These accounts made it very clear that the liver bleeds easily and heavily—a feature which would mount a formidable obstacle for the pioneers of liver transplantation. And thus the liver continued, until the end of the nineteenth century, to be viewed as inoperable.

A. X. Sang
Department of Surgery, Stanford University School of Medicine, Stanford, CA, USA

C. O. Esquivel (✉)
Division of Abdominal Transplantation, Department of Surgery, Stanford University School of Medicine, Stanford, CA, USA
e-mail: esquivel@stanford.edu

© Springer International Publishing AG, part of Springer Nature 2019
Y. Sher, J. R. Maldonado (eds.), *Psychosocial Care of End-Stage Organ Disease and Transplant Patients*,
https://doi.org/10.1007/978-3-319-94914-7_13

At the time, patients with ESLD universally had poor prognoses. The course of clinical decline—the ascites, peritonitis, variceal bleeding, and encephalopathy—seemed irreversible, and physicians were powerless to provide more than supportive care.

Overcoming the Early Surgical and Immunological Barriers of Transplantation

In the early twentieth century, there was a great interest in the scientific and medical communities for organ grafting. Isolated reports of attempts at animal solid-organ transplants emerged around this time, but they were largely unsuccessful.

The first attempt at *human* solid-organ transplantation came in 1906, when French surgeon Dr. Mathieu Jaboulay reported two cases of kidney xenotransplantation. The first was the left kidney of a pig that was transplanted into the antecubital space of a woman with nephrotic syndrome; the second was a goat kidney transplanted into a woman who had lost a kidney due to infection [4, 5]. Neither graft worked, which Jaboulay attributed to vascular thrombosis.

Around the same time, one of Jaboulay's students, Dr. Alexis Carrel, was making important contributions to organ transplantation by pioneering end-to-end suture techniques that could reconnect vessels. This included anastomosing fragile veins—a feat considered impossible at the time. Using these techniques, he then experimented on a variety of transplant operations in animals. In a landmark paper published in the Journal of the American Medical Association in 1908, Carrel described the transplantation of kidneys, spleens, and even faces in various animal models [6]. He also reported the use of cold fluids to preserve the tissue for transplantation, a practice which continues even today. In many cases, the cats and dogs who underwent these invasive surgeries had good outcomes months after the procedure. But consistent with previous findings, Carrel observed that organs transplanted between zoologically distant organisms underwent deterioration, which he termed "cytolysis." Altogether, Carrel's vascular surgery innovations and systematic transplantation experiments in animals cleared an important technical hurdle to transplantation in humans. Carrel was awarded the Nobel Prize in Physiology or Medicine in 1912.

Sophisticated experimental work in animal models continued for the next three decades. The technical hurdle of transplantation (i.e., the vascular anastomosis) appeared to have been mastered, but in many cases, the organs were still not surviving. No one understood why this was happening, short of the "biological incompatibility" described by Carrel and his predecessors. Many leaders in the field thus saw organ transplantation as ultimately nonviable, and interest began to wane. In addition, much of the focus in research and clinical care was now being shifted toward the World Wars.

It was Professor Peter Medawar, a British biologist, who eventually solved the mystery of biological incompatibility. He was recruited by the British Medical Research Council to work on skin allotransplantation, as necessitated by the trauma and burns from World War II. His work unveiled the immune system as the main vehicle of biological incompatibility and established many of the tenants of immunological tolerance and rejection. He and his student Dr. Frank Burnet even demonstrated that tolerance to foreign tissue could be "acquired" early during embryogenesis, which would then prevent the recipient from rejecting this foreign tissue in the future. Medawar and Burnet published extensively on this subject in the 1950s and eventually won a Nobel Prize in Physiology or Medicine in 1960. Medawar was knighted by the British government in 1965, and in 1968, he was elected as the first President of the Transplantation Society (TTS), which is one of the world's largest transplantation organizations today.

With Medawar's work showing that the immune system was at the core of organ rejection, interest in transplantation revived. Thus came a string of successes in the field of kidney transplantation, starting with the first successful kidney transplant in 1954.

The Preclinical Successes with Liver Transplantation

The liver was long considered an organ too complex to manipulate, with its dual blood supply and its venous drainage into the inferior vena cava (IVC), a vein most surgically unforgiving. Thus, successful liver transplants in humans lagged more than a decade behind kidney transplants.

The 1950s brought several breakthroughs in preclinical liver transplantation. Dr. Vittorio Staudacher from the University of Milan was (recently) credited with the first liver transplant procedure in canines, reported in 1952 [7, 8]. Previously, the achievement was credited to Dr. Cristopher Welch from Albany Medical College, who in 1955 published a one-page manuscript describing his work on transplanting auxiliary liver segments into the abdominal cavity of dogs [9]. Although using auxiliary segments bypassed the need for a hepatectomy, the transplanted segments nonetheless deteriorated, which was likely due to a combination of rejection and ischemia. One year later, Dr. Jack Cannon from the University of California, Los Angeles, described orthotopic liver transplantation, in which the animal's own liver (presumably a canine) was removed and replaced by a full-size donor liver into the correct anatomic position [10].

Work in the dog model was further expounded by three surgeons who all went on to become the fathers of human liver transplantation. In 1958, Dr. Francis Moore, the Chief of Surgery at the Brigham Hospital, was looking to extend their success with kidney transplantation into the field of liver transplantation. He established a formal canine liver transplantation program, which performed over 30 canine liver transplants and published extensively on various surgical aspects of the demanding procedure [11, 12].

Dr. Thomas Starzl, meanwhile, was working out of Northwestern University in Chicago. As a surgical resident, Starzl had a strong interest in the physiology of portal venous circulation and developed several surgical models to remove and replace the liver, including abdominal multi-visceral organ transplantation [13, 14]. He was then awarded a Markle Scholars in Medicine Fellowship, which funded him to formally study liver transplantation and engineer it into a viable clinical service [15]. Starzl and his team eventually performed over 80 liver transplants in dogs [16].

Both groups made progress in tackling what was then a substantial surgical roadblock. Clamping the portal vein and the IVC in their dog model, an essential step during the removal of the native liver, usually resulted in the death of the animal [17]. Moore and colleagues developed a veno-venous bypass system that shunted the blood from the IVC and the portal vein to the superior vena cava (SVC). Starzl's team, on the other hand, pioneered the strategy of using a portocaval shunt to first divert blood from the portal vein to the IVC and then draining the IVC to the SVC via an iliac vein cannula and avoiding the clamped liver [18].

The third individual who helped usher in the era of successful liver transplantation was an English surgeon Dr. Roy Calne. As a medical student in 1950, Calne was taking care of a patient with kidney failure and saddened by the reality that their entire team could not provide anything more than supportive care [19]. He was interested in unraveling the immune system to allow humans to benefit from transplants—something that even Medawar did not believe could happen [13]. Calne's early work as a faculty focused on developing strategies to suppress the immune system. The only tool available at that time was whole-body irradiation, which Calne found ineffective in the setting of solid-organ transplantation. He worked on a relatively novel drug—6-mercaptopurine (6-MP)—and demonstrated that it prolonged kidney graft survival in dogs [19].

Encouraged by Medawar, Calne applied for and received a Harkness Fellowship in 1960, which allowed him to travel to Harvard Medical School. He observed Moore and his canine liver transplant experiments, which were dubbed the "sputnik" procedures (again drawing a parallel between liver transplantation and the Space Race) [18]. He started a series of experiments with Murray in dogs to test the efficacy of several new immunosuppressive compounds. One of them—azathioprine—was found to be more effective than 6-MP and actually allowed for long-term graft survival [12]. Starzl also tested azathioprine in dogs and found the *combination* of azathioprine and steroids to be even more efficacious. Calne returned to England in 1961 and subsequently initiated the clinical use of azathioprine and steroids for his kidney transplant program. In 1965, Calne was promoted as the Chair of Surgery at the University of Cambridge.

The First Human Attempt and the Moratorium

In 1962, Starzl joined the University of Colorado in Denver as an Associate Professor of Surgery. Denver was one of the only centers outside of Boston that had a commitment to transplantation and also had one of the few dialysis units in the country at the time [1]. There, Starzl started a successful kidney transplant program [1, 20]. Given the increasingly successful worldwide experience with kidney transplantation, the opportunity was ripe for an attempt at liver transplantation [14].

On March 1, 1963, Starzl attempted a liver transplant for a 3-year-old boy with biliary atresia, a congenital defect in the bile ducts. To reduce the risk of organ rejection, the patient underwent a pre-transplant thymectomy, as well as 13 days of azathioprine treatment [21]. But as Starzl recalls, upon starting the operation: "Nothing we had done in advance could have prepared us for the enormity of the task. Several hours were required just to make the incision and enter the abdomen. Every piece of tissue that was cut contained the small veins under high pressure that had resulted from obstruction of the portal vein by the diseased liver. Inside the abdomen, Bennie's liver was encased in scar tissue left over from operations performed shortly after his birth. His intestine and stomach were stuck to the liver in this mass of bloody scar. To make things worse, Bennie's blood would not clot…he bled to death as we worked desperately to stop the hemorrhage. The operation could not be completed." [22]

Despite this adverse outcome, the effort continued, and several more liver transplants were attempted thereafter. Two were performed by Starzl for primary liver cancer. Both adult patients tolerated the initial surgery, but only survived for 7 and 22 days, succumbing to pulmonary embolism, likely from the veno-venous bypass tubing [23]. Among the next four attempts, including two by Starzl, and one by Moore, none survived beyond 23 days. In addition, several attempts at auxiliary liver transplantation in the United States (three by Starzl), Australia, and the United Kingdom were also unsuccessful [20]. Thus, liver transplantation continued to be viewed as an insurmountable challenge and an impractical risk, and a voluntary worldwide moratorium was placed on this procedure.

While kidney transplant programs continued to thrive, liver transplantation ceased. However, Starzl did not give up. He and others reexamined the early outcomes, returned to the laboratory, and worked to find solutions during this moratorium. Starzl continued experimentation on various aspects of transplantation, including xenotransplantation and tissue-type matching [13]. In 1966, a preservation chamber was developed in Denver which improved organ survival ex vivo [24]. Most importantly, Starzl and his team began preparing and testing antihuman antilymphocyte globulin (ALG), obtained from inoculated horses. It was the first time that antibodies targeted against the cells of the adaptive immune system were used as immunosuppression. Trials using ALG in combination with azathioprine and steroids, first in dogs and then in kidney transplant patients, demonstrated its clinical efficacy [15, 20].

In addition, several individuals, including Calne, Starzl, and, French surgeon, Dr. Henri Garnier, began observing an interesting immunological property of the liver. In some species, such as pigs, an orthotopic liver transplant could survive indefinitely without any immunosuppression. Furthermore, if *another* organ was transplanted at the same time as the liver, that organ would also have prolonged survival [18]. Unfortunately, the same observation could not be made in humans and dogs, which still rejected their grafts. However, a certain subset of the dogs in the transplant cohort continued to accept their graft long after immunosuppression was stopped. These observations suggested that the liver was an immune "privileged" organ and might eventually be immune-tolerated by the recipient, a discovery which renewed hope in successful liver transplantation.

The First Human Successes on Both Sides of the Atlantic

After 3 years of renewed focus, Starzl reopened the liver transplantation program in Denver. On July of 1967, Starzl performed what would be the first successful liver transplantation. The patient was a 19-month-old girl with hepatocellular carcinoma and ESLD. She underwent a successful liver transplant as well as a splenectomy, with the donor liver maintained in a preservation chamber for 3 hours [20]. She was treated postoperatively with azathioprine, prednisolone, and ALG. She had good liver function for a year but unfortunately succumbed to cancer recurrence [25].

Starzl went on to perform seven more liver transplants, all in the pediatric population (ages 13 months to 16 years). The most common indication was for biliary atresia. Of these first eight patients, four died within the first 6 months due to liver infarction and sepsis, two died of liver cancer recurrence after 1 year post-transplantation, and one died of chronic rejection [25]. The last patient, as of 2002, was still alive and off immunosuppression [23].

In Europe, a liver transplant had been attempted in 1964 by Dr. Jean Demirleau, but the patient only survived for 3 hours [26]. Calne, who had continued to perform experimental liver transplants in pigs in England, observed Starzl's program gaining momentum in Denver and was ready to attempt a liver transplant at his home institution of Addenbrooke's Hospital at the University of Cambridge.

A well-told story of Calne's first liver transplantation unfolded as such. In 1968, a lady with a primary liver malignancy was referred to Calne. She was anxious to proceed despite the dangers disclosed to her, because "she said she had nothing to lose" [18]. A few weeks later, a young child became irreversibly comatose due to a viral infection of the brain stem, and the parents gave permission for the child's kidneys and liver to be used to help other patients.

When Calne presented the potential donor and recipient to a council of his medical colleagues, they all swiftly opposed the operation, citing a spectrum of medical and ethical risks. But Calne had an ace card: he introduced the world-famous Moore, who happened to be in Cambridge visiting his son, to the council [17]. Moore affirmed his support by simply saying, "Roy, you have to do it." Suddenly, the tide of the room changed [18]. Calne, with Moore as the first assistant, proceeded immediately to the operating room.

Per Calne's accounts, that first operation went smoothly. He utilized a "piggyback" technique, in which the donor IVC was anastomosed directly to the side of the recipient's IVC (which is otherwise left intact), instead of the conventional method of replacing the recipient's retrohepatic IVC with the IVC of the graft. This technique was necessary because of the size mismatch between the pediatric donor and the adult recipient, but as Calne smugly notes, "this operation was re-invented years later by other teams, who had not read our 1968 report in the British Medical Journal." [18] Unfortunately, Calne's patient passed away 3 months later due to pneumonia, secondary to immunosuppression.

The First Decade: From Few to Many

In the first few years, the mortality associated with this experimental procedure remained dismal. A survey published by the American College of Surgeons and the National Institutes of Health Organ Transplant Registry in 1972 showed that, by 1969, 81 orthotopic and 32 heterotopic liver transplants had been performed, the majority of which were from either Denver (Starzl's group) or Cambridge (Calne's group) [27]. Only 9% of patients (13 patients, all with orthotropic liver grafts) survived beyond 1 year. For the next decade, outcomes had only marginally improved—1-year survival was 23.7% for the Cambridge group and 38% for the Denver group [28]. There was pressure to arrest liver transplantation programs—the procedure was dangerous as well as a huge drain of resources (e.g., a single liver transplant could consume the supply of an entire blood bank).

Several important evolutions in liver transplantation occurred in the next decade as the learning curve continued:

First, the pioneering centers developed pipelines to overcome the logistical demands of liver transplantation, which involved coordinating two operations (a donor operation and a recipient operation) that were often separated by time and space, and a vast multitude of nonsurgical providers who must act in perfect unison to keep patients stable and organs viable. In England, Calne partnered with former colleague Dr. Roger Williams, a liver failure expert from King's College Hospital in London. Williams was the rare internal medicine physician who shared Calne's enthusiasm for liver transplantation because Williams knew firsthand the poor prognosis of these patients without an operation. Whenever a prospective donor at any neighboring hospital became available, teams from both Addenbrooke and King's would be mobilized. An intensive care team from King's would bring the liver patient to the donor hospital, where a surgical team from Addenbrooke would converge at the same time. The surgical team would wait in sterile operating room attire, while the ventilator for the donor patient was turned off. After the anesthesiologist declared cessation of cardiac activity, the donor liver and kidneys were perfused surgically with cooling solution, removed, and further preserved with sterile ice. At this point, the recipient would be taken to the operating room. After recovering for 2 weeks, the patient would be transferred back to either King's or Addenbrooke [18].

Second, the concept of brain death ("coma depasse") became accepted. Previously, a patient with irreversible brain injury had to be disconnected from life support—usually artificial ventilation—and the heart allowed to fully stop on its own, before the patient was considered "deceased" and suitable to donate organs. In 1968, for the first time, donation after brain death but with a beating heart was allowed in France. Brain death was accepted in the United States that same year, and later in England in 1976 [29]. This change refined the organ donation procedures, allowed grafts to be more easily transported, and resulted in better graft and patient survival.

Third, the final breakthrough was the discovery of cyclosporine in 1972 by Swiss physician Dr. Jean Borel, which Calne called a "watershed moment" in transplantation [19]. Calne first used it in liver transplantation in 1978 [28]. Cyclosporine could specifically target lymphocytes, the main vehicles of immune rejection. The concomitant use of cyclosporine with steroids starting in the 1980s dramatically improved outcomes, leading to 1-year survival close to 70% [28, 30]. Cyclosporine was approved by the Food and Drug Administration (FDA) in 1983, and its use has led to lower toxicity and overall improved outcomes across both kidney and liver transplants.

In 1980, Starzl moved to the University of Pittsburgh. Immediately, their liver transplant program blossomed,

which Starzl attributed to the large supply of cyclosporine available [1]. Pittsburgh became the worldwide leader in liver transplantation, with many surgeons and physicians traveling there in the 1980s to receive training in this newly emerging field. Dr. Russell Strong, for example, trained there in 1984 and went on to not only start the first transplantation unit in Australia but also perform the first living donor liver transplant in 1989 [31]. Dr. Carlos Esquivel, one of our co-authors, also trained under Starzl during this period and subsequently founded a transplant program at the California Pacific Medical Center in San Francisco in 1988. By that time, Pittsburgh had already reached 1000 human liver transplants [30].

From an Experimental Procedure to a Mainstream Clinical Service

Despite this progress in the late 1970s, liver transplantation was still not widely accepted as a reliable treatment. Experience was limited to only a handful of centers in the United States and Europe. One particular area of challenge was transplanting livers in infants and young patients, for whom suitable donors were rare and technical aspects more daunting. The rate of mortality from vascular complications in these patients was unacceptably high, resulting in another self-imposed moratorium for young children. In 1984, after working with Starzl for a few years, Esquivel moved to the Children's Hospital of Pittsburgh and began focusing exclusively on young children. His group published the first series of liver transplants in patients younger than 1 year of age in 1987 [32]. While outcomes improved, the scarcity of donors remained a problem [33].

For the next few years, the surgical techniques continued to be refined, anesthesia support improved, and a second generation of surgeons slowly took on the mantle of liver transplantation, primarily by joining donor teams. In addition, newer preservation solutions became available which staved off ischemic injury and allowed more control over the logistics of transplantation. This culminated in the University of Wisconsin solution, developed by James Southard and Folkert Belzer in 1987 [34]. The UW solution mimics intracellular osmolarities using inert substances while scavenging free radicals and remains the gold standard for cold preservation solution even today.

On June 20, 1983, the US Surgeon General Everett Koop, encouraged by Starzl and President Ronald Reagan, called for a National Institutes of Health (NIH) Consensus Development Conference on liver transplantation in Bethesda, Maryland. Liver transplant teams from four countries—the United States, Germany, England, and the Netherlands—gathered to present their data. After reviewing the outcome of 531 liver transplant cases, including comparisons to ESLD patients who did not receive a liver transplant, the expert panel approved liver transplantation as a valid "clinical service" to aid patients with cirrhosis and liver failure [35]. Liver transplantation was no longer an experimental procedure reserved as a last-ditch effort, but a standard treatment that could be utilized electively. This shift was further bolstered by a large study in 1989, by Starzl and colleagues, which examined 1179 liver transplant patients, whom had 1- and 5-year survival rates of 73% and 64% on cyclosporine, exceeding that of ESLD [36].

Partially because of these findings and the NIH consensus, more and more transplant centers emerged across the world in the 1980s. This was followed by a liver transplant by Dr. Carl-Gustav Groth, a protégé of Starzl, in Sweden in 1984 [20]; in Brazil [37] and Australia [31] in 1985; and in France, by Dr. Henri Bismuth in 1993 [38].

In Asia, the first described attempt at liver transplantation was by Dr. Nakayama in Japan in 1964 [39]. The second case (1978) was in China for a patient with advanced hepatocellular carcinoma [40]. While liver transplantation took off rather slowly in Asia, several Asian countries were instrumental in pushing the frontiers of living donor liver transplantation (LDLT). This was driven by several region-unique factors such as cultural and religious views against organ harvesting, the late adoption of brain death criteria in 1987 [39], and the high incidence of hepatitis B and C infections and resultant liver cancer.

Governing Fair Organ Allocation

As the indications for liver transplantation and the centers that could safely perform them expanded, the demand quickly exceeded the availability of livers. In 1988, there were 616 patients on the waiting list in the United States. By 1998, the number had risen to 12,000. Along with increased transplant demands, the average wait times increased and mortality while waiting for a liver grew exponentially.

In the first two decades of liver transplantation in the United States, allocations were managed by the individual transplant centers themselves [35]. In 1984, Congress passed the National Organ Transplant Act (NOTA) giving the federal government broad oversight over organ allocation, including prohibiting the sale of organs (see Chap. 2).

Suddenly, the organ allocation policies in the United States underwent several major changes in the 1990s. Initially, organ allocation was based on the length of time on the wait list. However, this prompted clinicians to aggressively enlist their patients earlier and earlier, thus inflating the wait list. In 1998, UNOS introduced a system of stratifying patients into four levels of acuity. Status 1 was emergent need, status 2 was intensive care unit (ICU), status 3 was inpatient, and status 4 was outpatient. Available organs were given to status 1 patients first, and so forth. Several problems with this allocation strategy emerged, including the fact that within a specific UNOS geographic region, there were multiple patients with the same status. This led to the development of the Child–Turcotte–Pugh score, which attempted to further stratify patients based on disease severity using several metrics, some of which were subjective.

In 1998, the US Department of Health and Human Services, under pressure from both the public and Congress, issued a regulation known as "the Organ Procurement and Transplantation Network (OPTN) Final Rule." This provision called for more objective and uniform organ allocation policies that would eliminate some of the geographic variability in terms of wait times. After much work, the Model for End-Stage Liver Disease (MELD) and Pediatric End-Stage Liver Disease (PELD) systems were implemented in 2002 as the central component of organ allocation priority. The MELD and PELD scores are well-studied metrics which can be calculated based on objective laboratory data and have been shown to predict mortality while on wait list. Therefore, a patient with a higher MELD or PELD score would get higher priority than a patient with a lower score.

In Europe, allocation systems vary by country and even by institution. In the late 2000s, many European transplant centers shifted to incorporating MELD/PELD as part of the criteria, based on the experience from the United States [41].

Organ Shortage Drives Surgical Innovation

Increasing the organ supply is an important ongoing effort in the field of liver transplantation. Promoting the use of expanded criteria donors (ECD) (e.g., donors who are older, have comorbidities, or have blood-borne infection history) is one strategy. ECD also includes donation after cardiac death (DCD). DCDs grew from 0.5% of liver transplants in 1999 to over 4.5% in 2008 [42]. These factors make the graft suboptimal, and when obtaining consent from liver transplant recipients today, disclosure about the quality and nature of the graft constitutes a key component. By using ECDs, more patients are able to come off the wait list and receive a life-preserving organ.

In addition, newer surgical techniques have allowed for LDLT. Living donation for kidneys has been around since its inception, but the liver is a non-paired organ, and surgically splitting the liver safely into two functional units (and relying on the remaining liver to regenerate) is a much newer breakthrough. The first required step was to be able to reduce a cadaveric donor liver down to appropriate size for the recipient. Recently, it was reported that Dr. Henry Gans and colleagues from the New York Hospital-Cornell Medical Center performed the first reduced-size liver transplant in 1969 [43]. Gans had resected the left lobe of the donor liver for a 24-year-old patient with ESLD whose abdomen was not large enough to accommodate the entire graft. It was Dr. Bismuth who had been classically credited with the first successful downsizing of an adult deceased donor liver into just the left lobe and successfully transplanting this reduced liver into a pediatric recipient in 1984 [44]. These pioneering cases, although utilizing cadaveric livers, established the tenet that livers can be split along its lobar planes and still function well as grafts.

A few years later, the first reported attempt at LDLT was performed in 1988 by Dr. Silvana Raia and colleagues in Sao Paulo, Brazil [37]. The patient was a young 4-year-old girl whose mother donated her left lateral segment; unfortunately, the child died 6 days postoperatively from hemolytic anemia, secondary to blood type mismatch. The mother recovered well after her donor procedure and eventually became pregnant again.

In 1989, Dr. Strong, who had trained with Starzl, reported on using the left lateral segment in a LDLT in Brisbane for a pediatric recipient [45]. This was considered the first successful LDLT in the world. Later that year, Raia performed a second LDLT for a 19-month-old girl with Caroli's disease. In this case, a healthy 40-year-old altruistic man volunteered for organ donation [37]. Natural expansions of LDLT techniques came shortly thereafter. In 1993, the first successful left lobe living donor transplant between adults [46] and the first successful right liver graft from adult to child [47] were performed. This was followed in 1996 by the first successful extended right lobe for adult-to-adult liver transplantation, performed in Hong Kong [48].

The first LDLT in the United States was performed by Dr. Christoph Broelsch at the University of Chicago in 1989. However, the utilization of LDLT in the United States appears to have peaked in 2002, when around 10% of liver transplantations involved a living donor [49]. One primary reason was the medical and ethical concerns of subjecting a healthy individual to a surgical procedure and possible liver failure, without any direct benefit to that individual. Partial hepatectomies for living donors carry a reported mortality of 0.5–1% and a morbidity of 20%—one living donor even required a liver transplant himself [50, 51]!

Split cadaveric livers were another method developed to address the organ shortage. An adult-sized graft from a deceased donor would be split along anatomic planes—initially on a back table—and prepared for transplantation into two separate recipients, usually one adult (receiving the larger right lobe) and one child (left lobe). Dr. Rudolf Pichlmayr from Germany first performed and described this technique in 1988 [52]. Broelsch and Strong subsequently championed this technique at their respective institutions in Chicago and Brisbane. Broelsch published a series in 1989, detailing 9 whole livers that were split to treat 18 patients [53]. Patient and graft survival were similar to whole organ

transplantation, although biliary complications were higher in the split liver group. In 1996, a group from Germany published on splitting the liver in situ in a deceased donor [54]. This newer technique has the benefit of better hemostasis and reduced ischemia times. However, currently, the surgical complexity of splitting a liver and the prospect of sacrificing one good liver for two riskier grafts have prevented widespread adoption of this technique.

Despite these advanced techniques, however, the organ shortage crisis has persisted and appears to be worsening. In 2010, for example, 11,352 new patients were added to the liver wait list, but only 6291 patients underwent liver transplantation [55]. The outcomes of both LDLT and split livers will continue to improve until they are equivalent to that of cadaveric whole liver transplant, but it remains to be seen whether they can be adopted widely enough to put a dent on the organ shortage.

The Next Generation of Strategies to Protect the Liver Graft

Several important next-generation immunosuppressants have been introduced in the past two decades. In the late 1980s, many liver grafts continued to show signs of rejection even while on cyclosporine. After much preclinical work by Starzl and colleagues at Pittsburgh, tacrolimus (FK-506) was first used in liver transplantation in 1989 and was then fast-tracked by the FDA in 1993 [56]. Similar to cyclosporine, tacrolimus suppressed the calcineurin axis and modulated the ability of T cells to respond to and attack the allograft. By using tacrolimus, almost three quarters of grafts which were rejecting while on cyclosporine were rescued [57]. Another antimetabolite, mycophenolic acid mofetil, was approved for use in 1995 and has replaced azathioprine at many centers. Four years later, rapamycin, an mTOR inhibitor studied extensively by Calne since 1989, was approved for clinical use as an immunosuppressant.

As our understanding of immunology improved, the therapeutic potential of recombinant antibodies became apparent. Starzl's ALG was the first drug in this category. Since then, a multitude of others have appeared. Some of the "biologic" immunosuppressants in this category include basiliximab (targets IL-2 receptors on T cells), alemtuzumab (targets CD52 on mature lymphocytes), and the fusion proteins abatacept and belatacept (blocks CD80 and CD86, which are costimulation signals for T cells). These and other newer antibodies increase the arsenal for transplant physicians today in helping patients stave off rejection.

Next, strategies are being developed to help select patients taper off immunosuppression completely. This approach is based on earlier observations that the liver is more tolerogenic than other organs. Starzl and the Pittsburgh group showed that with careful selection and monitoring, complete withdrawal of immunosuppression appeared safe in some liver transplant patients. The same has been observed on some kidney cases [58]. Many of these instances of tolerance were discovered serendipitously after the patient had stopped taking their medications, with no apparent adverse effects.

A recent strategy to *induce* tolerance in liver recipients is also based on early observations by Starzl and Calne, specifically regarding the natural history of the recipient's immune system post-transplant. They found that some recipients had circulating immune cells which originated from the donor and termed it "microchimerism." In addition, these patients' own immune cells seemed less reactive toward the graft. Today, many academic centers around the world are piloting protocols to introduce donor bone marrow cells to the recipient *prior* to receiving the solid-organ transplant, as a means to induce chimerism. This strategy is used initially in conjunction with more traditional immunosuppressants, which are then tapered off over time.

Future

When a life-saving operation, despite an extremely high early mortality, is shown to be possible, it eventually becomes established, the errors are recognized and eliminated, and a new generation of surgeons wonders why the pioneers had such a hard time. (Sir Roy Calne, MD [18])

As of 2010, there are 142 liver transplant centers in Europe, 129 in the United States, and many more in over 80 countries around the world [35, 59]. Within the United States, there are more than 50,000 patients living with transplanted livers as of 2009. It is amazing what has been accomplished in just five decades since the first successful liver transplantation. In 2012, Starzl and Calne won the Lasker-DeBakey Clinical Medical Research Award, one of the most prestigious awards given in medicine, for their work in pioneering liver transplantation.

Organ shortage will continue to be a problem for the foreseeable future. Many leaders in the field have advocated for more LDLT, especially for the pediatric population [60]. Xenotransplantation, engineered tissues suitable for transplant, and liver replacement devices are other avenues which are being actively investigated.

As liver transplant outcomes continue to improve, patients are living longer, and we are now seeing many of the long-term complications associated with immunosuppression. This includes the metabolic diseases secondary to the drugs themselves, as well as de novo cancers. As a result, the aforementioned strategies to reduce or eliminate immunosuppression will continue to be studied exhaustively. There will also be more tolerance induction programs, utilizing more robust induction protocols.

Liver transplantation and transplantation as a whole have been one of the most remarkable therapeutic advances in the past century. Many giants of the field were acknowledged above, but we must also remember the countless patients and their families whom we will never be able to name and how their willingness to sacrifice at a time of desperation contributed just as much to the endeavor.

References

1. Gondolesi GE, Mazariegos G, Starzl TE. Thomas Starzl, Video Interview for his living legend award at the ISBTS 2015. Transplant Proc. 2016;48(2):444–9.
2. Lehmann K, Clavien P-A. History of hepatic surgery. Surg Clin North Am. 2010 Aug;90(4):655–64.
3. Hardy KJ. Liver surgery: the past 2000 years. Aust N Z J Surg. 1990;60(10):811–7.
4. Papalois VE, Hakim NS, Najarian JS. The history of kidney transplantation. In: The history of cell and organ transplantation. London: Imperial College Press; 2003. p. 76–99.
5. Reemtsma K. Xenotransplantation: a historical perspective. ILAR J. 1995;37(1):9–12.
6. Carrel A. Results of the transplantation of blood vessels, organs, and limbs. J Am Med Assoc. 1908;51:1662–7.
7. Busuttil RW, De Carlis LG, Mihaylov PV, Gridelli B, Fassati LR, Starzl TE. The first report of orthotopic liver transplantation in the Western world. Am J Transplant. 2012;12(6):1385–7.
8. Vilarinho S, Lifton RP. Liver transplantation: from inception to clinical practice. Cell. 2012;150(6):1096–9.
9. Welch C. A note on transplantation of the whole liver in dogs. Transplant Bull. 1955;2(54):54–5.
10. Cannon J. Brief report. Transplant Bull. 1956;3:7.
11. Moore FD, Smith LL, Burnap TK, Ballenbach FD, Dammin GJ, Gruber UF, et al. One-stage homotransplantation of the liver following total hepatectomy in dogs. Transplant Bull. 1959;6(1):103–7.
12. Moore FD, Wheele HB, Demissianos HV, Smith LL, Balankura O, Abel K, et al. Experimental whole-organ transplantation of the liver and of the spleen. Ann Surg. 1960;152:374–87.
13. Hurst J. A modern Cosmas and Damian: Sir Roy Calne and Thomas Starzl receive the 2012 Lasker~ Debakey Clinical Medical Research Award. J Clin Invest. 2012;122(10):3378.
14. Starzl TE. The long reach of liver transplantation. Nat Med. 2012;18(10):1489–92.
15. Starzl TE. The saga of liver replacement, with particular reference to the reciprocal influence of liver and kidney transplantation (1955–1967). J Am Coll Surg. 2002;195(5):587–610.
16. Starlz TE, Kaupp HAJ, Brock DR, Lazarus RE, Johnson RV. Reconstructive problems in canine liver homotransplantation with special reference to the postoperative role of hepatic venous flow. Surg Gynecol Obstet. 1960;111:733–43.
17. Calne RY. Early days of liver transplantation. Am J Transplant. 2008;8(9):1775–8.
18. Calne RY. The history of liver transplantation. In: The history of organ and cell transplantation. London: Imperial College Press; 2003. p. 100–19.
19. Calne RY. It can't be done. Nat Med. 2012;18(10):1493–5.
20. Groth CG. Forty years of liver transplantation: personal recollections. Transplant Proc. 2008;40(4):1127–9.
21. Starzl TE, Marchioro TL, Vonkaulla KN, Hermann G, Brittain RS, Waddell WR. Homotransplantation of the liver in humans. Surg Gynecol Obstet. 1963;117:659–76.

22. Eiseman B. The puzzle people: memoirs of a transplant surgeon. Arch Surg Chic Ill 1960. 1992;127(9):1009–11.

23. Otte JB. History of pediatric liver transplantation. Where are we coming from? Where do we stand? Pediatr Transplant. 2002;6(5):378–87.

24. Starzl TE, Marchioro TL, Faris TD, McCardle RJ, Iwaski Y. Avenues of future research in homotransplantation of the liver with particular reference to hepatic supportive procedures, antilymphocyte serum, and tissue typing. Am J Surg. 1966;112(3):391–400.

25. Starzl TE, Groth CG, Brettschneider L, Penn I, Fulginiti VA, Moon JB, et al. Orthotopic homotransplantation of the human liver. Ann Surg. 1968;168(3):392.

26. Maggi U, Azoulay D. Further details From the first human liver transplantation in Europe. Transplant J. 2013;96(6):e47–8.

27. The tenth report of the Human Renal Transplant Registry, Advisory Committee to the Renal Transplant Registry. JAMA 1972;221:1495–501.

28. Starzl TE, Iwatsuki S, Van Thiel DH, Gartner JC, Zitelli BJ, Malatack JJ, et al. Evolution of liver transplantation. Hepatol Baltim Md. 1982;2(5):614–36.

29. Kootstra G. The history of organ donation and sharing. In: The history of organ and cell transplantation. London: Imperial College Press; 2003. p. 55–63.

30. Gordon R, Iwatsuki S, Tzakis AG, Esquivel CO, Todo S, Makowka L, et al. The Denver-Pittsburgh liver transplant series. Clin Transpl. 1987;43–9.

31. Strong RW. Obstacles to the establishment of liver transplantation in Australia. J Gastroenterol Hepatol. 2009;24:S119–23.

32. Esquivel CO, Koneru B, Karrer F, Todo S, Iwatsuki S, Gordon RD, et al. Liver transplantation before 1 year of age. J Pediatr. 1987;110(4):545–8.

33. Esquivel CO, Iwatsuki S, Gordon RD, Marsh WW, Koneru B, Makowka L, et al. Indications for pediatric liver transplantation. J Pediatr. 1987;111(6):1039–45.

34. Jamieson NV, Sundberg R, Lindell S, Claesson K, Moen J, Vreugdenhil PK, et al. Preservation of the canine liver for 24–48 hours using simple cold storage with UW solution. Transplantation. 1988;46(4):517–22.

35. Sass DA, Doyle AM. Liver and kidney transplantation. Med Clin North Am. 2016;100(3):435–48.

36. Starzl TE, Todo S, Tzakis AG, Gordon RD, Makowka L, Stieber A, et al. Liver transplantation: an unfinished product. In: Transplantation proceedings [Internet]. NIH Public Access; 1989 [cited 2017 Jun 7]. p. 2197. Available from: https://www.ncbi.nlm. nih.gov/pmc/articles/PMC2950325/.

37. Raia S, Nery JR, Mies S. Liver transplantation from live donors. Lancet Lond Engl. 1989;2(8661):497.

38. He VJ. Professor Henri Bismuth: the past, present and future of hepatobiliary surgery. Hepatobiliary Surg Nutr. 2013;2(4):236–8.

39. Lo C-M. Deceased donation in Asia: challenges and opportunities. Liver Transpl. 2012;18(S2):S5–7.

40. Ng KK, Lo CM. Liver transplantation in Asia: past, present and future. Ann Acad Med Singap. 2009;38(4):322–31.

41. Song ATW. Liver transplantation: fifty years of experience. World J Gastroenterol. 2014;20(18):5363.

42. Thuluvath PJ, Guidinger MK, Fung JJ, Johnson LB, Rayhill SC, Pelletier SJ. Liver transplantation in the United States, 1999–2008. Am J Transplant. 2010;10(4p2):1003–19.

43. Gans H. Development of modern liver surgery. Lancet Lond Engl. 2002;360(9335):805.

44. Bismuth H, Houssin D. Reduced-sized orthotopic liver graft in hepatic transplantation in children. Surgery. 1984;95(3):367–70.

45. Strong RW, Lynch SV, Ong TH, Matsunami H, Koido Y, Balderson GA. Successful liver transplantation from a living donor to her son. N Engl J Med. 1990;322(21):1505–7.

46. Hashikura Y, Makuuchi M, Kawasaki S, Matsunami H, Ikegami T, Nakazawa Y, et al. Successful living-related partial liver transplantation to an adult patient. Lancet Lond Engl. 1994;343(8907):1233–4.

47. Yamaoka Y, Washida M, Honda K, Tanaka K, Mori K, Shimahara Y, et al. Liver transplantation using a right lobe graft from a living related donor. Transplantation. 1994;57(7):1127–30.

48. Lo C-M, Fan S-T, Liu C-L, Wei WI, Lo RJ, Lai C-L, et al. Adult-to-adult living donor liver transplantation using extended right lobe grafts. Ann Surg. 1997;226(3):261.

49. Northup PG, Berg CL. Living donor liver transplantation: the historical and cultural basis of policy decisions and ongoing ethical questions. Health Policy. 2005;72(2):175–85.

50. Chan SC, Fan ST, Lo CM, Liu CL, Wong J. Toward current standards of donor right hepatectomy for adult-to-adult live donor liver transplantation through the experience of 200 cases. Ann Surg. 2007;245(1):110–7.

51. Ringe B, Xiao G, Sass DA, Karam J, Shang S, Maroney TP, et al. Rescue of a Living Donor with liver transplantation: transplantation of a living liver donor. Am J Transplant. 2008;8(7):1557–61.

52. Pichlmayr R, Ringe B, Gubernatis G, Hauss J, Bunzendahl H. Transplantation of a donor liver to 2 recipients (splitting transplantation)—a new method in the further development of segmental liver transplantation. Langenbecks Arch Chir. 1988;373(2):127–30.

53. Emond JC, Whitington PF, Thistlethwaite JR, Cherqui D, Alonso EA, Woodle IS, et al. Transplantation of two patients with one liver. Analysis of a preliminary experience with "split-liver" grafting. Ann Surg. 1990;212(1):14–22.

54. Rogiers X, Malagó M, Gawad K, Jauch KW, Olausson M, Knoefel WT, et al. In situ splitting of cadaveric livers. The ultimate expansion of a limited donor pool. Ann Surg. 1996;224(3):331.

55. Dienstag JL, Cosimi AB. Liver transplantation—a vision realized. N Engl J Med. 2012;367(16):1483–5.

56. Starzl TE, Todo S, Fung J, Demetris AJ, Venkataramman R, Jain A. FK 506 for liver, kidney, and pancreas transplantation. Lancet Lond Engl. 1989;2(8670):1000–4.

57. Fung JJ, Todo S, Tzakis A, Demetris A, Jain A, Abu-Elmaged K, et al. Conversion of liver allograft recipients from cyclosporine to FK 506-based immunosuppression: benefits and pitfalls. Transplant Proc. 1991;23(1 Pt 1):14–21.

58. Mazariegos GV, Reyes J, Marino I, Flynn B, Fung JJ, Starzl TE. Risks and benefits of weaning immunosuppression in liver transplant recipients: long-term follow-up. In: Transplantation proceedings [Internet]. Elsevier; 1997 [cited 2017 May 26]. p. 1174–1177. Available from: http://www.sciencedirect.com/science/article/pii/S0041134596005350.

59. Dutkowski P, De Rougemont O, Müllhaupt B, Clavien P. Current and future trends in liver transplantation in Europe. Gastroenterology. 2010;138(3):802–809.e4.

60. Pham TA, Enns GM, Esquivel CO. Living donor liver transplantation for inborn errors of—an underutilized resource in the United States. Pediatr Transplant. 2016;20(6):770–3.

Medical Course and Complications After Liver Transplantation

14

Rajanshu Verma and Sanjaya K. Satapathy

Abbreviations

AASLD	American Association for the Study of Liver Diseases
ACEI	Angiotensin-converting enzyme inhibitor
ACR	Acute cellular rejection
AKI	Acute kidney injury
ARB	Angiotensin receptor blocker
AST	Aspartate aminotransferase
ATG	Antithymocyte globulin
BTA	Biliary tract abnormality.
CAUTI	Catheter-associated urinary tract infection.
CKD	Chronic kidney disease.
CLABSI	Central line-associated bloodstream infection.
CMV	Cytomegalovirus
CNI	Calcineurin inhibitor
CT	Computed tomography
DCD	Donation after cardiac death
DDLT	Deceased donor liver transplant
DEXA	Dual-energy X-ray absorptiometry
dTaP	Diphtheria, tetanus, acellular pertussis
EBV	Epstein-Barr virus
ENT	Ear, nose, throat
ERC	Endoscopic retrograde cholangiography
ERCP	Endoscopic retrograde cholangiopancreatography
ESRD	End-stage renal disease
HAT	Hepatic artery thrombosis
HbA1c	Hemoglobin A1c
HCV	Hepatitis C virus
HIV	Human immunodeficiency virus
HLA	Human leukocyte antigen
HPV	Human papillomavirus
HRQoL	Health-related quality of life
ICU	Intensive care unit
IL-2	Interleukin-2
INR	International normalized ratio
IVC	Inferior vena cava
LDL	Low-density lipoprotein
LDLT	Living donor liver transplant
LT	Liver transplant
MHC	Major histocompatibility complex
MRCP	Magnetic resonance cholangiopancreatography
MRI	Magnetic resonance imaging
mTOR	Mammalian target of rapamycin
NASH	Nonalcoholic steatohepatitis
NNRTI	Non-nucleoside reverse transcriptase inhibitors
PCV13	Pneumococcal conjugate vaccine 13
PJP	*Pneumocystis jirovecii* pneumonia
PNF	Primary Nonfunction
PPSV23	Pneumococcal polysaccharide vaccine 23
PTC	Percutaneous transhepatic cholangiography
PTLD	Post-transplant lymphoproliferative disorder
PVT	Portal vein thrombosis
SFSS	Small-for-size syndrome
SPF	Sun protection factor
TB	Tuberculosis
TIPS	Transjugular intrahepatic portosystemic shunt
UTI	Urinary tract infection
VAP	Ventilator-associated pneumonia

R. Verma
Division of Transplantation, Methodist University Hospital
Transplant Institute/University of Tennessee Health Sciences
Center, Memphis, TN, USA

S. K. Satapathy (✉)
Division of Transplantation, Methodist University Hospital
Transplant Institute/University of Tennessee Health Sciences
Center, Memphis, TN, USA
e-mail: ssatapat@uthsc.edu

© Springer International Publishing AG, part of Springer Nature 2019
Y. Sher, J. R. Maldonado (eds.), *Psychosocial Care of End-Stage Organ Disease and Transplant Patients*,
https://doi.org/10.1007/978-3-319-94914-7_14

Introduction

Liver transplantation outcomes have come a long way since the first successful transplant took place in the 1960s when 1-year survival was under 30% and 5-year survival was nonexistent [1]. Due to advancement in development of surgical techniques, proper selection of liver donor, availability of better preservative solutions, and more effective immunosuppressive agents, modern post-liver 1-year and 5-year transplant survival rates are above 90% and 75% (except in those transplanted for hepatocellular carcinoma), respectively [2]. However, this improvement in post-transplant longevity comes at a cost of a myriad of complications owing to early or late surgical complications, prolonged use of immunosuppressive agents, and their untoward side effects such as metabolic syndrome, opportunistic infections, de novo malignancies, and others. In addition, there is an ever-looming risk of allograft rejection either due to patient's nonadherence with immunosuppressive treatment or its premature cessation by an overzealous physician.

Medical Course and Recovery from Liver Transplantation

Liver transplant (LT) surgery is a major abdominal surgery where a complete liver (from deceased donor) or partial liver (from living donor) is harvested and transplanted in to a recipient. Surgery may be performed in two fashions: bicaval or piggyback (where IVC is left intact) technique. In former, allograft is anastomosed with recipient's suprahepatic IVC, infrahepatic IVC, portal vein, and hepatic artery and common bile duct; whereas latter involves ligating perforating veins from donor's right lobe to recipient's IVC [3]. LT typically requires a patient to have a short ICU stay post-transplantation when he/she may be endotracheally intubated, be mechanically ventilated, and require vasopressors for hemodynamic support. Theoretically, piggyback technique has lower odds of causing hemodynamic instability as blood flow through IVC is unperturbed. Average length of ICU stay after LT barring any complications is 1–3 days. Immediate signs of a successful liver transplant include correction of acidosis and coagulopathy, and normal bile production by the allograft. These signs are usually evident to the surgeon on the operating table itself. Like any major abdominal surgery, some of the complications that may be encountered during LT include bleeding and hemorrhage, fluid overload, cardiovascular instability, arrhythmias, abdominal compartment syndrome, acute tubular necrosis, pulmonary edema, and postoperative pneumonia [4]. Patients are started on induction immunosuppression therapy during surgery and are monitored for any related complications during their hospital stay.

The patient is typically transferred from ICU to a monitored medical bed after stabilization where he/she may spend another 4–7 days provided no untoward complications develop during the clinical course. Explanted liver is typically examined by a pathologist to provide histologic confirmation of patient's underlying illness and to look for incidental foci of hepatocellular carcinoma which may change post-LT management. In addition to checking basic serum chemistries such as electrolytes, renal function, liver profile, and coagulation profile, transplanted liver is imaged with a Doppler ultrasound to assess its echogenicity, portal vein patency, and presence of ascites and evaluated for any evidence of hepatic artery thrombosis.

Though every transplant center has a different protocol, it is quite common for patients to be very closely involved with their transplant surgeons and transplant hepatologists for the first year, after which primary care physician usually partakes in management of chronic metabolic complications and scheduling appropriate cancer screenings.

Immediate Surgical Complications

Small for Size Syndrome

Small-for-size syndrome (SFSS) is a complication which is by and large unique to living donor liver transplant recipients or where partial or split liver transplantation is performed. In this case, if allograft weighs less than 0.8% of recipient's body weight or is less than 40% the standard liver volume, it runs the risk of allograft dysfunction/nonfunction within first week of transplant [5]. SFSS is more of a diagnosis of exclusion where acute rejection and vascular, biliary, or infectious complications are either absent or unable to explain newly transplanted graft's dysfunction. It is hypothesized that hyperperfusion of a small graft from pre-existing portal hypertension and splenomegaly in recipient causes severe endothelial injury leading to new graft's dysfunction [6]. Clinically, it presents in the form of ascites, coagulopathy, hyperbilirubinemia, and encephalopathy. Since portal hyperperfusion is thought to be central to the pathogenesis of SFSS, the most popular strategies for prevention have focused on modulating inflow to the liver via inputs to the portal system. Surgical techniques, such as splenic artery ligation, splenectomy, creation of portocaval shunts, and preserving pre-existing collateral veins, help redirect blood flow coming toward the graft, thus helping to minimize the risk of developing SFSS [7–9]. Terlipressin has also been used in this setting to reduce portal venous flow and thus lower portal pressure in these patients [10].

Primary Graft Nonfunction

Primary allograft nonfunction (PNF) is one of the most serious, life-threatening complications in the immediate postoperative period where transplant surgeon notices lack of bile production by the allograft during the surgery. PNF is a true surgical emergency and requires immediate re-listing of the patient (status 1A) for a second liver transplant while hemodynamically supporting the patient. It is characterized by elevation of liver enzymes (AST > 3000 U/L), hepatic encephalopathy, severe acidosis, elevated INR and lactic acid, profound hypotension, hypothermia, and multi-organ failure requiring intensive care admission and monitoring. Fortunately, this complication is rare and occurs in 2–4% of liver transplants [11]. Precise mechanism behind the cause of PNF is not fully known; however, advanced donor age, graft from a female donor, hypernatremia, prolonged cold ischemia time, and higher percentage of hepatic macrovesicular steatosis in donor have all been identified as risk factors for PNF [11, 12].

Hepatic Artery Thrombosis

Hepatic artery thrombosis (HAT) is similar to acute cellular rejection in its timing: it can present in the immediate postsurgical period or may present several months to years after liver transplant. It is one of the dreaded surgical complications when it occurs in the immediate post-transplant period (<7 days). Akin to PNF, it requires re-listing of the patient for re-transplant (status 1A), especially if thrombolysis, stenting or repeat surgery, and anastomosis are not an option or have failed to salvage the allograft. HAT usually has a propensity to occur at the site of anastomosis of donor and recipient hepatic artery [13]. The injury gets compounded if there is a pre-existing or concurrent portal vein thrombosis. HAT is characterized by severe transaminitis occurring from focal allograft ischemia and/or infarction. On the other hand, late HAT may be quite asymptomatic and might be detected as an incidental radiographic finding. Other presentations of HAT include delayed bile leak, cholangitis, bacteremia, biloma/liver abscess formation, and biliary cast syndrome [14, 15]. HAT is diagnosed with a liver ultrasound with arterial Doppler or MRI, though angiogram may be necessary for confirmation. Late HAT (occurring after 4 weeks) is treated with stenting, focal liver resection, or biliary drainage depending on its presentation. HAT is seen in up to 10% of adult recipients and is associated with low donor weight in addition to technical surgical risk factors, such as higher number of anastomoses, anomalous anatomy, and use of bypass grafts [16]. The use of aortohepatic conduit may be a novel surgical approach to avoid artery-to-artery anastomosis and resulting HAT in patients with unsuitable hepatic artery anatomy [17].

Portal Vein Thrombosis

Earlier, portal vein thrombosis (PVT) used to be considered a contraindication for liver transplant. However, with advancement in surgical techniques (e.g., venous jump graft, using portal vein tributaries, thrombectomy), PVT is no longer considered an absolute contraindication [18]. PVT may either present with transaminitis or signs/symptoms of portal hypertension such as ascites, variceal bleeding, or both. Liver Doppler, CT abdomen, and MR venogram are modalities of choice for its diagnosis. It is seen in up to 8% of liver transplant surgeries and is associated with risk factors such as advanced age, underlying malignancy, TIPS, male gender, Child-Turcotte-Pugh class C cirrhosis, and alcoholic liver disease [18]. PVT may be treated with anticoagulation, catheter-directed thrombolysis, or surgical thrombectomy.

Late Surgical Complications

Hepatic Vein Stenosis

Hepatic vein stenosis is characterized by a pressure difference of greater than 10 mm Hg between hepatic vein and IVC and is usually seen several months after liver transplantation [19]. It is more common in patients who undergo living donor liver transplantation and may present with symptoms of portal hypertension in addition to deranged liver enzymes and pedal edema. It is a rare condition which occurs in less than 5% of post-transplant patients [19]. Diagnosis can be made with the help of Doppler ultrasound, MRI, CT abdomen, or venography. Treatment involves hepatic vein stenting or balloon angioplasty [20].

Biliary Tract Abnormalities

Biliary tract abnormalities (BTA) are quite common following liver transplantation and as many as one-third of the patients may develop them. In descending order of their frequency, BTA may include biliary strictures, biliary leaks, bile duct stones, biloma/abscess, and biliary cast formation. Though BTA (especially biliary leaks) can occur fairly early following transplant (<4 weeks), majority of BTA occur after the first month, but within 6 months of liver transplantation.

Early biliary strictures are largely due to surgical technical issues, such as difference in size of donor and recipient bile ducts, ABO incompatibility, prolonged cold ischemia time, acute HAT, and Roux-en-Y anastomosis, whereas late (>4 weeks) biliary strictures are usually the result of ischemia, abnormal healing, and fibrosis [21]. Widespread use of T-tubes during liver transplantation in earlier decades contributed significantly to development of a multitude of biliary complications in the postoperative period [22]. In general, biliary complications are somewhat more common and harder to manage in patients who undergo Roux-en-Y choledochojejunostomy than in patients with choledocho-choledochostomy due to the ease of access to the biliary tree via ERCP in latter. LT recipients with early anastomotic biliary strictures have inferior graft survival despite better response to endoscopic interventions [23]. The incidence of biliary complications (leaks or strictures) is twice in case of LDLT (60%) as compared to DDLT (30%), which is due to the fact that in former, leaks can occur from exposed hepatic parenchyma in addition to anastomoses [24]. Initial diagnostic modality in detecting a biliary stricture is an abdominal Doppler ultrasound; however, MRCP is usually the best noninvasive diagnostic test for detecting BTA owing to its higher specificity. It is a very reliable tool for ruling in or ruling out anastomotic as well as non-anastomotic strictures in post-LT patients [25, 26]. Biliary strictures may present with deranged liver enzymes and right upper quadrant abdominal pain. Biliary strictures are divided into anastomotic (those occurring at the junction of donor and recipient bile duct), non-anastomotic (occurring proximal or distal to donor/recipient junction), and diffuse biliary strictures.

Treatment of biliary strictures revolves around endoscopic retrograde cholangiography (ERC) in patients with choledochocholedostomy and double balloon endoscopy or PTC-based interventions in patients with choledochojejunostomy. Dilation, stenting, biliary sphincterotomy, conversion from choledochocholedochostomy to choledochojejunostomy or revision of the latter, or a combination of all of above may be required to treat a non-responding lesion depending on the clinical scenario [27, 28]. A combination algorithm comprising of hepatobiliary scan, peak aspartate transaminase, and peak total bilirubin values in immediate post-transplant patients with hepatocellular/cholestatic dysfunction has been shown to help identify patients in whom ERC may not be necessary [29]. Strictures have a tendency to recur, and so long-term monitoring is required in patients who have previously been treated for biliary strictures. Most patients require multiple ERC-guided (dilation/stenting) procedures over a course of year or two to guarantee a high rate of stricture resolution [28, 30]. A recent study showed that implantation of fully covered self-expanding metallic stents was more effective than repeated balloon dilatation of anastomotic strictures with subsequent plastic biliary stent placement, while both approaches had similar complication rates [31]. However, even though shorter treatment times and fewer ERCP procedures support the use of self-expanding metal stents, whether one technique has well-defined advantages over the other remains to be seen [32].

Non-anastomotic strictures tend to occur earlier than anastomotic strictures and are harder to treat [33]. They may not be amenable to ERC intervention alone and may progress to cause bacterial cholangitis and unremitting fibrosis requiring surgical intervention or re-transplantation. Non-anastomotic strictures may be seen in up to 10% of post-LT patients [33]. Diffuse biliary strictures are a result of ischemia and are seen in the setting of hepatic artery thrombosis, prolonged cold ischemia time, and DCD allograft donation. Given the long extent and diffuse nature of these strictures, endoscopic intervention is usually ineffective, and they require hepatic resection or re-transplantation to address the issue [34].

Biliary leaks are known risk factors for early as well as late strictures [28, 35]. Similar to bile duct strictures, biliary leaks also are divided into early and late subtypes. Early bile leak (after transplant) is usually due to technical surgical reasons. As bile is a peritoneal irritant, patients may present with symptoms of peritonitis, abdominal pain, or biliary ascites. Best diagnostic modality for detection of a bile leak is an ERC. Incidence of anastomotic bile leaks is estimated to be <10% [36]. Treatment involves endoscopic placement of a biliary stent with optional biliary sphincterotomy. Late bile leaks are associated with the use of T-tubes and are treated with papillary stenting via ERC [37]. Surgical exploration is necessary when endoscopic intervention fails.

Biloma or sterile collection of bile and hepatic abscesses in post-transplant state occur in the setting of ischemia (e.g., HAT) and require percutaneous drainage and treatment with antibiotics. Surgery may be required if nonsurgical approach fails to address the issue.

Biliary cast formation is an aftermath of allograft ischemia as well and may be precipitated by HAT or hepatic artery stenosis. Biliary casts may mimic symptoms of ascending cholangitis and can be challenging to treat. Joint collaboration of endoscopy, intervention radiology, and surgical teams may be required to manage biliary cast syndrome.

Bile stones and sludge are late complications of liver transplant and can be seen in up to 10% of patients [28]. Usually ERCP with biliary sphincterotomy is curative.

Immediate Medical Complications

Acute Immunosuppressive Induction Issues

Induction therapy with high-dose immunosuppressive agents begins right at the time of liver transplant surgery. High-dose corticosteroids, tacrolimus, antithymocyte globulin, and basiliximab are most commonly used induction agents [38, 39]. Steroids inhibit inflammation by multiple mechanisms, including decreased migration of neutrophils, decreased tissue accumulation and activation of macrophages, decreased production of interleukins (IL-1, IL-2, IL-6), and decreased transcription of proinflammatory genes [40, 41]. High-dose corticosteroids cause profound hyperglycemia which requires the use of intravenous insulin infusion for blood sugar control. High-dose steroids may also result in insomnia, delirium, psychosis, azotemia, and infections in the immediate post-transplant period. Tacrolimus is used with or without azathioprine for induction to minimize adverse effects associated with steroids. High-dose CNI is responsible for development of AKI in these patients [42]. Selective or nonselective T-cell-depleting agents (ATG or basiliximab) may be used to avoid side effects associated with high-dose steroids and CNIs. Some centers have adopted a steroid-free protocol with rabbit antithymocyte globulin induction demonstrating excellent outcomes, low complication rates, and preservation of renal function [43]. The use of these agents also lowers risk of development of CMV infection; however, infusion reactions have been reported with intravenous administration of ATG [44]. There is recent evidence to suggest that induction immunosuppression regimen may be customized to include mTOR inhibitors along with very low-dose CNI in patients who are at high risk of developing renal failure post-LT [45].

Acute Cellular Rejection

Acute cellular rejection (ACR) is a histologic diagnosis and is graded mild [4, 5], moderate [6, 7], or severe [8, 9] rejection based on Banff scoring system (maximum score 9) which is based on portal inflammation involving small lymphocytes/eosinophils, biliary ductulitis, and hepatic/portal venule endotheliitis [46, 47]. ACR can occur as early as <4 weeks (early ACR) after transplantation or as late as years after LT (late ACR). ACR occurs in 16.5–26.9% of liver transplant recipients [48]. Treatment of ACR usually involves giving high dose of pulsed steroids, if rejection is severe, or increasing existing immunosuppression for mild to moderate rejection. Patients who do not respond to corticosteroids may need to be treated with T-cell depleting agents (e.g., anti-T-cell antibodies) to salvage the allograft [49]. Risk factors for ACR include unmonitored interaction of or inadvertent intake of P-450 enzyme inducer (e.g., antiepileptic drugs, rifampin/rifabutin, NNRTI) which can lower efficacy of immunosuppressive agents, patient's nonadherence with immunosuppressive treatment, or its premature cessation by a physician.

Late Medical Complications

Chronic Allograft Rejection

The word "chronic" in chronic allograft rejection or chronic ductopenic rejection (also known as arteriopathic rejection based on pathognomonic foam cell obliterative arteriopathy seen in biopsy specimens) is a misnomer as "chronic rejection" may be seen <4 weeks of LT, though typically it presents >4 weeks after LT [50]. Chronic rejection is characterized by atrophy and loss of bile ducts along with obliterative arteriopathy and fibrosis in portal tracts [50]. Risk factors associated with chronic rejection include non-Caucasian race, recurrent ACR, CMV, HCV infection, and HLA/MHC donor/recipient mismatch. Treatment of this condition is challenging and may not respond to mere increase in dose of immunosuppressants [49]. Re-transplantation may be required in recalcitrant cases.

Late Complications from Use of Immunosuppressive Agents

Even though a liver allograft, unlike other solid-organ transplants, is less immunogenic, it still requires high-dose immunosuppression for at least first 6 months, after which intensity of immunosuppression may be lightened. Although theoretically it is possible for LT patients to completely come off of immunosuppression, a large majority of patients continue to require long-term immunosuppression to keep rejection at bay [51, 52]. As a result, patients tend to develop late complications (e.g., metabolic syndrome, bone density loss, de novo cancers, opportunistic infections, and others) from accruing adverse effects of chronic exposure to immunosuppressive drugs [51]. The goal of immunosuppression in post-LT care is to strike a fine balance between maintaining adequate allograft function while minimizing long-term toxicities of antirejection medications.

Immunosuppressive agents are used in LT during induction and maintenance and for treatment of rejection. Some of the commonly used classes of drugs include corticosteroids, CNIs (tacrolimus and cyclosporine), nucleotide synthesis inhibitors (azathioprine, mycophenolate mofetil, mycophenolic acid), mTOR inhibitors (sirolimus, everolimus), monoclonal antibody against IL-2 receptor (basiliximab), antithymocyte globulin, and costimulation blockers (belatacept) [38].

Diabetes Mellitus

Both corticosteroids and CNIs (especially tacrolimus) are diabetogenic and cause hyperglycemia and insulin resistance [53]. More and more centers are now using protocols which involve rapid tapering of corticosteroids which minimizes the risk of hyperglycemia and development of de novo diabetes in allograft recipients [43, 54]. Patients should be routinely monitored with fasting blood glucose and Hba1c monitoring, while they are on these immunosuppressive agents. Target goal for Hba1c in post-LT patients is ≤7%

[46]. Switching patients from tacrolimus to cyclosporine for better glycemic control is an acceptable practice [46]. The use of insulin to control hyperglycemia is the best approach during induction phase and when they are undergoing treatment for rejection [46, 55]. Diabetes has independently been shown to reduce survival in post-LT recipients [56].

Hypertension

Up to two-thirds of the patients develop hypertension after liver transplantation [57]. Corticosteroids as well as CNIs, especially cyclosporine, have been implicated in raising blood pressure. Patient should be advised to do self-monitoring of blood pressure at home every week and get blood pressure checked every month at a provider's office. Target goal for blood pressure in post-LT patients is 130/80 mmHg [46, 57]. Choice of antihypertensive agent should be based on drug's adverse effect profile, patient's pre-existing comorbidities, and interactions with other medications. However, dihydropyridine calcium channel blockers (i.e., felodipine, nicardipine, amlodipine) and cardioselective beta-blockers (e.g., metoprolol) are the recommended agents to counter CNI-associated vasoconstriction of afferent renal arteriole. ACEI/ARB are drugs of choice in patients with concurrent diabetes, proteinuria, or CKD stage 3 [46].

Dyslipidemia

Corticosteroids, CNIs, and mTOR inhibitors all have been associated with development of dyslipidemia in post-transplant patients. There is some emerging evidence that use of mycophenolate mofetil might help lower the risk of late cardiovascular morbidities and mortality in post-LT patients [58]. Patients with isolated hypertriglyceridemia may be given a trial of omega-3 fatty acids. Patients with an elevated LDL (>100 mg/dl) with or without hypertriglyceridemia should be treated with statins along with lifestyle modifications [46, 57]. Statin-intolerant patients may be treated with ezetimibe [46]. A strategy to follow up on lipid profile every 3–6 months should be adopted while emphasizing the importance of healthy eating and exercise.

Obesity

Though majority of patients with liver disease are malnourished due to impaired hepatic function, interestingly, obesity is not uncommon in post-LT patients [57]. This can be attributed to adverse effects of immunosuppressive agents (steroids, CNIs), return of appetite due to improvement in the sense of general well-being, and nonadherence to lifestyle modification practices. Morbid obesity is associated with a lower rate of survival in post-LT patients [59]. Much akin to the general population, it is imperative to emphasize the importance of healthy eating and regular exercise in post-LT patients. In patients who are obese to begin with, use of weight loss surgeries such as sleeve gastrectomy or adjustable gastric lap band at the time of transplantation is a reasonable option to avoid compounding the problem with adverse effects of immunosuppressants in the post-transplant period [60]. Bariatric surgery after LT remains a technically challenging procedure and has been often performed directly using an open approach [60]. The place of laparoscopy for these patients remains debatable, with few studies reporting its use in selected patients [60], although a recent study has shown potential feasibility with single-port sleeve gastrectomy [60].

Osteopenia and Osteoporosis

Bone density loss is a known side effect of long-term corticosteroid use. CNIs add to this problem as well. As per AASLD guidelines, starting 5 years after transplant, DEXA screening for osteoporosis should be done on an annual basis in osteopenic patients and every 2–3 years in patients with normal bone density [46]. Patients who undergo liver transplant for chronic cholestatic reasons (e.g., primary biliary cholangitis) are at even higher risk of bone loss given their pre-existing osteopenic state [61]. As about 25% of patients undergoing LT for chronic cholestatic liver disease develop de novo fractures post-LT, this situation warrants an ongoing search for more effective therapeutic agents for these patients [62]. Treatment of metabolic bone disease includes regular intake of calcium and vitamin D and participation in weight-bearing exercises [46]. Bisphosphonates are used to treat osteoporosis like in general population [46].

Worsening of Pre-existing CKD or Development of De Novo CKD

CKD has become one of the leading causes of morbidity and mortality after liver transplantation [63, 64]. Although CNI toxicity is typically considered a major contributor, other risk factors for CKD include perioperative acute kidney injury, diabetes mellitus, hypertension, and chronic hepatitis C infection [65–67]. Additionally, there is increasing knowledge of the association between HCV infection and glomerular disease in both native kidneys and after kidney or liver transplantation [68]. There is 8% incidence of CKD 1-year post-LT and incidence goes up to 18% at 5 years after LT [69]. Patients who are at highest risk of development of CKD should be treated with non-CNI-based immunosuppression

[69, 70]. Discontinuation of CNI and its replacement with either mycophenolate mofetil or sirolimus have shown to result in significant improvement in renal function even in patients with severe CKD [71]. Development of ESRD in post-LT patients decreases their survival, and renal transplant should be considered in these patients to improve survival [46].

Fertility, Sexuality, and Pregnancy

Fortunately, many women of reproductive age group regain their ovulation and menstruation as early as 4–6 weeks after LT [46]. On the other hand, however, men who had impotence prior to LT usually do not notice any improvement despite a "new" liver [72]. Mycophenolate mofetil, mycophenolic acid, and mTOR inhibitors due to their teratogenic potential are contraindicated in pregnant women and nursing mothers. Steroids, CNIs, and azathioprine are safer alternatives in post-LT women contemplating pregnancy [73]. In general, it is advisable to avoid pregnancy until allograft function and immunosuppression regimes are stable and it has been 1 year since LT [46]. These women should coordinate their prenatal and pregnancy care in conjunction with a high-risk obstetrician who is an expert in maternal-fetal medicine and their transplant hepatologist [46]. Sildenafil and other phosphodiesterase inhibitors are acceptable treatment options for erectile dysfunction in post-LT men.

Fatigue and Quality of Life of a Transplant Recipient

Though LT significantly improves quality of life of patients afflicted with chronic liver disease [74, 75], fatigue, unfortunately, is a significant yet unremitting symptom which impairs health-related quality of life (HRQoL) of post-LT patients [76]. Most LT recipients have other chronic comorbidities which contribute to persistence of fatigue despite LT. Use of modafinil, structured exercise program, improved nutrition, and sleep hygiene help mitigate the disabling effects of fatigue on the lifestyle of transplant recipients [77].

Development of De Novo Malignancies

Immunosuppressive agents increase the risk of development of new malignancies in post-LT patients. Thus, it is important for these patients to be up to date with their cancer screenings. Of all malignancies, development of non-melanoma skin cancer is the highest, and so patients should be advised to avoid prolonged sun exposure and use at least SPF 15 sunscreen when outdoors [46]. Use of wide-brim hats, long sleeve shirts, and pants reduces the incidence of development of skin cancers. Risk of melanoma is increased in this cohort as well [78]. A comprehensive annual skin exam by a dermatologist is in order for post-LT patients (who had LT > 5 yrs ago) for early detection and treatment of skin cancers [46].

Post-transplant lymphoproliferative disorder (PTLD) is a B-cell lymphoma seen in post-LT patients on immunosuppressants. It has been associated with use of muromonab for immunosuppression [79]. Symptoms of presentation might include fever, lymphadenopathy, weight loss, and pancytopenia. It is associated with EBV and requires treatment of EBV along with lightening the intensity of immunosuppression. Majority of PTLD develop within 1 year after transplant [79].

A fair share of post-LT patients has had tobacco and alcohol use disorders. This cohort of patients is at a very high risk of development of de novo head and neck cancers. Some centers recommend regular evaluation with an ENT physician in addition to low-dose annual chest CT for lung cancer screening.

Patients with primary sclerosing cholangitis and chronic ulcerative colitis are at heightened risk of development of colorectal carcinoma and so should undergo annual screening colonoscopy [46]. Rigorous cancer screening is of paramount importance in post-LT patients because due to their suppressed immune system, these patients tend to get advanced stage cancers that present at a younger age compared to general population.

Opportunistic Infections

Opportunistic infections are a major cause of morbidity and mortality in post-LT patients. In the immediate post-LT period, patients are at equal risk of contracting nosocomial infections (e.g., CAUTIs, CLABSIs, VAP, surgical site infections, clostridium difficile infection, infection with *Acinetobacter*, or pseudomonas in ICU) as the general population [4]. Standard precautions and infection prevention practices should be instituted to avoid these nosocomial infections. Any fever or symptoms of a simple urinary tract infection, sore throat, or cellulitis should be taken seriously and promptly evaluated in post-LT recipients as these patients have a tendency to quickly deteriorate and go in to septic shock with multi-organ failure.

First 6 months when the level of immunosuppression is highest is the most perilous times in terms of contracting opportunistic infections. Patients should avoid high-risk exposures (e.g., avoiding crowded places, exposure to soil, unpasteurized milk, travel to endemic countries) during this time [46].

Post-LT patients are started on trimethoprim-sulfamethoxazole for 6 months for prophylaxis against *Pneumocystis jirovecii* pneumonia (PJP). Those patients with concurrent HIV are placed on long-term PJP prophylaxis [46].

Invasive aspergillosis is frequently seen in immunosuppressed solid-organ transplant recipients. Treatment involves administration of a combination of voriconazole (azole) and caspofungin (echinocandin) for a minimum of 12 weeks. Other opportunistic fungal infections include *Candida* (*albicans, glabrata, krusei*), cryptococcosis, coccidioidomycosis, histoplasmosis, and blastomycosis. *Candida albicans*, cryptococcosis, and coccidioidomycosis are treated with fluconazole, whereas resistant *Candida* spp., histoplasmosis, and blastomycosis are treated with itraconazole for 4–6 weeks [46].

There is high incidence of CMV infection in post-transplant period. CMV has the potential to involve almost any organ and present with organ-specific symptoms; it commonly presents with fever and leukopenia. Risk is highest when CMV- recipient receives a CMV+ allograft. Valganciclovir (900 mg/day) is used for 6 months to treat CMV [46]. For recipients who already are CMV+, valganciclovir is used to treat resurgence of CMV for 3 months or till viremia subsides [46]. Successful treatment of CMV might require reducing the level of immunosuppression. Foscarnet is used in the event of ganciclovir/valganciclovir resistance.

It is prudent to identify patients with latent TB prior to LT and treat them with isoniazid for 9 months to minimize chances of development of active TB in post-transplant period.

Recurrence of Primary Disease

Metabolic diseases (e.g., alpha-1 antitrypsin deficiency, cystic fibrosis, hemochromatosis, tyrosinemia, Wilson's disease) and polycystic liver disease do not recur in the allograft. On the other hand, hepatitis (viral, autoimmune), cholestatic diseases, and NASH may recur in allograft posing management challenges and requiring a second transplant [80–82]. HCV recurrence occurs in almost all post-LT patients [49]. Management strategies to prevent or ameliorate the risk of development of recurrent autoimmune disease have recently been reviewed [83]. Some centers have adopted a dual immunosuppression protocol in LT recipients with autoimmune liver disease without corticosteroid maintenance and reported acceptable rates of survival and ACR without predisposing patients to the adverse effects of long-term steroid therapy [54]. For patients who undergo LT for HCC, mTOR inhibitors may be the immunosuppressants of choice as they are purported to have anti-oncogenic properties which might help to minimize the risk of HCC recurrence in these recipients. For first 5 years after transplant, patients should be screened with biannual AFP and liver ultrasound performed in tandem to detect HCC recurrence [46].

Immunization of LT Recipients

Live vaccines must be avoided in LT recipients [46]. It is recommended that all patients with LT should undergo vaccination against hepatitis B, hepatitis A, influenza, dTaP, HPV, varicella, and zoster prior to LT. Regarding pneumococcal vaccine, all adults who have previously received PCV13 vaccine should get PPSV23 vaccine 8 weeks later. On the other hand, adults who have received PPSV23 vaccination before should wait a year before receiving PCV13 vaccine [84]. Annual influenza vaccine and PPSV23 vaccine every 3–5 years are recommended in all post-LT patients [46].

Prognosis

Liver transplantation and its outcomes have seen some tremendous improvements in the last half century. It is the only definitive treatment for several hepatic diatheses. LT is curative in metabolic disorders affecting the liver. It adds several years to lives of patients with hepatocellular carcinoma who otherwise have a dismal prognosis. For patients with other chronic liver diseases, LT improves their quality of life [74]. Due to remarkable improvement in surgical techniques, improved immunosuppression, infection control, and donor/recipient selection, 1-year and 10-year post-transplant rates are above 90% and above 50%, respectively. As there remains a dearth of donors for LT as demand outstrips supply by manifold, all efforts should be made to increase public awareness on organ donation by working in collaboration with government and non-government organizations.

References

1. Starzl TE. History of liver and other splanchnic organ transplantation. In: Busuttil RW, Klintmalm GB, editors. Transplant liver. Philadelphia: W.B. Saunders; 1996. p. 3–22.
2. Kotlyar DS, Campbell MS, Reddy KR. Recurrence of diseases following orthotopic liver transplantation. Am J Gastroenterol. 2006;101(6):1370–8.
3. Ascher N. Liver transplantation. In: Townsend Jr CM, Beauchamp D, Evers M, Mattox KL, editors. Sabiston textbook of surgery. 20th ed. Philadelphia: Elsevier; 2017. p. 637–48.
4. Chung RT, Dienstag JL. Liver transplantation. In: Kasper D, Fauci A, Hauser S, Longo D, Jameson JL, Loscalzo J, editors. Harrison's principles of internal medicine. 19th ed. New York: McGraw-Hill Education; 2015.
5. Dahm F, Georgiev P, Clavien PA. Small-for-size syndrome after partial liver transplantation: definition, mechanisms of disease and clinical implications. Am J Transplant. 2005;5(11):2605–10.

6. Man K, Fan ST, Lo CM, Liu CL, Fung PC, Liang TB, et al. Graft injury in relation to graft size in right lobe live donor liver transplantation: a study of hepatic sinusoidal injury in correlation with portal hemodynamics and intragraft gene expression. Ann Surg. 2003;237(2):256–64.

7. Kim SH, Lee EC, Park SJ. Impact of preserved collateral veins on small-for-size grafts in living donor liver transplantation. Hepatol Res. 2018;48(4):295–302.

8. Raut V, Alikhanov R, Belghiti J, Uemoto S. Review of the surgical approach to prevent small-for-size syndrome in recipients after left lobe adult LDLT. Surg Today. 2014;44(7):1189–96.

9. Goldaracena N, Echeverri J, Selzner M. Small-for-size syndrome in live donor liver transplantation-Pathways of injury and therapeutic strategies. Clin Transplant. 2017;31(2):e12885.

10. Mukhtar A, Salah M, Aboulfetouh F, Obayah G, Samy M, Hassanien A, et al. The use of terlipressin during living donor liver transplantation: effects on systemic and splanchnic hemodynamics and renal function. Crit Care Med. 2011;39(6):1329–34.

11. Uemura T, Randall HB, Sanchez EQ, Ikegami T, Narasimhan G, McKenna GJ, et al. Liver retransplantation for primary nonfunction: analysis of a 20-year single-center experience. Liver Transpl. 2007;13(2):227–33.

12. Kulik U, Lehner F, Klempnauer J, Borlak J. Primary non-function is frequently associated with fatty liver allografts and high mortality after re-transplantation. Liver Int. 2017;37(8):1219–28.

13. Herrero A, Souche R, Joly E, Boisset G, Habibeh H, Bouyabrine H, et al. Early hepatic artery thrombosis after liver transplantation: what is the impact of the arterial reconstruction type? World J Surg. 2017;41(8):2101–10.

14. Gunsar F, Rolando N, Pastacaldi S, Patch D, Raimondo ML, Davidson B, et al. Late hepatic artery thrombosis after orthotopic liver transplantation. Liver Transpl. 2003;9(6):605–11.

15. Tzakis AG, Gordon RD, Shaw BW Jr, Iwatsuki S, Starzl TE. Clinical presentation of hepatic artery thrombosis after liver transplantation in the cyclosporine era. Transplantation. 1985;40(6):667–71.

16. Mourad MM, Liossis C, Gunson BK, Mergental H, Isaac J, Muiesan P, et al. Etiology and management of hepatic artery thrombosis after adult liver transplantation. Liver Transpl. 2014;20(6):713–23.

17. Jung DH, Park CS, Ha TY, Song GW, Park GC, Cho YP, et al. Placement of an aortohepatic conduit as an alternative to standard arterial anastomosis in liver transplantation. Ann Transplant. 2018;23:61–5.

18. Yerdel MA, Gunson B, Mirza D, Karayalcin K, Olliff S, Buckels J, et al. Portal vein thrombosis in adults undergoing liver transplantation: risk factors, screening, management, and outcome. Transplantation. 2000;69(9):1873–81.

19. Ko EY, Kim TK, Kim PN, Kim AY, Ha HK, Lee MG. Hepatic vein stenosis after living donor liver transplantation: evaluation with Doppler US. Radiology. 2003;229(3):806–10.

20. Yeh YT, Chen CY, Tseng HS, Wang HK, Tsai HL, Lin NC, et al. Enlarging vascular stents after pediatric liver transplantation. J Pediatr Surg. 2017;52(12):1934–9.

21. Pascher A, Neuhaus P. Biliary complications after deceased-donor orthotopic liver transplantation. J Hepato-Biliary-Pancreat Surg. 2006;13(6):487–96.

22. Scatton O, Meunier B, Cherqui D, Boillot O, Sauvanet A, Boudjema K, et al. Randomized trial of choledochocholedochostomy with or without a T tube in orthotopic liver transplantation. Ann Surg. 2001;233(3):432–7.

23. Satapathy SK, Sheikh I, Ali B, et al. Long-term outcomes of early compared to late onset choledochocholedochal anastomotic strictures after orthotopic liver transplantation. Clin Transplant. 2017;31:e13003. https://doi.org/10.1111/ctr.13003.

24. Wojcicki M, Milkiewicz P, Silva M. Biliary tract complications after liver transplantation: a review. Dig Surg. 2008;25(4):245–57.

25. den Dulk AC, Wasser MN, Willemssen FE, Monraats MA, de Vries M, van den Boom R, et al. Value of magnetic resonance cholangiopancreatography in assessment of nonanastomotic biliary strictures after liver transplantation. Transplant Direct. 2015;1(10):e42.

26. Katz LH, Benjaminov O, Belinki A, Geler A, Braun M, Knizhnik M, et al. Magnetic resonance cholangiopancreatography for the accurate diagnosis of biliary complications after liver transplantation: comparison with endoscopic retrograde cholangiography and percutaneous transhepatic cholangiography – long-term follow-up. Clin Transpl. 2010;24(5):E163–9.

27. Ostroff JW. Management of biliary complications in the liver transplant patient. Gastroenterol Hepatol (N Y). 2010;6(4):264–72.

28. Rerknimitr R, Sherman S, Fogel EL, Kalayci C, Lumeng L, Chalasani N, et al. Biliary tract complications after orthotopic liver transplantation with choledochocholedochostomy anastomosis: endoscopic findings and results of therapy. Gastrointest Endosc. 2002;55(2):224–31.

29. Nair S, Lingala S, Satapathy SK, Eason JD, Vanatta JM. Clinical algorithm to guide the need for endoscopic retrograde cholangiopancreatography to evaluate early postliver transplant cholestasis. Exp Clin Transplant. 2014;12(6):543–7.

30. Dai SC, Goldberg D, Agarwal A, Ma GK, Yam C, Ahmad NA, et al. Endoscopic therapy is effective for recurrent anastomotic biliary strictures after orthotopic liver transplantation. Ann Hepatol. 2017;16(6):924–31.

31. Zeair S, Butkiewicz F, Butkiewicz J, Stasiuk R. Application of fully covered self-expandable metallic stents with and without Antimigration waist versus repeated plastic biliary stent placement in management of anastomotic biliary strictures after orthotopic liver transplantation. Ann Transplant. 2017;22:719–24.

32. Landi F, de'Angelis N, Sepulveda A, Martinez-Perez A, Sobhani I, Laurent A, et al. Endoscopic treatment of anastomotic biliary stricture after adult deceased donor liver transplantation with multiple plastic stents versus self-expandable metal stents: a systematic review and meta-analysis. Transpl Int. 2018;31(2):131–51.

33. Guichelaar MM, Benson JT, Malinchoc M, Krom RA, Wiesner RH, Charlton MR. Risk factors for and clinical course of non-anastomotic biliary strictures after liver transplantation. Am J Transplant. 2003;3(7):885–90.

34. Lee HW, Suh KS, Shin WY, Cho EH, Yi NJ, Lee JM, et al. Classification and prognosis of intrahepatic biliary stricture after liver transplantation. Liver Transpl. 2007;13(12):1736–42.

35. Maheshwari A, Maley W, Li Z, Thuluvath PJ. Biliary complications and outcomes of liver transplantation from donors after cardiac death. Liver Transpl. 2007;13(12):1645–53.

36. Thuluvath PJ, Pfau PR, Kimmey MB, Ginsberg GG. Biliary complications after liver transplantation: the role of endoscopy. Endoscopy. 2005;37(9):857–63.

37. Thuluvath PJ, Atassi T, Lee J. An endoscopic approach to biliary complications following orthotopic liver transplantation. Liver Int. 2003;23(3):156–62.

38. Dhanasekaran R. Management of immunosuppression in liver transplantation. Clin Liver Dis. 2017;21(2):337–53.

39. Zhang GQ, Zhang CS, Sun N, Lv W, Chen BM, Zhang JL. Basiliximab application on liver recipients: a meta-analysis of randomized controlled trials. Hepatobiliary Pancreat Dis Int. 2017;16(2):139–46.

40. Vacca A, Felli MP, Farina AR, Martinotti S, Maroder M, Screpanti I, et al. Glucocorticoid receptor-mediated suppression of the interleukin 2 gene expression through impairment of the cooperativity between nuclear factor of activated T cells and AP-1 enhancer elements. J Exp Med. 1992;175(3):637–46.

41. Vacca A, Martinotti S, Screpanti I, Maroder M, Felli MP, Farina AR, et al. Transcriptional regulation of the interleukin 2 gene by glucocorticoid hormones. Role of steroid receptor and antigen-responsive 5'-flanking sequences. J Biol Chem. 1990;265(14):8075–80.

42. Hao JC, Wang WT, Yan LN, Li B, Wen TF, Yang JY, et al. Effect of low-dose tacrolimus with mycophenolate mofetil on renal function following liver transplantation. World J Gastroenterol. 2014;20(32):11356–62.

43. Yoo MC, Vanatta JM, Modanlou KA, Campos L, Nezakatgoo N, Nair S, et al. Steroid-free liver transplantation using rabbit antithymocyte globulin induction in 500 consecutive patients. Transplantation. 2015;99(6):1231–5.

44. Busani S, Rinaldi L, Begliomini B, Pasetto A, Girardis M. Thymoglobulin-induced severe cardiovascular reaction and acute renal failure in a patient scheduled for orthotopic liver transplantation. Minerva Anestesiol. 2006;72(4):243–8.

45. Herden U, Galante A, Fischer L, Pischke S, Li J, Achilles E, et al. Early initiation of everolimus after liver transplantation: a single-center experience. Ann Transplant. 2016;21:77–85.

46. Lucey MR, Terrault N, Ojo L, Hay JE, Neuberger J, Blumberg E, et al. Long-term management of the successful adult liver transplant: 2012 practice guideline by the American Association for the Study of Liver Diseases and the American Society of Transplantation. Liver Transpl. 2013;19(1):3–26.

47. Banff schema for grading liver allograft rejection: an international consensus document. Hepatology. 1997;25(3):658–63.

48. Levitsky J, Goldberg D, Smith AR, Mansfield SA, Gillespie BW, Merion RM, et al. Acute rejection increases risk of graft failure and death in recent liver transplant recipients. Clin Gastroen Hepatol. [Observational Study]. 2017;15(4):584–93 e2.

49. Fox AN, Brown RS Jr. Liver transplantation. In: Podolsky DK, Camilleri M, Fitz JG, Kalloo AN, Shanahan F, Wang TC, editors. Yamada's textbook of gastroenterology. Hoboken: Wiley; 2016. p. 2129–45.

50. Demetris A, Adams D, Bellamy C, Blakolmer K, Clouston A, Dhillon AP, et al. Update of the International Banff Schema for Liver Allograft Rejection: working recommendations for the histopathologic staging and reporting of chronic rejection. An international panel. Hepatology. 2000;31(3):792–9.

51. Levitsky J, Feng S. Tolerance in clinical liver transplantation. Hum Immunol. 2018;79(5):283–87.

52. Zhang CX, Wen PH, Sun YL. Withdrawal of immunosuppression in liver transplantation and the mechanism of tolerance. Hepatobiliary Pancreat Dis Int. 2015;14(5):470–6.

53. Haddad EM, McAlister VC, Renouf E, Malthaner R, Kjaer MS, Gluud LL. Cyclosporin versus tacrolimus for liver transplanted patients. Cochrane Database Syst Rev. 2006;18(4):CD005161.

54. Satapathy SK, Jones OD, Vanatta JM, Kamal F, Kedia SK, Jiang Y, et al. Outcomes of liver transplant recipients with autoimmune liver disease using long-term dual immunosuppression regimen without corticosteroid. Transplant Direct. 2017;3(7):e178.

55. Wilkinson A, Davidson J, Dotta F, Home PD, Keown P, Kiberd B, et al. Guidelines for the treatment and management of new-onset diabetes after transplantation. Clin Transpl. 2005;19(3):291–8.

56. Lv C, Zhang Y, Chen X, Huang X, Xue M, Sun Q, et al. New-onset diabetes after liver transplantation and its impact on complications and patient survival. J Diabetes. 2015;7(6):881–90.

57. Stegall MD, Everson G, Schroter G, Bilir B, Karrer F, Kam I. Metabolic complications after liver transplantation. Diabetes, hypercholesterolemia, hypertension, and obesity. Transplantation. 1995;60(9):1057–60.

58. D'Avola D, Cuervas-Mons V, Marti J, Ortiz de Urbina J, Llado L, Jimenez C, et al. Cardiovascular morbidity and mortality after liver transplantation: the protective role of mycophenolate mofetil. Liver Transpl. 2017;23(4):498–509.

59. Barone M, Viggiani MT, Losurdo G, Principi M, Leandro G, Di Leo A. Systematic review with meta-analysis: post-operative complications and mortality risk in liver transplant candidates with obesity. Aliment Pharmacol Ther. 2017;46(3):236–45.

60. Lazzati A, Iannelli A, Schneck AS, Nelson AC, Katsahian S, Gugenheim J, et al. Bariatric surgery and liver transplantation: a systematic review a new frontier for bariatric surgery. Obes Surg. 2015;25(1):134–42.

61. Guichelaar MM, Kendall R, Malinchoc M, Hay JE. Bone mineral density before and after OLT: long-term follow-up and predictive factors. Liver Transpl. 2006;12(9):1390–402.

62. Guichelaar MM, Schmoll J, Malinchoc M, Hay JE. Fractures and avascular necrosis before and after orthotopic liver transplantation: long-term follow-up and predictive factors. Hepatology. 2007;46(4):1198–207.

63. Allen AM, Kim WR, Therneau TM, Larson JJ, Heimbach JK, Rule AD. Chronic kidney disease and associated mortality after liver transplantation – a time-dependent analysis using measured glomerular filtration rate. J Hepatol. 2014;61(2):286–92.

64. Watt KD, Pedersen RA, Kremers WK, Heimbach JK, Charlton MR. Evolution of causes and risk factors for mortality post-liver transplant: results of the NIDDK long-term follow-up study. Am J Transplant. 2010;10(6):1420–7.

65. Kim JY, Akalin E, Dikman S, Gagliardi R, Schiano T, Bromberg J, et al. The variable pathology of kidney disease after liver transplantation. Transplantation. 2010;89(2):215–21.

66. McGuire BM, Julian BA, Bynon JS Jr, Cook WJ, King SJ, Curtis JJ, et al. Brief communication: Glomerulonephritis in patients with hepatitis C cirrhosis undergoing liver transplantation. Ann Intern Med. 2006;144(10):735–41.

67. Pillebout E, Nochy D, Hill G, Conti F, Antoine C, Calmus Y, et al. Renal histopathological lesions after orthotopic liver transplantation (OLT). Am J Transplant. 2005;5(5):1120–9.

68. Perico N, Cattaneo D, Bikbov B, Remuzzi G. Hepatitis C infection and chronic renal diseases. Clin J Am Soc Nephrol. 2009;4(1):207–20.

69. Gonwa TA, Mai ML, Melton LB, Hays SR, Goldstein RM, Levy MF, et al. End-stage renal disease (ESRD) after orthotopic liver transplantation (OLTX) using calcineurin-based immunotherapy: risk of development and treatment. Transplantation. 2001;72(12):1934–9.

70. Masetti M, Montalti R, Rompianesi G, Codeluppi M, Gerring R, Romano A, et al. Early withdrawal of calcineurin inhibitors and everolimus monotherapy in de novo liver transplant recipients preserves renal function. Am J Transplant. 2010;10(10): 2252–62.

71. Herlenius G, Felldin M, Norden G, Olausson M, Backman L, Gustafsson B, et al. Conversion from calcineurin inhibitor to either mycophenolate mofetil or sirolimus improves renal function in liver transplant recipients with chronic kidney disease: results of a prospective randomized trial. Transplant Proc. 2010;42(10):4441–8.

72. Sorrell JH, Brown JR. Sexual functioning in patients with end-stage liver disease before and after transplantation. Liver Transpl. 2006;12(10):1473–7.

73. Chelala L, Ilaiwy G, Hanouneh IA. A female liver transplant recipient asks: can I become pregnant? Cleve Clin J Med. 2016;83(7):498–9.

74. Grant D, Evans D, Hearn M, Duff J, Ghent C, Wall W. Quality of life after liver transplantation. Can J Gastroenterol Hepatol. 1990;4(2):49–52.

75. Duffy JP, Kao K, Ko CY, Farmer DG, McDiarmid SV, Hong JC, et al. Long-term patient outcome and quality of life after liver transplantation: analysis of 20-year survivors. Ann Surg. 2010;252(4):652–61.

76. van den Berg-Emons R, Kazemier G, van Ginneken B, Nieuwenhuijsen C, Tilanus H, Stam H. Fatigue, level of everyday physical activity and quality of life after liver transplantation. J Rehabil Med. 2006;38(2):124–9.

77. Abbas G, Jorgensen RA, Lindor KD. Fatigue in primary biliary cirrhosis. Nat Rev Gastroenterol Hepatol. 2010;7(6):313–9.
78. Watt KD, Pedersen RA, Kremers WK, Heimbach JK, Sanchez W, Gores GJ. Long-term probability of and mortality from de novo malignancy after liver transplantation. Gastroenterology. 2009;137(6):2010–7.
79. Kremers WK, Devarbhavi HC, Wiesner RH, Krom RA, Macon WR, Habermann TM. Post-transplant lymphoproliferative disorders following liver transplantation: incidence, risk factors and survival. Am J Transplant. 2006;6(5 Pt 1):1017–24.
80. Andrade AR, Bittencourt PL, Codes L, Evangelista MA, Castro AO, Sorte NB, et al. New onset diabetes and non-alcoholic fatty liver disease after liver transplantation. Ann Hepatol. 2017;16(6):932–40.
81. Martin EF, Levy C. Timing, management, and outcomes of liver transplantation in primary sclerosing cholangitis. Semin Liver Dis. 2017;37(4):305–13.
82. Wright TL, Donegan E, Hsu HH, Ferrell L, Lake JR, Kim M, et al. Recurrent and acquired hepatitis C viral infection in liver transplant recipients. Gastroenterology. 1992;103(1):317–22.
83. Montano-Loza AJ, Bhanji RA, Wasilenko S, Mason AL. Systematic review: recurrent autoimmune liver diseases after liver transplantation. Aliment Pharmacol Ther. 2017;45(4):485–500.
84. Use of 13-valent pneumococcal conjugate vaccine and 23-valent pneumococcal polysaccharide vaccine for adults with immunocompromising conditions: recommendations of the Advisory Committee on Immunization Practices (ACIP). MMWR Morb Mortal Wkly Rep. 2012;61(40):816–9.

Post-transplant Psychosocial and Mental Health Care of the Liver Recipient

Andrea F. DiMartini, Eric Golden, Andrew Matz,
Mary Amanda Dew, and Catherine Crone

Introduction

While the intent of liver transplantation (LT) is to restore health, vitality, and well-being in the recipient, the surgical process and subsequent recovery can be very stressful. Awareness of mental health issues is key to post-LT care as liver transplant patients have some of the highest rates of psychiatric disorders among all solid organ transplant patients. Additionally, evidence shows that untreated psychiatric disorders can impact post-transplant medical outcomes. As psychiatric and psychological disorders typically cross the pre- to post-transplant periods, early post-transplant identification and treatment will aid in the restoration of stable mental health and ultimately facilitate optimal recovery. Substance use issues, which are common in LT recipients,

are most often considered in post-LT studies. These studies provide ample evidence of post-transplant substance use outcomes. Beyond psychiatric disorders, awareness of psychosocial outcomes is critical to understanding overall outcomes for LT recipients. It is essential to consider whether LT recipients recover adequate physical and cognitive functioning, have good quality of life (QOL), and are able to resume normal pre-LT activities and employment. Data on these types of outcomes are limited, and many studies of mental health and psychosocial outcomes include recipient cohorts of a variety of organ types. In this chapter, we will review prospective findings to the extent they are available, although the bulk of the studies are either cross-sectional or retrospective. While we will focus on the post-transplant period, some studies considering pre- to post-transplant comparisons will be used to illustrate changes over time. We will also report on meta-analytic reviews relevant to LT recipient outcomes. Although this chapter covers return to substance use and briefly reviews pharmacotherapy, additional chapters in this book (Chap. 45 Substance Use Disorders and Chap. 42 Psychopharmacology) provide further information on these issues in liver transplant recipients.

Mental Health and Behavioral Issues

Depression and Anxiety

Mood and anxiety disorders, both new onset and recurrence of preexisting disorders, are common post-LT. Beyond the psychological stressors of the transplant experience, physiological changes and immunosuppression medications can contribute to mood and anxiety symptoms. Depression and anxiety pose significant clinical concern, as up to 30% of LT recipients experience depressive and/or anxious symptoms [1–4]. Post-traumatic stress disorder (PTSD) can occur specifically due to the life-threatening nature of the transplant process and has been identified in greater than 10% of LT patients

A. F. DiMartini (✉)
Departments of Psychiatry and Surgery and the Clinical and Translational Science Institute, University of Pittsburgh, Pittsburgh, PA, USA
e-mail: dimartiniaf@upmc.edu

E. Golden
Department of Psychiatry, University of Pittsburgh, Pittsburgh, PA, USA

A. Matz
Department of Psychiatry, Inova Fairfax Hospital, Falls Church, VA, USA

Department of Psychiatry, George Washington University Medical Center, Washington, DC, USA

M. A. Dew
Departments of Psychiatry, Psychology, Epidemiology, Biostatistics and the Clinical and Translational Science Institute, University of Pittsburgh, Pittsburgh, PA, USA

C. Crone
Department of Psychiatry, Inova Fairfax Hospital, Falls Church, VA, USA

Department of Psychiatry, George Washington University Medical Center, Washington, DC, USA

Department of Psychiatry, Virginia Commonwealth University, Richmond, VA, USA

© Springer International Publishing AG, part of Springer Nature 2019
Y. Sher, J. R. Maldonado (eds.), *Psychosocial Care of End-Stage Organ Disease and Transplant Patients*,
https://doi.org/10.1007/978-3-319-94914-7_15

[5]. The development of PTSD in LT recipients is associated with a greater severity of liver disease prior to LT, longer stay in intensive care post-transplant, acute rejection, and post-LT complications [6, 7]. PTSD symptoms are associated with poorer QOL across multiple domains [6, 7]. A history of major depressive episodes, as well as decreased availability of psychosocial support during the transplantation process, can increase risk for developing depressive and anxious symptoms following liver transplant [1, 6]. Screening for mood and anxiety symptoms and specifically PTSD is an essential part of the post-transplant follow-up for early identification and appropriate management. In the special case of patients transplanted for acetaminophen overdose, early involvement of the mental health team during the transplant hospitalization is critical to determining psychiatric care needs and whether inpatient psychiatric hospitalization is indicated (see [8] Crone 2014 for review and treatment recommendations).

Of particular importance, depression is associated with a number of adverse transplant-related outcomes. A meta-analysis of 27 transplant studies including 6 studies of liver transplant patients contributing over 1000 liver transplant subjects found that, regardless of transplant type, depression increased the relative risk of both post-transplant mortality and death-censored graft loss by 65% [9]. Although studies of liver transplant patients appeared to show a lesser relative risk compared to other organ types, this was not significant. The smaller number of studies on anxiety and transplant outcomes showed no effect between anxiety and mortality or morbidities [9].

Individual studies of LT recipients show that the presence of depression after a liver transplant predicts poorer survival in the post-transplant phase. Compared to post-LT patients without depression as measured by the Beck Depression Inventory, patients with high depression scores had a poorer survival rate after the first post-transplant year [1]. Further, depression at 3 months post-liver transplant predicts increased mortality in the long term, even after accounting for other variables which influence transplant survivability including age and recurrence of hepatitis C [2].

In a study of alcoholic liver disease (ALD) LT recipients, those with untreated or undertreated depression had a significantly higher number of encounters with healthcare providers, including hospital readmissions, and thus a higher utilization of healthcare resources, even after adjusting for variables such as MELD score and other donor/recipient characteristics known to influence post-transplant outcomes [10]. At the same time, adequate treatment of depression post-transplant normalizes use of healthcare resources to levels seen in transplant patients without a history of depression either pre- or post-transplant [10]. Thus, depression may be a modifiable risk factor and, not only may adequate treatment improve the patient's mental health outcome, some studies suggest it may reduce the risk of poorer medical outcomes.

Psychotic Disorders

Transplant teams can demonstrate significant reservations about considering patients with schizophrenia as candidates for organ transplantation. Much of this is related to concerns about these patients' ability to adhere to post-transplant immunosuppressive regimens and fears about their susceptibility to steroid-induced neuropsychiatric side effects. Nevertheless, individual case reports and small case series suggest that with good management, patients with serious mental health conditions can have successful outcomes [11]. Because of the rarity of psychotic disorders in the general population and the likely underrepresentation of persons with psychotic disorders referred for liver transplantation, it is difficult to study post-transplant outcomes. Much of available literature relies on mixed organ transplant samples. Despite this limitation, a case series of ten patients with pre-existing psychotic disorders who underwent transplantation, with four receiving livers and one combined kidney-liver, demonstrated that none had episodes of nonadherence to medical or psychiatric treatment after transplant and none suffered graft loss [12]. In another mixed organ transplant series from the Veterans Health Administration, 20 patients with psychotic disorders (schizophrenia or bipolar disorder) who received a transplant had no difference in survival rates over the first 3 years post-transplant compared to patients with no history of mental illness or other nonpsychotic mental illnesses [13].

Although post-transplant liver data are limited, it appears to indicate that persons with psychotic disorders can have comparable medical outcomes to those without psychosis. However, there may be a need to carefully consider potential risk factors pre-transplant and determine whether they can be addressed prior to transplant or managed following transplant. A survey of transplant programs identified 35 cases of patients with psychotic disorders, many of whom were liver transplant patients, and identified potential risk factors affecting post-transplant outcomes. Living alone or being homeless, positive psychotic symptoms 1 year prior to transplant, history of assault, family history of schizophrenia, and borderline or antisocial features appeared to be linked to post-transplant psychiatric complications and nonadherence [14]. In some cases, helping pre-transplant patients to establish stable housing, ongoing mental healthcare, and identifying an available support system may increase chances of successful post-transplant outcome. After transplant, teams should plan on closer follow-up for patients with psychotic disorders and make efforts to collaborate with patients' mental health providers and supports.

Despite concerns about the risk of administering steroids to patients with psychotic disorders, there is a lack of prospective studies identifying a clear increased risk of neuropsychiatric complications. While higher steroid doses contribute to increased risk for all patients, there is equivocal evidence as to whether patients with premorbid psychiatric disorders are at increased risk [15–17]. However, clinical experience reveals that some patients are highly sensitive to steroids and have repeated history of developing serious neuropsychiatric side effects. For such patients, prophylactic use of antipsychotic agents such as olanzapine or lithium may prove helpful [18].

Substance Use Disorders

Alcohol Use

Alcohol and other substance use disorders are common among LT recipients as excess alcohol and viral hepatitis incurred from illicit drug use are more likely to result in the need for LT than for other types of transplantation. Preparation for post-LT addiction stability begins during the pre-LT phase as potential candidates are carefully evaluated and addiction rehabilitation may be required to improve abstinence stability. However, because substance use disorders are chronic medical illnesses requiring long-term management, it should not be assumed that transplantation cures an addiction or that addiction issues are no longer relevant following transplantation. To the contrary, rates of alcohol use for ALD LT recipients are significant (see below), and optimal treatment planning should encompass a longitudinal perspective for which LT is not the terminus. Studies examining the timing of addiction treatment demonstrate that LT recipients with alcohol use disorders who receive addiction treatment both before *and after* LT have the lowest relapse rates compared to those who receive addiction treatment only prior to LT or not at all [19, 20]. At one LT center, the introduction of an embedded alcohol addiction unit that provided intensive treatment and monitoring across the pre- to post-LT period was associated with reduced post-LT relapse rates compared to those patients not in the program (16.4% vs. 35.1%) and an improvement in the 5-year mortality rate [20]. Ongoing addiction treatment is especially pertinent post-LT as the early recovery period can be very stressful and physical stress and emotional distress during this period are associated with increased risk for alcohol relapse [21]. In one study, the use of an "alcohol contract" signed prior to transplant confirming a commitment to abstinence following transplant and agreement to attend addiction rehabilitation did not reduce the rates or amounts of alcohol use following LT [22].

For these reasons, transplant clinicians should monitor for alcohol use early on and reengage recipients in psychiatric and/or addiction counseling as indicated. Optimally the recipient would resume addiction counseling therapy early post-LT as a preventative measure. However, this can be challenging as patients have many competing medical priori-

ties and may not feel fully recovered in the early postoperative period. Among these priorities, they may not see the need or value in resuming counseling. This is especially true if the patient was resistant to addiction counseling prior to LT. The intensity of the post-LT counseling will depend on where the patient is in their recovery treatment plan. Some may only require maintenance therapy, while others with short sobriety and little pre-LT counseling who proceeded to transplantation quickly due to the urgency of their condition may require intensive counseling post-LT. Motivational interviewing may facilitate reengagement in addiction counseling. Although most transplant programs do not have embedded addiction clinicians, if psychiatric consultants are available in the outpatient transplant clinic, these specialists may be able to see the patient during the early postoperative transplant clinic appointments and bridge the eventual transition back to community addiction services. Psychiatric consultation can provide a thorough post-LT reevaluation of the patient's recovery stability, understanding of his/her addiction, commitment to lifelong abstinence, family and social support for continued abstinence, and the presence of other psychiatric disorders.

Monitoring of alcohol use is commonly done through self-report during transplant team clinic appointments [23–25]. Maintaining an open, nonjudgmental approach during the interview can facilitate disclosure. In one study, three methods were used to monitor alcohol use post-LT (addiction specialist interview, hepatologist interview, and the Alcohol Use Disorders Identification Test-Consumption (AUDIT-C)). In patients who had not yet developed liver test abnormalities due to their drinking, the addiction specialist not only identified more patients drinking alcohol but also uncovered significantly higher consumption amounts than were discovered by the hepatologist interview or AUDIT-C [26]. The authors hypothesized this was in part due to the focus of the hepatologist interview more on transplant specific issues but also perhaps due to denial and shame on the part of the patient [26]. It was also suggested that the addiction specialist's expertise and the provision of confidentially without sharing information with the transplant program facilitated more open disclosure. However, whether transplant teams would agree to this arrangement for post-LT follow-up is unknown [27]. Following LT, while some disincentives to reveal alcohol use prior to transplant (e.g., fear of removal from transplant waitlist) may no longer exist, continued psychological obstacles of shame, guilt, and denial can make revelation of alcohol consumption to transplant clinicians difficult. Some patients may be concerned about how the transplant team will respond to their resumption of alcohol use and may need to know that the transplant team will not abandon them. Nevertheless, transplant teams should be careful not to condone or dismiss small amounts of alcohol use as these can quickly lead to a relapse as noted below. Although we found that our transplant clinical interviews with a psychiatrist who was part of the team at the University of Pittsburgh revealed the most episodes of post-LT alcohol use in comparison to other monitoring methods, using a combination of methods provides the greatest yield [28]. One study conducted in an LT clinic found among several biomarkers, urinary ethyl glucuronide was the strongest marker of alcohol consumption and provided a more accurate prediction rate of alcohol consumption than the AUDIT-C or carbohydrate-deficient transferrin [23]. Blood alcohol level is the most commonly used biomarker for monitoring alcohol use due to widespread availability of this test. In some cases, a review of liver enzymes and biopsy results along with a candid discussion with the LT recipient can provide opportunity to overcome denial of the damaging consequences of their alcohol use [29].

One of the most highly investigated outcomes for LT recipients is alcohol use after LT. A meta-analysis that included 50 LT studies of patients who received LT for ALD showed the cumulative incidence rate of any alcohol use was 5.6% of patients per year and heavy use was 2.5% per year [25]. Some studies identified return to alcohol use beginning many years after LT, suggesting that relapse rates are unlikely to level off over time [25]. While these rates may appear low cumulatively, by 10 years, over 50% will have had any alcohol, and 25% will have engaged in heavy drinking. Among 12 possible psychosocial risk factors for alcohol use (e.g., demographics and pre-LT characteristics), only 3 variables were significantly associated with relapse: poorer social support, family history of alcohol abuse/dependence, and pre-LT abstinence of less than 6 months [25]. However, a 6-month cut point for pre-LT sobriety, although used in clinical practice, is an arbitrary value. Cumulatively each additional month sober confers less risk to drink [30]. A study using cluster analysis of the DSM-IV criteria for alcohol abuse/dependence disorders found whereas the patient's subcategory of alcohol dependence identified by the cluster analysis was unimportant for risk stratification with respect to post-LT relapse, it was the diagnosis of alcohol dependence compared to alcohol abuse that most accurately predicted relapse [31].

A prospective study of 208 ALD LT recipients found that, of those who drank, 40% (20% of the total cohort) progressed to a binge episode (6 drinks or more on a single occasion)—many within 6 months of their first drink [30]. This suggests that any exposure to alcohol is dangerous with the recipient quickly losing control over their consumption. In addition, moderate to heavy persisting patterns of alcohol consumption were identified in 20% of the cohort. These recipients tended to resume alcohol early postoperatively within the first months following LT. They were also significantly more likely to experience poorer early outcomes, with more frequent evidence of acute rejection or steatohepatitis on biopsy, and higher likelihood of graft failure or death from recurrent ALD [21]. Those most likely to drink in these early problematic patterns also reported experiencing more stress, more pain, and less vitality, and they felt their health was worse after LT.

Overall patients transplanted for ALD as a group have survival comparable or better than patients transplanted for other types of liver diseases. However, not surprisingly, those who relapse, especially those who return to abusive drinking, have poorer 10-year survival rates (45.1% vs. 85.5%) [32] and decreased survival related to both recurrent ALD [33] and acute alcoholic hepatitis [34]. A meta-analysis of the impact of alcohol use on outcomes showed that, compared to those who did not drink, those who drank had nearly 4 times higher odds of graft steatosis, had 7 times higher odds of graft fibrosis, were 4.6 times more likely to develop worse histological findings on biopsy, and were 3.7 times more likely to die by 10 years [35].

Marijuana Use

In a recent survey, only 43% of liver transplant programs considered pre-LT marijuana use an absolute contraindication to transplantation [36], and thus LT programs may not require discontinuation as a prerequisite for transplantation. In addition, some states have passed laws protecting organ transplantation for medicinal marijuana users. For example, in 2015, the state of California passed the Medical Cannabis Organ Transplant Act prohibiting discrimination against patients using legally prescribed medical cannabis in the organ transplant process, unless a surgeon or other physician has determined that medical cannabis use is clinically significant to the transplant process. Consequently LT programs may be caring for recipients who are using marijuana following LT. Specific rates of post-LT marijuana use have not been investigated, and there are no large studies of marijuana use in transplant recipients to examine the actual impact on outcomes. However, a number of case reports of fungal lung infections in cannabis smoking transplant recipients indicate that smoked cannabis may expose immunocompromised patients to infectious agents [37, 38]. New evidence suggests inhaled/vaporized marijuana may be the source of these infections [39]. More worrisome is the fact that a recent study of medicinal dispensaries cultured multiple fungi (*Aspergillus* and *Penicillium* spp.) and bacteria (*Klebsiella*, *Enterobacter*, *Salmonella*, and *Bacillus*) from dispensary cannabis samples [39]. This underscores the fact that viable infectious organisms can be recovered from cannabis, even medicinal grade marijuana. Patients and clinicians are likely unaware that medicinal dispensaries do not have governmental quality or purity oversight [40], which raises risks specifically for immunocompromised patients. It is notable that clinical studies demonstrating the medicinal benefits of cannabinoids used synthetic pharmaceutical grade cannabinoids, not smoked marijuana [41]. Additionally the Institute of Medicine maintains there is no medicinal role for smoked marijuana and no other medication is smoked [41]. This suggests if medicinal cannabinoids are to be used, the best choice, to avoid these risks, would be the cannabinoid medications approved by the FDA (dronabinol and nabilone).

Other Non-alcohol Substance Use

While there is a limited literature on LT patients with other nonalcohol substance use disorders, the same post-LT clinical management and treatment as discussed above with alcohol use disorders would similarly apply to LT recipients with other substance use disorders. A few studies have addressed substance use in LT recipients who had comorbid alcohol and substance use. One study of ALD LT recipients with a median follow-up of 41 months found that 47% additionally used illicit drugs prior to LT with 17.2% of the total group using substances after LT [42]. Another study of LT patients with a pre-LT history of polysubstance use found that not only did polysubstance users have a higher rate of post-LT alcohol use but the majority also had ongoing substance use following LT [43]. The majority of post-LT substance use was marijuana, with pre-LT substance use being the only independent predictor of substance use after LT [42]. A meta-analysis including 4 studies of illicit drug use in LT recipients showed illicit drug relapse among all organ types averaged 3.7 cases per 100 patients per year, with a significantly lower rate in liver versus other recipients (1.9 vs. 6.1 cases) [25].

Tobacco Use

While there is no doubt of the well-established negative effect of tobacco use on post-LT outcomes, only a quarter of LT programs consider tobacco use to be an absolute contraindication to transplantation [36]. Both current and prior smokers have an increased risk of post-LT morbidity, including biliary and vascular complications, cardiovascular disease, increased rates of de novo cancer as well as recurrence of hepatocellular carcinoma, and poorer graft and patient survival [44–46]. Efforts toward tobacco use cessation, for both smoked and chewed tobacco, should be vigorously pursued. Unfortunately, many LT recipients who stopped smoking as a condition for transplant resume afterwards, $\geq$60% in two studies [47, 48]. In addition, a meta-analysis found that of patients with a prior substance use history, LT cohorts had the highest prevalence rate of post-LT tobacco use, with a rate of nearly 10% per year [25] as compared to 3.4% per year for all solid-organ transplant recipients [49].

Not surprisingly, those who resumed smoking had a shorter period of abstinence pre-LT and a longer history of smoking [48]. In addition those who smoked were also more likely to drink alcohol post-LT (OR, 1.79; 95% CI, 0.75–

4.27; $P = 0.026$) [48]. Resumption of smoking can occur very early on within the first months after LT and can quickly increase in amount and frequency of use [47]. Thus, close monitoring, assessment of relapse risk, and assistance with smoking cessation are essential parts of the post-LT clinical care. In addition to pharmacotherapies that transplant clinicians/psychiatrists can prescribe (see Chap. 42), many states have smokers assistance programs including free nicotine replacement therapies and health coaches. The American Lung Association has a web-based smoking cessation program with a number of assistance options (e.g., American Lung Association's Freedom From Smoking Online). Similar to alcohol and other substance use, random biochemical monitoring for nicotine and cotinine is suggested to supplement self-reported use [48].

Methadone-Maintained LT Recipients

For patients on methadone maintenance therapy (MMT), higher doses may be required after LT when hepatic metabolic function becomes normalized. In one study, the post-LT dose of methadone was increased an average of 60% from baseline [50]. LT teams often use methadone as the postoperative pain medication to avoid patient exposure to other narcotics that could precipitate relapse. MMT programs do not treat chronic pain, but following postoperative recovery when the patient transitions back to the MMT program, a methadone increase can be justified to provide adequate coverage for opioid addiction with improved liver functioning. Coordination of such dose increases with the MMT program is required so as not to interfere with the agreed upon treatment plan. Although MMT patients may see LT as a new chapter in their life and wish to discontinue methadone, in the stressful early recovery period, this should not be undertaken, as it can increase the risk for relapse. In a study of 36 MMT LT recipients, 4 (11%) relapsed to heroin, and 2 had their methadone increased to address their addiction [51]. Relapses were brief and did not appear to affect outcomes [51].

Although several small cohort studies have reported similar medical outcomes for MMT LT recipients compared to non-MMT recipients [51], several other studies suggest these patients may have higher perioperative morbidity, longer hospital stays, and more severe recurrent hepatitis C infections [50, 52].

Treatment Adherence

Lifelong adherence to medical treatment and self-management is crucial to successful liver transplantation. Unfortunately, nonadherence is emerging as a major cause of transplant patient morbidity and graft loss. Adherence includes perpetual daily self-administration of at least one antirejection medication, frequent self-monitoring (e.g., vital signs, weight) and reporting of symptoms as indicated to the transplant team, as well as follow-up appointments, laboratory testing, and general self-care. The concept of adherence also includes following prescribed diet and exercise regimens. A meta-analysis of adherence behaviors across all organ types showed that liver recipients had some of the lowest rates of nonadherence when compared to kidney, heart, pancreas, and lung recipients including the lowest rates of medication nonadherence; 6.7 cases per 100 persons per year of follow-up (PPY) compared to 14.5 PPY for heart and 35.6 PPY for kidney recipients [49]. Liver recipients were the least likely to be nonadherent to an exercise regimen and interestingly had similar, not higher, rates of substance use including alcohol, tobacco, and illicit drugs compared to other organ recipients [49].

While many liver transplant patients have a history of medical illness from which a pattern of adherence (or nonadherence) can be established, it remains difficult to predict based on pre-transplant evaluation which patients will have nonadherence behaviors and resulting complications post-transplant. Across all organ types, in addition to pre-transplant nonadherent behaviors, depression and anxiety, substance use, poor support, low health literacy, lower socio-economic status, and greater complexity of the treatment regimen have been associated with poorer adherence following transplant [53, 54]. A single study comparing adherence rates between kidney and liver recipients showed symptoms of depression were associated with lower rates of immuno-suppressive medication adherence in renal but not liver transplant recipients [55]. However, another study examining treated versus untreated depression in LT recipients found higher rates of acute rejection in the untreated depressed group suggesting acute rejection may have been mediated by depression-related nonadherence [56].

Transplant recipients tend to underestimate their level of nonadherence to medications [57]. Given that self-report of adherence is not always reliable, other methods are sometimes used to monitor adherence. Most commonly, immuno-suppressive medication blood levels are used. A higher variability in successive blood levels between blood draws indicates a non-steady state of immunosuppression coverage in the transplant recipient and can be used as a marker for nonadherence and can also be used as a predictor of graft rejection [58].

In a study of LT recipients' treatment, knowledge of prescribed medication regimen (defined as a patient's ability to describe each medication's indication and dosing schedule) showed factors correlated with lower treatment knowledge were lower income, less time since transplant, a higher number of medications in the regimen, and low health literacy. A higher level of treatment knowledge was associated with fewer rehospitalizations after transplant [59]. These findings highlight the importance of ongoing assessment of LT recipients' understanding of prescribed medication regimen as well as reeducation around the time of changes in the regimen. Possible measures toward increasing treatment knowledge would be complete medication reconciliation at every appointment, counseling with a pharmacist about medications at every refill visit and frequently providing the most up-to-date medication list for patients. The use of drug-reminder (blister pack) packaging was also shown to improve medication adherence and could be recommended and facilitated by providers for those patients at high risk of nonadherence [60].

A systematic review including three studies of LT recipients examined interventions intended to improve medication adherence [61]. A combination of cognitive, educational, counseling, and psychological interventions at the patient, provider, and system levels were more likely to be effective than single interventions [61]. Improving patient education and encouraging an active role in treatment may improve patient adherence [62]. In addition to education assessment of barriers, involving the patient in the selection of strategies to improve adherence, and allowing them with support to make their own decisions about their care, is most likely to produce the best results [63, 64]. Motivational interviewing or problem-solving therapies can be used to address barriers to adherence. However, because adherence tends to deteriorate over time [53], ongoing assessment of adherence behaviors with booster intervention sessions will likely be required over the long term.

Cognitive Recovery Post-Liver Transplantation

Cognitive impairment is common prior to LT due to physiological consequences of end-stage liver disease, specifically hepatic encephalopathy (HE), but comorbid diseases (e.g., diabetes, vascular disease), prior trauma, or the effects of substance use (e.g., alcohol or drugs) may also contribute to pre-LT deficits. Hepatic encephalopathy is common pre-LT with 70% of patients demonstrating subtle symptoms, but nearly 50% having overt motor and neuropsychological impairment [65]. While successful treatment of HE improves cognitive functioning, several studies show even one episode of overt HE can result in persistent cognitive deficits in the areas of working memory, response inhibition, and learning [66, 67]. Thus, the reversibility of cognitive impairment or the potential for worsening cognitive symptoms following LT depends on a variety of factors influencing the vulnerability of the brain including age, prior central nervous system damage, severity of pre-LT hepatic encephalopathy, homeostatic reserve of the brain, and the ability to withstand transplant-related stressors (e.g., hemodynamic changes, operative stresses, immunosuppressive medications).

The incidence of postoperative cognitive dysfunction, defined as a "more than expected" postoperative deterioration in cognitive areas such as short-term and long-term memory, consciousness, mood, and circadian rhythm, is estimated at 44% [68]. It is associated with several factors including the severity of hepatic failure before transplantation, alcohol abuse, use of immunosuppressants and corticosteroids, neuroinflammation, ischemia-reperfusion syndrome, and postoperative infections [68]. In terms of long-term cognitive recovery, the literature indicates that improvement in pre-LT cognitive deficits is possible, though complete resolution of these deficits may not be. Moreover, pre-LT cognitive status based largely on the presence of HE may play a significant role in post-LT cognitive outcomes. In a prospective study of 66 patients who underwent neuropsychological testing before and 6 months after LT, the percentage of patients who exhibited cognitive impairment as determined by psychometric hepatic encephalopathy scores was significantly reduced from 67% pre-transplant to 21% post-transplant. However, the researchers also found that patients with pre-LT cognitive impairment performed worst in almost all areas of cognitive testing except for block design and line tracing after LT compared to the cognitively unimpaired pre-transplant patients [69].

The connection between post-LT cognitive recovery and severity of pre-transplant HE was explored by comparing the post-LT cognitive functioning of three groups: those with HE pre-LT, those without HE pre-LT, and matched controls. Compared to the control group and those without HE pre-LT, patients who had HE pre-LT demonstrated significantly worse performance 18 months post-LT on several domains of the Repeatable Battery for the Assessment of Neuropsychological Status (RBANS) exam, Psychometric Hepatic Encephalopathy Score subtests, and critical flicker frequency test [70]. Additionally, a study involving 65 LT recipients found that 1-year post-transplant EEG normalization was similar between patients with and without history of overt HE. On neuropsychological testing though, patients with a history of overt HE showed the most improvement in cognitive functioning from their pre-transplant baseline but continued to perform worse on cognitive testing compared to those without a history of overt HE. In terms of predictors of cognitive dysfunction post-transplantation, only age was found to be significant predictor [71].

While most studies show global cognitive improvement, at least one study found discrepancies in specific areas of cognitive recovery. In a prospective study, patients with prior minimal HE failed to reach the functional level of controls on visuomotor performance testing conducted on average 21 months post-LT. In fact, 7 of the 14 patients with prior minimal HE showed no improvement in this cognitive area [72]. Knowledge that post-LT patients may have continued cognitive impairment should be shared with patients and their support system prior to LT to provide them with reasonable expectations. It may also suggest the need for continued engagement of patient's support system at post-LT follow-up, especially when significant medication adjustments or patient education need to be provided. In some cases, patients may also be considered for cognitive rehabilitation to help optimize their functioning post-LT.

Pharmacologic Considerations

In addition to psychotherapy (see Chap. 43), pharmacotherapy is an essential treatment component in the psychiatric care of LT recipients. Here we will briefly touch on liver-specific metabolic issues and refer the reader to Chap. 42 on psychopharmacology in transplant patients. Psychotropic medications are often inadvertently discontinued in the early post-LT recovery period due to oversight, lack of awareness of the need of ongoing treatment by nonpsychiatric providers, or concern over the patients' medical fragility and the potential risks of psychotropic medications. Although the treatment of transplant recipients can be complicated, withholding needed psychotropic medications can lead to onset/recurrence of psychiatric disorders and, as noted above, result in poorer patient outcomes.

As most psychotropic medications are hepatically metabolized, it is critical to establish the restoration of normal organ functioning during the early recovery period after LT. For the majority of recipients, the newly transplanted organ functions immediately, so that normal physiological parameters are quickly restored and pharmacokinetic abnormalities resolve. However delayed graft function (DGF) is the most common allograft complication affecting pharmacokinetics in the immediate post-transplantation period. DGF occurs in 10%–25% of liver recipients but can reach 50% if marginal organs are counted [73, 74]. Although the pharmacokinetics of psychotropic medications in DGF have not been examined, studies of immunosuppressive medication metabolism suggest recipients with DGF may require one-half of the typical dose [75, 76]. Acute cellular rejection with resulting transient graft dysfunction occurs in 20–70% of LT recipients, typically within the first 3 weeks post-transplant. Most cases are effectively treated, do not lead to clinically significant alteration in liver histology or architecture [77], and require no specific change to psychotropic dosages. However, chronic rejection that evolves over time in 5%–10% of liver recipients eventually leads to chronic liver dysfunction and loss of metabolic capacity [77]. In these cases, precautions similar to pre-LT cirrhosis should be taken.

In addition to graft status, the patient's total physiologic status should be considered in drug choice and dosing. Resolving hepatorenal syndrome, lingering ascites, or liver congestion can affect pharmacokinetics. In the absence of these issues within the first month following LT, patients with stable liver functioning can have the clearance and steady-state volume of distribution of drugs similar to healthy volunteers [75]. Following the surgical recovery and resolution of immediate postoperative complications (e.g., sedation, intestinal paralysis), patients can be treated with normal therapeutic dosing. An additional consideration is whether the pre-LT dosing of a psychotropic medication may require an increase to accommodate the improved functioning of the liver.

Post-transplant Quality of Life and Employment

Improving mental health outcomes requires not only understanding and lessening the impact of mental health disorders on transplant outcomes but also an awareness of the role of quality of life (QOL) and functional status. Ideally, following a period of postoperative recovery, rehabilitation, and adjustment to a new self-care regimen, patients would resume their roles within their family, community, and workplace. There is substantial evidence that QOL across many domains improves pre- to post-transplant [78]. Unfortunately, liver transplant recipients do not achieve the QOL of healthy controls [78]. The degree of improvement appears largely driven by the severity of illness at the point of transplant rather than the primary liver disease [78, 79]. While LT recipients' QOL can dramatically improve in the early period following transplant and largely be sustained over a decade following transplant, there are gradual and consistent decrements in QOL over time [80]. Additionally, those with combined ALD and hepatitis C reported the worst quality of life compared to others and had the greatest rate of physical decline compared to those with either etiology alone or other etiologies of liver disease [80]. Whether these outcomes will improve with the newer antiviral therapies is yet unknown.

Following LT, employment rates are significantly lower than the general population. Across studies, rates range from 22% to 60%, with an average employment rate of 37% from studies published after 2000 [81, 82]. A considerable portion of recipients pursue early retirement, but this does not fully explain the low rates among younger patients. Even compared against renal transplant recipients, rates are below expected, and efforts have been made to understand what factors influence post-LT employment [82, 83]. Results from several studies have shown that the most consistent factors associated with employment include pre-LT employment, younger age (18–40), higher education, functional/health status, and subjective work ability [82, 84, 85]. Although some report higher employment rates with males, it is unclear if this is due to females being more likely to be doing unsalaried work as homemakers [82, 84]. Racial differences have

also been suggested, but have not been adequately studied [84]. Interestingly, severity of pre-LT liver disease as measured by MELD has not seemed to influence post-LT employment [82]. A recent study looking at pre-LT hepatic encephalopathy suggested similar findings [86]. Even if there is a desire to return to work, patients may not be able to return to their pre-LT level of employment [87]. For others, fear of losing health insurance coverage tied to disability benefits dissuades efforts at seeking employment [82, 84].

Existing studies of post-LT employment are mostly cross-sectional and descriptive in nature. There is also considerable heterogeneity among studies regarding the definition of employment, approaches to assessing work experience, the time point of assessment, as well as other factors, making broad conclusions about findings challenging [82, 84]. Nonetheless, some studies bear greater attention due to large sample size or use of a control group [81, 85, 88]. Huda et al. obtained United Network for Organ Sharing (UNOS) employment data on recipients within 24 months after LT between 2002 and 2008. Of approximately 22,000 patients, only 24% were employed within 24 months after LT, and those employed had significantly better functional status than those not employed [81]. Another study examined UNOS data on approximately 13,000 recipients 5 years after LT and divided those employed based on level of continuity of post-LT employment and timing of return to work [85]. Lower socioeconomic status, higher local unemployment rates, and post-transplant complications and comorbidities were predictors of less than continuous post-LT employment. Of note, nearly half who resumed work within 2 years after LT later became unemployed [85]. A Finnish study utilized an age and gender-standardized community-based control group for comparison against 353 LT recipients [88]. Assessments included health-related quality of life (HRQOL), which was slightly lower than the control group. Recipients who were employed reported significantly better HRQOL compared to those unemployed. This finding is similar to an earlier study of 308 LT recipients that found better SF-36 scores on role physical and physical functioning, indicating less limitation in these areas due to health problems, were independently associated with post-LT employment [89]. Beyond a positive impact of physical well-being on post-LT employment, separate studies have reported a negative impact from depression [90, 91].

A recent review of post-LT employment studies stressed the need for transplant programs and clinical studies to incorporate efforts at providing job rehabilitation post-LT [82]. Additionally, as a consistent finding across studies is the positive influence of pre-LT employment, it was also recommended that transplant candidates be provided with assistance in maintaining employment. Reducing pre-LT disability by managing minimal HE, maintaining mobility, and helping to plan for work adjustments was encouraged.

Post-LT, physical rehabilitation, encouragement, self-efficacy measures, and depression management were recommended to facilitate recipients' return to employment [82]. Although social functioning is another factor contributing to post-LT QOL, studies are lacking. Usually mentioned in employment or QOL studies, there is indication that social functioning may not improve significantly post-LT [88, 91, 92].

Conclusions

Liver transplant recipients represent a complex patient population who among solid organ recipients have some of the highest prevalences of mental health disorders. Patients with mental health disorders can successfully undergo transplantation and have good outcomes, especially if they are identified and adequately psychiatrically managed. Those with serious mental health disorders can also achieve good outcomes, if expert management, good caregiver support, and collaboration with the transplant team are established. Substance use, especially alcohol and tobacco use, and nonadherence to medications continue to represent significant issues following LT. Clinicians should consistently monitor for these behaviors, including self-report and biochemical screening for substances and immunosuppressive medication levels. With all mental health disorders, continuity of psychiatric care from pre- to post-LT is essential for optimal mental health and medical outcomes to be achieved. In the early postoperative period assessment, identification and treatment of emerging psychiatric and behavioral issues are critical. Reinstitution and adjustment of psychotropic medications may be indicated. If nonadherent behaviors are identified, the use of psychotherapeutic techniques including education, motivation, and problem-solving may alleviate poor adherence behaviors. Beyond mental health outcomes, whether strategies to improve quality of life and social reintegration can additionally improve medical outcomes can be considered, but studies of such interventions are lacking.

References

1. DiMartini A, Dew MA, Chaiffetz D, Fitzgerald MG, Devera ME, Fontes P. Early trajectories of depressive symptoms after liver transplantation for alcoholic liver disease predicts long-term survival. Am J Transplant. 2011;11(6):1287–95. https://doi.org/10.1111/j.1600-6143.2011.03496.x.
2. Corruble E, Barry C, Varescon I, Falissard B, Castaing D, Samuel D. Depressive symptoms predict long-term mortality after liver transplantation. J Psychosom Res. 2011;71(1):32–7. https://doi.org/10.1016/j.jpsychores.2010.12.008.
3. Corbett C, Armstrong MJ, Parker R, Webb K, Neuberger JM. Mental health disorders and solid-organ transplant recipients. Transplantation. 2013;96:593–600.
4. Nickel R, Wunsch A, Egle UT, Lohse AW, Otto G. The relevance of anxiety, depression, and coping in patients after liver transplantation. Liver Transpl. 2002;8:63–71.
5. Annema C, Drent G, Roodbol PF, Metselaar HJ, Van Hoek B, Porte RJ, et al. A prospective cohort study on posttraumatic stress disorder in liver transplantation recipients before and after transplantation. J Psychosom Res. 2017;95:88–93.
6. Rothenhäusler HB, Ehrentraut S, Kapfhammer HP, Lang C, Zachoval R, Bilzer M, et al. Psychiatric and psychosocial outcome of orthotopic liver transplantation. Psychother Psychosom. 2002;71:285–97.
7. Jin SG, Yan LN, Xiang B, Li B, Wen TF, Zhao JC, et al. Posttraumatic stress disorder after liver transplantation. Hepatobiliary Pancreat Dis Int. 2012;11(1):28–33.
8. Crone C, DiMartini A. Liver transplant for intentional acetaminophen overdose: a survey of transplant clinicians experiences with recommendations. Psychosomatics. 2014;55(6):602–12. PMID: 25016353.
9. Dew MA, Rosenberger EM, Myaskovsky L, DiMartini AF, DeVito Dabbs AJ, Posluszny DM, et al. Depression and anxiety as risk factors for morbidity and mortality after organ transplantation: a systematic review and meta-analysis. Transplantation. 2015;100:988–1003.
10. Sebaaly JC, Fleming J, Pilch N, Meadows H, Finn A, Chavin K, Baliga P, et al. Depression, resource utilization, and outcomes following liver transplant. Prog Transplant. 2016;26(3):270–6.
11. Price A, Whitwell S, Henderson M. Impact of psychotic disorder on transplant eligibility and outcomes. Curr Opin Organ Transplant. 2014;19:196–200.
12. Zimbrean P, Emre S. Patients with psychotic disorders in solid-organ transplant. Prog Transplant. 2015;25:289–96.
13. Evans LD, Stock EM, Zeber JE, Morissette SB, MacCarthy AA, Sako EY, et al. Posttransplantation outcomes in veterans with serious mental illness. Transplantation. 2015;99:e57–65.
14. Coffman KL, Crone C. Rational guidelines for transplantation in patients with psychotic disorders. Curr Opin Organ Transpl. 2002;7:385–8.
15. Dubovsky AN, Arvikar S, Stern TA, Axelrod L. The neuropsychiatric complications of glucocorticoid use: steroid psychosis revisited. Psychosomatics. 2012;53:103–15.
16. Ross DA, Cetas JS. Steroid psychosis: a review for neurosurgeons. J Neuro-Oncol. 2012;109:439–47.
17. Fardet L, Pettersen I, Nazareth I. Suicidal behavior and severe neuropsychiatric disorders following glucocorticoid therapy in primary care. Am J Psychiatry. 2012;169:491–7.
18. West S, Kenedi C. Strategies to prevent the neuropsychiatric side-effects of corticosteroids: a case reports and review of the literature. Curr Opin Organ Transplant. 2014;19:201–8.
19. Rodrigue JR, Hanto DW, Curry MP. Substance abuse treatment and its association with relapse to alcohol use after liver transplantation. Liver Transpl. 2013;19:1387–95.
20. Addolorato G, Mirijello A, Leggio L, Ferrulli A, D'Angelo C, Vassallo G, et al. Liver transplantation in alcoholic patients: impact of an alcohol addiction unit within a liver transplant center. Alcohol Clin Exp Res. 2013;37(9):1601–8.
21. DiMartini A, Dew MA, Day N, Fitzgerald MG, Jones BL, deVera ME, Fontes P. Trajectories of alcohol consumption following liver transplantation. Am J Transplant. 2010;10(10):2305–12.
22. Masson S, Marrow B, Kendrick S, et al. An "alcohol contract" has no significant effect on return to drinking after liver transplantation for alcoholic liver disease. Transpl Int. 2014;27(5):475–81.
23. Piano S, Marchioro L, Gola E, Rosi S, Morando F, Cavallin M, et al. Assessment of alcohol consumption in liver transplant candidates and recipients: the best combination of the tools available. Liver Transpl. 2014;20:815–22.

24. DiMartini A, Dew MA. Monitoring alcohol use on the liver transplant wait list: therapeutic and practical issues. Liver Transpl. 2012;18(11):1267–9.

25. Dew MA, DiMartini AF, Steel J, De Vito DA, Myaskovsky L, Unruh M, Greenhouse J. Meta-analysis of risk for relapse to substance use after transplantation of the liver or other solid organs. Liver Transpl. 2008;14(2):159–72.

26. Donnadieu-Rigole H, Olive L, Nalpas B, Winter A, Ursic-Bedoya J, Faure S, Pageaux GP, Perney P. Follow-up of alcohol consumption after liver transplantation: interest of an addiction team? Alcohol Clin Exp Res. 2017;41:165–70.

27. Dom G. Confidentiality and the role of the addiction specialist team in liver transplantation procedures. Commentary on Donnadieu-Rigole et al., 2017, Follow-Up of alcohol consumption after liver transplantation: interest of an addiction team? Alcohol Clin Exp Res. 2017;41(3):504–6.

28. DiMartini A, Day N, Dew M, Lane T, Fitzgerald MG, Magill J, Jain A. Alcohol use following liver transplantation: a comparison of follow-up methods. Psychosomatics. 2001;42:55–62.

29. Weinrieb RM, Van Horn DH, McLellan AT, Lucey MR. Interpreting the significance of drinking by alcohol-dependent liver transplant patients: fostering candor is the key to recovery. Liver Transpl. 2000;6:769–76.

30. DiMartini A, Day N, Dew MA, Javed L, Fitzgerald MG, Jain AK, Fung JJ, Fontes P. Alcohol consumption patterns and predictors of use following liver transplantation for alcoholic liver disease. Liver Transpl. 2006;12:813–20.

31. DiMartini A, Dew MA, Fitzgerald MG, Fontes P. Clusters of alcohol use disorders diagnostic criteria and predictors of alcohol use following liver transplantation for alcoholic liver disease. Psychosomatics. 2008;49(4):332–40.

32. Cuadrado A, Fabrega E, Casafont F, Pons-Romero F. Alcohol recidivism impairs long-term patient survival after orthotopic liver transplantation for alcoholic liver disease. Liver Transpl. 2005;11(4):420–6.

33. Pfitzmann R, Schwenzer J, Rayes N, Seehofer D, Neuhaus R, Nussler NC. Long-term survival and predictors of relapse after orthotopic liver transplantation for alcoholic liver disease. Liver Transpl. 2007;13(2):197–205.

34. Conjeevaram HS, Hart J, Lissoos TW, et al. Rapidly progressive liver injury and fatal alcoholic hepatitis occurring after liver transplantation in alcoholic patients. Transplantation. 1999;67(12):1562–8.

35. Kaif M, Tariq R, Singal AK. Impact of recidivism after liver transplantation for alcoholic cirrhosis on liver graft and patient survival: a meta-analysis. Gastroenterology. 2015;148(4)S:S-1038–S-1039.

36. Butt FK, Earl TM, Anderson CD. Top ten facts you need to know: about liver transplantation. J Miss State Med Assoc. 2014;55(7):212–5.

37. Marks WH, Florence L, Lieberman J, Chapman P, Howard D, Roberts P, Perkinson D. Successfully treated invasive pulmonary aspergillosis associated with smoking marijuana in a renal transplant recipient. Transplantation. 1996 June 27;61(12):1771–177.

38. Coffman KL. The debate about marijuana usage in transplant candidates: recent medical evidence on marijuana health effects. Curr Opin Organ Transplant. 2008;13:189–95.

39. Thompson GR, Tuscano JM, Dennis M, Singapuri A, Libertini S, Gaudino R, et al. A microbiome assessment of medical marijuana. Clin Microbiol Infect. 2017;23(4):269–70.

40. Wilkinson ST, D'Souza DC. Problems with the medicalization of marijuana. JAMA. 2014;311(23):2377–8.

41. Schrot RJ, Hubbard JR. Cannabinoids: medical implications. Ann Med. 2016;48(3):128–41.

42. Gedaly R, McHugh PP, Johnston TD, Jeon H, Koch A, Clifford TM, Ranjan D. Predictors of relapse to alcohol and illicit drugs after liver transplantation for alcoholic liver disease. Transplantation. 2008;86(8):1090–5.

43. Fireman M. Outcome of liver transplantation in patients with alcohol and polysubstance dependence. Presented at Research Society on Alcoholism: Symposium on Liver Transplantation for the Alcohol Dependent Patient. Denver, June 2000.

44. Mangus RS, Fridell JA, Kubal CA, Loeffler AL, Krause AA, Bell JA, et al. Worse long term patient survival and higher cancer rates in liver transplant recipients with a history of smoking. Transplantation. 2015;99:1862–8.

45. Leithead JA, Ferguson JW, Hayes PC. Smoking-related morbidity and mortality following liver transplantation. Liver Transpl. 2008;14:1159–64.

46. Pungapong S, Manzarabeitia C, Ortiz J, Reich DJ, Araya V, Rothstein KD, Munoz SJ. Cigarette smoking is associated with an increased risk of vascular complications after liver transplant. Liver Transpl. 2002;8:582–7.

47. DiMartini A, Javed L, Russell S, Dew MA, Fitzgerald MG, Jain A, Fung JJ. Tobacco use following liver transplantation for alcoholic liver disease: an underestimated problem. Liver Transpl. 2005 June;11(6):679–83.

48. Ehlers SL, Rodrigue JR, Widows MR, Reed AI, Nelson DR. Tobacco use before and after liver transplantation: a single center survey and implications for clinical practice and research. Liver Transpl. 2004;10(3):412–7.

49. Dew MA, DiMartini A, De Vito DA, Myaskovsky L, Steel J, Unruh M, et al. Rates and risk factors for nonadherence to the medical regimen after adult solid organ transplantation. Transplantation. 2007 Apr 15;83(7):858–73.

50. Weinrieb R, Barnett R, Lynch K, De Piano M, Atanda A, Olthoff K. A matched comparison study of medical and psychiatric complications and anesthesia and analgesia requirements in methadone-maintained liver transplant recipients. Liver Transpl. 2004;10:97–106.

51. Liu LU, Schiano TD, Lau N, O'Rourke M, Min AD, Sigal SH, et al. Survival and risk of recidivism in methadone dependent patients undergoing liver transplantation. Am J Transplant. 2003;3:1273–7.

52. Kanchana TP, Kaul V, Manzarbeitia C, Reich DJ, Hails KC, Munoz SJ, Rothstein KD. Liver transplantation for patients on methadone maintenance. Liver Transpl. 2002;8(9):778–82.

53. De Geest S, Burkhalter H, Bogert L, Berben L, Glass TR, Denhaerynck K; Psychosocial Interest Group; Swiss Transplant Cohort Study. Describing the evolution of medication nonadherence from pre-transplant until 3 years post-transplant and determining pre-transplant medication nonadherence as risk factor for post-transplant nonadherence to immunosuppressives: the Swiss Transplant Cohort Study. Transpl Int. 2014;27(7):657–666.

54. DiMartini A, Sotelo J, Dew MA. Chapter 31-Organ transplantation. In: Levenson J, editor. The American Psychiatric Press textbook of psychosomatic medicine: psychiatric care of the medically ill. 2nd ed. Washington, DC: American Psychiatric Publishing; 2011. p. 725–58.

55. Gorevski E, Succop P, Sachdeva J, Cavanaugh TM, Volek P, Heaton P, et al. Is there an association between immunosuppressant therapy medication adherence and depression, quality of life, and personality traits in the kidney and liver transplant population? Patient Prefer Adherence. 2013;7:301–7.

56. Rogal S, Landsittel D, Surman O, Chung RT, Rutherford A. Pretransplant depression, antidepressant use, and outcomes of orthotopic liver transplantation. Liver Transpl. 2011;17(3):251–60. https://doi.org/10.1002/lt.22231.

57. Butler JA, Peveler RC, Roderick P, Mason JC. Measuring compliance with drug regimens after renal transplantation: comparison of self-report and clinician rating with electronic monitoring. Transplantation. 2004;77(5):786–9.

58. Supelana C, Annunziato R, Schiano T, Anand R, Viadya S, Chuang K, et al. Medication level variability index predicts rejection, possibly due to nonadherence, in adult liver transplant recipients. Liver Transpl. 2014;20(10):1168–77. https://doi.org/10.1002/lt.23930.

59. Serper M, Patzer RE, Reese PP, Przytula K, Koval R, Ladner DP, et al. Medication misuse, nonadherence, and clinical outcomes among liver transplant recipients. Liver Transpl. 2014;21(1):22–8.

60. Boeni F, Spinatsch E, Suter K, Hersberger KE, Arnet I. Effect of drug reminder packaging on medication adherence: a systematic review revealing research gaps. Syst Rev. 2014;3(1):1–15.

61. De Bleser L, Matteson M, Dobbels F, Russell C, De Geest S. Interventions to improve medication-adherence after transplantation: a systematic review. Transpl Int. 2009;22:780–97.

62. Faeder S, Moschenross D, Rosenberger E, Dew MA, DiMartini A. Psychiatric aspects of organ transplantation and donation. Curr Opin Psychiatry. 2015;28(5):357–64.

63. Popoola J, Greene H, Kyegombe M, MacPhee IA. Patient involvement in selection of immunosuppressive regimen following transplantation. Patient Prefer Adherence. 2014;8:1705–12.

64. Dobbels F, De Bleser L, Berben L, Kristanto P, Dupont L, Nevens F, et al. Efficacy of a medication adherence enhancing intervention in transplantation: the MAESTRO-Tx trial. J Heart Lung Transplant. 2017;36(5):499–508.

65. Teperman LW. Impact of pretransplant hepatic encephalopathy on liver posttransplantation outcomes. Int J Hepatol. 2013;2013:952828.

66. Umapathy S, Dhiman RK, Grover S, Duseja A, Chawla YK. Persistence of cognitive impairment after resolution of overt hepatic encephalopathy. Am J Gastroenterol. 2014;109:1011–9.

67. Bajaj JS, Schubert CM, Heuman DM, Wade JB, Gibson DP, Topaz A, et al. Persistence of cognitive impairment after resolution of overt hepatic encephalopathy. Gastroenterology. 2010;138:2332–40.

68. Aceto P, Perilli V, Lai C, Ciocchetti P, Vitale F, Sollazzi L. Postoperative cognitive dysfunction after liver transplantation. Gen Hosp Psychiatry. 2015;37:109–15.

69. Ahluwalia V, Wade JB, White MB, Gilles HG, Herman DM, Fuchs M, et al. Liver transplantation significantly improves global functioning and cerebral processing. Liver Transpl. 2016;22:1379–90.

70. Sotil EU, Gottstein J, Avala E. Impact of preoperative overt hepatic encephalopathy on neurocognitive function after liver transplantation. Liver Transpl. 2009;15:184–92.

71. Campagna F, Montagnese S, Schiff S, Biancardi A, Mapelli D, Angeli P, et al. Cognitive impairment and electroencephalographic alterations before and after liver transplantation. Liver Transpl. 2014;20:977–86.

72. Mechtcheriakov S, Graziadei IW, Mattedi M, Bodner T, Kugener A, Hinterhuber HH, et al. Incomplete improvement of visuo-motor deficits in patients with minimal hepatic encephalopathy after liver transplantation. Liver Transpl. 2004;10:77–83.

73. Angelico M. Donor liver steatosis and graft selection for liver transplantation: a short review. Eur Rev Med Pharmacol Sci. 2005;9:295–7.

74. Stockmann M, Lock JF, Malinowski M, Seehofer D, Puhl G, Pratschke J, Neuhaus P. How to define initial poor graft function after liver transplantation? – a new functional definition by the LiMAx test. Transpl Int. 2010;23(10):1023–32.

75. Hebert MF, Wacher VJ, Roberts JP, Benet LZ. Pharmacokinetics of cyclosporine pre- and post-liver transplantation. J Clin Pharmacol. 2003;43:38–42.

76. Luck R, Boger J, Kuse E, Klempnauer J, Nashan B. Achieving adequate cyclosporine exposure in liver transplant recipients: a novel strategy for monitoring and dosing using intravenous therapy. Liver Transpl. 2004;10:686–91.

77. Lake JR. Liver transplantation. In: Friedman SL, McQuaid KR, Grendell JH, editors. Current diagnosis and treatment in gastroenterology. 2nd ed. New York: McGraw-Hill; 2003. p. 813–34.

78. Tome S, Wells JT, Said A, Lucey MR. Quality of life after liver transplantation. A systematic review. J Hepatol. 2008;48:567–77.

79. Estraviz B, Quintana JM, Valdivieso A, Bilbao A, Padierna A, Ortiz de Urbina J, Sarabia S. Factors influencing change in health-related quality of life after liver transplantation. Clin Transplant. 2007;21:481–90.

80. Ruppert K, Kuo S, DiMartini A, Balan V. In a 12-year study, sustainability of quality of life benefits after liver transplantation varies with pretransplantation diagnosis. Gastroenterology. 2010;139:1619–29.

81. Huda A, Newcomer R, Harrington C, Blegen MG, Keeffe EB. High rate of unemployment after liver transplantation: analysis of the United Network for Organ Sharing database. Liver Transpl. 2012;18:89–99.

82. Aberg F. From prolonging life to prolonging working life: tackling unemployment among liver-transplant recipients. World J Gastroenterol. 2016;22:3701–11.

83. De Baere C, Delva D, Kloeck A, Remans K, Vanrenterghem Y, Verleden G, et al. Return to work and social participation: does type of organ transplantation matter? Transplantation. 2010;89:1009–15.

84. Huda A, Newcomer R, Harrington C, Keeffe EB, Esquivel CO. Employment after liver transplantation: a review. Transplant Proc. 2015;47:233–9.

85. Beal EW, Tumin D, Mumtaz K, Nau M, Tobias JD, Hayes D Jr, et al. Factors contributing to employment patterns after liver transplantation. Clin Transplant. 2017;31(6):1–6.

86. Pflugrad H, Tryc AB, Goldbecker A, Strassburg CP, Barg-Hock H, Klempnauer J, Weissenborn K. Hepatic encephalopathy before and neurological complications after liver transplantation have no impact on the employment status 1 year after transplantation. World J Hepatol. 2017;9:519–32.

87. Kelly R, Hurton S, Ayloo S, Cwinn M, De Coutere-Bosse S, Molinari M. Societal reintegration following cadaveric orthotopic liver transplantation. Hepatobiliary Surg Nutr. 2016;5:234–44.

88. Aberg F, Rissanen AM, Sintonen H, Roine RP, Höckerstedt K, Isoniemi H. Health-related quality of life and employment status of liver transplant patients. Liver Transpl. 2009;15(1):64–72.

89. Saab S, Wiese C, Ibrahim AB, Peralta L, Durazo F, Han S, et al. Employment and quality of life in liver transplant recipients. Liver Transpl. 2007;13:1330–8.

90. Gorevski E, Succop P, Sachdeva J, Scott R, Benjey J, Varughese G, Martin-Boone J. Factors influencing posttransplantation employment: does depression have an impact? Transplant Proc. 2011;43:3835–9.

91. Weng LC, Huang HL, Wang YW, Lee WC, Chen KH, Yang TY. The effect of self-efficacy, depression and symptom distress on employment status and leisure activities of liver transplant recipients. J Adv Nurs. 2014;70:1573–83.

92. Casanovas T, Herdman M, Chandia A, Peña MC MC, Fabregat J, Vilallonga JS. Identifying improved and non-improved aspects of health-related quality of life after liver transplantation based on the assessment of the specific questionnaire liver disease quality of life. Transplant Proc. 2016;48:132–7.

Part V

Cardiac Patient

End-Stage Heart Disease and Indications for Heart Transplantation

June Rhee and Randall Vagelos

Introduction

Heart failure (HF) affects more than 6 million people in the United States (US) and over 26 million worldwide [1]. It is the leading cause of hospitalizations in the United States and Europe [2], imposing a major economic burden with an estimated total cost of greater than $100 billion annually worldwide [3, 4]. While there have been significant breakthroughs in the management of HF, the current medical and device therapies more often delay or halt than reverse its progression. Consequently, the prevalence of symptomatic HF has continued to rise, resulting in more than one million hospitalizations in the United States annually due to HF [2]. As more patients progress to the advanced phase of the disease, there is a growing need for advanced HF therapies including mechanical circulatory support (MCS) and heart transplantation, the ultimate therapy for HF.

This chapter highlights the clinical manifestations and natural course of HF and the role of heart transplantation evaluation in the care of those with advanced HF. Specifically, we aim to describe the foundation of medical evaluations leading to heart transplantation consideration, summarize issues around risk assessment, and review a framework of pre-transplantation workup with specific reference to the decision-making process. Our goal is not to recreate currently available, published guidelines (2016) [5] but rather highlight the key considerations in heart transplantation evaluation and share our approach to managing and evaluating patients with advanced HF, based on our experiences at Stanford and the data from the International Society for Heart and Lung Transplantation (ISHLT) registry.

J. Rhee · R. Vagelos (✉)
Division of Cardiovascular Medicine, Department of Medicine, Stanford University School of Medicine, Stanford, CA, USA
e-mail: jwrhee@stanford.edu; rvagelos@stanford.edu

Definitions of Heart Failure

The American College of Cardiology (ACC)/American Heart Association (AHA) guidelines define HF as "a complex clinical syndrome that can result from any structural or functional cardiac disorder that impairs the ability of the ventricle to fill or eject blood [5–7]." It is important to note that HF is a clinical diagnosis based on a careful history and physical examination [8]. HF can be further classified into two groups according to the parameters of left ventricular (LV) function: (1) HF with reduced ejection fraction (HFrEF) or systolic HF and (2) HF with preserved ejection fraction (HFpEF) or diastolic HF. While variations in the threshold to define HFpEF exist (generally LVEF $\geq$ 50%), about half of the HF cases, especially in patients aged greater than 65 years, are due to HFpEF. Regardless of the underlying ventricular function, the diagnosis of acute decompensated HF is made when there is a "gradual or rapid change in heart failure signs and symptoms resulting in a need for urgent therapy [9]."

Symptoms of Heart Failure

Dyspnea is a cardinal symptom of HF. Typically it reflects pulmonary congestion due to elevated cardiac filling pressures but may represent restricted cardiac output. The absence of progressive dyspnea, however, does not necessarily exclude the diagnosis of HF, because patients may accommodate to symptoms by substantially modifying their lifestyle and limiting their physical activities. Additionally, patients may sleep with their head elevated (orthopnea) to relieve dyspnea or develop nocturnal cough, which is frequently overlooked as symptoms of HF. Other common congestive or "fluid overloaded" symptoms include weight gain, edema in dependent areas (e.g., extremities or scrotum), increasing abdominal girth from ascites, and early satiety. Fatigue is another important symptom of HF and may result from (1) reduced cardiac output either at rest or with physical exertion and (2) altered metabolic capacities of skeletal muscles due to cardiac limitation. The low cardiac output may also cause other generalized symptoms including lack of appetite or anorexia with resultant progressive malnutrition, depressive mood, and cognitive impairment, which are critical for clinicians to recognize and respond to urgently and appropriately.

Stages of Heart Failure

The severity of HF is frequently assessed by patients' exercise capacity and symptomatic status. The most commonly used classification system to quantify functional status was developed by the New York Heart Association (NYHA) which assigns patients to one of the four functional classes, depending on the degree of effort needed to elicit symptoms (Table 16.1). It is based solely on symptoms and can be variable and dynamic depending on one's dietary and medical compliance, temporary comorbidities (e.g., gastrointestinal bleed, renal dysfunction, etc.), or concurrent arrhythmias. On the other hand, American College of Cardiology/ American Heart Association (ACC/AHA) HF stages are based on risk factors and structural abnormalities of the heart as well as clinical symptoms of HF. The ACC/AHA HF stages are progressive. Once a patient advances to a higher stage of HF, there is no regression to an earlier stage. The HF stages also have prognostic implications—in a population cohort study, a 5-year survival rate for stage A, B, C, and D HF was 97%, 96%, 75%, and 20%, respectively [10].

The NYHA functional classification and the ACC/AHA stages of HF provide complementary information when assessing the severity of HF. While the NYHA classes focus on the functional limitation by HF that is both subjective and dynamic, the ACCF/AHA stages of HF emphasize the development and progression of the disease. Since a majority of the HF patients in the United States are older than 65 years, however, the symptom-based, functional classification can be limited by other comorbidities such as pulmonary or musculoskeletal limitations.

Advanced Heart Failure

Over time, if patients don't succumb to other comorbidities or to cardiac-related sudden death, patients progress to advanced HF, defined as a condition refractory to maximal medical and device therapies with persistent severe symptoms [11]. This corresponds to ACC/AHA HF stage D and NYHA classes III–IV. Patients with advanced HF are considered for special treatment strategies such as implantation of MCS; heart transplantation; other innovative, experimental procedures (e.g., cell therapy); or palliative care. Estimating prognosis in this population is challenging as the clinical course varies significantly across the spectrum of disease severity. Typically, the diagnosis of advanced HF leads to a 1-year mortality rate of 50% [12] and 5-year mortality rate of 80%, comparable to or even worse than those of metastatic cancer.

Etiologies of Heart Failures

About half of the HF cases among adult patients are due to ischemic insult from coronary artery disease, called ischemic cardiomyopathy. This typically results from obstruction of coronary flow due to atherosclerosis, which could be abrupt in the form of acute myocardial infarction, or occult in many cases where only the manifestations of HF rather than overt ischemic symptoms are present. In some cases, chronic ischemia from critically narrowed coronary arteries can also cause functionally reduced yet viable myocardium called hibernating myocardium, which may be reversible with coronary revascularization therapies such as percutaneous coronary interventions or coronary artery bypass graft surgeries.

The other half of the HF cases, collectively called non-ischemic cardiomyopathy, have wide-ranging etiologies, including but not limited to chronic hypertension, structural/ anatomical abnormalities (e.g., congenital heart diseases, valvular heart disease), primary myocardial processes (e.g., hypertrophic cardiomyopathy, dilated cardiomyopathy,

Table 16.1 Stages of HF

ACCF/AHA stages of HF		NYHA functional classification	
A	At risk for HF but without structural heart disease or symptoms of HF	None	
B	Structural heart disease but without signs or symptoms of HF	I	No limitation of physical activity. Ordinary physical activity does not cause symptoms of HF
C	Structural heart disease with prior or current symptoms of HF	II	Slight limitation of physical activity. Comfortable at rest, but ordinary activity results in symptoms of HF
		III	Marked limitation of physical activity. Comfortable at rest, but less than ordinary activity causes symptoms of HF
D	Refractory HF requiring specialized interventions	IV	Unable to carry on physical activity without symptoms of HF or symptoms of HF at rest

arrhythmogenic right ventricular cardiomyopathy, left ventricular non-compaction), infiltrative processes (e.g., hemochromatosis, amyloidosis, and sarcoidosis), drugs/toxins (e.g., alcohol, cocaine, amphetamine, chemotherapies, acute stress/catecholamine surge, and radiation), inflammation (e.g., idiopathic, infective, and autoimmune), and endocrine/metabolic abnormalities (e.g., thyrotoxicosis, diabetic cardiomyopathy, peripartum cardiomyopathy). Identifying the underlying causes of HF can help risk-stratify patients and customize treatments beyond conventional HF therapies. For instance, patients with amyloid cardiomyopathy have a grave prognosis if untreated (median survival approximately 13 months) and may benefit from chemotherapies to eradicate the plasma cells responsible for amyloid production. Or, if patients suffer from HF due to acute or chronic substance abuse in the form of alcohol or cocaine, abstinence from these substances itself can potentially lead to complete or partial recovery of the cardiac function.

Treatment Options for Advanced Heart Failure

The guideline-directed HF therapies are aimed to alleviate symptoms, prevent disease progression, and prolong survival. Once these treatments are no longer effective, alternative options may be considered such as heart transplantation, implantation of permanent MCS, and palliative therapy with or without continuous inotropic support. The decisions on these approaches are complex and depend on both what is medically reasonable for the patient and the patient's values and goals of care. Therefore, comprehensive medical and psychosocial evaluations are necessary when considering advanced therapies. In cases of acute presentation with cardiogenic shock where a patient's cognitive and communicative capacities can be compromised, it may not be possible to sufficiently assess the patient's psychological capacities to cope with illness or to comply with medical therapies required for the advanced HF intervention.

In general, heart transplantation is considered as the gold standard therapy for advanced HF. According to the 2016 33rd ISHLT Registry Report [13], more than 113,000 heart transplantations have been performed worldwide since 1983, with nearly 5000 heart transplantations performed every year. The actual number of transplantations is likely higher given the presence of under-reporting outside of the United States. The number of heart transplantations performed annually has largely plateaued since the early 1990s, reflective of the limited organ availability. With advancements in surgical techniques and the post-transplant care, the outcomes following heart transplantation has improved dramatically, with 1-year survival rate of 90% and 10-year survival rate greater than 50% [13].

However, the number of potential organ donors remains insufficient to meet the growing need for heart transplantation. In response to this mismatch, permanent MCS devices such as the left ventricular assist device (LVAD) have been developed to treat advanced systolic HF. The LVAD is a surgically implanted mechanical device that collects blood from the LV and delivers the blood to the aorta, providing circulatory support for the body without relying on intrinsic LV function (see Chap.18 for further details). The LVAD may be used as (1) destination therapy (DT) for patients in whom heart transplantation is not an option due to advanced age, significant comorbidities, or other inadequate social circumstances, (2) bridge-to-eligibility (BTE) for those who are not considered ideal transplant candidates at the time of the surgery (e.g., due to unresolved psychosocial issues, relatively recent cancer, significant but possibly reversible end-organ dysfunctions, etc.) or those with reversible cardiac pathology with a higher chance of recovery, or (3) bridge-to-transplant (BTT) for patients in whom heart transplantation is anticipated and planned but who require immediate intervention for impending clinical deterioration. Due to limited organ availability, BTT is increasingly used to provide hemodynamic stability for those awaiting heart transplantation. Approximately 5.6% of the heart transplant recipients were under MCS at the time of the surgery in 1998 versus 24.1% in 2011 [14]. However, it is important to point out that MCS devices are associated with high rates of complications, including infections, bleeding, thrombosis, and cerebrovascular accidents [15]. With more patients under MCS before transplantation, heart transplant candidates are at risk for increasing medical comorbidities.

Alternatively, for patients who are medically deemed inappropriate for advanced therapies or whose wishes are not consistent with the invasive surgical approaches, medical care can be directed at managing symptoms and improving the quality of life with palliative measures such as continuous intravenous inotropic support, supplemental oxygen, diuretics, and opioids to relieve dyspnea. These measures do not significantly prolong life expectancy and can be delivered at home with the help of hospice agency geared toward maximal comfort.

Indications for Heart Transplantation

ACC/AHA and ISHLT guidelines include the following indications for heart transplantation (Table 16.2) [5, 6, 16]: (1) cardiogenic shock requiring mechanical circulatory support or inotropic drugs; (2) refractory end-stage HF consistent with NYHA class 4 or ACC/AHA stage D despite optimal therapy; (3) recurrent life-threatening arrhythmias despite maximal interventions; or, rarely, (4) refractory angina without potential for revascularization. With increasing use of

Table 16.2 Indications for heart transplantation

Listing criteria for cardiac transplantation
Cardiogenic shock requiring continuous intavenous inotropic therapy or mechanical circulatory support
NYHA class IV HF symptoms despite maximized medical and resynchronization therapy AND VO₂: For patients intolerant of beta-blocker therapy, a peak VO$_2$ ≤ 14 mL/kg/min For patients on beta-blocker therapy, a peak VO$_2$ ≤ 12 mL/kg/min For patients who are young (<50 years old) or women, peak VO$_2$ < 50% predicted may be used as an alternative criterion
Selective NYHA class III or IV patients with restrictive or hypertrophic cardiomyopathies (including those with cardiac amyloidosis)
Recurrent, intractable life-threatening left ventricular arrhythmias despite an implantable cardiac defibrillator, antiarrhythmic therapy, or catheter-based ablation
Refractory angina without potential medical or surgical therapeutic options
End-stage congenital HF with no evidence of pulmonary hypertension

continuous LVAD as BTT, there is a growing number of post-LVAD patients on the transplant list. Additionally, as more patients with congenital heart disease are surviving to an older age, growing number of adult patients with repaired congenital heart defect and progressive heart failure are being considered for heart transplantation [17].

All patients who are actively considered for heart transplantation must undergo an extensive medical and psychosocial evaluation by a designated transplant team to stratify the overall medical and psychosocial risk and the urgency of heart transplantation. In this chapter, we will primarily focus on the medical evaluation required prior to the listing for heart transplantation.

Understanding the balance of HF-related risk and perioperative risk is critical in identifying patients who would derive the most benefit from heart transplantation. First, beyond the ACC/AHA and NYHA stages of HF, other objective data assessing one's cardiac function, such as echocardiographic and hemodynamic parameters, should be included when evaluating patients for transplantation candidacy. In particular, a noninvasive hemodynamic testing, often termed as cardiopulmonary exercise physiology test (CPX), is useful in screening and monitoring ambulatory patients with HF. It provides an objective assessment of a patient's functional and physiological capacities and also estimates cardiac output by measuring its surrogate marker, peak oxygen consumption rate (peak VO₂). A peak VO₂ less than 14 mL/kg/min or 12 mL/kg/min while on beta-blockade therapy indicates a poor prognosis with a survival rate that is less than that of a transplant (Table 16.2), thus warranting initiation of heart transplantation evaluation. Additionally, invasive right heart catheterization (RHC) should be performed in all transplant candidates

periodically (e.g., every 6 months at Stanford) to document their hemodynamic parameters (e.g., cardiac output, pulmonary artery pressures) and to evaluate for the presence of reversible or irreversible pulmonary hypertension (pHTN) which is relevant to both heart transplant and MCS candidacy.

To further determine the suitability of listing patients for heart transplantation, especially in cases where hemodynamic measures are ambiguous, risk models may be used. While estimating individual prognosis is difficult due to the large variability in clinical course even within the same HF stage, few scoring systems have been developed to predict outcomes in HF, such as the Seattle Heart Failure Model (SHFM) [18] and the Heart Failure Survival Score (HFSS) [19] that utilize the combination of clinical, echocardiographic, and laboratory data. Generally, estimated 1-year survival of less than 80% on SHFM or high−/medium-risk range on HFSS with a score of less than 8.1 correlating with a 1-year survival rate of less than 72% is considered to favor listing for heart transplantation. However, it is important to note that the results of these risk models alone should not be used as a sole determinant for heart transplantation listing.

Assessment of End Organs for Potential Multi-organ Transplantation

The end-organ functions (e.g., kidneys, lungs, and liver) depend on adequate perfusion from the heart. Impaired cardiac function may lead to temporary or irreversible damage to the organs. Inadequate function of these vital organs may lead to poor outcome following heart transplantation. Therefore, it is critical to accurately assess end-organs' status as a part of the heart transplant evaluation. To determine whether concurrent end-organ dysfunction would likely complicate the outcome of the heart transplant, careful evaluations should be performed to assess (1) how much of the observed dysfunction is related to cardiac limitation and (2) to what extent it is reversible, often assessed by preoperative interventions such as withdrawal of nephrotoxic medications or initiation of inotropic or circulatory support. In cases where significant, irreversible end-organ dysfunction is present, heart transplantation is generally considered contraindicated, unless concurrent listing for the transplant of those affected organs is planned. Therefore, it is necessary to distinguish patients with reversible end-organ failure from those patients with advanced, irreversible end-stage disease. Thus far, multi-organ transplantations including combined heart-kidney, heart-lung, and heart-liver have been successfully accomplished. However, these aforementioned combinations comprise only a minority of overall heart transplant operations.

Renal dysfunction is common among patients with HF and may be due to a combination of congestion from the high filling pressure and reduced perfusion from the low cardiac output (also known as the cardiorenal syndrome). It may also result from predisposed conditions such as diabetes, hypertension, or primary renal disease, all of which are risk factors for HF. Kidney function can be evaluated by creatinine clearance, the presence of significant protein in the urine (proteinuria), and ultrasound of the kidneys. To determine the reversibility of underlying renal dysfunction, medical or device manipulation can be attempted to temporarily augment cardiac output and correlate with changes in renal function. Generally, irreversible renal dysfunction with serum creatinine level > 2 mg/dL or creatinine clearance <30 (mL/min/1.73 m^2) is considered as a relative contraindication to cardiac transplantation without plans for concurrent listing for the kidney.

Pulmonary disease can be subdivided into the primary parenchymal disease (e.g., chronic obstructive lung disease, interstitial lung disease) or the pulmonary vascular disease (e.g., pulmonary hypertension (pHTN)). Primary parenchymal disease can be assessed by pulmonary function test and chest imaging such as chest X-ray and computerized tomography (CT) scan. Since infection or pulmonary congestion can transiently alter the results of these tests, it is important to optimize one's medical condition prior to the evaluation. Given the high arrhythmia burden among advanced HF population with subsequent increased use of amiodarone therapy, there is a relatively high incidence of amiodarone pulmonary toxicity (APT) in up to 2–5% of the cases. APT largely depends on cumulative exposure and can be reversible upon withdrawing the drug, highlighting the importance of detecting this side effect early in the clinical course.

The pulmonary vascular disease can be assessed by invasive hemodynamic studies (RHC) directly measuring pulmonary arterial pressures and pulmonary vascular resistance or by echocardiogram with Doppler studies estimating relevant pulmonary pressures. pHTN is most frequently caused by left-sided HF with chronic pressure overload, although other etiologies such as thromboembolic disease or primary pulmonary vascular disease should be considered when the degree of pHTN is out of proportion to the underlying HF. Generally, significant pulmonary dysfunction or advanced pHTN defined as pulmonary artery systolic pressure > 50 mmHg or pulmonary vascular resistance > 3 WU despite vasodilator challenge during RHC are considered a contraindication to heart transplantation without plans for concurrent listing for the lungs. See Chap. 22 for further discussion of heart-lung transplantation.

Abnormal liver function is also frequently seen in HF population and is a predictor of adverse outcome following heart transplantation. The liver disease may develop from chronic right-sided HF with resultant pressure overload to the liver, toxicities from cardiovascular drugs (e.g., amiodarone), genetic predisposition (e.g., hemochromatosis), or other comorbid conditions such as chronic hepatitis infections, alcohol use disorder, or metabolic syndrome. The initial assessment of the liver includes (1) blood tests with liver function tests and serum markers for its synthetic function including albumin and international normalized ratio (INR) and (2) imaging studies such as ultrasound or computed tomography (CT) scan. A disproportionately low albumin level (<2.5 g/dL) places patients at significant surgical risk and should prompt a workup for protein-losing enteropathy (PLE), a rare condition associated with right-sided HF especially in patients with congenital heart defects. If there is any concern for cirrhosis, a liver biopsy should be considered and can be performed at the same time of RHC via transjugular approach to assess the degree of liver damage. If there is evidence of biopsy-proven cirrhosis, transplant with heart alone is generally contraindicated. Alternatively in some cases, adequate synthetic function and minimal portal hypertension may allow recovery of the liver function after cardiac transplant. Clinical manifestations of end-stage liver disease, such as refractory ascites, impaired synthetic function, and the presence of varices, portend overall poor prognosis and warrant consideration for concurrent listing for the liver transplantation.

Assessment of Immunologic Status

Immunocompatibility is another important consideration when assessing patients for their transplant candidacy. Heart transplantation generally requires donor-recipient ABO blood group matching as well as human leukocyte antigen (HLA) histocompatibility. The recipient's pre-existing significant allosensitization to HLA has been associated with adverse outcomes including higher rates of acute rejection, premature graft failure, and allograft vasculopathy. Therefore, all transplant candidates must be screened for allosensitization, measured by % panel reactive antibodies (PRA). Significant allosensitization is most likely to be present in females with multiple pregnancies, patients who have received numerous blood transfusions, and those with prior extensive surgeries such as implantation of MCS or complex congenital heart reparative surgeries. Although a high PRA is not a contraindication to transplantation, it is associated with a marked decrease in suitable donor availability. Besides the efforts to "virtually cross-match" those highly sensitized patients (calculated PRA > 50%) with potential donors, strategies to reduce PRA are underway. Presently, these patients are often treated with plasmapheresis and/or intravenous immunoglobulin (IVIG) and sometimes more aggressive measures with immunosuppressives [20].

Contraindications to Heart Transplantation

Contraindications to heart transplantation besides concurrent end-organ failure continue to evolve, especially with advances in other medical therapies (e.g., development of antiviral drugs to treat human immunodeficiency virus (HIV) or hepatitis C virus (HCV)). Per 2016 ISHLT listing criteria [6], heart transplantation is contraindicated when patients (1) have any severe systemic illness (e.g., malignancy, inflammatory condition, or chronic infection) that would significantly reduce expected life expectancy despite heart transplantation, (2) suffer from severe symptomatic cerebrovascular disease, (3) are engaged in active substance (drug or alcohol) abuse, or (4) demonstrate inability to comply with drug therapy (Table 16.3). Considering 5-year post-transplant survival rates approaching 80% with a median survival of 11 years [21, 22], immediate identification, treatment, and monitoring of some of these conditions (e.g., substance use disorders, nonadherence) might make transplantation still possible and successful.

There are a number of relative contraindications to heart transplant; one of the most debated and variable among transplant centers is the upper age limit for consideration. In general, patients older than 70 years are considered ineligi-

Table 16.3 Contraindications to Heart Transplantation (Stanford)

Absolute contraindications
Systemic illness with a life expectancy <5 years despite heart transplantation.
Irreversible pulmonary hypertension with pulmonary vascular resistance >3 Wood Units (WU)
Clinically severe symptomatic cerebrovascular disease
Active substance (drug or alcohol) abuse
Inability to comply with drug therapy
Multisystem disease with severe and likely irreversible extracardiac organ dysfunction
Relative contraindications
Age > 70 years
Extremes of the weight (i.e., body mass index >35 or < 18 kg/m²)
Diabetes mellitus with poor glycemic control (HbA1c > 7.5%) despite optimal effort or end-organ damage other than nonproliferative retinopathy
Irreversible renal dysfunction (eGFR <30 ml/min/1.73 m²)
Neoplasm (requires individualized assessment of severity, treatment options, and prognosis)
Infection (requires individualized assessment of severity, treatment options, and prognosis)
Acute pulmonary embolism (within 6–8 weeks)
Tobacco use (within 6 months)
Recent past (within 6 months) substance (drug or alcohol) abuse
Frailty
Inadequate social support or cognitive-behavioral disability that would prevent compliant care
Other conditions that increase the risk of perioperative complications or limit tolerance of immunosuppression

ble due to their age-related comorbidities and limitations. Instead, they are more often managed with high-risk reparative surgery or permanent MCS implantation as DT. However, the recent heart transplant guidelines indicated that carefully selected patients aged > 70 years may be considered for heart transplantation. Thus, individual centers must determine their own age cutoff.

Extremes in weight, as measured by body mass index (BMI) either > 35 for severe obesity or <18 for cachexia, have also been shown to worsen post-transplant prognosis. Additionally, the presence of clinically severe symptomatic cerebrovascular disease, severe peripheral vascular disease interfering with rehabilitation potential, and poorly controlled diabetes also portends worse outcome and is therefore considered relative contraindications. Recently, frailty, defined as 3 and more of 5 possible symptoms, including unintentional weight loss of greater than 4.5 kg (10 lbs) within the past year, muscle loss, fatigue, slow walking speed, and low levels of physical activity, has been increasingly recognized as an important measure predicting poor outcome. Finally, psychological instability (e.g., untreated severe depression or anxiety) or any active or recent (within 6 months) substance abuse (alcohol, cocaine, opioids, tobacco products, etc.) are also considered potential contraindications given the concern for inability to comply with complex medical therapies following heart transplantation leading to the risk of early graft failure. Chronic mental illness, even when adequately treated, can influence patients' overall survival outcomes and therefore must be taken into consideration when assessing for patients' post-transplant mortality risk and needed treatment and follow-up. Some of the parameters specifically related to nutrition and frailty can progress after transplant listing and therefore should be monitored regularly with routine surveillance.

Besides indications and contraindications related to the patient's medical conditions, adequate cognitive and psychological status, as well as psychosocial support, are considered critical in predicting better outcomes after the heart transplant. Detailed psychosocial evaluation for transplant listing is addressed in Chap. 3.

Heart Transplant Listing

The ultimate decision on whether and when to place a patient on the heart transplantation waiting list is made after careful review of the indications and contraindications based on collected data and clinical judgment by a designated selection committee at a transplant center. For example, the transplant team at Stanford is comprised of cardiac transplant surgeons, heart failure and post-transplant physician specialists, psychiatrists, social workers, dieticians, pharmacists, occupational therapists, and nurses, all of whom have important contribution to the final decision. The team meets weekly to review newly presented patient cases as well as those already on the list and extensively discusses their eligibility for the heart transplant listing. If a concurrent listing of non-cardiac organs is considered, the relevant other transplant team(s) also participates in the review process. The overall heart

transplantation evaluation and decision-making process at Stanford is summarized in Fig. 16.1.

Once approved for listing, active heart transplantation candidates are further stratified based on their medical urgency. According to the United Network for Organ Sharing (UNOS) which was established in 1984 by an Act of Congress to facilitate equitable organ sharing within the United States, the current adult heart allocation system

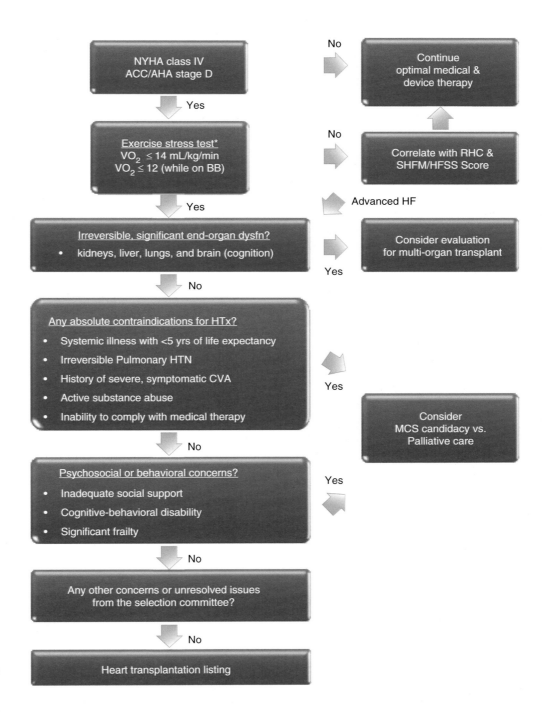

Fig. 16.1 Stanford pre-heart transplantation algorithm. *If ambulatory (outpatient setting). Abbreviations: BB beta-blockade, CVA cerebrovascular accident, HFSS Heart Failure Survival Score, HTN hypertension, HTx heart transplantation, MCS mechanical circulatory support, RHC right heart catheterization, SHFM Seattle Heart Failure Model

stratifies active candidates into three tiers: statuses 1A, 1B, and 2. Candidates qualify for status 1A, if they:

- Require a continuous infusion of a single high-dose intravenous inotrope or multiple intravenous inotropes *and* continuous hemodynamic monitoring (usually monitored in the intensive care unit in a hospital)
- Are supported by a total artificial heart, an intra-aortic balloon pump (IABP), extracorporeal mechanical oxygenation (ECMO), mechanical ventilation, or a ventricular assist device (VAD) (for a 30-day discretionary period)
- Are implanted with a permanent MCS device and are experiencing a device-related complication

Exceptions on the listing priority (denoted as 1AE or 1BE) may be granted if patients are:

- Suffering from poorly controlled life-threatening arrhythmia such as VT storm; or
- NOT candidates for inotropic and/or invasive monitoring because of arrhythmic potential or anatomical limitations (e.g. the anatomy of patients with adult congenital heart disease may not be amenable for pulmonary artery cannulation for hemodynamic monitoring)
- NOT candidates for MCS support as BTT (e.g. hypertrophic cardiomyopathy, infiltrative/restrictive cardiomyopathy, primary RV failure, or complex congenital heart disease)
- Highly allosensitized and have very low likelihood of getting an appropriate offer in a timely manner without prioritization

Candidates that are stable and either supported by MCS or continuous infusion of intravenous inotropes without meeting the criteria for status 1A qualify for status 1B. Candidates that are in need of a heart transplant but do not meet status 1A or 1B criteria qualify for status 2. If a previously listed patient is temporarily unsuitable to receive heart transplantation (e.g., due to active infection or bleeding), they would be placed on status 7 until the underlying cause is reversed.

Presently, due to prolonged waiting time, a greater percentage of heart transplantation candidates are prioritized as status 1A. In 2001, only 35% of all heart transplantation were performed on UNOS status 1A patients, while in 2011, 55 + % were performed on status 1A patients. Therefore, ongoing efforts have been made to further risk-stratify and identify those at the highest level of medical urgency. There will likely be a move toward a new prioritization scheme in the near future (Table 16.4), which establishes six new medical urgency status levels based on short-term mortality risk

Table 16.4 2017 Revised UNOS heart allocation status (proposed)

Status	Proposed criteria
1	ECMO (up to 14 days of support)
	Non-dischargeable Bi-VAD or RVAD
	Mechanical circulatory support with life-threatening ventricular arrhythmia
2	Intra-aortic balloon pump (up to 14 days of support)
	Acute percutaneous endovascular circulatory support device (up to 14 days of support)
	Ventricular tachycardia/ventricular fibrillation, mechanical support not required
	Mechanical circulatory support with device malfunction/mechanical failure
	Total artificial heart
	Dischargeable Bi-VAD or RVAD
3	LVAD for up to 30 days
	Multiple inotropes or single high-dose inotropes with continuous hemodynamic monitoring (up to 14 days of support)
	Mechanical circulatory support with device-related complications such as infection, hemolysis, or thromboembolism
	Mechanical circulatory support with device infection
	Mechanical circulatory support with thromboembolism
4	Diagnosis of congenital heart disease
	Diagnosis of ischemic heart disease with intractable angina
	Diagnosis of hypertrophic cardiomyopathy
	Diagnosis of restrictive cardiomyopathy
	Stable LVAD candidates after 30 days
	Inotropes without hemodynamic monitoring
	Diagnosis of amyloidosis
	Re-transplant
5	Combined organ transplants
6	All remaining active transplant candidates

Abbreviations: ECMO extracorporeal membrane oxygenation, Bi-VAD bi-ventricular assist device, RVAD right ventricular assist device, LVAD left ventricular assist device

without a transplant. In particular, the updated statuses provide more detailed criteria for when and how MCS treatments impact on the recipient's candidacy.

Conclusions

Heart failure is a major public health issue affecting more than 26 million worldwide. The prevalence of symptomatic HF has continued to rise, and increasingly more patients survive to the advanced phase of the disease with an overall prognosis of 1-year mortality approaching 50%. There is a growing need for advanced treatment strategies such as implantation of MCS and heart transplantation, the ultimate therapy for the HF. Unfortunately, the ability to perform heart transplantation remains largely limited by donor availability. Therefore, it is important to carefully screen and identify optimal candidates who would derive the most benefit while balancing an acceptable perioperative risk. To this end, all patients must undergo extensive medical and psychosocial evaluation as well as surveillance by a designated transplant selection committee to stratify overall risk and the urgency of transplant, examine the involvement of other non-cardiac organs for potential multi-organ listing, determine proper immunologic status, and exclude contraindications for transplant.

References

1. Mozaffarian D, et al. Heart disease and stroke statistics-2016 update a report from the American Heart Association. Circulation. 2016;133:e38–360.
2. Ambrosy AP, et al. The global health and economic burden of hospitalizations for heart failure: lessons learned from hospitalized heart failure registries. J Am Coll Cardiol. 2014;63:1123–33.
3. Cook C, Cole G, Asaria P, Jabbour R, Francis DP. The annual global economic burden of heart failure. Int J Cardiol. 2014;171:368–76.
4. Heidenreich PA, et al. Forecasting the impact of heart failure in the United States a policy statement from the american heart association. Circ Heart Fail. 2013;6:606–19.
5. Yancy CW, et al. 2013 ACCF/AHA guideline for the management of heart failure: a report of the American college of cardiology foundation/american heart association task force on practice guidelines. J Am Coll Cardiol. 2013;62:e147–239.
6. Mehra MR, et al. The 2016 International Society for Heart Lung Transplantation listing criteria for heart transplantation: a 10-year update. J Heart Lung Transplant. 2016;35:1–23.
7. Mehra MR, et al. Guidelines for listing candidates for heart transplant. JAMA Cardiol. 2016;34:1244–54.
8. Jessup M, et al. 2009 focused update: ACCF/AHA guidelines for the diagnosis and Management of Heart Failure in adults: a report of the American College of Cardiology Foundation/American Heart Association Task Force on Practice Guidelines: developed in collaboration with the International Society for Heart and Lung Transplantation. Circulation. 2009;119:1977–2016.
9. Gheorghiade M, et al. Acute heart failure syndromes: current state and framework for future research. Circulation. 2005;112: 3958–68.
10. Ponikowski P, et al. 2016 ESC Guidelines for the diagnosis and treatment of acute and chronic heart failure. Eur Heart J. 2016;37:2129–2200m.
11. Chaudhry S-P, Stewart GC. Advanced heart failure: prevalence, natural history, and prognosis. Heart Fail Clin. 2016;12: 323–33.
12. Friedrich EB, Böhm M. Management of end stage heart failure. Heart. 2007;93:626–31.
13. Yusen RD, et al. The registry of the International Society for Heart and Lung Transplantation: thirty-third adult heart transplantation report – 2016; Focus theme: primary diagnostic indications for transplant. J Heart Lung Transplant. 2016;35:1170–84.
14. Mancini DM, Schulze PC. Heart transplant allocation: in desperate need of revision. J Am Coll Cardiol. 2014;63:1179–81.
15. Gustafsson F, Rogers JG. Left ventricular assist device therapy in advanced heart failure: patient selection and outcomes. Eur J Heart Fail. 2017;19:1–8.
16. Mancini D, Lietz K. Selection of cardiac transplantation candidates in 2010. Circulation. 2010;122:173–83.
17. Doumouras BS, et al. Outcomes in adult congenital heart disease patients undergoing heart transplantation: a systematic review and meta-analysis. J Heart Lung Transplant. 2016;35:1337–47.
18. Levy WC, et al. The seattle heart failure model. Circulation. 2006;113:1424 LP–1433.
19. Aaronson KD, et al. Development and prospective validation of a clinical index to predict survival in ambulatory patients referred for cardiac transplant evaluation. Circulation. 1997;95: 2660 LP–2667.
20. Eckman PM, Hanna M, Taylor DO, Starling RC, Gonzalez-Stawinski GV. Management of the sensitized adult heart transplant candidate. Clin Transpl. 2010;24:726–34.
21. Politi P, et al. Ten years of 'extended' life: quality of life among heart transplantation survivors. Transp J. 2004;78:257–63.
22. Yusen RD, et al. The registry of the International Society for Heart and Lung Transplantation: thirty-second official adult lung and heart-lung transplantation report – 2015; Focus theme: early graft failure. J Heart Lung Transplant. 2015;34:1264–77.

Mental Health in Chronic and End-Stage Heart Disease

Mental Health in Chronic and End-Stage Heart Disease

17

Yelizaveta Sher

Introduction

Heart disease and psychiatric comorbidities have bidirectional relationships. While such psychiatric comorbidities as depression, anxiety, and tobacco dependence increase risk of heart disease, patients with heart disease have increased rates of depression, anxiety, and cognitive dysfunction. In fact, heart disease is one of the original playing fields of psychosomatic medicine with psychosomatic medicine physicians and researchers exploring the links between cardiac disease and personality types (such as "type D," distressed personality) [1]. Many studies have been conducted on the interplay between depression and heart disease, including its pathophysiology, epidemiology, and treatments. In this chapter, we will explore some of this knowledge and learn how it applies to patients struggling with heart disease and those being considered or preparing for heart transplantation.

Depression and Heart Disease

Epidemiology

Depression and heart disease have bidirectional influence. Depression increases the risk for the development of cardiovascular disease [2]. In fact, a meta-analysis by Wulsin and Singal demonstrated that depression is associated with a 60% increased risk of developing incident coronary artery disease (CAD) [3]. On the other hand, patients with heart disease have increased rates of depression as compared to those without heart disease. Moreover, depression in patients with heart disease worsens clinical outcomes and increases mortality [4–6].

While 17–27% of patients with heart disease have major depression at some point in their life, even greater numbers of patients experience minor depressive symptoms [7]. In addition, clinically significant depression is present in a fifth of heart failure (HF) patients, with higher incidence (35–70%) in hospitalized patients, as compared to outpatients (10–35%) [8]. Depression worsens quality of life and increases risk of hospitalization in patients with heart disease and HF [6, 9–15]. When depression is chronic and worsening, it is the single most important driver of healthcare-related costs in patients with HF over 3 years [16]. Depression is a more significant contributor to decreased quality of life in patients with HF, than the actual measures of HF severity, such as left ventricular ejection fraction, New York Heart Association (NYHA) functional status, and N-terminal prohormone of brain natriuretic peptide levels, which show only mild associations [6, 10].

Multiple studies have demonstrated that similar to more traditional risk factors for mortality (i.e., smoking, diabetes, and hypertension), depression increases the risk of mortality in patients with heart disease [17–19]. In a meta-analysis of 20 prospective studies of patients with stable ischemic heart disease, history of myocardial infraction (MI), coronary bypass graft (CABG) surgery, or percutaneous transluminal coronary angioplasty, depressive symptoms were associated with twice as high mortality during the 2-year follow-up period as compared to no depressive symptoms [20]. In patients who have undergone CABG surgery, depression was associated with progression of atherosclerotic disease in the graft and narrowing of the graft diameter [21].

Depression can remain a poor prognosticator even many years after its diagnosis. In a prospective study of patients admitted to a cardiology service for severe HF, 30.1% of patients were diagnosed with clinically significant baseline depression (i.e., Beck's Depression Inventory (BDI) ≥ 10) [22]. Patients were followed for up to 12 years after this admission (mean 1792.3 days). While 73% of non-depressed patients died during this time, 80% of

Y. Sher (✉)
Department of Psychiatry and Behavioral Sciences, Stanford University School of Medicine, Stanford, CA, USA
e-mail: ysher@stanford.edu

depressed patients died during the same period ($P = 0.01$; hazard ratio (HR) 1.35; 95% confidence interval (CI) 1.15–1.57) [22].

Mechanisms

Several mechanisms have been proposed and studied to explain the increased comorbidity of depression and heart disease. These mechanisms include serotonergic dysfunction, systemic inflammation and immune activation, hypothalamic-pituitary-adrenal axis and autonomic nervous system dysfunction, vascular changes, decreased heart rate variability, genetic changes in short allele of serotonin transporter gene-linked polymorphic region, and variations in von Willebrand factor (vWF) gene [5, 6]. In addition, psychosocial factors usually associated with depression, such as increased rates of smoking, nonadherence to medical regimens, sedentary lifestyle, and weight changes, including visceral fat accumulation, may exacerbate this connection [5]. Moreover, decreased concentrations of omega-3 fatty acids have been shown both in patients with cardiovascular disease and patients with depression [6].

Treatment

While there is some evidence that treatment of depression with selective serotonin reuptake inhibitors (SSRIs) might increase remission rates of depression in patients with coronary heart disease (CHD), these treatments have not produced an effect on reducing mortality in these patients [23–25]. Moreover, studies on treatment of depression with standard pharmacological agents in patients with HF have not produced consistent positive results [26–28].

Treatment of Depression in Patients with Heart Disease

In the Sertraline Antidepressant Heart Attack Randomized Trial (SADHART), 369 patients with MI or unstable angina and major depressive disorder (MDD) from the United States, Canada, Europe, and Australia were randomized to receive sertraline or placebo [23]. At the end of 24 weeks, there was no difference in the primary end point of change in left ventricular function or other cardiac parameters, including change in QTc interval. However, sertraline was more effective than placebo for treatment of depression, especially in patients with recurrent and more severe depression.

In the Enhancing Recovery in Coronary Heart Disease Patients (ENRICHD) trial, post-MI patients with depression or low social support were randomized to cognitive behavioral therapy (CBT) or treatment as usual [29]. Patients with more severe depression or not responding to CBT were also treated with an SSRI, in non-randomized fashion. While patients treated with CBT did better in terms of depression scores at 6 months, the difference between the groups disappeared by 30 months. There was also no difference in MI recurrence or mortality. Post-hoc analysis showed that patients who received SSRIs had lower rates of MI recurrence or mortality (HR 0.57) [30].

The Myocardial Infarction and Depression Intervention Trial (MIND-IT) randomized 331 patients with acute MI and depression to an antidepressant treatment (i.e., mirtazapine, citalopram) versus usual care (which included antidepressant for some patients) in an effectiveness trial [24]. There was no difference between two groups at 18 months in terms of depression outcomes or cardiac event rates. Medications were well-tolerated.

The Canadian Cardiac Randomized Evaluation of Antidepressant and Psychotherapy Efficacy (CREATE) randomized 284 patients with stable angina and depression in 2 × 2 factorial trial to citalopram and/or interpersonal therapy (IPT) [25]. While patients on citalopram did better with mean Hamilton Depression Rating Scale (HAM-D) difference of 3.3 points (14.9 vs 11.6 point reduction; $P = 0.05$), IPT did not show superiority over treatment as usual. Similar to SADHART study [23], the subgroup analysis demonstrated that citalopram had a significant effect on recurrent, and not the first episode, depression. The Escitalopram for DEPression in Acute Coronary Syndrome (EsDEPACS) study showed that escitalopram was well-tolerated and more effective for treatment of depression in a trial of 217 patients after a confirmed acute coronary syndrome, as compared to placebo [31].

A study of 248 patients with acute coronary artery disease evaluated the efficacy of bupropion for its safety and efficacy for smoking cessation in a 12-week, placebo-controlled trial [32]. Of note, patients with major depression were excluded. While there was no difference in smoking cessation between two groups, bupropion was found to be safe for cardiac patients with no statistically significant differences in mortality, blood pressure, or cardiovascular events between the two groups.

Additional studies have explored non-pharmacological interventions. Blumenthal et al. randomized patients with CHD and depression to either exercise versus sertraline versus placebo. The study found that both sertraline and exercise were associated with reductions in depressive symptoms as compared to placebo [33]. There was also a trend toward improvement in heart rate variability with both active treatments, with exercise having a greater effect compared to sertraline. A Stepwise Psychotherapy Intervention for Reducing Risk in Coronary Artery Disease (SPIRR-CAD) trial also demonstrated effectiveness of psychotherapy in patients with CAD [34].

Treatment of Depression in Patients with Heart Failure

While there is some evidence to support the treatment of depression with traditional pharmacological agents in patients with stable CAD or after acute coronary syndrome [23, 24, 31], randomized control trials (RCTs) evaluating SSRIs in patients with HF have not had the same success with treatment of depression.

Earlier small non-randomized studies have examined fluoxetine, paroxetine, and sertraline in patients with HF, demonstrating safety and improvement in depression and cognitive status [26]. However, larger RCTs with SSRIs have not been as encouraging.

In particular, the Sertraline Against Depression and Heart Disease in Chronic Heart Failure (SADHART-CHF), which included 469 patients, did not show sertraline's effectiveness in decreasing depression rates or adverse cardiovascular clinical outcomes [27]. However, a sub-study has demonstrated that patients whose depression remitted after 12 weeks, regardless of whether they received sertraline or placebo, had indeed improved mortality. Thus, while particular depression treatment is not associated with improved mortality, remission of depression is.

Similarly, a German study, the Morbidity, Mortality, and Mood in Depressed Heart Failure Patients (MOOD-HF), on treatment of depression in HF patients with escitalopram, did not demonstrate difference in the primary outcome of death or rehospitalization or in-between group difference in depression remission at 12 weeks [28]. However, the study demonstrated that escitalopram was safe in patients with HF.

Given these results, studies on non-pharmacological interventions, such as psychotherapy and exercise, have taken an even greater importance in patients with HF.

A study of CBT in patients with HF, patients were randomized to usual care ($n = 79$) versus CBT ($n = 79$) [35]. At 6 months of follow-up, depression scores were lower and remission rates higher in the CBT group as compared to usual care group, with the number needed to treat between 3 and 4. In addition, anxiety and fatigue scores were lower in the CBT arm, and health-related quality of life and social functioning were also improved. However, scores indicating HF self-care and physical functioning remained unchanged.

A large multicenter trial on group-based meta-cognitive therapy, PATHWAY Group MCT, is underway in the United Kingdom [36]. This trial is investigating the clinical outcomes and cost-effectiveness of this particular modality in patients with depression and anxiety attending cardiac rehabilitation and results are expected with great interest.

Exercise has been evaluated for the treatment of depression in HF patients. The Heart Failure – A Controlled Trial Investigating Outcomes of Exercise Training study (HF-ACTION) demonstrated that aerobic exercise resulted in a small, but significant, reduction in depressive symptoms

in HF patients (1.75 point reduction in BDI-II scores compared with 0.98 point reduction in usual care), with even larger reduction in patients with clinically significant depression (2.2 point reduction versus 1.3 in the usual care group) [37].

Of note, loss of energy and fatigue are the most common symptoms that persist after treatment of depression in patients with heart disease. This may be significant as somatic symptoms of depression are correlated with increased morbidity and mortality in this patient population to a greater degree compared to cognitive symptoms [38].

Given the prevalence of heart disease and depression, and recognition of the association and prognostication between the two, it is important to establish systems to effectively screen cardiac patients for depression and to allow easy and wide access to mental health services and interventions. Collaborative care models have been shown to be promising in provision of better care for patients with heart disease, leading to reduction in depressive symptoms [4, 39].

Safety of Antidepressants in Patients with Heart Disease and Drug-Drug Interactions

Although studies have demonstrated that antidepressants, in particular SSRIs, can be safely used in patients with CHD, clinicians should be aware about potential side effects.

One concern with certain psychotropic medications includes their contribution to QTc prolongation, which may lead to an increased risk of torsades de points, a potentially lethal arrhythmia. Most psychotropics have propensity to increase QTc with debatable translation into clinical relevance and risks [40]. While tricyclic antidepressants (TCAs) increase the QTc interval via blockage of sodium and calcium channels, SSRIs can prolong QTc via their effect on potassium rectifier channels [40]. Among TCAs, amitriptyline has the largest risk of prolonging the QTc interval [40, 41]. On the other hand, among SSRI agents, citalopram has the most prominent dose-dependent effect on QTc prolongation, leading the Federal Drug Administration (FDA) to issue warning against its use in doses higher than 40 mg per day, as well as caution in elderly patients [40, 41]. Citalopram's cousin, escitalopram, has a lesser QTc prolongation effects, thus far with no warning issued by the FDA [40, 41].

Since SSRIs and serotonin-norepinephrine reuptake inhibitors (SNRIs) can decrease platelet aggregation, via inhibition of serotonin reuptake in the presynaptic neuronal membrane and uptake by platelets, there is a theoretical increased risk for bleeding when using these agents. A recent meta-analysis of studies on patients undergoing CABG found that while SSRI use was associated with an increased risk for the need of red blood cell transfusion (odds ratio (OR) = 1.15; 95% CI 1.06–1.26), there was no documented change in the rate of reoperation due to bleeding (OR = 1.07; 95% CI 0.66–1.74), rates of platelet

(OR = 0.93; 95% CI 0.79–1.09) or fresh frozen plasma (OR = 0.96; 95% CI 0.74–1.24) transfusion, or the mortality rate (OR = 1.03; 95% CI 0.90–1.17) [42]. However, caution should be used in patients with low platelets or those on blood-thinning agents, such as aspirin, nonsteroidal anti-inflammatory agents, and clopidogrel. Of course, in patients with CAD, this mechanism of SSRIs has been also postulated to be therapeutic [43].

Since many cardiac medications, in particular beta-blockers (e.g., carvedilol, propranolol, and metoprolol) and antiarrhythmics, are metabolized via CYP-2D6, the use of antidepressant agents with potent CYP-2D6 inhibition (i.e., bupropion, fluoxetine, duloxetine, and paroxetine) may increase their levels leading to potential adverse drug-drug interactions and side effects (e.g., hypotension) [44]. On the other hand, some antidepressant medications are potent CYP-3A4 inhibitors (e.g., fluoxetine and fluvoxamine) which can cause increased levels and potential side effects when combined with agents that are metabolized via CYP-3A4 (e.g., statins). For more information, please refer to an excellent chapter by Shapiro in "Clinical Manual of Psychopharmacology in the Medically Ill" [44].

Treatment Algorithms

When treating patients with depression and cardiac disease, non-pharmacological interventions, such as exercise and therapy, should be implemented whenever possible. When considering pharmacological treatments, sertraline would likely be the first choice among psychotropic medication-naïve patients. Other SSRIs, such as escitalopram and citalopram, are good choices as well, with close consideration and monitoring for QTc, especially with citalopram. Citalopram, escitalopram, and sertraline (at lower doses) are also advantageous due to lack of significant CYP interactions [44]. Second-line agents include mirtazapine (especially in patients with loss of appetite and cachexia), bupropion (in patients with low energy, concentration, and amotivation), and duloxetine or venlafaxine (in patients with pain or diabetic neuropathy). Blood pressures should be monitored with the latter three agents. Nortriptyline is the third-line agent in patients with severe treatment-refractory depression, with close monitoring and follow-up [44].

Anxiety and Heart Disease

Epidemiology

Anxiety disorders and symptoms are common in patients with heart disease and HF; however, there is less literature on the associations, significance, and treatment of anxiety in cardiac patients, as compared to those of depression.

Relationship between anxiety disorders and heart disease is bidirectional, with anxiety contributing to the risk of heart disease development and heart disease increasing the odds of anxiety symptoms.

A variety of anxiety disorders and symptoms have been shown to increase the risk of heart disease. An earlier meta-analysis by Tully et al. evaluating different anxiety disorders and cardiovascular complications noted that there was a non-significant association between generalized anxiety disorder (GAD) and major adverse cardiac events (MACE) with significant effect size for outpatients (adjusted HR = 1.9; 95% CI 1.5–2.6; P < 0.001) [45]. This study did not find the associations between other anxiety disorders and MACE, but noted significant heterogeneity between studies' assessment methods. Another meta-analysis did show that individuals with anxiety were at increased risk for developing CHD (HR 1.3; 95% CI 1.2–1.4; p < 0.0001) and cardiac death (HR 1.5; 95% CI 1.1–1.9; p = 0.003) [46].

A meta-analysis of five studies by Edmonson et al. demonstrated that in patients first free of CHD, presence of post-traumatic stress disorder (PTSD) increases the risk of developing incident CHD, even after controlling for frequently comorbid depression (four studies: RR 1.3; 95% CI 1.1–1.5) [47]. This association might be even stronger for women, although more research needs to be done on the link between gender and this connection [47]. Tully et al. also conducted a meta-analysis of 12 studies on the association between panic disorder (PD) and incident CHD. The authors found that patients with PD had a 47% increased risk of developing CHD, a 36% increased risk of MI, and a 40% risk of MACE [48]. The associations and increased risks remained significant even after controlling for depression. Authors also noted heterogeneity between studies.

On the other hand, patients with established heart disease have increased rates of anxiety. For example, a meta-analysis of 73 studies by Easton et al. examined prevalence of anxiety in HF patients [49]. A variety of tools have been used between different studies. The authors reported a pooled prevalence of 13.1% (95% CI 9.3–16.9%) for anxiety disorders, 28.8% (95% CI 23.3–34.3%) for probable clinically significant anxiety, and 55.5% (95% CI 48.1–62.8%) for elevated symptoms of anxiety. Different screening tools can produce different results. In this meta-analysis, the Brief Symptom Scale-Anxiety scale led to the highest anxiety prevalence (72.3%), while the Generalized Anxiety Disorder-7 (GAD-7) led to the lowest prevalence (6.3%).

As already noted above, anxiety often co-exists with depression in medically healthy patients and in patients with heart disease and HF. In fact, one study of outpatients with HF with NYHA status III/IV determined that one-third of their sample had comorbid depression and anxiety, using Brief Symptom Inventory-anxiety subscale for anxiety and the Beck Depression Inventory-II (BDI) for depression measures [50]. Depressive symptoms were predictive of anxiety presence with a dose-dependent effect. Thus, cardiac patients should be evaluated for both depression and anxiety, and treatments should be considered given this comorbidity.

Similar to depression, anxiety in cardiac patients may be associated with adverse clinical events. Anxiety may predict hospitalizations in patients with chronic HF [51]. Anxiety is also associated with increased mortality in cardiac patients, although this association is not as strong or robust as it is for depression [52].

Treatment of Anxiety in Patients with Heart Disease

No pharmacological studies have been conducted specifically on treatment of anxiety in patients with heart disease. However, as discussed above, multiple SSRIs have been found to be safe in cardiac patients, and they are frequently used as the fist-line treatment for a variety of anxiety disorders, including GAD, PD, and PTSD. Benzodiazepines are used for short-term episodic relief, but caution should be used regarding cognitive side effects and dependency risks. If benzodiazepines are used, lorazepam, oxazepam, or temazepam are the safer options, given that they do not rely on Phase I metabolism and thus their metabolism is not affected by HF [44].

CBT has been shown to decrease symptoms of anxiety in patients with HF [35]. In addition, mindfulness-based programs and positive psychological interventions are promising for treatment of anxiety and reduction of distress in cardiac patients [4]. Finally, collaborative care has been shown to decrease anxiety symptoms for patients with comorbid anxiety and CHD [4, 39].

Severe Mental Illness in Heart Disease

Epidemiology

Patients with severe mental illness, such as schizophrenia, have increased rates of cardiovascular disease for many reasons [53]. First of all, the underlying psychopathology leads to many health behaviors contributing to the development and progression of heart disease: smoking, sedentary lifestyle, and nonadherence to medications, clinic visits, and other recommendations from the team. In addition, most low-potency first-generation and all second-generation antipsychotics are known to have significant metabolic side effects (i.e., dyslipidemia, glucose intolerance, hypertension, abdominal obesity), thus significantly contributing to an increased risk of heart disease [44, 53, 54]. This especially

applies to the antipsychotic agents olanzapine and clozapine. Patients with schizophrenia are also more likely to have lower socioeconomic status and decreased support systems, both factors limiting their access to care. These patients are also likely to present later to the medical care and their somatic symptoms be more likely dismissed as "psychosomatic." Thus, they are more likely to be misdiagnosed and offered fewer treatment options [53]. This is represented by a case report of a young man with schizophrenia who was diagnosed with heart disease only in end-stage and was initially turned down from heart transplant [55]. Only with lobbying and support from his mental health team did this young man receive his life-saving heart transplant, and with intact support system and treatment of his mental illness, he did well for at least over 3 years of follow-up by the time of the publication.

Patients with schizophrenia and comorbid heart disease have significantly higher mortality and die, on average, 25 years earlier as compared to general population, frequently from cardiovascular disease [53, 54]. In a Danish nationwide cohort study, Kugathasan et al. demonstrated that patients with comorbid schizophrenia and MI have higher mortality at 1 and 5 years post-MI, as compared to schizophrenia-only controls (HR 4.50; 95% CI 4.36–4.64), MI-only controls (HR 3.27; 95% CI 3.0–3.5), and individuals without schizophrenia or MI (HR 9.9; 95% CI 8.7–11.4) [56].

Close collaboration between the medical team and mental health providers is especially important for such complicated and vulnerable patients. While traditionally patients with severe mental illness were excluded from transplantation, more recent reports have suggested that with appropriate support systems and treatments in place, these patients can do well after cardiac transplant [57].

Treatment of Severe Mental Illness in Patients with Heart Disease

As discussed above, antipsychotics are associated with significant metabolic side effects and potential QTc prolongation. Of the novel antipsychotic agents, lurasidone and aripiprazole appear to have the least effect on QTc prolongation [40, 58] and thus are preferred agents in patients for whom this is a significant concern. In addition, orthostatic hypotension can be a side effect of low-potency first-generation antipsychotics (e.g., chlorpromazine) as well as some second-generation antipsychotics (i.e., olanzapine, clozapine, and quetiapine). Finally, clozapine is associated with a risk of myocarditis, usually occurring early in the course of treatment (e.g., in the first few weeks), and cardiomyopathy, usually occurring months to years after treatment initiation [44].

Of note, antipsychotics are used as adjuvants in the management of many other psychiatric conditions, such as delirium, augmentation of depression treatment, and treatment-resistant anxiety, and above cardiac considerations would apply to those applications as well.

Cognitive Impairment in Patients with Heart Disease

Epidemiology

Cognitive impairment is common, identified in up to 43% of patients enrolled in cohort HF studies [59]. The OR for cognitive impairment in patients with HF was 1.67 (95% CI 1.15–2.42) as compared to patients without HF in one study [59]. Possible etiologies contributing to this high prevalence of cognitive impairment include hypoperfusion and systemic inflammation. These high rates are concerning as patients are required to manage complex medical regimens, both before and after transplantation. Thus, it is important to identify cognitive impairment when present, address any contributing etiologies if possible, adapt education sessions to the patient's particular needs, and involve their support systems.

Treatment

Acetylcholinesterase inhibitors (ACHIs) and NMDA antagonists are often used to treat cognitive impairment. ACHIs are rarely associated with bradycardia, sick sinus rhythm, or QTc prolongation, which could lead to torsades de pointes [44, 60, 61]. Caution should be used when combining these agents with other QTc-prolonging medications, including antipsychotics and antidepressants.

Patients with Implantable Cardioverter Defibrillators and Mechanical Circulatory Support

Certain heart disease patient populations are at even greater risk for stress, depression, and anxiety, given the more invasive interventions their cardiac status requires. For example, while implantable cardioverter defibrillators (ICDs) decrease mortality with primary and secondary prevention of lethal arrhythmias (see Chap. 18 for more details), they can contribute to additional psychological distress in at least some of the patients [62, 63]. Approximately a quarter of patients with ICDs for secondary prevention suffer from depression, while 24–87% have increased symptoms of anxiety, and 13–35% are clinically anxious [62]. Younger age, female gender, and greater number of shocks may serve

as risk factors for psychopathology [62]. Significant numbers of patients (7.8–15%) might develop PTSD in relation to ICDs and shocks delivered, whether appropriately triggered or not [64, 65].

Non-pharmacological interventions have been studied for anxiety and depression in patients with ICDs. CBT, including home-based CBT, as well as psychoeducational interventions, have been found to be effective in the reduction of anxiety and depression symptoms [62].

Living with ventricular assistive devices (VADs) has its own emotional and psychological stressors. While perceived quality of life might improve and depression and anxiety actually lessen after VAD implantation [66–68], the emotional stress continues, and patients now live with more limitations and physical considerations (see Chap. 18). In fact, suicidal behavior manifested by medical nonadherence [69] and driveline disconnection [70] have been reported in patients with VADs. Of interest, while patients' quality of life improves after VAD implantation, that of their caregivers does not [66]. Caregivers of patients with VADs have also high rates of depression and anxiety [66, 71]. It is thus important that individuals with VADs are taken care of within multidisciplinary collaborative settings where their physical and psychosocial needs are anticipated and swiftly addressed. It is also important that if patients are bridged to heart transplant with a VAD, caregivers' burnout is carefully evaluated, and caregivers are maximally supported.

As discussed above, patients with HF are at increased risk for impaired cognition, partly due to hypoxia. Thus, implantation of VADs can improve cognition with better delivery of oxygen to brain [72, 73]. However, these patients are also at higher risk for cardiovascular events, in particular ischemic stroke and intracranial hemorrhage [74], and thus have increased risk for subsequent cognitive impairment (see Chap. 18).

Diagnosis of Psychiatric Syndromes in Cardiac Patients

While depression, anxiety, and cognitive dysfunction are common in patients with heart disease, it is important to accurately ascertain whether the symptoms have a psychiatric versus medical etiology [44]. Paroxysmal ventricular arrhythmias can present with anxiety, while pulmonary congestion and orthopnea can cause sleep disturbances. Both hypotension and arrhythmias may reduce cerebral blood flow and present with symptoms of organic mental disorders and/or cognitive dysfunction.

In addition, many cardiac medications can have neuropsychiatric side effects [44]. While it has been disproven that beta-blockers lead to depression, they do contribute to depressive-like symptoms (e.g., sexual dysfunction and fatigue). Alpha-adrenergic blockers can also cause sexual dysfunction and depressive-like symptoms [44]. Amiodarone can cause delirium [75, 76] and contribute to thyroid dysfunction, manifesting as mood disorders [77]. Antiarrhythmic agents and digoxin can lead to visual hallucinations/changes and delirium [77–79], while digoxin is also associated with depression [77]. Thus, it is important for cardiologists and psychiatrists to know the neuropsychiatric side effects of cardiac and related medications and to work collaboratively to disentangle patients' presentations to provide optimal care and treatment.

Effect of Pre-transplant Mental Health Conditions on Post-Heart Transplant Outcomes

Psychosocial evaluation for heart transplantation involves an evaluation of a patient's understanding of and motivation for transplant, history of psychiatric symptoms and disorders, history of substance use and abuse if relevant, prior adherence to treatments, and support system (see Chap. 2 for full description of psychosocial evaluation). Many pre-transplant psychosocial factors are associated with post-transplant outcomes and success [80, 81]. The role of heart transplant mental health clinicians includes identification of the psychosocial risk factors, so that ideally a treatment plan and needed support can be developed and implemented to strengthen patient's candidacy and chance of success.

Owen et al. followed 108 heart transplant recipients for an average of 970 days post-transplant [81]. The authors reported that pre-heart transplant suicide attempts, poor adherence to medical recommendations, previous drug or alcohol rehabilitation, and depression significantly predicted survival post-transplant. In addition, prior suicide attempt was associated with a greater risk for post-transplant infection in this patient cohort.

Pre-transplant and early post-transplant depression has been demonstrated to increase morbidity and mortality in a meta-analysis of 27 studies on solid-organ transplant recipients, including 10 studies on heart transplant patients [82]. In fact, depression increased the relative risk (RR) of mortality by 65% (RR 1.65; 95% CI 1.34–2.05), while it also increased the risk for death-censored graft loss (RR 1.65; 95% CI 1.21–2.26) [82]. Pre-transplant depression in heart disease patients is associated with increased nonadherence to medications and an increased rate of hospitalizations post-transplant [83].

A retrospective application of the Stanford Integrated Psychosocial Assessment for Transplantation (SIPAT) and chart review of 51 heart transplant recipients demonstrated that SIPAT had strong inter-rater reliability (ICC = 0.89; 95% CI = 0.76–0.96) in this patient population [84]. In addition, patients with "minimally acceptable/high-risk" ratings were more likely to miss clinic appointments after the transplant as compared to patients with "excellent/good" SIPAT ratings ($p = 0.004$).

Psychosocial and mental health challenges should be identified early in the process of the heart transplant evaluation. Connection with the mental health professionals can help identify psychosocial risks early and establish the relationships that will be important throughout the process of transplantation.

Waiting on the Heart Transplant List

While the evaluation for heart transplantation and waiting on the list can give patients hope, it is also very stressful. While patients hope for the new life with a new heart, they also prepare for the real possibility of death. They experience a sense of urgency, might feel that don't have "a real choice," contemplate a lot about death, and eagerly await "the Call" to move on to the next stage of life [85]. As time progresses and functionality decreases, patients become more home-bound and dependent on others, and depression and demoralization can increase as well [86]. Support from cardiologists, mental health teams, and palliative care become ever more important. Acceptance of uncertainty, focusing on small goals, and relinquishing control over what cannot be controlled become the themes in therapy and life.

Conclusions

Psychiatric disorders have bidirectional relationships with cardiac illness. Symptoms of depression and anxiety are common in heart disease and HF patients. Depression, anxiety, and severe mental illness are associated with worse clinical outcomes and increased mortality in patients with heart disease. Studies have demonstrated some effectiveness of antidepressants for depression in patients with heart disease, but this has not translated into pharmacological treatments of depression leading to decreased mortality. Pharmacological treatments of depression in HF patients have not demonstrated positive effect on depression treatment in large RCTs, but remission of depression has been shown to improve survival. Therapy, exercise, and collaborative care are all promising treatment modalities. Knowledge of medical etiologies of psychiatric symptoms, neuropsychiatric side effects of cardiac medications, and drug-drug interactions is important in care of these complex patients. Mental health professionals are crucial in their roles of providing support to cardiac patients, their families, and medical teams throughout the stages of heart disease, heart transplant evaluation, and awaiting for heart transplant.

References

1. Denollet J, Sys SU, Brutsaert DL. Personality and mortality after myocardial infarction. Psychosom Med. [Comparative Study Research Support, Non-U.S. Gov't]. 1995;57(6):582–91.

2. O'Neil A, Fisher AJ, Kibbey KJ, Jacka FN, Kotowicz MA, Williams LJ, et al. Depression is a risk factor for incident coronary heart disease in women: an 18-year longitudinal study. J Affect Disord. [Research Support, Non-U.S. Gov't]. 2016;196:117–24.

3. Wulsin LR, Singal BM. Do depressive symptoms increase the risk for the onset of coronary disease? A systematic quantitative review. Psychosom Med. [Meta-Analysis Review]. 2003;65(2):201–10.

4. Huffman JC, Adams CN, Celano CM. Collaborative care and related interventions in patients with heart disease: An update and new directions. Psychosomatics. [Review]. 2018;59(1):1–18.

5. Sher Y, Lolak S, Maldonado JR. The impact of depression in heart disease. Curr Psychiatry Rep. [Review]. 2010;12(3):255–64.

6. Newhouse A, Jiang W. Heart failure and depression. Heart Fail Clin. [Review]. 2014;10(2):295–304.

7. Rudisch B, Nemeroff CB. Epidemiology of comorbid coronary artery disease and depression. Biol Psychiatry. [Research Support, Non-U.S. Gov't Review]. 2003;54(3):227–40.

8. Rutledge T, Reis VA, Linke SE, Greenberg BH, Mills PJ. Depression in heart failure a meta-analytic review of prevalence, intervention effects, and associations with clinical outcomes. J Am Coll Cardiol. [Meta-Analysis]. 2006;48(8):1527–37.

9. Schowalter M, Gelbrich G, Stork S, Langguth JP, Morbach C, Ertl G, et al. Generic and disease-specific health-related quality of life in patients with chronic systolic heart failure: impact of depression. Clin Res Cardiol. [Research Support, Non-U.S. Gov't]. 2013;102(4):269–78.

10. Muller-Tasch T, Peters-Klimm F, Schellberg D, Holzapfel N, Barth A, Junger J, et al. Depression is a major determinant of quality of life in patients with chronic systolic heart failure in general practice. J Card Fail. [Comparative Study Research Support, Non-U.S. Gov't]. 2007;13(10):818–24.

11. Albert NM, Fonarow GC, Abraham WT, Gheorghiade M, Greenberg BH, Nunez E, et al. Depression and clinical outcomes in heart failure: an OPTIMIZE-HF analysis. Am J Med. [Research Support, Non-U.S. Gov't]. 2009;122(4):366–73.

12. Braunstein JB, Anderson GF, Gerstenblith G, Weller W, Niefeld M, Herbert R, et al. Noncardiac comorbidity increases preventable hospitalizations and mortality among Medicare beneficiaries with chronic heart failure. J Am Coll Cardiol. [Research Support, Non-U.S. Gov't]. 2003;42(7):1226–33.

13. Lesman-Leegte I, van Veldhuisen DJ, Hillege HL, Moser D, Sanderman R, Jaarsma T. Depressive symptoms and outcomes in patients with heart failure: data from the COACH study. Eur J Heart Fail. [Research Support, Non-U.S. Gov't]. 2009;11(12):1202–7.

14. Moraska AR, Chamberlain AM, Shah ND, Vickers KS, Rummans TA, Dunlay SM, et al. Depression, healthcare utilization, and death in heart failure: a community study. Circ Heart Fail. [Research Support, N.I.H., Extramural]. 2013;6(3):387–94.

15. Sherwood A, Blumenthal JA, Trivedi R, Johnson KS, O'Connor CM, Adams KF, Jr., et al. Relationship of depression to death or hospitalization in patients with heart failure. Arch Intern Med. [Multicenter Study Research Support, N.I.H., Extramural]. 2007;167(4):367–73.

16. Palacios J, Khondoker M, Mann A, Tylee A, Hotopf M. Depression and anxiety symptom trajectories in coronary heart disease: associations with measures of disability and impact on 3-year health care costs. J Psychosom Res. 2018;104:1–8.

17. Lichtman JH, Froelicher ES, Blumenthal JA, Carney RM, Doering LV, Frasure-Smith N, et al. Depression as a risk factor for poor prognosis among patients with acute coronary syndrome: systematic review and recommendations: a scientific statement from the American Heart Association. Circulation. [Meta-Analysis Review]. 2014;129(12):1350–69.

18. Nicholson A, Kuper H, Hemingway H. Depression as an aetiologic and prognostic factor in coronary heart disease: a meta-analysis of 6362 events among 146 538 participants in 54 observational studies. Eur Heart J. [Meta-Analysis Research Support, Non-U.S. Gov't]. 2006;27(23):2763–74.

19. Penninx BW, Beekman AT, Honig A, Deeg DJ, Schoevers RA, van Eijk JT, et al. Depression and cardiac mortality: results from a community-based longitudinal study. Arch Gen Psychiatry. [Research Support, Non-U.S. Gov't]. 2001;58(3):221–7.

20. Barth J, Schumacher M, Herrmann-Lingen C. Depression as a risk factor for mortality in patients with coronary heart disease: a meta-analysis. Psychosom Med. [Comparative Study Meta-Analysis]. 2004;66(6):802–13.

21. Wellenius GA, Mukamal KJ, Kulshreshtha A, Asonganyi S, Mittleman MA. Depressive symptoms and the risk of atherosclerotic progression among patients with coronary artery bypass grafts. Circulation. [Comparative Study Randomized Controlled Trial Research Support, N.I.H., Extramural Research Support, Non-U.S. Gov't]. 2008;117(18):2313–9.

22. Adams J, Kuchibhatla M, Christopher EJ, Alexander JD, Clary GL, Cuffe MS, et al. Association of depression and survival in patients with chronic heart failure over 12 Years. Psychosomatics. 2012;53(4):339–46. https://doi.org/10.1016/j.psym.2011.12.002.

23. Glassman AH, O'Connor CM, Califf RM, Swedberg K, Schwartz P, Bigger JT, Jr., et al. Sertraline treatment of major depression in patients with acute MI or unstable angina. JAMA. [Clinical Trial Multicenter Study Randomized Controlled Trial Research Support, Non-U.S. Gov't]. 2002;288(6):701–9.

24. van Melle JP, de Jonge P, Honig A, Schene AH, Kuyper AM, Crijns HJ, et al. Effects of antidepressant treatment following myocardial infarction. Br J Psychiatry. [Comparative Study Multicenter Study Randomized Controlled Trial Research Support, Non-U.S. Gov't]. 2007;190:460–6.

25. Lesperance F, Frasure-Smith N, Koszycki D, Laliberte MA, van Zyl LT, Baker B, et al. Effects of citalopram and interpersonal psychotherapy on depression in patients with coronary artery disease: the Canadian Cardiac Randomized Evaluation of Antidepressant and Psychotherapy Efficacy (CREATE) trial. JAMA. [Multicenter Study Randomized Controlled Trial Research Support, Non-U.S. Gov't]. 2007;297(4):367–79.

26. Echols MR, Jiang W. Clinical trial evidence for treatment of depression in heart failure. Heart Fail Clin. [Review]. 2011;7(1):81–8.

27. O'Connor CM, Jiang W, Kuchibhatla M, Silva SG, Cuffe MS, Callwood DD, et al. Safety and efficacy of sertraline for depression in patients with heart failure: results of the SADHART-CHF (Sertraline Against Depression and Heart Disease in Chronic Heart Failure) trial. J Am Coll Cardiol. [Randomized Controlled Trial Research Support, N.I.H., Extramural]. 2010;56(9):692–9.

28. Angermann CE, Gelbrich G, Stork S, Gunold H, Edelmann F, Wachter R, et al. Effect of escitalopram on all-cause mortality and hospitalization in patients with heart failure and depression: the MOOD-HF randomized clinical trial. JAMA. [Multicenter Study Randomized Controlled Trial Research Support, Non-U.S. Gov't]. 2016;315(24):2683–93.

29. Berkman LF, Blumenthal J, Burg M, Carney RM, Catellier D, Cowan MJ, et al. Effects of treating depression and low perceived social support on clinical events after myocardial infarction: the Enhancing Recovery in Coronary Heart Disease Patients (ENRICHD) Randomized Trial. JAMA. [Clinical Trial Multicenter Study Randomized Controlled Trial Research Support, U.S. Gov't, P.H.S.]. 2003;289(23):3106–16.

30. Taylor CB, Youngblood ME, Catellier D, Veith RC, Carney RM, Burg MM, et al. Effects of antidepressant medication on morbidity and mortality in depressed patients after myocardial infarc-

tion. Arch Gen Psychiatry. [Clinical Trial Comparative Study Multicenter Study Randomized Controlled Trial Research Support, N.I.H., Extramural Research Support, U.S. Gov't, P.H.S.]. 2005;62(7):792–8.

31. Kim JM, Bae KY, Stewart R, Jung BO, Kang HJ, Kim SW, et al. Escitalopram treatment for depressive disorder following acute coronary syndrome: a 24-week double-blind, placebo-controlled trial. J Clin Psychiatry. [Randomized Controlled Trial Research Support, Non-U.S. Gov't]. 2015;76(1):62–8.

32. Rigotti NA, Thorndike AN, Regan S, McKool K, Pasternak RC, Chang Y, et al. Bupropion for smokers hospitalized with acute cardiovascular disease. Am J Med. [Multicenter Study Randomized Controlled Trial Research Support, N.I.H., Extramural Research Support, Non-U.S. Gov't]. 2006;119(12):1080–7.

33. Blumenthal JA, Sherwood A, Babyak MA, Watkins LL, Smith PJ, Hoffman BM, et al. Exercise and pharmacological treatment of depressive symptoms in patients with coronary heart disease: results from the UPBEAT (Understanding the Prognostic Benefits of Exercise and Antidepressant Therapy) study. J Am Coll Cardiol. [Randomized Controlled Trial Research Support, N.I.H., Extramural Research Support, Non-U.S. Gov't]. 2012;60(12): 1053–63.

34. Herrmann-Lingen C, Beutel ME, Bosbach A, Deter HC, Fritzsche K, Hellmich M, et al. A stepwise psychotherapy intervention for reducing risk in coronary artery disease (SPIRR-CAD): results of an observer-blinded, multicenter, randomized trial in depressed patients with coronary artery disease. Psychosom Med. [Multicenter Study Randomized Controlled Trial]. 2016;78(6):704–15.

35. Freedland KE, Carney RM, Rich MW, Steinmeyer BC, Rubin EH. Cognitive behavior therapy for depression and self-care in heart failure patients: A randomized clinical trial. JAMA Intern Med. [Randomized Controlled Trial]. 2015;175(11):1773–82.

36. Wells A, McNicol K, Reeves D, Salmon P, Davies L, Heagerty A, et al. Improving the effectiveness of psychological interventions for depression and anxiety in the cardiac rehabilitation pathway using group-based metacognitive therapy (PATHWAY Group MCT): study protocol for a randomised controlled trial. Trials. 2018;19(1):215.

37. Blumenthal JA, Babyak MA, O'Connor C, Keteyian S, Landzberg J, Howlett J, et al. Effects of exercise training on depressive symptoms in patients with chronic heart failure: the HF-ACTION randomized trial. JAMA. [Comparative Study Multicenter Study Randomized Controlled Trial Research Support, N.I.H., Extramural]. 2012;308(5):465–74.

38. Carney RM, Freedland KE, Steinmeyer BC, Rubin EH, Rich MW. Residual symptoms following treatment for depression in patients with coronary heart disease. Psychosom Med. 2018;80(4): 385–92

39. Tully PJ, Baumeister H. Collaborative care for comorbid depression and coronary heart disease: a systematic review and meta-analysis of randomised controlled trials. BMJ Open. [Meta-Analysis Research Support, Non-U.S. Gov't Review]. 2015;5(12):e009128.

40. Beach SR, Celano CM, Noseworthy PA, Januzzi JL, Huffman JC. QTc prolongation, torsades de pointes, and psychotropic medications. Psychosomatics. [Review]. 2013;54(1):1–13.

41. Castro VM, Clements CC, Murphy SN, Gainer VS, Fava M, Weilburg JB, et al. QT interval and antidepressant use: a cross sectional study of electronic health records. BMJ. [Comparative Study Research Support, N.I.H., Extramural]. 2013;346:f288.

42. Eckersley MJ, Sepehripour AH, Casula R, Punjabi P, Athanasiou T. Do selective serotonin reuptake inhibitors increase the risk of bleeding or mortality following coronary artery bypass graft surgery? A meta-analysis of observational studies. Perfusion. 2018:267659118765933.

43. Ziegelstein RC, Parakh K, Sakhuja A, Bhat U. Platelet function in patients with major depression. Intern Med J. [Research Support,

N.I.H., Extramural Research Support, Non-U.S. Gov't Review]. 2009;39(1):38–43.

44. Shapiro PA. Cardiovascular disorders. In: Ferrando SJ, Levenson JL, Owen JA, editors. Clinical manual of psychopharmacology in medically ill. Washington, DC/New York: American Psychiatric Publishing; 2010. p. 181–212.

45. Tully PJ, Cosh SM, Baumeister H. The anxious heart in whose mind? A systematic review and meta-regression of factors associated with anxiety disorder diagnosis, treatment and morbidity risk in coronary heart disease. J Psychosom Res. [Research Support, Non-U.S. Gov't Review]. 2014;77(6): 439–48.

46. Roest AM, Martens EJ, de Jonge P, Denollet J. Anxiety and risk of incident coronary heart disease: a meta-analysis. J Am Coll Cardiol. [Meta-Analysis Research Support, Non-U.S. Gov't]. 2010;56(1):38–46.

47. Edmondson D, Kronish IM, Shaffer JA, Falzon L, Burg MM. Posttraumatic stress disorder and risk for coronary heart disease: a meta-analytic review. Am Heart J. [Meta-Analysis Review]. 2013;166(5):806–14.

48. Tully PJ, Turnbull DA, Beltrame J, Horowitz J, Cosh S, Baumeister H, et al. Panic disorder and incident coronary heart disease: a systematic review and meta-regression in 1131612 persons and 58111 cardiac events. Psychol Med. [Meta-Analysis Research Support, Non-U.S. Gov't Review]. 2015;45(14):2909–20.

49. Easton K, Coventry P, Lovell K, Carter LA, Deaton C. Prevalence and measurement of anxiety in samples of patients with heart failure: meta-analysis. J Cardiovasc Nurs. [Meta-Analysis]. 2016;31(4):367–79.

50. Dekker RL, Lennie TA, Doering LV, Chung ML, Wu JR, Moser DK. Coexisting anxiety and depressive symptoms in patients with heart failure. Eur J Cardiovasc Nurs. [Research Support, N.I.H., Extramural Research Support, Non-U.S. Gov't]. 2014;13(2): 168–76.

51. Vongmany J, Hickman LD, Lewis J, Newton PJ, Phillips JL. Anxiety in chronic heart failure and the risk of increased hospitalisations and mortality: a systematic review. Eur J Cardiovasc Nurs. [Review]. 2016;15(7):478–85.

52. Celano CM, Millstein RA, Bedoya CA, Healy BC, Roest AM, Huffman JC. Association between anxiety and mortality in patients with coronary artery disease: a meta-analysis. Am Heart J. [Meta-Analysis Review]. 2015;170(6):1105–15.

53. Newcomer JW, Hennekens CH. Severe mental illness and risk of cardiovascular disease. JAMA. [Research Support, N.I.H., Extramural]. 2007;298(15):1794–6.

54. Mangurian C, Newcomer JW, Modlin C, Schillinger D. Diabetes and cardiovascular care among people with severe mental illness: a literature review. J Gen. Intern Med. [Case Reports Review]. 2016;31(9):1083–91.

55. Le Melle SM, Entelis C. Heart transplant in a young man with schizophrenia. Am J Psychiatry. [Case Reports Clinical Conference]. 2005;162(3):453–7.

56. Kugathasan P, Laursen TM, Grontved S, Jensen SE, Aagaard J, Nielsen RE. Increased long-term mortality after myocardial infarction in patients with schizophrenia. Schizophr Res. 2018;199:103–8.

57. Zimbrean P, Emre S. Patients with psychotic disorders in solid-organ transplant. Prog Transplant. 2015;25(4):289–96.

58. Leucht S, Cipriani A, Spineli L, Mavridis D, Orey D, Richter F, et al. Comparative efficacy and tolerability of 15 antipsychotic drugs in schizophrenia: a multiple-treatments meta-analysis. Lancet. [Comparative Study Meta-Analysis Review]. 2013;382(9896):951–62.

59. Cannon JA, Moffitt P, Perez-Moreno AC, Walters MR, Broomfield NM, McMurray JJV, et al. Cognitive impairment and heart failure: systematic review and meta-analysis. J Card Fail. [Review]. 2017;23(6):464–75.

60. Kitt J, Irons R, Al-Obaidi M, Missouris C. A case of donepezil-related torsades de pointes. BMJ Case Rep. [Case Reports]. 2015;2015.

61. Takaya T, Okamoto M, Yodoi K, Hata K, Kijima Y, Nakajima H, et al. Torsades de pointes with QT prolongation related to donepezil use. J Cardiol. [Case Reports]. 2009;54(3):507–11.

62. Freedenberg V, Thomas SA, Friedmann E. Anxiety and depression in implanted cardioverter-defibrillator recipients and heart failure: a review. Heart Fail Clin. [Review]. 2011;7(1):59–68.

63. Thomas SA, Friedmann E, Kao CW, Inguito P, Metcalf M, Kelley FJ, et al. Quality of life and psychological status of patients with implantable cardioverter defibrillators. Am J Crit Care. [Research Support, N.I.H., Extramural Research Support, Non-U.S. Gov't Review]. 2006;15(4):389–98.

64. Habibovic M, van den Broek KC, Alings M, Van der Voort PH, Denollet J. Posttraumatic stress 18 months following cardioverter defibrillator implantation: shocks, anxiety, and personality. Health Psychol. 2012;31(2):186–93.

65. Kobe J, Hucklenbroich K, Geisendorfer N, Bettin M, Frommeyer G, Reinke F, et al. Posttraumatic stress and quality of life with the totally subcutaneous compared to conventional cardioverter-defibrillator systems. Clin Res Cardiol. [Controlled Clinical Trial]. 2017;106(5):317–21.

66. Bidwell JT, Lyons KS, Mudd JO, Gelow JM, Chien CV, Hiatt SO, et al. Quality of life, depression, and anxiety in ventricular assist device therapy: longitudinal outcomes for patients and family caregivers. J Cardiovasc Nurs. 2017;32(5):455–63.

67. Yost G, Bhat G, Mahoney E, Tatooles A. Reduced anxiety and depression in patients with advanced heart failure after left ventricular assist device implantation. Psychosomatics. 2017;58(4):406–14.

68. Reynard AK, Butler RS, McKee MG, Starling RC, Gorodeski EZ. Frequency of depression and anxiety before and after insertion of a continuous flow left ventricular assist device. Am J Cardiol. [Research Support, Non-U.S. Gov't]. 2014;114(3):433–40.

69. Balliet WE, Madan A, Craig ML, Serber ER, Borckardt JJ, Pelic C, et al. A ventricular assist device recipient and suicidality: multidisciplinary collaboration with a psychiatrically distressed patient. J Cardiovasc Nurs. [Case Reports]. 2017;32(2):135–9.

70. Tigges-Limmer K, Schonbrodt M, Roefe D, Arusoglu L, Morshuis M, Gummert JF. Suicide after ventricular assist device implantation. J. Heart Lung Transplant. [Case Reports]. 2010;29(6):692–4.

71. Brouwers C, Denollet J, Caliskan K, de Jonge N, Constantinescu A, Young Q, et al. Psychological distress in patients with a left ventricular assist device and their partners: an exploratory study. Eur J Cardiovasc Nurs. [Comparative Study Multicenter Study Observational Study Research Support, Non-U.S. Gov't]. 2015;14(1):53–62.

72. Bhat G, Yost G, Mahoney E. Cognitive function and left ventricular assist device implantation. J Heart Lung Transplant. 2015;34(11):1398–405.

73. Petrucci RJ, Wright S, Naka Y, Idrissi KA, Russell SD, Dordunoo D, et al. Neurocognitive assessments in advanced heart failure patients receiving continuous-flow left ventricular assist devices. J Heart Lung Transplant. [Clinical Trial]. 2009;28(6):542–9.

74. Cho SM, Moazami N, Frontera JA. Stroke and intracranial hemorrhage in HeartMate II and HeartWare left ventricular assist devices: a systematic review. Neurocrit Care. [Review]. 2017;27(1):17–25.

75. Yuppa DP, Nichols S. Amiodarone-induced delirium in advanced cancer: a case report. Psychosomatics. [Case Reports]. 2013;54(3):294–6.

76. Barry JJ, Franklin K. Amiodarone-induced delirium. Am J Psychiatry. [Case Reports Letter]. 1999;156(7):1119.

77. Keller S, Frishman WH. Neuropsychiatric effects of cardiovascular drug therapy. Cardiol Rev. [Review]. 2003;11(2):73–93.

78. Piltz JR, Wertenbaker C, Lance SE, Slamovits T, Leeper HF. Digoxin toxicity. Recognizing the varied visual presentations. J Clin Neuroophthalmol. [Case Reports]. 1993;13(4):275–80.

79. Renard D, Rubli E, Voide N, Borruat FX, Rothuizen LE. Spectrum of digoxin-induced ocular toxicity: a case report and literature review. BMC Res Notes. [Case Reports Review]. 2015;8:368.

80. Maldonado JR, Sher Y, Lolak S, Swendsen H, Skibola D, Neri E, et al. The Stanford Integrated Psychosocial Assessment for Transplantation: a prospective study of medical and psychosocial outcomes. Psychosom Med. [Research Support, Non-U.S. Gov't]. 2015;77(9):1018–30.

81. Owen JE, Bonds CL, Wellisch DK. Psychiatric evaluations of heart transplant candidates: predicting post-transplant hospitalizations, rejection episodes, and survival. Psychosomatics. 2006;47(3):213–22.

82. Dew MA, Rosenberger EM, Myaskovsky L, DiMartini AF, DeVito Dabbs AJ, Posluszny DM, et al. Depression and anxiety as risk factors for morbidity and mortality after organ transplantation: a systematic review and meta-analysis. Transplantation. 2015;100(5):988–1003.

83. Delibasic M, Mohamedali B, Dobrilovic N, Raman J. Pre-transplant depression as a predictor of adherence and morbidities after orthotopic heart transplantation. J Cardiothorac Surg. 2017;12(1):62.

84. Vandenbogaart E, Doering L, Chen B, Saltzman A, Chaker T, Creaser JW, et al. Evaluation of the SIPAT instrument to assess psychosocial risk in heart transplant candidates: a retrospective single center study. Heart Lung. [Evaluation Studies]. 2017;46(4):273–9.

85. Flynn K, Daiches A, Malpus Z, Yonan N, Sanchez M. 'A post-transplant person': narratives of heart or lung transplantation and intensive care unit delirium. Health. 2014;18(4):352–68.

86. Zipfel S, Lowe B, Paschke T, Immel B, Lange R, Zimmermann R, et al. Psychological distress in patients awaiting heart transplantation. J Psychosom Res. [Research Support, Non-U.S. Gov't]. 1998;45(5):465–70.

ICDs, VADs, and Total Artificial Heart Implantation

18

Jared J. Herr

Implantable Cardioverter-Defibrillator Use in Heart Failure

Ventricular arrhythmias are a common complication of structural heart disease and pose a considerable risk of mortality and morbidity for those patients who develop them. Patients with heart failure have a six- to nine-fold higher rate of sudden cardiac death (SCD) when compared to the general population. The presence of nonsustained ventricular tachycardia in patients with previous myocardial infarction and left ventricular systolic dysfunction is associated with a 2-year mortality rate approaching 30% [1]. Due to this considerable risk in heart failure patients, medical- and device-based therapies are utilized to reduce risk of sudden cardiac death. Unfortunately, trial results of medical therapy for prevention of ventricular arrhythmia have shown mixed results. The Cardiac Arrhythmia Suppression Trial evaluated the use of the antiarrhythmic drugs flecainide and encainide to prevent ventricular arrhythmia in patients with structural heart disease. This trial actually showed an increased risk of mortality compared to placebo with the use of these drugs [2]. Results like this have driven implantable cardioverter-defibrillators to become the treatment of choice in prevention of sudden cardiac death in patients with heart failure.

An implantable cardioverter-defibrillator (ICD) is a specialized pacemaker device with defibrillation capabilities for treating ventricular arrhythmias. ICDs are available in two basic forms based on implant technique, transvenous and subcutaneous. Transvenous devices are placed typically by accessing the subclavian or axillary vein and introducing small, flexible electrical leads directly into the heart. ICD leads follow the thoracic veins that course to the heart and

directly attach to the endocardium and are connected to a generator placed subcutaneously near the clavicle. The generator serves as a power source and a microcomputer for controlling the device. The intracardiac leads register electrical activity within the heart to identify and treat ventricular arrhythmia with either pacing or electrical defibrillation. The subcutaneous ICD (SICD) is a novel defibrillator that is placed under the tissue in the chest wall and does not enter the central veins or the heart. These devices therefore do not carry the same risk to intracardiac structures such as the development of tricuspid regurgitation or need for lead extraction. However, they carry their own downsides such as being unable to pace the heart or provide resynchronization therapy. Subcutaneous ICDs have a considerably larger generator and a shorter battery life compared to transvenous devices [3].

Indications for use of ICDs have expanded over the years and now encompass strategies for both primary and secondary prevention of sudden cardiac death. Secondary prevention refers to those patients who have survived a prior sudden cardiac arrest or sustained ventricular tachycardia or ventricular fibrillation (VT/VF). Primary prevention refers to those patients who are at high risk for developing but have not had a cardiac arrest or sustained VT. The American College of Cardiology (ACC) and the American Heart Association (AHA) publish joint evidence-based guidelines with recommendations for use of these [4].

Trials investigating secondary prevention of SCD with the use of ICD therapy have shown a significant risk reduction compared to antiarrhythmic drugs. A recent meta-analysis of multiple randomized, controlled trials in secondary prevention showed a 50% relative risk reduction for SCD and 25% risk reduction in all-cause mortality [5]. The majority of patients who undergo ICD implant for secondary prevention have a history of coronary artery disease (CAD), and most clinical trials have had a large portion of patients (upward of 80%) with CAD and impaired left ventricular systolic function. Patients with nonischemic cardiomyopathy, although

J. J. Herr (✉)
Sutter Health CPMC Center for Advanced Heart Failure Therapies, San Francisco, CA, USA
e-mail: herrjj@sutterhealth.org

© Springer International Publishing AG, part of Springer Nature 2019
Y. Sher, J. R. Maldonado (eds.), *Psychosocial Care of End-Stage Organ Disease and Transplant Patients*,
https://doi.org/10.1007/978-3-319-94914-7_18

having a smaller representation in these clinical trials, have shown a similar or greater benefit compared to those with ischemic heart disease. ICD implantation is now the preferred choice of treatment for patients who have survived cardiac arrest based on multiple clinical trial results showing clinical benefit [6–9]. Current guidelines give a Class I recommendation for ICD therapy in patients who have survived a cardiac arrest due to ventricular fibrillation (VF) or hemodynamically unstable sustained VT in the absence of completely reversible factors. ICD use is also a Class I recommendation in patients who have structural heart disease and spontaneous sustained VT regardless of hemodynamic stability as well as those who have unexplained syncope with inducible VT or VF during electrophysiology study [4].

Primary prevention of SCD with ICD therapy has also been shown to be highly effective in reducing risk in those patients who have not had a prior arrest, sustained VT, or VF episode. Chronic ischemic heart disease in the setting of reduced left ventricular ejection fraction (LVEF) poses a significant risk for sudden death. Results from multiple trials have shown a considerable reduction in risk with the use of ICD therapy in these patients. Clinical trials such as the Multicenter Automatic Defibrillator Implantation Trial I (MADIT-I) and MADIT-II investigated ICD use in patients with ischemic heart disease and LVEF less than or equal to 30–35%. Relative risk of mortality was reduced in these two trials by 31% in MADIT-II and 54% in MADIT-I. The MADIT-I trial required the presence of nonsustained VT and inducible sustained VT with electrophysiology study. These criteria were not required in MADIT-II and may account for some of the differences in risk reduction [10, 11]. The SCD-HeFT trial published in 2005 compared ICD therapy with amiodarone for primary prevention of SCD in patients with New York Heart Association (NYHA) functional Class II–III heart failure and LVEF less than or equal to 35%. This large trial included patients who had both ischemic and nonischemic cardiomyopathy and showed a reduction in overall mortality by 23%. Overall, strong evidence supports that ICD therapy for primary prevention of SCD in the setting of CAD and decreased LVEF reduces risk by 20–30%. In the SCD-HeFT patient population, relative risk reduction was similar in the nonischemic patients compared to ischemic, though absolute mortality was lower in nonischemic patients [12]. Myocardial dysfunction due to nonischemic etiologies can be reversible with optimal medical therapy for heart failure. Thus, the time dependence of risk for sudden death relative to the time of diagnosis of cardiomyopathy is important. Studies have been unable to determine an optimal timeframe for observation with medical therapy prior to device implant. Current heart failure management guidelines recommend 3–6 months of guideline-directed medical therapy prior to implantation in patients with NYHA Class I–III heart failure with LVEF less than or equal to 35% [13].

Cardiac Resynchronization Therapy in Heart Failure

Heart failure patients often develop atrioventricular and intraventricular conduction abnormalities, and prolonged QRS duration is associated with an increase in mortality. Conduction delays can lead to dyssynchronous ventricular activation and contraction leading to reductions in stroke volume, increased mitral regurgitation, and negative ventricular remodeling. Cardiac resynchronization therapy (CRT) is a specialized pacing strategy targeting optimization of atrioventricular (AV) and intraventricular conduction. CRT devices consist of three intracardiac pacing leads: right atrial, right ventricular, and a left ventricular lead placed through the coronary sinus into a cardiac vein. These devices are commonly coupled with an ICD function serving a dual purpose. Through optimization of electrical timing in the heart, these devices can shorten delays in AV conduction and coordinate timing of left and right ventricular contraction. CRT can lead to an improvement in ejection fraction, reduction in mitral regurgitation, and decrease in ventricular size, all of which are beneficial in heart failure. Data from multiple clinical trials have demonstrated that CRT therapy can improve quality of life and NYHA functional class and increase 6-min walk distance [14]. CRT has also been shown to reduce hospitalizations for heart failure and when coupled with ICD therapy can reduce the risk of death or heart failure events by over 30% [15].

However, not all patients with heart failure qualify for CRT, and even those who undergo placement may not respond to resynchronization. Those that respond to CRT typically show improvement in symptoms or ventricular function within 3–6 months after implantation. Current estimates indicate that about 30% of heart failure patients will not respond with clinical improvement to CRT. In addition, CRT is only beneficial in certain patient populations, and the indications for placement and potential for benefit vary based on electrocardiographic variables. CRT has been shown to have the best response in patients with a QRS duration greater than 150 ms and a left bundle-branch block pattern [15]. Recognition of patient variables that guide benefit has recently led to limitations in the indications for the use of CRT. Current guidelines give CRT a Class I recommendation only for patients with an LVEF less than or equal to 35%, sinus rhythm, left bundle-branch block, QRS duration greater than or equal to 150 ms, and NYHA Class II to ambulatory IV symptoms [4].

Complications and Considerations for the Use of ICD and CRT Devices

Although there is clear benefit from ICD placement in both primary and secondary prevention of sudden cardiac death, these procedures are not without risk. Complications that occur during the hospitalization for implant are most often procedure-related. The most common early, in-hospital complications are lead dislodgement or perforation (more common with left ventricular leads), pocket hematoma, pneumothorax, and arrhythmia. Mortality during implantation with transvenous systems varies but based on clinical trials is low and is generally less than 1% [16]. Pocket hematomas, while they are typically small-volume bleeds, do carry a risk of morbidity and are associated with a 15-fold increased risk of pocket infection [17].

After hospital discharge, long-term complications may also occur. The most common events include delivery of inappropriate shocks, infection, lead/device malfunction, and pacing−/lead-related hemodynamic effects.

Inappropriate shocks are unfortunately not uncommon and can affect a significant number of patients. Recently, a large sample of ICD patients from the Netherlands was evaluated and showed an event rate of 7% in the first year, 13% within 3 years, and 18% within 5 years post implant [18]. Delivery of inappropriate shocks is often caused by atrial tachyarrhythmia such as atrial fibrillation and is associated with usage of antiarrhythmic drugs. ICD discharges, whether appropriate or not, have a significant psychological impact on the patient and become a source of anxiety, depression, and even post-traumatic stress disorder (PTSD). Frequent ICD shocks are consistently associated with significant emotional distress and reduction in quality of life [19]. In one study, 7.6% of patients qualified for a PTSD diagnosis 18 months post implantation, with pre-existing anxiety being a significant risk factor [20]. Another study showed PTSD rate of almost 15% irrespective of subcutaneous or transvenous type of ICD [21].

Due to the morbidity associated with ICD shocks, device programming methods have become available to attempt to limit delivery of inappropriate therapies. A recent study evaluating one of such methods showed a reduction in all-cause mortality by 55% and reduction in the risk of first inappropriate shock delivery by more than 79% depending using a high-rate therapy method [22].

Device-related infections are an increasingly common complication and are associated with significant morbidity. Infections range from superficial incisional infections that can occur early after implant to more severe infections of the leads or pocket either from direct infection or secondary sources. These infections can be more serious requiring prolonged antibiotic courses and possibly complete removal of the device hardware. Device extraction when necessary is associated with significant morbidity [23]. Cardiac hemodynamics can also be affected by ICD function and lead placement. Tricuspid regurgitation frequently can develop as the leads traverse the valve leaflets and frequent right ventricular pacing may lead to worsening of heart failure due to dyssynchrony.

Patient survival in heart failure is tied to multiple variables, and despite the overall strong body of evidence to support the use of ICD therapy to prevent SCD, there are still patients that do not benefit. There is a very limited life expectancy in patients with end-stage heart failure who are not candidates for advanced therapies. These patients are likely to survive less than 6–12 months from diagnosis without the possibility of heart transplantation or mechanical circulatory support. The cause of death at this stage of disease is more frequently from progressive pump failure rather than from sudden death, and ICD implantation in this population is not indicated from a lack of clinical benefit. At times prognosis can be difficult to estimate, and careful consideration should be made by the treating physicians prior to implant where benefit is unclear [4, 13].

At the end of life, deactivation of an ICD is an important discussion that must be had with patients and their families. When patients are near death, ICD discharge is not beneficial. Delivery of therapies can be associated with significant pain and anxiety for patients and family members as well as interfere with the natural dying process.

Mechanical Circulatory Support for the Treatment of Advanced Heart Failure

Medical therapy for heart failure has decreased mortality, reduced hospitalizations, and improved quality of life for patients. However, despite these advances, some patients still progress to an advanced disease state. These patients require specialized interventions to improve mortality and quality of life such as mechanical circulatory support (MCS) or transplant. Treatment of advanced heart failure with MCS is a rapidly growing field that has evolved substantially since its beginnings. As survival from cardiovascular disease improves and the heart failure population grows, the proportion of patients that may benefit from MCS therapy expands. Previously, heart transplantation or palliative care were the only options for many with advanced heart failure. Despite a growing population, registry data indicates that the number of heart transplants has been largely unchanged over the last 10 years [24]. As a result of this and in conjunction with recent developments in device technology, MCS is rapidly becoming a preferred treatment option for patients with advanced heart failure. The Interagency Registry for

Mechanically Assisted Circulatory Support (INTERMACS) was established in 2005 as a partnership between industry, the National Heart, Lung, and Blood Institute (NHLBI), and the Food and Drug Administration (FDA) in order to collect clinical data relevant to patients who undergo implantation of mechanical circulatory support devices. This registry partnership has allowed for better clinical understanding of patient selection, risk stratification, and outcomes as they relate to MCS [25].

Ventricular Assist Devices

Mechanical circulatory support involves the use of surgically implanted mechanical pumps that assist or replace the failing ventricles by increasing cardiac output, optimizing hemodynamics, and improving end-organ perfusion. Ventricular assist devices (VAD) are used as a bridge to transplant and bridge to recovery and for those patients who do not qualify for transplant but are failing medical therapy, as a permanent treatment known as destination therapy. There are multiple different types of devices available, and they are described by the ventricle(s) they assist and their method/configuration of flow. Most pumps are left ventricular assist devices (LVAD) and provide partial support for the heart by assisting the left ventricular output and hemodynamics. LVADs account for the majority of devices currently implanted and require that the right ventricle functions well enough on its own without independent mechanical support. Available LVAD devices are designed with an inflow cannula that is implanted into the left ventricular apex that drains blood from the heart, through a mechanical pump, and delivers the blood through an outflow graft in the ascending aorta. Currently, most devices utilize continuous-flow technology as their method of support with pump rotors configured either axial or centrifugal (Figs. 18.1 and 18.2). Blood is drawn continuously from the heart through the pump which

in turn delivers it to the central circulation in a non-pulsatile manner. Early devices were external to the body; however, all currently available durable devices are almost completely implanted. The driveline is the only external portion of the

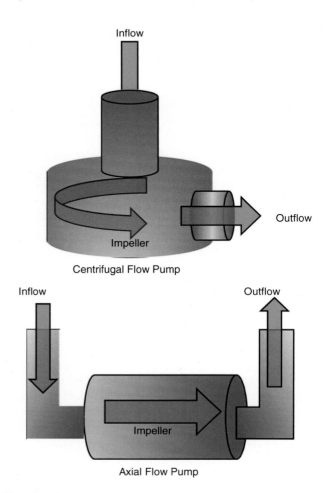

Fig. 18.1 Schematic representation of continuous-flow left ventricular assist device configurations, axial and centrifugal flow pumps. Red arrows indicate direction of blood flow through the impeller

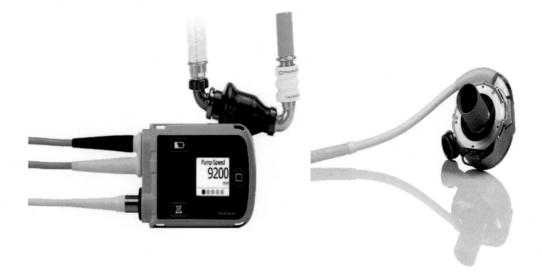

Fig. 18.2 HeartMate II axial continuous-flow LVAD (left) and HeartMate 3 centrifugal continuous-flow LVAD (right). HeartMate 3 utilizes a fully magnetically levitated impeller technology, and the small size allows for intra-pericardial placement. (Courtesy Thoratec/Abbott)

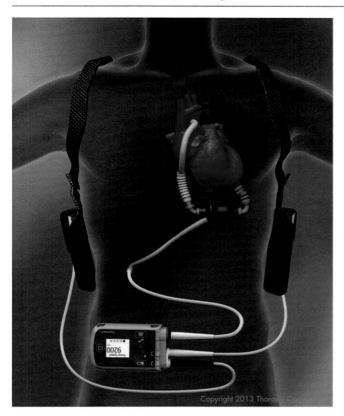

Fig. 18.3 HeartMate II LVAD implant orientation and patient peripherals. Percutaneous driveline exits the body and connects to device controller and power source. Battery power source illustrated here. (Courtesy Thoratec/Abbott)

Table 18.1 Description of INTERMACS profiles, considerations for the timing of implantation, and frequency of implant by profile based on data from Kirklin et al. [26]

Profile	Clinical characteristics	% of MCS implants	Implant timing
1	Cardiogenic shock "Crash and burn"	15	Min–hours
2	Progressive decline on inotropes	37.5	Hours–days
3	Stable and inotrope dependent	28.8	Days–weeks
4	Recurrent advanced HF, resting symptoms	13.7	Weeks–months
5	Exertion intolerant	2.7	Variable
6	Exertion limited NYHA IIIB	1.2	Variable
7	Advanced NYHA class III	0.6	Not indicated

device which exits the patient subcutaneously through the abdomen and is connected to a device controller and power source (Fig. 18.3).

Adequate patient selection for mechanical circulatory support is essential to maximizing patient benefit and outcomes. Clinical data from the INTERMACS registry has helped risk stratify patients based on severity of illness prior to implantation. INTERMACS profiles are used to describe illness severity and range from most severe (1 – critical cardiogenic shock) to least (7 – advanced NYHA Class III heart failure) (Table 18.1). Most patients that undergo implant of MCS devices are INTERMACS profiles 1–3, accounting for 81% of total implants in the registry from 2008 to 2014 with the majority being profile 2 and 3. Clinical outcomes are tied to INTERMACS profile with lowest survival and highest complication rates in patients with critical cardiogenic shock. Other important risk factors that predict poor early outcome post implant include older age, female sex, higher body mass index, prior stroke, renal failure, right ventricular dysfunction, and increased surgical complexity [26].

Publication of the RE-MATCH trial in 2001 highlighted the poor survival of patients with end-stage heart failure that do not qualify for cardiac transplantation. In this study, these patients had an observed 1- and 2-year survival with medical therapy of 23% and 8%, respectively. This trial evaluated the use of the HeartMate XVE (Thoratec/Abbott) implantable pulsatile-flow LVAD and showed a significant improvement in both 1- and 2-year survivals from death from any cause compared to medical therapy. Patients supported with an LVAD had an observed survival of 52% and 25% at 1 and 2 years, respectively, which was a 48% reduction in risk of death in the LVAD group. Quality-of-life indexes and functional capacity by NYHA functional class were also improved in the LVAD group at 1 year [27]. When compared to more recent trials and registry data, these outcomes are less than ideal; however, this study led to increased interest in MCS therapy as a viable treatment and introduced the concept of destination therapy. Subsequent development and success with the next generation in LVAD technology utilizing continuous-flow technology occurred with the introduction of the HeartMate II (Thoratec/Abbott). Patients awaiting cardiac transplant were initially studied, and data from the pivotal trial showed a 75% survival to transplant, recovery, or ongoing support while remaining eligible for transplant at 6 months post implantation [28]. The subsequent post-FDA approval study in this population showed continued improvement in patient outcomes with 90% survival at 6 months to transplant, recovery, or continued support [29]. This improvement in outcome illustrated the change in awareness and use of LVAD technology coupled with improved clinical care as centers became more experienced in their use. Continuous-flow LVAD technology has also been shown to be beneficial in prolonging and improving quality of life in patients who are not candidates for heart transplantation as destination therapy. The HeartMate II destination therapy trial compared the then already FDA-approved HeartMate XVE pulsatile-flow LVAD to the HeartMate II with a primary end point of survival free from disabling stroke and reoperation to repair or replace the pump at 2 years. The continuous-flow device performed better with an improved survival rate of 68% and 58% at 1 and 2 years compared to 55% and 24%

with the pulsatile LVAD [30]. Paralleling the bridge to transplant trial and refined experience in the management of these devices showed further improvement in outcomes with 1- and 2-year survivals of 74% and 61% in the post-FDA approval study [31]. Contemporary data from the 7th report of the INTERMACS registry indicates an overall 1-year survival of 80% in all patients supported with continuous-flow VADs, regardless of indication [26].

Device technology has continued to improve, and devices are now smaller allowing for intra-pericardial placement. Examples of third-generation centrifugal continuous-flow pumps include the FDA-approved HeartWare ventricular assist device (HVAD, HeartWare/Medtronic) and the FDA approved HeartMate 3 (Thoratec/Abbott). When compared to data from the INTERMACS registry in a bridge to transplant population, the HVAD was non-inferior to the currently approved axial-flow device with approximately 90% survival at 6 months to transplant, recovery, or ongoing support on the original device [32]. Long-term support outcomes in non-transplant candidates with the HVAD were recently published, and this device was also found to be non-inferior to the currently available axial-flow LVAD with respect to the combined end point of survival free from disabling stroke or device removal for malfunction or failure [33].

For many patients with heart failure, treatments that improve quality of life are equally important as those that extend life. End-stage heart failure patients have a poor quality of life as they experience significant symptoms at rest or with minimal activity. Qualification for VAD implantation as destination therapy requires severe left ventricular systolic dysfunction with significant functional limitation or dependence on inotropic agents or temporary mechanical support. VADs have consistently shown improvements in heart failure quality-of-life measures and functional status. In the destination therapy trial of the HeartMate II, 96% of patients were NYHA Class IIIB/IV at baseline, and 75% improved to Class I or II within 3 months of implant, and 80% improved to that level within 24 months after implant. Patients who underwent HeartMate II implant also showed sustained improvement in 6-min walk distance, doubling from baseline, within 24 months. Distance walked averaged 372 m, which is longer than the length of four football fields [30]. Improvements in functional status allow patients to regain independence, return to activities they previously enjoyed, and maintain a largely normal life. In reality there are few limits that are put on patients in regard to activities they can participate in, with the exception of those that require submerging in water and contact sports. After recovery, and per program preference, patients may be able to drive and can travel on planes. An important aspect of the use of MCS in treating advanced heart failure is the ability to regain a consistently high quality of life.

VAD placement is a major cardiac surgery, and patients are often debilitated from functional limitations prior to implant. During the recovery period after surgery, these patients require rehabilitation and psychosocial support. Early post implant, patients are seen in clinic for frequent assessment, and medications are adjusted often, as their bodies continue to adapt to their new physiology. Patients initially require a significant amount of help from a support person in managing their equipment, medications, and clinic visits. Program standards are variable in regard to the level of support necessary and length of time until complete independence. Given the fact that the first month post discharge is a high-risk period, many programs would require 24-h support for at least a period of 30 days post discharge. Patient self-management involves driveline exit-site care including sterile dressing changes which occur daily to weekly and maintenance of power supply including battery changes or external power sources. Patients also are required to develop an understanding of basic device function including alarms or malfunctions and how to manage them in an emergency.

As patients improve in their strength, medication regimens stabilize, many patients will be able to regain their near complete independence in their daily living. Care provided by the support system during this period of change and recovery is essential to attaining a positive outcome.

Total Artificial Heart: Cardiac Replacement Therapy

In contrast to VADs, the total artificial heart (TAH, SynCardia) is a cardiac replacement therapy. Placement of a TAH requires removal of the native ventricles and replacing their function with two separate pneumatically driven pumps. Mechanistically these pumps are different from continuous-flow VADs as they generate pulsatile blood flow. The artificial ventricles are placed orthotopically and contain four artificial mechanical heart valves [34]. TAH is available for use in the United States as a bridge to cardiac transplantation for transplant-eligible patients with biventricular heart failure who are at risk of imminent death from their disease. The pivotal trial for this device enrolled 81 patients and investigated the rate of survival to cardiac transplant compared to patients of similar clinical severity who did not receive mechanical circulatory support while awaiting transplant. Survival to transplant occurred in 79% of patients who received the device and 46% in the control group. Overall 1-year survival was also improved compared to controls with 70% alive at 1 year compared to 31%. Previously, this device required patients to remain in the hospital while awaiting transplantation as the controller required to power the device was unable to be used outside the hospital. However, through recent advances in driver technology, a smaller, portable device driver is now available allowing for safe hospital discharge for patients while awaiting transplantation [35]. An important consideration in the use of this device and the support it requires is that it is a *cardiac replacement* therapy. Patients who have undergone placement of this device are completely dependent on its function, and in the uncommon event of device malfunction or failure, they are at significant risk. Due to this risk, the level of independence gained after surgical recovery in patients with the TAH is significantly less than that of those with an LVAD. Patients require constant supervision by a caregiver when outside of the hospital, unlike a patient with an LVAD who may only require that level of supervision early in recovery. Despite this limitation, the mortality in patients considered for its use is significant enough that the overall benefit may outweigh the cost of the support necessary for its placement. Patient size is a consideration in selection of this device, as unfortunately due to the size of the device itself, it may be too large for some smaller patients. Currently, a clinical trial for a smaller size TAH device is being conducted and may lead to a further expansion of its potential patient population.

Mechanical Circulatory Support-Related Adverse Events

Mechanical circulatory support devices can be life-saving for patients with advanced heart failure; however, there are limitations and risks to these devices. Adverse events range from significant to minor, and many patients will experience an adverse event after implant. A majority of adverse events occur in the early period post implantation, and the frequency of certain events changes over time. The most clinically significant events that can occur include right ventricular failure, infection, bleeding, neurologic event, valvular disease, and pump thrombosis/hemolysis.

Right ventricular failure post-LVAD implantation is associated with increased morbidity and mortality. The native right ventricle (RV) must adapt to changes in hemodynamics and cardiac output accompanying LVAD implant, and if it is unable to compensate, it may fail. This often occurs early and may be noticed within the first few hours after implantation and can be severe. RV failure can lead to renal and hepatic failure as well as low LVAD flow due to left ventricular under filling. Treatment is aimed at optimization of right-sided pressures and function with diuresis, inotropes, and if needed temporary mechanical circulatory support. Optimal patient selection can reduce the risk of development of RV failure; however, currently available risk prediction models are based on data from older trials with variable definitions of RV failure and have suboptimal predictive accuracy [36]. It is now recognized that RV failure may also occur late within several months to years after implant and is associated with poor outcomes. Further studies are needed to determine risk factors and outcomes in larger populations for the development of late RV failure [37].

Infections post-MCS placement early post implant often are surgical or hospitalization related (i.e., wound or catheter-associated infections). Over time the rate of other infections increases in prevalence, most notably of the percutaneous driveline. Bacterial infections of the driveline can be either superficial at the exit site or extend more proximally along the course of the line. More extensive infections may ascend into and affect the device pocket or pump hardware. Infections affecting the device hardware are difficult to manage and often require extraction and replacement. Percutaneous driveline infections are most often associated with trauma to the line allowing an entry point for bacteria. Uncomplicated driveline infections can be managed with antibiotics; however, more extensive infections may require surgical debridement or long-term suppressive antibiotic therapy [38, 39].

Bleeding complications post implant are not infrequent and are typically surgery-related early post implant, though mucosal sources can complicate long-term care. Estimates of long-term bleeding complication rates are 13–30%, occurring more often with continuous-flow versus pulsatile devices. Cumulative bleeding risk associated with MCS is dependent on multiple factors. First, currently available devices all require systemic anticoagulation to prevent thrombotic events and therefore inherently increase bleeding tendency. All currently available MCS devices are mechanical with metallic components in constant contact with and generating a shear force on the circulating blood. Patients with continuous-flow LVADs have been shown to have a reduction in high molecular weight von Willebrand multimers that are essential in clot formation. This leads to the development of an acquired von Willebrand disease, and subsequently clot stabilization is decreased, and bleeding tendency is increased. Continuous-flow devices also predispose to the development of arteriovenous malformations (AVM) typically within the gastrointestinal tract. Coupled with increased tendency to bleed from anticoagulation and acquired von Willebrand disease, patients are at increased risk of gastrointestinal bleeding. Despite diligent monitoring and care, mucosal bleeding remains a common cause of hospital readmission and morbidity for these patients [40, 41].

The interface between the blood and device components carries a risk for development of thrombotic events such as stroke or pump thrombosis which can potentially lead to device malfunction. Neurologic events can be a devastating complication of MCS implant. Overall event rates are variable between the available devices; and outcomes often combine ischemic stroke, hemorrhagic stroke, and transient ischemic attack (TIA). Rates are device and population specific and generally range from 8% to 17% with continuous-flow devices to as high as 26% with the total artificial heart [30, 32, 34]. Initial trial data of the HeartMate II showed an event rate for ischemic stroke of 0.13 events per patient-year; however, with improved clinical management through the duration of the trial, a rate of 0.05 events per patient-year was observed. Rates of stroke appear to be higher in patients supported by the HVAD, and blood pressure control appears to be a significant risk factor [33]. Hemorrhagic stroke carries the highest risk of mortality for patients and are related to antiplatelet and anticoagulant medications required by the devices. Hemorrhagic stroke event rates also declined through the duration of the HeartMate II destination therapy trial from 0.07 events per patient-year to 0.03 [32, 34, 42]. Pump thrombosis and hemolysis can result from the changes in blood flow through the different components of the device. Pump thrombosis can lead to device malfunction and subsequently may require device exchange. Replacement of an LVAD pump in this setting is associated with significant morbidity and reduction in patient survival [43]. Recent data suggests that there has been an increase in the observed rate of pump thrombosis associated with the HeartMate II device. Analysis of registry data showed a small and progressive increase in thrombosis associated with the device and that early changes in markers of hemolysis may be a signal triggering intervention [44, 45].

Valvular heart disease may occur as a result of continuous-flow LVADs as well. Aortic regurgitation can develop as a consequence of continuous-flow and has the potential to cause deleterious hemodynamic effects. Presence of significant native aortic regurgitation at the time of implant needs to be addressed with either valve repair, closure, or replacement. Development of de novo aortic regurgitation is time dependent and can lead to reduced output, elevated left ventricular filling pressures, and symptomatic heart failure. Observational studies have estimated that as high as 37% of patients will develop at least moderate aortic regurgitation after 3 years of LVAD support who did not have surgical intervention at the time of initial implant. Non-opening of the aortic valve after implantation is strongly associated with development of de novo regurgitation. Treatment in symptomatic patients post implant is currently with surgical intervention [46–49].

Mechanical Circulatory Support at the End-of-Life and Advanced Care Planning

End-of-life decisions involving patients supported with MCS devices can often be very complex due to the nature of the support provided by the device. Several profiles of clinical course and decline to death have been described in LVAD patients. Some patients die rapidly very early post-surgery, while some others do not improve post implant and continue to struggle with heart failure or other organ dysfunction. Patients that do improve may have better quality of life

initially but later on develop a new life-limiting condition or organ failure leading to a slow decline or suddenly suffer an event leading to their death (e.g., hemorrhagic stroke) [50]. Due to these variable clinical courses, advanced care planning becomes an essential component to the informed decision-making process prior to MCS device implant. In order to fully understand goals of care and patient expectations, it is essential to discuss preferences for life-prolonging measures, including the possibility of device deactivation. These discussions optimally take place prior to implant and major clinical deterioration, when patients are still best able to express their preferences. Hospice is a commonly used treatment for patients with end-stage heart failure who are dying and do not qualify for advanced therapies. However, hospice appears to be less frequently used in patients who have undergone MCS device placement, as most of these patients die in the hospital due to multisystem organ failure, hemorrhagic stroke, or progressive heart failure [51]. Decision aids have been developed to attempt to best provide support for end-of-life decision-making. Proactive use of palliative care consultation has been shown to help patients in their decision-making [52, 53]. Overall, the decision to pursue MCS device placement, particularly for destination therapy, must take into consideration the psychosocial aspects involved in the care of the patient after implant as well as in the event of a life-limiting complication.

Conclusions

Device therapy for heart failure has evolved significantly over the years and now encompasses a range of potential treatments. ICDs and CRT have been able to reduce risk of sudden cardiac death and improve quality of life and functional status for patients. Mechanical circulatory support has provided treatment options for many who previously had none or were only limited. MCS devices can provide patients time to await transplantation or improve survival and quality of life of those who do not qualify for it. Despite the risks involved, MCS has changed the face of treatment of advanced heart failure. Overall, device therapy is a rapidly changing field, and continued advancements in technology will lead to the introduction of further novel treatments for heart failure.

References

1. Anderson KP, DeCamilla J, Moss AJ. Clinical significance of ventricular tachycardia (3 beats or longer) detected during ambulatory monitoring after myocardial infarction. Circulation. 1978;57:890–7.
2. Echt DS, Liebson PR, Mitchell LB, Peters RW, Obias-Manno D, Barker AH, et al. Mortality and morbidity in patients receiving encainide, flecainide, or placebo: the cardiac arrhythmia suppression trial. N Engl J Med. 1991;324:781–8.
3. Rowley CP, Gold MR. Subcutaneous implantable cardioverter defibrillator. Circ Arrhythm Electrophysiol. 2012;5:587–93.

4. Epstein AE, DiMarco JP, Ellenbogen KA, Estes M, Freedman RA, Gettes LS, et al. 2012 ACCF/AHA/HRS focused update incorporated into the ACCF/AHA/HRS 2008 guidelines for device based therapy for cardiac rhythm abnormalities. J Am Coll Cardiol. 2013;61:e6–75.

5. Connolly SJ, Hallstrom AP, Cappato R, Schron EB, Kuck KH, Greene HL, et al. Meta-analysis of the implantable cardioverter defibrillator secondary prevention trials. AVID, CASH and CIDS studies. Antiarrhythmics vs implantable defibrillator study. Cardiac arrest study Hamburg. Canadian implantable defibrillator study. Eur Heart J. 2000;21:2071–8.

6. Connolly SJ, Gent M, Roberts RS, et al. Canadian implantable defibrillator study (CIDS): a randomized trial of the implantable cardioverter defibrillator against amiodarone. Circulation. 2000;101:1297–302.

7. Powell AC, Fuchs T, Finkelstein DM, Garan H, Cannom DS, McGovern BA, et al. Influence of implantable cardioverter-defibrillators on the long-term prognosis of survivors of out-of-hospital cardiac arrest. Circulation. 1993;88:1083–92.

8. Kuck KH, Cappato R, Siebels J, Ruppel R. Randomized comparison of antiarrhythmic drug therapy with implantable defibrillators in patients resuscitated from cardiac arrest: the cardiac arrest study Hamburg (CASH). Circulation. 2000;102:748–54.

9. Wever EF, Hauer RN, van Capelle FL, Tijssen JG, Crijns HJ, Algra A, et al. Randomized study of implantable defibrillator as first-choice therapy versus conventional strategy in postinfarct sudden death survivors. Circulation. 1995;91:2195–203.

10. Moss AJ, Hall WJ, Cannom DS, Daubert JP, Higgins SL, Klein H, et al. Improved survival with an implanted defibrillator in patients with coronary disease at high risk for ventricular arrhythmia. Multicenter automatic defibrillator implantation trial investigators. N Engl J Med. 1996;335:1933–40.

11. Moss AJ, Zareba W, Hall WJ, Klein H, Wilber DJ, Cannom DS, et al. Prophylactic implantation of a defibrillator in patients with myocardial infarction and reduced ejection fraction. N Engl J Med. 2002;346:877–83.

12. Bardy G, Lee K, Mark D, Poole JE, Packer DL, Boineau R, et al. Amiodarone or an implantable cardioverter-defibrillator for congestive heart failure. N Engl J Med. 2005;352:225–37.

13. Yancy CW, Jessup M, Bozkurt B, Butler J, Casey DE, et al. 2013 ACCF/AHA guideline for management of heart failure: a report of the American College of Cardiology Foundation/American Heart Association task force on practice guidelines. J Am Coll Cardiol. 2013;62:e147–239.

14. Abraham WT, Fisher WG, Smith AL, Delurgio DB, Leon AR, Loh E, et al. Cardiac resynchronization in chronic heart Failure. N Engl J Med. 2002;246:1845–53.

15. Moss AJ, Hall WJ, Cannom DS, Klein H, Brown MW, Daubert JP, et al. Cardiac-resynchronization therapy for the prevention of heart-failure events. N Engl J Med. 2009;361:1329–38.

16. Van Rees JB, de Bie MK, Thijssen J, Borleffs CJ, Schalij MJ, van Erven L. Implantation-related complications of implantable cardioverter-defibrillators and cardiac resynchronization therapy devices: a systematic review of randomized clinical trials. J Am Coll Cardiol. 2011;58:995–1000.

17. Klug D, Balde M, Pavin D, Hidden-Lucet F, Clementy J, Sadoul N, et al. Risk factors related to infections of implanted pacemakers and cardioverter-defibrillators: results of a large prospective study. Circulation. 2007;116:1349–55.

18. Van Rees JB, Borleffs JW, de Bie MK, Stijnen T, van Erven L, Bax JJ, et al. Inappropriate implantable cardioverter-defibrillator shocks: incidence, predictors and impact on mortality. J Am Coll Cardiol. 2011;57:556–62.

19. Sears S, Conti J. Understanding implantable cardioverter defibrillator shocks and storms: medical and psychosocial considerations for research and clinical care. Clin Cardiol. 2003;26:107–11.

20. Habibovic M, van den Broek KC, Alings M, Van der Voort PH, Denollet J. Posttraumatic stress 18 months following cardioverter defibrillator implantation: shocks, anxiety and personality. Health Psychol. 2012;31(2):186–93.

21. Köbe J, Hucklenbroich K, Geisendörfer N, Bettin M, Frommeyer G, Reinke F, et al. Posttraumatic stress and quality of life with the totally subcutaneous compared to conventional cardioverter-defibrillator systems. Clin Res Cardiol. 2017;106:317–21.

22. Moss AJ, Schuger C, Beck CA, Brown MW, Cannom DS, Daubert JP, et al., for the MADIT-RIT Trial investigators. Reduction in inappropriate therapy and mortality through ICD programming. N Engl J Med. 2012;367:2275–83.

23. Greenspon AJ, Patel JD, Lau E, Ochoa JA, Frisch DR, Ho RT, et al. 16-year trends in the infection burden for pacemakers and implantable cardioverter-defibrillators in the United States: 1993–2008. J Am Coll Cardiol. 2011;58:1001–6.

24. Lund LH, Edwards LB, Dipchand AI, Goldfarb S, Kucheryavaya AY, Levvey RJ, et al. The registry of the international society for heart and lung transplantation: thirty-third adult heart transplantation report – 2016; focus theme: primary diagnostic indications for transplant. J Heart Lung Transplant. 2016;35(10):1149–205.

25. Interagency Registry for Mechanically Assisted Circulatory Support Website. http://www.uab.edu/medicine/intermacs/about-us. Accessed 26 Feb 2017.

26. Kirklin JK, Naftel DC, Pagani FD, Kormos RL, Stevenson LW, Blume ED, et al. Seventh INTERMACS annual report: 15,000 patients and counting. J Heart Lung Transplant. 2015;34:1495–504.

27. Rose EA, Gelijns AC, Moskowitz AJ, Heitjan DF, Stevenson LW, Dembitsky W, et al. Long-term use of a left ventricular assist device for end-stage heart failure. N Engl J Med. 2001;345:1435–43.

28. Miller LW, Pagani FD, Russell SD, John R, Boyel AJ Aaronson KD, et al., for the HeartMate II Clinical Investigators. Use of a continuous-flow device in patients awaiting heart transplantation. N Engl J Med. 2007;357:885–96.

29. Starling RC, Naka Y, Boyle AJ, Gonzalez-Stawinski G, John R, Jorde U, et al. Results of the post-US Food and Drug Administration-approval study with a continuous flow left ventricular assist device as a bridge to heart transplantation: a prospective study using the INTERMACS. J Am Coll Cardiol. 2011;57:1890–8.

30. Slaughter MS, Rogers JG, Milano CA, Russell SD, Conte JV, Feldman D, et al., for the HeartMate II Investigators. Advanced heart failure treated with continuous-flow left ventricular assist device. N Engl J Med. 2009;361:2241–51.

31. Jorde UP, Kushwaha SS, Tatooles AJ, Naka Y, Bhat G, Long JW, et al., for the HeartMate II Clinical Investigators. Results of the destination therapy post-food and drug administration approval study with a continuous flow left ventricular assist device: a prospective study using the INTERMACS registry. J Am Coll Cardiol. 2014;63:1751–7.

32. Aaronson KD, Slaughter MS, Miller LW, McGee EC, Cotts WG, Acker MA, et al., for the HeartWare Ventricular Assist Device (HVAD) Bridge to Transplant ADVANCE Trial Investigators. Use of an intrapericardial, continuous-flow, centrifugal pump in patients awaiting heart transplantation. Circulation. 2012;125:3191–200.

33. Rogers JG, Pagani FD, Tatooles AJ, Bhat G, Slaughter MS, Birks EJ, et al. Intrapericardial left ventricular assist device for advanced heart failure. N Engl J Med. 2017;376:451–60.

34. Copeland JG, Smith RG, Arabia FA, Nolan PE, Sethi GK, Tsau PH, et al. Cardiac replacement with a total artificial heart as a bridge to transplantation. N Engl J Med. 2004;351:859–67.

35. FDA Approves the Freedom Portable Driver that Powers the SynCardia Total Artificial Heart. http://www.syncardia.com/2014-press-releases/fda-approves-the-freedom-portable-driver-that-powers-the-syncardia-total-artificial-heart.html. Accessed 26 Feb 2017.

36. Lampert BC, Tueteberg JJ. Right ventricular failure after left ventricular assist devices. J Heart Lung Transplant. 2015;34:1123–30.

37. Kapelios CJ, Charitos C, Kaldara E, Malliaras K, Nana E, Pantsios C, et al. Late-onset right ventricular dysfunction after mechanical support by a continuous-flow left ventricular assist device. J Heart Lung Transplant. 2015;34:1604–10.

38. Schaffer JM, Allen JG, Weiss ES, Arnaoutakis GJ, Patel ND, Russell SD, et al. Infectious complications after pulsatile and continuous-flow left ventricular assist device implantation. J Heart Lung Transplant. 2011;30:164–74.

39. Gordon RJ, Weiberg A, Pagani F, Slaughter MS, Pappas PS, Naka Y, et al. Prospective multicenter study of ventricular assist device infections. Circulation. 2013;127:691–702.

40. Crow S, John R, Boyle A, Shumway S, Liao K, Colvin-Adams M, et al. Gastrointestinal bleeding rates in recipients of nonpulsatile and pulsatile left ventricular assist devices. J Thorac Cardiovasc Surg. 2009;137:208–15.

41. Suarez J, Patel CB, Felker M, Becker R, Hernandez AF, Rogers JG. Mechanisms of bleeding and approach to patients with axial-flow left ventricular assist devices. Circ Heart Fail. 2011;4: 779–84.

42. Park SJ, Milano CA, Tatooles AJ, Rogers JG, Adamson RM, Steidly E, et al., for the HeartMate II Clinical Investigators. Outcomes in advanced heart failure patients with left ventricular assist devices for destination therapy. Circ Heart Fail. 2012;5:214–48.

43. Kirklin JK, Naftel DC, Kormos RL, Pagani FD, Myers SL, Stevenson LW, et al. Interagency Registry for Mechanically Assisted Circulatory Support (INTERMACS) an analysis of pump thrombosis in the HeartMate II left ventricular assist device. J Heart Lung Transplant. 2014;33:12–22.

44. Starling RC, Moazami N, Silvestry SC, Ewald G, Rogers JG, Milano CA, et al. Unexpected abrupt increase in left ventricular assist device thrombosis. N Engl J Med. 2014;370:33–40.

45. Kirklin JK, Naftel DC, Kormos RL, Myers S, Acker MA, Rogers J, et al. Pump thrombosis in the Thoratec HeartMate II device: an update analysis of the INTERMACS registry. J Heart Lung Transplant. 2015;34:1515–26.

46. Cowger J, Pagani FD, Haft JW, Romano MA, Aaronson KD, Kolias TJ. The development of aortic insufficiency in left ventricular assist device-supported patients. Circ Heart Fail. 2010;3:668–74.

47. Jorde UP, Uriel N, Nahumi N, Bejar D, Gonzalez-Costello J, Thomas SS, et al. Prevalence, significance, and management of aortic insufficiency in continuous flow left ventricular assist device recipients. Circ Heart Fail. 2014;7:310–9.

48. Park SW, Uriel N, Takayama H, Cappleman S, Song R, Colombo PC, et al. Prevalence of de novo aortic insufficiency in left ventricular assist device-supported patients. J Heart Lung Transplant. 2010;29:1172–6.

49. Atkins BZ, Hashmi ZA, Ganapathi AM, Harrison JK, Hughes GC, Rogers JG, et al. Surgical correction of aortic valve insufficiency after left ventricular assist device implantation. Cardiovasc Surg. 2013;146:1247–52.

50. Rizzieri AG, Verheijde JL, Rady MY, McGregor JL. Ethical challenges with the left ventricular assist device as a destination therapy. Philos Ethics Humanit Med. 2008;3:20. https://doi. org/10.1186/1747-5341-3-20.

51. Dunlay SM, Strand JJ, Wordingham SE, Stulak JM, Luckhardt AJ, Swetz KM. Dying with a left ventricular assist device as destination therapy. Circ Heart Fail. 2016;9:e003096. https://doi.org/10.1161/ CIRCHEARTFAILURE.116.003096.

52. Thompson JS, Matlock DD, McIlvennan CK, Jenkins AR, Allen LA. Development of a decision aid for patients with advanced heart failure considering a destination therapy left ventricular assist device. JACC Heart Fail. 2015;3:965–76.

53. Swetz KM, Freeman MR, AbouEzzeddine OF, Carter KA, Boilson BA, Ottenberg AL, et al. Palliative medicine consultation for preparedness planning in patients receiving left ventricular assist devices as destination therapy. Mayo Clin Proc. 2011;86:493–500.

History of Heart Transplantation

19

Sharon A. Hunt

While very early surgical reports documented the feasibility and safety of creating vascular anastomoses and transplanting solid organs in animal models [1], excision of a normal heart and its implantation in a recipient necessarily involve denervating the donor heart. The clinical field of heart transplantation could not exist until it was proven that a denervated heart could provide adequate circulatory support to allow normal physical activity in a heart recipient. Documentation of such physiology was first published in the early 1960s by the surgical pioneers in the field Drs. Norman Shumway and Richard Lower working in their research laboratory at Stanford University. They used the canine model and measured quite normal physiologic function in dogs with transplanted denervated hearts. Their surgical procedure was fairly simple and involved midatrial excision of both the left and right atria and of the great vessels just above their semilunar valves. This procedure was performed on both the donor and the recipient dog, and the donor heart was implanted into the recipient in the orthotopic position using the same suture lines. The recipient dogs subsequently had standard measurements of hemodynamics which were shown to be normal at rest and with exercise [2]. Such dogs were then seen to run and play normally for weeks, much to the satisfaction of the laboratory staff.

Simultaneous with this pioneering work, the field of kidney transplantation was beginning to flourish and to demonstrate the effectiveness of pharmacologic suppression of the immune system (then with azathioprine and prednisone) to prevent what was otherwise the inevitable rejection of non-human leukocyte antigen (HLA)-identical donor organs. These two converging developments set the stage for the introduction of clinical heart transplantation. At Stanford, an appropriate recipient with end-stage heart disease was identified by the surgical team and awaited the availability of a compatible donor heart from a brain dead individual. Much to the surprise of the team (and the world), the first clinical heart transplant was actually announced to have been performed in South Africa by Dr. Christian Barnard on December 3, 1967. Dr. Barnard was a heart surgeon who had observed several of the canine procedures which were done by Dr. Lower, who was then at Virginia Commonwealth University. Louis Washkansky, the recipient, lived for 18 days after the groundbreaking surgery. Stanford found an appropriate donor for their patient a month later and performed the first heart transplant in the United States on January 6, 1968. Mike Kasperak, who had had a massive heart attack, lived for 15 days after the transplant. Although he regained consciousness, was able to communicate with his wife post-transplant, and provided hope for recovery, in retrospect, his other organs were too sick, and he died of severe hemorrhage and multisystem organ failure.

Subsequent to these two very well-publicized procedures, many cardiac surgical teams were excited and quickly started heart transplant programs. There were 101 heart transplants performed worldwide in the calendar year 1968. The outcomes were abysmal, however, with survival rates measured in weeks or months, and the procedure became quite contentious, and ultimately an unofficial moratorium on clinical heart transplantation was accepted in 1970. The one program that did not follow this moratorium was Stanford, and the group continued clinical activities virtually alone during the next decade, tackling the problems that limited survival rates. Many small incremental improvements occurred in the field of solid-organ transplantation over that decade, but the signal contributions of the Stanford team included introducing the use of the endomyocardial biopsy to definitively diagnose rejection and document the effectiveness of its treatment and the demonstration of safe cold ischemic donor heart times to permit distant heart procurement. During that decade a definition of donor brain death was also accepted societally and legally, the need for which had not previously been recognized [3].

S. A. Hunt (✉)
Division of Cardiovascular Medicine, Department of Medicine, Stanford University School of Medicine, Stanford, CA, USA
e-mail: hunts@stanford.edu

© Springer International Publishing AG, part of Springer Nature 2019
Y. Sher, J. R. Maldonado (eds.), *Psychosocial Care of End-Stage Organ Disease and Transplant Patients*,
https://doi.org/10.1007/978-3-319-94914-7_19

Prior to the introduction of the endomyocardial biopsy, the diagnosis of heart rejection was made by careful observation of the recipient developing heart failure signs and symptoms and a drop in the total amplitude of QRS complexes on the surface EKG, reflecting edema and inflammation of the graft. Both of these findings of rejection were well documented in the canine model but were unfortunately late developments in the clinical course. In 1973, Dr. Phillip Caves, a cardiac surgical resident on leave from the United Kingdom at Stanford, took an older Japanese bioptome instrument and modified it to allow access to the apex of the right ventricle in order to snip off and retrieve myocardial specimens to analyze for rejection. The instrument was inserted percutaneously into the right internal jugular vein and advanced under fluoroscopic guidance across the tricuspid valve and into the right ventricle. It proved to be safe and simple to perform, able to be performed repeatedly, and productive of very useful tissue for analysis [4]. A pathological system and scale for reproducibly grading rejection were developed at Stanford by Dr. Margaret Billingham. The system has undergone a variety of iterations and now stands as the international standard for grading heart rejection [5].

The initial need to have the donor patient in an adjoining operating room usually required transport of a brain dead individual to the transplant center and, understandably, posed a major limitation on the clinical expansion of heart transplantation. In the laboratory, both Lower and Shumway demonstrated that a donor heart could be preserved in iced saline for periods up to 3 hours and then implanted and have normal physiologic function [6]. The safety of such preservation opened the way for distant heart procurement at centers other than the transplant center which, ever since, has been the major means of procuring donor hearts.

The (then) new immunosuppressive agent cyclosporine was introduced into the field of renal transplantation in the 1970s and proved to be a major improvement over the older agents. In 1980, it was introduced to heart transplantation at Stanford with similar major improvement in outcomes [7] and helped rekindle interest in the field in the medical community. Subsequently, increasing numbers of centers restarted heart transplant programs, and increasing numbers of procedures were performed. In 1982, the International Society for Heart Transplantation was formed and started a Registry of such procedures and their outcomes. The Registry remains robust and continues activity to this day and reports results to the public annually. It currently includes data on over 118,000 recipient patients.

The burgeoning number of patients over these years has led to a need for clinicians trained to provide them with highly specialized care. In the year 2010, the American Board of Internal Medicine approved the field of Advanced Heart Failure and Transplant Cardiology as a distinct subspecialty, and certifying exams are now given every 2 years. It is a subspecialty which allows clinicians the opportunity to deal with the medical issues that these patients develop as well as the psychological issues involved in their return (usually from the brink of death) to a functional lifestyle, able to exercise and study and travel and have families. Although the return to normalcy is wonderful, the interactions with family, friends, and employers can be most challenging and are the subject of this book.

Since the donor supply is clearly finite and will not likely increase in the future, we now look forward to the continued "evolution" of the field of mechanical circulatory support to eventually provide not only durable but also safe non-biological replacement of the heart.

References

1. Carrel A, Guthrie CC. The transplantation of veins and organs. Am J Med. 1905;10:1101.
2. Lower RR, Shumway NE. Studies on orthotopic homotransplantation of the canine heart. Surg Forum. 1960;11:18.
3. Guidelines for the determination of death. Report of the medical consultants on the diagnosis of death to the President's Commission for the Study of Ethical Problems in Medicine and Biomedical and Behavioral Research. JAMA 1981;246:2184.
4. Caves PK, Stinson EB, Graham AF, et al. Percutaneous transvenous endomyocardial biopsy. JAMA. 1973;225:288.
5. Billingham ME, Cary MR, Hammond MR, et al. A working formulation for the standardization of nomenclature in the diagnosis of heart and lung rejection. Heart Rejection Study Group. The International Society for Heart and Lung Transplantation. J Heart Lung Transplant. 1990;9:587.
6. Thomas FC, Szentpetry SS, Mammanna RE, et al. Transportation of human hearts for transplantation. Ann Thorac Surg. 1978;26:344.
7. Oyer PE, Stinson EB, Jamieson SW, et al. One year experience with cyclosporine A in clinical heart transplantation. J Heart Transplant. 1982;1:285.

Medical Course and Complications After Heart Transplantation

Medical Course and Complications After Heart Transplantation

20

Ranjan Ray and Michael Pham

Introduction

Quality of life and prognosis for many patients with end-stage heart failure remain suboptimal despite recent advances in medical and device therapy. For these patients, cardiac transplantation and durable mechanical circulatory support (see Chap. 18) have become standard of care. These interventions provide mortality benefit and improve quality of life in carefully selected patients. Cardiac transplant is the preferred treatment of choice; however, the number of transplant procedures is limited by donor availability and has remained stable over the last 20 years [1]. Annually, there are approximately 4700 heart transplant procedures performed worldwide [1].

Indications for Heart Transplantation

Cardiac transplantation is indicated for patients with end-stage heart failure who experience severe functional limitations and heart failure symptoms that are refractory to management with medications, electrophysiologic device therapy such as cardiac resynchronization, or conventional surgical interventions. The most common indications for adult heart transplantation are nonischemic cardiomyopathy and coronary artery disease [1]. Please see Chap. 16 for more details on indications and contraindications.

Heart Transplant Surgery

Lower and Shumway originally described the biatrial surgical technique for orthotopic heart transplantation in 1960 [2]. In this procedure, both the donor and recipient hearts are removed by transecting the atria at the midatrial level, leaving the multiple pulmonary venous connections to the left atrium intact in the posterior wall of the left atrium, and then transecting the aorta and pulmonary artery just above their respective semilunar valves.

The donor heart is explanted by a surgical team at a hospital, typically remote from the transplant center. The heart procurement procedure needs to be coordinated with the requirements of the surgical teams procuring other organs for transplantation. The donor heart is first arrested with cardioplegic solution. It is then placed in a secure container and transported to the transplant center. Ischemic times average from 3 to 4 hours.

Implantation of the heart in the orthotopic position begins with reanastomosis at the midatrial level, beginning with the atrial septum (Fig. 20.1). Efforts are made to include a generous cuff of donor right atrium so that the sinoatrial node will be included. The great vessels are connected just above the semilunar valves. More recently, the bicaval technique (Fig. 20.2), a modification of the biatrial technique, has been utilized. This technique leaves the donor atria intact and makes the anastomoses at the level of the superior and inferior vena cava and pulmonary veins [3]. This results in less distortion of atrioventricular geometry, resulting in improved atrial and ventricular function, less AV valve regurgitation, decreased incidence of atrial arrhythmias, and decreased incidence of donor sinus node dysfunction and heart block [4–6].

Immediate postoperative care for the transplant patient is very similar to routine post-cardiac surgery management with the additional component of immunosuppression and the need for chronotropic support of the donor sinoatrial node for the first 2–3 postoperative days. Uncomplicated patients are discharged from the hospital within 2 weeks post-transplant.

Post-transplant Outcomes

Volume and outcomes data of thoracic organ transplantation are provided yearly by the Registry of the International Society for Heart and Lung Transplantation (ISHLT). Since

R. Ray (✉) · M. Pham
Center for Advanced Heart Failure Therapies, Palo Alto Foundation Medical Group, San Francisco, CA, USA
e-mail: RayR@Sutterhealth.org; PhamMX@sutterhealth.org

© Springer International Publishing AG, part of Springer Nature 2019
Y. Sher, J. R. Maldonado (eds.), *Psychosocial Care of End-Stage Organ Disease and Transplant Patients*,
https://doi.org/10.1007/978-3-319-94914-7_20

Fig. 20.1 Original biatrial technique for orthotopic heart transplantation. The left panel shows the completed recipient cardiectomy with the recipient atria transected at the midatrial level. The right panel shows the completed reanastomosis of the donor heart. (Used with permission)

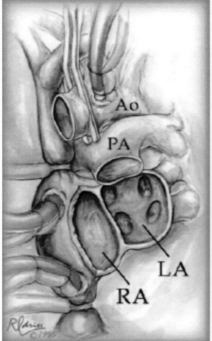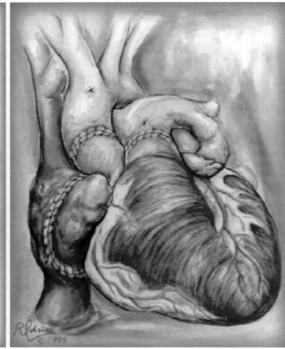

Fig. 20.2 Bicaval technique for orthotopic heart transplantation. The left panel shows the completed recipient cardiectomy. The recipient atria are completely removed except for a cuff of tissue around the pulmonary vein orifices. The superior and inferior venae cavae are transected at their junction with the right atrium. The right panel shows the completed anastomoses of the donor heart at the level of the superior and inferior venae cava and pulmonary veins. (Used with permission)

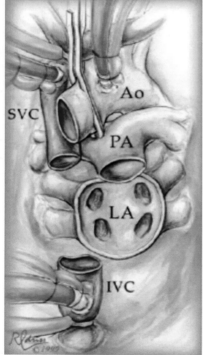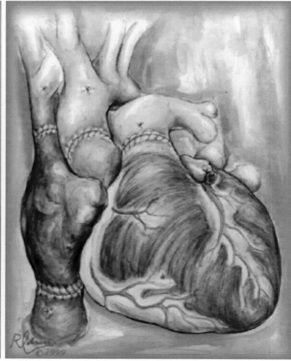

1994, the Registry has been administered by the US donor allocation organization, the United Network for Organ Sharing (UNOS), that includes data from US programs as well as non-US programs. The most recent Registry report includes data on over 100,000 heart transplants performed worldwide since 1982 and documents overall patient sur-vival rates of 85%, 79%, and 74%, at 1 year, 3 years, and 5 years, respectively (Fig. 20.3) [1]. There is an initial steep fall in survival during the first 6 months, followed by a linear attrition rate of 3–4% per year to a survival of approximately 50% at 10 years. The major causes of death during the first 30 days post-transplant are primarily due to graft failure,

Fig. 20.3 Actuarial survival for adult and pediatric heart transplants patients performed between January 1982 and June 2014. The half-life is the time at which 50% of those transplanted remain alive, and the conditional half-life is the time to 50% survival for those recipients surviving the first-year post-transplantation. (From Lund et al. [1]. Used with permission)

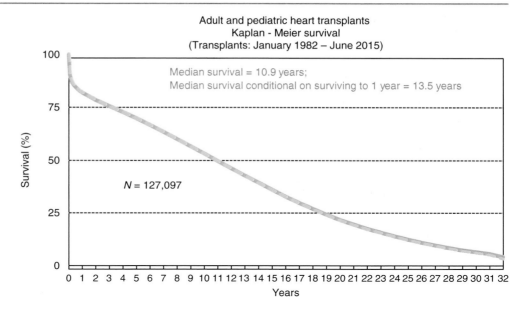

multi-organ failure, and infection. Within the first year, infection accounts for the leading cause of death, followed by graft failure and acute rejection. The majority of deaths after 5 years are primarily due to cardiac allograft vasculopathy and malignancy [1].

Quality of Life After Heart Transplantation

Although heart transplant patients require long-term immunosuppression, are exposed to long-term toxicities of these drug regimens, and are committed to ongoing long term medical follow-up, a majority of transplant patients experience improvement in their quality of life and level of well-being after transplantation [7–9].

Unique Physiologic Characteristics of the Transplanted Heart

At the time of transplant surgery, the transplanted heart is completely denervated. The donor sinus node function will usually recover within the first 2–3 postoperative days. The denervated donor heart typically maintains a faster resting heart rate (usually between 95 and 110 beats per minute) due to the intrinsic fast heart rate of the sinus node and absence of the counter-regulatory effects of the parasympathetic nervous system. Cardiac denervation has several important clinical manifestations. First, the cardiac allograft will be slower to increase its heart rate in response to exercise and will exhibit a slower heart rate recovery. At the onset of exercise, an increase in venous return results in an increase in stroke volume in accordance with the Frank-Starling prin-

ciple, in which increased stretch or tension on cardiac muscle results in an increased force of contraction. Later in exercise, circulating peripheral catecholamines provide chronotropic support. Second, many heart transplant patients will not experience angina with ischemia of the cardiac allograft and present instead with congestive heart failure, silent myocardial infarction, or sudden death. Reinnervation of the cardiac allograft is thought to occur after the first year, but the timing and degree of reinnervation are highly variable and not well understood. Despite cardiac denervation, most heart transplant patients report minimal functional limitations.

Immunosuppression

Post-transplant immunosuppression regimens are based on a set of general principles and combine several agents concurrently. First, the highest risk for graft rejection and immune reactivity is during the first 3–6 months after transplantation with subsequent decrease over time. Therefore, the highest levels of immunosuppression are utilized immediately after surgery. The levels are gradually decreased over the first year until the lowest maintenance levels of immunosuppression that are compatible with preventing graft rejection and minimizing drug toxicities are achieved. Second, a preferred strategy is the one using low doses of several drugs without overlapping toxicities in preference to higher (and more toxic) doses of fewer drugs whenever feasible. Third, it is important to achieve the correct balance between over- and under-immunosuppression as too much immunosuppression can lead to a number of undesirable effects such as susceptibility to infection and malignancy.

Induction Therapy

Approximately 50% of transplant programs utilize a strategy of augmented immunosuppression, or "induction" therapy, with antilymphocyte antibodies during the early postoperative period. The goal of induction therapy is to provide intense immunosuppression during a time when the risk of allograft rejection is highest. Additionally, induction therapy allows delayed initiation of nephrotoxic immunosuppressive drugs in patients with compromised renal function following surgery. Available agents for induction therapy include T-cell cytolytic agents such as polyclonal antithymocyte antibodies and anti-interleukin-2 (IL-2) receptor antagonists such as daclizumab or basiliximab.

Maintenance Therapy

Maintenance immunosuppression protocols typically consist of a three-drug regimen including a calcineurin inhibitor (cyclosporine or tacrolimus), an antimetabolite agent (mycophenolate mofetil or azathioprine), and tapering doses of corticosteroids over the first-year post-transplantation.

Calcineurin inhibitors (CNIs) act by inhibiting calcineurin, a phosphatase that is involved in the transcription of cytokines such as IL-2, TNF-alpha, granulocyte-macrophage colony-stimulating factor, and interferon gamma, thereby decreasing T-lymphocyte activation and proliferation in response to alloantigens. Both cyclosporine and tacrolimus are extremely effective and have comparable post-transplant survival. However, clinical trial data suggests that tacrolimus-based immunosuppression may decrease rates of acute rejection as compared with cyclosporine-based regimens [10, 11]. Additionally, cyclosporine and tacrolimus have different side effect profiles. Higher incidences of hypertension and dyslipidemia are associated with cyclosporine and more new-onset insulin-requiring diabetes with tacrolimus [12, 13].

The antimetabolites exert their immunosuppressive effects by blocking purine synthesis and inhibiting proliferation of both T and B lymphocytes. *Mycophenolate mofetil* (Cellcept) is associated with a significant reduction both in mortality and in the incidence of treatable rejection at 1 year when compared to azathioprine (Imuran) [14]. Thus, *Mycophenolate mofetil* has become the preferred antimetabolite agent.

The proliferation signal inhibitors, or mammalian target of rapamycin (mTOR) inhibitors, consist of two agents, *sirolimus* and *everolimus*. These drugs have been used in selected patients with renal insufficiency, cardiac allograft vasculopathy, or malignancies, in order to reverse or slow progression of these conditions. Their mechanism of action is through inhibition of proliferation of human T cells, B cells, and vascular smooth muscle cells in response to growth factor and cytokine signals.

Corticosteroids are non-specific anti-inflammatory agents that interfere with multiple steps in immune activation, including antigen presentation, cytokine production, and proliferation of lymphocytes. Steroids are highly effective for the prevention and treatment of acute rejection. However, long-term use is associated with several adverse side effects such as new-onset or worsening diabetes mellitus, hyperlipidemia, hypertension, fluid retention, myopathy, osteoporosis, and a predisposition toward opportunistic infections. Therefore, most immunosuppression regimens utilize corticosteroids at higher doses in the early postoperative period with a gradual taper to lower doses or discontinuation after the first 6–12 months post-transplant.

Complications of Immunosuppression

Hypertension, hyperlipidemia, and the development of post-transplant diabetes mellitus are among the most common metabolic complications associated with calcineurin inhibitors. Renal dysfunction occurs in up to one third of individuals and is related to the direct effects of the CNIs on the kidney tubules and from CNI-mediated vasoconstriction of the afferent arteriole, leading to decreased kidney perfusion. Due to their immunosuppressed state, in addition to experiencing drug- and class-specific toxicities, heart transplant patients have a higher risk of developing opportunistic infections and malignancies compared to the general population.

Infection

Infection is the major cause of death during the first postoperative year and remains a risk throughout the life of a chronically immunosuppressed patient. Infections in the first postoperative month are commonly bacterial and typically related to indwelling catheters and wound infections. These infections typically present in the form of pneumonias, urinary tract infections, sternal wound infections and mediastinitis, and bacteremia. Late infections (those occurring 2 months to 1 year post-transplant) are more diverse. In addition to typical pathogens, transplant patients are susceptible to viruses (particularly *Cytomegalovirus*), fungi (*Aspergillus*, *Candida*, and *Pneumocystis*), *Mycobacterium*, *Nocardia*, and *Toxoplasma*. Infection surveillance is mainly clinical, but routine surveillance chest radiography often detects infections, especially fungal and mycobacterial pulmonary infections that may be at an early and asymptomatic stage. Experience in recognizing common clinical presentations of these infections and an aggressive approach to obtain a specific diagnosis is crucial to effective management of infectious complications in transplant patients.

Malignancy

Solid-organ transplant recipients have an increased lifetime risk of cancer over the general population due to their chronic immunosuppressed state [1]. The risk of neoplasm correlates to the intensity and duration of immunosuppression. In heart transplant recipients surviving to 5 years, malignancies are the second most common cause of death, after cardiac allograft vasculopathy and graft failure. Skin cancers accounted for the majority (67%) of malignancies reported, followed by lymphomas (9%) [1]. The incidence of prostate, lung, bladder, breast, cervical, and colon cancers are similar in frequency as observed in the general population; however, these cancers may behave more aggressively in an immuno-compromised patient. Age-appropriate cancer screening, including dermatologic examination, screening colonoscopy for patients over the age of 50, mammography and Papanicolaou testing for women, and prostate-specific antigen (PSA) level measurements for men over the age of 40, should be undertaken according to published guidelines [14].

The most common non-cutaneous malignancies in organ transplant recipients are a heterogeneous group of lympho-proliferative malignancies collectively known as post-transplant lymphoproliferative disorder (PTLD). There is convincing evidence that most cases of PTLD are related to infection (either primary or reactivation) with the Epstein-Barr virus (EBV) [15, 16]. They frequently present as localized or disseminated B-cell proliferations, tend to occur in unusual, extranodal locations, and resemble classic nodal malignant lymphomas such as large-cell lymphoma and Burkitt lymphoma. Treatment involves reduction of immunosuppression, administration of standard chemotherapy, and use of the anti-CD20 monoclonal antibody rituximab [17, 18]. PTLDs are usually quite radiosensitive, and both radiotherapy and surgical resection can play a major role in therapy when the disease is localized to a single lesion.

Rejection

Classification

Cardiac allograft rejection is classified as hyperacute, acute cellular, acute antibody-mediated (humoral), or chronic. *Hyperacute rejection* is rare but can occur in the setting of circulating preformed antibodies to the ABO blood group (in cases of ABO blood group incompatibility) or to major histocompatibility antigens in the donor. Potential risk factors include presensitization following multiple blood transfusions, multiparity, and previous organ grafts [19]. Hyperacute rejection manifests as severe graft failure within the first few minutes to hours after transplantation. Without inotropic and

mechanical circulatory support, plasmapheresis, and emergent retransplantation, the recipient usually does not survive.

Acute cellular rejection (ACR) is the most common form of allograft rejection and occurs in 30–50% of heart transplant recipients in the first year following transplantation [20]. Most episodes of ACR occur within the first 3–6 months. Acute cellular rejection is primarily mediated by T-lymphocytes and is identified by examining histologic findings in surveillance endomyocardial biopsy (EMB) samples obtained from the right ventricle. The principal histo-pathologic features are the distribution and extent of inflammation and the presence or absence of myocyte damage. The severity of the rejection process reflects these features along a morphologic continuum. Biopsies are classified as 1R (mild), 2R (moderate), or 3R (severe) in accordance with a standardized ISHLT grading scheme [21].

Antibody-mediated rejection (AMR) is a B lymphocyte mediated process that is characterized by immunoglobulin deposition on the cardiac allograft microvasculature, complement activation, and graft dysfunction. It is more likely to be associated with hemodynamic instability compared with ACR, carries a worse prognosis, and is a strong risk factor for the early development of cardiac allograft vasculopathy [22, 23]. The prevalence of AMR has been reported to be between 15% and 20%, and it can occur independently of or in combination with cellular rejection [24]. More recently, diagnostic criteria for AMR have been suggested and include a combination of clinical, histologic, and immunopathologic findings, in addition to demonstration of circulating donor-specific antibodies in the serum [25, 26]. Risk factors for AMR include a history of pre-transplant sensitization to HLA antigens, positive pre-transplant cytotoxicity crossmatch, female gender, cytomegalovirus seropositivity, multiparity, retransplantation, and a previous history of AMR [22, 27].

Chronic rejection can occur months to years after transplantation and manifests as cardiac allograft vasculopathy and late graft failure. The mechanisms of chronic rejection is thought to involve a proliferative response to both immunologically and non-immunologically mediated endothelial injury with progressive intimal thickening within the coronary vessels.

Diagnosis of Rejection

The signs and symptoms of rejection are often non-specific and may only be clinically evident in the late stages of rejection. Common signs and symptoms are fatigue, low-grade fevers, heart failure symptoms, or hypotension. Rejection can occasionally present in the form of atrial arrhythmias or new pericardial effusions. Physical exam findings of heart failure such as elevated jugular venous pressure or a new gallop would be of concern. Most patients with acute rejection are asymptomatic and have no clinical findings of allograft dysfunction. Close surveillance of heart transplant recipients for acute rejection is critical. Patients are typically monitored for rejection using a combination of clinical assessment, imaging, and/or quantification of allograft function (echocardiography or right heart catheterization), in addition to surveillance EMB.

The endomyocardial biopsy is the gold standard for the diagnosis of acute allograft rejection. It is performed via the right internal jugular vein or femoral vein by introducing a bioptome into the right ventricle and obtaining three to five pieces of endomyocardium, typically from the right ventricular septum. More recently, the use of a blood test (AlloMap) based upon gene expression profiling of peripheral leukocytes has provided as a noninvasive option of monitoring for allograft rejection in clinically stable patients. The test uses real-time PCR to measure the expression of certain genes involved in immune activation and trafficking. In a multicenter observational study, the test was able to accurately detect the absence of moderate to severe cellular rejection and thus identify a state of "quiescence" in the allograft [28]. The IMAGE clinical trial evaluated the clinical outcomes associated with use of this test as part of a noninvasive strategy for rejection surveillance [29].

Protocols for the timing of rejection surveillance generally are chosen to match the observed frequency of rejection episodes, which is highest in the early postoperative period. Most programs perform surveillance biopsies on a weekly basis for the first 4–6 postoperative weeks and then with diminishing frequency in a stable patient but at a minimum of every 3 months for the first postoperative year. The need for continued surveillance biopsies after the first year in clinically stable patients has been debated [30, 31], and many centers continue to perform them on an every 4–6 months schedule during years 2–5 following transplantation [32].

Treatment of Acute Rejection

Rejection episodes are typically treated with augmentation of immunosuppression, the intensity of which is matched to the severity of the episode. Mild cellular rejection (Grade 1R) without associated hemodynamic compromise (defined as a decrease in left ventricular systolic function, decrease in cardiac output, or signs of hypoperfusion) does not typically require treatment. Moderate to severe cellular rejection (Grades 2R and 3R) is treated with high-dose intravenous methylprednisolone with or without cytolytic antibody therapy in the form of polyclonal antithymocyte globulin [33]. Antibody mediated rejection is treated with a combination of high-dose corticosteroids, plasmapheresis, intravenous immunoglobulin, cytolytic agents, and/or adjuvant therapy with the anti-CD20 monoclonal antibody rituximab [34–36].

Several strategies are employed as adjunctive therapy for repetitive or recalcitrant rejection episodes. They include the use of two modalities with proven efficacy in therapy for autoimmune disease: total lymphoid irradiation and low-dose methotrexate. Both have been shown to be of benefit in patients with frequent or difficult-to-treat cardiac allograft rejection [37–40]. If the aforementioned strategies are not successful and there is persistent severe graft dysfunction, then retransplantation is the only remaining option and is offered by some centers. However, the results of retransplantation in this setting are poor with significantly decreased survival at 1 year compared (30–40%) to patients undergoing retransplantation for cardiac allograft vasculopathy (80–90%) [41, 42].

Cardiac Allograft Vasculopathy

Cardiac allograft vasculopathy (CAV) is detected by coronary angiography and is a major cause of late graft failure and death in heart transplant patients. The incidence of CAV in heart transplant patients is approximately 10% by the first postoperative year and 30–50% by 5 years postoperatively [1]. Despite advances in immunosuppression and surveillance protocols, the incidence of CAV has not significantly decreased, and its development continues to limit long-term survival in patients undergoing cardiac transplantation.

Morphologic Features

In CAV, the major epicardial vessels, their branches, and often the intramyocardial divisions display uniform, diffuse involvement extending along their entire length (Fig. 20.4). The asymmetric and calcified plaques or lesions composed of cholesterol that are characteristic of conventional atherosclerosis are not found in uncomplicated lesions of vessels affected by transplant vasculopathy [43].

Diagnosis

Due to a persistent state of both afferent and efferent cardiac denervation, most heart transplant patients do not experience the subjective sensation of angina pectoris. Clinical presentations of ischemia in this patient population are typically related to the sequelae of allograft ischemia, including arrhythmias, myocardial infarction, and either systolic or diastolic heart failure. Some cardiac transplant recipients do have physiologic evidence of reinnervation [44, 45] and may experience angina pectoris [46].

Surveillance testing is typically performed with coronary angiography, but the diffuse and concentric nature of the disease process makes diagnosis challenging. Consequently, it

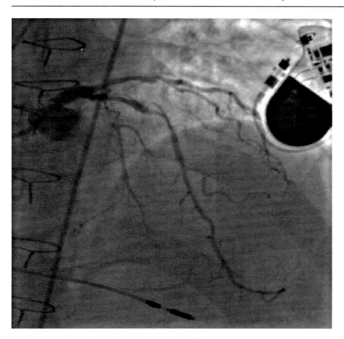

Fig. 20.4 Coronary angiogram in a patient with severe CAV showing diffuse disease of the left anterior descending (LAD) coronary artery, occlusion of the left circumflex coronary artery, and obliteration of the obtuse marginal branches

is easy to underestimate the severity of CAV angiographically. Recently, the use of intravascular ultrasound (IVUS) has gained acceptance as a sensitive and early detector of the intimal thickening that characterizes CAV [47]. IVUS measurements of the degree and progression of coronary intimal thickening at 1-year post-transplantation have prognostic significance with respect to future death, graft loss, and non-fatal major adverse cardiac events [48], and these measurements now serve as endpoints for early CAV in contemporary trials of immunosuppressive agents [49–51].

Prognosis

The prognosis for survival once angiographically significant graft vasculopathy is detected is generally poor. In one study, the 1- and 2-year survival rates ranged from 18–67% depending on the severity and extent of disease [52].

Prevention and Treatment

There are several approaches to the prevention of CAV. These include protecting against endothelial injury through decreased ischemic time, prevention of early rejection, modification of traditional cardiac risk factors such as

hyperlipidemia and hypertension, and pharmacologic therapy [53–55]. Additionally, the mTOR inhibitors sirolimus and everolimus have also shown promise in preventing the development of CAV when used in de novo heart transplant recipients [49, 50].

The choice of treatment for established CAV is often difficult and controversial. Due to the diffuse nature of CAV involvement, this disease is not typically amenable to standard revascularization procedures, such as percutaneous coronary interventions (PCI) and coronary artery bypass grafting (CABG). In heart transplant patients undergoing PCI, the rate of observed in-stent restenosis and vessel restenosis within 6 months was higher when compared to historically reported rates in PCI of native vessels [56]. Similarly, outcomes following CABG have been extremely poor, with a reported 33% operative mortality rate and 50% mortality rate at 2 months in one registry [57].

The most definitive form of therapy for graft failure resulting from severe vasculopathy is retransplantation for carefully selected patients who have advanced disease but otherwise good end-organ function. Historically, post-transplant survival rates in retransplant patients have been significantly lower in comparison with primary transplants [58]; however, due to improvements in surgical technique, immunosuppression and post-transplant care, survival rates after retransplantation have improved significantly and are now comparable to those after primary transplantation [1].

Conclusions

Apart for the mechanical circulatory support, heart transplant has become the standard care treatment for patients with end-stage heart failure refractory to medication management. Carefully selected patients survive on average 10 years, with those who are retransplanted are now doing as well as those who were transplanted for the first time. Patients are managed with intensive immunosuppressive regimens and experience associated complications, such as infections and malignancy. In addition, acute cellular rejection occurs in 30–50% of patients within first post-transplant year, and antibody-mediated rejection, which carries a worse prognosis, occurs in 10–20% of the patients. Chronic rejection occurs months to years after transplantation and manifests as cardiac allograft vasculopathy and late graft failure. Heart transplantation prolongs lives and improves quality of life and, however, requires ongoing intensive medication management, vigilance, and treatments of new complications and comorbidities. Knowledge of the associated complications allows providers to guide their patients along their post-transplant journey.

References

1. Lund LH, Edwards LB, Dipchang AI, et al. Registry of the International Society for Heart and Lung Transplantation: thirty-third official adult heart transplant report – 2016. J Heart Lung Transplant. 2016;35(10):1158–69.

2. Lower RR, Shumway NE. Studies on orthotopic homotransplantation of the canine heart. Surg Forum. 1960;11:18–9.

3. Dreyfus G, Jebara V, Mihaileanu S, Carpentier AF. Total orthotopic heart transplantation: an alternative to the standard technique. Ann Thorac Surg. 1991;52(5):1181–4.

4. El-Gamel A, Deiraniya AK, Rahman AN, Campbell CS, Yonan NA. Orthotopic heart transplantation hemodynamics: does atrial preservation improve cardiac output after transplantation? J Heart Lung Transplant. 1996;15(6):564–71.

5. Traversi E, Pozzoli M, Grande A, et al. The bicaval anastomosis technique for orthotopic heart transplantation yields better atrial function than the standard technique: an echocardiographic automatic boundary detection study. J Heart Lung Transplant. 1998;17(11):1065–74.

6. Meyer SR, Modry DL, Bainey K, et al. Declining need for permanent pacemaker insertion with the bicaval technique of orthotopic heart transplantation. Can J Cardiol. 2005;21(2):159–63.

7. Angermann CE, Bullinger M, Spes CH, Zellner M, Kemkes BM, Theisen K. Quality of life in long-term survivors of orthotopic heart transplantation. Z Kardiol. 1992;81(8):411–7.

8. Jones BM, Taylor F, Downs K, Spratt P. Longitudinal study of quality of life and psychological adjustment after cardiac transplantation. Med J Aust. 1992;157(1):24–6.

9. Salyer J, Flattery MP, Joyner PL, Elswick RK. Lifestyle and quality of life in long-term cardiac transplant recipients. J Heart Lung Transplant. 2003;22(3):309–21.

10. Grimm M, Rinaldi M, Yonan NA, et al. Superior prevention of acute rejection by tacrolimus vs. cyclosporine in heart transplant recipients – a large European trial. Am J Transplant. 2006;6(6):1387–97.

11. Kobashigawa JA, Miller LW, Russell SD, et al. Tacrolimus with mycophenolate mofetil (MMF) or sirolimus vs. cyclosporine with MMF in cardiac transplant patients: 1-year report. Am J Transplant. 2006;6(6):1377–86.

12. Taylor DO, Barr ML, Radovancevic B, et al. A randomized, multicenter comparison of tacrolimus and cyclosporine immunosuppressive regimens in cardiac transplantation: decreased hyperlipidemia and hypertension with tacrolimus. J Heart Lung Transplant. 1999;18(4):336–45.

13. Ye F, Ying-Bin X, Yu-Guo W, Hetzer R. Tacrolimus versus cyclosporine microemulsion for heart transplant recipients: a meta-analysis. J Heart Lung Transplant. 2009;28(1):58–66.

14. Smith RA, Cokkinides V, Eyre HJ. American Cancer Society guidelines for the early detection of cancer, 2006. CA Cancer J Clin. 2006;56(1):11–25; quiz 49–50.

15. Young L, Alfieri C, Hennessy K, et al. Expression of Epstein-Barr virus transformation-associated genes in tissues of patients with EBV lymphoproliferative disease. N Engl J Med. 1989;321(16):1080–5.

16. Hanto DW, Frizzera G, Gajl-Peczalska KJ, et al. Epstein-Barr virus-induced B-cell lymphoma after renal transplantation: acyclovir therapy and transition from polyclonal to monoclonal B-cell proliferation. N Engl J Med. 1982;306(15):913–8.

17. Jain AB, Marcos A, Pokharna R, et al. Rituximab (chimeric anti-CD20 antibody) for posttransplant lymphoproliferative disorder after solid organ transplantation in adults: long-term experience from a single center. Transplantation. 2005;80(12):1692–8.

18. Blaes AH, Peterson BA, Bartlett N, Dunn DL, Morrison VA. Rituximab therapy is effective for posttransplant lymphoproliferative disorders after solid organ transplantation: results of a phase II trial. Cancer. 2005;104(8):1661–7.

19. Kemnitz J, Cremer J, Restrepo-Specht I, et al. Hyperacute rejection in heart allografts. Case studies. Pathol Res Pract. 1991;187(1):23–9.

20. Hershberger RE, Starling RC, Eisen HJ, et al. Daclizumab to prevent rejection after cardiac transplantation. N Eng J Med. 2005;352(26):2705–13.

21. Stewart S, Winters GL, Fishbein MC, et al. Revision of the 1990 working formulation for the standardization of nomenclature in the diagnosis of heart rejection. J Heart Lung Transplant. 2005;24(11):1710–20.

22. Michaels PJ, Espejo ML, Kobashigawa J, et al. Humoral rejection in cardiac transplantation: risk factors, hemodynamic consequences and relationship to transplant coronary artery disease. J Heart Lung Transplant. 2003;22(1):58–69.

23. Kobashigawa J, Miller L, Renlund D, et al. A randomized active-controlled trial of mycophenolate mofetil in heart transplant recipients. Mycophenolate Mofetil Investigators. Transplantation. 1998;66(4):507–15.

24. Hammond EH, Yowell RL, Nunoda S, et al. Vascular (humoral) rejection in heart transplantation: pathologic observations and clinical implications. J Heart Transplant. 1989;8(6):430–43.

25. Subherwal S, Kobashigawa JA, Cogert G, Patel J, Espejo M, Oeser B. Incidence of acute cellular rejection and non-cellular rejection in cardiac transplantation. Transplant Proc. 2004;36(10):3171–2.

26. Reed EF, Demetris AJ, Hammond E, et al. Acute antibody-mediated rejection of cardiac transplants. J Heart Lung Transplant. 2006;25(2):153–9.

27. Taylor DO, Yowell RL, Kfoury AG, Hammond EH, Renlund DG. Allograft coronary artery disease: clinical correlations with circulating anti-HLA antibodies and the immunohistopathologic pattern of vascular rejection. J Heart Lung Transplant. 2000;19(6):518–21.

28. Deng MC, Eisen HJ, Mehra MR, et al. Noninvasive discrimination of rejection in cardiac allograft recipients using gene expression profiling. Am J Transplant. 2006;6(1):150–60.

29. Pham MX, Deng MC, Kfoury AG, Teuteberg JJ, Starling RC, Valantine H. Molecular testing for long-term rejection surveillance in heart transplant recipients: design of the Invasive Monitoring Attenuation Through Gene Expression (IMAGE) trial. J Heart Lung Transplant. 2007;26(8):808–14.

30. Sethi GK, Kosaraju S, Arabia FA, Roasdo LJ, McCarthy MS, Copeland JG. Is it necessary to perform surveillance endomyocardial biopsies in heart transplant recipients? J Heart Lung Transplant. 1995;14(6 Pt 1):1047–51.

31. White JA, Guiraudon C, Pflugfelder PW, Kostuk WJ. Routine surveillance myocardial biopsies are unnecessary beyond one year after heart transplantation. J Heart Lung Transplant. 1995;14(6 Pt 1):1052–6.

32. Stehlik J, Starling RC, Movsesian MA, et al. Utility of long-term surveillance endomyocardial biopsy: a multi-institutional analysis. J Heart Lung Transplant. 2006;25(12):1402–9.

33. Cantarovich M, Latter DA, Loertscher R. Treatment of steroid-resistant and recurrent acute cardiac transplant rejection with a short course of antibody therapy. Clin Transpl. 1997;11(4):316–21.

34. Keren A, Hayes HM, O'Driscoll G. Late humoral rejection in a cardiac transplant recipient treated with the anti-CD20 monoclonal antibody rituximab. Transplant Proc. 2006;38(5):1520–2.

35. Garrett HE Jr, Duvall-Seaman D, Helsley B, Groshart K. Treatment of vascular rejection with rituximab in cardiac transplantation. J Heart Lung Transplant. 2005;24(9):1337–42.

36. Crespo-Leiro MG, Veiga-Barreiro A, Domenech N, et al. Humoral heart rejection (severe allograft dysfunction with no signs of cellular rejection or ischemia): incidence, management, and the value of C4d for diagnosis. Am J Transplant. 2005;5(10):2560–4.

37. Hunt SA, Strober S, Hoppe RT, Stinson EB. Total lymphoid irradiation for treatment of intractable cardiac allograft rejection. J Heart Lung Transplant. 1991;10(2):211–6.

38. Levin B, Bohannon L, Warvariv V, Bry W, Collins G. Total lymphoid irradiation (TLI) in the cyclosporine era – use of TLI in resistant cardiac allograft rejection. Transplant Proc. 1989;21(1 Pt 2):1793–5.

39. Costanzo-Nordin MR, Grusk BB, Silver MA, et al. Reversal of recalcitrant cardiac allograft rejection with methotrexate. Circulation. 1988;78(5 Pt 2):III47–57.

40. Bouchart F, Gundry SR, Van Schaack-Gonzales J, et al. Methotrexate as rescue/adjunctive immunotherapy in infant and adult heart transplantation. J Heart Lung Transplant. 1993;12(3):427–33.

41. Dein JR, Oyer PE, Stinson EB, Starnes VA, Shumway NE. Cardiac retransplantation in the cyclosporine era. Ann Thorac Surg. 1989;48(3):350–5.

42. Radovancevic B, McGiffin DC, Kobashigawa JA, et al. Retransplantation in 7,290 primary transplant patients: a 10-year multi-institutional study. J Heart Lung Transplant. 2003;22(8):862–8.

43. Pucci AM, Forbes RD, Billingham ME. Pathologic features in long-term cardiac allografts. J Heart Transplant. 1990;9(4):339–45.

44. Kaye DM, Esler M, Kingwell B, McPherson G, Esmore D, Jennings G. Functional and neurochemical evidence for partial cardiac sympathetic reinnervation after cardiac transplantation in humans. Circulation. 1993;88(3):1110–8.

45. Bernardi L, Bianchini B, Spadacini G, et al. Demonstrable cardiac reinnervation after human heart transplantation by carotid baroreflex modulation of RR interval. Circulation. 1995;92(10):2895–903.

46. Stark RP, McGinn AL, Wilson RF. Chest pain in cardiac-transplant recipients. Evidence of sensory reinnervation after cardiac transplantation. N Eng J Med. 1991;324(25):1791–4.

47. Rickenbacher PR, Pinto FJ, Lewis NP, et al. Prognostic importance of intimal thickness as measured by intracoronary ultrasound after cardiac transplantation. Circulation. 1995;92(12):3445–52.

48. Kobashigawa JA, Tobis JM, Starling RC, et al. Multicenter intravascular ultrasound validation study among heart transplant recipients: outcomes after five years. J Am Coll Cardiol. 2005;45(9):1532–7.

49. Keogh A, Richardson M, Ruygrok P, et al. Sirolimus in de novo heart transplant recipients reduces acute rejection and prevents coronary artery disease at 2 years: a randomized clinical trial. Circulation. 2004;110(17):2694–700.

50. Eisen HJ, Tuzcu EM, Dorent R, et al. Everolimus for the prevention of allograft rejection and vasculopathy in cardiac-transplant recipients. N Engl J Med. 2003;349(9):847–58.

51. Kobashigawa JA, Tobis JM, Mentzer RM, et al. Mycophenolate mofetil reduces intimal thickness by intravascular ultrasound after heart transplant: reanalysis of the multicenter trial. Am J Transplant. 2006;6(5 Pt 1):993–7.

52. Keogh AM, Valantine HA, Hunt SA, et al. Impact of proximal or midvessel discrete coronary artery stenoses on survival after heart transplantation. J Heart Lung Transplant. 1992;11(5):892–901.

53. Schroeder JS, Gao SZ, Alderman EL, et al. A preliminary study of diltiazem in the prevention of coronary artery disease in heart-transplant recipients. N Eng J Med. 1993;328(3):164–70.

54. Kobashigawa JA, Katznelson S, Laks H, et al. Effect of pravastatin on outcomes after cardiac transplantation. N Eng J Med. 1995;333(10):621–7.

55. Wenke K, Meiser B, Thiery J, et al. Simvastatin reduces graft vessel disease and mortality after heart transplantation: a four-year randomized trial. Circulation. 1997;96(5):1398–402.

56. Bader FM, Kfoury AG, Gilbert EM, et al. Percutaneous coronary interventions with stents in cardiac transplant recipients. J Heart Lung Transplant. 2006;25(3):298–301.

57. Halle AA 3rd, DiSciascio G, Massin EK, et al. Coronary angioplasty, atherectomy and bypass surgery in cardiac transplant recipients. J Am Coll Cardiol. 1995;26(1):120–8.

58. Topkara VK, Dang NC, John R, et al. A decade experience of cardiac retransplantation in adult recipients. J Heart Lung Transplant. 2005;24(11):1745–50.

Post-transplant Psychosocial and Mental Health Care of the Cardiac Recipient

Peter A. Shapiro, Luis F. Pereira, Katherine E. Taylor, and Ilona Wiener

Life Course After Heart Transplantation and Its Psychological Correlates

The Experience Immediately After Surgery

While some patients arrive at the moment of heart transplantation after a long downhill course of heart failure, others present with an acute, catastrophic cardiac event. Thus, there is great variation in patients' medical status, cerebral function, understanding of what is entailed in having a transplant, motivation, and psychological readiness for transplantation [1, 2]. This variation sets the stage for a wide range of psychological responses in the immediate aftermath of heart transplantation.

Patients who were aware of their terminal prognosis before transplantation may view the transplant procedure as a miraculous rescue from death. They often speak of being reborn. These ideas are often accompanied by elation, euphoria, and intense feelings of gratitude. In these first few days, patients often express resolutions about changing their lives. Patients may also struggle with more or less consciously articulated feelings about incorporation of another person's heart into their body, body image, and sense of self, and may experience anxiety or guilt. The extent and lability of their emotional responses may be heightened by high-dose corticosteroid treatment. These reactions to surgery tend to wane over the first few weeks afterward.

P. A. Shapiro (✉) · L. F. Pereira · I. Wiener
Department of Psychiatry, Columbia University Irving Medical Center, New York, NY, USA
e-mail: pas3@cumc.columbia.edu

K. E. Taylor
Department of Psychiatry, Columbia University Irving Medical Center, New York, NY, USA

Department of Psychiatry, New York University Medical Center, New York, NY, USA

In rare cases, euphoria, irritability, and sleeplessness worsen and develop into a manic episode. Patients with a history of bipolar disorder may be particularly at risk. High steroid dosing in the first few weeks after surgery or in treatment of graft rejection also contributes to the risk of manic symptoms. Steroids, immunosuppressants, and other medications can cause delirium and other neuropsychiatric effects (discussed below).

Patients who are experiencing difficulty with recovery in the immediate postoperative course may be fearful, anxious, and depressed. The first complication occurring after transplantation often bursts the euphoric bubble. Post-traumatic stress disorder (PTSD) can occur when patients have recall of intraoperative events due to inadequate sedation, undergo painful procedures such as defibrillation or placement of central venous or intra-arterial lines, or experience frightening events in the intensive care unit (ICU) environment.

The Early Stage of Recovery After Discharge

At some point, often shortly after returning home, patients develop a deeper understanding that heart transplantation is not a rebirth, but rather a process in which some old problems are relinquished, while the new problems and tasks of living with a transplant must be managed. Surgery is not the end of illness but a milestone on the road of continuing adaptation to illness. In a review of studies of psychological well-being after heart transplantation, Conway and colleagues highlight the value of perceived control and the experience of good social support [3]. These aspects of the patient's experience become especially important after the patient has been discharged from the hospital. Early months after heart transplantation may be dominated by appointments, tests, medication adjustments, management of side effects, and rehabilitation, thereby reinforcing the patient role. Medical events may interrupt progress toward resumption of social, physical, and sexual activity and return to work. This phase of recovery may be complicated by feelings of anxiety, disappointment, or depression. Patients and families are often confronted by the failure of reality to live up to idealized expectations about quality of life after transplantation or length of recovery. Failure of the experience to meet expectations sometimes leads to overt family conflict and may in turn feed into the development of depression.

Guilt feelings may come to the fore as the patient recovers. In addition to the experience of recovery as insufficient to ease caregiving burden on loved ones, other guilt-laden themes include the idea that one has benefited from the death of another person, the recognition of the impossibility of adequately paying back a perceived debt, and survivor guilt when other transplant recipients die.

Later Stages of Recovery and Reintegration into the Regular World: The "New Normal" of Heart Transplant Survivorship

After several months, the intensity of medical follow-up tapers off, and medication regimens have been stabilized. Intensive cardiac rehabilitation is likely to have been completed. Patients might want to return to work, but many are unable, and some do not want to, although they are well enough. Because of requirements to avoid infection, some previously held work is unsuitable. Difficulty resuming work is associated with financial and psychological distress and reduced self-rated quality of life [4].

Many patients experience sexual dysfunction after heart transplantation, and it may persist even after recovery in other domains of health and functional status. Loss of libido and arousal may be due to psychological, interpersonal, and medical factors.

Patients at this stage are living with the chronic disease of heart transplant survivorship. They must manage medications and appointments, maintain diet and exercise regimens, and avoid cigarette smoking and harmful substance use. Many successfully navigate many years with excellent quality of life. Personality pathology, poor coping skills, and low social support may be particularly problematic for maintaining adherence and good self-care, with subsequent increased risk of medical complications [5–7]. Severe depression is uncommon at this stage after transplantation, but may be life-threatening via suicide or complications due to poor adherence to care, while mild to moderate symptoms are common [8–10]. Even in adherent patients, aging and adverse effects of the transplantation regimen lead to new health problems: the transplant fails, kidney function declines, and other medical issues arise. Re-transplantation, hemodialysis or renal transplantation, and treatment of malignancies may become necessary.

Psychiatric Disorders

Many patients have a mixture of psychiatric symptoms, including some combination of anxiety, mood, and cognitive problems. Careful differential diagnosis and individualized treatment are necessary [11].

It has been estimated that 40–60% of transplant recipients receiving calcineurin-inhibiting immunosuppressants experience mild neuropsychiatric side effects [12]. Steroid-related mild neuropsychiatric side effects are estimated to occur in 13–62% of transplant recipients, in a dose-dependent fashion [13]. Mild neuropsychiatric side effects can be managed by correction of any underlying metabolic disturbances or by decreasing the drug's blood level. More severe symptoms may require discontinuation of the offending agent.

Delirium

Delirium is a common occurrence after cardiac surgery, including heart transplantation, but little has been written specifically about post-heart transplant delirium. Studies, some using retrospective self-report, have reported incidence as high as 75% [14].

Delirium is often multifactorial, and it may not be possible to isolate a single causative factor. Side effects of immunosuppressive drugs, opioid analgesics, infections, hypoxia, periods of cerebral hypoperfusion, and other organ-related issues can be triggers for delirium [14–17]. Treatment of the underlying causes and discontinuation or antidoting of offending medications are key aspects of management. Haloperidol and atypical antipsychotic medications are commonly used in treatment of post-transplant delirium, despite the absence of evidence of their value from controlled clinical trials [15].

After an episode of delirium, some patients have recollections of having experienced confusion, paranoid ideation, or hallucinations. These experiences stimulate fear and anxiety [14]. In some patients, delirium experiences form the nidus for PTSD [18].

Mood Disorders

Depression and anxiety (including adjustment disorders with depressed or anxious mood) are the most common psychiatric conditions following heart transplantation [19, 20]. Transplant-related health issues are the most commonly identified stressors precipitating depression.

Prevalence of Depression in Heart Transplant Patients

Reported post-transplant lifetime prevalence rates for depression reach 58%, although these estimates have often been based on retrospective assessments, with small samples and without adjusting for time [21]. In a few studies with larger samples, the incidence of major depressive disorder (MDD) post-transplant ranged from 11% at 1 year [22] to 26% at 3 years [20]. Previous history of psychiatric illness and female gender were associated with increased risk [20].

Five to ten years after surgery, heart transplant recipients reported improved quality of life, functioning, and good overall health. However, depression continues to occur several years after transplantation, in part related to long-term complications and comorbidities [3, 23]. Other studies show 22–32% of patients surviving more than 10 years had self-reported depressive symptoms, along with a range of other signs of emotional distress. Patients' self-perception of inability to work and limitations on function and physical activity contributed to depression [24].

Several studies indicate that patients with depression following transplantation are more likely to suffer from allograft rejection and to die within 3 years after transplantation. Zipfel and colleagues found that preoperative depression was associated with increased post-transplant mortality in patients with ischemic cardiomyopathy but not in those with other causes of heart failure [25]. This study did not assess the persistence of depressive symptoms in these patients, after transplantation, as a factor mediating the association. In other studies, post-transplant depression was associated with diminished post-transplant adherence and with subsequent increased mortality [8, 10]. In a 2015 meta-analysis and systematic review, Dew and colleagues found that depression in the early post-transplant period among the solid organ transplant recipients increased the risks of death and graft loss by 65% over many years of follow-up [9].

Psychopharmacological Treatment of Depression in Heart Transplant Patients

Reported treatments for depression specifically in heart transplant recipients include antidepressants, psychotherapy, and electroconvulsive therapy (ECT). Tricyclic antidepressants (TCAs) can cause orthostatic hypotension and impaired cardiac conduction, but some, particularly nortriptyline, have been reported to be well tolerated in heart transplant recipients and to have little effect on immunosuppressant blood levels [26, 27]. Selective serotonin reuptake inhibitors (SSRIs) have minimal cardiovascular effects; concern about their use in heart transplant recipients is primarily about effects on immunosuppressant blood levels via inhibition of hepatic cytochrome P450 isoenzymes. Sertraline and fluoxetine are modest inhibitors of CYP450-3A4, which metabolizes cyclosporine and sirolimus. Paroxetine, escitalopram, and citalopram have less effect on the 3A4 isoenzyme. In actuality, however, there are only a few clinical reports of problematic interactions of immunosuppressants with SSRIs. In one case, cyclosporine level doubled after introduction of fluoxetine and fell by 50% after fluoxetine was discontinued [28], but in a case series of 13 heart transplant patients, fluoxetine did not affect cyclosporine level [29]. In another case series of three liver and two heart transplant patients, citalopram did not affect cyclosporine pharmacokinetics [30]. Nefazodone (a strong CYP3A4 inhibitor, not an SSRI) has also been reported to increase cyclosporine blood levels [31]. The sexual side effects of SSRIs may limit patients' enthusiasm for their use. Mirtazapine, which is less likely to cause sexual dysfunction and which has anxiolytic, sedative, and antiemetic properties, may be more useful, but its use has not been specifically studied in transplant recipients [32]. In the authors' clinical experience, stimulants are generally well-tolerated as adjunctive treatment for depression in heart transplant patents, despite their potential to increase heart rate, blood pressure, and arrhythmia risk [33]. ECT has also been used safely in heart transplant patients [34].

Non-pharmacological Treatment of Depression in Heart Transplant Patients

Limited data on exercise, social support, and mindfulness-based stress reduction techniques suggest that they may contribute to lowering anxiety and depression in heart transplant patients, although the effects have not been tested specifically in patients with clinically significant depressive symptoms [35]. For example, Dew and colleagues studied Internet-based psychoeducation and social support for 4 months in a group of 24 heart transplant recipients [36]. Anxiety and depression symptoms declined from pre- to post-intervention, but the mean level of anxiety and depression symptoms at baseline was only 1 on a 0–4 scale, indicating that this was not a very distressed or symptomatic cohort to begin with.

A recent uncontrolled pilot study found that a 6-week mindfulness-based stress reduction intervention reduced depression and anxiety symptoms in a small cohort of solid organ transplant recipients (who were not selected on the basis of high levels of symptoms) [37]. Likewise, a study of high-intensity interval exercise training found a beneficial effect on mood and anxiety symptoms in a cohort of heart recipients (not selected for high depression or anxiety) [38]. Whether these types of interventions would benefit heart transplant patients with mood or anxiety disorders is unknown.

Mania and Hypomania in Heart Transplant Patients

The main risk factors for manic and hypomanic episodes after heart transplantation are steroids and previous history of bipolar disorder. Large steroid doses may precipitate a manic episode, even in patients with no history of mood disorder. Apparent manic symptoms may also be a feature of delirium. Little empirical data is available to guide treatment. Valproic acid is a reasonable first-line treatment for mania, but caution is required due to its potential effects on liver function and platelets. Impaired renal function is a long-term complication of both lithium and calcineurin-inhibitor immunosuppressants; for this reason, lithium is best avoided if possible. Carbamazepine is relatively contraindicated due to potential for many drug-drug interactions through induction of cytochrome P450 system enzymes and its tendency to cause hyponatremia. Antipsychotic agents may be extremely helpful in management of acute mania after heart transplantation, as long as attention is paid to potential drug interactions [33, 39].

Cognitive Disorders

Cognitive impairment has been described in up to 77% of heart transplant candidates [40] and is thought to be caused by chronic central nervous system hypoperfusion, as seen in advanced stages of heart failure. The risk is especially high in older patients [41]. Restoration of normal cardiac output, with improved hepatic and renal function, improves at least some domains of cognitive function [42, 43]. However, deficits may take months to years to resolve [13] and a subset of patients remain impaired [44]. Undergoing cardiac surgery in and of itself may increase risk of subsequent cognitive dysfunction [45].

It is uncertain if immunosuppressants, or specific classes of immunosuppressants, contribute to persistent or long-term cognitive impairment. Using standard psychometric tests and evoked potential recording, Grimm et al. demonstrated that cardiac transplantation initially normalizes impaired brain function, followed by a relative long-term decline, hypothesized to be due to cumulative cyclosporine toxicity [46]. Burker and colleagues found no difference in cognitive function between heart transplant patients treated with everolimus-based versus calcineurin-inhibitor-based regimens [47].

There is no published data assessing pharmacological treatment of cognitive impairment after heart transplantation. If medications such as donepezil, galantamine, rivastigmine, and memantine are used by transplant recipients, drug-drug interactions must be considered. Donepezil, in particular, is a weak inhibitor of cytochrome P4503A4 and may increase serum levels of immunosuppressants [48–51]. Donepezil and galantamine are both substrates of CYP3A4 [50, 52].

Anxiety

Adjustment disorder with anxious mood and mixed presentations of generalized anxiety disorder symptoms with mood or behavioral disturbances are common in the first year after transplantation and may also occur in subsequent years [20]. In one study, significant anxiety symptoms were detected within 8 weeks after surgery in over 50% of heart transplant recipients [53]. Female sex, previous history of anxiety, and older age were associated with increased risk. Precipitating factors included transplant-related complications, medication side effects, unpleasant or risky medical procedures, and fears about returning to the home environment. Other concurrent life events may also trigger anxiety.

In their 2015 review and meta-analysis, Dew and colleagues found that, in contrast to depression, anxiety symptoms and anxiety disorders following transplantation were not significantly associated with increased morbidity or mortality [9].

Despite the substantial prevalence of anxiety symptoms, clinical studies on its treatment specifically in heart transplant recipients are lacking. Benzodiazepines and SSRIs are commonly employed, along with psychotherapy and behavioral interventions, such as relaxation training. Gabapentin, which is cleared by renal excretion without hepatic metabolism, is another option [54]. As noted above, small studies of mindfulness-based stress reduction [37] and exercise training [38] in solid organ transplant recipients both yielded reduction in reported anxiety symptoms, but neither study targeted patients with high baseline anxiety symptoms, and the benefit for patients with anxiety disorders is uncertain.

Post-traumatic Stress Disorder

PTSD is common after cardiac surgery and is a recognized complication of organ transplantation. Stukas and colleagues followed 126 heart transplant recipients and found that 14% developed transplant-related PTSD [55]. Many factors may contribute to the development of PTSD, including the life-threatening illness experienced during the waiting period, the transplant surgery, and the ICU stay. Delusions and hallucinations associated with post-transplant delirium have also been reported to provoke PTSD [18]. In a systematic review, pre-transplant psychiatric illness and poor social support post-transplant were consistent predictors of post-transplant PTSD [56]. PTSD symptoms were associated with worse mental health-related quality of life. In one prospective study, patients who experienced PTSD during the first year after the transplant were over 13 times more likely to die within 3 years of follow-up [55].

Standard treatments for PTSD include cognitive behavior therapy, especially prolonged exposure therapy, and SSRIs, sometimes augmented with antipsychotic medication. However, no controlled studies of PTSD treatment in solid organ transplant recipients, or specifically in heart transplant recipients, have been conducted [57].

Sexual Dysfunction

Most male and about half of female heart transplant recipients report sexual dysfunction, with associated impairment in self-rated quality of life [58]. Contributing factors include pre-existing comorbidities (e.g., atherosclerosis, diabetic neuropathy, and angiopathy), effects of medications (e.g., antihypertensive medicines, steroids, immunosuppressants, antidepressants), mobility and pain issues, fear, depression, stress, perceived changes in attractiveness and body image, and relationship conflicts. Impairments of the desire and arousal phases of normal sexual response may be due to physiological or primarily psychological difficulties. Impaired orgasm is most often related to medication (e.g., SSRI) or physiological effects. Therefore, a thorough investigation of both medical and psychological contributors to sexual dysfunction may be necessary in order to direct intervention. Furthermore, cardiac patients often avoid sex because of fear that it may cause excessive strain on the heart. In addition, cardiac surgery patients with large midline surgical incisions are warned to avoid tension on the incision during the healing process, in order to avoid wound dehiscence [59–62].

Post-heart transplant patients may benefit from explicit, focused counseling about resuming sexual behavior after transplantation [63], but no studies have specifically addressed treatment in heart transplant recipients. Phosphodiesterase type 5 (PDE5) inhibitors such as sildenafil, utilized in treatment of pulmonary hypertension, are used for treatment of erectile dysfunction and can be tolerated by heart transplant recipients as long as nitrates and alpha-adrenergic blocking agents are not co-administered [33].

Sleep Disorders

Sleep disorders are highly prevalent after heart transplantation and associated with poor health-related quality of life. Tseng and colleagues found 72% of post-cardiac transplant patients reported sleep disturbance [64]. Reilly-Spong and colleagues reported rates of clinically defined poor sleep in 41%, and decreased sleep efficiency in 69%, of solid organ recipients [65]. Physiological, psychological, and social factors contribute to the low quality of sleep in heart transplant recipients.

Physiological factors include obstructive sleep apnea (OSA), post-transplant physical symptoms, and medication side effects. A cross-sectional study found that 36% of cardiac transplant recipients had moderate to severe OSA [66].

Psychological and social factors that contribute to poor sleep include role shifts within the family, unemployment and loss of daily structure, and financial stress. Sleep disturbance can be symptomatic of an underlying mood or adjustment disorder, PTSD, or of pain or shortness of breath. These conditions must be addressed in order to improve sleep quality.

Sleep quality may be impacted directly or indirectly by post-transplantation medications. Calcineurin-inhibiting immunosuppressants and corticosteroids commonly cause insomnia, either as an independent symptom or as part of a constellation of neuropsychiatric symptoms [12]. Indirect medication side effects include nocturia secondary to diuretics and altered sleep-wake cycle due to use of sedating analgesic medications. When appropriate, medication timing and doses should be adjusted to maximize quality of sleep.

Although sedative-hypnotics are the most common treatment for insomnia, these medications often have little effect, and do not address underlying causes. For transplant recipients, these ancillary medications may additionally contribute to polypharmacy, raising risks of medication errors and nonadherence. Addressing underlying medical and psychiatric conditions and sleep hygiene education are important steps in managing sleep disorders. Although it is a plausible intervention, no studies of cognitive behavioral therapy for insomnia have been conducted in heart transplant patients.

Adherence After Heart Transplantation

Failure to adhere to the transplant regimen is an obvious risk factor for morbidity and mortality after transplantation, making psychosocial and behavioral factors associated with adherence problems an important topic for post-transplant psychosocial care. A recent review noted that pre-transplant medication nonadherence predicts post-transplant medication nonadherence and that nonadherence increases after the first few months following transplant, often in association with intercurrent life stressors, financial strain, and high cost of medication [67]. Negative attitudes and beliefs about transplant medications, for example, that the medications cause side effects, and are not actually important to protect against rejection, are also associated with nonadherence. Similarly, patients with poorer knowledge and understanding of transplantation have higher rates of nonadherence [68]. Structured evaluations conducted before placing a patient on the waiting list for transplantation that consider psychiatric disorders, personality, substance use, cognitive function, motivation and understanding, social supports, and intercurrent stressors can identify patients with increased risk of adherence problems following transplantation and of consequent morbidity [5–7]. These evaluations can provide opportunity for interventions to mitigate risk before adverse consequences ensue. To date, however, there has been little in the way of controlled trials to demonstrate benefits of interventions to promote adherence.

Another review highlights the paucity of controlled studies of interventions to improve adherence in heart transplant patients. Identified quasi-experimental intervention studies examined simplifying the medication dosing schedule, psychoeducation, and Internet-based interactive workshops; these studies provide very limited evidence for at least a modest benefit of such interventions [69].

Conclusions

Psychiatric disorders are common and contribute substantially to suffering and decreased quality of life in heart transplant recipients. Some disorders are associated with increased risk of poor adherence to the transplant regimen and increased morbidity and mortality. Careful differential diagnosis, appreciation of the potential psychiatric side effects of the transplant medication regimen, and awareness of drug interactions are important aspects of psychiatric care of heart transplant recipients. Many of these psychiatric problems can be successfully prevented or treated, but more controlled trials are needed to establish treatment effectiveness for many psychiatric disorders in heart transplant recipients.

Acknowledgement Supported in part by the Nathaniel Wharton Fund, New York, NY.

References

1. Shapiro PA. Life after heart transplantation. Prog Cardiovasc Dis. 1990;32:405–18.
2. Shapiro PA. The process of acquiring and keeping an organ transplant. In: O'Reilly-Landry M, editor. A psychodynamic understanding of modern medicine: placing the person at the center of care. London: Radcliffe; 2012. p. 149–61.
3. Conway A, Schadewaldt V, Clark R, Ski C, Thompson DR, Doering L. The psychological experiences of adult heart transplant recipients: a systematic review and meta-summary of qualitative findings. Heart Lung. 2013;42:449–55.
4. Paris W, Woodbury A, Thompson S, Levick M, Nothegger S, Slade-Hutkin L, Arbukle P, Cooper DKC. Social rehabilitation and return to work after cardiac transplantation-a multicenter survey. Transplantation. 1992;53:433–8.
5. Shapiro PA, Williams DL, Foray AT, Gelman IS, Wukich N, Sciacca R. Psychosocial evaluation and prediction of compliance problems and morbidity after heart transplantation. Transplantation. 1995;60:1462–6.
6. Shapiro PA. Psychiatric evaluation of potential heart transplant candidates as a predictor of post-heart transplant mortality. Paper presented at the annual meeting of the Academy of Psychosomatic Medicine, Nov. 19, 2011.
7. Maldonado J, Sher Y, Lolak S, Swendsen H, Skibola D, Neri E, David E, Sullivan C, Standridge K. The Stanford integrated psychosocial assessment for transplantation: a prospective study of medical and psychosocial outcomes. Psychosom Med. 2015;77:1018–30.
8. Dew MA, Kormos RL, Roth LH, Murali S, Dimartini A, Griffith BP. Early post-transplant medical compliance and mental health predict physical morbidity and mortality one to three years after heart transplantation. J Heart Lung Transplant. 1999;18:546–62.
9. Dew MA, Rosenberger EM, Myaskovsky L, DiMartini AF, DeVito Dabbs AJ, Posluszny DM, Steel J, Switzer GE, Shellmer DA, Greenhouse JB. Depression and anxiety as risk factors for morbidity and mortality after organ transplantation: a systematic review and meta-analysis. Transplantation. 2015;100:988–1003.
10. Dobbels F, De Geest S, van Cleemput J, Droogne W, Vanhaecke J. Effect of late medication non-compliance on outcome after heart transplantation: a 5-year follow-up. J Heart Lung Transplant. 2004;23:1245–51.
11. Stiefel P, Malehsa D, Bara C, Strueber M, Haverich A, Kugler C. Symptom experiences in patients after heart transplantation. J Health Psychol. 2013;18(5):680–92.
12. DiMartini AF, Crone CC, Fireman M. Organ transplantation. In: Ferrando SJ, Levenson JL, Owen JA, editors. Clinical manual of psychopharmacology in the medically ill. Washington, DC: American Psychiatric Publishing; 2010. p. 469–99.
13. DiMartini A, Crone C, Fireman M, Dew MA. Psychiatric aspects of organ transplantation in critical care. Crit Care Clin. 2008;24:949–81.
14. Flynn K, Daiches A, Malpus Z, Yonan N, Sanchez M. 'A post-transplant person': narratives of heart or lung transplantation and intensive care unit delirium. Health (London). 2014;18:352–68.
15. Sockalingam S, Parekh N, Bogoch II, Sun J, Mahtani R, Beach C, Bollegalla N, Turzanski S, Seto E, Kim J, Dulay P, Scarrow S, Bhalerao S. Delirium in the postoperative cardiac patient: a review. J Card Surg. 2005;20:560–7.
16. Dhar R. Neurologic complications of transplantation. Neurocrit Care. 2018 Feb;28(1):4–11. https://doi.org/10.1007/s12028-017-0387-6.
17. Senzolo M, Ferronato C, Burra P. Neurologic complications after solid organ transplantation. Transpl Int. 2009;22:269–78.
18. DiMartini A, Dew MA, Kormos R, McCurry K, Fontes P. Posttraumatic stress disorder caused by hallucinations and delusions experienced in delirium. Psychosomatics. 2007;48:436–9.
19. Shapiro PA, Kornfeld DS. Psychiatric outcome of heart transplantation. Gen Hosp Psychiatry. 1989;11:352–7.
20. Dew MA, Kormos RL, DiMartini AF, Switzer GE, Schulberg HC, Roth LH, Griffith BP. Prevalence and risk of depression and anxiety-related disorders during the first three years after heart transplantation. Psychosomatics. 2001;42:300–13.
21. Freeman AM, Folks DG, Sokol RS, Fahs JJ. Cardiac transplantation: clinical correlates of psychiatric outcome. Psychosomatics. 1988;29:47–54.
22. Dew MA, Roth LH, Schulberg HC, Simmons RG, Kormos RL, Trzepacz PT, Griffith BP. Prevalence and predictors of depression and anxiety-related disorders during the year after heart transplantation. Gen Hosp Psychiatry. 1996;18(6 Suppl):48s–61s.
23. Grady KL, Naftel DC, Kobashigawa J, Chait J, Young JB, Pelegrin D, Czerr J, Heroux A, Higgins R, Rybarczyk B, McLeod M, White-Williams C, Kirklin JK. Patterns and predictors of quality of life at 5 to 10 years after heart transplant. J Heart Lung Transplant. 2007;26:535–43.
24. Fusar-Poli P, Martinelli V, Klersy C, Campana C, Callegari A, Barale F, Vigano M, Politi P. Depression and quality of life in patients living 10 to 18 years beyond heart transplantation. J Heart Lung Transplant. 2005;24:2269–78.

25. Zipfel S, Schneider A, Wild B, Lowe B, Junger J, Haass M, Sack F, Bergmann G, Herzog W. Effect of depressive symptoms on survival after heart transplantation. Psychosom Med. 2002;64:740–7.

26. Shapiro PA. Nortriptyline treatment in depressed cardiac transplant recipients. Am J Psychiatry. 1991;148:371–3.

27. Kay J, Bienenfeld D, Slomowitz M, Burk J, Zimmer L, Nadolny G, Marvel NT, Geier P. Use of tricyclic antidepressants in recipients of heart transplants. Psychosomatics. 1991;32:165–70.

28. Horton R, Bonser R. Interaction between cyclosporine and fluoxetine. BMJ. 1995;311:422.

29. Strouse T, Fairbanks L, Skotzko C. Fluoxetine and cyclosporine in organ transplantation. Failure to detect significant drug interactions or adverse clinical events in depressed organ recipients. Psychosomatics. 1996;37:23–30.

30. Liston HL, Markowitz JS, Hunt N, DeVane CL, Boulton DW, Ashcraft E. Lack of citalopram effect on the pharmacokinetics of cyclosporine. Psychosomatics. 2001;42:370–2.

31. Vella J, Sayegh M. Interactions between cyclosporine and newer antidepressant medications. Am J Kidney Dis. 1998;31:320–2.

32. Fusar-Poli P, Picchioni M, Martinelli V, Bhattacharyya S, Cortesi M, Barale F, Politi P. Anti-depressive therapies after heart transplantation. J Heart Lung Transplant. 2006;25:785–93.

33. Shapiro PA. Cardiovascular disorders. In: Levenson J, Ferrando S, editors. Clinical manual of psychopharmacology in the medically ill. 2nd ed. Arlington: American Psychiatric Association; 2017. p. 233–70.

34. Lee HB, Jayaram G, Teitelbaum ML. Electroconvulsive therapy for depression in a cardiac transplant patient. Psychosomatics. 2001;42:362–4.

35. Conway A, Schadewaldt V, Clark R, Ski C, Thompson DR, Kynoch K, Doering L. The effectiveness of non-pharmacological interventions in improving psychological outcomes for heart transplant recipients: a systematic review. Eur J Cardiovasc Nurs. 2014;13:108–15.

36. Dew MA, Goycoolea JM, Harris RC, Lee A, Zomak R, Dunbar-Jacob J, Rotondi A, Griffith BP, Kormos RL. An internet-based intervention to improve psychosocial outcomes in heart transplant recipients and family caregivers: development and evaluation. J Heart Lung Transplant. 2004;23(6):745–58.

37. Stonnington CM, Darby B, Santucci A, Mulligan P, Pathuis P, Cuc A, Hentz JG, Zhang N, Mulligan D, Sood A. A resilience intervention involving mindfulness training for transplant patients and their caregivers. Clin Transpl. 2016;30:1466–72.

38. Yardley M, Gullestad L, Bendz B, Bjorkelund E, Rolid K, Arora S, Nytroen K. Long-term effects of high-intensity interval training in heart transplant recipients: a five-year follow-up of a randomized clinical trial. Clin Transplant. 2017;31:e12868. https://doi.org/10.1111/ctr.12868.

39. Beach SR, Celano CM, Noseworthy PA, Januzzi JL, Huffman JC. QTc prolongation, torsades de pointes, and psychotropic medications. Psychosomatics. 2013;54:1–13.

40. Putzke JD, Williams MA, Daniel JF, Foley BA, Kirklin JK, Boll TJ. Neuropsychological functioning among heart transplant candidates: a case control study. J Clin Exp Neuropsychol. 2000;22:95–103.

41. Festa JR, Jia X, Cheung K, Marchidann A, Schmidt M, Shapiro PA, Mancini DM, Naka Y, Deng M, Lantz ER, Marshall RS, Lazar RM. Association of low ejection fraction with impaired verbal memory in older patients with heart failure. Arch Neurol. 2011;68:1021–6.

42. DeShields TL, McDonough EM, Mannen RK, Miller LW. Psychological and cognitive status before and after heart transplantation. Gen Hosp Psychiatry. 1996;18(6 Suppl):62S–9S.

43. Schall RR, Petrucci RJ, Brozena SC, Cavarocchi NC, Jessup M. Cognitive function in patients with symptomatic dilated cardiomyopathy before and after cardiac transplantation. J Am Coll Cardiol. 1989;14:1666–72.

44. Cupples SA, Stilley CS. Cognitive function in adult cardiothoracic transplant candidates and recipients. J Cardiovasc Nurs. 2005;20(5 Suppl):S74–87.

45. Habib S, Khan A, Afridi MI, Saeed A, Jan AF, Amjad N. Frequency and predictors of cognitive decline in patients undergoing coronary artery bypass graft surgery. J Coll Physicians Surg Pak. 2014;24:543–8.

46. Grimm M, Yeganehfar W, Laufer G, Madl C, Kramer L, Eisenhuber E, Simon P, Kupilik N, Schreiner W, Pacher R, Bunzel B, Wolner E, Grimm G. Cyclosporine may affect improvement of cognitive brain function after successful cardiac transplantation. Circulation. 1996;94:1339–45.

47. Bürker BS, Gullestad L, Gude E, Relbo Authen A, Grov I, Hol PK, Andreassen AK, Arora S, Dew MA, Fiane AE, Haraldsen IR, Malt UF, Andersson S. Cognitive function after heart transplantation: comparing everolimus-based and calcineurin inhibitor-based regimens. Clin Transpl. 2017;31 https://doi.org/10.1111/ctr.12927.

48. Micuda S, Mundlova L, Anzenbacherova E, Anzenbacher P, Chladek J, Fuksa L, Martinkova J. Inhibitory effects of memantine on human cytochrome P450 activities: prediction of in vivo drug interactions. Eur J Clin Pharmacol. 2004;60:583–9.

49. Polinsky RJ. Clinical pharmacology of rivastigmine: a new-generation acetylcholinesterase inhibitor for the treatment of Alzheimer's disease. Clin Ther. 1998;20:634–47.

50. Farlow MR. Clinical pharmacokinetics of Galantamine. Clin Pharmacokinet. 2003;42:1383–92.

51. McEneny-King A, Edginton AN, Rao PP. Investigating the binding interactions of the anti-Alzheimer's drug donepezil with CYP3A4 and P-glycoprotein. Bioorg Med Chem Lett. 2015;25:297–301.

52. Jackson S, Ham RJ, Wilkinson D. The safety and tolerability of donepezil in patients with Alzheimer's disease. Brit J Clin Pharmacol. 2004;58(Suppl. 1):1–8.

53. Pudlo R, Piegza M, Zakliczyński M, Zembala M. The occurrence of mood and anxiety disorders in heart transplant recipients. Transplant Proc. 2009;41:3214–8.

54. Crone CC, Gabriel GM. Treatment of anxiety and depression in transplant patients: pharmacokinetic considerations. Clin Pharmacokinet. 2004;43:361–94.

55. Stukas AA, Dew MA, Switzer GE, DiMartini A, Kormos RL, Griffith BP. PTSD in heart transplant recipients and their primary family caregivers. Psychosomatics. 1999;40:212–21.

56. Davydow DS, Lease ED, Reyes JD. Posttraumatic stress disorder in organ transplant recipients: a systematic review. Gen Hosp Psychiatry. 2015;37:387–98.

57. Supelana C, Annunziato RA, Kaplan D, Helcer J, Stuber ML, Shemesh E. PTSD in solid organ transplant recipients: current understanding and future implications. Pediatr Transplant. 2016;20:23–33.

58. Phan A, Ishak WW, Shen BJ, Fuess J, Philip K, Bresee C, Czer L, Schwarz ER. Persistent sexual dysfunction impairs quality of life after cardiac transplantation. J Sex Med. 2010;7:2765–73.

59. Dew MA, DiMartini AF. Psychological disorders and distress after adult cardiothoracic transplantation. J Cardiovasc Nurs. 2005;20(5 Suppl):S51–66.

60. Rembek M, Tylkowski M, Piestrzeniewicz K, Goch JH. Problems connected with sexual activity in patients with heart disease. Pol Merkur Lekarski. 2007;23:151–4.

61. Holtzman S, Abbey SE, Stewart DE, Ross HJ. Pain after heart transplantation: prevalence and implications for quality of life. Psychosomatics. 2010;51(3):230–6.

62. Stein R, Sardinha A, Araújo CGS. Sexual activity and heart patients: a contemporary perspective. Can J Cardiol. 2016;32(4):410–20.

63. Steinke EE, Jaarsma T, Barnason SA, Byrne M, Doherty S, Dougherty CM, Fridlund B, Kautz DD, Mårtensson J, Mosack V, Moser DK, Council on Cardiovascular and Stroke Nursing of the American Heart Association and the ESC Council on Cardiovascular Nursing and Allied Professions (CCNAP). Sexual counselling for individuals with cardiovascular disease and their partners: a consensus document from the American Heart Association and the ESC Council on Cardiovascular Nursing and Allied Professions (CCNAP). Eur Heart J. 2013;34:3217–35.

64. Tseng PH, Shih FJ, Yang FC, Shih FJ, Wang SS. Factors contributing to poor sleep quality as perceived by heart transplant recipients in Taiwan. Transplant Proc. 2014;46:903–6.

65. Reilly-Spong M, Park T, Gross CR. Poor sleep in organ transplant recipients: self-reports and actigraphy. Clin Transpl. 2013;27:901–13.

66. Javaheri S, Abraham WT, Brown C, Nishiyama H, Giesting R, Wagoner LE. Prevalence of obstructive sleep apnoea and periodic limb movement in 45 subjects with heart transplantation. Eur Heart J. 2004;25:260–6.

67. Vitinius F, Ziemke M, Albert W. Adherence with immunosuppression in heart transplant recipients. Curr Opin Organ Transplant. 2015;20:193–7.

68. Kung M, Koschwanez HE, Painter L, Honeyman V, Broadbent E. Immunosuppressant nonadherence in heart, liver, and lung transplant patients: associations with medication beliefs and illness perceptions. Transplantation. 2012;93:958–63.

69. Marcelino CA, Díaz LJ, da Cruz DM. The effectiveness of interventions in managing treatment adherence in adult heart transplant patients: a systematic review. JBI Database System Rev Implement Rep. 2015;13:279–308.

End-Stage Lung Disease and Indications for Lung Transplantation

Joshua J. Lee and Laveena Chhatwani

Introduction

Lung transplantation remains the only therapeutic option for various end-stage lung diseases involving the lung parenchyma or vasculature. As discussed in Chap. 25 on History of Lung Transplantation, the first lung transplantation occurred in 1963, and significant advancements in surgical technique, immunosuppressive medications, and organ preservation techniques have improved postsurgical outcomes [1]. The most recent data from The International Society for Heart and Lung Transplantation (ISHLT) reports that there were over 4000 lung transplantations performed worldwide in 2015 [2]. Major indications for lung transplantation include idiopathic interstitial pneumonia (IIP), chronic obstructive pulmonary disease (COPD), cystic fibrosis (CF), and idiopathic pulmonary arterial hypertension (IPAH) (Fig. 22.1). Selection of appropriate candidates for lung transplantation involves a careful multidisciplinary approach. This includes assessing the severity of the underlying disease, other organ system function, and psychosocial aspects. Given the diverse nature of the underlying lung diseases, advanced lung failure affects people across all age groups and backgrounds. In this chapter, we provide an overview of the diseases and indications for lung transplantation and discuss the relative and absolute contraindications to lung transplantation.

Indications and Timing of Referral

In the broadest terms, lung failure of diverse etiologies which is progressive despite maximal medical therapy is an indication for lung transplantation. Lung transplantation is considered for those with advanced lung disease who have a high (>50%) risk of death from lung disease in 2 years along with a high (>80%) likelihood of short-term (90-day) and long-term (5-year) post-transplant survival from a general medical perspective, provided adequate lung allograft function [3]. Given the complexity of lung transplantation, it is correctly reserved as the treatment of last resort when medical therapy has failed. However, timely referral is key to providing the patient and the transplant center with adequate time to complete an evaluation and resolve barriers to transplantation.

Obstructive Lung Disease

Chronic obstructive pulmonary disease (COPD) accounted for 30% of all lung transplantations between 1996 and 2015 [2]. Other obstructive lung disease disorders for which lung transplantation is offered include α-1-antitrypsin deficiency (A1AT), Langerhans cell histiocytosis, and lymphangioleiomyomatosis (LAM).

The progression of COPD consists of a slow decline in lung function over several years [4]. Many patients have acceptable long-term survival outcomes with advanced COPD making the timing of lung transplantation challenging [4]. There are many clinical factors related to COPD that have been associated with poor outcomes including the degree of hypercapnia, coexisting pulmonary hypertension, lower post-bronchodilator force expiratory volume in the first second (FEV1), low body mass index (BMI), severity of emphysema, and exercise capacity [5, 6]. These factors alone are insufficient to use in determining the mortality risk in individual patients. In 2004, Celli et al. combined several of these factors to form a model predicting mortality known as the BODE (BMI, degree of airflow obstruction, dyspnea, exercise capacity) index [39]. The BODE score ranges from 0 to 10 with higher scores inferring a higher mortality risk (Table 22.1). The number of exacerbations per year is also associated with worsening mortality independent of the severity of the disease as measured by the BODE index [7, 8]. In addition,

J. J. Lee · L. Chhatwani (✉)
Division of Pulmonary and Critical Care, Department of Medicine, Stanford University, School of Medicine, Stanford, CA, USA
e-mail: laveena@stanford.edu

© Springer International Publishing AG, part of Springer Nature 2019
Y. Sher, J. R. Maldonado (eds.), *Psychosocial Care of End-Stage Organ Disease and Transplant Patients*,
https://doi.org/10.1007/978-3-319-94914-7_22

ISHLT 2017
ISHLT • INTERNATIONAL SOCIETY FOR HEART AND LUNG TRANSPLANTATION
JHLT. 2017 Oct; 36(10): 1037-1079

Diagnosis	SLT (N = 18,207)	BLT (N = 36,046)	Total (N = 54,253)
COPD	7266 (39.9%)	9539 (26.5%)	16,805 (31.0%)
IIP	6449 (35.4%)	6990 (19.4%)	13,439 (24.8%)
CF	218 (1.2%)	8266 (22.9%)	8484 (15.6%)
ILD-not IIP	1078 (5.9%)	1925 (5.3%)	3003 (5.5%)
A1ATD	797 (4.4%)	1,912 (5.3%)	2709 (5.0%)
Retransplant	922 (5.1%)	1269 (3.5%)	2191 (4.0%)
IPAH	88 (0.5%)	1481 (4.1%)	1569 (2.9%)
Non CF-bronchiectasis	67 (0.4%)	1413 (3.9%)	1480 (2.7%)
Sarcoidosis	312 (1.7%)	1026 (2.8%)	1338 (2.5%)
PH-not IPAH	135 (0.7%)	690 (1.9%)	825 (1.5%)
LAM/tuberous sclerosis	146 (0.8%)	381 (1.1%)	527 (1.0%)
OB	73 (0.4%)	395 (1.1%)	468 (0.9%)
CTD	140 (0.8%)	282 (0.8%)	422 (0.8%)
Cancer	7 (0.0%)	27 (0.1%)	34 (0.1%)
Other	509 (2.8%)	450 (1.2%)	959 (1.8%)

Fig. 22.1 Adult Lung Transplants (January 1995 - June 2016) Key: Chronic obstructive pulmonary disease (COPD), idiopathic interstitial pneumonia (IIP), cystic fibrosis (CF), interstitial lung disease (ILD), alpha-1 antitrypsin deficiency (A1ATD), idiopathic pulmonary arterial hypertension (IPAH), pulmonary hypertension (PH), lymphangioleiomyomatosis (LAM), obliterative bronchiolitis (OB), connective tissue disease (CTD), single-lung transplant (SLT), bilateral lung transplant (BLT)

Table 22.1 Predicting Mortality in Chronic Obstructive Pulmonary Disease: BODE Index

BODE index	12-month mortality (%)	24-month mortality (%)	52-month mortality (%)
0–2	2	6	19
3–4	2	8	32
4–6	2	14	48
7–10	5	31	80

patients admitted for hypercapnic respiratory failure have an inpatient mortality greater than 10%, and of those who survive the admission, 1- and 2-year mortality rates are 43% and 49%, respectively [9].

Post-transplant survival data in COPD patients include a median of 5.3 years, 2-year survival of 75% [2]. The most recent ISHLT consensus guidelines recommend that patients with obstructive lung disease be referred for lung transplantation with disease progression despite maximal medical therapy, not candidates for lung volume reduction surgery, BODE index of 5–6, $PaCo_2$ > 50 mmHg and/or PaO_2 < 60 mmHg, and FEV1 < 25% predicted [3]. Recommendations for listing for lung transplantation include BODE index >7, FEV1 < 15%–20% predicted, three or more severe exacerbations during the preceding year, one exacerbation with acute hypercapnic respiratory failure, and/or moderate to severe pulmonary hypertension [3].

One issue specific to the COPD population is the role of lung volume reduction surgery (LVRS) in a subset of patients. In 2003, the National Emphysema Treatment Trial (NETT) demonstrated that patients with an FEV1 between 20% and 25%, diffusing capacity for carbon monoxide (DLCO) > 20%, upper lobe predominant heterogeneous emphysema, and poor exercise capacity had improved exercise capacity, lung function, and quality of life after LVRS [10]. For those who meet the criteria for both LVRS and lung transplantation, it is reasonable to offer LVRS first, leaving lung transplantation as an option for those who do not respond to LVRS [4]. Successful LVRS can postpone lung transplantation allowing for further optimization of functional and nutritional status [11, 12].

A1AT deficiency is primarily seen in Northern European populations; however, it has been identified in all racial groups [13]. Alpha-1 antitrypsin (AAT) is a serine protease inhibitor designed to help preserve lung elasticity by neutralizing elastase. When levels of AAT decline below the protective threshold, neutrophil-mediated elastase activity is unopposed resulting in destruction of lung parenchyma and the development of emphysema [13]. Patients with A1AT deficiency are particularly vulnerable to developing early emphysema especially with tobacco exposure. The timing of listing for lung transplantation for A1AT deficiency is similar to the clinical guidelines for COPD [4]. Although A1AT deficiency is also known to cause end-stage liver disease, according to the United Network for Organ Sharing, only 1% of adult liver transplantations occurred in the United States in the setting of A1AT deficiency from 1995 to 2004 [14]. When both organs are severely affected, a combined liver-lung transplant may be an option for a select few. Data for combined liver-lung transplant for A1AT deficiency is limited to a few case reports [15, 16].

LAM is a rare cystic lung disease involving abnormal smooth muscle proliferation around small airways, pulmonary vasculature, and lymphatics [4]. It affects women of child-bearing years presenting with spontaneous pneumothoraces and chylothorax. LAM accounted for 1% of total lung transplants from 1996 to 2015 [2]. Due to the lack of data, prognostic parameters indicative of high mortality risks prompting listing for lung transplantation is limited. Population-based studies suggest that age of diagnosis, weight loss, and use of supplemental oxygen are independent predictors of mortality [17]. Patients with LAM are generally considered for listing when there is significant decline in pulmonary function, quality of life, and functional status [4]. Prior pleurodesis or pleurectomy for pneumothorax/chylothorax can result in adhesions, making the surgery more complicated with increased risk of severe hemorrhage. However, this should not be considered an absolute contraindication to transplantation [4]. Fifty percent of patients with LAM will develop renal angiomyolipomas which have a risk of spontaneous bleeding. In general, larger lesions are addressed with embolization prior to transplantation, and if renal function is not compromised, renal angiomyolipomas are not considered an absolute contraindication to lung transplantation [4]. Recurrence of LAM has been reported, although the exact incidence is not known.

Cystic Fibrosis and Non-cystic Fibrosis Bronchiectasis

Cystic fibrosis (CF) is an autosomal recessive genetic disorder that involves mutations in the cystic fibrosis transmembrane conductance regulator (CFTR) gene. This mutation causes a defective chloride channel expression in the membrane of apical epithelial cells. CF is a systemic disease affecting sweat glands, intestines, lungs, pancreas, liver, and sinuses, as well as reproductive organs in men [18]. From 1986 to 2012, the median survival of CF patients has increased to 36 years of age from 27. However, the primary morbidity and mortality results from respiratory failure [18]. CF accounted for 15% of total lung transplants from 1996 to 2015 [2].

There are no prospective, randomized studies that define the optimal timing for listing in CF patients. Thus, early referral of CF patients to transplant centers is encouraged to identify and correct potential barriers to transplantation [19]. Generally, the degree of lung function, decline in functional capacity, number of exacerbation, presence of refractory hemoptysis, and pneumothorax are clinical factors used when listing CF patients for transplantation. Kerem et al. reported that an FEV1 < 30% predicted was associated with a 2-year mortality of 40% in males and 55% in females [20]. Others have reported that FEV1 < 30% predicted, an ele-

vated $PaCO_2$ > 50 mmHg, and use of nutritional supplements were all associated with increased mortality [21]. Milla et al. looked at the rate of decline in lung function and found that the rate of decline, rather than the absolute values of FEV1, was associated with earlier mortality [22]. A 5-year survivorship model was developed using the Cystic Fibrosis Foundation database by Liou et al. They reported that female sex, diabetes mellitus, Burkholderia cepacia infection, and number of exacerbations were better indicators of mortality, as compared to FEV1 alone [23]. According to the 2014 ISHLT consensus guidelines, patients should be referred to transplant centers when FEV1 < 30%, or there is progressive decline in FEV1 despite optimal medical therapy, 6-min walk distance <400 m, presence of concomitant pulmonary hypertension, clinical deterioration with increased exacerbations associated with pneumothorax, life-threatening hemoptysis despite bronchial artery embolization, increasing antibiotic resistance organisms with slower recovery, or respiratory failure requiring noninvasive ventilation [2]. Indications for listing include chronic respiratory failure with PaO_2 < 60 mmHg, $PaCo_2$ > 50 mmHg, rapid progressive functional decline, New York Heart Association (NYHA) functional class IV, continued weight loss despite aggressive nutritional supplementation, and pulmonary hypertension [19]. Determining candidacy for lung transplantation varies among different centers based on program experience. Post-transplant survival statistics in CF patients include median survival of 12 years, the longest as compared to patients with other end-stage lung diseases; 5-year survival of 75%; and 10-year survival of 60% [2].

CF is a suppurative lung disease which has some specific issues to consider prior to lung transplantation. CF patients are often colonized or infected with multidrug-resistant organisms in their sinuses and respiratory tracts; thus post-transplant infections in the setting of immunosuppression are a major concern [24]. Typical organisms include multidrug-resistant pseudomonas, mycobacterium species, fungal organisms, and Burkholderia species. Most of these organisms can be treated post-transplant and do not appear to affect survival in CF patients when compared to other lung diseases [19]. However, Burkholderia cepacia is known to affect post-transplant survival. Patients with B. cenocepacia (genomovar III) have a very high post-transplant mortality rate and usually die from sepsis despite aggressive treatment [18]. Thus, most transplant programs will not offer lung transplantation to these patients.

Non-CF bronchiectasis has been linked to many different etiologies including inherited immunodeficiency disorders, human immunodeficiency virus (HIV), infections (aspergillus, non-TB mycobacterium), primary ciliary dyskinesia, inflammatory bowel disease, interstitial lung disease, and Young syndrome [25]. Similar to CF, patients with non-CF bronchiectasis have chronic airway inflammation, obstruction with mucus secretion, and bacterial infections in advanced disease. Non-CF bronchiectasis accounted for 2.7% of all lung transplantations from 1995 to 2015 [2]. Specific guidelines for referral of patients with non-CF bronchiectasis have not been established; thus similar clinical criteria used for CF patients are employed when considering for lung transplantation [40].

Idiopathic Interstitial Pneumonia (IIP)

The idiopathic interstitial pneumonias include a heterogeneous group of interstitial lung diseases (ILD) in which the underlying cause of lung inflammation and fibrosis is not known. Idiopathic pulmonary fibrosis (IPF) is the most common subtype of the IIPs. The revised classification scheme by the American Thoracic Society and European Respiratory Society is listed in Table 22.2. The main treatment modalities for most of the IIPs include immunosuppression and antifibrotic medications to slow down the progression of the disease. Lung transplantation remains an important option in patients with disease progression despite medical therapy and functional decline.

IIPs accounted for 24.8% of all lung transplants from 1996 to 2015 [2]. Over the past 13 years, the number of lung transplants performed for underlying IIP has increased (see Fig. 22.2). This is due to the implementation of the lung allocation score (LAS) in the United States in 2005 [26]. Prior to

Table 22.2 Classification of Idiopathic Interstitial Pneumonia (IIP)

Revised American Thoracic Society/European Respiratory Society classification of idiopathic interstitial pneumonias: Multidisciplinary diagnosis
Major idiopathic interstitial pneumonias
Idiopathic pulmonary fibrosis
Idiopathic nonspecific interstitial pneumonia
Respiratory bronchiolitis-interstitial lung disease
Desquamative interstitial pneumonia
Cryptogenic organizing pneumonia
Acute interstitial pneumonia
Rare idiopathic interstitial pneumonia
Idiopathic lymphoid interstitial pneumonia
Idiopathic pleuroparenchymal fibroelastosis
Unclassifiable idiopathic interstitial pneumonias[a]

[a]Causes of unclassifiable idiopathic interstitial pneumonia include (1) inadequate clinical, radiologic, or pathologic data and (2) major discordance between clinical, radiologic, and pathologic findings that may occur in the following situations: (a) previous therapy resulting in substantial alteration of radiologic or histologic findings (e.g., biopsy of desquamative interstitial pneumonia after steroid therapy, which shows only residual nonspecific interstitial pneumonia); (b) new entity or unusual variant of recognized entity, not adequately characterized by the current American Thoracic Society/European Respiratory Society classification (e.g., variant organizing pneumonia with supervening fibrosis); and (c) multiple high-resolution computed tomography and/or pathologic patterns that may be encountered in patients with idiopathic interstitial pneumonia

the LAS, lungs were allocated based on time on the waitlist. The LAS consists of a risk assessment of expected waitlist urgency and post-transplant survival.

Idiopathic pulmonary fibrosis (IPF) is one of the most common subtypes of the IIPs. It is characterized by persistent destruction of the lung parenchyma thought to be related to multiple injuries to the lung over a period of time, ultimately leading to fibrosis [27]. The median survival from diagnosis of IPF is 2.5–3.8 years [26]. The progression of IPF can be unpredictable, with many patients remaining stable for long periods of time, while others experience multiple exacerbations leading to respiratory failure and death [27]. Since there is no way of predicting which course the disease will follow, patients should be referred for lung transplantation at the time of diagnosis. Although clinical tools to predict mortality in IPF have limitations, there are a number of factors associated with poor prognosis. These include age, sex, smoking history, DLCO, forced vital capacity, degree of fibrosis seen on high-resolution CT scan, and the number of fibroblastic foci seen on histopathology [28–31].

Patients with IIP should undergo serial evaluations focusing on lung function, functional decline, impairment in gas exchange, and number of exacerbations. Current guidelines recommend referring all patients with radiographic or histopathologic evidence of usual interstitial pneumonia (UIP) regardless of lung function, forced vital capacity (FVC) <80% predicted or diffusion capacity <40% predicted, any oxygen requirement, any functional limitations or dyspnea secondary to lung disease, or failure to improve despite maximal medical therapy. Timing for listing includes a decline in FVC of more than 10% within a 6-month follow-up, decline in DLCO of greater than 15% within a 6-month follow-up, oxygen saturations of less than 88% on a 6-min walk, pulmonary hypertension on right heart catheterization or echocardiography, hospitalizations secondary to acute exacerbations, respiratory decline, or pneumothorax [3].

Pulmonary Hypertension

Pulmonary hypertension (PH) is characterized by an increase in the resistance of the pulmonary vasculature. PH is defined as a mean pulmonary artery pressure greater than 25 mmHg at rest, with a pulmonary capillary wedge pressure of less than 15 mmHg, and pulmonary vascular resistance greater than 3 Woods units as measured by cardiac catheterization [32]. The current World Health Organization classification scheme divides PH into five major categories with further subdivisions (Table 22.3). Abnormal pathways involving endothelial and smooth muscle cells and dysregulation of the pulmonary vasculature are thought to be the underlying mechanisms leading to increased pulmonary vascular resistance (PVR) [32]. In response to this increased PVR, the

Fig. 22.2 Major Indications for Adult Lung Transplants Over the Years Key: Chronic obstructive pulmonary disease (COPD), alpha-1 antitrypsin deficiency (A1ATD), cystic fibrosis (CF), idiopathic interstitial pneumonia (IIP), interstitial lung disease (ILD)

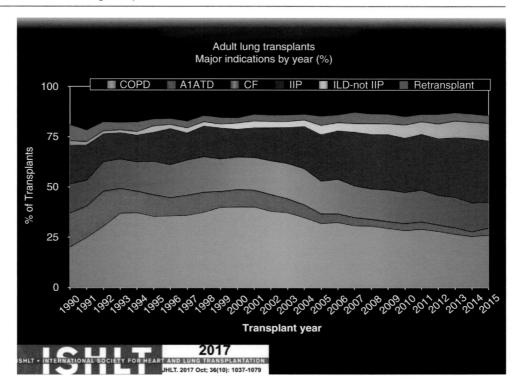

Table 22.3 Classification of Pulmonary Hypertension

Group	Category of PH	Associated disease
1	Pulmonary arterial hypertension	Idiopathic PH (IPAH) Inherited Drug/toxin associated Associated with HIV, connective tissue disease, schistosomiasis Pulmonary venous occlusive disease (PVOD)
2	PH secondary to left heart disease	Systolic dysfunction, diastolic dysfunction, valvular disease
3	PH secondary to lung disease or hypoxemia	COPD, interstitial lung disease
4	Chronic thromboembolic PH (CTEPH)	
5	PH with unclear multifactorial mechanisms	Sarcoid, LAM, hematologic disorders, fibrosing mediastinitis, glycogen storage disease, thyroid disorders, Gaucher disease

right ventricle becomes hypertrophic and dilated. Patients ultimately develop right ventricular failure with decreased cardiac output. The median survival rate for PH is 2.8 years when untreated [32]. Functional class is a strong predictor of survival with patients in NYHA functional class IV having a mean survival of less than 6 months [32].

Pharmacotherapy for PH includes targeting three different pathways that regulate pulmonary artery vasoconstriction. Endothelin-1 is a potent vasoconstrictor produced by endothelial cells, and it also promotes endothelial and smooth muscle cell proliferation [33]. Endothelin receptor antagonists have been developed to counteract this pathway. Phosphodiesterase type 5 inhibitors and guanylate cyclase stimulator also exert vasodilatory and antiproliferative effects on the pulmonary vasculature. Prostacyclin analogs and receptor agonists cause potent vasodilation with cytoprotective effects [33]. Current guidelines recommend referring patients with NYHA class III or IV symptoms during escalation of therapy, rapidly progressive disease, use of parenteral therapy regardless of symptoms or NYHA functional class, known or suspected pulmonary veno-occlusive disease, or pulmonary capillary hemangiomatosis [3]. Timing for listing patients for transplantation include NYHA functional class III or IV despite a trial of at least 3 months of combination of therapy including prostanoids, cardiac index of <2 L/min, mean right atrial pressure > 15 mmHg, 6 min walk test of <350 m, development of significant hemoptysis, pericardial effusion, or signs of progressive right heart failure [3].

Heart-Lung Transplantation

A combined dual-organ transplantation remains an option for a select few patients who have multi-organ failure and would not survive a single-organ transplantation. In patients with severe cardiopulmonary disease, a heart-lung transplant may be the only available therapeutic option. Indications for heart-lung transplantation include congenital heart disease with Eisenmenger syndrome, end-stage pulmonary disease with right ventricular failure, or refractory left ventricular failure [34]. According to the latest ISHLT registry data, the number of reported heart-lung transplants performed worldwide has declined to less than 75 in 2014 [35].

In patients with complex congenital heart disease with Eisenmenger syndrome, the presence of elevated pulmonary arterial systolic pressure > 50 mmHg and either pulmonary vascular resistance greater than 3 Woods units or transpulmonary pressure gradient of greater than 15 mmHg indicate a greater risk for right heart failure and death and, thus, are considered a relative contraindication to isolated heart transplantation [34]. If the pulmonary vascular resistance fails to improve with medical therapy, these patients may be considered for heart-lung transplantation.

PH used to be the most common indication for heart-lung transplantation until the early 1990s. Since then, several studies have shown that patients with PH have similar outcomes with bilateral lung transplantation compared to a combined heart-lung transplantation, even in the setting of severe right heart failure requiring inotropic or VA ECMO support [36, 37]. Thus, unless there is concomitant left ventricular failure, a double-lung transplant should be the procedure of choice in these patients. Cutoff values for right and left heart systolic function vary significantly from center to center. Based on published reports, these values can range from 10% to 25% for right ventricular ejection fraction and 32–50% for left ventricular ejection fraction [34].

Patients with end-stage lung disease and cardiac disease may be candidates for combined lung transplantation and cardiac surgery. This includes concomitant coronary artery bypass, valve repair or replacement, and repair of congenital defects [38]. Since single-organ transplant waitlist times are significantly shorter than combined organ and donor organs are a limited resource, all options are carefully considered for the individual case.

Contraindications to Lung Transplantation

In general, strong predictors of poor outcome after lung transplantation are considered contraindications to transplant. The following are considered absolute contraindications to lung transplantation, although there is considerable transplant center-specific variation in practice [3]:

- Recent history of cancer. A 2-year disease-free interval with a low predicted risk of recurrence may be reasonable in selected cases, although in general, a 5-year disease-free interval is considered prudent. This can be a challenging area since predicting risk of recurrence in the context of immunosuppression is difficult.

- Significant dysfunction of another major organ system that is not treatable (unless a multi-organ transplant can be considered)
- Coronary artery disease that is not amenable to revascularization
- BMI > 35
- Uncorrectable bleeding diathesis
- Acute medical instability
- Nonadherence to medical therapy and follow-up
- Psychiatric or psychologic conditions associated with inability to comply with complex medical therapy
- Substance abuse or dependence
- Absence of adequate social support
- Severely limited functional status with poor rehabilitation potential

Over the last several years, the lung transplant field has seen considerable change, such that several contraindications previously considered absolute contraindications have now moved to the relative contraindication list. Patients infected with hepatitis B, hepatitis C, and HIV are an example of this. Relative contraindications are outlined below:

- Age greater than 65 years. Although no particular age is considered an absolute cutoff or contraindication, advancing age is usually associated with development of other comorbidities, and an individual patient must be considered carefully as age advances.
- BMI 30–35
- Severe malnutrition
- Severe symptomatic osteoporosis
- Prior thoracic surgery
- Hepatitis B and/or C infection. These candidates should be carefully considered in centers with experienced hepatology teams.
- Patients with HIV infection with controlled disease and undetectable HIV RNA and no current AIDS defining illnesses may be considered at centers with expertise in HIV care.
- Patients with *Burkholderia cenocepacia*, *Burkholderia gladioli*, and MDR *Mycobacterium abscessus* may be considered if infection sufficiently treated preoperatively and at centers with appropriate infectious disease experience and expertise.
- Coronary artery disease. Carefully selected patients may be candidates for percutaneous coronary intervention pretransplant or, on occasion, for combined lung transplant and coronary artery bypass graft (CABG).

From a psychosocial standpoint, the evaluation comprises careful identification and assessment of risk factors for poor outcome and further considering whether these are modifiable or non-modifiable. In practice, this can present some vexing clinical scenarios, and collaboration between transplant pulmonologists, surgeons, and experienced transplant psychologists and psychiatrists is key to appropriate patient selection.

Conclusions

Patients with end-stage pulmonary disease who are being evaluated for lung transplantation require very careful and detailed evaluation aimed at selecting appropriate candidates in order to maximize the chances of a good outcome from transplantation. While medical contraindications can be a reason for decline, psychosocial barriers to transplantation can be particularly challenging for both the patient and the transplant team. On occasion, these may raise ethical dilemmas given the limited resource of donor organs.

References

1. Whitson BA, Hayes D Jr. Indications and outcomes in adult lung transplantation. J Thorac Dis. 2014;6(8):1018.
2. Yusen RD, Edwards LB, Dipchand AI, Goldfarb SB, Kucheryavaya AY, Levvey BJ, Lund LH, Meiser B, Rossano JW, Stehlik J. The registry of the International Society for Heart and Lung Transplantation: thirty-third adult lung and heart–lung transplant report 2016; focus theme: primary diagnostic indications for transplant. J Heart Lung Transplant. 2016;35(10):1149–276.
3. Weill D, Benden C, Corris PA, Dark JH, Duane Davis R, Keshavjee S, Lederer DJ, Mulligan MJ, Alexander Patterson G, Singer LG, Snell GI, Verleden GM, Zamora MR, Glanville AR. A consensus document for the selection of lung transplant candidates: 2014 – An update from the Pulmonary Transplantation Council of the International Society for Heart and Lung Transplantation. J Heart Lung Transplant. 2015;34(1):1–15.
4. Shah RJ, Kotloff RM. Lung transplantation for obstructive lung disease. Semin Respir Crit Care Med. 2013;34(03):288–96.
5. Martinez FJ, Kotloff R. Prognostication in chronic obstructive pulmonary disease: implications for lung transplantation. Semin Respir Crit Care Med. 2001;22(5):489–98.
6. Vestbo J, Edwards LD, Scanlon PD, et al. ECLIPSE Investigators. Changes in forced expiratory volume in 1 second over time in COPD. N Engl J Med. 2011;365(13):1184–92.
7. Soler-Cataluna JJ, Martinez-Garcia MA, Roman Sanchez P, Salcedo E, Navarro M, Ochando R. Severe acute exacerbations and mortality in patients with chronic obstructive pulmonary disease. Thorax. 2005;60:925–31.
8. Soler-Cataluna JJ, Martinez-Garcia MA, Sanchez LS, Tordera MP, Sanchez PR. Severe exacerbations and BODE index: two independent risk factors for death in male COPD patients. Respir Med. 2009;103:692–9.
9. Connors AF Jr, Dawson NV, Thomas C, et al. Outcomes following acute exacerbation of severe chronic obstructive lung disease. The SUPPORT investigators (Study to Understand Prognoses and Preferences for Outcomes and Risks of Treatments). Am J Respir Crit Care Med. 1996;154:959–67.
10. Fishman A, et al. A randomized trial comparing lung-volume-reduction surgery with medical therapy for severe emphysema. N Engl J Med. 2003;348(21):2059–73.
11. Senbaklavaci O, Wisser W, Ozpeker C, et al. Successful lung volume reduction surgery brings patients into better condition for later lung transplantation. Eur J Cardiothorac Surg. 2002;22(3):363–7.
12. Burns KE, Keenan RJ, Grgurich WF, Manzetti JD, Zenati MA. Outcomes of lung volume reduction surgery followed by lung transplantation: a matched cohort study. Ann Thorac Surg. 2002;73(5):1587–159.
13. Stan L, David S, Mark G. Aralast: a new α1- protease inhibitor for treatment of α-antitrypsin deficiency. Ann Pharmocother. 2005;39(11):1861–9.
14. Hadzic N. Therapeutic options in alpha-1 antitrypsin deficiency: liver transplantation. In: Borel F, Mueller C, editors. Alpha-1 antitrypsin deficiency. Methods in molecular biology, vol. 1639. New York: Humana Press; 2017.
15. Grannas G, Neipp M, Hoeper MM, et al. Indications for and outcomes after combined lung and liver transplantation: a single center experience on 13 consecutive cases. Transplantation. 2008;85:524–31.
16. Yi SG, Burroughs SG, Loebe M, et al. Combined lung and liver transplantation: analysis of a single center experience. Liver Transpl. 2014;20:46–53.
17. Oprescu N, McCormack FX, Byrnes S, et al. Clinical predictors of mortality and cause of death in lymphangioleiomyomatosis: a population-based registry. Lung. 2013;191:35. https://doi-org.laneproxy.stanford.edu/10.1007/s00408-012-9419-3
18. Braun A, Merlo C. Cystic fibrosis lung transplantation. Curr Opin Pulm Med. 2011;17(6):467–72.
19. Morrell M, Pilewski J. Lung transplantation for cystic fibrosis. Clin Chest Med. 2016;37:127–38.
20. Kerem E, Reisman J, Corey M, Canny GJ, Levison H. Prediction of mortality in patients with cystic fibrosis. N Engl J Med. 1992;326(18):1187–91.
21. Augarten A, Akons H, Aviram M, et al. Prediction of mortality and timing of referral for lung transplantation in cystic fibrosis patients. Pediatr Transplant. 2001;5(5):339–42.
22. Milla CE, Warwick WJ. Risk of death in cystic fibrosis patients with severely compromised lung function. Chest. 1998;113(5):1230–4.
23. Liou TG, Adler FR, Cahill BC, et al. Survival effect of lung transplantation among patients with cystic fibrosis. JAMA. 2001;286(21):2683–9.
24. Snell G, Reed A, Hadjiliadis D. The evolution of lung transplantation for cystic fibrosis: A 2017 update. J Cyst Fibros. 2017;16:553–64.
25. Hayes D, Meyer KC. Lung transplantation for advanced bronchiectasis. Semin Respir Crit Care Med. 2010;31(2):123–38.
26. Brown AW, Kaya H, Nathan SD. Lung transplantation in IIP: a review. Respirology. 2016;21(7):1173–84.
27. Caminanti A, Harari S. IPF: new insight in diagnosis and prognosis. Respir Med. 2010;104:S2–S10.
28. King TE Jr, Schwarz MI, Brown K, Tooze JA, Colby TV, Waldron JA Jr, et al. Idiopathic pulmonary fibrosis: relationship between histopathologic features and mortality. Am J Respir Crit Care Med. 2001;164:1025e32. 11.
29. Mogulkoc N, Brutsche MH, Bishop PW, Greaves SM, Horrocks AW, Egan JJ. Pulmonary function in idiopathic pulmonary fibrosis and referral for lung transplantation. Am J Respir Crit Care Med. 2001;164:103e8.
30. Flaherty KR, Mumford JA, Murray S, Kazerooni EA, Gross BH, Colby TV, et al. Prognostic implications of physiologic and radiographic changes in idiopathic interstitial pneumonia. Am J Respir Crit Care Med. 2003;168:543e8. 13.
31. Collard HR, King TE Jr, Bartelson BB, Vourlekis JS, Schwarz MI, Brown KK. Changes in clinical and physiologic variables predict survival in idiopathic pulmonary fibrosis. Am J Respir Crit Care Med. 2003;168:538e42. 14. Latsi PI, du Bois RM, Nicholson AG, Colby TV, Bisirtzoglou D, Nikolakopoulou A, et al. Fibrotic idio-

pathic interstitial pneumonia: the prognostic value of longitudinal functional trends. Am J Respir Crit Care Med 2003;168:531e7.

32. Long J, Russo M, Wickii V. Surgical treatment of pulmonary hypertension: lung transplantation. Pulm Circ. 2011;1(3):327–33.

33. Sahay S, Humbert M, Sitbon O. Medical treatment of pulmonary arterial hypertension. Semin Respir Crit Care Med. 2017;38:686–700.

34. Gadre S, Turowski T, Budev M. Overview of lung transplantation, heart-lung transplantation, liver-lung transplantation, and combined hematopoietic stem cell transplantation and lung transplantation. Clin Chest Med. 2017;38(4):623–40.

35. Mehra MR, Canter CE, Hannan MM, et al. The 2016 International Society for Heart Lung Transplantation listing criteria for heart transplantation: a 10-year update. J Heart Lung Transplant. 2016;35:1–23.

36. Fadel E, Mercier O, Mussot S, et al. Long-term outcome of double-lung and heart-lung transplantation for pulmonary hypertension: a comparative retrospective study of 219 patients. Eur J Cardiothorac Surg. 2010;38:277–84.

37. Hill C, Maxwell B, Boulate D, et al. Heart-lung vs. double-lung transplantation for idiopathic pulmonary arterial hypertension. Clin Transpl. 2015;29:1067–75.

38. Hoong CK, Sweet SC, Guthrie TJ, et al. Repair of congenital heart lesions combined with lung transplantation for the treatment of severe pulmonary hypertension: a 13-year experience. J Thorac Cardiovasc Surg. 2005;129:661–9.

39. Celli BR, Cote CG, Marin JM, et al. The body-mass index, airflow obstruction, dyspnea, and exercise capacity index in chronic obstructive pulmonary disease. N Engl J Med. 2004;350(10):1005–12.

40. Gottlieb J, et al. Lung transplantation for non-cystic fibrosis bronchiectasis. Respir Med. 2016;115:60–5.

Mental Health in Chronic and End-Stage Lung Disease

23

Yelizaveta Sher

Introduction

Pulmonary conditions most frequently leading to lung transplantation include chronic obstructive pulmonary disease (COPD), interstitial lung disease (ILD), pulmonary hypertension (PH), and cystic fibrosis (CF). These disorders have their unique challenges and psychological adaptations. CF is a genetic disease frequently diagnosed at birth; thus individuals grow up incorporating the knowledge about their expected decreased life span and eventual need of lung transplantation into their psyches. Growing up with a chronic condition like CF, which demands an extensive daily treatment routine, is not infrequently met with growing psychological pains and rebellion during adolescence and young adulthood. The notion of lung transplantation is frequently a part of life's expected course.

On the other hand, with COPD and IPF, the diagnosis and discussion of lung transplantation comes much later and more suddenly in life. Guilt, shame, and regret might accompany the psychological processing for some patients with COPD, especially when their disease may be, at least in part, be due to past or current psychosocial behaviors (i.e., smoking).

Patients with progressive pulmonary conditions are at increased risk for depression and anxiety, which not only increase suffering, decrease quality of life (QOL), and make adherence to medical treatments and tolerance of physical distress more challenging, but also might have a negative impact on overall morbidity and mortality before and after lung transplantation [1–4].

Chronic Obstructive Pulmonary Disease

COPD is the most common etiology leading to lung transplantation. It is a common respiratory disorder characterized by progressive airflow limitation, associated with increased inflammation in airways and lung tissue in response to noxious particles. COPD affects 5% of the population, is responsible for more than 20,000 deaths each year [5], and represents approximately 30% of patients undergoing lung transplantation (see Chap. 22 for details).

Epidemiology and Risk Factors of Psychiatric Conditions

Smoking and COPD

Tobacco use disorder has a complicated relationship with COPD and various psychiatric conditions. It is the most common psychiatric disorder in patients with COPD, with incidence of 47.3% in one diverse sample in the United States (USA) [6]. Smoking is indeed a significant risk factor for development of COPD. In a retrospective study of 8045 Swedish individuals followed for 25 years, odds ratio (OR) for developing clinically significant COPD in smokers as compared to non-smokers was 6.3 (95% confidence interval (CI) 4.2–9.5) [7]. In fact, 25% of smoking patients developed COPD over the 25 years [7].

Smoking also might moderate the relationship between other psychiatric disorders and COPD. Individuals who smoke are approximately twice as likely to develop major depression [8], which is common in patients with COPD. Anxiety predisposes some individuals to use smoking as a coping mechanism [9]. In addition, evidence suggests that patients with schizophrenia are more prone to develop COPD [10], likely due to high incidence of smoking in this population.

Y. Sher (✉)
Department of Psychiatry and Behavioral Sciences, Stanford University School of Medicine, Stanford, CA, USA
e-mail: ysher@stanford.edu

© Springer International Publishing AG, part of Springer Nature 2019
Y. Sher, J. R. Maldonado (eds.), Psychosocial Care of End-Stage Organ Disease and Transplant Patients,
https://doi.org/10.1007/978-3-319-94914-7_23

Depression in COPD

Depression is diagnosed in 10–57% of patients with stable COPD in primary care and respiratory clinics, depending on the tools used for screening and diagnosis [11]. In a recent systematic review and meta-analysis of 8 controlled studies with 5552 individuals with COPD and 5211 controls, 27.1% of COPD subjects had incident depression as compared to 10% of individuals in the control group (OR 3.74) [12]. In this meta-analysis, depression was diagnosed with a structured interview or a validated depression questionnaire.

Risk factors for depression in COPD include severity of COPD, current smoking, female gender, living alone, severity of dyspnea, and severity of physical functioning [11, 13]. Patients who require long-term oxygen, are hospitalized for COPD exacerbations or were recently discharged from hospital, or undergo palliative care also have increased rates of depression [11].

Several factors have been proposed to explain the increased prevalence of depression in COPD patients, including increased rates of smoking, inflammation, and hypoxia, while the strongest influences on development of depression in COPD are thought to be the severity of COPD and perceived quality of life (QOL) [11].

Depression increases healthcare utilization, worsens adherence to treatments, increases rates of COPD exacerbations and frequency and length of hospital stays, and decreases QOL [11, 14, 15]. Depression also decreases survival in patients with COPD [16, 17]. Of interest, the treatment of depression might decrease mortality in older patients with COPD [18].

Anxiety in COPD

Anxiety is also very common in patients with COPD. In a systematic review of 10 studies and 691 subjects, the prevalence of clinical anxiety ranged from 10% to 55% among hospitalized patients with COPD and from 13% to 46% among outpatients with COPD [9]. The reported prevalence of specific anxiety disorders varied significantly: generalized anxiety disorder was 6–33%, panic disorder (with and without agoraphobia) 0–41%, specific phobia 10–27%, and social phobia 5–11%. In this population, women were significantly more likely to have a clinical anxiety disorder, particularly specific phobia and panic disorder [9].

Several pathophysiological mechanisms have been proposed to explain the link between anxiety and COPD. First, smoking itself is associated with increased rates of anxiety [19] and COPD, as discussed above [7]. Second, symptoms of anxiety/panic overlap with physical symptoms of breathlessness or shortness of breath, such as heart palpitations and sensations of dyspnea [14]. For some patients, these physical sensations exacerbate their sense of anxiety and worry. The sympathetic nervous system is activated during episodes of anxiety [14]. In response, patients hyperventilate, which makes them feel more dyspneic and thus more anxious. This self-perpetuating cycle conceptualized as "dyspnea–anxiety–dyspnea cycle" highlights how patients' emotional response to breathlessness exacerbates their perception of breathlessness [14].

A parallel model explaining this link is the *carbon dioxide hyperventilation model*, proposing that patients with comorbid COPD and panic disorder might be sensitive to even mild variations in carbon dioxide [11]. An increase in carbon dioxide activates the ventrolateral medulla and locus coeruleus, the particular brain areas sensitive to carbon dioxide/hydrogen ions. In turn, this activation leads to increases in ventilatory rates and panic behavior in predisposed individuals.

Finally, the *cognitive behavior model* of panic disorder suggests that, in predisposed subjects, normal bodily sensations are misinterpreted, thus precipitating a panic attack [11]. Frequently preceding traumatic events have sensitized patients to misinterpretation of such sensations. COPD exacerbations can be traumatic and behaviorally sensitize predisposed individuals to panic responses. This manifests itself in patients struggling to discern between normal and dangerous bodily and respiratory responses, leading to increased anxiety.

Severe Mental Illness in COPD

As mentioned above, patients with schizophrenia have increased risk of developing COPD with OR of 1.88 [10], likely due to high incidence of smoking in this population. In a recent Taiwanese sample from medical database claims, patients with schizophrenia were found to have a higher annual incidence of COPD than that of the general population (2.21% vs. 1.43%, risk ratio 1.83; 95% CI, 1.62–2.07) [20]. Both extremes of age, as well as male gender, were risk factors. In addition to smoking, a sedentary lifestyle and the presence of metabolic dysfunction were postulated risk factors for this increased comorbidity.

Similarly, bipolar disorder might be a risk factor for COPD. Again, a Taiwanese medical claims study found that patients with bipolar disorder were approximately twice as likely to have comorbid COPD, as compared to the general population. In this population, risk factors included increased age, male gender, hypertension, and the use of second-generation antidepressant [21].

Cognitive Disorders in COPD

Cognitive functioning in patients with COPD has been investigated with a variety of study designs and neuropsychological tools [22, 23]. In general, patients with COPD have been found to have decreased cognitive functioning, especially in areas of attention and memory [24]. In a prospective study of 1425 participants with normal cognition at baseline and followed on average for 5 years, a diagnosis of COPD significantly increased the risk for non-amnestic mild cognitive impairment (MCI) by 83% (hazard ratio (HR) 1.83; 95% CI, 1.04–3.23) [25]. There was a dose-response relationship:

patients who had COPD for longer than 5 years at baseline had the greatest risk for MCI development (HR 1.58; 95% CI, 1.04–2.40) and non-amnestic-MCI (2.58; 95% CI 1.32–5.06). Studies have demonstrated that the prevalence of cognitive impairment is associated with a number of factors, including severity of COPD, presence of hypoxemia, and duration of illness [22–24].

In addition, cognitive dysfunction can influence information processing and treatment adherence [26, 27], both important considerations when evaluating patients for lung transplantation. It is important to appreciate the patients' cognitive functioning and potential limitations in order to adapt transplant teaching to their needs and to timely and appropriately engage support systems pre-transplant.

Treatment of Psychiatric Comorbidities in COPD

Tobacco Use Disorders

One of the most important psychopharmacological interventions in patients with COPD is treatment of tobacco use disorders. In addition to nicotine replacement therapy (NRT), varenicline and bupropion can be effective for smoking cessation. Reassuringly, an English retrospective cohort study identified patients with COPD who received a prescription of NRT ($N = 10,426$), bupropion ($N = 350$), or varenicline ($N = 3574$) for smoking cessation [28]. At 6-month follow-up, neither bupropion nor varenicline was associated with any increased risk of cardiovascular (i.e., ischemic heart disease, stroke, heart failure, peripheral vascular disease, and cardiac arrhythmias) or psychiatric (i.e., developing or worsening depression or self-harm) side effects as compared with NRT. In addition, varenicline was associated with a significantly reduced risk of both heart failure (HR = 0.56, 95% CI 0.34–0.92) and depression (HR = 0.73, 95% CI 0.61–0.86).

Depression and Anxiety

As is true with many other medical conditions, there is a lack of randomized controlled trials (RCTs) on the effectiveness of psychopharmacological agents for the treatment of depression and anxiety in patients with COPD. Small studies have been conducted on the use of tricyclic antidepressants (i.e., nortriptyline, doxepin, desipramine) [29–31] and newer antidepressants (i.e., paroxetine, citalopram, bupropion) [14, 32, 33] in patients with comorbid COPD and depression/anxiety with conflicting results. While a small study on doxepin in patients with COPD did not lead to changes in depression or anxiety [30], nortriptyline was found to be safe and effective [29]. A small study of paroxetine did not demonstrate its benefits in intention-to-treat analysis for quality of life measures in patients with COPD, but paroxetine was not associated with adverse respiratory events [32]. Yet another small randomized study of 27 COPD patients did not show differ-

ence between citalopram or placebo arms for measures of depression, anxiety, or physical functioning; however, citalopram was safe in this patient population [33]. More recently, an RCT of 120 patients with COPD and moderate to severe depression in China demonstrated improvements in depression scores on Hamilton Depression Scale (HAM-D), walking capacity, and QOL measures in patients randomized to sertraline as compared to placebo, but it did not demonstrate any improvement in lung function [34]. There is also some suggestion that sertraline might be helpful in managing the sensation of dyspnea in patients with COPD, in subjects with or without psychiatric comorbidities [35]. Moreover, a retrospective cohort study of Medicare beneficiaries has suggested that adhering to antidepressant treatment in patients with newly diagnosed COPD and new-onset depression increased adherence to COPD treatments [36].

When selecting agents for treatment of depression and anxiety in COPD, it is important to be careful with psychotropic agents that might promote carbon dioxide retention or decrease respiratory drive (e.g., benzodiazepines, certain tricyclic antidepressants (TCAs), sedating antipsychotics) [37]. Selective serotonin inhibitors (SSRIs) are usually first-line treatments (e.g., sertraline, citalopram, escitalopram) due to their favorable side effect profile, tolerability, minimal drug-drug interactions, and effectiveness for both depression and anxiety in general psychiatric patients [34, 38]. Mirtazapine can be helpful for depression, anxiety, sleep, and appetite, but should be monitored for sedation and caution should be used in patients who retain carbon dioxide [39]. If needed, benzodiazepines with shorter half-life (i.e., lorazepam) can be employed on a short-term basis with attention paid to the potential risk of respiratory depression, risk of dependence, and cognitive side effects [37]. Buspirone can be also considered given its lack of respiratory depression [37, 39]. In addition, gabapentin and hydroxyzine can be helpful in patients with respiratory conditions for treatment of anxiety [39] while monitoring for sedation especially in patients who retain carbon dioxide, and with attention to renal clearance.

Dyspnea often presents or is misdiagnosed as anxiety in respiratory patients. Those who struggle with treatment-resistant dyspnea can have some relief with opioid medications, if the treatment of underlying pathology is not helpful [37, 38, 40]. Although there is concern for respiratory depression with opioids, the judicious use of low-dose opioids in respiratory patients has not translated into deleterious effects on blood gases, oxygen saturation, or clinical adverse events [40, 41]. In fact, in a study examining co-management of lung transplant candidates with the palliative care team treating patients for dyspnea (most patients had ILD in this cohort), 92% ($N = 59$) of referred patients were prescribed opioids for dyspnea [41]. Out of these patients, 55/59 used the opioids more than once, and 38/59 were maintained on standing opioids. No opioid toxicity or respiratory depression was reported. In addition, of the 30 patients who underwent lung transplantation, only 23% still used opioids 1 month after discharge from the hospital.

Non-pharmacological interventions have been studied in this patient population. Pulmonary rehabilitation and multicomponent exercise can be helpful not only in physical conditioning, which is very important for transplant preparation, but also for anxiety and depression treatment [42, 43]. Pulmonary and physical therapists frequently are able to teach patients techniques on proper breathing to prevent hyperventilation, which allows patients to gain greater control over their anxiety.

Mindfulness-based cognitive therapy, as an adjunct to pulmonary rehabilitation, has been shown to decrease anxiety on the Hospital Anxiety and Depression Scale (HADS), but had no effect on physical symptoms on the COPD Assessment Test [44].

Several studies incorporating cognitive behavioral therapy (CBT) have been conducted in patients with COPD and comorbid depression and/or anxiety. A meta-analysis including four studies showed a small decrease in symptoms for both anxiety and depression [45].

Interstitial Lung Disease

ILD is a diverse group of conditions resulting in chronic inflammation and fibrosis of lung parenchyma. There are many forms of ILD, including idiopathic pulmonary fibrosis (IPF), hypersensitivity pneumonitis, sarcoidosis, and ILD complicating connective tissue diseases (CTD-ILD) [46]. ILD is a chronic condition with distressing dyspnea, progressive worsening of exercise tolerance, and decreased life expectancy [46]. Symptoms are disabling and invariably lead to decreased QOL. Dyspnea in particular is a very distressing symptom, associated with increased rates of depression and decreased functional status [46]. Approximately a quarter of patients undergoing lung transplantation have this group of conditions (see Chap. 22).

Epidemiology and Risk Factors of Psychiatric Conditions

Depression and Anxiety

One of the first studies of depression in subjects with ILD identified that 21% of patients had depression using the Center for Epidemiological Study Depression (CES-D) measure, with most patients continuing to experience depression symptoms at follow-up, indicating the chronic nature of depression in individuals afflicted by ILD [47]. The independent predictors of depressive symptoms at baseline included dyspnea severity, pain severity, sleep quality, and forced vital capacity. A recent study by Matsuda et al. evaluated the effects of depression on health-related quality of life (HRQOL) with the St. George's Respiratory Questionnaire (SGRQ) [48]. Out of 121 patients, 22.3% patients had depressive symptoms according to HADS. In a stepwise multiple regression model, Baseline Dyspnea Index, 6-minute walk distance (6MWD) test, and HADS-D were found to be independent determinants of the total SGRQ score.

In a Korean sample of 112 patients with IPF evaluated with HADS, symptoms of depression and anxiety were present in 25.9% and 21.4% of patients, respectively [49]. While the rate of hospitalization and survival was not different between patients with or without depression and/or anxiety (possibly due to short period of follow-up and/or lack of effective treatments for ILD in general at the time of study), patients with depression or anxiety reported poorer QOL.

Cognitive Disorders

Patients with ILD might also have worse cognitive performance, similar to that of other older patients with pulmonary conditions, such as COPD. In a study by Bors et al., patients with severe IPF had a significantly longer mean trail making test B time and lower number of correctly identified colors in the Stroop 3 test, as compared to patients with mild IPF or healthy controls. Accordingly, these results suggest inferior performance on tasks requiring speed divided attention and slower processing speed [50].

Treatment of Psychiatric Comorbidities

Pulmonary rehabilitation programs involving aerobic exercises to improve breathing, education about a patient's condition, muscle strength improvement, and psychological support are important components of treatment in this patient population [47].

There have been no studies done on the pharmacological treatment of depression or anxiety in patients with ILD. However, antidepressants can be used, taking into consideration their side effect profile and drug-drug interactions, similar to the guidelines for patients with COPD listed above. In general, depressed subjects report more severe dyspnea, poorer sleep quality, and worse pain, suggesting that treating these symptoms might improve depressive symptoms [46, 51]. Treatment with antidepressants can be combined with psychotherapy [51].

Cystic Fibrosis

Cystic fibrosis (CF) is the most common autosomal recessive life-shortening condition among Caucasians, affecting approximately 30,000 individuals in the United States and over 70,000 people worldwide [52]. It is caused by a mutation in CF transmembrane conductance regulator (CFTR) gene, with resulting deficiency of sodium, chloride, and bicarbonate transport, leading to impairment of mucociliary clearance, pulmonary infections, chronic inflammation, and progressive lung function deterioration [53]. While the average life expectancy was just a few months of life in 1950s, with significant scientific and clinical advances, the median life expectancy now exceeds 40 years [53]. CF represents approximately 15% of patients undergoing lung transplantation (see Chap. 22).

In addition to pulmonary manifestations, CF presents with gastrointestinal symptoms (i.e., meconium ileus shortly after birth and distal intestinal obstruction syndrome (DIOS) in adulthood), pancreatic insufficiency (90% of patients), CF-related diabetes (20%), biliary cirrhosis (10%), and infertility (most men and 50% of women) [52]. This multisystem involvement can have a profound effect on QOL, self-image, and psychiatric comorbidities [52].

Epidemiology and Risk Factors of Psychiatric Conditions

Depression and Anxiety

Increased depression and anxiety have been long suspected in patients with CF; however, it is the work of Quittner and colleagues via The International Depression Epidemiological Study (TIDES) that has finally demonstrated its true incidence and effects. TIDES was conducted in 154 CF centers spanning nine countries across Europe and the United States [54]. In this study, 6088 patients with CF (12 years old and older) and 4102 caregivers of children with CF (birth to 18 years old) were screened for depression and anxiety during regular clinic visits using self-report measures (i.e., HADS or CES-D). Depressive scores were elevated in 10% of adolescents, 19% of adults, 37% of mothers, and 31% of fathers of patients with CF. Similarly, anxiety scores were elevated in 22% of adolescents, 32% of adults, 48% of mothers, and 36% of fathers. The incidences of these psychiatric disorders were 2–3 times of those seen in community samples. In addition, patients with anxiety were also more likely to report depression. Of note, adolescents whose parents reported their own depression or anxiety were also more likely to report depression or anxiety, accordingly.

Psychological distress in CF has been shown to correlate with worse adherence, decreased pulmonary function, increased hospitalization risk, reduced health-related QOL, and increased healthcare costs [54]. In response to these findings, the International Committee on Mental Health in CF (ICMH) in the United States and Europe has created guidelines advising the screening for depression and anxiety of all adolescent and adult patients with CF, as well as the

caregivers of adolescent patients using the Patient Health Questionnaire-9 (PHQ-9) and Generalized Anxiety Disorder-7 (GAD-7) screening tools [55]. They recommend further evaluation and provision of or referral to appropriate mental health services for patients with elevated scores and/or clinical concerns.

Treatment

ICMH recommends CBT as one of the first-line treatment approaches for the management of depression and anxiety in patients with CF [55]. Limited but promising evidence has demonstrated efficacy of behavioral interventions for improving adherence and nutritional status in child and adolescent patients with CF [56]. A web CBT-based writing therapy has been found to be helpful in reducing symptoms of depression and anxiety in caregivers of child CF patients in a small pilot study [57].

No pharmacological studies on treatment of depression or anxiety have been done in the CF patient population so far. Of interest, amitriptyline, a TCA and functional acid sphingomyelinase inhibitor, was studied in few small case-control trials on its effect on degradation of ceramide in lung cells of patients with CF (patients with depression were excluded). The use of amitriptyline was well tolerated at a daily dose of 50 mg and had a favorable effect on increased lung functioning and weight gain [58].

Despite the lack of evidence-based treatments of psychiatric syndromes in the CF population, the ICMH recommends the use of SSRIs (i.e., sertraline, fluoxetine, citalopram, or escitalopram) as first-line pharmacological agents in patients requiring pharmacotherapy for depression or anxiety [55]. Lorazepam is recommended for distressing anxiety, such as anxiety associated with procedures (e.g., intravenous line placement), on as needed basis. In addition to these recommendations, mirtazapine can be considered given its minimal gastrointestinal side effect profile and favorable effect on weight gain, often needed in this patient population, especially when approaching lung transplantation [59]. In addition, there is decreased concern for serotonergic toxicity when mirtazapine is coadministered with linezolid [60], a monoamine oxidase inhibitor (MAOI) antibiotic, used for treatment of some CF exacerbations.

Light therapy has been shown to be helpful for patients with depression in general. Of note, not infrequently, patients with CF have prolonged hospitalizations, with an associated reduction in light exposure, which can further exacerbate depressive symptoms. Light therapy has recently been studied in 30 patients with CF hospitalized for pulmonary exacerbation with the use of a light box emitting 10,000 lx for 30 min each day for 7 consecutive days [61]. The authors noted that depressive symptom severity (using Quick

Inventory of Depressive Symptomatology, Clinician Rating) and QOL factors (Cystic Fibrosis Questionnaire-Revised) were decreased with the use of light therapy. In addition, these patients had a significantly shorter length of hospital stay (11.0 ± 3.6 days) compared to a historical cohort from the year prior (13.3 ± 4.4 days, $p = 0.038$).

An important source of anxiety for patients with CF is having to make a decision regarding lung transplantation. Although many patients realize that lung transplantation will likely be a part of their lives, when the time comes, it is a very difficult reality. Some patients may be very conflicted about their choice. In a study of 149 patients with advanced CF lung disease in Canada and Australia, patients were provided usual education and counseling about lung transplantation and then randomized to a lung transplantation decision aid that they worked through on their own to further understand the benefits versus risks of a referral to lung transplantation, or to usual care [62]. Three weeks after randomization, those randomized to the decision tool had more realistic expectations about their level of risk for surgery and the probabilities of survival with and without surgery, as well as decreased total decisional conflict, compared to subjects randomized to usual care. Thus, empowering patients with greater knowledge, encouraging further reflection on their reality and choices, and taking a systematic approach to this decision-making might decrease anxiety regarding consideration of lung transplantation.

Pulmonary Hypertension

Pulmonary hypertension (PH) is characterized by persistent elevation of pressure in the pulmonary arteries and pulmonary vascular resistance leading to right heart failure. These patients usually present with exertional shortness of breath, fatigue, and chest palpitations. The course is progressive and fatal, if untreated.

Epidemiology and Risk Factors of Psychiatric Conditions

Depression and Anxiety
Patients with PH have many life stressors, including physical disability, unemployment, uncertain nature of the disease process, and complex, invasive, and costly medical treatments. Important and pervasive themes of living with uncertainty and coping with illness were highlighted in a qualitative study by Flattery et al. [63]. Not surprisingly, PH is associated with significantly elevated depression and anxiety, with approximately a third of patients suffering from some mental disorder [64–66]. In fact, in a prospective study of 172 patients with PH, most subjects endorsed some degree of

psychological distress on measures of PHQ-9 and GAD-7: on PHQ-9, 34.8% endorsed mild symptoms (score 5–9), 13.3% - moderate symptoms (score 10–14), and 7% - serious/severe symptoms (score 15 and above); and on GAD-7, 34.8% - mild symptoms (score 5–9), 8.2% - moderate symptoms (score 10–14), and 2.5% - serious/severe symptoms (score 15 and above) [66]. As expected, the prevalence of mental disorders increases with functional impairment and is associated with worse QOL in patients with PH [65].

A recent study by Von Visger et al. of 108 PH patients found that any psychiatric disorder, major depression, and "other depressive disorder" were present in 29.6%, 15.7%, and 9.3% of patients, respectively [67]. In this sample, time since diagnosis of PH was positively associated with greater perceived social support and greater perceived stress.

Cognitive Disorders
A small study by White et al. performed neuropsychological testing in 46 patients with PH [68]. Cognitive impairment was found in 58% of patients, with 57% of patients demonstrating impaired motor abilities, 40% impaired memory, 17% slow mental processing speed, 15% executive dysfunction, and 13% impaired attention. Anxiety, but not depression, was correlated with worse cognitive functioning. Not surprisingly, patients described challenges with activities requiring attention, executive functioning, and memory, such as mixing medications (i.e., Flolan).

Treatment

No studies have been done to evaluate the effectiveness of pharmacological treatments for depression and anxiety in PH; however, interesting literature regarding the effect of SSRIs on PH has been emerging.

Given its role in vasoconstriction, some have postulated a role of serotonin in the pathophysiology of PH, in particular, the serotonin transporter (SERT) [69]. SERT inhibitors, such as SSRIs, have been postulated to have a beneficial effect on protection against PH and its progression [70]. Animal studies have lent support to this hypothesis [70]. In addition, a retrospective study of 84 patients with PH, 15% of whom were taking high affinity SSRIs, reported a 50% reduction in mortality in patients on SSRIs, although this was not a statistically significant finding [71]. To further explore this hypothesis, Sadoughi et al. analyzed the association between SSRI use and PH outcomes using the Registry to Evaluate Early and Long-term pulmonary arterial hypertension (PAH) Disease Management (REVEAL Registry) [70]. They found an elevated risk of death (HR 1.74) and clinical worsening of PH in new users of SSRIs. Conversely, a more recent nested case-control study from the United Kingdom found a 67% increased risk of idiopathic PH in patients using any antidepressant, irrespective of the antidepressant class, serotonin receptor affinity, or duration of use [72]. The study authors warned that this effect was thus not causal and may represent a common genetic dysregulation in serotonin signaling, thus predisposing patients to both conditions (i.e., PH and depression) and thus leading to the use of antidepressant agents. This remains an area where current studies are not yet able to guide our treatment and where ongoing active investigaion is urgently needed. In clinical practice, SSRIs remain the first line of pharmacological treatment for depressive and/or anxiety disorders.

Few studies have explored the use of behavioral interventions for emotional disorders and symptoms in PH. Given that these are safe, non-pharmacological interventions should be enlisted whenever possible. Progressive muscle relaxation has been shown to be effective on decreasing depression and anxiety and improving QOL in a 12-week study with PH patients [73]. A combination of carefully monitored aerobic and strength-training exercise and respiratory training has been shown to increase exercise capacity and QOL of patients with PH [74]. CBT and support groups may be also helpful with adjustment to a chronic illness and its uncertainties.

Mental Disorders in Patients Evaluated for Lung Transplant and Their Effect on Post-Lung Transplant Outcomes

Given the high levels of anxiety and depression in patients with pulmonary disorders, it is not surprising that the distress remains high as patients approach and undergo the lung transplant evaluation. In a Norwegian sample of 118 patients, 74% of whom had COPD, current and lifetime prevalence for mental disorders was 41.5% and 61.0%, respectively, using the DSM-IV version of the Mini-International Neuropsychiatric Interview (MINI) [75]. In particular, current anxiety disorders were diagnosed in 39.8% of patients, mood disorders in 11.8%, and subsyndromal disorders in 8.7%. In addition, depression was correlated with worse results on lung function tests ($P = 0.0012$) and 6MWD test ($P = 0.030$).

Overall Psychosocial Risk

A study by Hitschfeld et al. evaluated the correlation between pre-transplant psychosocial risk, as reflected in the Psychosocial Assessment of Candidates for Transplantation (PACT) score, and post-transplant survival in lung transplant recipients [3]. This study included 110 lung transplant recipients evaluated with PACT, 7 of whom (6.4%) initially received a score <2, indicating high psychosocial risk.

Although all these patients received psychosocial interventions (e.g., smoking cessation, psychiatric treatment, social support stabilization) and demonstrated subsequent improvement in PACT score, thus suggesting an improved psychosocial risk, their risk of death was still 2.7 times higher at any point post-transplant, as compared to patients with initially lower psychosocial risk (PACT 2 and above), over 12 years they were followed.

Depression and Anxiety

An important question in the research and clinical care of transplant patients relates to the effect of pre-transplant depression and anxiety on post-transplant outcomes. Depression and anxiety may make it challenging to process important information communicated to patients by their healthcare providers, alienate support systems, decrease motivation, and impede adherence to complex medical treatments.

Courtwright et al. conducted a meta-analysis of six prospective longitudinal cohort studies of lung transplant patients [1]. The meta-analysis included a total of 711 lung transplant recipients of whom 345 (48.5%) died during the follow-up period (mean follow-up time of 7.8 years). Most of the studies included in this analysis treated depression and anxiety as a continuous variable measured by such tools as the Beck Depression Inventory (BDI) or the State-Trait Anxiety Inventory (STAI). The authors concluded that in this patient population, pre-transplant anxiety and depression were not associated with post-transplant survival with a hazard ratio of 1.009 (95% CI, 0.998–1.019). However, there are important limitations to these findings. First, authors were unable to assess whether, as part of the listing process, patients with anxiety and/or depression were required to engage in appropriate mental health treatment, which could have then lessened or negated the effect of these disorders on post-transplant survival. In practice, patients identified as having anxiety or depression during the pre-transplant evaluation process are referred to an appropriate mental health practitioner and expected to receive necessary support and interventions. In addition, as the authors of the study indicated, no data was available on patients whose anxiety or depression were so severe as to prohibit lung transplant candidacy altogether. A separate retrospective study by Courtwright did find that pre-transplant anxiety was associated with an increased number of hospitalizations within the first year after lung transplantation [2].

A later study of 273 lung transplant recipients by Smith et al. found that pre-transplant clinical depressive symptoms, as measured by BDI-II scores, were present in 21% of patients [76]. They also found that greater pre-transplant depressive symptoms, as well as lower social support, were associated with longer post-transplant hospital stay. In patients with hospital stay greater than 1 month, pre-transplant depression tripled the risk of mortality (HR = 2.97). In addition, patients with pre-transplant depression who had persistent symptoms 3 months after lung transplant surgery also experienced greater mortality (HR = 1.85; 95% CI, 1.04, 3.28; $P = 0.036$) [4].

This study illustrates what likely plays out in the clinical practice of lung transplant patients. When patients do well postoperatively from a surgical and medical perspective, they experience an emotional "honeymoon phase." However, if medical complications occur with an associated prolonged hospital stay, patients with pre-transplant depression are more likely to experience demoralization, which further dampens their motivation and complicates recovery, with potential adverse effects on their survival. Poor social support further exacerbates this negative connection.

In addition, pre-transplant depression and anxiety have been shown to increase levels of post-lung transplant surgery pain [77]. Therefore, patients with pre-transplant anxiety and depression should have access to vigilant ongoing evaluation and mental health support during the post-transplant period.

Tobacco and Alcohol Use in Patients Evaluated for Lung Transplant

A study by Evon et al. evaluated 219 patients (116 CF, 103 non-CF) to assess tobacco and alcohol use during and immediately post-lung transplant evaluation, using patient self-report and corroboration by transplant coordinators [78]. The results indicated that 72% of non-CF patients and 16% of CF patients reported a remote history of cigarette smoking, while no CF and only one non-CF patient reported smoking at the time of the pre-transplant evaluation. In CF patients, past smoking was related to higher depression scores, while in non-CF patients, it was associated with being Caucasian and older. Of note, in this study, 100% of lung transplant recipients in a parallel separate sample reported abstinence from tobacco 2–7 years post-transplant.

A different picture is painted by a Czech Republic study of lung transplant candidates and recipients who were monitored with urinary cotinine levels (163 patients prior to inclusion on lung transplant list and 53 lung transplant recipients) [79]. Prior to listing, 4.9% of patients had at least one positive urinary cotinine test, while 6.1% of patients had borderline results. During post-transplant follow-ups, 15.1% had positive cotinine test, with an additional 3.8% of patients having borderline results. Patients with COPD were 35 times more likely to resume smoking post-transplant, with 38.5% (10/26) having positive or borderline urinary cotinine levels.

In a study by Vos et al., several factors were associated with a risk of smoking resumption post-lung transplant, including shorter cessation period prior to transplantation,

lower socioeconomic status, exposure to secondhand smoke, emphysema, and death of a spouse [80]. A shorter pre-transplant abstinence from tobacco corresponding to higher risk of tobacco relapse post-lung transplant was corroborated by a different study, where patients who relapsed on tobacco post-lung transplant had on average 1 year of abstinence pre-transplant as compared to 6 years of abstinence for patients who did not relapse ($p < 0.0001$) [81]. These findings highlight the importance of psychosocial interventions pre-transplant and of continued monitoring and ready availability of resources and ready availability of resources during the post-transplant period.

Alcohol use and its effects on outcomes have not been well studied in the lung transplant population. Evon et al. demonstrated that the majority of patients (80% and above) consumed alcohol in the past, and a third of all patients consumed alcohol at the time of evaluation [78]. For CF patients, past alcohol consumption was associated with more education and less social support, while alcohol consumption at the time of transplant evaluation was associated with being older and being less depressed. Non-CF patients who were consuming alcohol at the time of their evaluation tended to be more educated and had marginally less social support. In a parallel separate sample within this study, 60% of lung transplant recipients reported abstinence from alcohol 2–7 years after transplantation.

Lowery et al. recently conducted a study on alcohol use among lung transplant candidates, using self-report measures at the time of pre-transplant evaluation, as well as the Alcohol Use Disorders Identification Test (AUDIT) and alcohol biomarkers at the time of lung transplant surgery [82]. The study included 86 patients, 34% of whom reported current alcohol use at the time of evaluation, 13% having AUDIT scores >3 at the time of lung transplant surgery, and 10% having positive results for alcohol biomarkers at the time of transplantation. Only one patient had an AUDIT score > 8 [12], indicating serious alcohol misuse. The authors found that patients with recent alcohol use, as evidenced by biomarkers, had 1.5 times longer hospital stay, 3 times longer ventilation time, and 3 times longer ICU stay. Although there was no difference in primary graft dysfunction between those with and without recent alcohol use, several patients with recent use had post-LT surgery atrial arrhythmias, acute kidney injury, and acute cellular rejection.

Cognitive Disorders in Lung Transplant Candidates

In a study of 47 lung transplant recipients who received pre- and post-transplant neuropsychological examinations, on average participants performed in the 30th percentile on the Repeatable Battery for the Assessment of Neuropsychological

Status (RBANS), in the 30th percentile on the Trail Making Test part B, and in the 31st percentile on Trail Making Test part A on their pre-transplant evaluation. Twenty-one patients (45%) were determined to have neurocognitive impairment before transplant based on MoCA scores <26, which occurred exclusively in patients without CF [83]. Lower executive function (hazard ratio [HR] = 1.09, P = 0.012) and memory performance (HR = 1.11, P = 0.030) were independently associated with greater mortality following lung transplantation [4].

Some of the mechanisms leading to increased cognitive disorders in patients with progressive lung conditions include hypoxemia, hypercapnia, age, severity of respiratory disease, frequency of respiratory exacerbations, smoking, and inflammation [23]. It is important to appreciate these cognitive deficits in lung transplant candidates to ensure that patients have the appropriate education, organization, and psychosocial support needed. It is also important to understand that these patients are at increased risk for post-lung transplant delirium [84], thus allowing for the use of appropriate prophylactic measures and the education of patients and their families.

Other

An interesting study evaluated whether a history of childhood physical or sexual abuse was associated with post-lung transplant survival [85]. Thirty-three lung transplant recipients (35.5% male; median age, 55 years) were included in this study. A history of childhood physical or sexual abuse (grouped together) was present in 24.2% and was associated with decreased survival following lung transplantation (P = 0.003). Although there was no difference in sex, marital status, or smoking history between patients who reported history of abuse versus those who did not, abuse survivors had a higher Personality Assessment Screener total score, a measure of maladaptive personality traits (P = 0.02). This finding requires further study but alerts clinicians to potentially high history of abuse in lung transplant candidates and recipients and its important link to formation of maladaptive personality traits and increased mortality. History of prior trauma, such as abuse, also predisposes patients to greater risk of developing PTSD if another traumatic event occurs [86]. Thus, patients with prior abuse history should be more vigilantly monitored for PTSD-T after the transplant.

Conclusions and Recommendations

Anxiety and depression are common in patients with chronic and end-stage pulmonary disorders and individuals undergoing lung transplant evaluation. They affect the patient's

QOL, morbidity pre-lung transplant, and potentially outcomes after lung transplantation. Tobacco use disorders are prevalent, especially in a specific subset of lung transplant candidates (i.e., patients with COPD), and some characteristics (i.e., COPD, shorter abstinence from tobacco) are risk factors for post-transplant recurrence. Finally, cognitive dysfunction can accompany progressive respiratory deterioration.

Thus, few recommendations can be made based on above literature and clinical experience:

1. Patients with progressive respiratory conditions and those being evaluated for lung transplantation should be evaluated for depression and anxiety. Non-pharmacological treatments, such as pulmonary rehabilitation and psychotherapy, should be utilized whenever possible. Psychopharmacological treatments should be considered with careful risk-benefit analysis, paying attention to the available evidence base, potential of medications to suppress respiration in those who retain carbon dioxide, side effects, drug-drug interactions, and additional positive effects of the medications.
2. Patients should be asked about and monitored for the use of tobacco. Those with tobacco use disorders should be referred to appropriate behavioral and pharmacological interventions. Monitoring should be continued postoperatively, and again patients should be offered needed education and support.
3. Patients should be evaluated for cognitive disorders. Reversible additional contributing factors should be evaluated and eliminated (e.g., medications, hypoxia, deconditioning, thyroid dysfunction, vitamin B12 deficiency, etc.). Education should be tailored according to patient's cognitive status. Family and support system should be engaged and educated. Patients and their families should be in particular educated on the risk of postoperative delirium, increased in patients with pre-transplant cognitive dysfunction.

References

1. Courtwright AM, Salomon S, Lehmann LS, Wolfe DJ, Goldberg HJ. The Effect of Pretransplant Depression and Anxiety on Survival Following Lung Transplant: A Meta-analysis. Psychosomatics. [Meta-Analysis Review]. 2016;57(3):238–45.
2. Courtwright AM, Salomon S, Lehmann LS, Brettler T, Divo M, Camp P, et al. The association between mood, anxiety and adjustment disorders and hospitalization following lung transplantation. Gen Hosp Psychiatry. [Research Support, N.I.H., Extramural]. 2016;41:1–5.
3. Hitschfeld MJ, Schneekloth TD, Kennedy CC, Rummans TA, Niazi SK, Vasquez AR, et al. The psychosocial assessment of candidates for transplantation: a cohort study of its association with survival among lung transplant recipients. Psychosomatics. 2016;57(5):489–97.

4. Smith PJ, Blumenthal JA, Carney RM, Freedland KE, O'Hayer CV, Trulock EP, et al. Neurobehavioral functioning and survival following lung transplantation. Chest. [Multicenter Study Randomized Controlled Trial Research Support, N.I.H., Extramural Research Support, U.S. Gov't, P.H.S.]. 2014;145(3):604–11.

5. Committee TGS. Global strategy for the diagnosis, management and prevention of COPD, global initiative for chronic obstructive lung disease (GOLD) 2016.

6. Schauer GL, Wheaton AG, Malarcher AM, Croft JB. Smoking prevalence and cessation characteristics among U.S. adults with and without COPD: findings from the 2011 behavioral risk factor surveillance system. COPD. 2014;11(6):697–704.

7. Lokke A, Lange P, Scharling H, Fabricius P, Vestbo J. Developing COPD: a 25 year follow up study of the general population. Thorax. [Research Support, Non-U.S. Gov't]. 2006;61(11):935–9.

8. Flensborg-Madsen T, von Scholten MB, Flachs EM, Mortensen EL, Prescott E, Tolstrup JS. Tobacco smoking as a risk factor for depression. A 26-year population-based follow-up study. J Psychiatr Res. [Research Support, Non-U.S. Gov't]. 2011;45(2):143–9.

9. Willgoss TG, Yohannes AM. Anxiety disorders in patients with COPD: a systematic review. Respir Care. [Review]. 2013;58(5):858–66.

10. Carney CP, Jones L, Woolson RF. Medical comorbidity in women and men with schizophrenia: a population-based controlled study. J Gen Intern Med. [Comparative Study Controlled Clinical Trial Research Support, N.I.H., Extramural Validation Studies]. 2006;21(11):1133–7.

11. Pumar MI, Gray CR, Walsh JR, Yang IA, Rolls TA, Ward DL. Anxiety and depression-Important psychological comorbidities of COPD. J Thorac Dis. [Review]. 2014;6(11):1615–31.

12. Matte DL, Pizzichini MM, Hoepers AT, Diaz AP, Karloh M, Dias M, et al. Prevalence of depression in COPD: a systematic review and meta-analysis of controlled studies. Respir Med. [Review]. 2016;117:154–61.

13. Hanania NA, Mullerova H, Locantore NW, Vestbo J, Watkins ML, Wouters EF, et al. Determinants of depression in the ECLIPSE chronic obstructive pulmonary disease cohort. Am J Respir Crit Care Med. [Multicenter Study Research Support, Non-U.S. Gov't]. 2011;183(5):604–11.

14. Tselebis A, Pachi A, Ilias I, Kosmas E, Bratis D, Moussas G, et al. Strategies to improve anxiety and depression in patients with COPD: a mental health perspective. Neuropsychiatr Dis Treat. [Review]. 2016;12:297–328.

15. Atlantis E, Fahey P, Cochrane B, Smith S. Bidirectional associations between clinically relevant depression or anxiety and COPD: a systematic review and meta-analysis. Chest. [Meta-Analysis Review]. 2013;144(3):766–77.

16. Stage KB, Middelboe T, Pisinger C. Depression and chronic obstructive pulmonary disease (COPD). Impact on survival. Acta Psychiatr Scand. 2005;111(4):320–3.

17. Ng TP, Niti M, Tan WC, Cao Z, Ong KC, Eng P. Depressive symptoms and chronic obstructive pulmonary disease: effect on mortality, hospital readmission, symptom burden, functional status, and quality of life. Arch Intern Med. [Multicenter Study Research Support, Non-U.S. Gov't]. 2007;167(1):60–7.

18. Qian J, Simoni-Wastila L, Langenberg P, Rattinger GB, Zuckerman IH, Lehmann S, et al. Effects of depression diagnosis and antidepressant treatment on mortality in Medicare beneficiaries with chronic obstructive pulmonary disease. J Am Geriatr Soc. [Comparative Study Research Support, N.I.H., Extramural]. 2013;61(5):754–61.

19. Moylan S, Jacka FN, Pasco JA, Berk M. Cigarette smoking, nicotine dependence and anxiety disorders: a systematic review of population-based, epidemiological studies. BMC Med. [Research Support, Non-U.S. Gov't Review]. 2012;10:123.

20. Hsu JH, Chien IC, Lin CH, Chou YJ, Chou P. Increased risk of chronic obstructive pulmonary disease in patients with schizophrenia: a population-based study. Psychosomatics. 2013;54(4):345–51.

21. Hsu JH, Chien IC, Lin CH. Increased risk of chronic obstructive pulmonary disease in patients with bipolar disorder: a population-based study. J Affect Disord. 2017;220:43–8.

22. Kakkera K, Padala KP, Kodali M, Padala PR. Association of chronic obstructive pulmonary disease with mild cognitive impairment and dementia. Curr Opin Pulm Med. 2018;24(2):173–8.

23. Ouellette DR, Lavoie KL. Recognition, diagnosis, and treatment of cognitive and psychiatric disorders in patients with COPD. Int J Chron Obstruct Pulmon Dis. [Review]. 2017;12:639–50.

24. Schou L, Ostergaard B, Rasmussen LS, Rydahl-Hansen S, Phanareth K. Cognitive dysfunction in patients with chronic obstructive pulmonary disease – a systematic review. Respir Med. [Research Support, Non-U.S. Gov't Review]. 2012;106(8):1071–81.

25. Singh B, Mielke MM, Parsaik AK, Cha RH, Roberts RO, Scanlon PD, et al. A prospective study of chronic obstructive pulmonary disease and the risk for mild cognitive impairment. JAMA Neurol. [Randomized Controlled Trial Research Support, N.I.H., Extramural Research Support, Non-U.S. Gov't]. 2014;71(5):581–8.

26. Hayes TL, Larimer N, Adami A, Kaye JA. Medication adherence in healthy elders: small cognitive changes make a big difference. J Aging Health. [Research Support, N.I.H., Extramural Research Support, Non-U.S. Gov't Research Support, U.S. Gov't, Non-P.H.S.]. 2009;21(4):567–80.

27. Vinyoles E, De la Figuera M, Gonzalez-Segura D. Cognitive function and blood pressure control in hypertensive patients over 60 years of age: COGNIPRES study. Curr Med Res Opin. [Multicenter Study Research Support, Non-U.S. Gov't]. 2008;24(12):3331–9.

28. Kotz D, Viechtbauer W, Simpson CR, van Schayck OCP, West R, Sheikh A. Cardiovascular and neuropsychiatric risks of varenicline and bupropion in smokers with chronic obstructive pulmonary disease. Thorax. [Research Support, Non-U.S. Gov't]. 2017;72(10):905–11.

29. Borson S, McDonald GJ, Gayle T, Deffebach M, Lakshminarayan S, VanTuinen C. Improvement in mood, physical symptoms, and function with nortriptyline for depression in patients with chronic obstructive pulmonary disease. Psychosomatics. [Clinical Trial Randomized Controlled Trial Research Support, U.S. Gov't, Non-P.H.S.]. 1992 Spring;33(2):190–201.

30. Light RW, Merrill EJ, Despars J, Gordon GH, Mutalipassi LR. Doxepin treatment of depressed patients with chronic obstructive pulmonary disease. Arch Intern Med. [Clinical Trial Controlled Clinical Trial]. 1986;146(7):1377–80.

31. Gordon GH, Michiels TM, Mahutte CK, Light RW. Effect of desipramine on control of ventilation and depression scores in patients with severe chronic obstructive pulmonary disease. Psychiatry Res. [Clinical Trial]. 1985;15(1):25–32.

32. Lacasse Y, Beaudoin L, Rousseau L, Maltais F. Randomized trial of paroxetine in end-stage COPD. Monaldi archives for chest disease = Archivio Monaldi per le malattie del torace. [Clinical Trial Randomized Controlled Trial Research Support, Non-U.S. Gov't]. 2004;61(3):140–7.

33. Silvertooth EJ, Doraiswamy PM, Clary GL, Babyak MA, Wilkerson N, Hellegars C, et al. Citalopram and quality of life in lung transplant recipients. Psychosomatics. [Clinical Trial Letter Randomized Controlled Trial]. 2004;45(3):271–2.

34. He Y, Zheng Y, Xu C, Yang H, Wang Z, Zhou L, et al. Sertraline hydrochloride treatment for patients with stable chronic obstructive pulmonary disease complicated with depression: a randomized controlled trial. Clin Respir J. [Randomized Controlled Trial]. 2016;10(3):318–25.

35. Smoller JW, Pollack MH, Systrom D, Kradin RL. Sertraline effects on dyspnea in patients with obstructive airways disease. Psychosomatics. [Case Reports]. 1998;39(1):24–9.

36. Wei YJ, Simoni-Wastila L, Albrecht JS, Huang TY, Moyo P, Khokhar B, et al. The association of antidepressant treatment with COPD maintenance medication use and adherence in a comorbid Medicare population: a longitudinal cohort study. Int J Geriatr Psychiatry. 2018;33(2):e212–e20.

37. Thompson WL, Smolin YL. Respiratory disorders. In: Ferrando S, Levenson J, Owen JA, editors. Clinical manual of psychopharmacology in the medically ill. 1st ed. Washington, DC: American Psychiatric Publishing; 2010. p. 213–36.

38. Yohannes AM, Kaplan A, Hanania NA. Anxiety and depression in chronic obstructive pulmonary disease: recognition and management. Cleve Clin J Med. 2018;85(2 Suppl 1):S11–S8.

39. Sher Y. Psychiatric aspects of lung disease in critical care. Crit Care Clin. [Review]. 2017;33(3):601–17.

40. Jennings AL, Davies AN, Higgins JP, Gibbs JS, Broadley KE. A systematic review of the use of opioids in the management of dyspnoea. Thorax. [Meta-Analysis Research Support, Non-U.S. Gov't Review]. 2002;57(11):939–44.

41. Colman R, Singer LG, Barua R, Downar J. Outcomes of lung transplant candidates referred for co-management by palliative care: a retrospective case series. Palliat Med. 2015;29(5):429–35.

42. Tselebis A, Bratis D, Pachi A, Moussas G, Ilias I, Harikiopoulou M, et al. A pulmonary rehabilitation program reduces levels of anxiety and depression in COPD patients. Multidiscip Respir Med. 2013;8(1):41.

43. Coventry PA, Bower P, Keyworth C, Kenning C, Knopp J, Garrett C, et al. The effect of complex interventions on depression and anxiety in chronic obstructive pulmonary disease: systematic review and meta-analysis. PLoS One. [Meta-Analysis Research Support, Non-U.S. Gov't Review]. 2013;8(4):e60532.

44. Farver-Vestergaard I, O'Toole MS, O'Connor M, Lokke A, Bendstrup E, Basdeo SA, et al. Mindfulness-based cognitive therapy in COPD: a cluster randomised controlled trial. Eur Respir J. 2018;51(2)

45. Smith SM, Sonego S, Ketcheson L, Larson JL. A review of the effectiveness of psychological interventions used for anxiety and depression in chronic obstructive pulmonary disease. BMJ Open Respir Res. 2014;1(1):e000042.

46. Ryerson CJ, Berkeley J, Carrieri-Kohlman VL, Pantilat SZ, Landefeld CS, Collard HR. Depression and functional status are strongly associated with dyspnea in interstitial lung disease. Chest. [Research Support, Non-U.S. Gov't]. 2011;139(3):609–16.

47. Ryerson CJ, Arean PA, Berkeley J, Carrieri-Kohlman VL, Pantilat SZ, Landefeld CS, et al. Depression is a common and chronic comorbidity in patients with interstitial lung disease. Respirology. 2012;17(3):525–32.

48. Matsuda T, Taniguchi H, Ando M, Kondoh Y, Kimura T, Kataoka K, et al. Depression is significantly associated with the health status in patients with idiopathic pulmonary fibrosis. Intern Med. 2017;56(13):1637–44.

49. Lee YJ, Choi SM, Cho YJ, Yoon HI, Lee JH, Lee CT, et al. Clinical impact of depression and anxiety in patients with idiopathic pulmonary fibrosis. PLoS One. 2017;12(9):e0184300.

50. Bors M, Tomic R, Perlman DM, Kim HJ, Whelan TP. Cognitive function in idiopathic pulmonary fibrosis. Chron Respir Dis. [Research Support, Non-U.S. Gov't]. 2015;12(4):365–72.

51. Verma S, Cardenas-Garcia J, Mohapatra PR, Talwar A. Depression in pulmonary arterial hypertension and interstitial lung diseases. N Am J Med Sci. [Review]. 2014;6(6):240–9.

52. Quittner AL, Saez-Flores E, Barton JD. The psychological burden of cystic fibrosis. Curr Opin Pulm Med. [Review]. 2016;22(2):187–91.

53. Elborn JS. Cystic fibrosis. Lancet. 2016;388(10059):2519–1531.

54. Quittner AL, Goldbeck L, Abbott J, Duff A, Lambrecht P, Sole A, et al. Prevalence of depression and anxiety in patients with cystic fibrosis and parent caregivers: results of The International Depression Epidemiological Study across nine countries. Thorax. [Multicenter Study Research Support, Non-U.S. Gov't]. 2014;69(12):1090–7.

55. Quittner AL, Abbott J, Georgiopoulos AM, Goldbeck L, Smith B, Hempstead SE, et al. International Committee on Mental Health in Cystic Fibrosis: Cystic Fibrosis Foundation and European Cystic Fibrosis Society consensus statements for screening and treating depression and anxiety. Thorax. [Consensus Development Conference Research Support, Non-U.S. Gov't]. 2016;71(1):26–34.

56. Goldbeck L, Fidika A, Herle M, Quittner AL. Psychological interventions for individuals with cystic fibrosis and their families. Cochrane Database Syst Rev. [Meta-Analysis Research Support, N.I.H., Extramural Research Support, Non-U.S. Gov't Review]. 2014(6):CD003148.

57. Fidika A, Herle M, Lehmann C, Weiss C, Knaevelsrud C, Goldbeck L. A web-based psychological support program for caregivers of children with cystic fibrosis: a pilot study. Health Qual Life Outcomes. [Comparative Study Research Support, Non-U.S. Gov't]. 2015;13:11.

58. Adams C, Icheva V, Deppisch C, Lauer J, Herrmann G, Graepler-Mainka U, et al. Long-term pulmonal therapy of cystic fibrosis-patients with amitriptyline. Cell Physiol Biochem. [Observational Study]. 2016;39(2):565–72.

59. Chinuck RS, Fortnum H, Baldwin DR. Appetite stimulants in cystic fibrosis: a systematic review. J Hum Nutr Diet. [Research Support, Non-U.S. Gov't Review]. 2007;20(6):526–37.

60. Gillman PK. A review of serotonin toxicity data: implications for the mechanisms of antidepressant drug action. Biol Psychiatry. [Review]. 2006;59(11):1046–51.

61. Kopp BT, Hayes D, Jr., Ghera P, Patel A, Kirkby S, Kowatch RA, et al. Pilot trial of light therapy for depression in hospitalized patients with cystic fibrosis. J Affect Disord. [Clinical Trial]. 2016;189:164–8.

62. Vandemheen KL, O'Connor A, Bell SC, Freitag A, Bye P, Jeanneret A, et al. Randomized trial of a decision aid for patients with cystic fibrosis considering lung transplantation. Am J Respir Crit Care Med. [Randomized Controlled Trial Research Support, Non-U.S. Gov't]. 2009;180(8):761–8.

63. Flattery MP, Pinson JM, Savage L, Salyer J. Living with pulmonary artery hypertension: patients' experiences. Heart Lung. 2005;34(2):99–107.

64. Vanhoof JMM, Delcroix M, Vandevelde E, Denhaerynck K, Wuyts W, Belge C, et al. Emotional symptoms and quality of life in patients with pulmonary arterial hypertension. J Heart Lung Transplant. 2014;33(8):800–8.

65. Lowe B, Grafe K, Ufer C, Kroenke K, Grunig E, Herzog W, et al. Anxiety and depression in patients with pulmonary hypertension. Psychiatr Med. [Comparative Study Research Support, Non-U.S. Gov't]. 2004;66(6):831–6.

66. Harzheim D, Klose H, Pinado FP, Ehlken N, Nagel C, Fischer C, et al. Anxiety and depression disorders in patients with pulmonary arterial hypertension and chronic thromboembolic pulmonary hypertension. Respir Res. [Comparative Study]. 2013;14:104.

67. Von Visger TT, Kuntz KK, Phillips GS, Yildiz VO, Sood N. Quality of life and psychological symptoms in patients with pulmonary hypertension. Heart Lung. 2018;47(2):115–21.

68. White J, Hopkins RO, Glissmeyer EW, Kitterman N, Elliott CG. Cognitive, emotional, and quality of life outcomes in patients with pulmonary arterial hypertension. Respir Res. [Comparative Study Research Support, Non-U.S. Gov't]. 2006;7:55.

69. MacLean MR, Dempsie Y. Serotonin and pulmonary hypertension – from bench to bedside? Curr Opin Pharmacol. [Research Support, Non-U.S. Gov't Review]. 2009;9(3):281–6.

70. Sadoughi A, Roberts KE, Preston IR, Lai GP, McCollister DH, Farber HW, et al. Use of selective serotonin reuptake inhibitors and outcomes in pulmonary arterial hypertension. Chest. [Comparative Study Research Support, N.I.H., Extramural Research Support, Non-U.S. Gov't]. 2013;144(2):531–41.

71. Kawut SM, Horn EM, Berekashvili KK, Lederer DJ, Widlitz AC, Rosenzweig EB, et al. Selective serotonin reuptake inhibitor use and outcomes in pulmonary arterial hypertension. Pulm Pharmacol Ther. [Comparative Study Research Support, N.I.H., Extramural Research Support, Non-U.S. Gov't]. 2006;19(5):370–4.

72. Fox BD, Azoulay L, Dell'Aniello S, Langleben D, Lapi F, Benisty J, et al. The use of antidepressants and the risk of idiopathic pulmonary arterial hypertension. Can J Cardiol. [Multicenter Study Research Support, Non-U.S. Gov't]. 2014;30(12):1633–9.

73. Li Y, Wang R, Tang J, Chen C, Tan L, Wu Z, et al. Progressive muscle relaxation improves anxiety and depression of pulmonary arterial hypertension patients. Evid Based Complement Alternat Med. 2015;2015:792895.

74. Mereles D, Ehlken N, Kreuscher S, Ghofrani S, Hoeper MM, Halank M, et al. Exercise and respiratory training improve exercise capacity and quality of life in patients with severe chronic pulmonary hypertension. Circulation. [Randomized Controlled Trial Research Support, Non-U.S. Gov't]. 2006; 114(14):1482–9.

75. Soyseth TS, Lund MB, Bjortuft O, Heldal A, Soyseth V, Dew MA, et al. Psychiatric disorders and psychological distress in patients undergoing evaluation for lung transplantation: a national cohort study. Gen Hosp Psychiatry. 2016;42:67–73.

76. Smith PJ, Snyder LD, Palmer SM, Hoffman BM, Stonerock GL, Ingle KK, Saulino CK, Blumenthal JA. Depression, social support, and clinical outcomes following lung transplantation: a single-center cohort study. Transpl Intern. 2018;31(5):495–502.

77. Farquhar JM, Smith PJ, Snyder L, Gray AL, Reynolds JM, Blumenthal JA. Patterns and predictors of pain following lung transplantation. Gen Hosp Psychiatry. 2018;50:125–30.

78. Evon DM, Burker EJ, Sedway JA, Cicale R, Davis K, Egan T. Tobacco and alcohol use in lung transplant candidates and recipients. Clin Transpl. [Research Support, Non-U.S. Gov't]. 2005;19(2):207–14.

79. Zmeskal M, Kralikova E, Kurcova I, Pafko P, Lischke R, Fila L, et al. Continued smoking in lung transplant patients: a cross sectional survey. Zdravstveno varstvo. 2016;55(1):29–35.

80. Vos R, De Vusser K, Schaevers V, Schoonis A, Lemaigre V, Dobbels F, et al. Smoking resumption after lung transplantation: a sobering truth. Eur Respir J. [Letter Research Support, Non-U.S. Gov't]. 2010;35(6):1411–3.

81. Ruttens D, Verleden SE, Goeminne PC, Poels K, Vandermeulen E, Godderis L, et al. Smoking resumption after lung transplantation: standardised screening and importance for long-term outcome. Eur Respir J. [Letter Research Support, Non-U.S. Gov't]. 2014;43(1):300–3.

82. Lowery EM, Yong M, Cohen A, Joyce C, Kovacs EJ. Recent alcohol use prolongs hospital length of stay following lung transplant. Clin Transpl. 2018;5:e13250.

83. Smith PJ, Rivelli S, Waters A, Reynolds J, Hoyle A, Flowers M, et al. Neurocognitive changes after lung transplantation. Ann Am Thorac Soc. 2014;11(10):1520–7.

84. Smith PJ, Rivelli SK, Waters AM, Hoyle A, Durheim MT, Reynolds JM, et al. Delirium affects length of hospital stay after lung transplantation. J Crit Care. 2015;30(1):126–9.

85. Kennedy CC, Zubair A, Clark MM, Jowsey-Gregoire S. Childhood abuse is associated with worse survival following lung transplantation. Prog Transplant. [Research Support, Non-U.S. Gov't]. 2016;26(2):178–82.

86. DiGangi JA, Gomez D, Mendoza L, Jason LA, Keys CB, Koenen KC. Pretrauma risk factors for posttraumatic stress disorder: a systematic review of the literature. Clin Psychol Rev. [Review]. 2013;33(6):728–44.

Extracorporeal Membrane Oxygenation: Medical and Psychological Considerations

24

Joshua J. Lee and Joshua J. Mooney

Introduction

Extracorporeal membrane oxygenation (ECMO) is a form of extracorporeal life support (ECLS) for patients with severe respiratory and/or cardiac failure. It consists of an extracorporeal system that allows for carbon dioxide removal, oxygen delivery, and/or cardiac support. While first successfully used in 1971 for the treatment of refractory hypoxemic respiratory failure, its acceptance as a salvage therapy for respiratory failure was slowed by early trials that demonstrated no benefit compared to conventional management [1–3]. However, technological advancements and later demonstration of improved mortality in acute respiratory failure with specialty center-directed ECMO use have led to increased use of ECMO worldwide as a supportive therapy for severe respiratory and/or cardiac failure [4]. As of 2016, the extracorporeal life support registry reported 10,601 cases of adults receiving ECLS with a record 2,046 cases reported in 2015 [5].

Indications for Use

With advancement in ECMO technology and increased experience, the role of ECMO has evolved, and it is currently used to support patients with advanced respiratory and/or cardiac failure to either recovery, cardiothoracic transplant, or a decision on transplant candidacy.

Respiratory Failure

ECMO can be employed in cases of severe hypoxemic or hypercapnic respiratory failure, including cases of acute respiratory distress syndrome (ARDS), post-transplant primary graft dysfunction (PGD), obstructive lung disease-related hypercapnic respiratory failure, decompensated pulmonary hypertension, acute pulmonary embolism, and progression or exacerbation of end-stage lung disease such as pulmonary fibrosis. Criteria for ECMO consideration vary by center, but $PaO_2/FIO_2 < 100$ despite receiving appropriate positive end-expiratory pressure (PEEP), uncompensated hypercapnic respiratory failure (pH < 7.15), and high end-inspiratory plateau pressure (>35–45 cm of water) are general indications for ECMO use [6]. Relative contraindications to ECMO use include advanced age greater than 65 years, limited vascular access, multi-organ dysfunction, advanced malignancy or neurologic impairment, contraindication to systemic anticoagulation, frailty with poor rehabilitation potential, or an irreversible terminal condition not amenable to transplant [6–8].

In select cases, ECMO is used as a bridge to lung recovery if the etiology of the respiratory failure is thought to be reversible (i.e., ARDS, PGD, acute pulmonary embolism). Early data for the use of ECMO as a bridge to lung recovery in refractory respiratory failure demonstrated no survival benefit and frequent complications [2]. However, data from the Conventional Ventilatory Support Versus Extracorporeal Membrane Oxygenation for Severe Adult Respiratory Failure (CESAR) trial in patients with severe ARDS suggested increased survival and lung recovery with referral to an ECMO specialty center for ECMO consideration [4]. Notably, the CESAR study was limited by the fact that not all patients in the ECMO therapy arm received ECMO support and that no standard mechanical ventilation strategy was used in the conventional control arm. Additional worldwide experience from ECMO use in influenza-related ARDS supports potential efficacy of ECMO in severe hypoxemic respiratory failure, particularly in younger and more severely hypoxemic patients [9–11]. The improved outcomes, compared to historic studies, are likely secondary to better ECMO technology, greater center expertise in ECMO and non-ECMO medical care, and careful patient selection.

J. J. Lee · J. J. Mooney (✉)
Division of Pulmonary and Critical Care, Department of Medicine, Stanford University School of Medicine, Stanford, CA, USA
e-mail: jjmooney@stanford.edu

© Springer International Publishing AG, part of Springer Nature 2019
Y. Sher, J. R. Maldonado (eds.), *Psychosocial Care of End-Stage Organ Disease and Transplant Patients*,
https://doi.org/10.1007/978-3-319-94914-7_24

Therefore, while ECMO should be carefully considered as a salvage therapy in severe ARDS, further work is needed to confirm the efficacy of ECMO in severe ARDS and other causes of acute respiratory failure and in what patient population it is most appropriate.

Others cases of severe respiratory failure are secondary to irreversible progression of an underlying advanced lung disease. With the scarcity of donor lungs and the growing number of patients on the lung transplant waitlist, ECMO can serve as a bridge to lung transplant in patients who have progressive respiratory failure while actively on the transplant waitlist or while determining their lung transplant candidacy [7, 8, 12]. A number of single-center studies support the use of ECMO as a bridging strategy to lung transplant with centers who routinely employ awake and/or ambulatory ECMO demonstrating comparable post-transplant outcomes to non-ECMO bridged recipients [13–15]. US lung transplant registry data have also provided insight into candidate and center factors associated with post-transplant outcomes following pre-transplant ECMO use. The busyness of a lung transplant center is associated with the risk of post-transplant mortality after an ECMO bridge to transplant with a higher risk of 1-year mortality at low-volume transplant centers compared to high-volume centers [16]. Advanced age was also associated with an increased risk for post-transplant mortality following ECMO support with candidates ≥60 years of age demonstrating an increased mortality risk, while no increased risk was noted in those <40 years [17]. A recommended approach to determining lung transplant candidacy from ECMO support is to first assess whether they meet generally acceptable lung transplant criteria and then second to assess whether they are also a reasonable transplant candidate from ECMO. The International Society of Heart and Lung Transplantation has produced a consensus document that highlights recipient criteria along with absolute and relative contraindications to lung transplant and provides additional recommendations on generally reasonable candidates for an ECMO bridge to transplant [7]. Younger age patients with good rehabilitation potential and without multi-organ dysfunction, septic shock, vascular occlusive disease, contraindication to systemic anticoagulation, prior prolonged ventilation or immobility, or obesity are preferred candidates for an ECMO bridge to transplant [7, 8]. The acceptable duration of ECMO support prior to lung transplant is unclear, and the allowed duration should be determined by assessment of baseline and current medical contraindications, nutritional status, and physical rehabilitation status.

ECMO in the post-lung transplant setting is most frequently used in patients with significant PGD. PGD is an ischemia-reperfusion-related lung injury that results in bilateral radiographic lung infiltrates and hypoxemia, with the severity of PGD determined by the degree of hypoxemia [18]. In PGD with severe hypoxemia ($PaO_2/$ $FIO_2 < 100$ mmHg) not responsive to standard mechanical ventilation and pulmonary vasodilation therapy, ECMO is generally recommended, particularly in the presence of concurrent hypercapnia and/or right ventricular dysfunction [19]. Single-center use of ECMO for post-lung transplant PGD reported that 96% of patients were successfully weaned off ECMO with 64% alive at 1 year and 88% of survivors free from chronic lung allograft dysfunction at 3 years [20].

Cardiac Failure

ECMO can be used to provide hemodynamic support in cardiac failure or cardiogenic shock that is refractory to inotropic support or unsuitable for other mechanical circulatory support devices. Similar to respiratory failure, ECMO can be used to facilitate bridge to recovery, to long-term mechanical circulatory support (MCS) device implant, to cardiothoracic transplant, or to a decision on heart transplant candidacy. The indications for ECMO in cardiac failure continue to evolve and range from supporting those with a failure to wean from cardiopulmonary bypass after cardiac surgery to use for supporting cardiopulmonary resuscitation (CPR) [21]. The use of ECMO-supported CPR has been associated with improved survival following in-hospital cardiac arrest as compared to use of conventional CPR alone [22]. Despite the availability of long-term MCS devices for cardiac failure, ECMO is often preferable in the acute setting to stabilize the patient and allow assessment of transplant or MCS candidacy, particularly if multi-organ or pulmonary involvement is present.

ECMO Configurations and Gas Exchange

Although a number of possible configurations exist, the extracorporeal system is characterized by a drainage cannula(s) where blood flows via a pump from the patient to a gas exchange device, a membrane gas exchange device where oxygen delivery and carbon dioxide removal occur, and a reinfusion cannula(s) that returns blood to the patient. The configurations largely differ based upon whether the reinfusion cannula returns blood to the arterial (venoarterial, VA) or venous (venovenous, VV) circulation and how many cannulas are used to achieve cardiorespiratory support.

Venovenous (VV) ECMO

Venovenous (VV) ECMO is most commonly used in the setting of hypoxemic or hypercarbic respiratory failure without cardiac dysfunction as VV ECMO only provides gas exchange support, and any circulatory support is augmented as needed by conventional therapies. In this configuration deoxygenated blood is withdrawn from the central venous system and returned to the central venous system after passing through an oxygenator for oxygen uptake and carbon dioxide removal. Traditional venovenous ECMO involves multisite cannulation, commonly a femoral vein drainage cannulation located within the inferior vena cava and an internal jugular reinfusion cannula that returns oxygenated blood to the right atrium. This cannulation configuration can result in a recirculation phenomenon where the reinfused oxygenated blood is drawn immediately into the drainage cannulation instead of the systemic circulation. A newer single-site dual-lumen cannula has been developed that allows for a single internal jugular cannula that spans from the superior vena cava to the inferior vena cava. This cannula has drainage ports in the superior and inferior vena cava and a reinfusion port in the right atrium directed at the tricuspid valve. The advantages of this catheter include the lower theoretical risk for recirculation phenomenon and easier facilitation of physical therapy and ambulation given the absence of femoral cannulation.

Venoarterial (VA) ECMO

Venoarterial (VA) ECMO provides both respiratory and circulatory support. In VA ECMO, blood is traditionally withdrawn by a femoral vein drainage cannula, passed through a membrane oxygenator, and returned through a femoral arterial reinfusion cannula. This approach is limited by the need for retrograde flow of blood from the reinfusion cannula up the descending aorta, which can increase afterload and worsen cardiac function or ultimately be inadequate to reach the aortic arch for coronary and cerebral circulation. In this setting, the addition of venous reinfusion cannulas to deliver oxygenated blood (venoarterial-venous, VAV) or the use of more centrally located cannulation can be used.

ECMO Gas Exchange

Gas exchange occurs within the membrane oxygenator, which consists of a semipermeable membrane separating the extracorporeal blood from a sweep gas. Oxygen transfer is determined by the amount of blood flow across the oxygenator and the fraction of oxygen delivered in the sweep gas (FDO_2). While the FDO_2 can be readily adjusted to deliver 100% oxygen, further maximization of systemic oxygenation focuses on improving cardiac output, ensuring an adequate hemoglobin level for oxygen delivery, and maximizing blood flow through the circuit. Factors that influence the circuit blood flow, including cannula size and location, pump revolutions per minute, pressure within the venous drainage

cannula, and resistance within the reinfusion cannula, are carefully assessed and optimized to enable optimal circuit blood flow. Given the efficiency for carbon dioxide diffusion across the membrane, the removal of carbon dioxide is principally determined by the sweep gas flow rate with higher flow rates allowing greater carbon dioxide removal.

Management of the Patient on ECMO

Ventilator Strategies

The ability to minimize or even discontinue mechanical ventilation support should be assessed once on stable ECMO support. The use of mechanical ventilation in respiratory failure can directly contribute to lung injury through overdistension of lung alveoli and atelectrauma from the repeated opening and closing of lung alveoli [23]. The use of lung protective ventilation, specifically a tidal volume of less than 6 ml/kg of predicted body weight and a plateau pressure of 30 cm of water or less, reduces mortality in patients with ARDS [24]. While the optimal ventilation strategy for ECMO patients remains controversial, the majority of ECMO programs target a tidal volume of ≤6 ml/kg of predicted body weight with a positive end-expiratory pressure of 6–10 cm of water while decreasing the fraction of inhaled oxygen as clinically allowed [25]. The use of even more conservative lung protective strategies, including tidal volumes of ≤4 ml/kg of predicted body weight, was reported by 31% of ECLS registry programs and has been reported in the literature [26–28]. Those with an ongoing need for mechanical ventilation support should be considered for early tracheostomy to help facilitate active rehabilitation and minimize sedation.

Anticoagulation

Patients on ECMO require systemic anticoagulation to prevent thrombosis formation within the circuit and are carefully monitored for bleeding and thrombosis. Guidelines by the Extracorporeal Life Support Organization (ELSO) recommend a bolus of unfractionated heparin at the time of cannulation followed by a continuous infusion of heparin during ECMO support [29]. There are several tests that measure the efficacy of anticoagulation, including the activated clotting time (ACT), activated partial thromboplastin time (aPTT), thromboelastography, and anti-factor Xa levels, with the monitoring method and therapeutic range varying by center and tailored to the individual risk of thrombosis and bleeding. In the setting of contraindications to unfractionated heparin, direct thrombin inhibitors have been used.

Rehabilitation

Patients on mechanical ventilation and/or ECMO support are at risk for development of neuromuscular weakness and deconditioning from prolonged immobility. Exercise capacity pre-lung transplant is an established predictor of waitlist survival irrespective of the underlying lung disease and is associated with post-transplant outcomes including length of stay and survival [30–34]. Thus, optimizing physical conditioning prior to lung transplantation is an important component of maximizing post-transplant success. ECMO can support the transition of a patient to an awake state through a reduction in sedation and mechanical ventilator support and thereby facilitate a physical rehabilitation program consisting of active ambulation and strengthening exercises. Ambulatory ECMO programs that provide active rehabilitation and physical therapy support have reported favorable outcomes including reduced mortality and length of stay in single-center studies [14, 15, 35–39]. Implementing an ambulatory ECMO program requires multidisciplinary teamwork with support from physical therapists, nurses, respiratory therapists, physicians, and perfusionists. Although ambulatory ECMO is associated with reduced hospital costs compared to non-ambulatory ECMO [40], the heavy resource utilization and multidisciplinary effort to maintain an ambulatory ECMO program has limited widespread adoption of ambulatory ECMO, particularly in lower volume ECMO centers.

Psychological Considerations

Delirium is commonly encountered in critically ill patients and is associated with adverse short-term and long-term outcomes. Similarly delirium is frequently encountered in ECMO-supported patients, and the prevention, recognition, and management of delirium are important for optimizing alertness and facilitating rehabilitation [41, 42]. Delirium prevention and management strategies are extrapolated from other critical care settings and include limiting benzodiazepines use; normalizing sleep-wake cycle; removing unnecessary support devices, catheters, and restraints; and correcting electrolyte and nutritional deficiencies.

The experience of being on ECMO, along with the morbid medical circumstances that necessitate using this rescue intervention and the ICU environment, can be very anxiety producing and terrifying to patients. In a qualitative study of ten long-term ECMO survivors, subjects described their traumatic memories of rapid deterioration and crisis before the initiation of ECMO. Six themes were summarized including dealing with crisis, critical care, memory, role of significant others, and existence today and tomorrow. Patients reported deconditioning and patchy factual memories contrasting with detailed delirious memories and paranoid ideations [43].

Psychological considerations and management in ECMO patients also extend beyond the critical care setting to long-term care. Long-term psychiatric assessment of ECMO survivors has identified that 71% have a chronic mental health disorder with 39% developing a new psychiatric disorder following ECMO support [44]. These disorders included organic mental (18%), obsessive-compulsive disorders (OCD) (15%), and/or post-traumatic stress disorder (PTSD) (11%). On follow-up, ECMO patients reported high levels of distress, physical aggression, anger, and alexithymic traits. Similarly, other observational studies have demonstrated high rates of adverse mental health outcomes following ECMO, including the development of post-traumatic stress symptoms and PTSD, perhaps related to increasing emphasis on maintaining an awake state and ongoing exposure to a number of PTSD risk factors [43, 45]. In fact, one observational study noted PTSD symptom burden has been reported in up to 41% of long-term survivors of ECMO [43]. Notably, the risk for PTSD following ECMO support was seen in both patients and their caregivers [43]. The role of a psychiatrist and other mental health providers in the multidisciplinary management of ECMO patients and the utility of psychological interventions to improve short- and long-term outcomes warrant ongoing study.

Conclusions

Extracorporeal membrane oxygenation can provide advanced life support to those with severe cardiac or respiratory failure. The indications for ECMO have evolved over time and can be implemented in carefully selected patients with acute reversible cardiorespiratory failure as a bridge to recovery or as a bridge to long-term mechanical circulatory support or cardiothoracic transplant in select patients with irreversible cardiorespiratory disease. Optimal use of ECMO requires a multidisciplinary team to monitor and manage comorbidities and complications, including frequently encountered psychological disorders, and to facilitate active rehabilitation.

References

1. Hill JD, O'Brien TG, Murray JJ, Dontigny L, Bramson ML, Osborn JJ, et al. Prolonged extracorporeal oxygenation for acute posttraumatic respiratory failure (shock-lung syndrome). Use of the Bramson membrane lung. N Engl J Med. 1972;286(12):629–34.
2. Zapol WM, Snider MT, Hill J, et al. Extracorporeal membrane oxygenation in severe acute respiratory failure: a randomized prospective study. JAMA. 1979;242(20):2193–6.
3. Morris AH, Wallace CJ, Menlove RL, Clemmer TP, Orme JF Jr, Weaver LK, et al. Randomized clinical trial of pressure-controlled inverse ratio ventilation and extracorporeal CO_2 removal for

adult respiratory distress syndrome. Am J Respir Crit Care Med. 1994;149(2 Pt 1):295–305.

4. Peek GJ, Mugford M, Tiruvoipati R, Wilson A, Allen E, Thalanany MM, et al. Efficacy and economic assessment of conventional ventilatory support versus extracorporeal membrane oxygenation for severe adult respiratory failure (CESAR): a multicentre randomised controlled trial. Lancet. 2009;374(9698):1351–63.

5. Thiagarajan RR, Barbaro RP, Rycus PT, McMullan DM, Conrad SA, Fortenberry JD, et al. Extracorporeal life support organization registry international report 2016. ASAIO J. 2017;63(1):60–7.

6. Brodie D, Bacchetta M. Extracorporeal membrane oxygenation for ARDS in adults. N Engl J Med. 2011;365(20):1905–14.

7. Weill D, Benden C, Corris PA, Dark JH, Davis RD, Keshavjee S, et al. A consensus document for the selection of lung transplant candidates: 2014 – an update from the Pulmonary Transplantation Council of the International Society for Heart and Lung Transplantation. J Heart Lung Transplant. 2015;34(1):1–15.

8. Loor G, Simpson L, Parulekar A. Bridging to lung transplantation with extracorporeal circulatory support: when or when not? J Thorac Dis. 2017;9(9):3352–61.

9. Chan KK, Lee KL, Lam PK, Law KI, Joynt GM, Yan WW. Hong Kong's experience on the use of extracorporeal membrane oxygenation for the treatment of influenza A (H1N1). Hong Kong Med J. 2010;16(6):447–54.

10. Pham T, Combes A, Roze H, Chevret S, Mercat A, Roch A, et al. Extracorporeal membrane oxygenation for pandemic influenza A(H1N1)-induced acute respiratory distress syndrome: a cohort study and propensity-matched analysis. Am J Respir Crit Care Med. 2013;187(3):276–85.

11. The Australia and New Zealand Extracorporeal Membrane Oxygenation Influenza Investigators. Extracorporeal membrane oxygenation for 2009 influenza A (H1N1) acute respiratory distress syndrome. JAMA. 2009;302(17):1888–95.

12. Sharma NS, Hartwig MG, Hayes D Jr. Extracorporeal membrane oxygenation in the pre and post lung transplant period. Ann Transl Med. 2017;5(4):74.

13. Toyoda Y, Bhama JK, Shigemura N, Zaldonis D, Pilewski J, Crespo M, et al. Efficacy of extracorporeal membrane oxygenation as a bridge to lung transplantation. J Thorac Cardiovasc Surg. 2013;145(4):1065–70; discussion 70–1.

14. Hoopes CW, Kukreja J, Golden J, Davenport DL, Diaz-Guzman E, Zwischenberger JB. Extracorporeal membrane oxygenation as a bridge to pulmonary transplantation. J Thorac Cardiovasc Surg. 2013;145(3):862–7; discussion 7–8.

15. Biscotti M, Gannon WD, Agerstrand C, Abrams D, Sonett J, Brodie D, et al. Awake extracorporeal membrane oxygenation as bridge to lung transplantation: a 9-year experience. Ann Thorac Surg. 2017;104(2):412–9.

16. Hayanga JW, Lira A, Aboagye JK, Hayanga HK, D'Cunha J. Extracorporeal membrane oxygenation as a bridge to lung transplantation: what lessons might we learn from volume and expertise? Interact Cardiovasc Thorac Surg. 2016;22:406.

17. Hayes D Jr, Whitson BA, Black SM, Preston TJ, Papadimos TJ, Tobias JD. Influence of age on survival in adult patients on extracorporeal membrane oxygenation before lung transplantation. J Heart Lung Transplant. 2015;34(6):832–8.

18. Snell GI, Yusen RD, Weill D, Strueber M, Garrity E, Reed A, et al. Report of the ISHLT Working Group on Primary Lung Graft Dysfunction, part I: Definition and grading-A 2016 Consensus Group statement of the International Society for Heart and Lung Transplantation. J Heart Lung Transplant. 2017;36(10):1097–103.

19. Van Raemdonck D, Hartwig MG, Hertz MI, Davis RD, Cypel M, Hayes D, et al. Report of the ISHLT Working Group on primary lung graft dysfunction Part IV: Prevention and treatment: A 2016 Consensus Group statement of the International Society

for Heart and Lung Transplantation. J Heart Lung Transplant. 2017;36(10):1121–36.

20. Hartwig MG, Walczak R, Lin SS, Davis RD. Improved survival but marginal allograft function in patients treated with extracorporeal membrane oxygenation after lung transplantation. Ann Thorac Surg. 2012;93(2):366–71.

21. Shekar K, Mullany DV, Thomson B, Ziegenfuss M, Platts DG, Fraser JF. Extracorporeal life support devices and strategies for management of acute cardiorespiratory failure in adult patients: a comprehensive review. Crit Care. 2014;18(3):219.

22. Chen Y-S, Lin J-W, Yu H-Y, Ko W-J, Jerng J-S, Chang W-T, et al. Cardiopulmonary resuscitation with assisted extracorporeal life-support versus conventional cardiopulmonary resuscitation in adults with in-hospital cardiac arrest: an observational study and propensity analysis. Lancet. 2008;372(9638):554–61.

23. Slutsky AS, Ranieri VM. Ventilator-induced lung injury. N Engl J Med. 2013;369(22):2126–36.

24. The Acute Respiratory Distress Syndrome Network. Ventilation with lower tidal volumes as compared with traditional tidal volumes for acute lung injury and the acute respiratory distress syndrome. N Engl J Med. 2000;342(18):1301–8.

25. Marhong JD, Telesnicki T, Munshi L, Del Sorbo L, Detsky M, Fan E. Mechanical ventilation during extracorporeal membrane oxygenation. An international survey. Ann Am Thorac Soc. 2014;11(6):956–61.

26. Pavot A, Mallat J, Vangrunderbeeck N, Thevenin D, Lemyze M. Rescue therapeutic strategy combining ultra-protective mechanical ventilation with extracorporeal CO_2 removal membrane in near-fatal asthma with severe pulmonary barotraumas: a case report. Medicine (Baltimore). 2017;96(41):e8248.

27. Terragni PP, Del Sorbo L, Mascia L, Urbino R, Martin EL, Birocco A, et al. Tidal volume lower than 6 ml/kg enhances lung protection: role of extracorporeal carbon dioxide removal. Anesthesiology. 2009;111(4):826–35.

28. Bein T, Weber-Carstens S, Goldmann A, Muller T, Staudinger T, Brederlau J, et al. Lower tidal volume strategy (approximately 3 ml/kg) combined with extracorporeal CO_2 removal versus 'conventional' protective ventilation (6 ml/kg) in severe ARDS: the prospective randomized Xtravent-study. Intensive Care Med. 2013;39(5):847–56.

29. Extracorporeal Life Support Organization (ELSO). General guidelines for all ECLS cases 2017. Available from: https://www.elso.org/Portals/0/ELSO Guidelines General All ECLS Version 1_4.pdf.

30. Tuppin MP, Paratz JD, Chang AT, Seale HE, Walsh JR, Kermeeen FD, et al. Predictive utility of the 6-minute walk distance on survival in patients awaiting lung transplantation. J Heart Lung Transplant. 2008;27(7):729–34.

31. Lederer DJ, Arcasoy SM, Wilt JS, D'Ovidio F, Sonett JR, Kawut SM. Six-minute-walk distance predicts waiting list survival in idiopathic pulmonary fibrosis. Am J Respir Crit Care Med. 2006;174(6):659–64.

32. Castleberry AW, Englum BR, Snyder LD, Worni M, Osho AA, Gulack BC, et al. The utility of preoperative six-minute-walk distance in lung transplantation. Am J Respir Crit Care Med. 2015;192(7):843–52.

33. Martinu T, Babyak MA, O'Connell CF, Carney RM, Trulock EP, Davis RD, et al. Baseline 6-min walk distance predicts survival in lung transplant candidates. Am J Transplant. 2008;8(7):1498–505.

34. Li M, Mathur S, Chowdhury NA, Helm D, Singer LG. Pulmonary rehabilitation in lung transplant candidates. J Heart Lung Transplant. 2013;32(6):626–32.

35. Lehr CJ, Zaas DW, Cheifetz IM, Turner DA. Ambulatory extracorporeal membrane oxygenation as a bridge to lung transplantation: walking while waiting. Chest. 2015;147(5):1213–8.

36. Rehder KJ, Turner DA, Hartwig MG, Williford WL, Bonadonna D, Walczak RJ Jr, et al. Active rehabilitation during extracorporeal

membrane oxygenation as a bridge to lung transplantation. Respir Care. 2013;58(8):1291–8.

37. Turner DA, Cheifetz IM, Rehder KJ, Williford WL, Bonadonna D, Banuelos SJ, et al. Active rehabilitation and physical therapy during extracorporeal membrane oxygenation while awaiting lung transplantation: a practical approach. Crit Care Med. 2011;39(12):2593–8.

38. Fuehner T, Kuehn C, Hadem J, Wiesner O, Gottlieb J, Tudorache I, et al. Extracorporeal membrane oxygenation in awake patients as bridge to lung transplantation. Am J Respir Crit Care Med. 2012;185(7):763–8.

39. Garcia JP, Iacono A, Kon ZN, Griffith BP. Ambulatory extracorporeal membrane oxygenation: a new approach for bridge-to-lung transplantation. J Thorac Cardiovasc Surg. 2010;139(6):e137–9.

40. Bain JC, Turner DA, Rehder KJ, Eisenstein EL, Davis RD, Cheifetz IM, et al. Economic outcomes of extracorporeal membrane oxygenation with and without ambulation as a bridge to lung transplantation. Respir Care. 2016;61(1):1–7.

41. Zwischenberger JB, Pitcher HT. Extracorporeal membrane oxygenation management: techniques to liberate from extracorporeal membrane oxygenation and manage post–intensive care unit issues. Crit Care Clin. 2017;33(4):843–53.

42. Acevedo-Nuevo M, Gonzalez-Gil MT, Romera-Ortega MA, Latorre-Marco I, Rodriguez-Huerta MD. The early diagnosis and management of mixed delirium in a patient placed on ECMO and with difficult sedation: a case report. Intensive Crit Care Nurs. 2018;44:110–4.

43. Tramm R, Ilic D, Murphy K, Sheldrake J, Pellegrino V, Hodgson C. A qualitative exploration of acute care and psychological distress experiences of ECMO survivors. Heart Lung. 2016;45(3):220–6.

44. Risnes I, Heldal A, Wagner K, Boye B, Haraldsen I, Leganger S, et al. Psychiatric outcome after severe cardio-respiratory failure treated with extracorporeal membrane oxygenation: a case-series. Psychosomatics. 2013;54(5):418–27.

45. Tramm R, Hodgson C, Ilic D, Sheldrake J, Pellegrino V. Identification and prevalence of PTSD risk factors in ECMO patients: a single centre study. Aust Crit Care. 2015;28(1):31–6.

History of Lung Transplantation

Kapil Patel and David Weill

Early Surgical History

In 1947, Vladimir P. Demikhov performed the first experimental lung transplant in dogs. Over the next few decades, numerous accomplished surgeons performed experimental lung transplants which resulted in improved surgical techniques and better understanding of cardiopulmonary physiology. Hardy et al. [2] performed approximately 400 experimental canine lung transplants before performing the first lung transplant on June 13, 1963, at the Medical Center of the University of Mississippi. The patient survived 17 days, dying from renal failure and infectious complications. Until 1983, approximately 40 lung transplants were performed with survival varying from hours to days. However, on November 14, 1968, Derom et al. [3] performed a single left lung transplant in a 23-year-old man with silicosis, surviving 10 months and dying from infectious complications (pneumonia from *Pseudomonas* and *Candida*). In 1983, Dr. Cooper of Toronto General Hospital performed the first single-lung transplant resulting in long-term survival of approximately 7 years, in a patient with pulmonary fibrosis [4]; in 1986, Dr. Patterson performed a double-lung transplant in a patient with emphysema [5], with a survival of nearly 16 years.

In the 1990s, Starnes [6] performed the first living (right lobar) donor transplant in a 12-year-old child with bronchopulmonary dysplasia at Stanford University Medical Center.

Heart-lung transplantation was first performed in 1968 by Cooley at Texas Children's Hospital [7] in a 2.5-month-year-old girl with pulmonary hypertension, surviving only 14 hours. At various institutions, three combined heart-lung transplants were performed over years with poor survival.

The first long-term survivor from a combined heart-lung transplantation was performed at Stanford on March 9, 1981, by Reitz [8] for primary pulmonary hypertension surviving 5 years.

Over the decades, the field of lung transplantation has overcome major obstacles including surgical techniques, immunosuppressant regimen, lung donor preservation, and infectious prophylaxis. However, lung transplantation as a viable treatment option for end-stage lung diseases lagged behind other organ transplantations for many years.

Airway Complications and Immunosuppression

During the initial years of lung transplantation, dating back to the 1940s, experimental lung transplants were unsuccessful primarily related to airway dehiscence, reported at a 60–80% complication rate [9, 10]. Airway complications, primarily due to dehiscence of the bronchial anastomosis, continued to be a leading issue related to significant morbidity and mortality. The initial theory was that ischemia of the donor bronchus was due to the lack of restoration of the arterial systemic blood supply (bronchial arteries) at the time of transplantation. Therefore, it became clear that the viability of the donor bronchus was initially dependent upon retrograde collaterals from the pulmonary arteries (less oxygenated blood). Various centers introduced the possibility of bronchial artery revascularization with successful outcomes [11, 12]. However, given the technical difficulties leading to longer operative time, this technique has not been universally accepted, and large series are lacking. In addition, bronchial artery regeneration was evident in experimental lung transplants in canine models [13, 14].

Over the ensuing decades, other complications, including infections and lack of proper immunosuppressant regimen, continued to plague the field of lung transplantation [15]. With the advent and success with the use of cyclosporine in

K. Patel
Center for Advanced Lung Disease, Division of Pulmonary and Critical Care Medicine, Morsani College of Medicine, University of South Florida, Tampa, FL, USA
e-mail: kapilpatel@health.usf.edu

D. Weill
Weill Consulting Group, New Orleans, LA, USA

© Springer International Publishing AG, part of Springer Nature 2019
Y. Sher, J. R. Maldonado (eds.), *Psychosocial Care of End-Stage Organ Disease and Transplant Patients*,
https://doi.org/10.1007/978-3-319-94914-7_25

renal transplant, there was a renewed interest in advancing the field to lung transplant [16]. The Toronto Lung Transplant Group, led by Cooper and colleagues, began canine experimental lung transplants to investigate risk factors that were felt to be major contributors to bronchial dehiscence [17]. Initial immunosuppressant regimens included azathioprine and corticosteroids. In 1981, early practitioners discovered that steroids led to poor bronchial healing with no effect from the azathioprine [18]. Reitz and colleagues performed the first successful heart-lung transplantation using cyclosporine, azathioprine, and prednisone [8]. Introduction of cyclosporine to the standing regimen of azathioprine and lower dosing of prednisone allowed the success of five single-lung transplants with idiopathic pulmonary fibrosis with no patients dying of airway complications [19]. In addition, Cooper and colleagues used omentopexy, a surgical procedure whereby the suture of the omentum to another organ increases arterial circulation, to improve bronchial collateral circulation and possibly alleviate narrowing distal to the airway anastomosis which was thought to be related to ischemia.

With success from single-lung transplants, Patterson et al. evaluated the possibility of en bloc double-lung transplant using omentum wrapped around the tracheal anastomosis [20, 21]. However, due to high rate of tracheal anastomosis necrosis, there was a 25% mortality, and 20% of patients developed delayed airway stenosis requiring intervention. This technique was, therefore, abandoned. Complications related to gastrointestinal ischemia with omental wraps, and other alternative surgical techniques using intercostal muscle or peribronchial tissue anastomosis wrap, did not gain traction within the field. With the advent of end-to-end anastomosis with excision of the donor bronchus just proximal to the takeoff of the upper lobe bronchus, near the secondary carina, airway complications were significantly reduced [22, 23]. Bilateral sequential lung transplantation was introduced by Kaiser and colleagues with minimal airway complications and significantly reduced early morbidity and mortality, similar to single-lung transplant procedures [24].

Preservation Solutions

Since the beginning of lung transplantation, donor lung preservation has been an instrumental element leading to more successful outcomes. Proper preservation of organs resulted in full physiological and biochemical function after transplantation by maintaining the anatomical barriers (e.g., alveolar-capillary barrier). Historically, intracellular fluid (e.g., Euro-Collins solution and University of Wisconsin solution) composition had been utilized for the preservation of donor lungs, as derived from the kidney and liver transplant experience. Through experimental animal models, Fukuse et al. concluded that standard Euro-Collins solution, containing high potassium concentration, compared to modified Euro-Collins

solution (low potassium concentration) resulted in significant elevation in pulmonary vascular resistance, leading to possible damage to the vascular endothelium, further increasing the risk for ischemic reperfusion injury [25]. Further studies concluded that low-potassium dextran solution leads to improved preservation solution organ flush and ischemic storage [26]. Improvements in preservation solutions have led to reduced primary graft dysfunction. Okada et al. reviewed five clinical trials (four retrospective and one prospective non-randomized study) and concluded that low-potassium dextran solution was superior to Euro-Collins solution in graft preservation and early graft function [27].

Cytomegalovirus Prophylaxis

Historically, cytomegalovirus (CMV) has been an important contributor to morbidity and mortality in lung transplant recipients. It is important to differentiate CMV infection, defined as virus isolation or detection of viral proteins (antigens) or nucleic acid in any body fluid or tissue specimen, versus CMV disease, defined by the presence of CMV infection with attributable symptoms and signs or evidence of tissue invasion, as this aids in the approach of treatment and outcomes. The incidence of CMV infection and disease in other solid organs (e.g., heart, liver and kidney) is approximately 9–35% [28]. In contrast, the incidence of both CMV infection and disease is higher in lung transplant population, approximately 40% [29]. Major risk factors associated with CMV disease are the serostatus (donor positive, recipient negative [D+/R−] being at the highest risk), the type of organ transplanted, and the immunosuppressive regimen used, including induction therapy [30]. In the absence of prophylactic antiviral therapy in renal transplant recipients, median time of onset of CMV infection (CMV pp65 antigenemia) was 35 days in all serostatus groups (except, seronegative donor and recipient, D−/R−) [31]. Through indirect, induced systemic inflammation from CMV replication within in the host (e.g., transplant recipient) and direct deleterious effects of CMV, CMV disease has been shown to be associated with acute and chronic allograft dysfunction [32–35].

Rubin et al. evaluated the optimal prophylaxis in solid organ transplant recipients (e.g., kidney, liver, and heart) for the prevention of primary cytomegalovirus with oral ganciclovir or oral acyclovir. The incidence of CMV infection or disease was significantly reduced in the ganciclovir group (32% vs. 50%, $P < 0.05$), within the first 6 months post-transplant [36]. Similar results were seen in lung transplant recipients comparing intravenous (IV) ganciclovir versus oral acyclovir until 90 days post-transplant. Cumulative incidence of all CMV infections (including seroconversion) was significantly reduced in the IV ganciclovir group (15% vs. 75%, $P < 0.033$) [37]. In an open, comparative study of 22 patients, Speich et al. evaluated the efficacy of oral ($n = 9$) vs. IV ganciclovir (*n* = 5) for CMV prophylaxis in lung transplant recipients and comparative historical non-prophylaxed control (*n* = 8) group. One patient developed cytomegalovirus disease in the oral ganciclovir group, none in the IV group, and six in the non-prophylaxed group [38]. Limitations associated with ganciclovir formulations, including the low bioavailability of the oral preparation [39] and the patient inconvenience, cost, and catheter-related infections of the IV delivery route [40], led to the development of valganciclovir, an ester prodrug of ganciclovir. Valganciclovir, 900 mg/day, provides comparable plasma ganciclovir levels compared to those achieved with 5 mg/kg IV ganciclovir [39]. Its bioavailability (60%) is approximately tenfold higher than that of oral ganciclovir [39]. Studies have demonstrated the safety and efficacy of valganciclovir for CMV prophylaxis in solid organ transplant patients excluding lung transplant recipients [41]. Zamora et al. evaluated the efficacy and appropriate length of prophylaxis with valganciclovir for the primary prevention of CMV infection and disease in seropositive lung transplant recipients [42]. Consecutive lung transplant recipients (*n* = 90) received prophylaxis with valganciclovir (450 mg twice daily) to complete 180, 270, or 365 days, compared to historical group (*n* = 140) who received high-dose acyclovir (800 mg three times daily). Both groups initially received prophylaxis with IV ganciclovir (5 mg/kg daily) and cytomegalovirus immune globulin (CMV-IVIG), 30 days for seropositive recipients (D+/R+ and D−/R+), and 90 days for seropositive donors (D+/R−). CMV disease was significantly reduced in the valganciclovir group compared to acyclovir group (2.2% vs. 20%, *P* < 0.001).

Another evolution in the prophylaxis and treatment of CMV has been the use of cytomegalovirus immune. In 2010, Palmer et al. showed a decrease in CMV disease (4% vs. 32%, *P* < 0.001) and infection (10% vs. 64%, *P* 0.001), extending the valganciclovir prophylaxis period to 12 months versus standard 3 months. During the 6 months after study completion, a low incidence of CMV disease was observed in both groups [43].

Future understanding of the recipient's CMV-specific immunity may aid in developing the optimal duration of antiviral prophylaxis and sustaining prevention of CMV in this high-risk patient population [44]. However, the evolution of therapy to prevent and treat CMV-related complications has been an important step forward in improving the outcomes following lung transplantation.

Lung Allocation Score

Prior to May 2005, the allocation of lungs was based on accrued time on the waiting list. This resulted in disproportionately high mortality rates on the waiting list, mostly because there were no medical urgency parameters within the allocation system. Because the allocation system did not fac-

tor in severity of illness, patients with idiopathic pulmonary fibrosis (IPF) had an especially high mortality rate while on the waiting list. Recognizing this issue with respect to the IPF patients, in 1995 an exemption was put into effect that led to an additional 90-day wait-list credit for patients with IPF.

In response to the persistently increasing number of deaths on the transplant list, the US Department of Health and Human Services published in 1998 and implemented in March 2000 – the "Final Rule," which required the Organ Procurement and Transplantation Network (OPTN) to emphasize the broader sharing of organs, reducing waiting time as an allocation criterion and structuring a system for equitable organ allocation using objective medical criteria and urgency for allocation [45]. As a result, in 1998, the Lung Allocation Subcommittee of the OPTN Thoracic Organ Transplantation Committee was formed to structure an alternative lung allocation system in keeping with the goals of the Final Rule: (1) reduction of mortality on the lung waiting list, (2) prioritization of candidates based on urgency while avoiding futile transplants, and (3) reducing the importance of waiting time and geography in lung allocation within the limits of ischemic time [46].

In May 2005, OPTN changed the policy for donor lung allocation from a system that previously allocated based primarily on accrued waiting time on the list to a system that allocated lungs based primarily on a lung allocation score (LAS). The LAS is calculated from objective clinical data that predicts 1 year survival on the waiting list (without transplantation) and post-transplantation. Multiple factors, predictive of wait-list mortality and post-transplant survivability including diagnoses, were included in the LAS formula. The ultimate goals of the LAS are to (1) reduce the number of deaths on the lung transplant list, (2) increase transplant benefit for lung transplant recipients (avoiding futile transplants), and (3) ensure the efficient and equitable allocation of the lungs to active transplant candidates [46].

Donation After Cardiac Death and Ex Vivo Lung Perfusion

The relative scarcity of traditional brain-dead organ donors remains a most critical obstacle to ensuring the availability of organs to recipients with end-stage organ disease. Traditionally, the lungs are the lowest procured organs, approximately 15–25%, compared to all other transplanted organs [47]. As a result, several studies have shown that liberalization of the current standard lung donor criteria, also known as "marginal donor lungs," could achieve similar outcomes [48–50]. Emerging techniques for further increasing donor lungs include donation after cardiac death (DCD) and ex vivo lung perfusion (EVLP).

The first successful human lung transplant was performed by Hardy and colleagues in 1963 using an allograft from a

DCD [2]. Over the ensuing decades, the primary reason for the slow adoption of DCD lungs has been the concern for graft injury from prolonged warm ischemia time. Mason et al. reported on the retrospective review of the UNOS registry, from 1987 to 2007, analyzing the outcomes of 36 lung transplantations performed using DCD. Overall survival at 1 year post-transplantation was 94%, equivalent to the traditional donation after brain death [51]. Subsequently, single-center experience revealed similar outcomes [52–54]. Love and coworkers published long-term follow-up in a single-center experience [55]. Between 1993 and 2009, 18 recipients received lungs from DCD. Outcomes were compared with those recipients who received organs from brain-dead donors ($n = 406$). One, 3-, and 5-year survival rates ($P = 0.66$) and freedom from bronchiolitis obliterans syndrome ($P = 0.59$) were similar between groups. Incidence of primary graft dysfunction were similar ($P = 0.59$). Overall, DCD can expand the donor pool with similar outcomes compared to the traditional brain-dead donors.

In 2001, the utilization of EVLP in human lung transplantation using DCD was published [56]. Despite good physiological function of the transplanted lung until 5 months post-transplant, patient died from CMV infection. The University of Toronto published the largest series of lung transplants performed using EVLP with 58 EVLP cases resulting in 50 lung transplantations. The incidence of primary graft dysfunction was 2% in the EVLP group and 8.5% in the conventional transplant group ($P = 0.14$) with 87% survival at 1 year [57]. The development of EVLP systems allows for prolonged preservation of organ, ongoing assessment of physiological function (e.g., gas exchange, hemodynamics, ventilation), and reconditioning of injured organs. The latter is performed through high oncotic perfusate solution (dehydrating the lungs) and recruitment of the atelectatic lungs. Finally, EVLP can aid in the evaluation of DCD organs following procurement with assessment of graft function. The Toronto Lung Transplant Group published a detailed review of the step-by-step technique and assessment of donor pulmonary grafts placed on EVLP [58].

Conclusions

Although much progress has been made in the field of lung transplantation, there is still much that needs to be addressed. While surgical technique and basic early post-operative care has largely been well established, by far the biggest challenge to long-term success of lung transplantation continues to be how best to prevent the development of the bronchiolitis obliterans syndrome (BOS) and, when it occurs, how to slow the progressive loss of lung function associated with it. Although BOS research has focused on several different angles, some immunologic and some non-immunologic, no one single factor seems to explain its occurrence and the devastating effect it has

on patient survival. Until BOS can be better understood, the long-term survival of lung transplant recipients will be less assured than that seen in other solid organ transplant recipients.

References

1. Hertz MI, Aurora P, Christie JD, et al. Registry of the international society for heart and lung transplantation: a quarter century of thoracic transplantation. J Heart Lung Transplant. 2008;27:937–42.
2. Hardy JD, Webb WR, Dalton ML Jr, Walker GR. Lung homotransplantation in man. JAMA. 1963;186:1065–74.
3. Derom F, Barbier F, Ringoir S, et al. Ten-month survival after lung homotransplantations in man. J Thorac Cardiovasc Surg. 1971;61:835–46.
4. Cooper JD, Pearson FG, Patterson GA, et al. Technique of successful lung transplantation in humans. J Thorac Cardiovasc Surg. 1987;93:173–81.
5. Patterson GA, Cooper JD, Barr JH, Jones MT. Experimental and clinical double lung transplantation. J Thorac Cardiovasc Surg. 1988;95:70–4.
6. Starnes VA, Barr ML, Cohen RG. Lobar transplantation: indications, technique and outcome. J Thorac Cardiovasc Surg. 1994;108:403–10.
7. Cooley DA, Bloodwell RD, Hallman GL, et al. Organ transplantation for advanced cardiopulmonary disease. Ann Thorac Surg. 1969;8:30–42.
8. Reitz BA, Wallwork JL, Hunt SA, et al. Heart-lung transplantation: successful therapy for patients with pulmonary vascular disease. N Engl J Med. 1982;306:557–64.
9. Kshettry VR, Kroshus TJ, Hertz MI, et al. Early and late airway complications after lung transplantation: incidence and management. Ann Thorac Surg. 1997;63:1576–83.
10. Alvarez A, Algar J, Santos F, et al. Airway complications after lung transplantation: a review of 151 anastomoses. Eur J Cardiothorac Surg. 2001;19:381–7.
11. Couraud L, Baudet E, Nashef SAM, et al. Lung transplantation with bronchial revascularization. Eur J Cardiothorac Surg. 1992;6:490–5.
12. Pettersson GB, Karam K, Thuita L, et al. Comparative study of bronchial artery revascularization in lung transplantation. J Thorac Cardiovasc Surg. 2013;146:894–900.
13. Siegelman SS, Hagstrom JW, Koerner SK, et al. Restoration of bronchial artery circulation after canine lung allotransplantation. J Thorac Cardiovasc Surg. 1977;73:792–5.
14. Pearson FG, Goldberg M, Stone RM, Colapinto RF. Bronchial arterial circulation restored after reimplantation of canine lung. Can J Surg. 1970;13:243–50.
15. Wildevuur CR, Benfield JR. A review of 23 human lung transplantations by 20 surgeons. Ann Thorac Surg. 1970;9:489–515.
16. Calne RY, White DJ, Thiru S, et al. Cyclosporine a in patients receiving renal allografts from cadaver donors. Lancet. 1978;2:1323–7.
17. Cooper JD. Herbert Sloan lecture. Lung transplantation. Ann Thorac Surg. 1989;47:28–44.
18. Lima O, Cooper JD, Peters WJ, et al. Effects of methylprednisone and azathioprine on bronchial healing following lung autotransplantation. J Thorac Cardiovasc Surg. 1981;82:211–5.
19. Cooper JD, Pearson FG, Patterson GA, et al. Technique of successful lung transplants in humans. J Thorac Cardiovasc Surg. 1987;93:173–81.
20. Patterson GA, Cooper JD, Goldman B, et al. Technique of successful clinical double-lung transplantation. Ann Thorac Surg. 1988;45:626–33.

21. Patterson GA, Todd TR, Cooper JD, et al. Airway complications after double lung transplantation. Toronto lung transplant group. J Thorac Cardiovasc Surg. 1990;99:14–20.

22. Garfein ES, Ginsberg ME, Gorenstein L, et al. Superiority of end-to-end versus telescoped bronchial anastomosis in single lung transplantation for pulmonary emphysema. J Thorac Cardiovasc Surg. 2001;121:149–54.

23. Vieth FJ, Kambolg SL, Mollenkopf FP, Montefusco CM. Lung transplantation 1983. Transplantation. 1983;35:271–8.

24. Kaiser LR, Pasque MK, Trulock EP, et al. Bilateral sequential lung transplantation: the procedure of choice for double-lung replacement. Ann Thorac Surg. 1991;52:438–46.

25. Fukuse T, Albes JM, Brandes H, et al. Comparison of low potassium Euro-Collins solution and standard Euro-Collins solution in an extracorporeal rat heart-lung model. Eur J Cardiothorac Surg. 1996;10:621–7.

26. Yamazaki F, Yokomise H, Keshavjee SH, et al. The superiority of an extracellular fluid solution over Euro-Collins' solution for pulmonary preservation. Transplantation. 1990;49:690–4.

27. Okada Y, Kondo T. Impact of lung preservation solutions, Euro-Collins vs low-potassium dextran, on early graft function: a review of five clinical studies. Ann Thorac Cardiovasc Surg. 2006;12:10–4.

28. Roman A, Manito N, Campistol JM, et al. The impact of the prevention strategies on the indirect effects of CMV infection in solid organ transplant recipients. Transplant Rev (Orlando). 2014;28:84–91.

29. McDevitt LM. Etiology and impact of cytomegalovirus disease on solid organ transplant recipients. Am J Health Syst Pharm. 2006;63(19 Supple 5):S3–9.

30. Meylan PR, Manuel O. Late onset cytomegalovirus disease in patients with solid organ transplant. Curr Opin Infect Dis. 2007;20:412–8.

31. Sagedal S, Nordal KP, Hartman A, et al. A prospective study of the natural course of cytomegalovirus infection and disease in renal allograft recipients. Transplantation. 2000;70:1166–74.

32. Manuel O, Kralidis G, Mueller NJ, et al. Impact of antiviral preventive strategies on the incidence and outcome of cytomegalovirus disease in solid organ transplant recipients. Am J Transplant. 2013;13:2402–10.

33. Freeman RB. The 'indirect' effects of cytomegalovirus infection. Am J Transplant. 2009;9:2453–8.

34. Kroshus TJ, Kshettry VR, Savik K, et al. Risk factors for the development of bronchiolitis obliterans syndrome after lung transplantation. J Thorac Cardiovasc Surg. 1997;114:195–202.

35. Synder LD, Finlen-Copeland AF, Turbyfill WJ, et al. Cytomegalovirus pneumonitis is a risk factor for bronchiolitis obliterans syndrome in lung transplantation. Am J Respir Crit Care Med. 2010;181:1391–6.

36. Rubin RH, Kemmerly SA, Conti D, et al. Prevention of primary cytomegalovirus disease in organ transplant recipients with oral ganciclovir or oral acyclovir prophylaxis. Transpl Infect Dis. 2000;2:112–7.

37. Duncan SR, Grgurich WF, Iacono AT, et al. A comparison of ganciclovir and acyclovir to prevent cytomegalovirus after lung transplantation. Am J Respir Crit Care Med. 1994;150:146–52.

38. Speich R, Thurnheer R, Gaspert A, et al. Efficacy and cost effectiveness of oral ganciclovir in the prevention of cytomegalovirus disease after lung transplantation. Transplantation. 1999;67:315–20.

39. Pescovitz MD, Rabkin J, Merion RM, et al. Valganciclovir results in improved oral absorption of ganciclovir in liver transplant recipients. Antimicrob Agents Chemother. 2000;44:2811–5.

40. Hertz MI, Jordan C, Savik SK, et al. Randomized trial of daily versus three-times weekly prophylactic ganciclovir after lung and heart-lung transplantation. J Heart Lung Transplant. 1998;17:913–20.

41. Paya C, Humar A, Dominguez E, et al. Efficacy and safety of valganciclovir vs. oral ganciclovir for prevention of CMV disease in solid organ transplant recipients. Am J Transplant. 2004;4:611–20.

42. Zamora MR, Nicolls MR, Hodges TN, et al. Following universal prophylaxis with intravenous ganciclovir and cytomegalovirus immune globulin, valganciclovir is safe and effective for prevention of CMV infection following lung transplantation. Am J Transplant. 2004;4:1635–42.

43. Palmer SM, Limaye AP, Banks M, et al. Extended valganciclovir prophylaxis to prevent cytomegalovirus after lung transplantation. Ann Intern Med. 2010;152:761–9.

44. Schoeppler KE, Lyu DM, Grazia TJ, et al. Late-onset cytomegalovirus (CMV) in lung transplant recipients: can CMV serostatus guide the duration of prophylaxis? Am J Transplant. 2013;13:376–82.

45. Department of Health and Human Services. Organ Procurement and Transplantation Network; final rule. In: Federal Register 42 CFR, Part 121, October 20, 1999:56649–56661.

46. Egan TM, Murray S, Bustami RT, et al. Development of the new lung allocation system in the United States. Am J Transplant. 2006;6(Part 2):1212–27.

47. Fisher AJ, Donnelly SC, Pritchard G, et al. Objective assessment of criteria for selection of donor lungs suitable for transplantation. Thorax. 2004;59:434–7.

48. Bhorade SM, Vigneswaran W, McCabe MA, et al. Liberalization of donor criteria may expand the donor pool without adverse consequence in lung transplantation. J Heart Lung Transplant. 2000;19:1199–204.

49. Kron IL, Tribble CG, Kern JA, et al. Successful transplantation of marginally acceptable thoracic organs. Ann Surg. 1993;217:518–22.

50. Sundaresan S, Semenkovich J, Ochoa L, et al. Successful outcome of lung transplantation is not compromised by the use of marginal donor lungs. J Thorac Cardiovasc Surg. 1995;109:1075–9.

51. Mason DP, Thuita L, Alster JM, et al. Should lung transplantation be performed using donation after cardiac death? The United States experience. J Thorac Cardiovasc Surg. 2008;136:1061–6.

52. Snell GI, Levvey BJ, Oto T, et al. Early lung transplantation success utilizing controlled donation after cardiac death donors. Am J Transplant. 2008;8:1282–9.

53. De VS, Van RD, Vanaudenaerde B, et al. Early outcome after lung transplantation from non-heart-beating donors is comparable to heart-beating donors. J Heart Lung Transplant. 2009;28:380–7.

54. Mason DP, Murthy SC, Gonzalez-Stawinski GV, et al. Early experience with lung transplantation using donors after cardiac death. J Heart Lung Transplant. 2008;27:561–3.

55. De Oliveira NC, Osaki S, Maloney JD, et al. Lung transplantation with donation after cardiac death donors: long-term follow up in a single center. J Thorac Cardiovasc Surg. 2010;139:1306–15.

56. Steen S, Sjoberg T, Pierre L, et al. Transplantation of lungs from a non-heart-beating donor. Lancet. 2001;357:825–9.

57. Van Raemdonck D, Neyrinck A, Cypel M, Keshavjee S. Ex-vivo lung perfusion. Transpl Int. 2015;28:643–56.

58. Machuca TN, Cypel M. Ex vivo lung perfusion. J Thorac Dis. 2014;6:1054–62.

Medical Course and Complications After Lung Transplantation

26

Guillermo Garrido and Gundeep S. Dhillon

Overview

Lung transplantation for patients with end-stage lung disease is associated with improved survival and quality of life [1, 2]. The median post-lung transplant survival in the current era is approximately 6 years, as compared to a median survival of 4 years among those transplanted between 1990 and 1998 [3]. However, the survival following lung transplantation remains significantly worse as compared to other solid organ transplants. There are certain unique features of lung transplantation that predispose recipients to a multitude of surgical and medical complications.

Specific Relevant Features of the Lung Allograft

The lungs normally have a dual blood supply, consisting of 1) large pulmonary arteries that provide desaturated blood under low pressure for alveolar gas exchange and 2) smaller bronchial arteries that provide oxygenated blood under systemic pressure for nutrition and oxygenation of the bronchi and lung tissue. As the only solid organ transplant that does not undergo primary systemic (i.e., bronchial) arterial revascularization at the time of surgery, lung transplants rely on the deoxygenated pulmonary arterial circulation and are especially vulnerable to the effects of injury and ischemia [4].

It has been hypothesized that the absence of the bronchial system in the lung allograft increases susceptibility to microvascular injury and chronic airway ischemia, which may be implicated in the genesis of chronic rejection and other complications [5]. Similarly, the native lymphatics and the neural supply to lung allografts are disrupted at the time of trans-

plantation. The impact of these disruptions on lung transplant outcomes remains unclear, though it is possible that these changes lead to higher susceptibility to the development of pulmonary edema and infections, worse airway clearance, and ineffective cough [6]. Lastly, the lung allografts have higher exposure to immunogenic compounds, as compared to other organs, by ventilation. The ongoing exposure to various inhaled injurious agents may also predispose lung allografts to develop chronic rejection.

Post-Lung Transplantation Complications

There is a vast array of complications from lung transplantation. Broadly these complications can be divided into noninfectious and infectious complications and have been summarized in Table 26.1. These complications arise at different times in the postoperative period [7]. The understanding of timing of various complications post-lung transplant can lead to early recognition and management of these complications.

Noninfectious Complications

Primary Graft Dysfunction (PGD)

PGD is a syndrome of acute lung injury that ensues within the first 72 hours after lung transplant. It is manifested by the early development of bilateral pulmonary infiltrates, hypoxemia with a reduced PaO2/FiO2 ratio (<300), without an identifiable cause. The diagnosis of PGD is one of the exclusions. The other causes of graft dysfunction such as infection, hyperacute rejection, cardiogenic pulmonary edema, and pulmonary venous anastomotic obstruction should be excluded [8]. PGD is thought to be due to overexuberant infiltration of monocytes, neutrophils, and T cells in response to transplant-mediated immune signals from endothelium,

G. Garrido (✉) · G. S. Dhillon
Division of Pulmonary and Critical Care, Department of Medicine, Stanford University School of Medicine, Stanford, CA, USA
e-mail: gdhillon@stanford.edu

© Springer International Publishing AG, part of Springer Nature 2019
Y. Sher, J. R. Maldonado (eds.), *Psychosocial Care of End-Stage Organ Disease and Transplant Patients*,
https://doi.org/10.1007/978-3-319-94914-7_26

Table 26.1 Noninfectious and infectious complications post-lung transplant

Noninfectious complications	Infectious complications
Primary graft dysfunction (PGD)	Bacterial infections
	Pseudomonas aeruginosa
Venous thromboembolism (VTE)	*Burkholderia cepacia*
	Staphylococcus aureus
Nerve injury	(including methicillin-resistant),
Diaphragmatic dysfunction (phrenic nerve)	other gram-negative organisms
	Streptococcus pneumoniae
Gastroparesis (vagus nerve)	*Clostridium difficile*
	Nocardia
Pleural	Fungal infections
Effusions	*Aspergillus*
Pneumothorax, hemothorax, chylothorax	*Fusarium*
	Scedosporium
Bronchopleural fistula	Mucormycosis
Pleural fibrosis	*Candida, Pneumocystis jiroveci*
Vascular anastomotic complications	*Cryptococcus*
Airway anastomotic complications	Endemic fungi: *Histoplasma capsulatum, Coccidioides immitis, Blastomyces dermatitidis*
Rejection	Viral infections
Acute cellular rejection	*Cytomegalovirus* (CMV)
Antibody-mediated rejection	*Herpesviruses*
	JC virus
Chronic lung allograft dysfunction	*BK virus*
Bronchiolitis obliterans syndrome (BOS)	Respiratory syncytial virus (RSV), parainfluenza, and other respiratory viruses
Restrictive allograft syndrome (RAS)	
Post-transplant malignancies	
Metabolic	
Hyperammonemia	
Diabetes mellitus	
Acute kidney injury, chronic kidney disease	
Osteoporosis	
Dyslipidemia	
Cardiovascular (arrhythmias, coronary artery disease)	
Miscellaneous issues (psychiatric, gastrointestinal, sarcopenia)	

epithelium, and alveolar macrophages. The interaction between these cells leads to release of cytokines, reactive oxygen intermediates, and proteolytic enzymes leading to graft dysfunction [9]. The severity of PGD falls along a spectrum, ranging from mild dysfunction to severe lung injury. PGD can affect 10–25% of transplanted patients, and the 30-day mortality can be as high as 50%. Furthermore, severe PGD after lung transplantation has been associated with development of subsequent chronic rejection and graft dysfunction [10].

The management of PGD is largely supportive and includes lung-protective ventilation strategies (low tidal volume, high positive end-expiratory pressure), judicious fluid management, inhaled nitric oxide or other inhaled pulmonary vasodilators to improve oxygenation, and extracorporeal life

support (ECLS) for the most severe cases. Re-transplantation is an option for highly selected cases, but it is generally not recommended due to suboptimal outcomes [11].

Venous Thromboembolism (VTE)

Lung transplant recipients are at increased risk of VTE. The risk factors include major surgery status, hypercoagulable state, high dose of corticosteroids, immobility, and indwelling vascular access. The reported incidences of pulmonary embolism (PE) and deep venous thrombosis (DVTs) post-lung transplantation are approximately 5–15% and 20–45%, respectively [12]. The pulmonary embolism in setting of limited pulmonary reserve due to PGD, postoperative atelectasis, and single-lung transplantation can have catastrophic consequences, thus underscoring the need for early and appropriate VTE prophylaxis after lung transplantation [13].

The diagnosis can be made with computed tomography (CT) pulmonary angiography, ventilation-perfusion scan, or by documentation of DVT by Doppler ultrasonography. The treatment is the same as for VTEs in general, although the risk of postoperative bleeding needs to be weighed against the risk of PE. The choice of anticoagulant is based on kidney function, periprocedural reversibility of anticoagulant effect, and drug interactions, with unfractionated heparin, low-molecular-weight heparin, and/or warfarin being by far the most common agents used. In case of ongoing bleeding or high risk of bleeding, inferior vena cava filters can be used as a temporizing measure.

Nerve Injury

Inadvertent injury to various intrathoracic nerves during lung transplantation is a well-recognized and common complication. The most commonly affected structures are the phrenic and vagus nerves.

The reported rates of phrenic nerve injury have ranged from 3% to 9% in lung transplant cases. This rate can be as high as 40% in combined heart-lung transplantation [14, 15]. Diaphragmatic dysfunction as a consequence of phrenic nerve injury can present clinically with dyspnea, hypoventilation and hypercapnia, and hypoxemia or as difficult wean from the ventilator. Diaphragmatic paralysis can lead to increased length of stay and ventilator dependence. Diagnosis can be confirmed by documenting paradoxical movement of affected diaphragm during quiet and deep breathing, using fluoroscopy or ultrasound visualization.

The vagal nerve injury post-lung transplantation can lead to gastroparesis with associated risk of gastroesophageal reflux (GERD) and aspiration events. These in turn can place lung allograft at risk for recurrent infections, bronchiectasis, and possibly chronic allograft dysfunction [16–18]. Common symptoms of gastroparesis include early satiety, decreased appetite, abdominal pain, and bloating. A diagnosis is usually made by a nuclear medicine gastric emptying study. The potential management strategies include minimizing transit delaying medications (e.g., opioids), the use of pro-motility agents, placement of post-pyloric feeding tubes, botulinum toxin injection to the pylorus, and surgical fundoplication in conjunction with pyloroplasty [17].

Pleural Complications

The pleural complications in early post-lung transplantation period include pleural effusions, hemothorax, pneumothorax, empyema, chylothorax, and interpleural communication. These complications usually arise as a result of the pleural disruption from the surgery itself, though rejection and immunosuppressive regimens may also play a role. The risk factors for the development of pleural complications include previous thoracic surgery, pleural adhesions, and donor-recipient size mismatch [19, 20].

Pleural effusions are extremely common in the early post-lung transplant period. The reported incidence has been 100% in some series [19, 20]. All patients have chest tubes in place immediately post-operation to allow lung re-expansion, pleural air, and fluid drainage. The increased amount of pleural fluid post-lung transplantation is related to capillary leak due to allograft ischemia reperfusion, fluid overload, bleeding, and surgical interruption of allograft lymphatics at the time of explantation [19, 20].

Late pleural effusions can be a consequence of infection, acute rejection, trapped lung physiology from pleural fibrosis, or malignancy [21, 22].

In general, all pleural effusions need to be evaluated to rule out complicated effusions such as hemothorax, empyema, and chylothorax. These entities have all been associated with negative patient outcomes and are treated with a range of medical and surgical procedures depending on the condition and severity. For example, a chylothorax might necessitate mechanical interruption of thoracic duct, or hemothorax may need thoracotomy for control of bleeding.

Pneumothoraxes are common after lung transplantation. They can result from donor-recipient size mismatch, bronchopleural fistulas that occur secondary to operative injury or bronchial anastomoses dehiscence, or as a consequence of transbronchial biopsies performed in the course of allograft evaluation. Small and stable pneumothoraxes after lung transplantation can be managed by watchful waiting, though larger or symptomatic pneumothorax may require chest tube drainage. An inadequately drained, hemodynamically significant pneumothorax can be a medical emergency necessitating urgent drainage [23, 24]. In patients who have undergone sequential bilateral lung transplantation (BSLT) or heart-lung transplantation (HLT), interpleural communication due to surgical severance of the pleural recesses that separate the left and right pleural spaces can develop. This entails that pleural issues in these patients must be managed aggressively as pneumothoraxes can be bilateral and life threatening, and empyema can spread quickly.

Vascular Anastomotic Complications

Vascular anastomotic complications can arise either early or late in the post-transplant course and can have very severe adverse consequences. Pulmonary artery stenosis can be secondary to mechanical kinking, disruption, or narrowing of the anastomosis, sometimes due to the particulars of donor anatomy or due to thrombosis [25]. The clinical picture is usually consistent with pulmonary hypertension and right ventricular failure. Diagnosis can be made through pulmonary angiography and can be managed with interventions such as balloon dilation and stent deployment. Occasionally, patients may require surgery for definitive management of the stenosis.

Pulmonary vein occlusion post-lung transplantation is a rare but serious complication. The commonest cause of pulmonary vein occlusion is the development of thrombosis at the anastomotic junction of the pulmonary veins and the left atrium, though inadvertent narrowing or ligation of pulmonary veins has also been reported. The potential clinical consequences include hypoxic respiratory failure, pulmonary edema, and cardio-embolic events. This entity should be included in the differential diagnosis of a patient with acute pulmonary edema post-lung transplantation. Diagnosis is usually made by transesophageal echocardiography or CT angiography [26, 27].

Airway Anastomotic Complications

The airway complications after lung transplantation can be classified by time of occurrence. Early anastomotic complications, usually within 1 month of transplantation, include infection, dehiscence, and necrosis at the anastomotic sites. Later complications include bronchopleural, bronchovascular and bronchomediastinal fistulae, excessive granulation tissue, bronchomalacia, and airway stenosis. Airway anastomotic complications do not seem to be associated with decreased survival; however, they do negatively impact quality of life and significantly increase healthcare resource utilization [28].

The risk factors for airway anastomotic complications include colonization with *Burkholderia cepacia* and *Aspergillus fumigatus*, PGD, acute rejection, prolonged mechanical ventilation, and sirolimus use prior to anastomotic healing [29, 30].

Bronchial necrosis and dehiscence occur 1–2 weeks after transplant. They can present with dyspnea, difficulty weaning from the ventilator, persistent air leak on the water seal, pneumomediastinum, and subcutaneous emphysema and infection, with symptoms ranging from mild to severe. Depending on the severity, management can range from observation and antibiotics to minimally invasive or surgical repair.

Bronchial stenosis is the narrowing of the airway lumen, usually at the site of the anastomosis. Patients can present with wheezing, cough, post-obstructive pneumonias, decline in pulmonary function tests (PFTs), and stridor. The bronchial narrowing can also present distal to the anastomosis causing lobar lobe collapse. This syndrome occurs 2–6 months post-transplant but can present as late as 12 months. Treatment options include close monitoring, bronchial dilatation with or without stent placement, and re-transplantation [31].

Rejection

Allograft rejection is a major cause of morbidity and mortality post-lung transplantation. At least a third of patients are reported to have acute rejection in the first year after transplant. Acute rejection in itself seldom leads to mortality, but it is a main risk factor for the development of chronic rejection. The chronic rejection of lung allograft is the major hurdle to long-term survival after transplantation. Despite the use of potent and novel immunosuppressive regimens, the incidence of chronic rejection and long-term survival post-transplant has remained essentially unchanged over the last two decades [1, 32].

Acute Cellular Rejection

Acute cellular rejection (ACR) is the most common kind of acute lung transplant rejection and is mediated by T lymphocytes. Symptoms and signs of ACR include dyspnea, cough, fever, and hypoxia. High-grade rejection may be associated with respiratory failure. Mild ACR can be asymptomatic and frequently detected on surveillance pulmonary function testing and/or transbronchial biopsies. Current imaging modalities are not diagnostic but may reveal useful findings such as infiltrates and ground-glass opacities [32, 33]. Flexible bronchoscopy with transbronchial biopsies is the gold standard for diagnosis. Histologically, ACR is characterized by the presence of perivascular and/or peribronchiolar (grade B) lymphocytes in the absence of infectious etiologies [32, 34, 35]. Risk factors for ACR include the number of HLA mismatches between donor and recipient, although it is unclear which specific HLAs have more impact. Other reported risk factors are age, with older patients having more rejection, immunosuppressive regimen used (tacrolimus regimens reject less), other genetic factors such as IL-10 production,

and documented GERD. ACR has also been documented following infections with certain viruses, such as rhinovirus, parainfluenza virus, influenza virus, human metapneumovirus, coronavirus, and respiratory syncytial virus.

The treatment for ACR is not uniform, and high-quality randomized controlled trials are lacking. There is wide agreement that severe cases of ACR must be treated, but there is variability among transplant centers on whether to treat milder cases. The mainstay of therapy is high-dose corticosteroids. In cases that are refractory or recurrent, usually the immunosuppressive regimen gets intensified or altered, and medications such as anti-thymocyte globulin (ATG), anti-interleukin 2-receptor (IL-2R) antagonists, muromonab-CD3 (OKT3), and alemtuzumab (anti-CD52 monoclonal antibody), among others, can be used [36, 37].

Antibody-Mediated Rejection

Antibody-mediated rejection (AMR) is believed to be mediated by donor-specific antibodies (DSA) against human leukocyte antigens (HLA) and other donor antigens. These antibodies may have been present in the recipient prior to transplant, although most appear to develop after transplantation. AMR is described as the combination of the following: donor-specific anti-HLA antibodies, evidence of complement deposition in allograft biopsies, histologic tissue injury, and clinical allograft dysfunction [38]. Once the aforementioned antibodies bind their receptors in the graft, they are capable of binding complement, specifically C1q. This can trigger complement-mediated cell destruction and inflammation. The development of de novo anti-HLA antibodies is associated with poor prognosis [39, 40].

The mainstay of AMR management involves depletion and/or neutralization of anti-HLA antibodies by plasma exchange or intravenous immunoglobulin (IVIG), followed by rituximab infusion. Rituximab is an anti-CD-20 chimeric antibody that targets B-cell function and can decrease production of antibodies. In cases of refractory AMR, newer agents such as bortezomib (anti-proteasome 26s) and the anticomplement antibody eculizumab have been tried with limited success. Successful clearance of anti-HLA antibodies has been associated with decreased risk of development of chronic rejection following AMR [32].

Chronic Lung Allograft Dysfunction

The term chronic lung allograft dysfunction (CLAD) encompasses pathologies that lead to chronic dysfunction of lung allograft. CLAD is predominantly a consequence of chronic rejection and is a major hurdle to long-term survival. The two major phenotypes of CLAD include (i) bronchiolitis obliterans syndrome (BOS) and (ii) restrictive allograft syndrome (RAS) [41, 42].

BOS is the predominant form of CLAD and is the number one cause of death after 1 year of transplantation. It is reported to occur in up to 76% of lung transplant recipients at 10 years post-transplant, and it is a major cause of morbidity, negative impact in quality of life, and increased costs. BOS is defined by a sustained (>3 weeks) decline in the forced expiratory volume in the first second of expiration (FEV1); provided alternative causes of pulmonary dysfunction have been excluded. At the tissue level, the hallmark of BOS is obliterative bronchiolitis (OB), which is an inflammatory/fibrotic process affecting the small non-cartilaginous airways (membranous and respiratory bronchioles) characterized by subepithelial fibrosis causing partial or complete luminal occlusion [43, 44].

Risk factors include prior episodes of acute rejection, cytomegalovirus infection (CMV), community-acquired respiratory viruses (CARV) infection, history of PGD, isolation of *Aspergillus fumigatus* and *Pseudomonas aeruginosa*, the presence of GERD, and other immune-mediated factors [44]. The diagnosis can be made conditionally without histopathology (BOS) or definitively with histopathology (BO). Transbronchial biopsy is an insensitive method for detecting BO, and the clinical use of BOS is the favored method for diagnosis and monitoring.

The treatment of BOS is disappointing in terms of outcomes; often success is measured in slowing the decline or stabilizing it. Beyond augmentation of immunosuppression, azithromycin, extracorporeal photopheresis, montelukast, methotrexate, aerosolized cyclosporine, alemtuzumab, and total lymphoid irradiation have been used with limited success [44, 45].

RAS has been more recently described and occurs in less than a third of patients with CLAD. These patients present with predominant restriction, and the survival is worse as compared to patients with BOS. The median survival post-diagnosis is 8 months. CT scan shows interstitial opacities, ground-glass opacities, upper lobe-dominant fibrosis, and honeycombing. The only identified risk factor for the development of RAS is late-onset diffuse alveolar damage (DAD), occurring later than 3 months after lung transplant. There is no proven treatment for this condition, and re-transplantation remains technically challenging [46, 47].

Post-transplant Malignancies

Lung transplant and associated immunosuppression are an established risk factor for development of cancer [48]. The commonest malignancy post-lung transplant is the squamous cell cancer of the skin. The single-lung transplant recipients are at higher risk of development of lung cancer in their native lungs. This increased risk is in part related to the increased risk of cancer due to underlying disease (e.g., emphysema, idiopathic pulmonary fibrosis) [49, 50]. Similarly, the transplant recipients with cystic fibrosis remain

at an elevated risk for development of gastrointestinal malignancies [49]. It is imperative that transplant recipients adhere to age-appropriate health screening after transplant. Additionally, all lung transplant recipients should undergo skin cancer screening annually.

The risk is especially high for of viral infection associated malignancies such as lymphoma, Kaposi sarcoma, and anogenital cancers [49]. Post-transplant lymphoproliferative disorders (PTLD) encompass an array of diseases involving clonal expansion of B lymphocytes, ranging from polyclonal benign disorders to aggressive malignant lymphomas. The reported incidence of non-Hodgkin lymphoma post-lung transplant has been as high as 28 cases/100,000 person-years [49]. There is a significant association between PTLD and Epstein-Barr virus (EBV) infection, especially in patients who acquire infection the novo after being transplanted. PTLD is managed by reducing the intensity of immunosuppression if possible, with specific chemotherapy for more severe and refractory cases.

Metabolic Complications

Hyperammonemia

Hyperammonemia affects 1–4% of the lung transplant population; it is a rare but potentially fatal complication. It can be secondary to systemic infection with *Mycoplasma hominis* and *Ureaplasma*, which break down urea as an energy source, generating ammonia as a waste product. This likely represents a donor-derived infection and can respond to early appropriate antibiotic treatment [51]. Postoperative liver dysfunction and urea-cycle enzyme deficiencies can also cause hyperammonemia.

Diabetes Mellitus

Diabetes mellitus (DM) is common in lung transplant recipients, with 25–30% of patients developing it in the first year post-transplant and up to 40% at 5 years. The use of glucocorticoids, calcineurin inhibitors, obesity, and advanced age is a significant risk factor for the development of DM. The development of DM in lung transplant recipients is associated with decreased survival. A close and judicious glycemic control is indicated in this patient population [52, 53].

Acute Kidney Injury and Chronic Kidney Disease

Patients who undergo lung transplantation have multiple risk factors to develop acute kidney injury (AKI) post-transplant, including decreased renal perfusion before, during, and/or after surgery, drug toxicities, and systemic infections. AKI affects as many as 70% of patients with approximately 8% patients requiring renal replacement therapy (RRT). The postoperative renal failure necessitating the use of RRT is associated with increased risk of early mortality [54, 55].

By 3 years, 25% of surviving lung transplant recipients develop severe renal dysfunction (serum creatinine >2.5 mg/dl), and that percentage rises to 40% at 10-year mark [1]. The risk factors for development of chronic kidney disease (CKD) include older age, DM, hypertension, smoking history, and use of nephrotoxic drugs. CKD is also associated with higher mortality in lung transplant recipients [56].

Other Metabolic Complications

Recipients of lung transplant are at risk for development of osteopenia and osteoporosis due to multiple factors such as malnutrition, immobility, chronic corticosteroid use, calcineurin inhibitor use (e.g., tacrolimus), and other comorbidities. The strategies to prevent and reverse bone losses after transplant need to be proactively implemented. Treatment includes adequate supplementation of calcium, vitamin D, use of bisphosphonates, enhancing physical activity, and minimizing contributing medications, if possible [57, 58].

Dyslipidemia is also very common in lung transplant recipients, as high as 59%, and it may be related to the aforementioned metabolic risk factors. Treatment usually entails lifestyle modifications and cholesterol lowering medications.

Cardiovascular Complications

There are multiple cardiac complications after lung transplantation, both short and long term. Atrial dysrhythmias are very frequent in the early postoperative period, likely related to stress of major surgery, catecholamine surge, medication side effects, and mechanical stresses related to vascular anastomoses. The reported incidence has been as high as 25–35% [59, 60]. These arrhythmias are usually managed with medications aimed at rate and rhythm control. Hemodynamically significant and/or refractory arrhythmias may require electric cardioversion. Atrial dysrhythmias are associated with increased length of hospital stay and increased mortality [59, 60].

Over the long term, lung transplant recipients are at increased risk for developing coronary artery disease (CAD). As they progress into long-term survival, these patients have cumulative impact from risk factors previously discussed in this chapter, namely, DM, dyslipidemia, CKD, hypertension, chronic corticosteroid use, and other immunosuppressive medication. These risk factors should be carefully managed to decrease the impact of CAD and related complications, with a combination of lifestyle modifications and specific medical therapies [61].

Miscellaneous Issues

Lung transplant recipients experience a decrease in skeletal muscle strength and function, including respiratory and limb muscles. This is likely related to reduced activity postoperatively and deconditioning, corticosteroid-induced myopathy, critical illness-related weakness (neuropathy/myopathy), and in the case of the diaphragm, phrenic nerve injury. This issue seems to be consistent in lung transplant recipients and independent of pre-transplant diagnosis and surgery type. Muscle weakness, deconditioning, and sarcopenia are associated with adverse outcomes and decrease in quality of life. Aggressive rehabilitation is standard and important in the post-transplant care [62, 63].

Infectious Complications

Lung transplant recipients are at an increased risk for acquiring infections due to the immunosuppressed state, constant environmental pathogen exposure, decreased cough reflex, impaired mucociliary clearance, and lymphatic disruption. Infectious complications are responsible for about a quarter of post-transplant deaths [64].

Bacterial Infections

Pneumonias are the most significant bacterial infection in lung transplant recipients, and the highest risk is in the first 30 days post-transplant. In the early period, they are more likely to be caused by hospital-acquired organisms, which tend to be more virulent and more resistant to antibiotics. The patients with cystic fibrosis are frequently colonized by multidrug-resistant organisms and are at increased risk of pneumonia post-transplant. In later stages, community-acquired organisms become more prevalent. Moreover, throughout the post-transplant period, the patients are susceptible to numerous opportunistic infections [65].

Other commonly encountered bacterial infections in this patient population include pleural space infections, blood stream infections (BSIs), and soft tissue infections. The BSIs and empyema carry a high risk of morbidity and mortality [66, 67].

Pseudomonas aeruginosa, Burkholderia cepacia, Staphylococcus aureus (including methicillin-resistant), and other gram-negative organisms are common causes of serious infections in post-lung transplant period. These organisms have high rates of antibiotic resistance and are associated with worse outcomes [68–70]. *Streptococcus pneumoniae* is the most common cause of community-acquired pneumonia, and immunosuppressed patients have increased risk of disseminated infection [71]. *Clostridium difficile* associated diarrhea is a major complication in hospitalized, immunosuppressed and debilitated patients and is associated with increased hospital length of stay and mortality [72].

Fungal Infections

Molds are common fungal entities affecting lung allografts. *Aspergillus spp.* are the most common and have a predilection for the respiratory tract [73]. Lung transplants have the highest incidence of invasive aspergillosis among solid organ transplant recipients, and it is the most common invasive fungal infection in lung transplant. Aspergillus is ubiquitous in the environment and is acquired by inhalation. There are three main described presentations: invasive pulmonary disease, tracheobronchial aspergillosis, and disseminated disease, all of which are associated with varying degrees of increased mortality. Other implicated molds include *Fusarium, Scedosporium*, and Mucormycosis. These infections are difficult to treat and are associated with poor clinical outcomes [73]. *Candida* spp. are another common pathogen in lung transplant setting. Oral candidiasis is the most common manifestation of this infection. However, candida infections can also manifest as candidemia, empyema, surgical wound infection, and disseminated disease. Serious candida infections have been associated with increased mortality, though rates have been declining over time [74]. Other fungal infections in this patient population include opportunistic infections, such as *Pneumocystis jiroveci and Cryptococcus,* as well as endemic fungi, such as *Histoplasma capsulatum, Coccidioides immitis*, and *Blastomyces dermatitidis* [75, 76].

Viral Infections

Viral infections contribute to morbidity and mortality from acute infection and have been associated with an increased risk of rejection, chronic allograft dysfunction, lymphoproliferative and other neoplastic diseases, and other extra pulmonary organ damage [77].

Cytomegalovirus (CMV) is the most significant viral infection occurring in solid organ transplant recipients and is the second most common infection, after bacterial pneumonia. CMV infection can range from latent infection, to asymptomatic viremia, to CMV disease manifested with clinical symptoms and end-organ involvement. Severity of disease may range from mild to life threatening. When there is organ damage, affected organs can include the lungs, pancreas, intestines, retina, kidney, liver, and brain. CMV disease is associated with increased mortality [77, 78]. Other notable DNA viruses from the Herpesviridae family include Epstein-Barr virus (EBV), which is associated with increased risk of PTLD and other malignancies, *herpes simplex virus* (HSV) 1 and 2, *varicella-zoster virus* (VZV), and human *Herpesvirus* 6, 7, and 8 [77].

Community-acquired respiratory viruses, including influenza, are a major source of respiratory symptoms and morbidity after lung transplantation. These infections may also be associated with development of chronic allograft dysfunction [79].

Survival, Overall Prognosis, and Follow-Up Care

Currently, the median survival for all adult lung transplant recipients is 6 years [1]. Bilateral lung recipients appear to have a better median survival compared to single-lung recipients (7 versus 4.5 years) [1]. Overall lung transplantation confers clinically meaningful and statistically significant improvements in health-related quality of life (HRQOL). Greater than 80% of lung transplant recipients report no activity limitations [80].

The care of lung transplant recipients is multidisciplinary, labor intensive, and comprehensive. It includes management of immunosuppression regimen, opportunistic infection prophylaxis, prevention and management of various comorbidities, and complications. A typical medication regimen consists of three classes of immunosuppression drugs (i.e., calcineurin inhibitor, cell-cycle inhibitor, and corticosteroids), as well as opportunistic infection prophylaxis against *Pneumocystis jiroveci, other fungal infections, and CMV.*

In early postoperative period and after hospital discharge, the recipients are closely monitored in outpatient setting. Typical clinic visits include thorough medication reconciliation, clinical exam, pulmonary function testing, chest radiographs, and laboratory examinations. The role of surveillance bronchoscopies with transbronchial biopsies in monitoring of lung allograft remains unclear.

Conclusions

While lung transplantation improves survival and quality of life in patients with end-stage lung disease, it is associated with multitude of noninfectious and infectious complications. Lung transplant recipients have one of the shortest survival rates among other solid organ recipients, due to some unique characteristics of the lung allograft, including its unique blood supply and risk for ischemia, disruption of the native lymphatics and the neural supply during the transplant surgery, and exposure to immunogenic entities via ventilation. Among noninfectious complications, PGD, VTE, and rejection are the most important ones. CLAD affects most patients long term and remains a significant clinical concern and contributor to early mortality in lung transplant recipients. Lung transplant recipients are also at increased risk for a variety of malignancies, due to their underlying disease, comorbidities, and immunosuppressed status; thus they require vigilant monitoring and screening for cancer. Infectious complications (i.e., bacterial, fungal, viral) are also important contributors to morbidity and mortality, with bacterial pneumonias and CMV most commonly seen. Patients require multidisciplinary and intensive follow-up and aftercare, ongoing vigilance, early recognition and treatment, and open and frequent communication between recipients, caregivers, and healthcare team providers.

References

1. Yusen RD, Christie JD, Edwards LB, Kucheryavaya AY, Benden C, Dipchand AI, et al. The registry of the International Society for Heart and Lung Transplantation: thirtieth adult lung and heart-lung transplant report--2013; focus theme: age. J Heart Lung Transplant. 2013;32(10):965–78.
2. Gross CR, Savik K, Bolman RM 3rd, Hertz MI. Long-term health status and quality of life outcomes of lung transplant recipients. Chest. 1995;108(6):1587–93.
3. Lund LH, Khush KK, Cherikh WS, Goldfarb S, Kucheryavaya AY, Levvey BJ, et al. The registry of the International Society for Heart and Lung Transplantation: thirty-fourth adult heart transplantation Report-2017; focus theme: allograft ischemic time. J Heart Lung Transplant. 2017;36(10):1037–46.
4. Contreras AG, Briscoe DM. Every allograft needs a silver lining. J Clin Invest. 2007;117(12):3645–8.
5. Dhillon GS, Zamora MR, Roos JE, Sheahan D, Sista RR, Van der Starre P, et al. Lung transplant airway hypoxia: a diathesis to fibrosis? Am J Respir Crit Care Med. 2010;182(2):230–6.
6. Nicolls MR, Dhillon GS, Daddi N. A critical role for airway microvessels in lung transplantation. Am J Respir Crit Care Med. 2016;193(5):479–81.
7. Ahmad S, Shlobin OA, Nathan SD. Pulmonary complications of lung transplantation. Chest. 2011;139(2):402–11.
8. Snell GI, Yusen RD, Weill D, Strueber M, Garrity E, Reed A, et al. Report of the ISHLT working group on primary lung graft dysfunction, part I: definition and grading-a 2016 consensus group statement of the International Society for Heart and Lung Transplantation. J Heart Lung Transplant. 2017;36(10):1097–103.
9. Gelman AE, Fisher AJ, Huang HJ, Baz MA, Shaver CM, Egan TM, et al. Report of the ISHLT working group on primary lung graft dysfunction part III: mechanisms: a 2016 consensus group statement of the International Society for Heart and Lung Transplantation. J Heart Lung Transplant. 2017;36(10):1114–20.
10. Diamond JM, Arcasoy S, Kennedy CC, Eberlein M, Singer JP, Patterson GM, et al. Report of the International Society for Heart and Lung Transplantation working group on primary lung graft dysfunction, part II: epidemiology, risk factors, and outcomes-a 2016 consensus group statement of the International Society for Heart and Lung Transplantation. J Heart Lung Transplant. 2017;36(10):1104–13.
11. Van Raemdonck D, Hartwig MG, Hertz MI, Davis RD, Cypel M, Hayes D Jr, et al. Report of the ISHLT working group on primary lung graft dysfunction part IV: prevention and treatment: a 2016 consensus group statement of the International Society for Heart and Lung Transplantation. J Heart Lung Transplant. 2017;36(10):1121–36.
12. Evans CF, Iacono AT, Sanchez PG, Goloubeva O, Kim J, Timofte I, et al. Venous thromboembolic complications of lung transplantation: a contemporary single-institution review. Ann Thorac Surg. 2015;100(6):2033–9; discussion 9–40.
13. Noda S, Sundt TM 3rd, Lynch JP, Trulock EP, Sundaresan S, Patterson GA. Pulmonary embolectomy after single-lung transplantation. Ann Thorac Surg. 1997;64(5):1459–61.
14. Maziak DE, Maurer JR, Kesten S. Diaphragmatic paralysis: a complication of lung transplantation. Ann Thorac Surg. 1996;61(1):170–3.
15. Ferdinande P, Bruyninckx F, Van Raemdonck D, Daenen W, Verleden G. Leuven lung transplant G. Phrenic nerve dysfunction after heart-lung and lung transplantation. J Heart Lung Transplant. 2004;23(1):105–9.
16. Shafi MA, Pasricha PJ. Post-surgical and obstructive gastroparesis. Curr Gastroenterol Rep. 2007;9(4):280–5.
17. Hooft N, Smith M, Huang J, Bremner R, Walia R. Gastroparesis is common after lung transplantation and may be ameliorated by botulinum toxin-a injection of the pylorus. J Heart Lung Transplant. 2014;33(12):1314–6.
18. Au J, Hawkins T, Venables C, Morritt G, Scott CD, Gascoigne AD, et al. Upper gastrointestinal dysmotility in heart-lung transplant recipients. Ann Thorac Surg. 1993;55(1):94–7.
19. Ferrer J, Roldan J, Roman A, Bravo C, Monforte V, Pallissa E, et al. Acute and chronic pleural complications in lung transplantation. J Heart Lung Transplant. 2003;22(11):1217–25.
20. Arndt A, Boffa DJ. Pleural space complications associated with lung transplantation. Thorac Surg Clin. 2015;25(1):87–95.
21. Judson MA, Handy JR, Sahn SA. Pleural effusion from acute lung rejection. Chest. 1997;111(4):1128–30.
22. Chhajed PN, Bubendorf L, Hirsch H, Boehler A, Weder W, Tamm M. Mesothelioma after lung transplantation. Thorax. 2006;61(10):916–7.
23. Paranjpe DV, Wittich GR, Hamid LW, Bergin CJ. Frequency and management of pneumothoraces in heart-lung transplant recipients. Radiology. 1994;190(1):255–6.
24. Engeler CE, Olson PN, Engeler CM, Carpenter BL, Crowe JE, Day DL, et al. Shifting pneumothorax after heart-lung transplantation. Radiology. 1992;185(3):715–7.
25. Anaya-Ayala JE, Loebe M, Davies MG. Endovascular management of early lung transplant-related anastomotic pulmonary artery stenosis. J Vasc Interv Radiol. 2015;26(6):878–82.
26. Schulman LL, Anandarangam T, Leibowitz DW, Ditullio MR, McGregor CC, Galantowicz ME, et al. Four-year prospective study of pulmonary venous thrombosis after lung transplantation. J Am Soc Echocardiogr. 2001;14(8):806–12.
27. Gonzalez-Fernandez C, Gonzalez-Castro A, Rodriguez-Borregan JC, Lopez-Sanchez M, Suberviola B, Francisco Nistal J, et al. Pulmonary venous obstruction after lung transplantation. Diagnostic advantages of transesophageal echocardiography. Clin Transpl. 2009;23(6):975–80.
28. Meyers BF, de la Morena M, Sweet SC, Trulock EP, Guthrie TJ, Mendeloff EN, et al. Primary graft dysfunction and other selected complications of lung transplantation: a single-center experience of 983 patients. J Thorac Cardiovasc Surg. 2005;129(6):1421–9.
29. Santacruz JF, Mehta AC. Airway complications and management after lung transplantation: ischemia, dehiscence, and stenosis. Proc Am Thorac Soc. 2009;6(1):79–93.
30. Herrera JM, McNeil KD, Higgins RS, Coulden RA, Flower CD, Nashef SA, et al. Airway complications after lung transplantation: treatment and long-term outcome. Ann Thorac Surg. 2001;71(3):989–93; discussion 93–4.
31. Hasegawa T, Iacono AT, Orons PD, Yousem SA. Segmental non-anastomotic bronchial stenosis after lung transplantation. Ann Thorac Surg. 2000;69(4):1020–4.
32. McManigle W, Pavlisko EN, Martinu T. Acute cellular and antibody-mediated allograft rejection. Semin Respir Crit Care Med. 2013;34(3):320–35.
33. De Vito DA, Hoffman LA, Iacono AT, Zullo TG, McCurry KR, Dauber JH. Are symptom reports useful for differentiating between acute rejection and pulmonary infection after lung transplantation? Heart Lung. 2004;33(6):372–80.

34. Trulock EP, Ettinger NA, Brunt EM, Pasque MK, Kaiser LR, Cooper JD. The role of transbronchial lung biopsy in the treatment of lung transplant recipients. An analysis of 200 consecutive procedures. Chest. 1992;102(4):1049–54.

35. Stewart S, Fishbein MC, Snell GI, Berry GJ, Boehler A, Burke MM, et al. Revision of the 1996 working formulation for the standardization of nomenclature in the diagnosis of lung rejection. J Heart Lung Transplant. 2007;26(12):1229–42.

36. Martinu T, Pavlisko EN, Chen DF, Palmer SM. Acute allograft rejection: cellular and humoral processes. Clin Chest Med. 2011;32(2):295–310.

37. Levine SM. Transplant/immunology network of the American College of Chest P. A survey of clinical practice of lung transplantation in North America. Chest. 2004;125(4):1224–38.

38. Levine DJ, Glanville AR, Aboyoun C, Belperio J, Benden C, Berry GJ, et al. Antibody-mediated rejection of the lung: a consensus report of the International Society for Heart and Lung Transplantation. J Heart Lung Transplant. 2016;35(4):397–406.

39. Witt CA, Gaut JP, Yusen RD, Byers DE, Iuppa JA, Bennett Bain K, et al. Acute antibody-mediated rejection after lung transplantation. J Heart Lung Transplant. 2013;32(10):1034–40.

40. Morrell MR, Patterson GA, Trulock EP, Hachem RR. Acute antibody-mediated rejection after lung transplantation. J Heart Lung Transplant. 2009;28(1):96–100.

41. Verleden SE, Vos R, Vanaudenaerde BM, Verleden GM. Chronic lung allograft dysfunction phenotypes and treatment. J Thorac Dis. 2017;9(8):2650–9.

42. Gauthier JM, Hachem RR, Kreisel D. Update on chronic lung allograft dysfunction. Curr Transplant Rep. 2016;3(3):185–91.

43. Weigt SS, DerHovanessian A, Wallace WD, Lynch JP 3rd, Belperio JA. Bronchiolitis obliterans syndrome: the Achilles' heel of lung transplantation. Semin Respir Crit Care Med. 2013;34(3):336–51.

44. Meyer KC, Raghu G, Verleden GM, Corris PA, Aurora P, Wilson KC, et al. An international ISHLT/ATS/ERS clinical practice guideline: diagnosis and management of bronchiolitis obliterans syndrome. Eur Respir J. 2014;44(6):1479–503.

45. Benden C, Haughton M, Leonard S, Huber LC. Therapy options for chronic lung allograft dysfunction-bronchiolitis obliterans syndrome following first-line immunosuppressive strategies: a systematic review. J Heart Lung Transplant. 2017;36(9):921–33.

46. Verleden SE, Vandermeulen E, Ruttens D, Vos R, Vaneylen A, Dupont LJ, et al. Neutrophilic reversible allograft dysfunction (NRAD) and restrictive allograft syndrome (RAS). Semin Respir Crit Care Med. 2013;34(3):352–60.

47. Sato M, Waddell TK, Wagnetz U, Roberts HC, Hwang DM, Haroon A, et al. Restrictive allograft syndrome (RAS): a novel form of chronic lung allograft dysfunction. J Heart Lung Transplant. 2011;30(7):735–42.

48. Collett D, Mumford L, Banner NR, Neuberger J, Watson C. Comparison of the incidence of malignancy in recipients of different types of organ: a UK registry audit. Am J Transplant. 2010;10(8):1889–96.

49. Engels EA, Pfeiffer RM, Fraumeni JF Jr, Kasiske BL, Israni AK, Snyder JJ, et al. Spectrum of cancer risk among US solid organ transplant recipients. JAMA. 2011;306(17):1891–901.

50. Arcasoy SM, Hersh C, Christie JD, Zisman D, Pochettino A, Rosengard BR, et al. Bronchogenic carcinoma complicating lung transplantation. J Heart Lung Transplant. 2001;20(10):1044–53.

51. Bharat A, Cunningham SA, Scott Budinger GR, Kreisel D, DeWet CJ, Gelman AE, et al. Disseminated ureaplasma infection as a cause of fatal hyperammonemia in humans. Sci Transl Med. 2015;7(284):284re3.

52. Ye X, Kuo HT, Sampaio MS, Jiang Y, Bunnapradist S. Risk factors for development of new-onset diabetes mellitus after transplant in adult lung transplant recipients. Clin Transpl. 2011;25(6):885–91.

53. Hackman KL, Snell GI, Bach LA. Prevalence and predictors of diabetes after lung transplantation: a prospective, longitudinal study. Diabetes Care. 2014;37(11):2919–25.

54. Wehbe E, Brock R, Budev M, Xu M, Demirjian S, Schreiber MJ Jr, et al. Short-term and long-term outcomes of acute kidney injury after lung transplantation. J Heart Lung Transplant. 2012;31(3):244–51.

55. Fidalgo P, Ahmed M, Meyer SR, Lien D, Weinkauf J, Cardoso FS, et al. Incidence and outcomes of acute kidney injury following orthotopic lung transplantation: a population-based cohort study. Nephrol Dial Transplant. 2014;29(9):1702–9.

56. Paradela de la Morena M, De La Torre BM, Prado RF, Roel MD, Salcedo JA, Costa EF, et al. Chronic kidney disease after lung transplantation: incidence, risk factors, and treatment. Transplant Proc. 2010;42(8):3217–9.

57. Yu TM, Lin CL, Chang SN, Sung FC, Huang ST, Kao CH. Osteoporosis and fractures after solid organ transplantation: a nationwide population-based cohort study. Mayo Clin Proc. 2014;89(7):888–95.

58. Shane E, Papadopoulos A, Staron RB, Addesso V, Donovan D, McGregor C, et al. Bone loss and fracture after lung transplantation. Transplantation. 1999;68(2):220–7.

59. Raghavan D, Gao A, Ahn C, Torres F, Mohanka M, Bollineni S, et al. Contemporary analysis of incidence of post-operative atrial fibrillation, its predictors, and association with clinical outcomes in lung transplantation. J Heart Lung Transplant. 2015;34(4):563–70.

60. Orrego CM, Cordero-Reyes AM, Estep JD, Seethamraju H, Scheinin S, Loebe M, et al. Atrial arrhythmias after lung transplant: underlying mechanisms, risk factors, and prognosis. J Heart Lung Transplant. 2014;33(7):734–40.

61. Silverborn M, Jeppsson A, Martensson G, Nilsson F. New-onset cardiovascular risk factors in lung transplant recipients. J Heart Lung Transplant. 2005;24(10):1536–43.

62. Maury G, Langer D, Verleden G, Dupont L, Gosselink R, Decramer M, et al. Skeletal muscle force and functional exercise tolerance before and after lung transplantation: a cohort study. Am J Transplant. 2008;8(6):1275–81.

63. Lands LC, Smountas AA, Mesiano G, Brosseau L, Shennib H, Charbonneau M, et al. Maximal exercise capacity and peripheral skeletal muscle function following lung transplantation. J Heart Lung Transplant. 1999;18(2):113–20.

64. Aguilar-Guisado M, Givalda J, Ussetti P, Ramos A, Morales P, Blanes M, et al. Pneumonia after lung transplantation in the RESITRA cohort: a multicenter prospective study. Am J Transplant. 2007;7(8):1989–96.

65. Clark NM, Reid GE, Practice ASTIDCo. Nocardia infections in solid organ transplantation. Am J Transplant. 2013;13(Suppl 4):83–92.

66. Palmer SM, Alexander BD, Sanders LL, Edwards LJ, Reller LB, Davis RD, et al. Significance of blood stream infection after lung transplantation: analysis in 176 consecutive patients. Transplantation. 2000;69(11):2360–6.

67. Nunley DR, Grgurich WF, Keenan RJ, Dauber JH. Empyema complicating successful lung transplantation. Chest. 1999;115(5):1312–5.

68. van Duin D, van Delden C, Practice ASTIDCo. Multidrug-resistant gram-negative bacteria infections in solid organ transplantation. Am J Transplant. 2013;13(Suppl 4):31–41.

69. Dobbin C, Maley M, Harkness J, Benn R, Malouf M, Glanville A, et al. The impact of pan-resistant bacterial pathogens on survival after lung transplantation in cystic fibrosis: results from a single large referral Centre. J Hosp Infect. 2004;56(4):277–82.

70. Garzoni C, Vergidis P, Practice ASTIDCo. Methicillin-resistant, vancomycin-intermediate and vancomycin-resistant Staphylococcus aureus infections in solid organ transplantation. Am J Transplant. 2013;13(Suppl 4):50–8.

71. de Bruyn G, Whelan TP, Mulligan MS, Raghu G, Limaye AP. Invasive pneumococcal infections in adult lung transplant recipients. Am J Transplant. 2004;4(8):1366–71.

72. Dubberke ER, Riddle DJ, Practice ASTIDCo. Clostridium difficile in solid organ transplant recipients. Am J Transplant. 2009;9(Suppl 4):S35–40.

73. Bhaskaran A, Hosseini-Moghaddam SM, Rotstein C, Husain S. Mold infections in lung transplant recipients. Semin Respir Crit Care Med. 2013;34(3):371–9.

74. Silveira FP, Husain S. Fungal infections in lung transplant recipients. Curr Opin Pulm Med. 2008;14(3):211–8.

75. Miller R, Assi M, Practice ASTIDCo. Endemic fungal infections in solid organ transplantation. Am J Transplant. 2013;13(Suppl 4):250–61.

76. Husain S, Wagener MM, Singh N. Cryptococcus neoformans infection in organ transplant recipients: variables influencing clinical characteristics and outcome. Emerg Infect Dis. 2001;7(3):375–81.

77. Clark NM, Lynch JP 3rd, Sayah D, Belperio JA, Fishbein MC, Weigt SS. DNA viral infections complicating lung transplantation. Semin Respir Crit Care Med. 2013;34(3):380–404.

78. Zamora MR. Cytomegalovirus and lung transplantation. Am J Transplant. 2004;4(8):1219–26.

79. Gottlieb J, Schulz TF, Welte T, Fuehner T, Dierich M, Simon AR, et al. Community-acquired respiratory viral infections in lung transplant recipients: a single season cohort study. Transplantation. 2009;87(10):1530–7.

80. Singer JP, Singer LG. Quality of life in lung transplantation. Semin Respir Crit Care Med. 2013;34(3):421–30.

Post-transplant Psychosocial and Mental Health Care of the Lung Recipient

Yelizaveta Sher

Introduction

Patients with advanced lung disease approaching lung transplantation (LTx) have increased rates of depression and anxiety, as well as cognitive dysfunction. Evaluation for LTx and the process of waiting on the transplant list evoke great hopes and anxieties. On one hand, patients are hopeful that they will be able to breathe again, be untethered from oxygen, regain their independence, and continue to live their normal lives. On the other hand, they are fearful of suffocating and not making it to the transplant surgery. Patients simultaneously hope for continued life and prepare for death. While some patients wait for a long time until "the Call" comes, others decompensate rapidly and are on life support in the intensive care unit (ICU) before they get their new set of lungs. Recovery can be brisk or excruciating. If patients do well, they experience a "honeymoon period" and rejoice in their recovery and newfound quality of life (QOL). However, for others the pace of the recovery and ongoing complications are frustrating and demoralizing. As medical setbacks after transplant develop (e.g., infections, rejection, and renal insufficiency), depression and anxiety sink in once again. Transplant-related post-traumatic stress disorder (PTSD-T) may develop in relation to the peri-transplant process. Existential questions about life and death continue.

Patients' Qualitative Experiences of Post-lung Transplantation

In their narrative analysis of four heart and seven lung transplant recipients, all of whom have experienced delirium post-transplant, Flynn et al. shared themes that these patients had lived through [1]. Participants had been on the waiting list between 3 weeks and 2.5 years, and the interviews took place between 6.5 months and 14 years after their transplant. Individuals shared that during the pre-transplant period, their medical decompensation was accompanied with a sense that life was taken away and death became a central character. As one participant shared, "You live all the time with Mr. Death on your shoulder." "The Call" was expected with both fear and reverence. After the transplant surgery, participants described their distressing experiences of delirium in the ICU: disorganization, hallucinations and delusions, lack of control and trust, feeling threatened, fear, and finally embarrassment following realization of their false perceptions. After transplantation, during the initial recovery phase, patients dealt with merging their initial belief of transplant being "a miracle cure" with the reality that this "second chance" is limited and can be taken away by rejection or any of the other potential complications associated with transplantation. They described the tremendous pressure from the society after having been given this "gift." They sensed immense responsibility for success or failure of their transplanted organ. For some patients, symptoms of PTSD-T were setting in, with flashbacks and nightmares, as they were confronted with their ICU memories of delusions and hallucinations. Finally, patients described the evolution of the "post-transplant person" as they worked on coming to grips with ever-looming death, dealing with uncertainty, and attempting to integrate their complex stories.

This narrative captivates the themes that mental health professionals frequently witness in patients' hospital rooms and the outpatient clinics as they work with LTx recipients. Helping patients to navigate through their hopes and fears of being on the transplant list, into the immediate post-transplant experience not infrequently marked by delirium and/or anxiety, and then to the long-term ongoing integration of the new reality, is both challenging and rewarding. It is important to know the clinical psychological conditions that patients might experience at different stages post-transplantation, as

Y. Sher
Department of Psychiatry & Behavioral Sciences, Stanford University School of Medicine, Stanford, CA, USA
e-mail: ysher@stanford.edu

© Springer International Publishing AG, part of Springer Nature 2019
Y. Sher, J. R. Maldonado (eds.), *Psychosocial Care of End-Stage Organ Disease and Transplant Patients*,
https://doi.org/10.1007/978-3-319-94914-7_27

well as to listen to the unique themes and concerns that each individual person experiences and voices.

Neuropsychiatric Disorders Post-lung Transplant

Delirium

Delirium is common among critically ill patients in ICUs [2]. It is a distressing experience for patients and families, with negative effects on patients' morbidity and mortality [2]. While neurologists have been reporting on high incidences of post-transplant encephalopathy in LTx recipients [3–5], parallel studies have also emerged on its psychiatric counterpart – delirium – and its significance.

The first study on delirium in LTx patients consisted of a retrospective analysis of 30 recipients. It found a 73% incidence of delirium within 2 weeks of LTx surgery [6]. In their population, delirium was associated with the use of cardiopulmonary bypass, higher cyclosporine levels, and physical relocation closer to the transplant center while awaiting surgery. A prospective study of 21 LTx recipients reported a 19% incidence of delirium within 96 hours of LTx surgery, associated with an increased time to extubation [7]. Smith et al. prospectively evaluated 63 LTx recipients with the Confusion Assessment Method (CAM) and found a 37% incidence of delirium in the immediate postoperative period [8]. The authors found that poor preoperative cognitive functioning was associated with delirium occurrence, while the presence and duration of delirium were associated with longer hospital stay [8]. In addition, they identified that lower cerebral perfusion pressure during LTx surgery doubled the risk and increased the duration and severity of delirium [9].

In the largest retrospective sample to date, Sher and colleagues analyzed the medical records and applied DSM-IV criteria to extracted information of 163 LTx recipients [10]. The authors found that 36% of patients developed early-onset (within 5 days of surgery) and 44% developed ever-onset (within 30 days or duration of hospitalization, whichever was shortest) delirium. Obesity (OR 6.35) and the use of benzodiazepines within the first postoperative day (OR 2.28) were associated with early-onset delirium. Patients with early-onset delirium were more likely to have longer duration of ventilation and hospital stay. In fact, patients with delirium were hospitalized on average 10 days longer after their LTx surgery compared to those without delirium [8, 10]. Although there was a trend, after adjusting for clinical variables, delirium was not significantly associated with 1-year mortality in this study (early-onset HR 1.65, 95% CI 0.67–4.03; ever-onset HR 1.70, 95% CI 0.63–4.55) [10].

Finally, a more recent retrospective study of 155 LTx recipients from the Lung Transplant Outcomes Group (LTOG) cohort similarly found the incidence of postoperative delirium to be 36.8% via a chart review delirium ascertainment method [11]. Identified independent risk factors for delirium included pre-transplant benzodiazepine prescription (relative risk [RR] 1.82), total ischemic time (RR 1.10 per 30-min increase), duration of time with intraoperative mean arterial pressure < 60 mmHg (RR 1.07 per 15-min increase), and Grade 3 primary graft dysfunction (RR 2.13). In addition, higher neuron-specific enolase (NSE) plasma levels were associated with delirium (risk difference 15.1% comparing 75th and 25th percentiles), suggesting that cerebral injury may contribute to delirium development. Similar to the findings in the Stanford study [10], 1-year mortality appeared higher among delirious patients in this study, 12.3% compared with 7.1%, but the difference was not statistically significant ($p = 0.28$).

These studies clearly indicate that delirium is not only common among LTx recipients, but that it is also associated with poor medical outcomes. Although the association with poorer survival is only now being examined with early follow-up time, it is a worrisome trend. Contributing etiologies that should be considered for post-LTx surgery delirium include primary graft dysfunction, brain hypoxia, neuroinflammation, infections, metabolic and electrolyte disturbances, renal insufficiency, ICU environment, and medications (e.g., opioids, benzodiazepines, steroids, immunosuppressants, voriconazole, lidocaine) [2, 5, 6, 10–12]. Additional etiologies to consider for altered mental status in this period include seizures and strokes [3–5, 13], as well as posterior reversible encephalopathy syndrome (PRES) [14–18].

As of now, there are no studies on treatment or prevention of delirium in LTx recipients. One suggested area for delirium prevention is optimization of brain perfusion during the LTx surgery [11]. Identifying patients with preoperative benzodiazepine use and tapering them off these agents if possible, as well as avoiding postoperative benzodiazepine use during the immediate post-transplant period, may be helpful with delirium prevention and consistent with identified risk factors [10, 11]. In addition, general non-pharmacological prophylaxis and treatment (e.g., early mobilization, reorientation, maintenance of sleep-wake cycle) are indicated and helpful. Antipsychotic agents (e.g., haloperidol, risperidone, quetiapine, or aripiprazole) can be used in LTx recipients, based on the presenting delirium motor type, associated comorbid factors, and medication benevit versus risk analysis. The safe use of high-dose intravenous (IV) haloperidol in an agitated delirium following LTx has been described in the literature [19].

Prevention and management of post-LTx delirium might be a much needed and important area of study in the near future.

Neurologic Events

Shigemura et al. retrospectively examined 759 LTx recipients for major neurologic complications (i.e., defined in the study as "potentially life-threatening events requiring urgent treatment/intubation or admission to ICU") within 2 weeks of transplant surgery [5]. The authors found that the majority of these events included stroke (41%) or severe toxic-metabolic encephalopathy, frequently induced by tacrolimus (37%). Of note, although criteria for *toxic-metabolic encephalopathy* diagnosis were not defined in the report, in clinical practice, this term is frequently synonymous with delirium. In general, patients with neurologic complications after LTx had shorter survival with a 90-day mortality of 15% in patients who developed neurologic complications versus 4% in patients who did not ($P = 0.03$). Similarly, the 5-year survival was 51.1% in patients who developed neurologic complication versus 62.1% in patients who did not ($P < 0.05$).

Mateen et al. studied 120 patients with a median survival of 4.8 years in a retrospective cohort [4]. They reported that 95 patients (79.2%) developed a neurologic complication at some point during the post-LTx period, with median time to complication of 0.8 years. Neurologic complications were severe to the point of requiring hospitalization or urgent evaluation and care in 46 patients (38.3%), most often including perioperative stroke or encephalopathy (defined in this study as "decreased attention and orientation with variable restlessness… [which was] prolonged (lasting at least 24 h) and/or clinically severe resulting in prolonged hospitalization or warranting a specialty consultation"). Age was a significant risk factor for any neurologic complication. Neurologic complications of any severity (HR 4.3) and high severity (HR 7.2) were associated with increased risk of death.

PRES is a rare (0.5–6% of solid organ transplant recipients) but significant neuropsychiatric complication that can be precipitated by the immunosuppressants, presumed to be caused by a disruption of the blood-brain barrier integrity [20]. The clinical presentation includes altered mental status, headaches, visual disturbances, seizures, and autonomic instability [20]. The diagnosis is usually confirmed by the classic radiologic findings involving edema of the white matter in the posterior regions of the brain, although this may not always be the case, and edema may affect other brain areas [20]. There have been several reports of PRES in LTx recipients [14–18]. Although PRES is classically associated with the use of calcineurin inhibitors (CNIs) [18], it has also been reported in context of non-CNI immunosuppressant use, such as sirolimus, in LTx recipients [17]. The condition is usually treated with prompt recognition, supportive measures, and most importantly decreasing or removing the offending immunosuppressant. This usually requires switching to a different immunosuppressant agent, which may itself cause PRES.

Seizures are relatively common, both in the immediate postoperative period and later on. Vaughn et al. published the first report of seizures in 81 LTx recipients who underwent 85 lung transplantations [13]. Eighteen of 81 (22%) patients experienced seizures. Most patients with seizures were young (i.e., <25 years old) and suffered from cystic fibrosis (CF). CF appeared to be a risk factor for post-LTx seizures in another report as well [3]. Most seizures occurred within 3 months post-transplant. Only one patient required long-term antiepileptic therapy. Sixty-seven percent of patients had seizures during episodes of rejection; in 11 cases patients were also receiving high-dose steroids.

In Živković et al. retrospective study of 132 patients followed for up to 4 years, seizures were reported in 10 allograft recipients (8%) [3]. In this sample, contributing causes included tacrolimus neurotoxicity (three events), other medication toxicity (n = 2; imipenem and cefepime), anoxic brain injury (n = 3), stroke (n = 2), and the cause was unknown in five patients. Mateen et al. reported that in their sample of 120 LTx recipients, seven patients experienced generalized seizures, including three patients who had postoperative seizures (range 1–17 days after LTx) [4].

Additional distressing complications after LTx include headaches and tremors. Headaches have been reported in 20% of recipients in one study, with etiologies including exacerbation of pre-existing migraines, CNI neurotoxicity, and chronic sinusitis [3]. Tremors are present in up to 70% of LTx recipients [21, 22], likely related to the use of immunosuppressant agents and more apparent in the first months after LTx [22]. Tremors can impair patients' activities of daily living and be quite distressing to some patients.

Cognition After Lung Transplantation

Many LTx recipients experience ongoing impairments in cognition, months and even years after LTx [23–25]. In a retrospective cohort study, Cohen et al. evaluated cognitive functioning in 42 post-transplant patients (median follow-up, 8 months; interquartile range, 2–16 months) with the Montreal Cognitive Assessment (MoCA) [24]. Mild cognitive impairment (MoCA score 18–25) was observed in 67% of patients, while moderate cognitive impairment (score 10–17) was observed in 5%. Prolonged graft ischemic time was independently associated with worse cognitive performance. A functional gain in 6-min-walk distance achieved at the end of post-transplant physical rehabilitation was associated with improved cognitive performance. Another study identified that older age and less education were associated with decline in cognitive functioning post LTx [23].

A study by Smith et al. found that among their cohort of 47 patients, neurocognitive impairment is common among lung transplant candidates and worsens in some recipients [25]. As compared to 45% of patients with neurocognitive impairment (MoCA <26) before LTx, 57% had impairment both immediately on discharge and at 3-month follow-up. Patients who developed delirium after LTx surgery had worse post-transplant neurocognitive performance.

Persistent neurocognitive impairment has been associated with worse QOL and medication nonadherence in other medical populations; in fact, it might also be associated with decreased survival after LTx [26]. In a cohort of 49 patients followed for 13 years, better neurocognitive performance was associated with longer survival (hazard ratio [HR] = 0.49) [26]. Unadjusted analyses suggested that worse performance on memory tests specifically was associated with greater risk for chronic lung allograft dysfunction.

Depression Post-transplant

Depression remains a clinically significant concern after LTx, and it is a leading cause of poorer QOL and worse clinical outcomes [27–31]. Multiple etiologies can contribute to the recurrence or new onset of depression in LTx recipients. Fusar-Poli described the following: type of end-stage disease, personality disorders, dysfunctional coping strategies, stressful events, physical complications, immunosuppressant medications, limitations in job performance, sexual dysfunctions, and lack of psychosocial support [27].

Dew et al. demonstrated that 30% of patients had at least one episode of major depressive disorder (MDD) within 2 years of LTx [31]. Post-transplant depression was associated with pre-transplant depression or anxiety, poor social support, and particular coping styles, such as high expression of emotions [31]. Another study demonstrated that higher resilience correlated with less psychological distress in the domains of depression [24].

Post-transplant depression has been shown to have a significant effect on clinical outcomes in all solid organ recipients [32], and in particular in LTx recipients. As presented below, at any stage evaluated, post-LTx depression has been shown to be associated with increased mortality. Patients who had persistently elevated depressive scores from pre-transplant evaluation into 3 months post-transplant period and followed up to 12 years (a mean follow-up of 10.2 years) had greater mortality (HR = 1.85) [33].

In another study, depression, but not anxiety, at 6 months post-transplant was associated with increased mortality in a study of 132 LTx recipients followed for up to 13.5 years (median 7.4 years) following transplantation [28]. Similarly,

in the Investigational Study of Psychological Intervention in Recipients of Lung Transplant (INSPIRE) clinical trial, depressive symptoms identified at 18 months post-transplant were associated with increased risk of mortality (HR = 1.07), while anxiety was not [33]. Rosenberger et al. studied 155 recipients who survived at least 1 year after LTx and followed for up to 15 years [29]. Patients with post-transplant depression had an elevated risk of bronchiolitis obliterans syndrome (BOS) (HR 1.91), graft loss (HR 1.75), and patient death (HR, 1.65, 95% CI 1.01–2.71).

Even very early post-LTx depression is associated with increased post-LTx mortality. Smith et al. demonstrated that greater depressive symptoms assessed approximately 2 weeks after LTx surgery were associated with subsequent mortality (HR = 2.17) during a median follow-up of 2.8 years [30]. This relationship persisted even after controlling for primary graft dysfunction, duration of transplant hospitalization, and gender.

These findings are consistent with a meta-analysis by Dew et al. of 27 studies in solid organ transplant recipients which demonstrated that the occurrence of post-transplant depression was associated with a 65% increased mortality (relative risk [RR], 1.65; 20 studies) and death-censored graft loss risk (RR, 1.65; 3 studies) [32].

These are important and alarming findings, suggesting the need for screening and treatment of depression in LTx recipients to not only improve their QOL and enjoyment from life, but also to improve their clinical outcomes and survival after LTx.

Treatment

No pharmacological studies have been done on treatment of depression in LTx recipients. Selective serotonin reuptake inhibitors (SSRIs), such as sertraline, citalopram, and escitalopram, are frequently first choices in medically complicated patients. A case report of a LTx recipient on tacrolimus, sotalol, omeprazole, and escitalopram for the treatment of depression highlighted the need for vigilance, given the multiple possible drug-drug interactions in these complex patients [34]. In this case report, a patient presented with a prolonged QTc and associated torsades de pointes, thought to be due to inhibition of potassium rectifier channel by various agents (i.e., tacrolimus, sotalol, and escitalopram). Although the dose of administered escitalopram was low, it accumulated due to the blockade of its metabolism by omeprazole and tacrolimus.

Mirtazapine has been suggested as a good choice in LTx recipients [27, 35]. Mirtazapine has minimal drug-drug interactions and may be helpful for depression, anxiety, sleep, and nausea, all problems which are prevalent in lung transplant recipients. Mirtazapine side effects include sedation and weight gain. For further details on treatment of mood and anxiety disorders in transplant recipients, please refer to Chap. 42 on Psychopharmacology.

Anxiety

Dew et al. demonstrated that within 2 years of LTx, 4% of recipients had experienced generalized anxiety disorder, 22% adjustment disorder, and 18% panic disorder among 178 subjects [31]. Of note, LTx recipients were more likely to have panic disorder as compared to heart transplant recipients within the same follow-up period (8%). Female gender, prior history of depression or anxiety, and high avoidance coping were all associated with post-LTx panic disorder.

While post-transplant depression has been shown to be a risk factor for mortality after LTx, post-transplant anxiety has not been associated with an increased mortality risk [28, 29, 32]. Of interest, in patients who survived at least 1 year post-LTx and observed for up to 15 years after surgery, a trend toward reduced risk of BOS was observed in recipients with post-transplant anxiety (HR, 0.61; 95% CI, 0.37–1.00) [25].

Treatment

The SSRIs and mirtazapine can be used for long-term pharmacological treatment of anxiety in LTx recipients. Although benzodiazepines are frequently used in the short-term management of anxiety, caution should be used in LTx patients. In addition to psychological and physical dependence and potential cognitive side effects, benzodiazepines may reduce upper airway muscle tone and blunt the arousal response to hypercapnia, which may lead to respiratory depression [27]. Both gabapentin and hydroxyzine can be considered for the short-term treatment of anxiety. In severe cases, low dose of quetiapine may be considered, especially in acute settings. Caution is recommended, as the use of any of these agents may be associated with respiratory depression and sedation. As always, all psychotropic agents should be started at low doses, and patients should be closely monitored.

Post-traumatic Stress Disorder

Post-traumatic stress disorder associated with transplantation (PTSD-T) deserves special attention. Lung transplant recipients may experience many traumatic events as they go through their journey: from life-threatening deterioration and dyspnea due to their primary lung disease, to the LTx surgery itself, to the environment of ICU, to life-threatening post-LTx complications, such as rejections and infections [36]. The occurrence of PTSD-T can make routine clinic visits anxiety provoking and rehospitalizations emotionally overwhelming. Some patients might postpone appointments or avoid necessary procedures and interventions, such as surveillance bronchoscopies, as they are trying to avoid reminders associated with the clinical environment. Others may find that engaging in activities that previously were considered normal is now anxiety triggering, and thus they avoid them. Examples include watching a movie where someone is drowning, wearing a tie around the neck, and talking and hearing other patients' post-LTx experiences.

Dew et al. estimated that PTSD-T occurs in up to 15% of patients by the end of the first post-LTx year [31]. Gries et al. performed a cross-sectional study of 210 LTx recipients using PTSD checklist to determine the burden of PTSD symptomatology after the transplant (median time since transplant interquartile range 2.4 years (0.7–5.3)) [36]. The authors found that 12.6% of patients had symptoms of PTSD, with re-experiencing (29.5%) and arousal (33.8%) symptoms being more common than avoidant symptoms (18.4%). Risk factors for the development of PTSD symptoms included younger age, lack of private insurance, prior exposure to trauma, and diagnosis of BOS.

Based on other solid organ transplant studies, the two main factors consistently predicting the development of PTSD-T are a history of psychiatric illness prior to transplantation and poor social support post-transplantation [37]. In turn, the development of PTSD-T has been consistently associated with poor mental health-related QOL (HRQOL) and potentially associated with worse physical HRQOL [37]. In addition, studies of ICU survivors indicate that the development of ICU delirium and greater ICU benzodiazepine administration also increases the risk for post-ICU PTSD [38, 39].

The use of ICU diaries for critical illness survivors, where healthcare providers and families document occurring events, allow patients to process their frightening experiences and may be helpful in the prevention of post-ICU PTSD [40]. In addition, inquiring about these experiences, normalizing them to some degree, helping patients to process these memories and events, and referring to mental health professionals for further help can all be important interventions to decrease the risk and burden of PTSD-T.

Substance Use Disorders

Tobacco

As discussed in detail in Chap. 23, a history of tobacco use is common in at least some groups of patients undergoing LTx, such as those with chronic obstructive pulmonary disease (COPD). Therefore, there is a realistic concern for the risk of tobacco use relapse in these patients post-LTx. The emerging literature indicates that tobacco use in LTx recipients is not uncommon and is associated with worse clinical outcomes.

Vos et al. surveyed 276 LTx recipients with 11% of patients reporting post-LTx smoking [41]. Patients on average relapsed a year after LTx and smoked three cigarettes per day. Risk factors for relapse included a history of emphysema associated with COPD (i.e., 23% of COPD patients relapsed), shorter cessation period prior to transplant, lower socioeconomic status, exposure to second-hand smoke, and being widowed. Similarly, Ruttens et al. reported a 12% smoking relapse rate in LTx recipients with such risk factors as COPD, shorter cessation of smoking, and peer smoking [42]. Smoking post-LTx was associated with an increased risk of oncologic events, specifically lung cancer. Also, Mateen et al. reported that 11% of LTx patients returned to smoking post-LTx; moreover, current smoking status was associated with increased risk of death (HR 2.1) [4].

The use of self-report questionnaires demonstrated good sensitivity (85%) and specificity (100%) in screening patients for smoking post-LTx, as compared to urinary cotinine tests [42]. Inquiries regarding smoking should be done in non-judgmental manner. In addition to self-report, patients may be monitored with toxicology screening of urine cotinine, a nicotine metabolite which has a longer half-life (10-25 hours) as compared to nicotine (2 hours). If it is determined that patients are smoking, further motivational interviewing can be conducted to elicit change talk and help patients arrive at health-promoting behaviors [43]. Patients should be offered support and smoking cessation with both pharmacological and non-pharmacological approaches.

Alcohol

Few studies have been conducted regarding alcohol use disorder among LTx candidates. The impact on post-transplant outcomes is discussed in Chap. 23. Overall, more studies need to be conducted to better understand the relationship between post-LTx alcohol use and transplant outcomes.

Other Substances

In terms of other substance use disorders, including intravenous (IV) drug use, there is a paucity of data in LTx patients. Several interesting reports have been published on patients with talc granulomatosis (TG) among IV drug users. Talc (magnesium silicate) is used as a filler in many oral medications; it is insoluble in blood, and when administered intravenously, it gets trapped in the lung, leading to granulomatous inflammation, interstitial fibrosis, airflow obstruction, and pulmonary arterial occlusion [44]. A single center in Alberta, Canada, reported on their experience with this patient population [44]. They described that pentazocine (Talwin) and methylphenidate (Ritalin) are common oral medications which are dissolved and abused intravenously in their geographic region. On the other hand, IV heroin use can also lead to the development of TG. In their study, out of 73 patients referred for LTx for this indication to their center, 34 (46.6%) were listed, and 19 (26%) were transplanted [44]. Selected patients were required to go through rehabilitation program, had a letter of support from their addiction counselor, and signed an abstinence contract. As compared to patients who underwent LTx for other indications, patients with TG were more likely to be ex-smokers and to have comorbid hepatitis C. Post-LTx, there was no difference in 1 and 5-year survival or rates of BOS between patients with TG and patients transplanted for other indications. The authors reported that no patients relapsed on IV drug use, but they had higher rates of post-transplant opioid dependence. An earlier case report did present a patient with TG who relapsed on IV drug use post-LTx [45], while yet another case report presented a successful case [46]. Thus, patients with IV drug use who are carefully screened and selected and undergo intensive rehabilitation treatments can do well after lung transplantation with necessary supports in place. It is important to closely collaborate with transplant and addiction psychiatrists when treating patients with history of IV drug use and to ensure appropriate supports are in place.

Adherence

Adherence to post-LTx regimen, including medications, diet, exercise, clinic appointments, blood draws, and other recommendations from the treatment team, is very important to maintain patients' health and well-being. Lower immunosuppressive levels in LTx recipients are associated with increased incidence of chronic allograft dysfunction, including BOS [47]. There is an increasing literature on adherence in LTx recipients, although more work needs to be done. Adherence is a complex construct with multiple contributors at play, including patients, their support systems, healthcare systems, insurance, finances, and others.

Dew et al. prospectively studied adherence in 9 areas of care among 178 LTx recipients, over a 2-year period after transplantation, and compared it to that of 126 heart transplant (HTx) recipients [48]. Compared to HTx recipients, the cumulative incidence of nonadherence (found during at least two consecutive visits) was lower for LTx recipients in areas of medication taking (21% for HTx versus 13% for LTx), diet (56% versus 34%), and smoking (8% versus 1%). On the other hand, LTx recipients had higher nonadherence in the areas of completing blood work (17% for HTx versus 28%

for LTx) and monitoring blood pressure (59% versus 70%). LTx recipients had high rates of nonadherence to spirometry, which is not done in HTx (63%). Nonadherence to clinic attendance (27%), exercise (44%), and alcohol limitations (7%) were reported at similar rates between the two groups of cardiothoracic transplant recipients. Poor caregiver support and having only public insurance increased nonadherence.

A systematic review on adherence among LTx patients, which included 30 articles, commented on the variability on adherence definitions, methodologies employed, and time to follow up among the studies, thus making comparison analyses challenging [49]. The authors did report that nonadherence rates varied greatly across different areas and that no single risk factor was consistently identified. For example, medication-taking nonadherence ranged from 2.3% to 72.2% between the studies, with observation period varying from 2 weeks to 4 years. Mortality was not affected by adherence in these studies.

Castleberry et al. analyzed the United Network for Organ Sharing (UNOS) database-reported data on lung (single organ) transplantations from October 1996 through December 2006 [50]. The study included 7284 patients who had a follow-up visit after transplantation documenting the degree of adherence to immunosuppressant agents during the first 4 years post-LTx. Nonadherence was termed "early" for events reported within the first year and "late" for events reported during years 2 through 4. The authors reported a 3.1% and 10.6% for early and late nonadherence, respectively [50]. Medicaid insurance and race (i.e., African-American) were associated with early and late nonadherence; while ages 18–20 and grade school or lower education were associated with late nonadherence. Early and late nonadherence were both associated with significantly shorter unadjusted survival ($p < 0.001$). Others have found that patients who experience disturbing side effects from their immunosuppressant regimen are more likely to take "drug holidays," postpone taking medications, or decrease doses on their own [21]. These findings highlight the many factors that contribute to the complexity of nonadherence. Access to healthcare, education, and other societal factors are important contributors. The authors note that racial factors might relate to differences in biology and human leukocyte antigen status observed between different racial groups and/or bias introduced by the providers documenting the nonadherence who might misinterpret clinical status as nonadherence. Young age has been demonstrated as a risk factor for nonadherence in prior studies [50] and might represent a developmental stage or biological factors at play. Understanding all of these factors and tailoring appropriate interventions is important to support posttients and maximize their success.

Several interventions aimed at improving adherence to different aspects of LTx care have been investigated. The Pocket Personal Assistant for Tracking Health (Pocket PATH) is a mobile device developed for LTx patients for data maintenance, tracking, and reporting back to transplant providers. Its use has shown to increase performance of self-care behaviors, as well as improve ratings of self-care agency and HRQOL during the first post-LTx year 1 [51, 52]. On a median follow-up of 5.7 years after transplant (range 4.2–7.2 years), while pocket PATH exposure was not associated directly with improved clinical outcomes, self-monitoring behaviors promoted by PATH in the first post-transplant year were associated with reduced mortality risk, and reporting abnormal health indicators to transplant clinicians was associated with reduced BOS and mortality risks [53].

Quality-of-Life Studies

As discussed above, LTx recipients deal with complex medical regimens, treatment complications, psychological processing, depression and anxiety, and ongoing existential quest after the LTx surgery. The surgery demarcates an important part of their life experience: it does not erase their struggles, just changes them. Beyond improving longevity, lung transplantation aims to improve patients' QOL, which is influenced by a variety of factors. QOL represents a patient-centered outcome defined as an individual's perceived well-being based on multiple factors affecting one's life: health, finances, social relationships, housing, and others [54]. HRQOL pertains to those aspects dealing with health and disease that affect a person's perception of their well-being. Lung transplantation has demonstrated to improve multiple domains contributing to QOL, such as physical functioning, general health, social functioning, dependency level, and dyspnea [54, 55]. One study found that most significant improvements happened within the first 3 months post-LTx and peaked at 6 months [56]. Among LTx recipients, CF patients had the greatest improvements [56]. Another study showed that age was not associated with meaningful differences in the HRQOL after LTx, but there was less HRQOL benefit in patients with interstitial lung disease as compared to patients with CF [55].

One study reported frequent side effects to immunosuppressants in LTx recipients, including tremor in 70% and hirsutism in 68.1% [21]. These symptom experiences decreased reported QOL in patients [21]. Another study reported that compared to HTx recipients, lung patients took longer time to recover in terms of HRQOL, depression, and stress [57]. In addition, their social support team also experienced higher burden and more stress 1 year after LTx as compared to social support of HTx recipients.

An interesting study by Fox et al. looked at posttraumatic growth (PTG) in 64 LTx recipients who survived on average 8 years at the time of evaluation [58]. PTG is defined as "positive psychological change conferred after a major life event or traumatic experience" [58]. Researchers found that levels of growth were high for this group of patients and exceeded those observed in other chronic disease patient groups. Female gender, lower level of education, history of post-transplant panic disorder, great friend support, and better perceived health were all associated with greater reported PTG. Interestingly, medical comorbidities, such as the presence of BOS, were not associated with high levels of PTG, indicating that this construct of meaning is different from medical clinical outcome and that despite how well or poorly someone does medically after LTx, they can still experience psychological growth.

Conclusions

Lung transplantation is just as much a psychological, as it is physical experience. Understanding what patients go through, anticipating what psychologically might lie ahead, and offering them the needed psychological support are paramount to their overall experience as a LTx recipient. Mental health clinicians play a large role in the well-being of LTx patients. There is a lot of interesting research that has been done and is still ongoing on the mental health aspects of LTx, and much more is needed. Specifically we need studies on preventative and treatment interventions for delirium, anxiety, depression, nonadherence, and other psychological and psychosocial experiences. As commentators Knezevik and Zalar noted [59], a lot of research money and resources are spent on medical causes to reduce post-LTx mortality, including figuring out the most effective induction and maintenance immunosuppressant therapies and ways to avoid or stop progression of BOS. As these authors point out, however, necessary recognition, priority, and resources are not given to ongoing psychosocial monitoring, interventions, and support to address post-transplant depression and adherence, which are definitely associated with post-LTx mortality. Hopefully, this will be changed soon.

Below are some conclusions and recommendations that the author shares given the above literature review.

Recommendations

1. Delirium develops in at least one third of LTx recipients. All lung transplant recipients should be provided with non-pharmacological delirium prophylactic measures during the post-transplant period. Patients should be closely monitored for the development of delirium, its etiologies addressed, and treatment suggested.
2. LTx patients are at high risk for depression, which has been linked to reduced survival. Anxiety and PTSD-T are also common and distressing in this patient population. All patients should be screened for depression and anxi-

ety, as well as for PTSD-T, post-LTx. Screening can be done similarly to what is advised and done in CF clinics thanks to the guidelines from CF Foundation: Patients are screened at least once per year with Patient Health Questionnaire-9 (PHQ-9) and Generalized Anxiety Disorder-7 (GAD-7) [60]. Patients with elevated scores or clinical concerns should undergo further evaluation and be referred to the appropriate mental health services and treatments. Screening should be ongoing for those at risk.
3. Patients should be screened for tobacco use pre- and post-LTx. Self-report questionnaires are simple and have good sensitivity and excellent specificity, although urine cotinine tests are also readily available and eliminate the risk of nondisclosure. Patients who smoke post-LTx should be promptly treated, given the effects of smoking on increased morbidity and decreased survival.
4. Nonadherence is common and multifactorial. Patients should be asked about nonadherence in nonjudgmental fashion, factors contributing should be understood, and patients supported with tailored approaches.

References

1. Flynn K, Daiches A, Malpus Z, Yonan N, Sanchez M. 'A post-transplant person': narratives of heart or lung transplantation and intensive care unit delirium. Health. 2014;18(4):352–68.
2. Maldonado JR. A cute brain failure: pathophysiology, diagnosis, management, and sequelar of delirium. Crit Care Clin. 2017;33(3):461–519.
3. Zivkovic SA, Jumaa M, Barisic N, McCurry K. Neurologic complications following lung transplantation. J Neurol Sci. 2009;280(1–2):90–3.
4. Mateen FJ, Dierkhising RA, Rabinstein AA, van de Beek D, Wijdicks EF. Neurological complications following adult lung transplantation. Am J Transplant. 2010;10(4):908–14.
5. Shigemura N, Sclabassi RJ, Bhama JK, Gries CJ, Crespo MM, Johnson B, et al. Early major neurologic complications after lung transplantation: incidence, risk factors, and outcome. Transplantation. 2013;95(6):866–71.
6. Craven JL. Postoperative organic mental syndromes in lung transplant recipients. Toronto lung transplant group. J Heart Transplant. 1990;9(2):129–32.
7. Santacruz JEE, Guzman Zavala E, Diaz-Gomez J, Budev M, Pettersson G, et al. Post-operative delirium in lung transplant recipients: incidence and associated risk factors and morbidity chest. Chest. 2009;136(4_MeetingAbstracts):18S-a-18S.
8. Smith PJ, Rivelli SK, Waters AM, Hoyle A, Durheim MT, Reynolds JM, et al. Delirium affects length of hospital stay after lung transplantation. J Crit Care. 2015;30(1):126–9.
9. Smith PJ, Blumenthal JA, Hoffman BM, Rivelli SK, Palmer SM, Davis RD, et al. Reduced cerebral perfusion pressure during lung transplant surgery is associated with risk, duration, and severity of postoperative delirium. Ann Am Thorac Soc. 2016;13(2):180–7.
10. Sher Y, Mooney J, Dhillon G, Lee R, Maldonado JR. Delirium after lung transplantation: association with recipient characteristics, hospital resource utilization, and mortality. Clin Transpl. 2017. 31(5).
11. Anderson BJ, Chesley CF, Theodore M, Christie C, Tino R, Wysoczanski A, et al. Incidence, risk factors, and clinical

implications of post-operative delirium in lung transplant recipients. J Heart Lung Transplant. 2018;37:755–62.

12. Maldonado JR. Neuropathogenesis of delirium: review of current etiologic theories and common pathways. Am J Geriatr Psychiatry. 2013;21(12):1190–222.

13. Vaughn BV, Ali II, Olivier KN, Lackner RP, Robertson KR, Messenheimer JA, et al. Seizures in lung transplant recipients. Epilepsia. 1996;37(12):1175–9.

14. Thyagarajan GK, Cobanoglu A, Johnston W. FK506-induced fulminant leukoencephalopathy after single-lung transplantation. Ann Thorac Surg. [Case Reports]. 1997;64(5):1461–4.

15. Arimura FE, Camargo PC, Costa AN, Teixeira RH, Carraro RM, Afonso JE Jr, et al. Posterior reversible encephalopathy syndrome in lung transplantation: 5 case reports. Transplant Proc. [Case Reports]. 2014;46(6):1845–8.

16. Hayes D Jr, Adler B, Turner TL, Mansour HM. Alternative tacrolimus and sirolimus regimen associated with rapid resolution of posterior reversible encephalopathy syndrome after lung transplantation. Pediatr Neurol. [Case Reports]. 2014;50(3):272–5.

17. Bodkin CL, Eidelman BH. Sirolimus-induced posterior reversible encephalopathy. Neurology. [Case Reports]. 2007;68(23):2039–40.

18. Rosso L, Nosotti M, Mendogni P, Palleschi A, Tosi D, Montoli M, et al. Lung transplantation and posterior reversible encephalopathy syndrome: a case series. Transplant Proc. 2012;44(7):2022–5.

19. Levenson JL. High-dose intravenous haloperidol for agitated delirium following lung transplantation. Psychosomatics. [Case Reports]. 1995;36(1):66–8.

20. Lamy C, Oppenheim C, Mas JL. Posterior reversible encephalopathy syndrome. Handb Clin Neurol. [Review]. 2014;121:1687–701.

21. Kugler C, Fischer S, Gottlieb J, Tegtbur U, Welte T, Goerler H, et al. Symptom experience after lung transplantation: impact on quality of life and adherence. Clin Transpl. 2007;21(5):590–6.

22. Lanuza DM, Lefaiver CA, Brown R, Muehrer R, Murray M, Yelle M, et al. A longitudinal study of patients' symptoms before and during the first year after lung transplantation. Clin Transpl. [Comparative Study Research Support, N.I.H., Extramural Research Support, Non-U.S. Gov't]. 2012;26(6):E576–89.

23. Hoffman BM, Blumenthal JA, Carney RC, O'Hayer CV, Freedland K, Smith PJ, et al. Changes in neurocognitive functioning following lung transplantation. Am J Transplant. 2012;12(9):2519–25.

24. Cohen DG, Christie JD, Anderson BJ, Diamond JM, Judy RP, Shah RJ, et al. Cognitive function, mental health, and health-related quality of life after lung transplantation. Ann Am Thorac Soc. [Research Support, N.I.H., Extramural Research Support, Non-U.S. Gov't]. 2014;11(4):522–30.

25. Smith PJ, Rivelli S, Waters A, Reynolds J, Hoyle A, Flowers M, et al. Neurocognitive changes after lung transplantation. Ann Am Thorac Soc. 2014;11(10):1520–7.

26. Smith PJ, Blumenthal JA, Hoffman BM, Davis RD, Palmer SM. Postoperative cognitive dysfunction and mortality following lung transplantation. Am J Transplant. 2018;18(3):696–703.

27. Fusar-Poli P, Lazzaretti M, Ceruti M, Hobson R, Petrouska K, Cortesi M, et al. Depression after lung transplantation: causes and treatment. Lung. [Review]. 2007;185(2):55–65.

28. Smith PJ, Blumenthal JA, Trulock EP, Freedland KE, Carney RM, Davis RD, et al. Psychosocial predictors of mortality following lung transplantation. Am J Transplant. [Randomized Controlled Trial Research Support, N.I.H., Extramural]. 2016;16(1):271–7.

29. Rosenberger EM, DiMartini AF, DeVito Dabbs AJ, Bermudez CA, Pilewski JM, Toyoda Y, et al. Psychiatric predictors of long-term transplant-related outcomes in lung transplant recipients. Transplantation. [Research Support, N.I.H., Extramural]. 2016;100(1):239–47.

30. Smith PJ, Blumenthal JA, Snyder LD, Mathew JP, Durheim MT, Hoffman BM, et al. Depressive symptoms and early mortality following lung transplantation: a pilot study. Clin Transpl. 2017;31(2):e12874.

31. Dew MA, DiMartini AF, DeVito Dabbs AJ, Fox KR, Myaskovsky L, Posluszny DM, et al. Onset and risk factors for anxiety and depression during the first 2 years after lung transplantation. Gen Hosp Psychiatry. 2012;34(2):127–38.

32. Dew MA, Rosenberger EM, Myaskovsky L, DiMartini AF, DeVito Dabbs AJ, Posluszny DM, et al. Depression and anxiety as risk factors for morbidity and mortality after organ transplantation: a systematic review and meta-analysis. Transplantation. 2015;100(5):988–1003.

33. Smith PJ, Blumenthal JA, Carney RM, Freedland KE, O'Hayer CV, Trulock EP, et al. Neurobehavioral functioning and survival following lung transplantation. Chest. [Multicenter Study Randomized Controlled Trial Research Support, N.I.H., Extramural Research Support, U.S. Gov't, P.H.S.]. 2014;145(3):604–11.

34. Van Asbroeck PJ, Huybrechts W, De Soir R. Case report, aetiology, and treatment of an acquired long-QT syndrome. Acta Clin Belg. [Case Reports]. 2014;69(2):132–4.

35. Fusar-Poli P, Martinelli V, Politi P, Hobson R. Successful antidepressive treatment with mirtazapine following lung transplantation. Prog Neuro-Psychopharmacol Biol Psychiatry. [Case Reports Letter]. 2008;32(7):1745–6.

36. Gries CJ, Dew MA, Curtis JR, Edelman JD, DeVito DA, Pilewski JM, et al. Nature and correlates of post-traumatic stress symptomatology in lung transplant recipients. J Heart Lung Transplant. [Research Support, N.I.H., Extramural Research Support, Non-U.S. Gov't]. 2013;32(5):525–32.

37. Davydow DS, Lease ED, Reyes JD. Posttraumatic stress disorder in organ transplant recipients: a systematic review. Gen Hosp Psychiatry. [Research Support, N.I.H., Extramural Review]. 2015;37(5):387–98.

38. Davydow DS, Gifford JM, Desai SV, Needham DM, Bienvenu OJ. Posttraumatic stress disorder in general intensive care unit survivors: a systematic review. Gen Hosp Psychiatry. 2008;30(5):421–34.

39. Wade D, Hardy R, Howell D, Mythen M. Identifying clinical and acute psychological risk factors for PTSD after critical care: a systematic review. Minerva Anestesiol. 2013;79(8):944–63.

40. Parker AM, Sricharoenchai T, Raparla S, Schneck KW, Bienvenu OJ, Needham DM. Posttraumatic stress disorder in critical illness survivors: a metaanalysis. Crit Care Med. [Meta-Analysis Research Support, N.I.H., Extramural Review]. 2015;43(5):1121–9.

41. Vos R, De Vusser K, Schaevers V, Schoonis A, Lemaigre V, Dobbels F, et al. Smoking resumption after lung transplantation: a sobering truth. Eur Respir J. [Letter Research Support, Non-U.S. Gov't]. 2010;35(6):1411–3.

42. Ruttens D, Verleden SE, Goeminne PC, Poels K, Vandermeulen E, Godderis L, et al. Smoking resumption after lung transplantation: standardised screening and importance for long-term outcome. Eur Respir J. [Letter Research Support, Non-U.S. Gov't]. 2014;43(1):300–3.

43. Lindson-Hawley N, Thompson TP, Begh R. Motivational interviewing for smoking cessation. Cochrane Database Syst Rev. [Meta-Analysis Research Support, Non-U.S. Gov't Review]. 2015;2(3):CD006936.

44. Weinkauf JG, Puttagunta L, Nador R, Jackson K, LaBranche K, Kapasi A, et al. Long-term outcome of lung transplantation in previous intravenous drug users with talc lung granulomatosis. Transplant Proc. 2013;45(6):2375–7.

45. Cook RC, Fradet G, English JC, Soos J, Muller NL, Connolly TP, et al. Recurrence of intravenous talc granulomatosis following single lung transplantation. Can Respir J. [Case Reports]. 1998;5(6):511–4.

46. Shlomi D, Shitrit D, Bendayan D, Sahar G, Shechtman Y, Kramer MR. Successful lung transplantation for talcosis secondary to intravenous abuse of oral drug. Int J Chron Obstruct Pulmon Dis. [Case Reports]. 2008;3(2):327–30.

47. Husain AN, Siddiqui MT, Holmes EW, Chandrasekhar AJ, McCabe M, Radvany R, et al. Analysis of risk factors for the development of bronchiolitis obliterans syndrome. Am J Respir Crit Care Med. 1999;159(3):829–33.

48. Dew MA, Dimartini AF, De Vito DA, Zomak R, De Geest S, Dobbels F, et al. Adherence to the medical regimen during the first two years after lung transplantation. Transplantation. [Comparative Study Research Support, N.I.H., Extramural]. 2008;85(2):193–202.

49. Hu L, Lingler JH, Sereika SM, Burke LE, Malchano DK, DeVito DA, et al. Nonadherence to the medical regimen after lung transplantation: a systematic review. Heart Lung. [Review]. 2017;46:178–86.

50. Castleberry AW, Bishawi M, Worni M, Erhunmwunsee L, Speicher PJ, Osho AA, et al. Medication nonadherence after lung transplantation in adult recipients. Ann Thorac Surg. [Observational Study]. 2017;103(1):274–80.

51. DeVito DA, Dew MA, Myers B, Begey A, Hawkins R, Ren D, et al. Evaluation of a hand-held, computer-based intervention to promote early self-care behaviors after lung transplant. Clin Transpl. [Randomized Controlled Trial]. 2009;23(4):537–45.

52. DeVito DA, Song MK, Myers BA, Li R, Hawkins RP, Pilewski JM, et al. A randomized controlled trial of a mobile health intervention to promote self-management after lung transplantation. Am J Transplant. [Randomized Controlled Trial Research Support, N.I.H., Extramural]. 2016;16(7):2172–80.

53. Rosenberger EM, DeVito Dabbs AJ, DiMartini AF, Landsittel DP, Pilewski JM, Dew MA. Long-term follow-up of a randomized controlled trial evaluating a mobile health intervention for self-Management in Lung Transplant Recipients. Am J Transplant. [Randomized Controlled Trial]. 2017;17(5):1286–93.

54. Kolaitis NA, Singer JP. Defining success in lung transplantation: from survival to quality of life. Semin Respir Crit Care Med. 2018;39(2):255–68.

55. Singer LG, Chowdhury NA, Faughnan ME, Granton J, Keshavjee S, Marras TK, et al. Effects of recipient age and diagnosis on health-related quality-of-life benefit of lung transplantation. Am J Respir Crit Care Med. [Clinical Study Research Support, Non-U.S. Gov't]. 2015;192(8):965–73.

56. Finlen Copeland CA, Vock DM, Pieper K, Mark DB, Palmer SM. Impact of lung transplantation on recipient quality of life: a serial, prospective, multicenter analysis through the first posttransplant year. Chest. [Multicenter Study Randomized Controlled Trial Research Support, Non-U.S. Gov't]. 2013;143(3):744–50.

57. Agren S, Sjoberg T, Ekmehag B, Wiborg MB, Ivarsson B. Psychosocial aspects before and up to 2 years after heart or lung transplantation: experience of patients and their next of kin. Clin Transpl. 2017;31(3).

58. Fox KR, Posluszny DM, DiMartini AF, DeVito Dabbs AJ, Rosenberger EM, Zomak RA, et al. Predictors of post-traumatic psychological growth in the late years after lung transplantation. Clin Transpl. [Clinical Trial Research Support, N.I.H., Extramural Research Support, Non-U.S. Gov't]. 2014;28(4):384–93.

59. Knezevic I, Zalar B. Pre-transplant depression in lung recipients – a lost battle? Transpl Int. 2018;31(5):481–3.

60. Quittner AL, Abbott J, Georgiopoulos AM, Goldbeck L, Smith B, Hempstead SE, et al. International committee on mental health in cystic fibrosis: Cystic Fibrosis Foundation and European cystic fibrosis society consensus statements for screening and treating depression and anxiety. Thorax. [Consensus Development Conference Research Support, Non-U.S. Gov't]. 2016;71(1):26–34.

Intestinal Failure and Indications for Visceral Transplantation

Yelizaveta Sher

Introduction

The term *intestinal failure* was first coined in 1981 by Fleming and Remington to describe "a reduction in the functioning gut mass below the minimal amount necessary for adequate digestion and absorption of food" [1]. Over time, the term has undergone several transformations [2]. At this time, intestinal failure (IF) is understood as the inability of the gut to absorb necessary macronutrients (protein, carbohydrates, and fat), micronutrients (minerals, vitamins, and electrolytes), and fluid required to maintain health and/or growth, resulting in necessity for parenteral nutrition (PN) [2–4]. The basic defect results from the decrease of absorptive length of the small intestine and reduction of the enterocyte mass. An international consensus group recently attempted to address this issue by proposing that intestinal failure results from obstruction, dysmotility, surgical resection, congenital defect, or disease-associated loss of absorption and is characterized by the inability to maintain protein, energy, fluid, electrolyte, or micronutrient balance [5].

Different portions of the intestine perform different functions (see Table 28.1). Depending on the potential etiologies, the particular segment that is lost or resected, and the health and length of the remaining gut, nutritional autonomy can be attained [6, 7]. If autonomy is not attained, patients are diagnosed with IF. IF is a rare condition, with chronic IF which requires long-term PN, affecting 50 per million people [8]. This condition has significant healthcare-related as well as individual costs.

Etiologies of Intestinal Failure

IF can have childhood or adult onset, be congenital or acquired, and be acute or chronic [2]. The most common etiologies in infants are necrotizing enterocolitis (14%) and congenital intestinal anomalies (e.g., gastroschisis (22%), volvulus (16%), and motility disorder (18%)) [9]. The most common etiologies in adults include mesenteric ischemia/thrombosis (24%), inflammatory bowel disease (i.e., Crohn's disease) (11%), tumors (13%), volvulus (8%), and trauma (7%) [9]. The most common umbrella etiology in both children and adults is short bowel syndrome (SBS), resulting from the extensive bowel loss and accounting for two thirds of the cases in both children and adults [9, 10].

IF is classified into three categories based on the acuity of presentation and duration [2]. "Type 1" IF often occurs following abdominal surgery, such as postoperative ileus, and is self-limiting. "Type 2" IF usually follows significant surgical bowel resection with the remnant intestine of less than 200 cm in length in patients with Crohn's disease (CD) or mesenteric vascular disease, although there may be other causes. Type 2 IF is usually associated with significant septic, metabolic, and complex nutritional complications [4, 11]. The resulting SBS leads to electrolyte and metabolic derangements, and patients require PN support. "Type 3" IF is a chronic form of intestinal failure requiring long-term nutritional support [4, 11].

Mesenteric Ischemia

Mesenteric ischemia is a rare condition associated with high mortality, in up to 80% of patients, if not addressed in timely fashion [12]. Since the small intestine has very little collateral circulation, acute arterial occlusions from emboli (responsible for approximately 50% of such cases) lead to SBS in those who survive such an event [10]. The left ventricle from cardiac dysrhythmias, cardiac valves from endo-

Y. Sher (✉)
Department of Psychiatry and Behavioral Sciences, Stanford University School of Medicine, Stanford, CA, USA
e-mail: ysher@stanford.edu

© Springer International Publishing AG, part of Springer Nature 2019
Y. Sher, J. R. Maldonado (eds.), *Psychosocial Care of End-Stage Organ Disease and Transplant Patients*,
https://doi.org/10.1007/978-3-319-94914-7_28

Table 28.1 Functions of the gastrointestinal tract structures and effects of their loss

Structures of gastrointestinal tract	Length	Function	Effect of loss/resection
Duodenum Jejunum	20–25 cm ~2.5 m	Duodenum receives gastric chyme from the stomach, digestive enzymes from the pancreas, and bile from the liver. The digestive enzymes break down proteins, and bile emulsifies fats into micelles.	
		First 150 cm of the small intestine absorb calcium, magnesium, phosphorus, iron, and folic acid.	Severe metabolic derangements
		Initial 100–200 cm of the jejunum absorb macronutrients, (i.e., carbohydrates and protein), and micronutrients, (i.e., water-soluble vitamins). Jejunum absorbs water.	Malnutrition Dehydration
Ileum	~3 m	Absorbs fluid. Absorbs vitamin B12 and bile salts. Produces hormones (i.e., cholecystokinin, peptide YY, glucagon-like peptide).	Pernicious anemia Rapid gastric emptying and increased intestinal transit, resulting in hypertonic intestinal contents, diarrhea and dehydration
Ileocecal valve (ICV)		Regulates the delivery of contents into the colon and serves as a mechanical barrier preventing reflux of colonic contents and bacteria.	Preservation allows return of oral diet and nutritional autonomy
Colon	~1.5 m	Absorption: Fluids and electrolytes. Absorbs 1 and up to 6 L of water per day. Also is a site of bacterial fermentation, aiding in conversion of undigested carbohydrates to absorbable short-chain fatty acids.	Dehydration Malnutrition

Adapted from Bharadwaj et al. [2] and Lal et al. [4]

carditis, and aortic atherosclerotic plaque are responsible for the majority of emboli. In 10% of patients, venous occlusion is responsible for mesenteric ischemia and is usually related to a hypercoagulable state. Patients with venous mesenteric thrombosis require thrombophilia workup and hematologic evaluation to decrease risk of future events in the remaining or transplanted gut [10]. Mesenteric ischemia accounts for 24% of adult patients undergoing intestinal transplantation [9].

Crohn's Disease

CD is an inflammatory disease characterized by transmural inflammation of the gastrointestinal tract; it may involve the entire gastrointestinal tract from mouth to the perianal area. CD is the second largest indication for intestinal transplant in adults, responsible for approximately 11% of such transplants [9]. Common complications of CD, such as perforation, stricture, obstruction, and abscess, lead to multiple surgical procedures, which over the time may result in IF and dependence on PN [10].

Acute Volvulus

In children typical cases of volvulus present due to classic congenital mesenteric anatomic defects [10]. However, in adults, acute volvulus is usually due to surgically altered mesenteric anatomy, for example, following the Roux-en-Y gastric bypass surgery, leading to intestinal ischemia and necessitating a life-saving total enterectomy [10].

Adult Motility Disorders

Motility disorders of the intestine are characterized by obstructive gastrointestinal symptoms without any evidence of obstruction [10]. Patients present with nausea and vomiting, abdominal bloating, diffuse chronic abdominal pain, and weight loss. Patients develop IF and require PN. Patients do not respond to intestinal rehabilitation and frequently undergo multiple futile explorative abdominal surgeries. These disorders account for approximately 11% of adult patients undergoing intestinal transplantation [10].

Intraabdominal Malignancy

Majority of the abdominal tumors in adults leading to intestinal transplantation are desmoid tumors, which are benign fibromatous neoplasms which can be infiltrative and invasive leading to the entrapment of the mesenteric vasculature, obstruction, and fistula formation [10]. These tumors frequently do not respond to conventional chemotherapy and thus require complete surgical resection, leading to ultra-short bowel syndrome, due to their location. Tumors account for 13% of intestinal transplants in adults [9].

Re-transplantation

Re-transplantation has grown as an indication for intestinal transplant in the recent years and accounts for 7% of patients undergoing this transplant [9, 10]. However, the prognosis of patients with isolated intestinal re-transplant is poor as compared to patients with their first intestinal transplant, due to high rates of rejection, primarily owing to the increased allosensitization in the candidate [10]. Patients with liver-intestine re-transplant have better outcomes likely due to the immunogenic protective effects of the liver allograft [10].

Parenteral Nutrition and Associated Complications

Although required to sustain life in IF, PN is associated with a variety of significant adverse effects. The most important complications of PN are venous access-related problems, including catheter-related bloodstream infections (CRBSI), IF-associated liver disease (IFALD), metabolic bone disease, and a negative effect on quality of life [2, 13].

CRBSI

Patients with IF require venous access for ongoing parenteral nutrition. For those in need of long-term PN at home, tunneled catheters and infusion ports are mostly used; for patients who will likely require PN for not longer than 12–18 months, peripherally inserted central venous catheters (PICCs) are the method of access [14]. The most common complications related to venous access are infections, thrombosis, occlusions, and pneumothorax [14]. CRBSI represent the most serious threat, usually requiring hospital admission, elevating care costs, and leading to increased morbidity and mortality [13]. In a systematic analysis of 39 studies with noted variability in terminology and definitions observed, the overall rate of CRBSI ranged between 0.38 and 4.58 episodes/1000 catheter days (median 1.31) [14]. Half of the infections identified were caused by gram-positive bacteria (i.e., human skin flora), such as *Staphylococcus* spp. Patient-related factors have been investigated by various groups. For example, O'Keefe et al. demonstrated that some of the risk factors for recurrent infections included CD (potentially due to immunologic defects), younger age, poor hand hygiene, and smoking status [15]. Others have suggested that taking opiods or sedative medications might contribute to this risk [16]. CRSBI are responsible for 5% of all deaths in patients on PN [3].

IF-Associated Liver Disease (IFALD)

IFALD is a significant complication of PN. Between 25% and 100% of patients on long-term PN develop liver enzyme abnormalities, while end-stage liver disease may develop in 15–40% of these patients [13]. IFALD is more common in children (25–50%) [8, 17], as compared to adults (<5%) [8, 18]. The pathophysiology of IFALD is multifactorial and includes intrahepatic inflammation associated with steatohepatitis, sepsis, nutrient deficiencies (i.e., choline, taurine, and essential fatty acids), nutrient excesses (i.e., lipid, glucose, and protein), dysfunctional biliary system (i.e., gall stones and bile acidification), medications, bacterial overgrowth, and some PN components [8].

It has been noted that when a modest amount of total energy but minimal amount of fat is given via PN, severe liver dysfunction is uncommon despite abnormal liver function tests [18]. Risk factors for IFALD include excess carbohydrates, excess fat, and longer duration of PN [13]. Based on the degree of liver function test elevations, patients are assessed for overfeeding, medications are reviewed, fat emulsion use is decreased, ultrasonography of gallbladder is performed, and eventually patients are referred to hepatology, if indicated [13].

Metabolic Bone Disease

Patients on long-term home PN are at risk for developing metabolic bone disease (i.e., osteoporosis and osteomalacia) [13]. In fact, 41–46% of patients on chronic PN develop osteoporosis on bone densitometry [8]. The etiologies leading to metabolic bone disease include vitamin D deficiency, the underlying condition (e.g., CD), and the mishandling of calcium and phosphate [8]. It is recommended that patients undergo a dual-energy, x-ray absorptiometry scan in their first year. If test results are abnormal, they should be referred to an endocrinologist for possible treatment with calcium, vitamin D, bisphosphonates, and teriparatide. Those who have normal bone scan results should continue monitoring with dual-energy, x-ray absorptiometry scan every 2 years, in addition to regular serum and urine monitoring of calcium, phosphorus, and magnesium [13].

Other Complications

Other complications of PN include fluid overload, electrolyte imbalances, and renal disease [8]. Renal dysfunction results from chronic dehydration as well as nephrolithiasis [8].

Outcomes

Due to the underlying diseases, as well as the above listed complications, patients requiring long-term PN commonly experience increased mortality [2]. In fact, in one study of 437 patients cared for in an academic medical center and requiring first-time use of TPN for an average of 1.5 years had a mortality rate of 42% [19]. The average age of this cohort was 60 years of age and 43% had an underlying malignancy [19]. In this cohort, risk factors for mortality included older age, admission to an intensive care unit or a nonsurgical department, lower body mass index, and an underlying malignancy [19].

Intestinal Adaptation

The bowel undergoes significant adaptation, even years after resection, in order to increase its absorptive area [13, 20]. Intestinal adaptation is a natural compensatory process where structural and functional changes in the intestine occur to improve nutrient and fluid absorption [20]. With time, the diameter and height of the villi increase to allow for more absorption in the remaining intestine. The factors that are important for intestinal adaptation include health of the remaining bowel, residual colonic length, location of resection (duodenum, jejunum, or ileum), enteral nutrients, and enterotrophic factors [20]. Enteral nutrients are very important for this process to stimulate gastric secretion, gastric emptying, and intestinal transit, eventually leading to epithelial surface area increase [20]. Two intestinotrophic growth factors, the glucagon-like peptide 2 analog teduglutide and recombinant growth hormone (somatropin), have been approved by the FDA and are used in patients with SBS, enhancing fluid absorption and decreasing requirements for PN and intravenous fluids in these patients [20]. Although it has been thought that intestinal adaptation is limited to 1–2 years after bowel loss or resection, it has been shown that patients can achieve nutritional autonomy after many years of being on PN [20].

Intestinal Rehabilitation

The main goal of the intestinal rehabilitation program is to wean patients off or avoid the long-term use of PN [13, 20]. Success in weaning from PN depends on many factors, including the length and anatomy of the remaining bowel. In general, patients with a remaining small bowel length greater than 100 cm and with a part of the colon, or a length of remaining small bowel greater than 150 cm without an intact and functional colon, can succeed with intestinal adaptation and be weaned off PN [13, 20]. Intestinal rehabilitation con-

sists of specific dietary interventions (e.g., modified oral diet or enteral nutrition [EN]), fiber supplementation, pharmacological measures, and surgical techniques with the goal to wean patients off PN therapy and attain complete nutritional autonomy (CNA) [6]. In fact, 50–75% of patients can wean off PN within 2 years of intestinal rehabilitation. In one study of 61 patients with SBS undergoing intestinal rehabilitation with EN, 85% of patients were weaned off PN when the follow-up took place at an average of 50 months [21]. Overall patient survival at 50 months of follow-up in this study was 95% [21]. Those patients who cannot be weaned off PN are deemed to have permanent IF and will need a referral for a potential intestinal or multivisceral transplantation.

Evaluation for Transplant

Intestinal and multivisceral transplant emerged as a lifesaving surgical intervention that can prolong lives and improve quality of life for patients with permanent IF who are unable to tolerate PN [3]. The Centers for Medicare and Medicaid Services-approved indications for intestinal transplantation consist of complications of PN, such as severe IFALD, loss of central venous access due to thrombosis, recurrent line infection and sepsis, and recurrent dehydration [2, 22]. In addition, the American Society of Transplantation recommends that the following patients are also considered and referred to the intestinal transplantation: patients at high risk of death from their primary disease (e.g., abdominal desmoid tumors, congenital mucosal disorders), patients with severe SBS (e.g., gastrotomy, duodenostomy, residual small bowel <10 cm in infants and < 20 cm in adults), patients who have frequent hospitalizations, narcotic dependency, or pseudo-obstruction, and patients who are unwilling to accept long-term home PN [3, 10, 23].

Some experts argue that patients should be referred earlier to intestinal transplantation and preferably transplanted before development of IFALD and within 1 year of initiation of long-term PN [3].

Contraindications to intestinal transplant are similar to those listed for liver transplantation, including active infection, aggressive malignancy, multisystem organ failure, cerebral edema, and overt acquired immune deficiency syndrome [24].

Evaluation for potential intestinal transplant is customarily conducted by a multidisciplinary team, usually consisting of a transplant surgeon, hepatologist/gastroenterologist, social worker, financial coordinator, pharmacist, infectious disease specialist, cardiologist, dietician, and a mental health expert. In addition to obtaining detailed past medical and surgical histories, and reviewing laboratory, serologic, endoscopic, and radiologic results, patients may require a liver biopsy, if significant liver disease is suspected. The evaluation will determine what type of intestinal transplant will be required. The particular types, history, management, and outcomes of intestinal transplant are discussed in Chaps. 29 and 32.

Conclusions

Intestinal failure is a rare but debilitating condition that can affect children and/or adults. After loss of intestinal tissue, the remaining bowel can undergo intestinal adaptation, and eventually some patients can return to nutritional anatomy via oral intake. Intestinal rehabilitation, consisting of specific dietary interventions, fiber supplementation, pharmacological measures, and surgical techniques, allows patients to attain such autonomy. However, others require lifelong PN, which is associated with its own set of complications, including venous access-related problems, such as catheter-related bloodstream infections, IF-associated liver disease, metabolic bone disease, and decreased quality of life. Intestinal transplant is an option for these patients and can decrease risk of such complications, allow reestablishment of oral diet, and improve quality of life.

References

1. Fleming CR, Remington M. Intestinal failure. In: HIll GL, editor. Nutrition and the surgical patient. Edinburgh: Churchill Livingstone; 1981. p. 219–35.
2. Bharadwaj S, Tandon P, Meka K, Rivas JM, Jevenn A, Kuo NT, et al. Intestinal failure: adaptation, rehabilitation, and transplantation. J Clin Gastroenterol. [Review]. 2016;50(5):366–72.
3. Bharadwaj S, Tandon P, Gohel TD, Brown J, Steiger E, Kirby DF, et al. Current status of intestinal and multivisceral transplantation. Gastroenterology report. [Review]. 2017;5(1):20–8.
4. Lal S, Teubner A, Shaffer JL. Review article: intestinal failure. Aliment Pharmacol Ther. 2006;24(1):19–31.
5. O'Keefe SJ, Buchman AL, Fishbein TM, Jeejeebhoy KN, Jeppesen PB, Shaffer J. Short bowel syndrome and intestinal failure: consensus definitions and overview. Clin Gastroenterol Hepatol. 2006;4(1):6–10.
6. Kappus M, Diamond S, Hurt RT, Martindale R. Intestinal failure: new definition and clinical implications. Curr Gastroenterol Rep. [Review]. 2016;18(9):48.
7. Nightingale J. Definition and classification of intestinal failure. In: Nightingale J, editor. Intestinal failure. London: Greenwich Medical Media Limited; 2001.
8. Allan P, Lal S. Intestinal failure: a review. F1000Research. [Review]. 2018;7:85.
9. Grant D, Abu-Elmagd K, Mazariegos G, Vianna R, Langnas A, Mangus R, et al. Intestinal transplant registry report: global activity and trends. Am J Transplant Off J Am Soc Transplant Surg. [Research Support, Non-U.S. Gov't]. 2015;15(1):210–9.
10. Matsumoto CS, Subramanian S, Fishbein TM. Adult intestinal transplantation. Gastroenterol Clin N Am. [Review]. 2018;47(2):341–54.
11. Howard L, Ashley C. Management of complications in patients receiving home parenteral nutrition. Gastroenterology. 2003;124(6):1651–61.
12. Bala M, Kashuk J, Moore EE, Kluger Y, Biffl W, Gomes CA, et al. Acute mesenteric ischemia: guidelines of the World Society of Emergency Surgery. World J Emerg Surg. [Review]. 2017;12:38.
13. Shatnawei A, Parekh NR, Rhoda KM, Speerhas R, Stafford J, Dasari V, et al. Intestinal failure management at the Cleveland Clinic. Arch Surg. [Review]. 2010;145(6):521–7.
14. Dreesen M, Foulon V, Spriet I, Goossens GA, Hiele M, De Pourcq L, et al. Epidemiology of catheter-related infections in adult patients receiving home parenteral nutrition: a systematic review. Clin Nutr. [Review]. 2013;32(1):16–26.
15. O'Keefe SJ, Burnes JU, Thompson RL. Recurrent sepsis in home parenteral nutrition patients: an analysis of risk factors. JPEN J Parenter Enteral Nutr. [Case Reports Comparative Study]. 1994;18(3):256–63.
16. Richards DM, Scott NA, Shaffer JL, Irving M. Opiate and sedative dependence predicts a poor outcome for patients receiving home parenteral nutrition. JPEN J Parenter Enteral Nutr. [Comparative Study]. 1997;21(6):336–8.
17. Lauriti G, Zani A, Aufieri R, Cananzi M, Chiesa PL, Eaton S, et al. Incidence, prevention, and treatment of parenteral nutrition-associated cholestasis and intestinal failure-associated liver disease in infants and children: a systematic review. JPEN J Parenter Enteral Nutr. [Research Support, Non-U.S. Gov't Review]. 2014;38(1):70–85.
18. Salvino R, Ghanta R, Seidner DL, Mascha E, Xu Y, Steiger E. Liver failure is uncommon in adults receiving long-term parenteral nutrition. JPEN J Parenter Enteral Nutr. [Research Support, Non-U.S. Gov't]. 2006;30(3):202–8.
19. Oterdoom LH, Ten Dam SM, de Groot SD, Arjaans W, van Bodegraven AA. Limited long-term survival after in-hospital intestinal failure requiring total parenteral nutrition. Am J Clin Nutr. [Observational Study]. 2014;100(4):1102–7.
20. Tappenden KA. Intestinal adaptation following resection. JPEN J Parenter Enteral Nutr. [Research Support, Non-U.S. Gov't Review]. 2014;38(1 Suppl):23S–31S.
21. Gong JF, Zhu WM, Yu WK, Li N, Li JS. Role of enteral nutrition in adult short bowel syndrome undergoing intestinal rehabilitation: the long-term outcome. Asia Pac J Clin Nutr. 2009;18(2):155–63.
22. Pironi L, Forbes A, Joly F, Colomb V, Lyszkowska M, Van Gossum A, et al. Survival of patients identified as candidates for intestinal transplantation: a 3-year prospective follow-up. Gastroenterology. [Research Support, Non-U.S. Gov't]. 2008;135(1):61–71.
23. Kaufman SS, Atkinson JB, Bianchi A, Goulet OJ, Grant D, Langnas AN, et al. Indications for pediatric intestinal transplantation: a position paper of the American Society of Transplantation. Pediatr Transplant. [Consensus Development Conference Review]. 2001;5(2):80–7.
24. Abu-Elmagd K, Bond G. Gut failure and abdominal visceral transplantation. Proc Nutr Soc. [Research Support, U.S. Gov't, Non-P.H.S. Research Support, U.S. Gov't, P.H.S. Review]. 2003;62(3):727–37.

History of Visceral Transplantation

29

Sherif Armanyous, Mohammed Osman, Neha Parekh,
Masato Fujiki, Raffaele Girlanda, Guilherme Costa,
and Kareem M. Abu-Elmagd

Abbreviations

CMS	Centers for Medicare and Medicaid Services
CMV	Cytomegalovirus
DSA	Donor-specific antibodies
EBV	Epstein-Barr virus
GVHD	Graft-versus-host disease
HRQOL	Health-related quality of life
PTLD	Post-transplant lymphoproliferative disease
PTLD	Post-transplant lymphoproliferative disorders
rATG	Rabbit antithymocyte globulin
SGS	Short gut syndrome
TPN	Total parenteral nutrition

Introduction

For many decades, the abdominal viscera were considered a forbidden organ for clinical transplantation because of the associated massive lymphoid tissue, high antigenicity, and microbial colonization [1, 2]. However, the practical clinical application of the procedure was only feasible after the clinical introduction of Tacrolimus in 1989 with history of sporadic attempts under cyclosporine-based immunosuppression during the late 1980s [3, 4]. With waves of enthusiasm and disappointment, the continual evolution of the procedure was achievable as a result of continuous interplay between innovative surgical techniques, novel immunosuppressive strategies, and improved postoperative care [1, 2, 5].

In 2000, the Centers for Medicare and Medicaid Services (CMS) qualified intestinal and multivisceral transplanta-tion as the standard of care for patients with irreversible gut failure who no longer can be maintained on total parenteral nutrition (TPN) [6]. With the subsequent increase in the worldwide experience, practical guidelines including expansion of the initial indications have evolved in recent years [7, 8]. Despite the continual improvement in outcomes, the procedure is still limited to patients with nutritional failure who no longer can be maintained on TPN. In addition, a few healthcare providers currently mandate failure of gut rehabilitative efforts as a prerequisite for transplantation. However, it is imperative to emphasize that early transplantation, at centers of excellence, has been associated with many therapeutic advantages including better survival, full restoration of nutritional autonomy, and improved quality of life [5]. Furthermore, halting the TPN-associated irreversible damage to the native liver with early transplantation reduces the need for simultaneous hepatic replacement.

This chapter focuses on the 50-year evolution of intestinal and multivisceral transplantation with special reference to nomenclature, indications, surgical techniques, management strategies, and therapeutic efficacy. The types of the visceral allograft are addressed in the milieu of newly introduced surgical techniques, and immunosuppression is discussed according to the era of transplantation. Evolution of postoperative management and long-term outcomes are featured according to the multifaceted continual improvement in the different aspects of the field.

Nomenclature and Type of Visceral Allograft

Nearly a decade ago, controversies were raised concerning the existing nomenclature of the different types of visceral transplantation [9, 10]. Such a dispute was emanated from the continual technical advances in the donor and recipient operation and the lack of better understanding of the historic evolution of the field [3, 10]. Establishment of the

S. Armanyous · M. Osman · N. Parekh · M. Fujiki · R. Girlanda · G. Costa · K. M. Abu-Elmagd (✉)
Center for Gut Rehabilitation and Transplantation, Department of Surgery, Digestive Disease and Surgery Institute, Cleveland Clinic, Cleveland, OH, USA
e-mail: abuelmk@ccf.org

© Springer International Publishing AG, part of Springer Nature 2019
Y. Sher, J. R. Maldonado (eds.), *Psychosocial Care of End-Stage Organ Disease and Transplant Patients*,
https://doi.org/10.1007/978-3-319-94914-7_29

current distinctive nomenclature has largely stemmed from the historic anatomic and surgical principles described with the original multivisceral transplant procedure [11, 12]. The intestine has always been the central core of any abdominal visceral allograft, and the nomenclature is based upon the type and number of donor organs that are included en bloc with the intestine (Table 29.1) [10]. Accordingly, the three main prototypes of visceral transplantation are isolated: intestinal (Fig. 29.1a), liver-intestinal (Fig. 29.1b), and multivisceral including the stomach, duodenum, pancreas, intestine, and liver (Fig. 29.1c).

The terms "isolated intestinal" and "multivisceral" originated more than half a century ago. The "liver-intestinal" was introduced in 1990 and subsequently modified to include the donor pancreaticoduodenal complex [14, 15]. In 1993, a subtype of the full multivisceral procedure was introduced with exclusion of the donor liver in patients with normal hepatic functions and named a "modified" multivisceral transplantation (Fig. 29.1d) [16]. It is important to emphasize that the term "multivisceral" is a distinctive nomenclature that describes the stomach-contained abdominal visceral allograft with (full) and without (modified) inclusion of the liver [10]. The term "cluster" transplant is a misnomer since it does not include the intestine as part of the allograft (Fig. 29.2). The "multi-organ" transplantation is also a common mis-nomenclature and should only be used when multiple solid abdominal or thoracic organs are transplanted simultaneously or sequentially without en bloc inclusion of the intestine.

Current Indications

Despite continual improvement in survival, the current utilization of the isolated intestinal transplant procedure is still limited to patients with irreversible intestinal failure who no longer can be maintained on artificial intravenous nutrition and those with ultrashort gut syndrome [6, 17]. Accordingly, the operation is mostly used as a rescue therapy for patients with TPN-associated life-threatening complications including frequent catheter-related infection, vanishing of the central venous access, and development of significant hepatic injury as fully defined by the senior author (KAE) in the CMS memorandum [6]. With short gut syndrome (SGS) being the major cause of irreversible intestinal failure, the underlying causes are mostly vascular thrombosis and Crohn's disease in adults and congenital disorders in children (e.g., gastroschisis, necrotizing enterocolitis, volvulus, microvillous inclusion disease). Other indications include motility disorders, neoplastic syndromes, trauma, enterocyte functional disorders, and other primary gastrointestinal diseases [17]. See Chap. 28 for further descriptions of intestinal failure and indications for intestinal transplant. Patients with intestinal failure and beta-cell failure commonly require combined intestinal and pancreatic transplantation. The coexistence of renal failure dictates the need for simultaneous or subsequent kidney transplantation.

Composite visceral transplantation utilizing the combined liver-intestinal and multivisceral allografts is commonly indicated for patients with multiple abdominal visceral organ failure and those with complex abdominal pathology [2, 5, 8, 17]. The liver-intestinal allograft is mostly given to the intestinal failure patients with end-stage liver disease due to long-term TPN therapy and other associated primary hepatic pathology [6]. The procedure is also indicated for patients with hepatic failure combined with other splanchnic vascular disorders that precludes isolated liver transplantation [6, 18].

The full and modified multivisceral transplantation has been increasingly utilized for patients with diffuse gut disorders and complex abdominal pathology [8]. The common indications include global gut dysmotility, neoplastic syndromes with extensive gut involvement, and diffuse porto-mesenteric venous thrombosis [8, 17]. The full multivisceral procedure is primarily indicated for patients with concomitant liver failure and those with diffuse thrombosis [18]. The modified procedure with exclusion of the liver is commonly utilized for those with preserved native hepatic functions [16]. In patients with hostile abdomen and complex upper abdominal pathology, the native liver is replaced as part of the full multivisceral procedure regardless of the status of the hepatic functions particularly among the pediatric population and those who are undergoing re-transplantation due to allograft rejection with and without the use of the domino procedure [5, 8].

The contraindications for all of the above types of visceral transplantation are fully addressed elsewhere [5]. They include severe cardiopulmonary insufficiency, incurable malignancy, and persistent significant systemic and/or abdominal infections. In addition to these universal standard contraindications, poor psychosocial support has been recently identified as a major risk factor for successful long-term outcome [19]. Accordingly, the coexistence of nonfunctional social support should be considered a relative contraindication to transplantation. On the contrary, the presence of controlled neuropsychiatric disorders should not preclude transplantation because successful rehabilitation after surgery has been recently demonstrated [8]. Another evolving contraindication is the coexistence of acquired immune deficiencies due to the prohibitive risk of graft-versus-host disease (GVHD) [8]. Without innovative immune-modulatory approaches including stem cell transplantation, the procedure should not be considered in the presence of acquired or hereditary immune deficiency syndromes.

Table 29.1 Types of composite visceral allografts

Types of composite visceral allografts

Intestine-pancreas	Liver-intestine[a]	Multivisceral	
		Full	Modified
		Stomach + duodenum + pancreas + intestine + liver	Stomach + duodenum + pancreas + intestine
Descriptive			
En bloc with the colon and/or kidney.	En bloc with the colon and/or kidney.	En bloc with the colon and/or kidney. With preserved pancreaticoduodenal complex and/or spleen.	

Adapted with permission of Abu-Elmagd [10]

[a]Inclusion of the pancreaticoduodenal complex is optional and commonly utilized for technical reasons

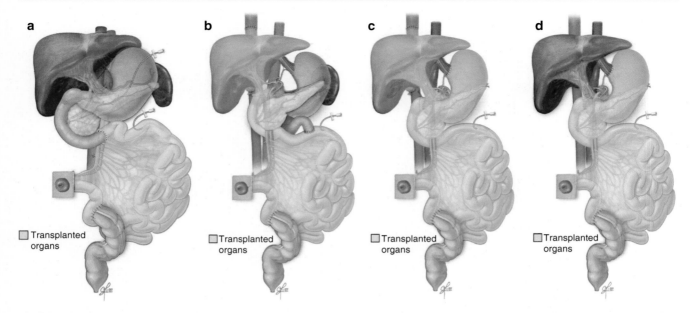

Fig. 29.1 The three main prototypes of visceral transplantation: (**a**) the isolated intestine, (**b**) the liver plus intestine with inclusion of the duodenopancreatic complex, and (**c**) full multivisceral that includes the stomach, duodenum, pancreases, intestine, and liver. The full multivis-ceral graft can be modified by retraining the native liver and transplanting the stomach, duodenum, pancreas, and intestine allografts (**d**). (Adapted with permission of Abu-Elmagd et al. [13])

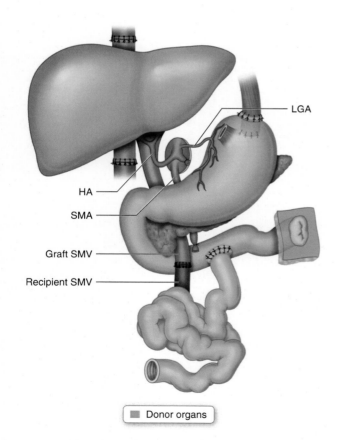

Fig. 29.2 Cluster graft with en bloc inclusion of the stomach, pancreas, and duodenum with the donor liver. (Used with permission from Starzl et al. [12])

Innovative Surgical Techniques

Modifications of the donor operation and introduction of innovative transplant surgical techniques have significantly contributed to the recent evolution of intestinal and multivisceral transplantation. With standard techniques described elsewhere, the donor operation witnessed novel techniques including simultaneous retrieval of the intestine and pancreas from the same donor to be given to two different recipients (Fig. 29.3a), en bloc retrieval of the intestine and pancreas (Fig. 29.3b), preservation of the pancreaticoduodenal complex with the combined liver-intestinal allograft (Fig. 29.3c), and en bloc retrieval of the small and large intestine (Fig. 29.3d) [6, 15, 20, 22]. The free vascular pedicle abdominal wall allograft (Fig. 29.3e) has also been introduced but with less frequent utilization [20]. These innovative approaches increased deceased organ utilization and reduced the recipient technical complications with increased practicality and improved outcome.

The previously published recipient operation with the different types of visceral transplantation has also received various modifications involving the evisceration and implantation techniques [6, 23, 24]. When medically and technically feasible, the native left upper quadrant organs are preserved, particularly of the spleen with (Fig. 29.4a) and without (Fig. 29.4b) the duodenopancreatic complex, in patients who are in need of full and modified multivisceral transplantation [23, 24]. The procedure is introduced with the premise to reduce risk of post-transplant lymphoproliferative disorders

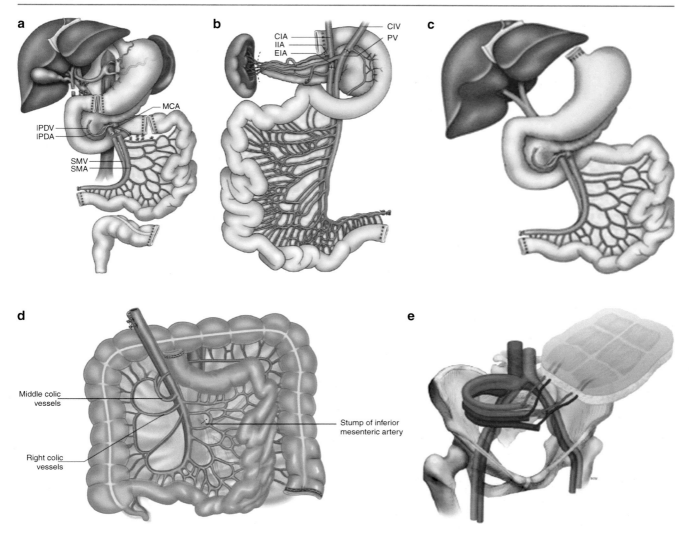

Fig. 29.3 (**a**) Simultaneous procurement of the intestine, pancreas, and liver from the same donor to be given to three different recipients. (Adapted with permission from Abu-Elmagd et al. [20]). (**b**) En bloc retrieval of the intestine and pancreas with back-table vascular reconstruction to be given to the same recipient. (Adapted with permission from Abu-Elmagd et al. [6]). (**c**) En bloc preservation of the donor duodenopancreatic complex with the liver and intestine to maintain integ- rity of the vascular axis and continuity of the biliary pancreatic system. (**d**) En bloc retrieval of the small and large intestine. Note the preservation of the middle colic vessels. (**e**) The abdominal wall graft with bilateral epigastric vessels retrieved in continuity with the external iliac vessels that are anastomosed into the recipient's common iliac vessels. (Reprinted from Cipriani et al. [21]; with permission)

(PTLD) and GVHD. The procedure also reduces the risk of post-transplant diabetes by retaining the native beta-cell mass in addition to the transplanted pancreas. Other important modifications include placement of free arterial (Fig. 29.5a) and venous (Fig. 29.5b) interposition grafts with all types of transplantation to ease the vascular reconstruction at the time of implantation. The native colon has also been recently utilized as an alimentary conduit in the isolated intestinal (Fig. 29.6a) and modified multivisceral (Fig. 29.6b) recipients [25, 26]. For patients who are suitable candidates for hindgut reconstruction, a pull-through operation is performed with a segment of the allograft colonic en bloc with the small intestine (Fig. 29.7) [28]. These various technical advances

unequivocally improved surgical outcomes, long-term outcomes, and quality of life [5].

Advanced Management Strategies

Management of intestinal and multivisceral transplantation has evolved over the last few decades with innovative immunosuppressive protocols, better allograft monitoring, and improved postoperative care including antimicrobial prophylaxis [2, 5, 8]. The high immunogenicity of the gut was behind the delayed clinical introduction of the procedure and the 1990s early disappointment with high graft loss due to

Fig. 29.4 Preservation of the native spleen in patients undergoing multivisceral transplantation with (**a**) and without (**b**) the pancreaticoduodenal complex

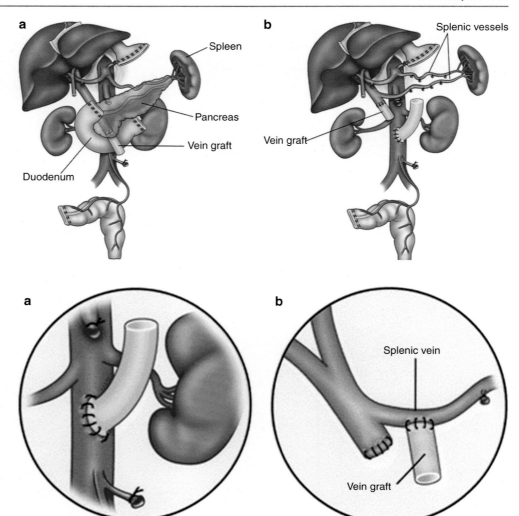

Fig. 29.5 Placement of free interposition arterial (**a**) and vein (**b**) graft before implantation of the visceral allograft. The arterial graft is commonly placed on the infrarenal native aorta, and the vein graft is placed on the main portal, superior mesenteric or splenic vein. In selected cases the vein graft is placed on the infrarenal inferior vena cava

rejection despite the use of tacrolimus-steroid-based immunosuppression, namely, Era-I [1, 5, 15, 29]. As a result, induction therapy with pharmacological and biologic agents such as cyclophosphamide and anti-IL2 receptor humanized antibodies was added to the immunosuppressive regimen during the second half of the 1990s and ushered in Era-II [5, 30]. In subsequent years, the anti-lymphocyte depleting agents, namely, rabbit antithymocyte globulin (rATG) and alemtuzumab, were used as an alternative induction treatment [1, 5, 31]. Meanwhile, azathioprine, mycophenolate mofetil, and mammalian target of rapamycin (mTOR) inhibitors have been widely used by most centers as an adjunct maintenance therapy [1]. Donor pretreatment with OKT3 and later with rATG was also used by one or two centers [8].

The immune-modulatory strategy was solely introduced and frequently utilized by the Pittsburgh group [1, 5, 22]. Bone marrow augmentation and allograft irradiation were introduced during the late 1990s to further improve outcome and reduce the long-term burden of heavy immunosuppression on long-term survival outcome. With new insights into the mechanism of allograft acceptance and transplant tolerance, the protocol was modified in 2001 to recipient pretreatment using a single dose of thymoglobulin (5 mg/Kg) or alemtuzumab (30 mg) with post-transplant minimal immunosuppression marking the beginning of Era-III [1, 5, 32–34]. The aim was to improve allograft stability with minimal post-transplant long-term immunosuppression achieving a state of partial "prope" tolerance. With such a novel protocol, further improvement in outcome was achieved with more survival advantage utilizing alemtuzumab compared to rabbit antithymocyte globulin (thymoglobulin) [5, 34]. Reduction in the incidence of intractable rejection and fatal opportunistic infections including PTLD partially contributed to better long-term survival. Minimization of maintenance immunosuppression was unprecedented among long-term survivors supporting the clinical feasibility of achieving partial tolerance in these immunologically challenging recipients [1, 5].

Immunologic monitoring of the visceral allograft response has been the Achilles heel and most challenging

Fig. 29.6 Utilization of the native colon as an alimentary conduit in isolated intestine (**a**) and modified multivisceral (**b**) recipients. The recipient colonic segment is used to connect the second part of the native duodenum to the allograft jejunum and the esophagus to the transplanted stomach, respectively

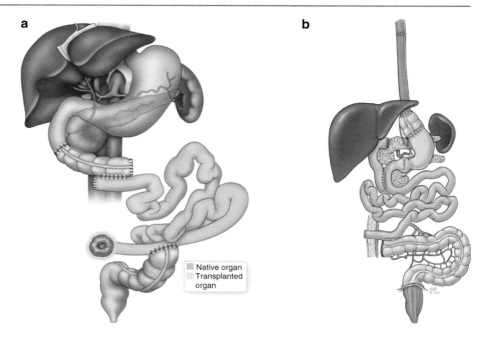

aspect of postoperative care [1, 5]. Little progress has been made concerning the early detection of graft-versus-host response (intestinal allograft rejection). Protocol ileoscopy with multiple random intestinal biopsies continued to be the standard of care for the diagnosis and management of acute rejection [5]. The diagnostic criteria of acute cellular, humoral, and chronic rejection have been established over the last two decades [5, 35, 36]. Rejection of the pancreatic allograft is suspected in patients with significant elevation of serum amylase and lipase without evident causes of non-immunologic pancreatitis. Rejection of the liver allograft among the composite visceral allograft recipients is very uncommon, and the diagnosis can be easily made utilizing the well-established biochemical and histopathologic criteria. With the recent technological advances in detection and serial measurement of circulating donor-specific antibodies (DSA), the detrimental impact of such a sinister problem on allograft survival has been well documented with the introduction of innovative management strategies to reduce the long-term risk of humeral and chronic rejection [37].

The dynamic process of graft-versus-host reaction has been recently monitored by the serial detection of circulating donor cells in the recipient peripheral blood [5]. The diagnosis of GVHD is usually confirmed by histopathologic and immunocytochemical studies that allow identification of donor leukocytes in the peripheral blood and targeted organs. The utilized methodology includes PCR techniques, in situ hybridization using Y-chromosome-specific probe, and the immunohistologic staining of donor-specific HLA antigens. In addition, the short tandem repeat technique has been more frequently utilized in recent years [5].

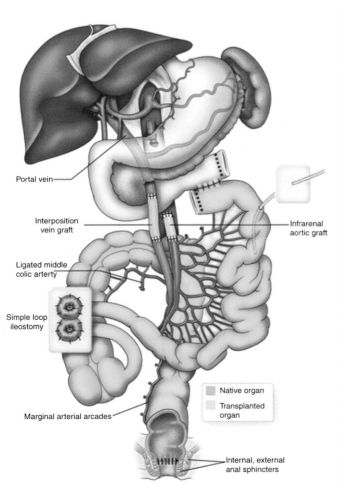

Fig. 29.7 Hindgut pull-through reconstruction with en bloc colon and intestinal transplantation (Adapted with permission from Eid et al. [27])

The short- and long-term nutritional care has also improved over time with speedy use of elementary enteral feeding due to better early graft function. With such an enhanced allograft recovery and proper discontinuation of TPN therapy, the time and cost of the initial hospitalization were reduced with better value of heath care. However, the achievement of full nutritional autonomy requires flexible and complex management strategies. Enteric feeding is commonly initiated within the first 2 weeks after transplantation with stepwise reduction in intravenous nutrition with the goal to completely discontinue TPN therapy within the first 4 weeks after transplantation. Temporary and intermittent reinstitution of TPN support is often required in patients with severe allograft rejection and protracted allograft dysfunction [8]. See Chap. 31 for more details on nutrition.

With cumulative clinical experience, advanced molecular diagnostic techniques, and new antimicrobial drugs, the outcome after multivisceral transplantation has substantially improved with reduced risk of lethal viral, bacterial, and fungal infections [5]. The availability of the PCR assay prompted early detection and serial monitoring of peripheral blood viremia with Epstein-Barr virus (EBV) and cytomegalovirus (CMV). The introduction of new antimicrobial agents has also improved the efficacy of infection prophylaxis, preemptive therapy, and active treatment. Along with stepwise judicious reduction in maintenance immunosuppression, these developments have considerably reduced the risks of PTLD, CMV, and fungal infections that were observed with the initial multivisceral transplant clinical experience [5].

The longitudinal follow-up has been essential to maintain the long-term success after intestinal and multivisceral transplantation [5, 19]. The multivisceral recipients are at a relatively high risk of PTLD and de novo malignancies and require a careful follow-up [38]. Such formidable threats are most probably due to prolonged exposure to different environmental and non-environmental oncogenes with a foreseeable acquired state of impaired immune surveillance [38]. Kidney function, glucose homeostasis, skeletal health, and cardiovascular integrity are also monitored closely in patients with suboptimal allograft function and chronic need for heavy maintenance immunosuppression. Regular tumor surveillance and other pertinent screening protocols have been effective in the early diagnosis and prompt management of these unique recipients with sustained improvement in outcome and quality of life [19].

Improved Therapeutic Efficacy

The recently reported growing global experience with visceral transplantation is a testimony of the continual improvement in the procedure's short- and long-term therapeutic efficacy [39]. Such an achievement is a result of the earlier underscored innovative surgical techniques, novel immunosuppressive protocols, and better postoperative management as comprehensively discussed above. These advances undoubtedly justify the recent elevation of the procedure status with the privilege to permanently reside in a respected place in the surgical armamentarium [8].

Survival

The worldwide and largest single-center cumulative experience has repeatedly demonstrated steady improvement in 1-year and 5-year actuarial patient and allograft survival with current rates comparable to other abdominal and thoracic allografts (Fig. 29.8) [5, 19, 39]. Beyond the 5-year milestone, the longest and largest single-center series documented a 10-year patient survival of 75% and 60% at 15 years with a respective graft

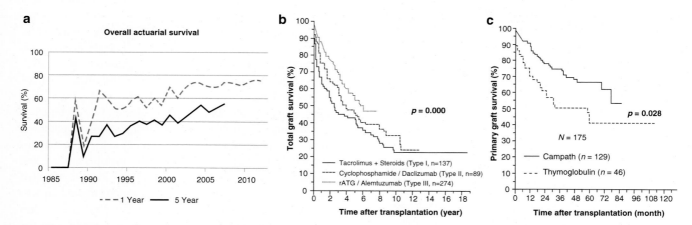

Fig. 29.8 (**a**) A time series analysis of the 1- and 5-year actuarial graft survival shows significant improvement over time ($p < 0.001$) (Grant et al. [39]). (**b**) Improvement of visceral allograft survival according to the type of immunosuppression (Data from Abu-Elmagd et al. [5]), (**c**) Better graft survival in patients pretreated with alemtuzumab (Campath-1H) compared to those pretreated with antithymocyte globulin (thymoglobulin) (Data from Abu-Elmagd et al. [34])

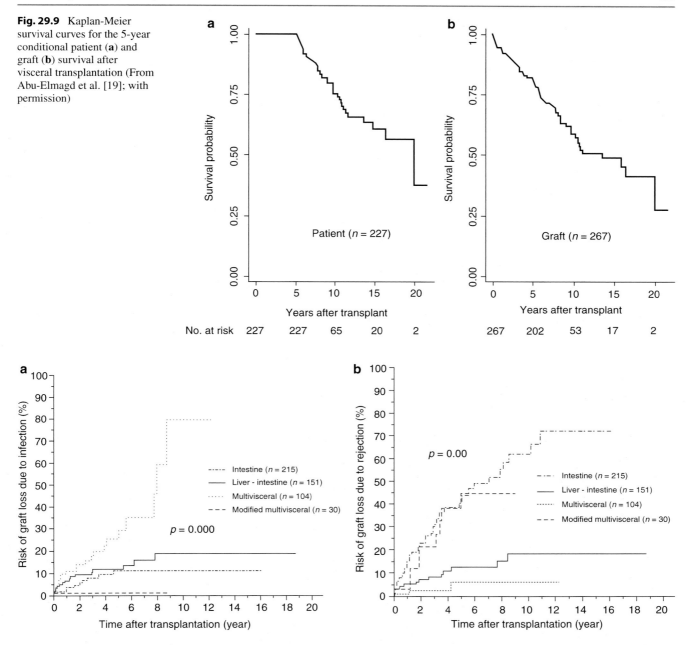

Fig. 29.9 Kaplan-Meier survival curves for the 5-year conditional patient (**a**) and graft (**b**) survival after visceral transplantation (From Abu-Elmagd et al. [19]; with permission)

Fig. 29.10 Cumulative risk of graft loss due to (**a**) infection and (**b**) acute and chronic rejection according to type of visceral allograft. (Used with permission of Abu-Elmagd et al. [5])

survival of 59% and 50% (Fig. 29.9) [19]. Of note, the data from worldwide experience as reported by ITR demonstrates lower survival rates (see Chap. 32). Loss of graft function and complications of immunosuppression continue to be the major threat to long-term survival with rejection, infection, and renal failure being the leading causes of death. Interestingly, the cumulative risk of infection has been significantly higher among the multivisceral recipients compared to other visceral allograft patients (Fig. 29.10a) [5, 19]. Meanwhile, the liver-free visceral allografts experienced a significantly higher risk of cumulative graft loss due to rejection (Fig. 29.10b) [5].

Several predictors of survival outcome for both patient and allograft have been recently published [19]. The lack of social support and absence of the liver as part of the composite and multivisceral grafts have emerged as highly significant risk factors for patient and graft survival, respectively (Table 29.2) [19]. The immunoprotective effect of the liver can be potentially explained in the context of ameliorating the detrimental effect of donor-specific antibodies (DSA) on the visceral allograft survival (Fig. 29.11) [37]. Other important risk factors include early rejection, recipient sex and age, splenectomy, re-transplan-

Table 29.2 Long-term survival risk factors for visceral transplantation

Risk factor	P value	Hazard ratio	95% CI
Patient			
Lack of social support	0.000	6.132	3.370–11.160
Rejection <90 days	0.016	2.363	1.172–4.765
Female recipient	0.025	1.992	1.089–3.646
Recipient age > 20 year	0.025	2.014	1.093–3.711
Re-transplantation	0.026	2.053	1.089–3.873
No preconditioning	0.046	2.013	1.013–4.997
Graft			
Liver-free allograft	0.000	3.224	2.026–5.132
Splenectomy	0.001	2.212	1.396–3.506
HLA mismatch	0.040	1.258	1.011–1.565
Rejection <90 days	0.046	1.601	1.008–2.541
PTLD	0.085	1.638	0.934–2.872

Abbreviations: *HLA* human leukocyte antigen, *PTLD* post-transplant lymphoproliferative disease. (Used with permission of Abu-Elmagd et al. [19])

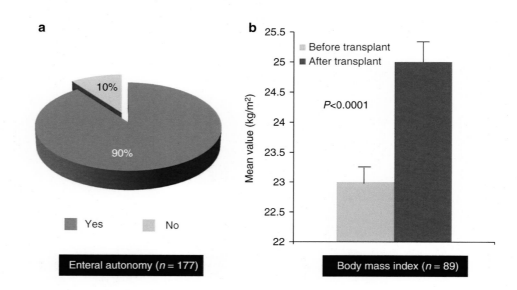

Fig. 29.11 The immunoprotective effect of the liver has been recently explained by ameliorating the detrimental effect of donor-specific antibodies (DSA) on the visceral allograft survival. (Used with permission of Abu-Elmagd et al. [37])

Fig. 29.12 Nutritional autonomy after visceral transplantation. (**a**) Achievement of enteric autonomy defined by freedom from intravenous nutrition and fluid supplement. (**b**) Body mass index before and after transplantation. (Used with permission of Abu-Elmagd et al. [19])

tation, HLA mismatch, and type of immunosuppression with variable weight of statistical significance [19].

Graft Function

The ability to restore nutritional autonomy is the second most important metric of successful visceral transplantation. A high rate of freedom from intravenous nutrition with maintained nutritional status and significant improvement in body mass index (BMI) has been documented after transplantation including long-term survivors for more than 20 years (Fig. 29.12) [19]. The adult recipients maintain normal serum albumin and trace elements with improved skeletal health (Fig. 29.13) [19]. Most children experience fairly normal linear growth with a few requiring hormonal replacement.

The failure to achieve full nutritional autonomy in a few of the composite and multivisceral recipients is mainly due to persistent allograft dysmotility and steatorrhea resulting from allograft denervation and lymphatic disruption inherent to the transplant procedure. With the clinical availability of normothermic ex vivo perfusion technology, the unwanted effect of ischemia reperfusion could be ameliorated [8]. It is also reasonable to believe that the altered allograft microbiota may play a major role in allograft dysfunction and recipient well-being.

Quality of Life

With improved survival outcome, quality of life has become one of the primary therapeutic end points. A few scattered

Fig. 29.13 (**a**) Physiological biochemical measures and (**b**) skeletal health in a large single-center series before and after visceral transplantation. Skeletal health was measured by dual-energy x-ray absorptiometry (DXA). (Used with permission of Abu-Elmagd et al. [19])

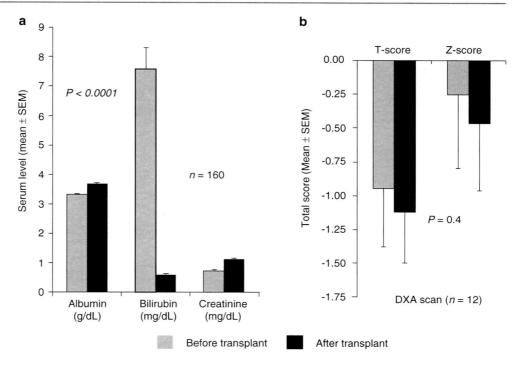

Fig. 29.14 Reversal of the depressed effect of PN on most quality of life domains, except depression, after visceral transplantation. (Used with permission of Abu-Elmagd et al. [19])

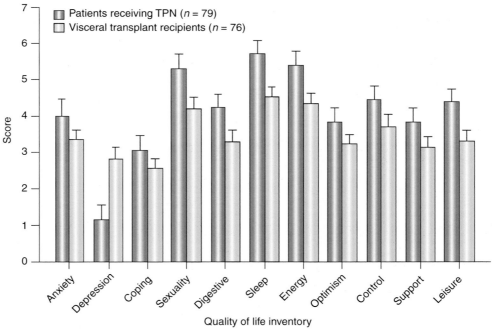

reports have been recently published among both children and adults [40–46]. Studies among children demonstrated physical and psychosocial functions similar to healthy normal children. However, the parental proxy assessments were different with lower responses in certain categories than that given by children. In addition, lower values in the school functioning subcategories and psychological health summary score were reported compared with healthy children. In

adults, most published studies on health-related quality of life (HRQOL) have demonstrated improvements in many of the domains with better rehabilitative indices than TPN. Except for depression, successful transplantation offsets the deprived effect of both PN and disease gravity in most domains (Fig. 29.14) [19].

The socioeconomic milestones have also been used to assess the rehabilitative efficacy of visceral transplantation in all age groups [19]. A high education score was reported with sustained cognitive, psychosocial, and physical functions. In addition, the ability to create a nuclear family along with high Lansky and Karnofsky performance scores is demonstrated and comprehensively reported [19]. The data has also been in favor of early consideration for visceral transplantation to further improve quality of life by reducing the risk of organic brain-dysfunction-related morbidities associated with brain atrophy, cerebral vascular insufficiency, micronutrient deficiencies, trace element toxicities, and liver failure. Accordingly, early consideration of transplantation is strongly recommended for patients with irreversible gut failure who are not suitable candidates for autologous gut rehabilitation.

Conclusions

Visceral transplantation continues to evolve as a life-saving therapy for patients with irreversible anatomic, parenchymal, and functional gut failure. The procedure has also been utilized to rescue patients with complex abdominal pathology that is not amenable to current conventional medical and surgical treatment modalities. Despite all efforts, the field continues to face the challenges of immunologic monitoring and longevity of the liver-free visceral allografts. With new insights into the biology of gut immunity and mechanisms of transplant acceptance, the establishment of less complex postoperative care and the achievement of a drug-free allograft acceptance are within reach.

References

1. Abu-Elmagd KM, Costa G, Bond GJ, et al. Evolution of the immunosuppressive strategies for the intestinal and multivisceral recipients with special reference to allograft immunity and achievement of partial tolerance. Transpl Int. 2009;22:96–109.
2. Grant D, Abu-Elmagd K, Reyes J, et al. 2003 report of the intestine transplant registry: a new era has dawned. Ann Surg. 2005;241:607–13.
3. Abu-Elmagd KM. The history of intestinal transplantation. In: Hakim NS, Papalois VE, editors. History of organ and cell transplantation. London: Imperial College Press; 2003. p. 171–93.
4. Starzl TE, Todo S, Fung J, et al. FK 506 for human liver, kidney, and pancreas transplantation. Lancet. 1989;2:1000–4.
5. Abu-Elmagd KM, Costa G, Bond GJ, et al. Five hundred intestinal and multivisceral transplantations at a single center: major advances with new challenges. Ann Surg. 2009;250:567–81.
6. Abu-Elmagd K, Bond G, Reyes J, et al. Intestinal transplantation: a coming of age. Adv Surg. 2002;36:65–101.
7. Grant D. Intestinal transplantation: 1997 report of the international registry: intestinal transplant registry. Transplantation. 1999;67:1061–4.
8. Abu-Elmagd K. The concept of gut rehabilitation and the future of visceral transplantation. Nat Rev Gastroenterol Hepatol. 2015;12:108–20.
9. Mazariegos GV, Steffick DE, Horslen S, et al. Intestine transplantation in the United States, 1999-2008. Am J Transplant. 2010;10:1020–34.
10. Abu-Elmagd KM. The small bowel contained allografts: existing and proposed nomenclature. Am J Transplant. 2011;11:184–5.
11. Starzl TE, Kaupp HA Jr. Mass homotransplantations of abdominal organs in dogs. Surg Forum. 1960;11:28–30.
12. Starzl TE, Todo S, Tzakis A, et al. The many faces of multivisceral transplantation. Surg Gynecol Obstet. 1991;172:335–44.
13. Abu-Elmagd K, Khanna A, Fujiki M, et al. Surgery for gut failure: auto-reconstruction and allo-transplantation. In: Fazio V, Church JM, Delaney CP, Kiran RP, editors. Current therapy in colon and rectal surgery. Philadelphia: Elsevier, Inc; 2017. p. 372–84.
14. Grant D, Wall W, Mimeault R, et al. Successful small-bowel/liver transplantation. Lancet. 1990;335:181–4.
15. Abu-Elmagd K, Reyes J, Todo S, et al. Clinical intestinal transplantation: new perspectives and immunologic considerations. J Am Coll Surg. 1998;186:512–25.
16. Cruz RJ Jr, Costa G, Bond G, et al. Modified "liver-sparing" multivisceral transplant with preserved native spleen, pancreas, and duodenum: technique and long-term outcome. J Gastrointest Surg. 2010;14:1709–21.
17. Abu-Elmagd KM. Intestinal transplantation: indications and patient selection. In: Langnas AN, Goulet O, Quigley EM, editors. Intestinal failure: diagnosis, management and transplantation. Oxford: Wiley-Blackwell; 2008. p. 245–53.
18. Vianna RM, Mangus RS, Kubal C, et al. Multivisceral transplantation for diffuse portomesenteric thrombosis. Ann Surg. 2012;255:1144–50.
19. Abu-Elmagd KM, Kosmach-Park B, Costa G, et al. Long-term survival, nutritional autonomy, and quality of life after intestinal and multivisceral transplantation. Ann Surg. 2012;256:494–508.
20. Abu-Elmagd K, Fung J, Bueno J, et al. Logistics and technique for procurement of intestinal, pancreatic, and hepatic grafts from the same donor. Ann Surg. 2000;232:680–7.
21. Cipriani R, Contedini F, Santoli M, et al. Abdominal wall transplantation with microsurgical technique. Am J Transplant. 2007;7:1304–7.
22. Abu-Elmagd K, Reyes J, Bond G, et al. Clinical intestinal transplantation: a decade of experience at a single center. Ann Surg. 2001;234:404–16.
23. Abu-Elmagd KM. Preservation of the native spleen, duodenum, and pancreas in patients with multivisceral transplantation: nomenclature, dispute of origin, and proof of premise. Transplantation. 2007;84:1208–9.
24. Cruz RJ Jr, Costa G, Bond GJ, et al. Modified multivisceral transplantation with spleen-preserving pancreaticoduodenectomy for patients with familial adenomatous polyposis "Gardner's syndrome". Transplantation. 2011;91:1417–23.
25. Fujiki M, Hashimoto H, Khanna A, Quintini C, Costa G, Abu-Elmagd K. Technical innovation and visceral transplantation. In: Subramaniam K, Sakai T, editors. Anesthesia and perioperative care for organ transplantation. New York: Springer; 2017. p. 497–511.
26. Abu-Elmagd KM, Costa G, McMichael D, et al. Autologous reconstruction and visceral transplantation for management of patients with gut failure after bariatric surgery: 20 years of experience. Ann Surg. 2015;262:586–601.
27. Eid KR, Costa G, Bond GJ, Cruz RJ, Rubin E, Bielefeldt K, et al. An innovative sphincter preserving pull-through technique with en bloc colon and small bowel transplantation. Am J Transplant. 2010;10:1940–6.
28. Abu-Elmagd K, Costa G. Intestinal lengthening and transplantation surgery: candidacy, logistics, and techniques. In: Oniscu G, et al., editors. Springer surgery atlas series: transplantation surgery. Milan: Springer; 2018. (In press.).

29. Todo S, Reyes J, Furukawa H, et al. Outcome analysis of 71 clinical intestinal transplantations. Ann Surg. 1995;222:270–80.

30. Abu-Elmagd K, Fung J, McGhee W, et al. The efficacy of daclizumab for intestinal transplantation: preliminary report. Transplant Proc. 2000;32:1195–6.

31. Tzakis AG, Kato T, Nishida S, et al. Preliminary experience with campath 1H (C1H) in intestinal and liver transplantation. Transplantation. 2003;75:1227–31.

32. Starzl TE, Zinkernagel RM. Transplantation tolerance from a historical perspective. Nat Rev Immunol. 2001;1:233–9.

33. Starzl TE, Murase N, Abu-Elmagd K, et al. Tolerogenic immunosuppression for organ transplantation. Lancet. 2003;361:1502–10.

34. Abu-Elmagd KM, Costa G, Bond GJ, et al. A decade of experience with a single dose of rabbit antithymocyte globulin or alemtuzumab pretreatment for intestinal and multivisceral transplantation. Clin Transplant. 2012;13:155–66.

35. Lee RG, Nakamura K, Tsamandas AC, et al. Pathology of human intestinal transplantation. Gastroenterol. 1996;110:2009–12.

36. Wu T, Abu-Elmagd K, Bond G, Demetris AJ. A clinic pathologic study of isolated intestinal allografts with preformed IgG lymphocytotoxic antibodies. Hum Pathol. 2004;35:1332–9.

37. Abu-Elmagd KM, et al. Preformed and de novo donor specific antibodies in visceral transplantation: long-term outcome with special reference to the liver. Am J Transplant. 2012;12:3047–360.

38. Abu-Elmagd KM, Mazariegos G, Costa G, et al. Lymphoproliferative disorders and de novo malignancies in intestinal and multivisceral recipients: improved outcomes with new outlooks. Transplantation. 2009;88:926–34.

39. Grant D, Abu-Elmagd K, Mazariegos G, et al. Intestinal transplant registry report: global activity and trends. Am J Transplant. 2015;15:201–19.

40. Sudan D, Iyer K, Horslen S, et al. Assessment of quality of life after pediatric intestinal transplantation by parents and pediatric recipients using the child health questionnaire. Transplant Proc. 2002;34:963–4.

41. Ngo KD, Farmer DG, McDiarmid SV, et al. Pediatric health-related quality of life after intestinal transplantation. Pediatr Transplant. 2011;15:849–54.

42. DiMartini A, Rovera GM, Graham TO, et al. Quality of life after small intestinal transplantation and among home parenteral nutrition patients. J Parenter Enteral Nutr. 1998;22:357–62.

43. Rovera GM, DiMartini A, Schoen RE, et al. Quality of life of patients after intestinal transplantation. Transplantation. 1998;66:1141–5.

44. Rovera GM, DiMartini A, Graham TO, et al. Quality of life after intestinal transplantation and on total parenteral nutrition. Transplant Proc. 1998;30:2513–4.

45. Stenn PG, Lammens P, Houle L, et al. Psychiatric psychosocial and ethical aspects of small bowel transplantation. Transplant Proc. 1992;24:1251–2.

46. Cameron EA, Binnie JA, Jamieson NV, et al. Quality of life in adults following small bowel transplantation. Transplant Proc. 2002;34:965–6.

Mental Health in Patients Requiring Pancreas and Visceral Transplantation

30

Catherine Crone and Jacqueline Posada

Pancreas Transplant

Depression in Patients with Type 1 Diabetes

Type 1 diabetes (T1D) is a chronic disorder involving autoimmune destruction of pancreatic beta cells resulting in lifelong insulin dependence. Disease onset primarily occurs in childhood or adolescence, though it can also develop during adulthood. Once diagnosed, patients face long-term dependence on insulin injections or continuous infusion, as well as a number of lifestyle modifications, including frequent daily blood glucose monitoring, dietary restrictions, increased self-monitoring, and ongoing medical care. Concerns about hypoglycemic episodes, diabetic ketoacidosis, hospitalizations, and long-term complications, such as nephropathy, retinopathy, neuropathy, cardiovascular disease, as well as a shortened life-span, accompany the diagnosis of diabetes. Under these circumstances, reports of increased psychological distress among this patient population are perhaps not surprising. For T1D patients referred for pancreas transplantation, greater awareness of their psychological needs may help providers to better assess candidates and facilitate care when concerns are identified.

Prevalence rates for depression are elevated among patients with T1D, with estimates up to three times higher than the general population [1]. This is primarily related to the presence of depressive symptoms, as formally diagnosed mood disorders are reported in approximately 10–15% of patients [2]. While fewer studies have focused on children and adolescents, the pooled prevalence of depressive symptoms is reportedly 30% [3]. The psychological burden of living with and managing diabetes is considered to be a significant contributor to the increased rate of depression observed in adults and children with T1D [4]. However, there is also evidence suggesting contributions from biologic factors, including hypothalamic–pituitary–adrenal (HPA) axis dysfunction, chronic inflammation, prefrontal cortical changes, and hippocampal atrophy potentially affecting neuroplasticity [2, 5–7].

Comorbid depression negatively impacts adherence to diabetes self-management, including glucose monitoring, dietary modifications, and foot care. Reduced glycemic control has been observed across studies in patients with comorbid depression, although the effect size is considered small to moderate [8]. In children and adolescents, depressive symptoms are more clearly linked with poorer glycemic control [9]. The impact of depression on the risk of developing diabetes complications has been apparent, as significant associations have been found with both microvascular and macrovascular complications [10]. These findings also suggest that increases in depressive symptomatology are associated with increased number and severity of complications [10]. Additional evidence points to increased healthcare costs, reduced quality of life (QOL), functional disability, and early mortality [11–13]. Depression is also predictive of a greater need for rehospitalization and retinopathy [2, 14].

Screening and Diagnosis of Depression in Patients with Type 1 Diabetes

Due to the increased prevalence and negative impact of depression, recommendations have been made to incorporate depression screening into routine diabetes care [15]. While

C. Crone (✉)
Department of Psychiatry, Inova Fairfax Hospital, Falls Church, VA, USA

Department of Psychiatry, Virginia Commonwealth University School of Medicine, Richmond, VA, USA

Department of Psychiatry, George Washington University School of Medicine, Washington, DC, USA
e-mail: Cathy.crone@inova.org

J. Posada
Department of Psychiatry, George Washington University School of Medicine, Washington, DC, USA

© Springer International Publishing AG, part of Springer Nature 2019
Y. Sher, J. R. Maldonado (eds.), *Psychosocial Care of End-Stage Organ Disease and Transplant Patients*,
https://doi.org/10.1007/978-3-319-94914-7_30

perhaps desirable, lack of consensus on the particular screening tool to use complicates matters [16]. Commonly used instruments include the Beck Depression Inventory, the Center for Epidemiological Studies Depression Scale, and the Patient Health Questionnaire, but there is limited data on reliability and validity in this patient population [17]. Whichever is chosen, raising the cutoff score and following up a positive screen with a formal assessment have been recommended to reduce the risk of overdiagnosis of depression [16].

Treatment of Depression in Patients with Type 1 Diabetes

Randomized clinical trials utilizing psychotherapy have yielded moderate reduction in depressive symptoms, with most utilizing cognitive behavioral therapy (CBT) or problem solving techniques [16, 18].

Antidepressants have also produced a positive effective, particularly selective serotonin reuptake inhibitors (SSRIs) [16, 18]. A recent study comparing a 12-week course of CBT to sertraline, with sertraline prescribed for an additional 12 months, showed that both treatments improved depression severity, but sertraline was more effective in preventing relapse at 1-year follow-up [19]. No benefits to glycemic control were observed with either approach, although mixed effects on glycemic control have been reported in other clinical trials [16, 18, 19]. Collaborative care aimed at addressing diabetes and depression has shown promise. While the Pathways study reported reduced depression, but lack of improvement in glycemic control, application of TeamCare, which combined behavioral and pharmacological approaches with diabetes management, showed positive effects on depression, glycemic control, blood pressure, lipids, and reduced costs [20, 21].

Diabetes Distress

Despite efforts to examine the relationship between diabetes and depression, the lack of a consistent definition of depression and its measurement has contributed to inconsistent findings across studies (e.g., depression and glycemic control) [22]. Instead of relying on a symptom-based diagnosis of depression, arguments have been made to apply an alternate concept that includes the psychological demands of living with diabetes. *Diabetes distress* is defined as the emotional distress caused by the ongoing worries, burdens, and concerns associated with this chronic disease [22]. It is not considered a substitute for "clinical" depression but serves as a continuous dimension encompassing distress ranging from subclinical depression to major depressive disorder [22]. When identified, diabetes distress links directly to reduced treatment adherence, poor glycemic control, higher complication rates, and impaired QOL [23]. Though most studies of diabetes distress focus on T2D patients, some center on T1D and include efforts to discern areas of distress unique to T1D. A qualitative survey that was developed and tested in two T1D patient populations identified seven areas of distress including powerlessness, negative social perceptions, physician distress, family/friend distress, hypoglycemia distress, self-management distress, and eating distress [24]. Subsequent application of the 28-item T1-Diabetes Distress Scale to patients at baseline and at 9 months demonstrated a prevalence of 42% and 54%, respectively [25]. Those identified as distressed at baseline tended to remain so over time. Distress related to a sense of powerlessness was a significant and persistent contributor to overall diabetes distress [25]. Another study assessing the relationship between diabetes distress and self-management showed that elevated baseline distress was associated with higher HbA1C levels and greater percentage of missed insulin doses [26]. Over time, elevated baseline distress was related to increases in missed insulin, while reduced distress was connected to decreases in HbA1C. On the other hand, depression symptoms were not associated with missed insulin, HbA1C levels, or hypoglycemic episodes. Identification of this risk for missed insulin over time was felt to be a potential intervention target [26]. The concept of diabetes distress has also been applied to parents of T1D children and teens, facilitating the identification of factors contributing to their distress [27]. Among adolescents, elevated diabetes distress has been found to be strongly related to poorer glycemic control [28].

Anxiety in Patients with Type 1 Diabetes

Although research on anxiety and diabetes is relatively limited, elevated rates of anxiety and anxiety disorders have been reported, and the presence of anxiety is associated with negative effects on treatment adherence, glycemic control, symptom burden, and QOL as well as increased complications and pain, depression, BMI, disability, and increased mortality [29]. Adults have a 20% increased prevalence of anxiety disorders, with generalized anxiety disorder being the most common diagnosis [29]. Women, younger individuals, those with longer disease duration, and those with diabetic complications appear to be at greater risk for an anxiety disorder [30]. Given the unique challenges of living with diabetes, specific sources of fear and anxiety have been identified. These include fear of complications, hypoglycemia, and invasive procedures (e.g., injections, blood glucose monitoring, insulin pump, continuous glucose monitors) [30]. While lifetime prevalence of phobias is not more common in diabetic patients, its presence, such as fear of needles, can complicate care [31]. Fear of invasive self-care behaviors includes the need for patients to rotate insulin injection sites to limit subcutaneous scarring which interferes with insulin absorption [30]. Small uncontrolled studies suggest benefits from systematic desensitization, while small controlled trials using mindfulness-based cognitive therapy, diabetes education, self-management training, and psychoeducation have proven helpful [30, 32, 33].

Efforts to maintain tighter glycemic control in order to reduce the risk of microvascular complications put T1D patients at higher risk of hypoglycemia. Fear of hypoglycemia is a diabetes-specific source of anxiety and refers to "fear associated with episodes of hypoglycemia and their negative consequences," which includes acute health consequences (e.g., loss of consciousness, impaired cognition), loss of control, and social reprisal [34]. Negative consequences of this fear include poorer glycemic control and increased complications if patients reduce their insulin usage in order to maintain a higher blood glucose level [35]. Fear of hypoglycemia is associated with the frequency of severe hypoglycemic episodes in past 12 months, perceived risk of future episodes, hypoglycemic unawareness, number of hypoglycemic symptoms, frequency of mild hypoglycemia, and presence of non-diabetes anxiety [36, 37]. As hypoglycemia tends to occur more often at night, associated fear may contribute to poor sleep quality [34]. Among adults and adolescents, females have been found to have higher levels of fear [34]. Group and individual interventions have been developed utilizing techniques such as CBT, blood glucose awareness training, and a behavioral approach aimed at improving in hypoglycemic unawareness [38–41]. Though limited in number and results are not consistent, some have noted a reduction in fear and improvement in glucose control.

Disordered Eating Behavior and Eating Disorders in Patients with Type 1 Diabetes

In addition to anxiety and depression, T1D patients appear to be at elevated risk for disordered eating behavior (DEB) and eating disorders (ED). The presence of ED is associated with impaired metabolic control, more frequent episodes of ketoacidosis, and early onset of microvascular complications, particularly retinopathy and neuropathy [42]. An estimated 30–40% of diabetic adolescents and young adults skip or reduce insulin doses in order to lose weight, a DEB known as diabulimia [42]. Consequences of this behavior include increased risk of dehydration, muscle tissue breakdown, and heightened risk for infection and fatigue [42]. There may also be an increased risk for early mortality [43]. Compared with normal peers, adolescents with T1D tend to gain significant amounts of weight as they move toward young adulthood. Additionally, the metabolic effects of insulin promote a slightly higher body weight [44]. This tendency for weight gain, along with typical adolescent concerns about appearance, contributes to DEBs such as insulin restriction or binging and purging to facilitate weight loss. The presence of low self-esteem, higher concerns about physical appearance, and

lower diabetes-related QOL appear to be risk factors for DEB [45–47].

Research regarding T1D patients suggests that female gender, elevated BMI, body dissatisfaction, fluctuations in body weight from repeated dieting, dietary restrictions associated with glycemic control, and skip or reduction of insulin doses for weight control purposes are risk factors for ED [44, 48, 49]. Avoidant coping styles and depressive symptoms may also be predictors [44]. Average age of onset is 23 years [50]. Experts suggest maintaining a high index of suspicion for DEB and ED among those with chronic poor metabolic control, repeated episodes of diabetic ketoacidosis, recurrent hypoglycemic episodes, and/or weight and body shape concerns [51]. The use of the 16-item self-report screening tool for disordered eating, the Diabetes Eating Problem Survey, which has good internal consistency, construct validity, and external validity, can assist in detection of abnormal behaviors needing attention [52]. Treatment of ED among T1D patients is complicated due to the need to focus on dietary intake as a normal part of diabetes management. Loosening of glycemic parameters may be necessary. Existing evidence suggests that the course of EDs tends to be chronic and recurrent among T1D patients, with continued use of insulin omission not uncommon [43, 50, 53, 54].

Multivisceral-Intestinal Transplant

An increasing number of multivisceral and intestinal (MV/I) transplants are performed, and the survival rates continue to improve with the 10-year graft survival rate ranging from 26% to 40% depending on whether the transplant is solely intestinal or multivisceral with the intestine, liver, and/or pancreas. According to the Centers of Medicare and Medicaid Services (CMS)-approved indications for MV/I transplantation, it is considered a rescue therapy for patients with intestinal failure who have maximized other gut rehabilitation techniques, failed parenteral nutrition (PN), or have high risk of death from their underlying disease [55]. Before their MV/I transplant, most patients encounter complications related to the underlying cause of intestinal failure or struggle with their dependence on PN. Patients dependent on PN often show impressive resilience in the face of daily hardships and hazards related to their life-sustaining nutritional support, and specifics of these challenges will be detailed later in this chapter. To put the choice of MV/I transplant in perspective, adults stable on long-term PN are more likely to die from the underlying disease causing their intestinal failure rather than from complications related to PN [56]. When electing MV/I transplant, patients weigh the potential of a PN-free existence against a high-risk transplant procedure accompanied by new challenges of graft rejection and complications related to immunosuppression.

Adult causes of intestinal failure leading to consideration of MV/I transplant varied: vascular, traumatic, congenital, and acquired [55]. Short bowel syndrome is the most common indication for MV/I transplant. Ischemia (24%) is the leading cause of short bowel syndrome followed by Crohn's disease (11%) and trauma (10%) [57]. Chronic and acute causes of intestinal failure differ in their psychological impact. During the pre-transplant psychosocial assessment of MVI/I transplant candidates, it is important to touch upon the following points: (1) severity and chronicity of pre-transplant illness and subsequent psychiatric sequelae, (2) duration of pre-transplant dependence on PN, (3) education about postoperative complications including continued substance use and risk of developing psychiatric disorders, and (4) extent of social support available [58].

For a holistic understanding of the patient choosing MV/I transplant, it is helpful to examine the pre-transplant life of a candidate and how it was influenced by dependency on PN, the primary long-term treatment for individuals with irreversible intestinal failure. While PN is life-saving, it also is invasive and degrades the QOL of individuals dependent on this form of nutrition. A helpful analogy to consider is: "parenteral nutrition is akin to MV/I transplant as hemodialysis is to kidney transplant." Like hemodialysis patients, individuals on PN may be ambivalent toward the medical technology that sustains and dictates their life [59]. As summarized by Winkler et al., "Despite the physiological benefits, home parenteral nutrition is also a high-risk, high expenditure, potentially problem prone therapy" [60].

Psychological Considerations in Patients Dependent on PN

PN takes a logistical, financial, physical, and emotional toll on patients. PN is administered overnight for 12 h at a time, and depending on gut function, patients require feedings two to seven times per week [61]. Estimated annual cost of PN ranges from $100,000 to $250,000 including cost of supplies, infusion solutions, and hospitalizations related to PN complications. Families suffer financial strain from unreimbursed and out-of-pocket costs and lost income related to the schedule demands of PN [62]. Unlike hemodialysis, in-home-based PN is common. Home parenteral nutrition is often abbreviated as HPN; for consistency in this chapter, it will be referred to as home PN. Although available at home, the treatment remains invasive in terms of time, physical constraints, and dependence on technology. The physical risks include catheter-related bloodstream infections (CRBSIs) which are associated with 5% of PN-related deaths, venous thrombosis, metabolic bone disease, and intestinal failure-associated liver disease (IFALD) [55]. IFALD progressing to liver failure carries the greatest risk of death caused by PN, with a mortality rate up to 15% [56].

Patients are continuously exposed to physical complications and risks of PN. Furthermore, psychosocial stressors of long-term PN pervade patients' QOL [60, 61, 63]. Poor sleep, fatigue, depression, and negative emotions related to the catheter, including fear, anxiety, and body image concerns, are common complaints [64]. Loss of autonomy and dependence on technology erode QOL as patients refer to being "hooked up" or "tethered" to machinery. Dependence on equipment restricts travelling and how patients spend their recreation and leisure time [60]. Ability to work and stable employment are hindered by reduced strength for physical activity and fatigue; some patients rely on disability insurance to fund their home PN [65].

As with any GI disturbance or illness, a person's relationship with food and eating changes. For some with short bowel syndrome and intestinal failure, they face "eating for survival" which means hypervigilance regarding number of meals and calorie intake and amount and osmolality of fluids; they manage the balance between getting enough nutrition and risking abdominal pain, diarrhea, and dehydration [66]. PN allows for nutrition without oral intake and alleviates some anxiety accompanying eating for survival. For others, dependency on PN means losing food as a means of experiencing pleasure, whether socially or alone, and this can be a cause of significant distress [67]. Decline in frequency and importance of social activities surrounding eating and drinking leads to social impairment. Every type of relationship suffers from family and friends to romantic or sexual relationships. Patients report their sexual desire and activity are diminished by PN [68]. In light of the cumbersome nature of PN and repercussions on functioning, a mental health clinician can contextualize the risks a patient is willing to face for MV/I transplant. A desire for autonomy and potential return to "normal socializing" are motivating factors.

Psychiatric Evaluation and Comorbidities in Pre-transplant MV/I Patients

The psychiatric evaluation for MV/I transplant should account for existing mental health issues related to PN including disrupted sleep, anxiety, depression, body image issues, and behaviors related to catheters. Though uncommon, some patients have used their venous access devices to engage in self-injurious behaviors of contamination, cutting the line or deliberate neglect [69]. Mental health providers can evaluate for contributing mood, anxiety, or personality disorders and abnormal illness behaviors that influence the patient's relationship with their chronic illness and by physical extension their catheter. These existing disorders, especially abnormal illness behaviors, may influence transplant outcomes such as adherence and rapport with the treatment team. Specific to pre-transplant mental status, some patients cite fear and anxiety accompanying the physical attachment to the PN apparatus; patients worry about catheter infection, pump malfunction, or air embolism [70]. In a vicious cycle, poor sleep and subsequent fatigue negatively impact QOL and functioning. Sleep often improved after MV/I transplant by virtue of no longer being connected to PN apparatus [70].

Depression was found in 10–80% of patients reliant on home-based PN [70]. Depressive disorder and social impairment were associated with venous access device-related complications such as occlusion and infection, as well as number of hospital readmissions related to these complications [71]. Depression alone can increase the risk of post-transplant mortality [72]. Clinicians can mitigate the impact of psychiatric comorbidity by addressing psychological issues and symptoms that occur before transplant (related to PN or not) and can monitor their development or resolution post-transplant.

As previously stated, the psychiatric care of MV/I transplant patients is informed by the severity and chronicity of pre-transplant illness. For example, a person may struggle adjusting to sudden loss of normal bowel function from more acute causes of intestinal failure such as ischemia caused by mesenteric vascular thrombosis or trauma. Gunshot wounds or abdominal trauma from a motor vehicle accident is a physically traumatic event that could lead to MV/I transplant [73]. A sudden, unexpected, and life-threatening event, like trauma associated with eventual organ transplant, is considered particularly pathogenic and may contribute to development of pre-transplant post-traumatic stress disorder (PTSD) [74]. Currently, no studies have examined the prevalence of PTSD in patients undergoing MV/I transplant. In solid organ transplant, previous exposure to trauma and existing psychiatric diagnoses contributed to post-transplant diagnosis of PTSD [75]. Decreased mental and physical QOL scores, along with diminished psychosocial functioning, were related to PTSD diagnosis or subclinical symptoms of PTSD.

Patients with chronic etiologies of their short bowel syndrome, such as Crohn's disease, often have psychiatric comorbidities ranging from substance use disorder influenced by chronic pain to depression and anxiety [76]. As discussed in terms of the etiology of intestinal failure, short bowel syndrome has several causes including Crohn's disease but extending to ischemia or malignancy. The confluence of a disordered gastrointestinal tract and the sensitive brain-gut axis adds to the complexity of pre-transplant psychological symptoms [77]. Before undergoing MV/I transplant, individuals with short bowel syndrome experience changes in their gut either due to inflammation in Crohn's disease, changes in flora as PN places them at risk for bacterial overgrowth, or resections leading to shortening of the bowel. Though speculative, changes in the brain-gut axis likely occur with each bowel resection [66, 78]. Pooled incidence values for depression and anxiety in inflammatory bowel disease (IBD) are reported, respectively, as 21% and 19%. These values rise with active disease, and both psychiatric comorbidities occur at a higher rate in Crohn's disease as compared to ulcerative colitis [79]. Psychiatric comorbidities aside, IBD is associated with fatigue, even when in clinical remission as measured by inflammatory markers such as ESR, CRP, and other interleukins. In a study of outpatients with IBD, fatigue in general was correlated with depression as measured by the Beck Depression Inventory, and severe fatigue was correlated with depression, anxiety, and lower QOL. Female patients with Crohn's disease were more likely to report fatigue [80]. Short bowel syndrome, due to Crohn's disease or not, causes troublesome GI symptoms, especially diarrhea, and fatigue contributing to psychological distress. Compared to patients with IBD in remission (and an intact gut), individuals with short bowel syndrome have higher daily use of analgesics and opioids. There is likely psychological and physical overlap in using opioids for pain and discomfort from GI symptoms, opioids as relief from diarrhea, and the resulting fatigue related to GI symptoms, opioids or both [80].

Chronic disease states before transplant pose the risk of narcotic use and development of dependence or a substance use disorder. IBD alone has a 6% point prevalence of active opioid use after 1 year of diagnosis, and comorbid depression increases risk of heavy opioid use [81]. Psychiatrists should maintain clinical suspicion for substance use disorders and withdrawal syndromes as possible complicating factors of MV/I transplant. The clinical overlap of organic gastrointestinal illness, abdominal pain syndromes, and psychiatric disorders warrants a physical and psychological evaluation of pain with attention to psychiatric disorders comorbid with chronic pain [82, 83]. Substance use disorders influence quality of life before and after transplant. In liver transplant recipients, pre-transplant opioid use was associated with pain-related hospital readmission at 30 days and 1-year post-transplant [84]. Despite the clinical relevance of pain and opioid use, only one study of six patients examined pain treatment during and after MV/I transplant surgery [85].

Psychopharmacology in Pre-transplant MV/I Patients

Even before transplant, pharmacological intervention and behavioral therapies can alleviate distress and improve transplant outcomes by treating anxiety, depression, poor sleep, and fatigue related to TPN or pre-transplant illness. Psychotropic medications such SSRI/selective norepinephrine reuptake inhibitor (SNRI) and tricyclic antidepressants used to treat anxiety and depression can mitigate physical pain [86]. Sleep is of paramount importance before and after transplant, and the impact of home TPN on sleep was emphasized earlier. For pre-transplant MV/I transplant candidates, their extent of bowel dysfunction, intestinal absorptive capacity, and any existing hepatic disease, such as IFALD, affects treatment with medications. Absorption of medication is impacted by length of the functioning small intestine and condition of the mucosal surface, gastric emptying, small bowel transit time, pancreato-biliary secretions, alteration in GI flora, and nutritional intake; realistically, a patient with intestinal failure may have alterations in several of these domains. Loperamide is administered with other medications to slow intestinal transit [87]. Of note, loperamide can be abused as an opioid medication. As a general tenet, barring any drug interactions, an oral psychotropic medication can be continued or initiated, with the presumption that absorption and metabolism may be affected by the condition of a patient's pre-transplant bowel and MV/I transplant. Dosage adjustments can be made in discussion with the patient and based on a clinical and mental status exam [88].

Few studies and case reports examine the use of psychotropic medications in patients with either intestinal failure or surgery involving the small intestine; most data is collected from patients undergoing bariatric surgery [88]. The authors of a systematic review regarding the treatment of mood disorders in patients with a history of intestinal surgery conclude that citalopram and escitalopram are a good choice for first-line therapy in these patients. Their conclusion is bolstered by a study of eight patients with short bowel syndrome who received citalopram and escitalopram. Patients with 80 centimeters of small bowel and 50% of remaining colon reached therapeutic drug levels, as measured by concentration-dose ratios that are effective in treatment of major depressive disorder [89].

For a comprehensive review of alternative routes of medication administration, the *Clinical Manual of Psychopharmacology in the Medically Ill* reviews the psychotropic medications available as dissolvable, intravenous, intramuscular, and suppository forms [90]. Here we have a limited discussion of medications most useful in regard to the psychological and psychiatric issues already presented. As a route of administration, orally disintegrating tablets (ODT) dissolve when exposed to saliva and the drug is absorbed in the esophageal and gastric mucosa when saliva is swallowed [90]. For treatment of depressive and anxiety disorders, mirtazapine, alprazolam, and clonazepam exist as ODT. Second-generation antipsychotic medications are more commonly available in ODT formulation including risperidone, olanzapine, aripiprazole, and clozapine. Sublingual administration, in which the tablet is dissolved under the tongue and saliva is not swallowed, avoids first-pass metabolism. For treatment of depression and anxiety, selegiline (MAO-B) is available as a sublingual tablet and a transdermal patch. The hypnotic and sleep aid zolpidem is available in the United States as a low-dose sublingual tablet (brand name Intermezzo) and indicated for treatment for middle-of-the-night wakefulness but could be used to initiate sleep in the context of impaired intestinal absorption. As opiod use disorder has been a topic of importance in our discussion, it is worth noting that buprenorphine/naloxone is available as a sublingual film, though contraindicated not only because of opioid use after surgery but also because of the use of loperamide for diarrhea and slowing intestinal transit. Buccal absorption can occur for ODTs or other tablets held under the tongue. In one case report, a woman with only 40 centimeters of proximal small bowel achieved normal therapeutic levels of amitriptyline with buccal administration of amitriptyline 125 mg given as tablets crushed into a powder [91]. Tricyclics have the advantage of therapeutic blood monitoring levels in patients whose absorption may be erratic pre- or post-transplant [92]. Citalopram is the only SSRI available intravenously, with a starting dose of 20 mg/day and transition to oral formulation in approximately 14 days [93]. However, this formulation is not available in the United States.

Conclusions

For patients being considered for pancreatic or MV/I transplantation, most have faced a variety of challenges brought on by chronic disease including the demands of ongoing medical follow-up, testing, medications, repeat hospitalizations, dietary and other lifestyle restrictions, as well as reduced QOL. Changes in body image, fear of complications, reduced long-term survival, and chronic pain are additional concerns confronting many. In light of these challenges, transplant teams need to be alert to the potential for psychological distress or diagnosable comorbid psychiatric disorders such as depression, anxiety, eating disorder, or substance use. Early identification of these conditions prior to transplant listing can allow them to be adequately addressed and, in turn, potentially improve post-transplant adherence and QOL.

References

1. Roy T, Lloyd CE. Epidemiology of depression and diabetes: a systematic review. J Affect Disord. 2012;142(Suppl):S8–21.
2. Holt RIG, de Groot M, Lucki I, et al. NIDDK international conference report on diabetes and depression: current understanding and future directions. Diabetes Care. 2014;37:2067–77.
3. Buchberger B, Huppertz H, Krabbe L, et al. Symptoms of depression and anxiety in youth with type 1 diabetes: a systematic review and meta-analysis. Psychoneuroendocrinology. 2016;70:70–84.
4. Nouwen A, Nefs G, Caranlau I, et al. Prevalence of depression in individuals with impaired glucose metabolism or undiagnosed diabetes: a systematic review and meta-analysis of the European Depression in Diabetes (EDID) research consortium. Diabetes Care. 2011;34:752–62.
5. Lyoo IK, Yoon S, Jacobson AM, et al. Prefrontal cortical deficits in type 1 diabetes mellitus: brain correlates of comorbid depression. Arch Gen Psychiatry. 2012;69:1267–76.

6. Ho N, Sommers MS, Lucki I. Effects of diabetes on hippocampal neurogenesis: links to cognition and depression. Neurosci Biobehav Rev. 2013;37:1346–62.

7. Rustad JK, Musselman DL, Nemeroff CB. The relationship of depression and diabetes: pathophysiological and treatment implications. Psychoneuroendocrinology. 2011;36:1276–86.

8. Lustman PJ, Anderson RJ, Freedland KE, et al. Depression and poor glycemic control. Diabetes Care. 2000;23:934–42.

9. Reynolds KA, Helgeson VS. Children with diabetes compared to peers: depressed? Distressed? A meta-analytic review. Ann Behav Med. 2011;42:29–41.

10. De Groot M, Anderson R, Freedland KE, et al. Association of depression and diabetes complications: a meta-analysis. Psychosom Med. 2001;63:619–30.

11. Molosankwe I, Patel A, Gagliardino J, et al. Economic aspects of the association between diabetes and depression: a systemic review. J Affect Disord. 2012;142:S42–55.

12. Park M, Katon WJ, Wolf FM. Depression and risk of mortality in individuals with diabetes: a meta-analysis and systemic review. Gen Hosp Psychiatry. 2013;35:217–25.

13. Katon W, Fan MY, Unutzer J, et al. Depression and diabetes: a potentially lethal combination. J Health Psychology. 2008;23:1571–5.

14. Stewart SM, Rao U, Emslie GJ, et al. Depressive symptoms predict hospitalization for adolescents with type 1 diabetes. Pediatrics. 2005;115:1315–9.

15. Ducat L, Rubenstein A, Philipson L, Anderson BJ. A review of the mental health issues of diabetes conference. Diabetes Care. 2015;38:333–8.

16. Petrak F, Baumeister H, Skinner TC, et al. Depression and diabetes: treatment and health-care delivery. Lancet Diabetes Endocrinol. 2015;3:472–485a.

17. Roy T, Lloyd CE, Pouwer F, et al. Screening tools used for measuring depression among people with type 1 and type 2 diabetes: a systematic review. Diabet Med. 2012;29:164–75.

18. Baumeister H, Hutter N, Bengel J. Psychological and pharmacological interventions for depression in patients with diabetes mellitus: an abridged Cochrane review. Diabet Med. 2014;31:773–86.

19. Petrak F, Herpertz S, Albus C, et al. Cognitive behavioral therapy versus sertraline in patient with depression and poorly controlled diabetes mellitus. Diabetes Care. 2015;38(5):767–75.

20. Simon GE, Katon WJ, Lin EHB, et al. Cost-effectiveness of systematic depression treatments among people with diabetes mellitus. Arch Gen Psychiatry. 2007;64:65–72.

21. Katon W, Russo J, Lin EH, et al. Cost-effectiveness of a multicondition collaborative care intervention: a randomized controlled trial. Arch Gen Psychiatry. 2012;69:506–14.

22. Fisher L, Gonzalez JS, Polonsky WH. The confusing tale of depression and distress in patients with diabetes: a call for greater clarity and precision. Diabet Med. 2014;31:764–72.

23. Gonzalez JS. Depression. In: Type 1 diabetes sourcebook. Alexandria: American Diabetes Association; 2013. p. 169–79.

24. Fisher L, Polonsky WH, Hessler DM, et al. Understanding the sources of diabetes distress in adults with type 1 diabetes. J Diabetes Complicat. 2015;29:572–7.

25. Fisher L, Hessler D, Polonsky W, et al. Diabetes distress in adults with type 1 diabetes: prevalence, incidence and change over time. J Diabetes Complicat. 2016;30:1123–8.

26. Hessler DM, Fisher L, Polonsky WH, et al. Diabetes distress is linked with worsening diabetes management over time in adults with type 1 diabetes. Diabet Med. 2017; https://doi.org/10.1111/dme.13381.

27. Hessler D, Fisher L, Polonsky W, et al. Understanding the areas and correlates of diabetes-related distress in parents of teens with type 1 diabetes. J Ped Psychol. 2016;41:750–8.

28. Weissberg-Bencehll J, Antisdel-Lomaglio J. Diabetes-specific emotional distress among adolescents: feasibility, reliability, and validity of the problem areas in diabetes-teen version. Pediatr Diabetes. 2011;12:341–4.

29. Smith KJ, Beland M, Clyde M, et al. Association of diabetes with anxiety: a systematic review and meta-analysis. J Psychosom Res. 2013;74:89–99.

30. De Groot M, Golden SH, Wagner J. Psychological condition in adults with diabetes. Am Psychol. 2016;71:552–62.

31. Cemeroglu AP, Can A, Davis AT, et al. Fear of needles in children with TID mellitus on multiple daily injections (MDI) and continuous subcutaneous insulin infusion (CSII). Endocr Pract. 2015;21:46–53.

32. Van Son J, Nyklicek I, Pop VJ, et al. The effects of a mindfulness-based intervention on emotional distress, quality of life, and HbA (1c) in outpatients with diabetes (DiaMind): a randomized controlled trial. Diabetes Care. 2013;36:823–30.

33. Hopkins D, Lawrence I, Mansell P, et al. Improved biomedical and psychological outcomes 1 year after structured education in flexible insulin therapy for people with type 1 diabetes: the UK DAFNE experience. Diabetes Care. 2012;35:1638–42.

34. Martyn-Nemeth P, Farabi SS, Mihailescu D, et al. Fear of hypoglycemia in adults with type 1 diabetes: impact of therapeutic advances and strategies for prevention: a review. J Diabetes Complicat. 2016;30:167–77.

35. Wild D, Von Maltzahn R, Brohan E, et al. A critical review of the literature on fear of hypoglycemia in diabetes: implications for diabetes management and patient education. Patient Educ Couns. 2007;68:10–5.

36. Anderbro T, Gonder-Frederick L, Bolinder J, et al. Fear of hypoglycemia: relationship to hypoglycemic risk and psychological factors. Acta Diabetol. 2015;52:581–9.

37. Anderbro T, Amsberg S, Adamson U, et al. Fear of hypoglycemia in adults with type 1 diabetes. Diabet Med. 2007;27:1151–8.

38. Amsberg S, Anderbro T, Wredling R, et al. A cognitive behavioral therapy-based intervention among poorly controlled adult type 1 diabetes patients: a randomized controlled trial. Patient Educ Couns. 2009;77:72–80.

39. George JT, Vadovinos AP, Russell I, et al. Clinical effectiveness of a brief educational intervention in type I diabetes: results from the BITES (Brief Intervention in Type I Diabetes. Education for Self-efficacy) trial. Diabet Med. 2008;25:1447–53.

40. Cox DJ, Gonder-Frederick L, Polonsky W, et al. Blood glucose awareness training (BGAT-2): long-term benefits. Diabetes Care. 2001;24:637–42.

41. Cox DJ, Ritterband L, Magee J, et al. Blood glucose awareness training delivered over the internet. Diabetes Care. 2008;31:1527–8.

42. Larranaga A, Docet MF, Garcia-Mayor RV. Disordered eating behaviors in type 1 diabetic patients. World J Diabetes. 2011;11:189–95.

43. Goebbel-Fabbri AE, Fikkan J, Franko DL, et al. Insulin restriction and associated morbidity and mortality in women with type 1 diabetes. Diabetes Care. 2008;31:415–9.

44. Gagnon C, Aime A, Belanger C. Predictors of comorbid eating disorders and diabetes in people with type 1 and type 2 diabetes. Can J Diabetes. 2017;41:52–7.

45. Racicka E, Brynska A. Eating disorders in children and adolescents with type 1 and type 2 diabetes- prevalence, risk factors, warning signs. Psychiatr Pol. 2015;49:1017–24.

46. Olmsted MP, Colton PA, Daneman D, et al. Prediction of the onset of disturbed eating behavior in adolescent girls with type 1 diabetes. Diabetes Care. 2008;31:1978–82.

47. Goebel-Fabbri AE. Disturbed eating behaviors and eating disorders in type 1 diabetes: clinical significance and treatment recommendations. Curr Diab Rep. 2009;9:133–9.

48. Gibbons CH, Goebel-Fabbri A. Microvascular complications associated with rapid improvement in glycemic control in diabetes. Curr Diab Rep. 2017;17:48. https://doi.org/10.1007/s11892-017-0880-5.

49. Goncalves S, Barros V, Gomes AR. Eating disordered behavior in adolescents with type 1 diabetes. Can J Diabetes. 2016;40:152–7.

50. Colton P, Olmsted M, Daneman D, et al. Eating disorders in girls and women with type1 diabetes: a longitudinal study of prevalence, onset, remission, and recurrence. Diabetes Care. 2015a;38:1212–7.

51. Pinhas-Hamiel O, Hamiel U, Levy-Shraga Y. Eating disorder in adolescents with type 1 diabetes: challenges in diagnosis and treatment. World J Diabetes. 2015;6:517–26.

52. Markowitz JT, Butler DA, Volkening LK, et al. Brief screening tool for disordered eating in diabetes: internal consistency and external validity in a contemporary sample of pediatric patients with type 1 diabetes. Diabetes Care. 2010;33:495–500.

53. Colton PA, Olmsted MP, Wong H, Rodin GM. Eating disorders in individuals with type 1 diabetes: case series and day hospital treatment outcome. Eur Eat Disord Rev. 2015b;23:312–7.

54. Custal N, Arcelus J, Aguera Z, et al. Treatment outcome of patients with comorbid type 1 diabetes and eating disorders. BMC Psychiatry. 2014;14:40. https://doi.org/10.1186/1471-224x-14-140.

55. Bharadwaj S, Tandon P, Gohel TD, et al. Current status of intestinal and multivisceral transplantation. Gastroenterol Rep (Oxf). 2017;5:20–8.

56. Pironi L, Goulet O, Buchman A, et al. Outcome on home parenteral nutrition for benign intestinal failure: a review of the literature and benchmarking with the European prospective survey of ESPEN. Clin Nutr. 2012;31:831–45.

57. Grant D, Abu-Elmagd K, Mazariegos G, et al. Intestinal transplant registry report: global activity and trends. Am J Transplant. 2015;15:210–9.

58. Stenn PG, Lammens P, Houle L, Grant D. Psychiatric psychosocial and ethical aspects of small bowel transplantation. Transplant Proc. 1992;24:1251–2.

59. Jeppesen PB, Langholz E, Mortensen PB. Quality of life in patients receiving home parenteral nutrition. Gut. 1999;44(6):844–52.

60. Winkler MF, Smith CE. Clinical, social, and economic impacts of home parenteral nutrition dependence in short bowel syndrome. JPEN J Parenter Enteral Nutr. 2014;38(1 Suppl):32S–7S.

61. Huisman-de Waal G, Schoonhoven L, Jansen J, Wanten G, van Achterberg T. The impact of home parenteral nutrition on daily life-a review. Clin Nutr. 2007;26:275–88.

62. Hofstetter S, Stern L, Willet J. Key issues in addressing the clinical and humanistic burden of short bowel syndrome in the US. Curr Med Res Opin. 2013;29:495–504.

63. Howard LJ. Length of life and quality of life on home parenteral nutrition. JPEN J Parenter Enteral Nutr. 2002;26(5 Suppl):S55–9.

64. Persoon A, Huisman-de Waal G, Naber TA, et al. Impact of long-term HPN on daily life in adults. Clin Nutr. 2005;24:304–13.

65. Winkler MF. Quality of life in adult home parenteral nutrition patients. JPEN J Parenter Enteral Nutr. 2005;29:162–70.

66. Kelly DG, Tappenden KA, Winkler MF. Short bowel syndrome: highlights of patient management, quality of life, and survival. JPEN J Parenter Enteral Nutr. 2014;38:427–37.

67. Stern J. Home parenteral nutrition and the psyche: psychological challenges for patient and family. Proc Nutr Soc. 2006;65:222–6.

68. Baxter JP, Fayers PM, McKinlay AW. The clinical and psychometric validation of a questionnaire to assess the quality of life of adult patients treated with long-term parenteral nutrition. JPEN J Parenter Enteral Nutr. 2010;34:131–42.

69. Stern JM, Jacyna N, Lloyd DA. Review article: psychological aspects of home parenteral nutrition, abnormal illness behaviour and risk of self-harm in patients with central venous catheters. Aliment Pharmacol Ther. 2008;27:910–8.

70. Huisman-de Waal G, Naber T, Schoonhoven L, et al. Problems experienced by patients receiving parenteral nutrition at home: results of an open interview study. JPEN J Parenter Enteral Nutr. 2006;30:215–21.

71. Huisman-de Waal G, Versleijen M, van Achterberg T, et al. Psychosocial complaints are associated with venous access-device related complications in patients on home parenteral nutrition. JPEN J Parenter Enteral Nutr. 2011;35:588–95.

72. Dew MA, Rosenberger EM, Myaskovsky L, et al. Depression and anxiety as risk factors for morbidity and mortality after organ transplantation: a systematic review and meta-analysis. Transplantation. 2015;100:988–1003.

73. Nishida S, Kato T, Levi D, Nery J, Madariaga J, Mittal N, et al. Intestinal transplantation for trauma patients. Transplant Proc. 2002;34:913.

74. McNally RJ. Special areas of interest: post traumatic stress disorder. In: Sadock BJ, Sadock VA, editors. Kaplan and Sadock's comprehensive textbook of psychiatry. 9th ed. Philadelphia: LWW; 2009. p. 2654.

75. Davydow DS, Lease ED, Reyes JD. Posttraumatic stress disorder in organ transplant recipients: a systematic review. Gen Hosp Psychiatry. 2015;37(5):387–98.

76. Regueiro M, Greer JB, Szigethy E. Etiology and treatment of pain and psychosocial issues in patients with inflammatory bowel diseases. Gastroenterology. 2017;152:430–9.

77. Sherwin E, Rea K, Dinan TG, Cryan JF. A gut (microbiome) feeling about the brain. Curr Opin Gastroenterol. 2016;32:96–102.

78. Nyabanga C, Kochhar G, Costa G, et al. Management of Crohn's disease in the new era of gut rehabilitation and intestinal transplantation. Inflamm Bowel Dis. 2016;22:1763–76.

79. Mikocka-Walus A, Knowles SR, Keefer L, Graff L. Controversies revisited: a systematic review of the comorbidity of depression and anxiety with inflammatory bowel diseases. Inflamm Bowel Dis. 2016;22:752–62.

80. Villoria A, Garcia V, Dosal A, et al. Fatigue in out-patients with inflammatory bowel disease: prevalence and predictive factors. PLoS One. 2017;12(4):e0181435.

81. Targownik LE, Nugent Z, Singh H, et al. The prevalence and predictors of opioid use in inflammatory bowel disease: a population-based analysis. Am J Gastroenterol. 2014;109(10):1613–20.

82. Mayer EA, Tillisch K. The brain-gut axis in abdominal pain syndromes. Annu Rev Med. 2011;62:381–96.

83. Halpin SJ, Ford AC. Prevalence of symptoms meeting criteria for irritable bowel syndrome in inflammatory bowel disease: systematic review and meta-analysis. Am J Gastroenterol. 2012;107:1474–82.

84. Rogal S, Mankaney G, Udawatta V, et al. Association between opioid use and readmission following liver transplantation. Clin Transpl. 2016;30(10):1222–9.

85. Siniscalchi A, Begliomini B, De Pietri L, et al. Pain management after small bowel/multivisceral transplantation. Transplant Proc. 2002;34:969–70.

86. Marazziti D, Mungai F, Vivarelli L, et al. Pain and psychiatry: a critical analysis and pharmacological review. Clin Pract Epidemiol Ment Health. 2006;2:31.

87. Ward N. The impact of intestinal failure on oral drug absorption: a review. J Gastrointest Surg. 2010;14:1045–51.

88. Lloret-Linares C, Bellivier F, Heron K, Besson M. Treating mood disorders in patients with a history of intestinal surgery: a systematic review. Int Clin Psychopharmacol. 2015;30:119–28.

89. Faye E, Corcos O, Lancelin F, et al. Antidepressant agents in short bowel syndrome. Clin Ther. 2014;36:2033.e3.

90. Owen JA, Crouse EL. Alternative route of drug administration. In: Levenson JL, Ferrando S, editors. Clinical manual of psychopharmacology in the medically ill. 2nd ed. Arlington: American Psychiatric Association Publishing; 2017. p. 101–25.

91. Robbins B, Reiss RA. Amitriptyline absorption in a patient with short bowel syndrome. Am J Gastroenterol. 1999;94:2302–4.

92. DiMartini A, Fitzgerald MG, Magill J, et al. Psychiatric evaluations of small intestine transplantation patients. Gen Hosp Psychiatry. 1996;18(6 Suppl):25S–9S.

93. Crone CC, Gabriel GM. Treatment of anxiety and depression in transplant patients: pharmacokinetic considerations. Clin Pharmacokinet. 2004;43(6):361–94.

Enteral and Parenteral Nutrition: Considerations for Visceral Transplant Patients

Neha D. Shah and Michelle Stroebe

Intestinal Failure

Intestinal failure (IF) is defined as the reduction of gut function below that necessary for absorption of macronutrients and micronutrients, such that intravenous nutrition supplementation is required to sustain health and growth [1]. The five major pathophysiological conditions that lead to IF are short bowel syndrome, intestinal fistula, intestinal dysmotility, mechanical obstruction, and extensive small bowel mucosal disease. Short bowel syndrome, intestinal fistula, and extensive small bowel mucosal disease cause a reduction in intestinal absorptive area. Intestinal dysmotility and mechanical obstruction may arise from altered gastrointestinal motility, extensive adhesions, or malignancy. The complications associated with IF manifest as malabsorption of oral nutrients, intestinal losses, electrolyte imbalances, altered transit time, and disease-associated hypophagia [2].

Patients with IF experience an intolerance to both an oral diet and enteral nutrition (EN) and are unable to meet their nutrition needs by either method. They are, therefore, primarily dependent on parenteral nutrition (PN) as the intravenous method of receiving nutrient provision. The Sustain Registry Report collected data on 1251 patients on home PN in the United States from 2011 to 2014 and showed that the primary indications for PN included short bowel syndrome (24%), gastrointestinal obstruction (23%), gastrointestinal fistula (19%), or gastrointestinal dysmotility (10%), in which all diagnoses are reflective of IF [3]. The extent of IF can vary among individuals and, depending on the severity, will determine if the patient is capable of weaning from PN. The management of IF necessitates interdisciplinary medical and nutrition care due to its complexity. Specialized rehabilitation programs that include a core team of surgeons, gastroenterologists, nurses, dietitians, pharmacists, and social workers for interdisciplinary management of IF have shown to reduce complications associated with long-term IF and PN [2].

For patients with irreversible IF who failed medical management and are experiencing complications with PN, multivisceral and intestinal (MV/I) transplantation may be necessary. The recent worldwide Intestinal Transplant Registry (ITR) Report collected outcome data on 2887 MV/I transplant cases completed before 2013 and showed there is now a decline seen in the annual case volume for MV/I transplantation [4]. This is likely due to the advancement in specialized care leading to improved survival outcomes in IF. Despite improvements in IF care, MV/I transplantation will continue to serve as an important therapeutic intervention to assist with long-term survival for some patients. The long-term utilization of PN significantly increases a patient's risk of developing metabolic and infectious complications, which can be potentially life-threatening. In addition, MV/I transplantation can improve quality of life (QOL), as it may provide the ability to restore complete nutritional autonomy through the opportunity to wean from PN and transition to EN or to an oral diet [5].

Identifying and Diagnosing Protein–Calorie Malnutrition

Due to the numerous metabolic and infectious complications that may arise in the IF patient, the development of protein-calorie malnutrition (PCM) should be monitored closely. The basic characteristics of PCM include insufficient energy intake, unintentional weight loss, and/or evidence of muscle/fat wasting. The tools used to identify and diagnose PCM range from simple ones evaluating for changes in appetite and unintentional weight loss to more complex methods that may include a combination of multiple anthropometric and

N. D. Shah, MPH, RD, CNSC (✉)
Intestinal Transplant Program, Digestive Health Center,
Stanford Health Care, Palo Alto, CA, USA
e-mail: neshah@stanfordhealthcare.org

M. Stroebe, MS, RD
Center for Advanced Lung Disease,
Stanford Health Care, Palo Alto, CA, USA
e-mail: mstroebe@stanfordhealthcare.org

© Springer International Publishing AG, part of Springer Nature 2019
Y. Sher, J. R. Maldonado (eds.), *Psychosocial Care of End-Stage Organ Disease and Transplant Patients*,
https://doi.org/10.1007/978-3-319-94914-7_31

laboratory measurements. The absence of standardization in the diagnosis of PCM may lead to an underestimation of its prevalence and incidence and an exclusion of the diagnosis. Appropriately identifying PCM in a timely manner may overall assist to optimize interventions, resources, and outcomes for patients with end-stage disease and transplantation [6–8].

Patients identified with PCM in end-stage organ disease are overall at a higher risk for post-transplant infections, morbidity, mortality, and increased length of hospital stay as compared with solid organ transplant recipients who had been well nourished prior to transplant. Additionally, the development of sarcopenia, characterized by a loss of muscle tissue and function, in patients with end-stage organ disease anticipating transplantation, has been associated with poor post-transplant outcomes [9, 10]. The data is minimal on the prevalence and incidence of PCM in IF patients on the transplant waitlist or those undergoing MV/I transplantation. Although the ITR collects data on patient and graft survival, the registry does not collect data on nutritional status or management of pre- and post-transplant patients; therefore, it is not known to what extent PCM or other nutritional parameters truly impact outcomes.

Currently, there is also no validated tool to identify and diagnose PCM in pre- and post-MV/I transplant patients. However, in the pre- and post-liver transplant patient population, the subjective global assessment (SGA) has been successfully used to identify PCM. The SGA has been shown to be an independent predictor of post-transplant outcomes in patients undergoing liver transplantation [11, 12]. The SGA evaluates subjective data as reported by the patient for weight changes in the past 6 months and in the past 2 weeks, alterations in nutritional intake, presence of gastrointestinal symptoms for greater than 2 weeks, and level of functional capacity. In addition, SGA evaluates physical signs of malnutrition, loss of subcutaneous fat, muscle mass wasting, and/or presence of edema. Based on the results from the SGA scores, patients are classified either as well nourished (SGA grade A), moderately malnourished (SGA grade B), or severely malnourished (SGA grade C) [13].

The Academy of Nutrition and Dietetics (AND) and the American Society of Parenteral and Enteral Nutrition (ASPEN) also recently developed a set of characteristics to standardize the process of identifying PCM in adults [7]. According to ASPEN guidelines, characteristics of PCM include insufficient energy intake, weight loss, loss of muscle mass, loss of subcutaneous fat, localized or generalized fluid accumulation, and decreased functional status as measured by handgrip strength. If a patient demonstrates two or more of the aforementioned characteristics, then the etiology and severity must be further evaluated to verify the diagnosis of PCM. Specific parameters within each characteristic are

also established to help determine whether the PCM is in the setting of an acute or chronic illness and whether it is moderate or severe PCM. Despite its frequent use in the general adult patient population, there are limited studies to assess the utilization of this tool in the transplant patient population. Further studies are warranted to look at the identification and diagnosis of PCM in solid organ transplant patients and MV/I transplant patients in particular, specifically looking at post-transplant outcomes.

Nutrition Assessment

It is recommended that patients evaluated for MV/I transplantation are referred to a registered dietitian (RD) to undergo a comprehensive nutritional assessment to improve nutrition and to provide a thorough individualized medical nutrition therapy plan. Nutrition assessments completed in a timely manner may allow early intervention and improve post-transplant outcomes [9].

Nutrition assessment has been defined by AND as a systematic process of obtaining, verifying, and interpreting data to assist with decision-making regarding the nature and cause of nutrition-related problems [14]. An evaluation of patient goals, patient history, anthropometric measurements, nutrition-focused physical findings, biochemical data, tests and procedures, and food/nutrition history is an essential component of the nutrition assessment.

Patient's history includes pertinent medical and social conditions that may be relevant nutritionally, including medications and comorbidities. Anthropometric measurements involve an evaluation of weight trends and body mass index (BMI). Weight changes are evaluated for nutritional significance; contributing factors to any weight change are determined through nutrition assessment. A system-based nutrition-focused physical examination should be conducted utilizing techniques to inspect the skin, nails, head, hair, eyes, nose, oral cavity, and musculoskeletal system to identify any overt nutrition deficiencies [14, 15]. A review of laboratory data, diagnostic tests, and procedures assists with identifying nutrition-related abnormalities. Relevant laboratory values and assessments include the complete metabolic panel, micronutrient labs, 72-hour fecal fat test, intake and output measurements, and indirect calorimetry. Food/nutrition history involves obtaining information about energy intake, restrictions, and potential challenges of oral diet and/or EN and PN regimens. Regardless of the mode of feeding, an evaluation of carbohydrate, protein, fat, and micronutrient intake is evaluated for adequacy. An individual's knowledge level and readiness to change are also assessed to determine any deficits or barriers to implementation. See Table 31.1 for the elements of a nutrition assessment.

Table 31.1 Elements of a nutrition assessment [14, 15]

Patient history
Personal history
Age
Language
Occupation
Education
Family role
Medical history
Signs/symptoms
Medical/surgical history
Psychological state
Quality of life
Medication/supplement history
Prescription/OTC drugs
Vitamin/herbal supplements
Probiotics
Use of illegal drugs
Social history
Socioeconomic status
Social support system
Housing situation
Cultural/religious beliefs
Anthropometric measurements
Evaluation of weight changes

$$\%\,\text{Weight Change} = \frac{\text{Usual Body Weight} - \text{Current Body Weight}}{\text{Usual Body Weight}} \times 100$$

Nutritional significance:
2% weight change in 1 week   5% weight change in a month
7% weight change in 3 months 10% weight change in 6 months
Body mass index (BMI)
BMI < 18: underweight   BMI 30–40: obese
BMI 19–25: normal   BMI >40: morbid obese
BMI 25–29: overweight
Nutrition-focused physical examination
Skin
Nails
Head
Hair
Eyes
Nose
Oral cavity
Musculoskeletal appearance
Biochemical data, tests, and procedures
Complete metabolic panel
Micronutrient labs
72-hour fecal fat test
Intake and output
Indirect calorimetry
Food/nutrition history
Food/nutrient intake
Feeding mode (*oral/enteral/parenteral*)
Food allergies
Food intolerances
Carbohydrate/protein/fat intake
Vitamin/mineral intake
Fluid intake
Food consistencies
Size, timing, and # of meals
Eating environment(s)
Sensory/environmental cues

Table 31.1 (continued)

Nutrition knowledge/beliefs
Level and accuracy
Food availability
Access to food purchasing
Ability of food preparation
Use of community nutrition programs
Physical activity level
Level of activity

A nutrition care plan is developed once the nutrition assessment is complete. The nutrition care plan may involve adjustments to the oral diet, PN or EN regimen, nutrition education to address knowledge deficits, or nutrition counseling to promote behavioral change to optimize adherence.

Nutrition Requirements

Successful nutrition management of the IF patient requires an accurate estimate and provision of nutrient requirements to reduce the risk of developing complications associated with underfeeding and overfeeding. Each patient's nutrition regimen is individualized to meet specific nutrition requirements, as well as to reduce the risk of further aggravation of complications, especially with PN. Underfeeding can lead to weight loss, PCM, delayed recovery, and the risk of refeeding syndrome. Overfeeding has several detrimental health consequences, ranging from metabolic acidosis to hypercapnia [16].

The European Society for Clinical Nutrition and Metabolism (ESPEN) has established nutrition recommendations for adult patients on home PN, which suggest a caloric provision between 20 and 35 calories/kg/day [17]. Predictive calorie equations that factor in parameters of age, sex, weight, and height of the patient are used to estimate basal metabolic rate (BMR), also known as resting energy expenditure (REE). The most commonly used predictive equations are the Harris-Benedict, Ireton-Jones, Johnstone, Mifflin St. Jeor, and Owen equations. Indirect calorimetry (IC) is the gold standard for measuring REE. IC studies, however, are challenging to obtain due to the extensive time and resources needed to complete. Therefore, its use is not always feasible in a clinical setting. It is unclear how accurate nutrition estimates are for the patient with IF as absorption of nutrients typically does not meet physiological demands [18]. Several IF studies showed that the Harris-Benedict and Johnstone equations, using actual body weight and ideal body weight as parameters, were the most accurate predictors of REE when IC studies were not able to be completed [18, 19].

ESPEN recommendations for the unstressed adult on home PN suggest a protein provision of 0.8–1.0 g/kg/day [17]. Additional protein – up to 2.0 g/kg/day – may be required in the stressed patient due to increased needs for malabsorption and/or losses from surgically placed drains, stomas, and wounds. Fluid requirements also factor in losses from surgically placed drains and stomas, renal function, and electrolyte balance. The electrolyte provision in the home PN regimen should reflect fluid losses to assist with replenishment.

Pre-transplant Care and PN Complications

The primary pre-intestinal transplant nutrition goal for the MV/I patient is to optimize the nutrition status of the patient, reduce complications from IF and PN, and ensure the patient is nutritionally prepared for transplantation. Monitoring of nutrition therapy is needed on an ongoing basis to prevent and manage metabolic and infectious complications of PN. This close and meticulous monitoring requires an interdisciplinary team for successful management [17].

Metabolic complications from the chronic use of PN include fluid alterations, electrolyte derangements, and long-term complications including hepatobiliary disorders, metabolic bone disease, and iron-deficiency anemia [20]. In the IF patient, fluid alterations may manifest as dehydration due to intestinal losses from malabsorption, stomas, or venting of gastrostomy tubes and drains. Dehydration may also arise from insufficient fluid volume and electrolyte provision in

PN. Intake and output records are useful to help appropriately adjust the infusion volume of PN and intravenous fluids. There are often significant gastrointestinal losses in the IF patient, requiring a high volume of PN. Additional intravenous fluids may be needed to meet fluid requirements to optimize hydration. Electrolyte disturbances, especially hyponatremia, hypokalemia, and hypomagnesemia are common in the IF patient due to ongoing intestinal losses. Patients on PN regularly complete scheduled laboratory tests for therapeutic adjustment of the electrolyte provision in their PN regimen. IF-associated liver disease (IFALD), also known as PN-associated liver disease (PNALD), is a serious complication of long-term PN use. Nutritional risk factors that may contribute to IFALD include PN that is run over a duration of 24 hours (continuous PN), deficiency of amino acids and essential fatty acids, minimal enteral stimulation, excess nutrient provision of carbohydrates and lipids, and mineral toxicity [21]. Treatment options for IFALD include running the PN nocturnally, over a specific duration of hours (cyclic PN), to allow hepatic rest, correcting nutritional deficiencies, adjusting the carbohydrate dose (goal for 4–6 mg/kg/day), adjusting the lipid dose (goal for 1 g/kg/day), and/or trial of fish oil-based lipid emulsion [17, 21]. See Table 31.2 for nutrition management options for IFALD.

Table 31.2 Nutritional deficiencies and excesses in intestinal failure associated liver disease

Nutrient deficiencies	Management options (adults)
Amino acid deficiency	
Carnitine	Measure plasma total and free carnitine and acylcarnitine concentrations Maintain age-specific carnitine levels within normal range

	Supplementation
	  Inconsistent data on the efficacy of supplementation on hepatic dysfunction
	  Titrate the dose based on individual needs of the patient and age-specific reference ranges
	  Parenteral dosing requirements
	    Consider 400 mg/day for 7 days, followed by a maintenance dose of 60 mg/day
	  More studies are needed

Choline	Measure choline as part of serum amino acid profile Maintain normal plasma choline levels

	Supplementation
	  Oral dosing requirements
	    >13 years: 550 mg/day (male), 425 mg/day (female), 450 mg/day (pregnant), 550 mg/day (lactation)
	  Consider IV 1–4 g/day choline chloride for 6 weeks

Methionine	Measure methionine as part of serum amino acid profile
	Supplementation More studies needed for recommendations on oral and parenteral supplementation
Taurine	Measure taurine as part of serum amino acid profile Maintain normal plasma taurine levels
	Supplementation More controlled studies needed on its hepatoprotective effect and dosing recommendations

Essential fatty acid deficiency	Measure triene/tetraene ratio (TTR)
	  Biochemical essential fatty acid deficiency: TTR > 0.2
	  Clinical essential fatty acid deficiency: TTR > 0.4
	Avoid prolonged use of lipid-free PN

	Supplementation
	  Cautiously increase dose and/or frequency of lipids
	  For soybean oil-based lipid emulsions, maintain lipid dose around 1 g/kg/day
	  Consider fish oil-based or mixed (soybean oil, medium-chain triglycerides, olive oil, fish oil) lipid emulsion at higher dose or frequency

Lack of enteral intake	Initiate a trial of trophic feeding

Table 31.2 (continued)

Nutrient deficiencies	Management options (adults)
Nutrient excesses	
Excess calories and carbohydrates	Reduce carbohydrate dose to maintain a glucose infusion rate <4–6 mg/kg/min
Lipid emulsions	Reduce dose of lipids to around 1 g/kg/day Reduce frequency of lipids Consider switch to fish oil-based or mixed (soybean oil, medium-chain triglycerides, olive oil, fish oil) lipid emulsion
Mineral toxicity	

Aluminum	Evaluate risk factors
	  Renal compromise
	  Age-related weakening of gastrointestinal mucosal barrier
	  Burns
	Measure serum aluminum level for those who are at risk
	As aluminum is not routinely included in PN, consider etiologies of toxicity, such as contamination from the manufacturing process, renal compromise, prematurity, age-related weakening of the gastrointestinal barrier, and burns
	Limit contamination of aluminum levels in PN additives to ≤5 mcg/kg/day

Copper	Check serum copper every 6 months in patients with cholestasis or liver dysfunction Parenteral dosing requirements 0.3–0.5 mg/day; 0.4–0.5 mg/day in presence of high gastrointestinal fluid loss One daily dose of multi-trace element. Reduce copper by 0.15 mg in the presence of severe cholestasis or high copper levels Limit copper contamination to <0.1 mg/day total in a typical adult PN formulation
Manganese	Monitor for signs and symptoms of manganese toxicity (e.g., neurologic symptoms) every 1–3 months if a multi-trace element product is used Check whole blood manganese levels every 3–4 months in presence of signs and symptoms of toxicity and monthly with significant cholestasis Parenteral dosing requirements 55 mcg/day Limit manganese contamination to <40 mcg/day total in a typical adult on PN Omit manganese when whole blood manganese is high Individual dosing of manganese is not required Recheck within 3 months of provision and discontinuation of manganese in PN.

Adapted with permission: Limketkai et al. [21]
PN parenteral nutrition, *TTR* triene/tetraene ratio

Acute Post-transplant Care

In the acute post-transplant phase, the primary nutrition goal is to provide sufficient calories and protein to enhance postoperative recovery, optimize the transition from PN to EN, and eventually to have an unrestricted oral diet [9]. PN will continue post-operatively during this transition and will be gradually weaned as tolerance to EN and oral diet is established. Post-operative PN regimens are generally lower in total fluid volume as compared to pre-operative regimens. Generally, PN is discontinued when complete nutrition needs are achieved through EN by post-operative week four [5].

EN is an integral component to the post-operative regimen. Experience shows that the intestinal allograft should be used as soon as is medically feasible – once motility is established – through either oral diet or EN. Contraindications to the initiation of EN post-operatively include severe preservation injury, transplantation rejection, post-operative complications, ileus, and/or persistent lymphatic leak [5, 22]. EN is typically initiated 3–7 days post-operatively with a full-strength EN formula at a trickle rate of 5–10 mL/hour and is very slowly increased with close monitoring of GI symptoms and stoma output. As tolerance to EN is established and the rate is increased, PN is tapered gradually [23, 24].

The choice of EN formula varies widely and depends on the method of delivery, the patient's medical history, and clinical judgment. Either during surgery or immediately after, a feeding tube is generally placed distal to the anastomosis. Jejunostomy tubes are frequently used for patient comfort and acceptance and also to reduce the possibility of aspiration [5]. A gastrostomy tube or nasogastric tube is also frequently placed in addition to the jejunostomy to help with decompression. Polymeric, standard EN formulas with intact proteins can be administered post-operatively as they do not appear to undergo significant malabsorption with the intestinal allograft and thus can be tolerated well [24].

There are, however, certain post-operative complications that may exclude a patient from tolerating a standard formula, including gastroparesis, diarrhea, malabsorption, chyle leak, and/or drug-induced hyperkalemia. In these circumstances, specialized formulas and medications may be used depending on the complication. For diarrhea or high effluent output, the administration of opioids, antidiarrheal medications, soluble fiber supplements, or fiber-containing EN formulas is common. Prokinetics and a fiber-free EN formula are used in patients with symptoms of gastroparesis. If a chyle leak is suspected, a low fat, elemental EN formula is recommended. In patients for whom malabsorption is suspected, isotonic, elemental EN formulas with peptide-based proteins are recommended [5, 24].

Chronic Post-transplant Care

In the chronic post-transplant phase, the primary nutrition goal is to transition from PN to EN and, eventually, to meet nutrition needs through an oral diet alone [9]. As tolerance to an oral diet and calorie intake by the mouth improves, EN is weaned accordingly. EN regimens are generally transitioned from continuous to nocturnal feeds as oral intake improves to encourage daytime oral intake and to allow independence from the EN pump. EN may be discontinued completely when the patient is able to meet total daily nutrition goals through oral intake alone (mean of 57 ± 36 days post-MV/I transplantation) [23]. Once the patient is eating, the ability to sustain and tolerate an oral diet alone is determined by ongoing evaluation of nutritional parameters such as weight maintenance and normal electrolyte and micronutrient levels without dependence on EN. Due to the high risk of infection with the use of immunosuppressive medications post-transplant, ongoing education on food safety should be provided to the patient and caregivers to reduce the risk of foodborne illness [25]. With suspicion of graft rejection, PN may be reinitiated, either as a full or partial complement to the oral diet.

Weight gain, along with potential development of obesity, can occur with the optimization of digestion and absorption of oral nutrients in the setting of established nutritional autonomy of the gastrointestinal tract [23]. Post-transplant nutrition goals include reducing the risk of developing obesity as well as other complications such as hypertension, hyperlipidemia, osteoporosis, and diabetes mellitus. See Table 31.3 for goals in pre-transplant and-post transplant nutrition care.

Transition from Hospital to Home

Post-transplant, the goal is to send the patient home free from nutrition support. If needed, EN is the preferred post-transplant home regimen and would hopefully only serve as a short-term nutrition bridge, while attempts are made to optimize intake with an oral diet. Once the patient is ready to be discharged home, planning must take place to ascertain a safe transition ensuring the patient and caregiver are

Table 31.3 Nutrition goals for pre-transplant and post-transplant care

Common goals		
Individualize nutrition requirements to prevent under and overfeeding of nutrients		
Manage nutrition-related complications associated with PN, EN, and oral diet		
Pre-transplant	**Acute post-transplant**	**Chronic post-transplant**
Reduce complications from IF Reduce complications from PN Ensure the nutrition status of the patient is optimized for transplantation	Discontinue PN with optimal transition to EN and eventually to an unrestricted oral diet	Meet nutrition needs through an oral diet alone Reduce risk of obesity, hypertension, hyperlipidemia, osteoporosis, and diabetes mellitus

proficient in safely administering the home care regimen. Prior to discharging the patient home on EN, a home provider must be identified to provide the patient with the appropriate tools to implement the nutrition plan autonomously. Additionally, a patient must meet insurance criteria to allow coverage of the EN therapy, and a physician that can serve as the long-term ordering provider must be determined. Finally, the patient and caregivers must be provided with ongoing education regarding the nutrition plan.

Medicare insurance is one of the major government payers for home PN and EN therapy and sets specific criteria for its coverage consideration. These criteria should be included in documentation in the patient's medical chart by the ordering medical provider. The coverage for EN and PN falls under Medicare Part B, in which the therapies and their associated supplies are deemed to be prosthetic devices [26]. Objective documentation and diagnostic tests supporting that the patient meets criteria for EN or PN is also needed for approval (e.g., operative reports, radiology reports, fecal fat test). The criteria for coverage of EN and PN therapy state that the length of permanence must be defined and it must be necessary for 90 days or longer to establish permanence of therapy. Additionally, a qualifying diagnosis per Medicare criteria must be included, and the therapy must serve as primary source of nutrition.

Impact on Quality of Life

The desire to eat and enjoy variety in the diet is one of the great pleasures in life, and it derives from our most basic needs for survival. When the pleasure of consuming an oral diet becomes devoid and one becomes dependent on PN as a primary source of nutrition, it often impacts QOL through the loss of one of the most innate human instincts: eating [27, 28].

For patients with irreversible IF, PN is a lifelong requirement due to ongoing risk for metabolic abnormalities, PCM, and/or death in the setting of significant malabsorption of oral nutrients and electrolytes, and the patients are no longer able to nutritionally sustain themselves through an oral diet alone [29]. Although PN is a life-saving therapy, its long-term use carries the potential to negatively impact one's QOL due to the emotional and physical demands it places on the patient. A patient who is fully reliant on PN for nutrition support may become dependent on others to assist with the day-to-day administration needs of this demanding therapy. Additionally, dependency on PN may interfere with leisure and social activities due to the need to be frequently connected to the PN pump, which may or may not be portable. Through use of QOL surveys, patients with IF on home PN have reported increased symptoms of anxiety, depression, distorted body image, gastrointestinal symptoms, frequent urination, abnormal sleep patterns, and the inability to consume oral diet [27, 28].

For IF patients who experience significant complications due to the chronic use of PN, MV/I transplantation may assist with achieving independence from the demands associated with PN. The ITR report showed that 67% of post-MV/I transplant patients worldwide have completely stopped the use of PN and have been able to return to an oral diet within 6 months post-transplant [4]. Patients who survived 5 years post-MV/I transplant have been shown to achieve complete nutritional autonomy evidenced by discontinuation of PN and to be able to sustain health through an unrestricted oral diet [30]. Significant improvement in QOL after MV/I transplantation has been demonstrated with reductions in anxiety, depression, gastrointestinal symptoms; improved perception of body image and sleep patterns; and increased engagement in leisure and social activities [27, 28, 31].

The majority of QOL studies for MV/I transplantation focused on the evaluation of non-nutritional aspects of QOL post-transplant. Further studies are warranted to evaluate alterations of oral diet and dietary habits in pre- and post-MV/I transplant patients.

Conclusions

MV/I transplantation can serve as an option for patients with irreversible IF to establish full nutritional autonomy and to provide an opportunity to wean completely from PN. As PCM has a high potential to adversely impact post-transplant outcomes, nutrition assessments and ongoing medical nutrition therapy are important to meet caloric and nutrient requirements in the pre-transplant and post-transplant phases. The overarching goal of MV/I transplantation is to improve the patient's quality of life through a complete wean from PN and transition to EN and oral diet, allowing patient to enjoy one of the essential joys of life, reassert control over their lives, and have more flexibility in their routines. An expert RD is an essential member of the MV/I transplantation team, providing the patient with necessary tools and support for nourishment and medical and psychological well-being.

References

1. Pironi L, Arends J, Baxter J, et al. ESPEN endorsed recommendations. Definition and classification of intestinal failure in adults. Clin Nutr. 2015;34:171–80.
2. Pironi L, Arends J, Bozzetti F, et al. ESPEN guidelines on chronic intestinal failure in adults. Clin Nutr. 2016;35:247–307.
3. Winkler M, DiMaria-Ghalili R, Guenter P, Resnick H, Robinson L, Lyman B, Ireton-Jones C, Banchik L, Steiger E. Characteristics of a cohort of home parenteral nutrition patients at the time of enrollment in the sustain registry. J Parenter Enter Nutr. 2016;40:1140–9.
4. Grant D, Abu-Elmagd K, Mazariegos G, Vianna R, Langnas A, Mangus R, Farmer D, Lacaille F, Iyer K, Fishbein T. Intestinal transplant registry report: global activity and trends. Am J Transplant. 2014;15:210–9.
5. Matarese L, Costa G, Bond G, Stamos J, Koritsky D, O'Keefe S, Abu-Elmagd K. Therapeutic efficacy of intestinal and multivisceral transplantation: survival and nutrition outcome. Nutr Clin Pract. 2007;22:474–81.
6. Jensen G, Bistrian B, Roubenoff R, Heimburger D. Malnutrition syndromes: a conundrum vs continuum. J Parenter Enter Nutr. 2009;33:710–6.
7. White J, Guenter P, Jensen G, Malone A, Schofield M. Consensus statement of the academy of nutrition and dietetics/American Society for Parenteral and Enteral Nutrition: characteristics recommended for the identification and documentation of adult malnutrition (undernutrition). J Acad Nutr Diet. 2012;112:730–8.
8. Jensen G, Compher C, Sullivan D, Mullin G. Recognizing malnutrition in adults. J Parenter Enter Nutr. 2013;37:802–7.
9. Hasse J. Nutrition assessment and support of organ transplant recipients. J Parenter Enter Nutr. 2001;25:120–31.
10. Carey E. Sarcopenia in solid organ transplantation. Nutr Clin Pract. 2014;29:159–70.
11. Stephenson G, Moretti E, El-Moalem H, Clavien P, Tuttle-Newhall J. Malnutrition in liver transplant patients. Transplantation. 2001;72:666–70.
12. Merli M, Giusto M, Giannelli V, Lucidi C, Riggio O. Nutritional status and liver transplantation. J Clin Exp Hepatol. 2011;1:190–8.
13. Makhija S, Baker J. The subjective global assessment: a review of its use in clinical practice. Nutr Clin Pract. 2008;23:405–9.
14. Lacey K, Pritchett E. Nutrition care process and model: ADA adopts road map to quality care and outcomes management. J Am Diet Assoc. 2003;103:1061–72.
15. Esper D. Utilization of nutrition-focused physical assessment in identifying micronutrient deficiencies. Nutr Clin Pract. 2015;30:194–202.
16. Klein C, Stanek G, Wiles C. Overfeeding macronutrients to critically ill adults. J Am Diet Assoc. 1998;98:795–806.
17. Staun M, Pironi L, Bozzetti F, et al. ESPEN guidelines on parenteral nutrition: home parenteral nutrition (HPN) in adult patients. Clin Nutr. 2009;28:467–79.
18. Skallerup A, Nygaard L, Olesen S, Vinter-Jensen L, Køhler M, Rasmussen H. Can we rely on predicted basal metabolic rate in patients with intestinal failure on home parenteral nutrition? J Parenter Enter Nutr. 2016;41:1139–45.

19. Araújo E, Suen V, Marchini J, Vannucchi H. Ideal weight better predicts resting energy expenditure than does actual weight in patients with short bowel syndrome. Nutrition. 2007;23:778–81.

20. Davila J, Konrad D. Metabolic complications of home parenteral nutrition. Nutr Clin Pract. 2017;32:753–68.

21. Limketkai B, Choe M, Patel S, Shah N, Medici V. Nutritional risk factors in the pathogenesis of parenteral nutrition-associated liver disease. Curr Nutr Rep. 2017;6:281–90.

22. Weimann A, Braga M, Harsanyi L, et al. ESPEN guidelines on enteral nutrition: surgery including organ transplantation. Clin Nutr. 2006;25:224–44.

23. Matarese LE. Nutrition interventions before and after adult intestinal transplantation: the Pittsburgh experience. Pract Gastroenterol. 2010;34(11):11–30.

24. Rovera G, Schoen R, Goldbach B, Janson D, Bond G, Rakela J, Graham T, O'Keefe S, Abu-Elmagd K. Intestinal and multivisceral transplantation: dynamics of nutritional management and functional autonomy. J Parenter Enter Nutr. 2003;27:252–9.

25. Obayashi P. Food safety for the solid organ transplant patient. Nutr Clin Pract. 2012;27:758–66.

26. Bonnes S, Salonen B, Hurt R, McMahon M, Mundi M. Parenteral and enteral nutrition—from hospital to home: will it be covered? Nutr Clin Pract. 2017;32:730–8.

27. DiMartini A, Rovera G, Graham T, Furukawa H, Todo S, Funovits M, Lu S, Abu-Elmagd K. Quality of life after small intestinal transplantation and among home parenteral nutrition patients. J Parenter Enter Nutr. 1998;22:357–62.

28. Avitzur Y, Miserachs M. Quality of life on long-term parenteral nutrition. Curr Opin Organ Transplant. 2018;23:1–8.

29. Richards D, Irving M. Assessing the quality of life of patients with intestinal failure on home parenteral nutrition. Gut. 1997;40:218–22.

30. Abu-Elmagd K, Kosmach-Park B, Costa G, et al. Long-term survival, nutritional autonomy, and quality of life after intestinal and multivisceral transplantation. Ann Surg. 2012;256:494–508.

31. Pironi L, Baxter J, Lauro A, Guidetti M, Agostini F, Zanfi C, Pinna A. Assessment of quality of life on home parenteral nutrition and after intestinal transplantation using treatment-specific questionnaires. Am J Transplant. 2012;12:S60–6.

Medical Course and Complications After Visceral Transplantation

32

Waldo Concepcion and Lung-Yi Lee

Introduction

Until relatively recently, in patients with intestinal failure who were unable to achieve intestinal adaptation through surgical or medical therapies, long-term parenteral nutrition was the only option. Early attempts at intestinal transplantation (ITx) were unsuccessful due to technical problems, infectious complications, and the inadequacy of the only types of immunosuppression available at the time. Fortunately, surgical innovations and standardization of surgical techniques, advances in immunosuppression and induction protocols, improved understanding of gut physiology and mucosal immunology, and improved transplant medical management, including monitoring for possible complications, have now led to the possibility of successful ITx.

Although the nomenclature used in this field varies, in general it can be considered that the main types of ITx are the following: isolated intestinal transplantation, which may or may not include the colon, combined liver-intestine transplantation, and multivisceral transplantation (MVTx) which along with the small intestine may include any combination of the stomach, large intestine, liver, spleen, and, especially in patients with cystic fibrosis, chronic pancreatitis, or type 1 diabetes mellitus, the pancreas. A modified MVTx (MMVTx) does not include the liver. As discussed in Chap. 29, which organs are included in MVTx will depend on patient anatomy and disease process.

In comparison to transplantation of other solid organs, MVTx is performed the least. The Intestinal Transplant Registry (ITR) reports that worldwide between 2001 and 2011, there were 458 multivisceral, 117 modified multivis-

ceral, and 572 liver-small intestine transplants, with significant improvement in both graft and patient survival rates over time [1]. MVTx is a very complex procedure that presents multiple challenges for proper post-transplantation management, with a substantial risk of complications including rejection, infection, de novo malignancy, renal dysfunction, graft-versus-host disease, and others. Such medical complications combined with the demands on patients for strict adherence to medications, hygiene rules, specific dietary regimens, and other health behaviors as well as long-term management of all other aspects of a chronic illness can result in significant anxiety, depression, and emotional distress requiring psychosocial and mental health care. A team approach including transplant surgeons, gastroenterologists, infectious disease specialists, child development specialists, and occupational, speech, and physical therapists as well as mental health clinicians is absolutely required for optimal post-transplantation management.

Medical Course and Complications After Visceral Transplantation

Rejection

In simple terms, rejection occurs because the allogeneic intestinal tissue triggers both adaptive immune responses (through T cells and B-cell-derived alloantibodies) and innate immune responses (through natural killer cells, dendritic cells, innate lymphoid cells, and macrophages), the combination of which ultimately results in graft damage. Clinically, this may manifest as fever, malabsorption, dysmotility, and ischemia, but there may also be an absence of symptoms in what is termed subclinical rejection [2]. In the earliest days of ITx, the risk of rejection was extremely high, with an estimated 85% risk of any type of rejection from 1990 to 1994. Although optimal approaches to induction therapy and immunosuppression are still evolving, multiple advances have yielded substantial improvements in recent years.

W. Concepcion (✉)
Division of Abdominal Transplantation,
Departments of Surgery and Pediatrics,
Stanford University School of Medicine, Stanford, CA, USA
e-mail: Waldo1@stanford.edu

L.-Y. Lee
Division of Abdominal Transplantation, Department of Surgery,
Stanford University School of Medicine, Stanford, CA, USA

© Springer International Publishing AG, part of Springer Nature 2019
Y. Sher, J. R. Maldonado (eds.), *Psychosocial Care of End-Stage Organ Disease and Transplant Patients*,
https://doi.org/10.1007/978-3-319-94914-7_32

The induction/immunosuppression regimen that is currently most commonly used includes the immunosuppressant tacrolimus (TAC), with or without corticosteroids, along with anti-interleukin-2 (IL-2) receptor antibodies (Simulect) or an antilymphocyte globulin such as Thymoglobulin (Sanofi Genzyme, Cambridge, Massachusetts, USA) or ATGAM (Pfizer, New York, New York, USA) or the monoclonal antibody to CD52 alemtuzumab (Sanofi Genzyme, Cambridge, Massachusetts, USA). Based on the most recent Organ Procurement and Transplantation Network (OPTN) data, in 2016 over half (52.9%) of intestine transplant recipients received T-cell depleting agents; 16.2% received IL-2 receptor antagonists; and 34.6% reported no induction therapy [3]. The most common initial immunosuppressants used in 2016 were tacrolimus (97.8%), steroids (73.5%), and mycophenolate (38.2%) [3]. Among those who had reached 1 year post-transplant in 2016, steroids were used in 80.2% [3]. At Stanford, Thymoglobulin is used for induction at 1.5 mg/kg × 5 doses. TAC is given intravenously until normal intestinal function is restored, after which it is switched to oral dosing. During the first 3 months post-transplant, the TAC target trough level at 12 h is 15–20 ng/ml; after 3 months, the target trough is reduced to 5–10 ng/mL. If corticosteroids are used, a bolus is given at the time of transplantation, after which the dose is tapered down over 5 days to the dose used for maintenance. When alemtuzumab or Thymoglobulin is used as part of the induction regimen, corticosteroids are not used. Mycophenolate mofetil may be used to reduce the dose-related toxicity of calcineurin inhibitor agents. Sirolimus is used at Stanford 1 month post-transplant surgery.

Despite use of more advanced drug therapies in recent years, the risk of acute rejection is still substantial. Based on OPTN data, the incidence of acute rejection by 1 year post-transplant from 2013 to 2014 was 23.9% in adult intestine-liver recipients and even higher in pediatric recipients, affecting approximately one in three patients [4]. Acute rejection can range from mild to severe. With severe exfoliative rejection, there is a very high risk of intestinal graft loss and mortality. Acute rejection most commonly occurs early, within the first 3 months post-transplant, but may occur much later, especially when there is reduced immunosuppression or patient nonadherence.

Diagnosis of rejection requires combining the findings of endoscopic examination, clinical observation, mucosal biopsies, and other factors. The complete approach to diagnosis that can distinguish between the various forms of rejection has been well reviewed by experts in the field [2, 5]. A unified grading system for assessing acute rejection through endoscopically derived small intestine allograft biopsy samples first proposed in 2003 [6] was later validated in a study that showed it to be reliable and useful for clinical decision-making [7]. Multiple centers currently use this grading sys-

tem. Experts in the field strongly recommend that biopsies be taken from both native tissues (such as the esophagus, rectum, or skin) and from multiple allografts in order to help determine if findings are the result of alloimmune responses indicating rejection or are changes originating in the graft possibly indicating graft-versus-host disease or are the result of indiscriminate and global pathologies indicating, for example, infection or post-transplant lymphoproliferative disease [2]. In combination with the biopsy results, endoscopic findings are used to estimate the extent of damage to the mucosal layer. In addition, our understanding of biomarkers that may be useful for a more complete understanding of the rejection process is growing, and these may be more widely used in the near future. At Stanford, we are currently using the Pleximmune™ test (Plexision Inc., Pittsburgh, PA, USA), a test which predicts acute cellular rejection in children with liver or intestine transplantation by assessing T-cell reactivity toward HLA from the donor.

Antibody-mediated acute rejection can fall in one of two categories: (1) acute antibody-mediated (humoral) rejection (AMR) and (2) hyperacute (the graft is rejected within minutes to hours) or accelerated acute (the graft is rejected within days) rejection [2]. Hyperacute and accelerated acute rejection have become much less common with the institution of cross-match testing in ITx. AMR occurs when antibodies directed to alloantigens trigger a graft-damaging combination of inflammation, coagulation, and other events. The most common form of acute rejection with ITx, including MVTx, is T-cell-mediated acute cellular rejection (ACR) [2]. ACR is thought to result when donor alloantigens activate an immune response in which the damaging effects of cytotoxic (CD8+) T cells and helper (CD4+) T cells are not sufficiently countered by the protective response of immunoregulatory T cells (Tregs) that could suppress ACR [8].

For ACR, increased immunosuppression may be an effective therapy. However, with AMR, standard therapy is generally ineffective [9]. In one of the only large series published to date, acute AMR developed in 10.3% of ITx recipients [10]. Although a combination of steroids and T-cell-targeted OKT3 resulted in initial improvement, the majority of grafts (61%) ultimately failed as the result of the later occurrence of severe ACR or chronic rejection; at an average follow-up of almost 3 years, mortality was high (44%). At Stanford, we treat acute mild rejection with steroid pulses. For severe acute rejection, we use ATG. For antibody-mediated rejection, we use plasmapheresis, IVIG, and rituximab (Rituxan and others). If there is complement activation, we use eculizumab (Soliris). For chronic ulcers, we use infliximab (Remicade) for treatment.

Chronic rejection that can lead to graft loss also occurs in some patients. In one large series, chronic rejection occurred in 15% of visceral allografts [11]. With chronic rejection, graft loss occurs in almost all patients [12]. Symptoms of chronic rejection include diarrhea, weight loss, failure to thrive, chronic abdominal pain, and protein-losing enteropathy [5], symptoms that are generally unresponsive to treatment [2]. Repeated episodes of acute rejection and the duration and severity of rejection episodes are associated with the risk of developing chronic rejection.

Multiple aspects of rejection and the immunosuppressant medications used to prevent it may result in the need for patients to be referred for psychosocial care. Neurotoxic adverse effects of immunosuppressants may include anxiety, depression, agitation, sleep disturbances, cognitive impairment, and other symptoms. Rejection episodes can result in anxiety and distress in transplant recipients. In addition, although specific findings on the association between rejection and medication adherence have differed between various populations studied and the various adherence measures used, it is generally accepted that there is a substantial risk of post-transplant medication nonadherence that confers a substantial risk for rejection and graft loss [13–18]. Systematic reviews have shown that nonadherence is associated with approximately half (range 20–73%) of late acute rejections and 15% (range 3–35%) of graft losses [16–18].

Risk factors for nonadherence that have been identified include age from adolescent through young adult, old age, previous nonadherence, minority ethnicity/race, inadequate social supports, limited literacy, frequent medication changes, perception of symptom burden related to immunosuppressant medications, presence of psychological or psychiatric illness, and poor perceived health [13, 14, 19–21]. In a large meta-analysis of 61 studies of nonadherence in pediatric transplantation, it was shown that poorer family functioning, including poor family cohesion and increased parental distress, poor child behavioral functioning, and increased child distress are important risk factors for nonadherence [19, 21].

With so many factors contributing to nonadherence, simple solutions for improving adherence are lacking. However, systematic reviews of solid organ transplant recipients support an individually designed approach that focuses on each recipient's specific needs, barriers to adherence, and motivations [22]. Thus, referral for psychosocial support aimed at optimizing medication adherence through this type of individualized approach may be an important component of a total approach to improving adherence and reducing associated rejection and graft loss.

Infection and De Novo Malignancy

The leading cause of post-transplant mortality is infection, with up to 94% of patients developing a bacterial infection. Sepsis occurs in almost 70% of those who have received an intestine transplant, most commonly in the first 3 months post-transplant, with the most common sources of sepsis being the central venous catheter (49%) and intra-abdominal infections (33%) [23]. Sepsis related to bacterial translocation from the graft may also occur. Along with broad-spectrum antibiotics to treat the bacterial infection, treatment of these infections may require catheter removal, gut decontamination, and cytomegalovirus (CMV) treatment.

CMV and other opportunistic viral infections are a significant cause of graft loss, morbidity, and mortality. With an incidence of 16–24%, CMV is the most common. Several important risk factors have been identified [24]: (1) CMV donor/recipient mismatch; because the majority of pediatric patients are seronegative for CMV, they are at higher risk for this; (2) bacterial and fungal infections; the inflammation and cytokine release induced by these may increase CMV reactivation; (3) human herpes virus 6 (HHV-6) and HHV-7 infections affect immune responses in ways that may reactivate CMV; (4) induction therapy with lymphocyte-depleting antibodies; and (5) the use of steroids or polyclonal antibodies to address rejection can increase risk for CMV reactivation [24]. The effects of CMV infection can range from relatively mild flu-like symptoms to severe pneumonia and gastrointestinal tract involvement. With the latter, nausea, vomiting, abdominal pain, and diarrhea are common. Most centers now do CMV prophylaxis in patients who are CMV donor-positive/recipient-negative or recipient-positive, with the choice of agent dependent on the ability to absorb oral medication [24]. In patients who can absorb oral drugs, valganciclovir, an oral prodrug of ganciclovir, is recommended for 3–6 months post-transplant; intravenous ganciclovir is often used immediately post-transplant until absorption is normalized and in any patient with nausea/vomiting or diarrhea or who is otherwise intolerant of oral medications.

Post-transplant lymphoproliferative disorder (PTLD) is the most common de novo malignancy that occurs after intestine transplantation. It is almost always associated with Epstein-Barr virus (EBV). The presence of EBV viremia is a major risk factor for development of this proliferation of B cells resulting from immunosuppression. PTLD occurs more commonly in pediatric than adult patients. As with CMV, children are more likely to be EBV-negative and thus more likely to acquire the infection from a graft from an EBV-positive donor. PTLD most commonly develops within the first 6 months post-transplant. According to OPTN data, for recipients who underwent transplant between 2003 and 2013, PTLD developed within 5 years post-transplant in 9.2% of intestine recipients and 6.8% of intestine-liver recipients [4].

Because the calcineurin inhibitors adversely affect the function of T cells that might otherwise control proliferation of B cells, the use of these agents increases PTLD risk. However, rather than singling out specific agents as PTLD risk factors, it appears clear that a higher total amount of immunosuppression, including that from maintenance therapies as well as induction and rejection therapies, confers the highest risk. Frequent measurement of EBV viral load in order to monitor the possible need for immunosuppression adjustment is important. Where possible, reduction of immunosuppression will often result in PTLD remission.

Primarily as the result of immunosuppression, other non-lymphoid malignancies may also occur post-transplant, with incidence increasing with each additional year of immunosuppression. Multiple other viral infections may also occur, and knowledge of these is crucial for proper management of patients. Florescu and colleagues have provided an excellent review of the viral infections that may occur in intestinal transplant recipients, including clinical manifestations and approaches to prophylaxis and management [24].

Invasive fungal infections are also major causes of morbidity and mortality in this population, occurring in 25.5–59% of intestinal transplantation recipients [25]. According to data from the Transplant-Associated Infection Surveillance Network (TRANSNET), *Candida* species account for the majority (53%) of fungal infections in all organ transplant recipients [26]. However, other invasive fungal infections also occur, including aspergillosis (19%), cryptococcosis and infection with non-*Aspergillus* molds (8% each), infection with endemic fungi (5%, including histoplasmosis, coccidioidomycosis, and blastomycosis), and zygomycosis (2%) [26]. Data to show the incidence of these specifically in MVTx recipients is largely missing. One study showed that in comparison with isolated intestine transplant recipients, *Candida* infection occurs less often in MVTx recipients, possibly because of the transplanted liver's immunomodulatory effects [25]. Florescu and colleagues have provided an excellent review of these fungal infections that may occur in intestinal transplant recipients, including recommendations for the management of the various syndromes caused by *Candida* species and the prophylaxis used to prevent them [25].

Another fungal infection that may occur in intestinal transplant recipients is Pneumocystis pneumonia (PCP) caused by *P. jirovecii*. Recommendations for routine PCP prophylaxis for 6–12 months post-transplant have lowered the occurrence of this pneumonia during that time period. However, studies that have shown PCP occurring in the years after prophylaxis was discontinued, particularly in patients who had been treated for rejection, were relatively more immunosuppressed, or were lymphopenic [27, 28], have led to the recommendation that prophylaxis duration should be chosen based on known risk factors [28].

The multiple medications used both for prophylaxis and for treatment of infections add to the burden of medication adherence that is already present with the immunosuppressant medications; see discussion above under *Rejection* for a discussion of approaches to improving adherence.

Graft-Versus-Host Disease

Graft-versus-host disease (GVHD) has been reported to occur in 5.6–9.1% of recipients of intestinal/multivisceral transplants, more commonly in children than adults [10, 28] and in recipients of MVTx compared to isolated intestine [10]. Patients with GVHD most commonly present with a macular erythematous rash, mild pruritus, and mouth or tongue lesions. There may also be blisters, most commonly on the abdominal skin, palms, and soles, native gastrointestinal tract ulcers, diarrhea, and bone marrow suppression [29]. The reported outcome has differed substantially, with one series reporting 73% mortality [10] and another noting GVHD resolution in most patients with optimization of tacrolimus immunosuppression and steroid treatment [29]. In general, when only the skin is involved, GVHD can be successfully treated with steroids. However, with more extensive involvement, particularly of the recipient bone marrow, there is significant morbidity and mortality [5].

Renal Dysfunction

Compared to other transplants, intestinal transplantation confers a higher risk of renal failure, although the reported incidence decreased from 21.3% in 2003 [30] to 16% in 2008 [31]. The renal toxicity caused by the calcineurin inhibitors may develop as either acute azotemia or as chronic progressive renal disease. Because the overall total exposure to calcineurin inhibitors is related to renal insufficiency, dose reduction to limit the adverse renal effects is used. However, this reduction may be associated with increased graft rejection and loss, so the balance between these must be carefully considered. The reduced target levels for tacrolimus associated with increased use of induction therapies are expected to result in a reduction in the renal disease associated with this class of drugs. The initial lack of normal colonic absorption of water that follows intestinal transplants results in dehydration that also contributes to renal disease.

Challenges in Maintaining Nutrition, Fluids, and Electrolyte Homeostasis

During the immediate post-transplant period, scrupulous monitoring of renal function, electrolytes, and fluid intake and output are crucial, with appropriate adjustments in intravenous fluids made as necessary to maintain fluid and electrolyte balance. After this initial postoperative period, dehydration, hyponatremia, and metabolic acidosis still occur as the result of the water, sodium, magnesium, and bicarbonate loss associated with increased stool output. Thus, careful monitoring and appropriate replacement via intravenous fluids will still be important. Initially, nutrition will be maintained with total parenteral nutrition (TPN), but this will be weaned as the return of intestinal function allows the gradual introduction of enteral nutrition. Both the concentration and type of enteral nutrition will be adjusted based on clinical response (see Chap. 31).

In some cases, particularly with pediatric patients, there will be food aversion. In these cases, the history of long-term TPN has left these children unaccustomed to a large gastric content volume. Many other factors may also contribute to oral aversion and referral to child development specialists, psychiatrists and psychologists, and speech and occupational therapists may be needed as part of the overall approach to transitioning the child to normal feeding. Team members may also need to work with parents to teach them the parent-child interactions that will support the child's transition to a normal oral feeding routine and to counsel them on the importance of this.

Outcomes and Survival

Based on the most recent ITR data [1, 32] at 1, 5, and 10 years post-transplant, survival of intestinal transplant recipients was 77%, 58%, and 47%, respectively, worldwide. Intestinal graft survival is still lower as compared to other major organs. The multiple components of intestinal immunogenicity still threaten long-term allograft stability and survival [12]. Based on ITR data, at 1, 5, and 10 years worldwide, graft survival was 71%, 50%, and 41%, respectively [1, 32].

Based on OPTN data on US patients:

- Patient survival was better overall for intestine recipients compared with intestine-liver recipients. It was lowest for adult intestine-liver recipients with 68.6% and 35.7% survival at 1 and 5 years, respectively, and highest for pediatric intestine recipients with 88.1% and 74.6% survival at 1 and 5 years, respectively [4].
- In pediatric patients (younger than age 18) who received intestine transplants (with or without a liver) in 2009–2011, graft survival at 1 and 5 years was 72.0% and 54.1%, respectively; for adult recipients, graft survival was 70.5% and 44.1%, respectively [3].
- For patients receiving the intestines without a liver from 2009 to 2011, graft survival at 1 and 5 years was 70.9% and 47.6%, respectively [3].
- For patients receiving both the intestine and liver from 2009 to 2011, graft survival at 1 and 5 years was 70.2% and 50.6%, respectively [3].

Compared to other transplant types, hospital readmission is more common after intestinal transplant. A recent single-center study of 65 adult patients who were recipients of an isolated intestinal (51 patients) or multivisceral (14 patients) transplant found that 68% required early (<1 month) and 91% required late rehospitalization [33]. Readmission is most commonly due to dehydration, infection, surgical complications, gastrointestinal complications, and rejection.

Although data is very limited, compared to patients on parenteral nutrition, significantly improved quality of life and functional status have been reported in both pediatric [34] and adult [35] intestinal transplant patients. The most recent systematic review found that, in comparison with pre-transplant quality of life, adult intestinal transplant recipients experienced improvements in anxiety, sleep, social support, and leisure and that quality of life improved with longer follow-up [35]. Compared to home parenteral nutrition patients, post-transplant patients had significantly better energy, social functioning, and travel ability. In an important cross-sectional study of 227 visceral allograft recipients (both adults and children) who survived beyond 5 years, Abu-Elmagd and colleagues showed that nutritional autonomy had been achieved in 90% of survivors, most of whom had been reintegrated to society and had achieved self-sustained socioeconomic status [36]. Quality-of-life inventories showed that most of the psychological, emotional, and social measures had significantly improved.

Conclusions

As is made clear by the discussion of the typical medical course of intestinal transplant patients and the many complications that they may experience, there are many challenges that are present in patients' post-transplant lives. In the most fundamental way, these patients' lives have permanently changed. Although quality of life may improve in multiple ways, most patients (and in the case of pediatric patients, their parents) will need help addressing all these challenges and will benefit from the assistance of the team members providing psychosocial care.

References

1. Grant D, Abu-Elmagd K, Mazariegos G, Vianna R, Langnas A, Mangus R, et al. Intestinal transplant registry report: global activity and trends. Am J Transplant. 2015;15(1):210–9.
2. Ruiz P. Updates on acute and chronic rejection in small bowel and multivisceral allografts. Curr Opin Organ Transplant. 2014;19(3):293–302.
3. Smith JM, Weaver T, Skeans MA, Horslen SP, Harper AM, Snyder JJ, et al. OPTN/SRTR 2016 annual data report: intestine. Am J Transplant. 2018;18(Suppl 1):254–90.
4. Smith JM, Skeans MA, Horslen SP, Edwards EB, Harper AM, Snyder JJ, et al. OPTN/SRTR 2015 annual data report: intestine. Am J Transplant. 2017;17(Suppl 1):252–85.
5. Kubal CA, Mangus RS, Tector AJ. Intestine and multivisceral transplantation: current status and future directions. Curr Gastroenterol Rep. 2015;17(1):427.

6. Ruiz P, Bagni A, Brown R, Cortina G, Harpaz N, Magid MS, et al. Histological criteria for the identification of acute cellular rejection in human small bowel allografts: results of the pathology workshop at the VIII international small bowel transplant symposium. Transplant Proc. 2004;36(2):335–7.

7. Ruiz P, Takahashi H, Delacruz V, Island E, Selvaggi G, Nishida S, et al. International grading scheme for acute cellular rejection in small-bowel transplantation: single-center experience. Transplant Proc. 2010;42(1):47–53.

8. Franzese O, Mascali A, Capria A, Castagnola V, Paganizza L, Di Daniele N. Regulatory T cells in the immunodiagnosis and outcome of kidney allograft rejection. Clin Dev Immunol. 2013;2013:852395.

9. Valenzuela NM, Reed EF. Antibody-mediated rejection across solid organ transplants: manifestations, mechanisms, and therapies. J Clin Invest. 2017;127(7):2492–504.

10. Wu G, Selvaggi G, Nishida S, Moon J, Island E, Ruiz P, et al. Graft-versus-host disease after intestinal and multivisceral transplantation. Transplantation. 2011;91(2):219–24.

11. Abu-Elmagd KM, Costa G, Bond GJ, Soltys K, Sindhi R, Wu T, et al. Five hundred intestinal and multivisceral transplantations at a single center: major advances with new challenges. Ann Surg. 2009;250(4):567–81.

12. Abu-Elmagd KM, Wu G, Costa G, Lunz J, Martin L, Koritsky DA, et al. Preformed and de novo donor specific antibodies in visceral transplantation: long-term outcome with special reference to the liver. Am J Transplant. 2012;12(11):3047–60.

13. Prendergast MB, Gaston RS. Optimizing medication adherence: an ongoing opportunity to improve outcomes after kidney transplantation. Clin J Am Soc Nephrol. 2010;5(7):1305–11.

14. Schulz KH, Kroencke S. Psychosocial challenges before and after organ transplantation. Transpl Res Risk Manage. 2015;7:45–58.

15. De Bleser L, Matteson M, Dobbels F, Russell C, De Geest S. Interventions to improve medication-adherence after transplantation: a systematic review. Transpl Int. 2009;22(8):780–97.

16. De Geest S, Dobbels F, Fluri C, Paris W, Troosters T. Adherence to the therapeutic regimen in heart, lung, and heart-lung transplant recipients. J Cardiovasc Nurs. 2005;20(5 Suppl):S88–98.

17. Denhaerynck K, Dobbels F, Cleemput I, Desmyttere A, Schafer-Keller P, Schaub S, et al. Prevalence, consequences, and determinants of nonadherence in adult renal transplant patients: a literature review. Transpl Int. 2005;18(10):1121–33.

18. Dobbels F, Van Damme-Lombaert R, Vanhaecke J, De Geest S. Growing pains: non-adherence with the immunosuppressive regimen in adolescent transplant recipients. Pediatr Transplant. 2005;9(3):381–90.

19. Dew MA, Dabbs AD, Myaskovsky L, Shyu S, Shellmer DA, DiMartini AF, et al. Meta-analysis of medical regimen adherence outcomes in pediatric solid organ transplantation. Transplantation. 2009;88(5):736–46.

20. Dew MA, DiMartini AF, De Vito DA, Myaskovsky L, Steel J, Unruh M, et al. Rates and risk factors for nonadherence to the medical regimen after adult solid organ transplantation. Transplantation. [Research Support, N.I.H., Extramural Research Support, Non-U.S. Gov't]. 2007;83(7):858–73.

21. Shellmer DA, Dabbs AD, Dew MA. Medical adherence in pediatric organ transplantation: what are the next steps? Curr Opin Organ Transplant. 2011;16(5):509–14.

22. Nevins TE, Nickerson PW, Dew MA. Understanding medication nonadherence after kidney transplant. J Am Soc Nephrol. 2017;28(8):2290–301.

23. Florescu DF, Qiu F, Langnas AN, Mercer DF, Chambers H, Hill LA, et al. Bloodstream infections during the first year after pediatric small bowel transplantation. Pediatr Infect Dis J. 2012;31(7):700–4.

24. Florescu DF, Langnas AN, Sandkovsky U. Opportunistic viral infections in intestinal transplantation. Expert Rev Anti-Infect Ther. 2013;11(4):367–81.

25. Florescu DF, Sandkovsky U. Fungal infections in intestinal and multivisceral transplant recipients. Curr Opin Organ Transplant. 2015;20(3):295–302.

26. Pappas PG, Alexander BD, Andes DR, Hadley S, Kauffman CA, Freifeld A, et al. Invasive fungal infections among organ transplant recipients: results of the transplant-associated infection surveillance network (TRANSNET). Clin Infect Dis. 2010;50(8):1101–11.

27. McKinnell JA, Cannella AP, Kunz DF, Hook EW 3rd, Moser SA, Miller LG, et al. Pneumocystis pneumonia in hospitalized patients: a detailed examination of symptoms, management, and outcomes in human immunodeficiency virus (HIV)-infected and HIV-uninfected persons. Transpl Infect Dis. 2012;14(5):510–8.

28. Yeap S, Gkrania-Klotsas E, Sharkey LM, Middleton SJ, Woodward JM, Butler AJ, et al. Incidence of pneumocystis jiroveci pneumonia in patients following intestinal transplantation. Transplantation. 2017;101(6S2):S49.

29. Mazariegos GV, Abu-Elmagd K, Jaffe R, Bond G, Sindhi R, Martin L, et al. Graft versus host disease in intestinal transplantation. Am J Transplant. 2004;4(9):1459–65.

30. Ojo AO, Held PJ, Port FK, Wolfe RA, Leichtman AB, Young EW, et al. Chronic renal failure after transplantation of a nonrenal organ. N Engl J Med. 2003;349(10):931–40.

31. Watson MJ, Venick RS, Kaldas F, Rastogi A, Gordon SA, Colangelo J, et al. Renal function impacts outcomes after intestinal transplantation. Transplantation. 2008;86(1):117–22.

32. Huard G, Schiano T, Moon J, Iyer K. Choice of allograft in patients requiring intestinal transplantation: a critical review. Can J Gastroenterol Hepatol. 2017;2017:1069726.

33. Kwon YK, Etesami K, Sharp AL, Matsumoto CS, Fishbein TM, Girlanda R. Hospital readmissions after intestinal and multivisceral transplantation. Transplant Proc. 2016;48(6):2186–91.

34. DiMartini A, Rovera GM, Graham TO, Furukawa H, Todo S, Funovits M, et al. Quality of life after small intestinal transplantation and among home parenteral nutrition patients. JPEN J Parenter Enteral Nutr. 1998;22(6):357–62.

35. Ceulemans LJ, Lomme C, Pirenne J, De Geest S. Systematic literature review on self-reported quality of life in adult intestinal transplantation. Transplant Rev (Orlando). 2016;30(2):109–18.

36. Abu-Elmagd KM, Kosmach-Park B, Costa G, Zenati M, Martin L, Koritsky DA, et al. Long-term survival, nutritional autonomy, and quality of life after intestinal and multivisceral transplantation. Ann Surg. 2012;256(3):494–508.

Post-transplant Psychosocial and Mental Health Care of Pancreas and Visceral Transplant Recipients

Jaqueline Posada and Catherine Crone

Pancreas Post-transplant

As discussed in Chap. 30, the diagnosis of type 1 diabetes (T1D) marks the beginning of a changed existence. These changes include reliance on insulin; lifestyle modifications including dietary changes, frequent blood glucose monitoring, and time-consuming medical care; and the psychological sequelae such as depression, anxiety, diabetes distress, fear of hypoglycemia, and long-term prospect of diabetes-related complications of nephropathy, neuropathy, and retinopathy. The psychological evaluation of a pancreas transplant recipient should consider the individual in the context of T1D, as a lifelong, often debilitating illness that undoubtedly shapes the identity and expectations of the recipient. Pancreas transplant is not classified as a life-saving procedure, yet if successful, the transplant is a potential cure for diabetes as it restores normoglycemia and limits the progression of the complications associated with diabetes [1].

Indications for Pancreas Transplant

Pancreas transplant is offered in several forms: simultaneous pancreas kidney transplant (SPK), pancreas after kidney transplant (PAK), pancreas transplant alone (PTA), and allogeneic islet transplant alone (ITA). ITA is a minimally invasive procedure for treatment of problematic hypoglycemia

J. Posada
Department of Psychiatry, George Washington University School of Medicine, Washington, DC, USA

C. Crone (✉)
Department of Psychiatry, Inova Fairfax Hospital, Falls Church, VA, USA

Department of Psychiatry, Virginia Commonwealth University School of Medicine, Richmond, VA, USA

Department of Psychiatry, George Washington University School of Medicine, Washington, DC, USA
e-mail: Cathy.crone@inova.org

and glycemic lability. Since the year 2000 with the publication of the Edmonton protocol by Shapiro et al., more than 1000 successful allogeneic islet transplants have been performed worldwide [2]. As of 2017, in the USA, ITA is pending a biologics license application to the FDA which would allow broader distribution of allogeneic islets and thus greater access to the procedure. Individuals with T1D and end-stage renal disease (ESRD) are candidates for SPK and PAK. The American Diabetes Association (ADA) recommends pancreas transplant for individuals with T1D without substantial renal disease but with frequent, acute, severe complications such as hypoglycemia, marked hyperglycemia or ketoacidosis, and failure of insulin-based treatment to prevent these acute metabolic complications [3]. A second ADA criterion focuses on psychological impact of T1D citing "clinical and emotional problems with exogenous insulin therapy that are so severe as to be incapacitating" [4].

It is important to examine the differences between whole organ PTA and ITA and assess patient expectations before and after transplant. The procedural specifics are beyond the scope of this chapter; however, we discuss related risks and benefits with each choice and how these might impact the recipient after their transplant. Lasting insulin independence is more likely in whole organ pancreas transplant compared to ITA [5], and for this reason, PTA is offered to individuals who have nonadherence with their exogenous insulin therapy contributing to the aforementioned complications of diabetes [1]. PTA carries a greater risk of postsurgical complications, such as hemorrhage and vascular graft thrombosis requiring re-laparotomy [6], and has a higher percent of death after 1 year when compared to SPK and PAK [7]. As with any transplant, the immunosuppressive agents confer their own post-transplant risks. PTA has relatively high cumulative incidence of post-transplant lymphoproliferative disorders (PTLD) of 2.3% at 5 years, as the intensive immunotherapy lends itself to higher risk of developing lymphoma [7]. Compared to whole organ PTA, allogeneic islet transplantation has lower procedure-related morbidity [8]. Yet ITA also demands lifelong immunosuppression and usually requires more than one infusion of islets to achieve insulin independence, and insulin independence is not guaranteed, with only 27–50% of patients remaining insulin independent after 5 years [5, 9]. For most recipients, ITA results in improved glycemic control as measured by HbA1C and prevents episodes of hypoglycemia and if not freedom from insulin; recipients can expect a reduced insulin requirement [10].

Fear of Hypoglycemia and QOL Peri-pancreas Transplant

Fear of hypoglycemia is a distressing condition which illustrates the all-encompassing nature of T1D as it touches on a person's physical well-being, living with daily risk of harm or even death from hypoglycemia and impact on identity and social interactions. ITA is a treatment option for patients with optimal insulin therapy, as with continuous glucose monitoring or a subcutaneous pump, who still experience hypoglycemic episodes [10]. Specifically ITA has demonstrated effect in reducing worry and behaviors associated with fear of hypoglycemia and resulted in patient-perceived improvement of mental and social functioning domains as measured by quality-of-life (QOL) instruments [11, 12]. Unfortunately, even in a 5-year follow-up after ITA, recipients did not show significant improvement when assessed by the diabetes distress scale which asks about the emotional burden of diabetes, distress related to the insulin regimen, physician perception and involvement in a patient's diabetes care, and interpersonal relationships such as friends and family [13]. A small Swedish study completed interviews with 11 patients about their fear of hypoglycemia before and after ITA, and qualitative analysis identified the following themes [14]. Before ITA, patients reported struggle for control over their social life due to unpredictability of their disease, and physical and mental limitations related to fluctuating blood glucose levels. After transplant, patients felt they regained power and control over their social life and improved well-being. These themes were echoed in similar qualitative analysis of interviews with Spanish patients pre-and post- SPK transplant. Although after transplant, patients reported fear of graft loss and suffered from complications of both T1D and surgery, these individuals reevaluated their priorities and approached life with renewed effort to remain healthy and savor the present moment [15]. Additional focus was placed on tempering patient expectations of being "insulin free" after ITA and how to cope with disappointment that follows when a patient requires exogenous insulin after a period of insulin independence [16].

Most QOL data related to pancreas transplant is gathered from studies examining SPK recipients. Overall, pancreas transplant, either alone or in addition to a kidney, leads to sustained improvement in patient-reported QOL outcomes, particularly those related to diabetes [17]. Patients with T1D and ESRD, after SPK or KTA, report improved QOL, largely related to correction of uremia and liberation from the demands of dialysis [18, 19]. When weighing the option of SPK or PAK transplant, patients should reflect on their personal diabetes-related illness burden in terms of QOL and existing diabetes complications. PTA and SPK transplants show the strongest evidence for reversing or stabilizing diabetic complications such as neuropathy, retinopathy, cardiovascular disease, and protection against future diabetes-related renal damage, although the calcineurin inhibitors (CNIs) pose their own risks of nephrotoxicity, glaucoma, and cataracts [20, 21]. Ideally for a patient, if either type of pancreas transplant is considered with a kidney transplant, it should be performed before diabetes complications are too far gone to be affected by pancreas transplant.

After pancreas transplant, patients report improvement in fear of hypoglycemia, diabetes-related QOL, and general health measures. Speight et al. comment that some patients consider their diabetes cured after pancreas transplant, and this perception may skew the patient-reported scores on diabetes-specific QOL tools [22]. Post-transplant, mental health providers can help the patient articulate their thoughts and feelings about living a life without diabetes and transitioning to post-transplant life, a different but perhaps more hopeful chronic medical condition. Recipients of combined pancreas and kidney grafts report improvement in T1D-specific outcomes such as diet flexibility, no longer having to manage insulin and diabetes-related health issues, in addition to generally better perceptions of physical and social functioning and recovery of control and independence [19]. Pancreas transplant recipients also cite specific benefits related to resolution of their diabetes, such as preventing further kidney disease, improving cardiovascular outcomes related to diabetes, and slowing or improving neuropathy and ophthalmologic outcomes. In the short term, SPK recipients reported significantly more hospitalizations within 1 year of their transplant, when compared to their KTA peers. However, after 3 years, there was no significant difference in reported emergency department visits or hospitalizations between SPK and KTA recipients [23]. A study of 126 patients after SPK transplant reported improvement in all domains on a QOL survey including enhanced mobility, self-care, usual activity, and less pain, discomfort, gastrointestinal symptoms, anxiety, and depression with a large effect size in psychological and social functioning. Especially encouraging for this cohort was the significant decrease in unemployment, from 51% unemployed before transplant to 37% remaining unemployed after transplant [24].

Psychiatric Comorbidities, Sexual Dysfunction, and Cognitive Disorders Post-pancreas Transplant

Currently, limited research exists examining psychiatric comorbidities after pancreas transplant. Some QOL studies use the Beck Depression Inventory (BDI) or the Profile of Mood State (POMS) to assess mood and generally report a decline in depressive symptoms after transplant [13, 25, 26]. A study of 27 individuals who received ITA was assessed using the BDI before transplant and annually for 5 years after transplant. The mean pre-transplant BDI score was 13.57, and transplant recipients reported a statistically significant decrease in their BDI scores at 6 months and up to 3 years post-transplant; the nadir of depression was reported at 1 year post-transplant. At 4 and 5 years out from transplant, the patients still had a lower BDI score than before transplant; however, the difference no longer reached statistical significance [13]. Two Italian studies used the POMS in their psychological assessment, and patients who received either ITA or kidney-pancreas transplant reported a lower score in the depression-dejection category as compared to patients with T1D with and without ESRD [25, 26]. Review of the literature resulted in information on two domains arguably important to mood and psychosocial functioning: cognition and sexual function. Whether pancreas alone, pancreas in combination with a kidney transplant or ITA, studies report improvement in cognitive functioning. Compared to individuals with T1D and controls with ESRD, patients who received ITA reported less confusion. Patients also reported lower error rate on the Stroop test and higher scores on the Paced Auditory Serial Addition tests, suggesting that improved glucose control leads to normalization of attention abilities and information processing speeds [25]. A similar effect on cognitive capabilities was found in patients after SPK transplant compared to peers who underwent solely kidney transplant [26, 27].

Multiple factors in T1D influence sexual performance and activity including neuropathy, vascular complications, ESRD, and hemodialysis. Erectile dysfunction (ED) in T1D patients, pre- or post-transplant, should not be overlooked as ED is associated with psychological stress as well as coronary artery disease and cardiovascular morbidity [28, 29]. Highlighting the importance of sexual function, a qualitative study of interviews with SPK recipients identified sexual dysfunction as an assault on masculinity for men, while both sexes expressed concerns related to diabetes, their reproductive function, and how transplant restored hope of fertility and ability to have a family [15]. Two studies examined ED and sexual satisfaction after SPK transplant. This research reminds clinicians to ask about intimacy, sexual function, and satisfaction, as these issues influence identity and close relationships and may be lost in the discussion of other clini-

cal outcomes. A study of 101 men with T1D and ESRD was evaluated for ED after SPK transplant. Before transplant, 79% rated themselves as having mild to severe ED. After SPK transplant, 41% reported improvement in their ED, and 51% reported unchanged sexual function; these findings were considered equivocal. The authors of this study suggest that long-standing diabetes and subsequent macrovascular complications have a sustained negative impact on sexual function [30]. In 20 patients with T1D and ESRD, the authors compared the effect of the two types of transplant, as the group was split evenly between SPK and KTA recipients. The SPK recipients reported a significant improvement and less ED after transplant; items related to sexual satisfaction were comparable between groups [31].

Multivisceral/Intestinal Post-transplant

Overall, patients undergoing MV/I transplant follow the pattern of other solid organ transplant recipients in which mood and anxiety disorders are the most common psychiatric illnesses [32]. Currently, no studies focus explicitly on psychiatric comorbidities after MV/I transplant, though it is helpful to examine the few studies that directly examine psychiatric diagnoses in patients both before and after MV/I transplant. For example, DiMartini et al. described pre- and postoperative psychiatric evaluation of 19 MV/I transplant patients. Polysubstance use, personality disorder, and anxiety disorder were reported as the most common pre-transplant diagnoses, with three patients admitting to continued polysubstance abuse as a continued problem post-transplant. In response to prolonged hospitalizations and medical complications after transplant, five patients developed adjustment disorders with anxious and depressive features [33]. As already emphasized, some patients undergoing MV/I transplant present with pre-transplant substance (e.g., opioid) use disorder related to their underlying chronic illness [34]. After transplant surgery, pain and appropriate management in either the context of a substance use disorder or psychological distress after surgery will arise as reasons for psychiatric consultation.

In a more recent study regarding psychiatric disorders in 25 patients undergoing MV/I transplant at a center in the UK, pre-transplant psychiatric diagnoses were frequent in patients whose chronic illness required transplant, such as Crohn's disease [35]. At the time of transplant, almost 50% of candidates had a single psychiatric disorder, most often depression; however, in four of the patients, depression remitted after their transplant. One explanation could be that transplant itself confers relief from symptoms precipitated by dependence on PN. In the same sample, other post-transplant psychological concerns included chronic pain, body image issues related to a stoma, and recreational drug use. A prolonged inpatient stay leading to social isolation and stress on relationships affects general well-being and mental health of a patient post-transplant. Social supports or partnership status can change with relationship breakdown after transplant. Notably, the presence of a double psychiatric diagnosis did not extend the length of postoperative hospital stay [35].

Based on self-reported QOL outcomes, MV/I transplant is generally perceived as improving the QOL of individuals with intestinal failure on PN, and gains in QOL continue with longer follow-up [36]. Even in the first study of QOL after MV/I transplant, patients described marked improvement in psychological, social, and physical domains [34]. For most MV/I transplant patients, interpreting gains or losses in QOL is based on comparisons of life while dependent on PN. Most QOL studies comparing PN-dependent patients to transplant patients use generic QOL questionnaires or questionnaires designed for other solid organ transplants. For the pre- and postoperative evaluation of MV/I transplant patients, a QOL questionnaire designed for long-term PN patients can help the evaluator focus on resolution of PN-specific issues. This would include questions regarding the impact of a catheter on body image; whether PN equipment interrupts sleep; ability to eat and drink; pain, nausea, or vomiting related to food intake; GI symptoms like bloating or bowel movements; care of a stoma; and clarification if QOL is impacted by TPN or the underlying illness. Data collected using a PN-specific QOL questionnaire demonstrated post-transplant improvement of statistical significance in five areas: ability to travel, fatigue, gastrointestinal symptoms, stoma management and bowel movements, and general quality of life [37].

A 2012 study by Abu-Elmagd et al. from the University of Pittsburgh presents the most comprehensive data on QOL measured using a Quality of Life Inventory (QOLI) which contained 125 questions addressing 25 domains; 76 patients were evaluated pre- and post-MV/I transplant with a mean follow-up of 6.5 +/− 4 years [38]. As measured by the QOLI, depression and financial obligations were considered worse after transplant, with the change reaching statistical significance for both of these domains. Patients also reported negative impact in terms of needing sleep medication, feeling forgetful, as well as physical impairments such as occasional loss of balance, involuntary body movements, and joint pain. The authors suggest tacrolimus and other maintenance medications contribute to the physical ailments. For many patients, MV/I transplant promises improvement in psychosocial and physical domains that suffered before transplant. The psychosocial impact of MV/I transplant is broad with improvement in symptoms such as anxiety, nervousness, mood, stress, cognitive ability, negative body issues, sleep pattern, and impulsiveness. Socially, patients report better coping skills and social support, more time for

hobbies and leisure, and enhancement of sexuality and quality of relationships [38, 39]. Despite overall optimism after transplant, for some the new identity of "transplant patient" is no easier to bear than "TPN dependent." In a study focused on psychological adaptation after transplant, patients emphasized positive personal growth while also reporting lower scores in autonomy and positive relationships with others [40]. Physical domains of weight, nausea/vomiting, energy, and medical satisfaction also improve [38, 39]. Post-transplant patients still face challenges of pain and discomfort, greater need for medications and drugs, and decreased mobility [41, 42].

Pediatric MV/I Transplant: From Developmental Concerns to Quality of Life Post-transplant

In children, anatomically short gut and motility disorders are causes of IF. Underlying diagnoses include gastroschisis, necrotizing enterocolitis, pseudo-obstruction, Hirschsprung's disease, and microvillus inclusion disease [43, 44]. The majority of developmental, psychological, and QOL issues continue after transplant and will be discussed from a post-transplant perspective. Counseling families before choosing MV/I transplant surgery is also examined, though in the context of QOL after MV/I transplant.

Challenges arise as children requiring MV/I transplant have not learned how to eat. Pre-transplant dependency on PN can lead to oral feeding delays of difficulty swallowing, chewing, and weak development of the oral cavity muscles contributing to speech and language delays [45]. Attention must be paid to oral intake and the development of disordered eating influenced by early dependency on PN. After transplant, some children may continue PN for nutritional support, while others may develop moderate to severe anorexia, as in loss of appetite and difficulty eating. Compliance to an immunosuppressive regimen and long-term graft function helps children attain normal growth or experience catch-up growth [46, 47]. Hyperphagia and intensive attention to nutrition compensate for subnormal energy absorption.

Nutritional deficits from IF and dependence on PN contribute to developmental delays. The risk of continued developmental delays should be communicated to parents who may expect a developmental recovery in parallel with medical recovery. A few small studies by Thevenin characterized the neurodevelopmental delays before and after MV/I transplant. Before liver or MV/I transplant, children are unlikely to function at normal mental or motor development. Of the MV/I transplant candidates studied, the majority were considered significantly delayed [48]. Infants receiving MV/I transplant experienced more cognitive and physical delays compared to peers who underwent liver transplant. Even with early transplant, before 3 years of age, the MV/I transplant group experienced mental delays, and over 90% had severe motor developmental delays [49].

Pediatric MV/I patients will need access to special education services, physical therapy, or speech therapy as developmental delays persist after transplant. With access to rehabilitative services, children have the potential to return to age-appropriate activities at daycare or school [47]. In a cohort of 26 patients who were children at the time of transplant, 66% completed high school or some college, while the remainder attended special skill class or attended high school with an Individualized Education Program (IEP). The 2012 study by Abu-Elmagd et al. from the University of Pittsburgh followed 59 children who were 5 months to 11 years of age at the time of transplant; 37% (n = 22) were diagnosed with a neuropsychiatric impairment including developmental delay, attention deficit hyperactivity disorder (ADHD), and autism [38]. As with developmental delays, pediatric intestinal transplant patients fared worse than their liver transplant peers in terms of performance of daily living skills, communication, and socialization [50]. However, female gender and having caregivers with higher educational levels (more than a high school degree) were identified as factors with a positive impact in resumption of these skills.

As families decide to pursue MV/I transplant, they will weigh survival statistics, functional assessments, and nonmedical outcomes measured by QOL evaluations. Though data remains limited, several studies have examined nonmedical outcomes in the pediatric population. Generally patient perceptions of QOL improve with age and time from transplant [51]. After MV/I transplant, children often rated their QOL similar to normal controls. Yet parents of children post-transplant, both intestinal and liver, rated their child as having a lower QOL including physical functioning and general health and social limitations due to physical functioning [52]. Discrepancy between child and parent perceptions of QOL was reflected in separate two studies [53]. Both studies reflected the child's desire to be perceived as healthy manifested in the divergence of children's answers from their parents.

Information about post-transplant QOL and nonmedical outcomes can assist families considering MV/I transplant as well as physicians who advise them. Pediatric surgeons and neonatologists were surveyed on their counseling practices regarding management of severe short bowel syndrome and recommendations of maintenance with PN, bowel adaptation or rehabilitation, and surgical options of bowel lengthening or intestinal transplant [54]. Long-term burden to the child and their family was listed as a QOL concern and reason for not offering intestinal transplant to parents of these infants. Undoubtedly, families will weigh survival data and QOL

factors according to their values. As with adults, certain QOL domains improve after intestinal transplant, though MV/I pediatric transplant patients do not show the same degree of improvement compared to peers receiving other solid organ transplants such as liver transplant. Even after transplant, children and their families endure chronic illness and risk continued dependence on TPN, difficulties surrounding eating, and emotional and behavioral problems established earlier periods of illness.

Conclusions

Pancreas and MV/I transplants are treatment options for patients who have struggled with chronic illness, whether T1D or IF, for considerable periods of time. The patients who choose these transplants are used to depending on something external, whether insulin or PN, to survive. MV/I and pancreas transplant carry risks of surgical and medical complications with prolonged hospitalizations, and patients should be counseled that neither transplant is a cure for all of their symptoms of underlying illness. For patients with T1D, ITA or PTA can relieve worry and behaviors associated with fear of hypoglycemia as well as improve symptoms of depression. Specifically, ITA is particularly useful for patients with hypoglycemia and reduces insulin burden but does not guarantee insulin independence in the long term. MV/I transplant typically results in freedom from PN dependence, and post-transplant patients report improvement of psychosocial domains such as anxiety, mood, sleep, and body issues. They now have the time and ability to pursue personal interests such as relationships, hobbies, and travel. Most importantly, pancreas and MV/I transplants provide relief to the underlying diseases that led to transplant and a sense of freedom from dependency on medical devices to survive. Mental health providers should approach these patients as chronically ill, often since childhood, and susceptible to distress and mental illness, but ultimately adaptable and resilient, particularly to medical challenges.

References

1. Dholakia S, Mittal S, Quiroga I, Gilbert J, Sharples EJ, Ploeg RJ, et al. Pancreas transplantation: past, present, future. Am J Med. 2016;129(7):667–73.
2. Chang CA, Lawrence MC, Naziruddin B. Current issues in allogeneic islet transplantation. Curr Opin Organ Transplant. 2017;22(5):437–43.
3. Dean PG, Kukla A, Stegall MD, Kudva YC. Pancreas transplantation. BMJ. 2017;357:j1321.
4. Robertson RP, Davis C, Larsen J, Stratta R, Sutherland DE, American Diabetes Association. Pancreas and islet transplantation in type 1 diabetes. Diabetes Care. 2006;29(4):935.
5. Lehmann R, Graziano J, Brockmann J, Pfammatter T, Kron P, de Rougemont O, et al. Glycemic control in simultaneous islet-kidney

versus pancreas-kidney transplantation in type 1 diabetes: a prospective 13-year follow-up. Diabetes Care. 2015;38(5):752–9.

6. Page M, Rimmele T, Ber CE, Christin F, Badet L, Morelon E, et al. Early relaparotomy after simultaneous pancreas-kidney transplantation. Transplantation. 2012;94(2):159–64.

7. Kandaswamy R, Stock PG, Gustafson SK, Skeans MA, Curry MA, Prentice MA, et al. OPTN/SRTR 2015 annual data report: pancreas. Am J Transplant. 2017;17(Suppl 1):117–73.

8. Shapiro AM, Ricordi C, Hering BJ, Auchincloss H, Lindblad R, Robertson RP, et al. International trial of the Edmonton protocol for islet transplantation. N Engl J Med. 2006;355(13):1318–30.

9. Lombardo C, Perrone VG, Amorese G, Vistoli F, Baronti W, Marchetti P, et al. Update on pancreatic transplantation on the management of diabetes. Minerva Med. 2017;108(5):405–18.

10. Lablanche S, Borot S, Wojtusciszyn A, Bayle F, Tetaz R, Badet L, et al. Five-year metabolic, functional, and safety results of patients with type 1 diabetes transplanted with allogenic islets within the Swiss-French GRAGIL network. Diabetes Care. 2015;38(9):1714–22.

11. Johnson JA, Kotovych M, Ryan EA, Shapiro AM. Reduced fear of hypoglycemia in successful islet transplantation. Diabetes Care. 2004;27(2):624–5.

12. Barshes NR, Vanatta JM, Mote A, Lee TC, Schock AP, Balkrishnan R, et al. Health-related quality of life after pancreatic islet transplantation: a longitudinal study. Transplantation. 2005;79(12):1727–30.

13. Radosevich DM, Jevne R, Bellin M, Kandaswamy R, Sutherland DE, Hering BJ. Comprehensive health assessment and five-year follow-up of allogeneic islet transplant recipients. Clin Transpl. 2013;27(6):715.

14. Haggstrom E, Rehnman M, Gunningberg L. Quality of life and social life situation in islet transplanted patients: time for a change in outcome measures? Int J Organ Transplant Med. 2011;2(3):117–25.

15. Isla Pera P, Moncho Vasallo J, Guasch Andreu O, Ricart Brulles M, Torras RA. Impact of simultaneous pancreas-kidney transplantation: patients' perspectives. Patient Prefer Adherence. 2012;6:597–603.

16. Speight J, Woodcock AJ, Reaney MD, Amiel SA, Johnson P, Parrott N, et al. Well, I wouldn't be any worse off, would I, than I am now? A qualitative study of decision-making, hopes, and realities of adults with type 1 diabetes undergoing islet cell transplantation. Transplant Direct. 2016;2(5):e72.

17. Sureshkumar KK, Patel BM, Markatos A, Nghiem DD, Marcus RJ. Quality of life after organ transplantation in type 1 diabetics with end-stage renal disease. Clin Transpl. 2006;20(1):19–25.

18. Matas AJ, McHugh L, Payne WD, Wrenshall LE, Dunn DL, Gruessner RW, et al. Long-term quality of life after kidney and simultaneous pancreas-kidney transplantation. Clin Transpl. 1998;12(3):233–42.

19. Gross CR, Limwattananon C, Matthees BJ. Quality of life after pancreas transplantation: a review. Clin Transpl. 1998;12(4):351–61.

20. Jenssen T, Hartmann A, Birkeland KI. Long-term diabetes complications after pancreas transplantation. Curr Opin Organ Transplant. 2017;22(4):382–8.

21. Gremizzi C, Vergani A, Paloschi V, Secchi A. Impact of pancreas transplantation on type 1 diabetes-related complications. Curr Opin Organ Transplant. 2010;15(1):119–23.

22. Speight J, Reaney MD, Woodcock AJ, Smith RM, Shaw JA. Patient-reported outcomes following islet cell or pancreas transplantation (alone or after kidney) in type 1 diabetes: a systematic review. Diabet Med. 2010;27(7):812–22.

23. Gross CR, Limwattananon C, Matthees B, Zehrer JL, Savik K. Impact of transplantation on quality of life in patients with diabetes and renal dysfunction. Transplantation. 2000;70(12):1736–46.

24. Martins LS, Outerelo C, Malheiro J, Fonseca IM, Henriques AC, Dias LS, et al. Health-related quality of life may improve after transplantation in pancreas-kidney recipients. Clin Transpl. 2015;29(3):242–51.

25. D'Addio F, Maffi P, Vezzulli P, Vergani A, Mello A, Bassi R, et al. Islet transplantation stabilizes hemostatic abnormalities and cerebral metabolism in individuals with type 1 diabetes. Diabetes Care. 2014;37(1):267–76.

26. Fiorina P, Vezzulli P, Bassi R, Gremizzi C, Falautano M, D'Addio F, et al. Near normalization of metabolic and functional features of the central nervous system in type 1 diabetic patients with end-stage renal disease after kidney-pancreas transplantation. Diabetes Care. 2012;35(2):367–74.

27. Ziaja J, Bozek-Pajak D, Kowalik A, Krol R, Cierpka L. Impact of pancreas transplantation on the quality of life of diabetic renal transplant recipients. Transplant Proc. 2009;41(8):3156–8.

28. Ponholzer A, Temml C, Mock K, Marszalek M, Obermayr R, Madersbacher S. Prevalence and risk factors for erectile dysfunction in 2869 men using a validated questionnaire. Eur Urol. 2005;47(1):6.

29. Gazzaruso C, Giordanetti S, De Amici E, Bertone G, Falcone C, Geroldi D, et al. Relationship between erectile dysfunction and silent myocardial ischemia in apparently uncomplicated type 2 diabetic patients. Circulation. 2004;110(1):22–6.

30. Jurgensen JS, Ulrich C, Horstrup JH, Brenner MH, Frei U, Kahl A. Sexual dysfunction after simultaneous pancreas-kidney transplantation. Transplant Proc. 2008;40(4):927–30.

31. Salonia A, D'Addio F, Gremizzi C, Briganti A, Deho F, Caldara R, et al. Kidney-pancreas transplantation is associated with near-normal sexual function in uremic type 1 diabetic patients. Transplantation. 2011;92(7):802–8.

32. DiMartini A, Dew MA, Crone C. Organ transplantation. In: Sadock BJ, Sadock VA, editors. Kaplan and Sadock's comprehensive textbook of psychiatry. 9th ed. Philadelphia: LWW; 2009. p. 2450.

33. DiMartini A, Fitzgerald MG, Magill J, Funovitz M, Abu-Elmagd K, Furukawa H, et al. Psychiatric evaluations of small intestine transplantation patients. Gen Hosp Psychiatry. 1996;18(6 Suppl):29S.

34. DiMartini A, Rovera GM, Graham TO, Furukawa H, Todo S, Funovits M, et al. Quality of life after small intestinal transplantation and among home parenteral nutrition patients. JPEN J Parenter Enteral Nutr. 1998;22(6):357–62.

35. Pither C, Green J, Butler A, Chukaulim B, West S, Gao R, et al. Psychiatric disorders in patients undergoing intestinal transplantation. Transplant Proc. 2014;46(6):2136–9.

36. Ceulemans LJ, Lomme C, Pirenne J, De Geest S. Systematic literature review on self-reported quality of life in adult intestinal transplantation. Transplant Rev (Orlando). 2016;30(2):109–18.

37. Pironi L, Baxter JP, Lauro A, Guidetti M, Agostini F, Zanfi C, et al. Assessment of quality of life on home parenteral nutrition and after intestinal transplantation using treatment-specific questionnaires. Am J Transplant. 2012;12(Suppl 4):60.

38. Abu-Elmagd KM, Kosmach-Park B, Costa G, Zenati M, Martin L, Koritsky DA, et al. Long-term survival, nutritional autonomy, and quality of life after intestinal and multivisceral transplantation. Ann Surg. 2012;256(3):494–508.

39. Cameron EA, Binnie JA, Jamieson NV, Pollard S, Middleton SJ. Quality of life in adults following small bowel transplantation. Transplant Proc. 2002;34(3):965–6.

40. Golfieri L, Lauro A, Tossani E, Sirri L, Venturoli A, Dazzi A, et al. Psychological adaptation and quality of life of adult intestinal transplant recipients: University of Bologna experience. Transplant Proc. 2010;42(1):42–4.

41. Pither C, Duncan S, Gao R, Butler A, West S, Gabe SM, et al. Quality of life and performance status before and after small intestinal transplantation. Transplant Proc. 2014;46(6):2109–13.

42. O'Keefe SJ, Emerling M, Koritsky D, Martin D, Stamos J, Kandil H, et al. Nutrition and quality of life following small intestinal transplantation. Am J Gastroenterol. 2007;102(5):1093–100.

43. Bharadwaj S, Tandon P, Gohel TD, Brown J, Steiger E, Kirby DF, et al. Current status of intestinal and multivisceral transplantation. Gastroenterol Rep (Oxf). 2017;5(1):20–8.

44. Mazariegos GV, Superina R, Rudolph J, Cohran V, Burns RC, Bond GJ, et al. Current status of pediatric intestinal failure, rehabilitation, and transplantation: summary of a colloquium. Transplantation. 2011;92(11):1173–80.

45. Thevenin DM, Baker A, Kato T, Tzakis A, Fernandez M, Dowling M. Neurodevelopmental outcomes of infant multivisceral transplant recipients: a longitudinal study. Transplant Proc. 2006;38(6):1694–5.

46. Lacaille F, Vass N, Sauvat F, Canioni D, Colomb V, Talbotec C, et al. Long-term outcome, growth and digestive function in children 2 to 18 years after intestinal transplantation. Gut. 2008;57(4):455–61.

47. Sudan DL, Iverson A, Weseman RA, Kaufman S, Horslen S, Fox IJ, et al. Assessment of function, growth and development, and long-term quality of life after small bowel transplantation. Transplant Proc. 2000;32(6):1211–2.

48. Thevenin DM, Mittal N, Kato T, Tzakis A. Neurodevelopmental outcomes of infant intestinal transplant recipients. Transplant Proc. 2004;36(2):319–20.

49. Thevenin DM, Baker A, Kato T, Tzakis A, Fernandez M, Dowling M. Neuodevelopmental outcomes for children transplanted under the age of 3 years. Transplant Proc. 2006;38(6):1692–3.

50. Shellmer DA, DeVito DA, Dew MA, Terhorst L, Noll RB, Kosmach-Park B, et al. Adaptive functioning and its correlates after intestine and liver transplantation. Pediatr Transplant. 2013;17(1):48–54.

51. Andres AM, Alameda A, Mayoral O, Hernandez F, Dominguez E, Martinez Ojinaga E, et al. Health-related quality of life in pediatric intestinal transplantation. Pediatr Transplant. 2014;18(7):746–56.

52. Ngo KD, Farmer DG, McDiarmid SV, Artavia K, Ament ME, Vargas J, et al. Pediatric health-related quality of life after intestinal transplantation. Pediatr Transplant. 2011;15(8):849–54.

53. Sudan D, Horslen S, Botha J, Grant W, Torres C, Shaw B Jr, et al. Quality of life after pediatric intestinal transplantation: the perception of pediatric recipients and their parents. Am J Transplant. 2004;4(3):407–13.

54. Cummings CL, Diefenbach KA, Mercurio MR. Counselling variation among physicians regarding intestinal transplant for short bowel syndrome. J Med Ethics. 2014;40(10):665–70.

Vascularized Composite Allotransplantation (VCA)

Psychological and Psychosocial Aspects of Face Transplantation

34

Kathy L. Coffman

Introduction

In 2005, the first partial face transplant was done, illuminating ethical and psychological issues that were only conjectured prior to that time [1].

Siemionov proposed the concept of the face as an organ with key functions, including communication, consumption of food, and conveying emotion [2]. Furr et al. noted that the face also contributed social information (age, ethnicity, gender identity, and biological sex) [3].

After traditional reconstructive techniques have failed to restore function and more normal appearance, face transplantation (FT) is considered a last resort intervention, not only for cosmetic purposes alone but also for restoration of function, sensation, and movement of important structures, such as the lips. Due to concerns about how much the recipient would resemble the donor, potentially upsetting to the donor family, appearance transfer was studied using cadavers [4] and computer simulation [5]. In these studies, the recipient looked like a blend of the donor and recipient as the donor face is applied over the recipient's bone structure.

Prevalence of Facial Disfigurement and Facial Transplantation

An estimated 10% of the US population has some degree of facial disfigurement that severely impacts their ability to lead a normal life [6].

The support group Changing Faces views the terms *disfigurement* or *deformity* as harsh and stigmatizing and has suggested using the terms *visible difference* or *visible distinction*. This group estimated those affected by visible difference in the United Kingdom at 400,000 in 2001 [7]. The etiologies of visible difference include acquired (disease and trauma) and congenital conditions [8, 9].

Since 2005 and to date, there have been 39 transplants in 8 countries, including Belgium (1), China (1), France (10), Spain (4), Turkey (7), and the United States (13). The median age of FT recipients was around 35 years old, ranging from 19 to 59 years old. Face transplantation has been done overwhelmingly for male patients, with 79.5% of FT recipients being male. Candidates may have a high rate of alcohol and opioid use disorders (60% in Cleveland Clinic series) and suicide attempts via gunshot wounds (GSW) (40% in Cleveland Clinic series). Worldwide mortality has been 6 out of 39 individuals, equaling 15.4% through May 2017, with the last 2 recipients less than 1 year post-transplant (Table 34.1).

The indications for face transplant have included:

- Animal attacks – 3
- Arteriovenous malformation – 1
- Ballistic injuries – 17
- Blunt trauma – 2
- Burn injuries – 10

Table 34.1 Indication for transplant, cause of death, and survival of patients who died after FT

Patient	Location	Indication	Cause of death	Survival
1[a]	France	Dog bite	Small-cell lung cancer	10 year 5 month
2	China	Bear bite	Nonadherence, sepsis	2 year 3 month
6	France	Burn injury	Sepsis	2 month
9[b]	Spain	Cancer	Cancer	3 year 11 month
16	France	Gunshot wound	Suicide	3 year
29	Turkey	Gunshot wound	Lymphoma, respiratory failure	1 year

[a]60.56
[b]Cavadas [60]

K. L. Coffman
Department of Psychiatry and Psychology,
Cleveland Clinic, Cleveland, OH, USA

© Springer International Publishing AG, part of Springer Nature 2019
Y. Sher, J. R. Maldonado (eds.), *Psychosocial Care of End-Stage Organ Disease and Transplant Patients*,
https://doi.org/10.1007/978-3-319-94914-7_34

- Cancer – 1
- Neurofibromatosis – 4
- Vascular tumor – 1

Facial Disfigurement and Psychological Comorbidity

Depending on the cause, duration, and age of onset of the facial disfigurement, the psychological comorbidities in these patients may differ. There is a broad spectrum of adaptation to facial reconstruction in adulthood [10].

Facial trauma in urban centers tends to be more prevalent in single unemployed young males in their 30s, with high levels of anxiety, depression, hostility, poor impulse control, and substance use disorders [11]. Determinants of post-traumatic stress disorder (PTSD) symptoms in the year following an injury include the level of stress the year before the injury, severity of pain, poor social supports, and previous trauma history. About 23% of patients will have PTSD symptoms 1 year after injury [12]. Other factors predisposing to PTSD after facial injury include older age and female sex [13, 14].

Factors predicting better adjustment in facial burn patients include less avoidant coping, lower functional disability in men, more involvement in recreational activities, more reliance on problem-solving for women, and higher levels of social support [15].

Patients with facial disfigurement from head and neck cancers typically have low levels of depression and report high levels of life happiness with positive feelings of well-being. Women show more depression and less happiness, but social support buffered the impact of disfigurement [15]. Quality of life (QOL) is not necessarily lower in these patients as compared to normal populations [16, 17].

After facial surgery, dysfunction may manifest as either denial or obsession with the defect, depression, nonadherence with follow-up visits, and social isolation. Dropkin observed that effective coping preoperatively predicted coping well postoperatively. Successful reintegration of body image was indicated by reduced anxiety, attending to self-care, and resuming socialization [18, 19].

Newell and Marks observed more psychological disturbance in those with facial disfigurement than the general population, as measured by the General Health Questionnaire and the Hospital Anxiety and Depression Scale [20]. Disfiguring conditions may result in more addiction, anxiety, altered body image, depressed mood, marital stress, PTSD, social anxiety and withdrawal, and worse quality of life [21, 22]. However, extent, severity, or type of facial disfigurement may not predict adjustment [23–26].

The impact of facial disfigurement may vary with the patient's developmental stage in life [26]. Bonding with parents may be altered by congenital facial disfigurement, especially if facial expression is affected [27, 28] as in Moebius syndrome (i.e., a rare congenital neurological disorder affecting muscles that control facial expression and eye movement) or if language development is affected. Behavioral problems in children may result from craniofacial conditions; these challenges include aggression, hyperactivity, learning disorders, oppositional defiant disorder, or social inhibition, with anxiety and depression continuing into adulthood [29, 30].

Teasing about facial differences may happen at any age but is more typical in the 4- to 12-year-old cohort. Adults with craniofacial conditions have experienced discrimination, may have interpersonal problems and marry later, and may have panic attacks [31–35]. Leaving familiar surroundings for new schools, jobs, or neighborhoods is more difficult for those with facial differences and may require developing new coping strategies for interacting with people that are unfamiliar with them [36, 37]. Rumsey and Harcourt have written in detail about treatment of developmental issues in children with visible differences and their families [9].

Psychiatrists should also be aware of trephine syndrome, once thought to be psychological, seen in some patients with traumatic midface injury resulting in a large craniectomy. In 1939, Grant proposed that the sense of vulnerability due to lack of an intact skull resulted in apprehension and insecurity, depressed mood, discomfort at the site of the defect, dizziness, fatigability, and intolerance to vibration [38]. Clues to the diagnosis of this syndrome include arrest of rehabilitation or acute deterioration, with aphasia, behavioral or cognitive deficits, paresis, and tremor [39]. Symptoms may include focal weakness, headache, neuropsychiatric disturbance, midbrain syndromes [40], and parkinsonian symptoms [41]. Other presenting symptoms may include altered level of consciousness, cranial nerve deficits, psychosomatic disturbance, and seizures. Cognitive deficits may include decreased attention, problems with executive function, and memory impairment. Headache may be positional, exacerbated by sitting up and relieved by the horizontal position. These symptoms may occur on average 5 months after craniectomy, with rapid improvement after cranioplasty in approximately 4 days. Roughly 55% of patients recover independence with activities of daily living within 3–6 months of rehabilitation [42]. Although verbal fluency may return within days to weeks, the spasticity in gait and weakness may persist in some patients requiring prolonged rehabilitation. The deficits in executive functioning and memory may delay the ability of the patient to retain information on facial transplantation in order to have capacity to consent the procedure. This

syndrome has also been called *syndrome of the sunken skin flap* [43], *the motor trephined syndrome,* and "neurological susceptibility to a skull defect," which has been suggested as a neutral descriptive term [44].

Comparing Face Transplantation with Solid Organ Transplantation

In comparing FT with solid organ transplantation (SOT), there are similarities and differences. The differences include:

- Face transplant, like hand transplant, has not been shown to improve survival but is performed to enhance QOL [45].
- Patients with FT have higher mortality compared to some SOT, total 15.4% to date.
- Rejection may occur later in FT, as compared to SOT, between days 7 and 120.
- Patients potentially have prolonged, up to 6 months, hospital stays, much longer than most SOT, other than small bowel transplant recipients [46].
- There is an increased emphasis on informed consent for an experimental procedure that is not life-saving, but hopefully life-enhancing [47].
- A demanding speech therapy regimen is needed to enhance facial mobility and to clarify speech, so patients must be motivated.
- Long-standing tracheotomy care and percutaneous endoscopic gastrostomy (PEG) tube feeding may be needed pre- and post-FT.
- Potential substance use and chronic pain disorders can arise from injury and multiple facial surgeries.
- A rescue plan must be in place in case the face transplant fails; the recipient must have enough skin available to do another flap to cover the facial structures.
- An increased focus on societal reintegration after surgery is a measure of success.
- Media training and tight security postoperatively are helpful for recipients, due to intense interest of the media and public.

Course and Complications After Facial Transplantation

Facial transplantation surgery duration has ranged from 15 to 53 h, with as little as 500 milliliters of blood loss up to 27 units of pack red blood cells needed for transfusion for a patient with neurofibromatosis [46]. Facial sensation may return within 2–6 months, with motor function recovering by 1 year after the transplant [46, 48]. In terms of social functioning, Lantieri documented that four of seven recipients

returned to work thus far [49]. The ethical issues relevant to FT have been addressed elsewhere at length and were considered at the Cleveland Clinic 5 years before the first face transplant was done [50–52].

Immunosuppression for FT resembles standard immunosuppression for solid organs. For facial transplantation, a target level of 12–15 ng/ml for tacrolimus is used for the first 3 months and 10–12 ng/ml thereafter, in combination with mycophenolate mofetil (MMF) and prednisone. Weekly biopsies are done on the skin and oral mucosa for 1 month, then biweekly for 2 months, and then monthly during the first 6 months. Mucosal biopsy may be more likely to show rejection than skin. Speech therapy may be daily for the first 6 weeks, including static and dynamic exercises, gentle massage, and sensory reeducation.

Patients must be educated about the potential risks inherent with transplantation, including infection, rejection, length of hospital stay and recuperation, surgical risks, and risk of cancers with long-term immunosuppression. In addition, there may be a need for revision procedures, averaging 2.6 per patient (range 0–5 procedures) [53]. Sosin and Rodrigues described at length the type and extent of revisions done by various teams, ranging from major to minor procedures [54] (Table 34.2).

In 2007 Vasilic et al. attempted to quantitate risks for FT based on 10-year data reported for kidney transplantation and 5-year data for hand transplantation using standard immunosuppression with tacrolimus, MMF, and corticosteroids. Estimates of risk for FT were as follows [58]:

- Acute rejection – 10–70% risk.
- Acute rejection reversibility – 100% with steroids alone.
- Chronic rejection – <10% over 5 years.
- Hypertension – 5–10%.
- Renal failure – <5%.
- Diabetes – 5–15%.

These predictions were fairly accurate; though there have been no cases of frank renal failure requiring dialysis, Lantieri reported decreased, but higher than 60 ml/min, glomerular filtration rate (GFR) in all recipients. He also reported hypertension in three out of seven patients, hypercholesterolemia in three out of seven patients, and hypertriglyceridemia in one recipient [49]. Diabetes has been reported in FT recipients [59, 60].

Acute rejection is nearly universal with worldwide teams reporting two to eight episodes of acute rejection per recipient

Table 34.2 Infections in facial transplant recipients [54–57]

Bacteria	*Pseudomonas, Staphylococcus*
Fungus	*Aspergillus, Candida*
Virus	CMV, EBV, HSV+, MCV+

[59, 60]. Two cases of chronic rejection have been reported as well [61]. With composite allografts, the skin is the primary target for rejection, and generally muscle and bone are spared. With FT rejection, mild rejection is seen only on biopsy, though with more severe rejection, this is readily apparent as the face appears sunburned. Topical tacrolimus has been used, but the efficacy has not yet been proven in FT [62].

Of note, the first FT recipient developed class II donor-specific antibodies, later had sentinel graft necrosis, and subsequently showed decreased flow in the right facial artery with C4d deposits on the endothelium of some dermal vessels in the graft. She was treated with plasmapheresis, three cycles of bortezomib, and rescue therapy with eculizumab. However, necrosis of the lips and perioral area developed, and surgical excision of the lower lip, labial commissures, and partial right cheek was needed [61].

To date, there are no reports of graft-versus-host disease with FT [63]. Infections transmitted to FT recipients from the donor include cytomegalovirus, oral herpes simplex virus, molluscum contagiosum, and treponema pallidum [46]. Fatigue due to CMV transmission may compromise QOL [64]. CMV resistant to current antiviral drugs has been seen in FT recipients [49]. Since face transplant is not a life-saving procedure, it may be prudent to require the donor to be CMV negative if the recipient is CMV negative, as is the case in hand transplantation [58]. However, requiring donors to be CMV negative for CMV negative recipients may unnecessarily prolong the waiting period.

Certain risks are difficult to quantitate for face transplantation, for example, neurological side effects with tacrolimus; osteonecrosis, cardiovascular risks, cataract, or glaucoma with corticosteroids; or gastrointestinal side effects and leukopenia from MMF. The experience with immunosuppression is still not sufficient to know whether minimizing protocols, with gradual steroid withdrawal and low levels of calcineurin inhibitors (CNIs), will be possible in FT recipients. There is some evidence with other grafts that mTor inhibitors may prevent chronic rejection. The risks of nonadherence to immunosuppression with grafts that are not life sustaining may be higher than with other organs, as evidenced by the high rates of acute rejection [61].

The risk of cancers postoperatively with hand transplant was estimated by extrapolation from kidney data and thought to be about 3%, with one third of these being skin cancers, some of which are preventable with good sunscreen prophylaxis [45]. To date, 10.3% of FT recipients have had cancer [54]. One patient, in particular, developed with EBV-related B-cell lymphoma 14 months after transplantation which recurred 9 months after treatment with rituximab [54]. After treatment with rituximab, cyclophosphamide, doxorubicin, prednisone, and vincristine, cancer went into remission. However, 3 months later, he was diagnosed with EBV-related smooth muscle cell tumor of the liver [54].

Another FT recipient was found to have a squamous cell carcinoma on his arm and 1 month later was diagnosed with stage III non-Hodgkin's lymphoma. After treatment with rituximab, cyclophosphamide, doxorubicin, prednisone, and vincristine, he developed aspergillus pneumonia that spread to the brain. His immunosuppression was discontinued, and the facial graft rejected 16 days later and was removed and replaced with an anterolateral thigh flap. A second episode of respiratory failure ensued after extubation, and he succumbed 11 months later to cardiac arrest [54].

Two other FT recipients developed cancer. One HIV-positive recipient had a relapse of squamous cell cancer, which he initially had 11 years prior to his FT [54]. Finally, the first FT recipient in France was found to have a small cell lung cancer during her reevaluation for re-transplant after diagnosis of chronic rejection and surgical excision of part of the graft. The lung cancer was resected, but the patient continued to smoke; the cancer recurred and led to patient's death in April 2016 [61].

EBV-mismatched transplants (donor+/recipient-) are thought to have a higher incidence of post-transplant lymphoproliferative disorder (PTLD) [65, 66]. To extrapolate from SOT, the incidence of non-Hodgkin's lymphoma is estimated at 0.3–0.4% in the first year post-transplant with SOT and 0.06–0.09% per year thereafter, but PTLD has been seen years after the original transplantation [65, 66]. Kaposi's sarcoma can occur in SOT recipients but is generally treatable by switching from CNI to sirolimus, which inhibits mTOR and has anticancer properties. There has been no increase in other common types of cancer seen among transplant recipients, such as breast, colon, lung, and prostate cancers [65, 66].

Assessment and Communication Strategies

Preoperative assessment of FT candidates may be hampered as many patients have severe speech impediments that impair communication if they lack midface structures such as the maxilla, upper and lower incisors, palate, nose, and lips. Surgical attachment of an artificial palate or using an obturator to close the gap in the palate can markedly improve intelligibility of speech. Writing boards may help but may be difficult to use post-transplant with visual impairment and tremor due to CNIs. A reading machine can be used for teaching about transplantation for patients that are legally blind but retain some vision. Cellular phone alarms and watch alarms can be set for the times medications are due. Visual impairment may result in some mistakes in adherence to the immunosuppression medication regimen. Total blindness was initially considered an absolute contraindication for FT, but totally blind patients have now been transplanted successfully despite the challenges [67, 68].

Eye Transplantation

Eye transplantation may one day remedy the dilemma of FT in totally blind patients. The ethical considerations were reviewed by Sivak et al. in 2016 [69]. Davidson et al. reported that surgical protocols are underway using the rat model, noting that the technical feasibility was established and that with advances in immunosuppression and new therapies in neuroregeneration, human surgical protocols are needed to promote momentum toward the goal of eye transplantation [70]. As novel as the idea of whole eye transplantation seems, the first report of an eye transplant in humans was in 1885 when Dr. Chibret replaced a girl's eye with a rabbit's eye which failed by postoperative day 15 due to lack of effective immunosuppression in that era [71]. Since that time, both cold-blooded animals (e.g., salamanders and frogs) and mammals (e.g., canine, rabbit, rat, sheep, and swine) have been used as models for eye transplantation [71].

Patient Selection and Psychiatric Evaluation of Face Transplant Surgery Candidates

The timing of evaluation for FT must allow for:

- Time to grieve losses and coming to grips with the injuries sustained,
- Treatment of PTSD and any depression,
- Rehabilitation.

Goals of psychiatric evaluation for FT include (1) selecting motivated patients, (2) deliberating options besides face transplant, (3) discussing risks and benefits of transplantation, (4) describing the success rate and rescue procedures, (5) providing education about immunosuppression regimen, (6) recognizing need for smoking or substance abuse rehabilitation, and (7) identifying psychiatric disorders requiring treatment for better outcomes.

In order to establish a registry of prospective face transplant candidates, a rating scale was developed, the Cleveland Clinic FACES score which is analogous to the MELD score for liver transplant candidates [72].

Psychiatric contraindications to face transplant surgery include [73, 74]:

- Active bulimia nervosa
- Active psychotic disorder
- Severe personality disorders
- Active substance use disorders
- Nonadherence to the medical regimen
- Mental retardation without adequate social support
- Suicide attempts or psychiatric admission within the past year

Many predictions were made before the first FT occurred, anticipating what personality traits and behaviors would typify the successful candidate [75]. The need for high levels of self-esteem based on factors other than physical appearance was thought to be necessary for successful FT [75]. In our two first recipients at Cleveland Clinic, the first had high self-esteem based on factors other than appearance. This patient continued to have fairly consistent high self-esteem after FT, with resumption of more social activities, and FT resulting in less teasing and verbal abuse in public. Our second recipient has not achieved his goal of resuming work with FT, namely, a corneal transplant. He also was more dependent on physical appearance for self-esteem, and his self-esteem initially diminished after transplantation, with poor satisfaction in social activities and strain in relationships. The FT did not lead to increased intimacy as he had hoped.

Taking an active approach to the comments made by the public about the patient's disfigurement is good preparation for handling the intense media attention and comments by the public after a face transplant [75]. Avoidant strategies can decrease anxiety but may delay the rehabilitation needed prior to successful FT.

Some predictions about FT were unrealistic. Patients who believe others judge them on appearance are accurately perceiving reality [76]. Studies show that opinions are formed within minutes of an introduction, and much of this assessment is based on appearance, involving encoding social information in the amygdala and posterior cingulate cortex [76].

Key to patient selection is the distinction between assertive coping strategies in handling the injury and social encounters and long-term avoidant strategies. Lazarus described this dilemma as the conflict between *protection of the self* versus *presentation of the self* [77]. Avoidant strategies may be used temporarily for some months to decrease anxiety and allow recovery; however, long-term passivity predicts poor adjustment after craniofacial injury [78].

Avoidant strategies include:

- Social withdrawal.
- Not talking about the extent of the injuries.
- Not mourning the losses due to the injuries.
- Not touching or looking at the facial injuries in the mirror.
- Covering the injuries habitually with makeup, masks, or hats.
- Excessive and repeated verbal denial that the injury occurred.
- Not confronting the functional losses (eating, drinking, speech, vision).

Assertive coping strategies include:

- Taking the initiative in social interactions.
- Educating others about facial disfigurement.

- Calmly confronting negative reactions from others.
- Use of social skills (firm handshake, good eye contact, smiling, and nodding).

Callahan describes the paradox that the injured bodily part is the same tool needed for reintegration of the sense of self [79].

Candidates may have some anxiety, depression, and social anxiety, especially if prior reconstructive surgeries have failed. Patients may have minor residual symptoms of PTSD that need to be treated to help patients tolerate interventions without severe exacerbation and to assist sleep. Depression or anxiety compromising functioning should be treated prior to listing for transplantation.

Patients often have undergone multiple surgical procedures in attempts to ameliorate disfigurement, and this is not necessarily a contraindication to FT. However, this may limit options for rescue procedures due to loss of skin suitable for grafting.

Girotto et al. noted many chronic sequelae after complex facial fractures, and these symptoms are often seen in face transplant candidates with facial disfigurement [80]. These include painful dentition, chronic headache, facial numbness or pain, shifting orofacial structures, diplopia or decreased vision, mastication problems or drooling, epiphora (uncontrolled watering eyes), anosmia or change in olfactory and gustatory sensation, chronic pain disorder related to the initial injury, and/or subsequent and reconstructive surgeries requiring large amounts of opioids for pain management.

At this time creating composite structures, such as the nose, eyelids, and lips, is beyond the scope of surgical interventions, though some envision applications of selective tissue engineering in vitro for craniofacial regeneration [81].

Lack of confidence in social situations may not be an absolute contraindication to face transplant. Social confidence may vary based on the time since injury and with the type of social situation. Patients with facial disfigurement often perceive reactions from the public ranging from avoidance, fear, revulsion, or staring to physical or verbal abuse [82–84].

We must be cautious about raising false hopes in potential candidates and continue to provide compassionate psychological support to those who are not deemed to be suitable candidates for FT [63]. Many candidates may be evaluated in order to find several that are suitable, ranging from 30% to 50% acceptance rate in adults, based on surgical, medical, and psychiatric factors [63, 85].

Pediatric Face Transplantation

A recent article by Marchac et al. raised the ethical issue of whether FT should be done in children [86]. Upon screening for inclusion criteria, including age under 18 years old and

severe facial disfigurement due to burns, malformation, neurofibromatosis, trauma, or vascular malformation, 12 candidates were identified. Candidates that did not have complete destruction of the orbicularis oris muscle or orbicularis oculi, along with a large central facial defect, or who had poor parental support or insurance problems were excluded, leaving three potential candidates. These children had diagnoses including third-degree burn of the entire face, Sturge-Weber syndrome, and neurofibromatosis type 1 with problems with breathing, feeding, and speech. When screening was extended, only 7 of 25 candidates were deemed psychologically stable enough to proceed. Growth of the facial graft is a specific issue, though nerve growth is faster in children than adults. Adherence with immunosuppression is a potential area of concern in children, particularly with adolescents. No ethical barriers to FT in children were found by this team.

Psychological screening tools suggested for children and adolescents included:

- Coping Strategies Inventory
- Parent Medication Barrier Scale
- Adolescent Medication Barrier Scale
- Parental Coping Strategies Inventory
- Body Image Disturbance Questionnaire
- Perceived Stigmatization Questionnaire
- Youth Quality of Life-Facial Differences Model
- Multidimensional Scale of Perceived Social Support

The expectations of the child and parents must be realistic. The patient's issues regarding QOL, body image, coping, and adherence are important areas to explore. The parents must be aware of the need for adherence in preventing acute and chronic rejection and be educated to monitor the facial graft for signs of infection or rejection. Clearly parents must consent for the child, but the child's assent is necessary for continuing long-term cooperation, and chronological age may not reflect maturity. Considerations for the donor family are also addressed including making an acrylic mask molded from the donor's face for restoring the appearance of the donor [87]. Marchac et al. mention the future possibility of 3-D printing to make a donor face mask, as this was recently done in Finland for their first facial transplant [86].

Psychological Tasks in Adjusting to Face Transplantation

The face is intimately connected with our identity and sense of individuality. In an ancient Persian poem, Attar observed, "You can never see your own face, only a reflection, not the face itself" [88].

Contemporary authors surmised that "wearing another person's face may raise complex issues of identity." [89]

Having a new face restores the person's ability to move in society inconspicuously, without comments and questions from others about their visual difference. Symbolic interaction theory hypothesized that people form identity and self-esteem through interpreting how others behave toward them [90, 91]. This was observed to be true in our first Cleveland Clinic FT recipient who was legally blind. She learned that her appearance was now acceptable by the comments from her daughter, who thought they looked more alike after the FT [92].

Every organ transplant recipient has the psychological task of incorporating the new organ. Muslin theorized in the 1970s that the transplant recipient may go through several steps to incorporate the organ including:

1. Perceiving the organ as a foreign object.
2. Perceiving the organ and donor as transitional objects.
3. Perceiving the organ as a personal belonging.
4. Letting go of the donor as a transitional object.
5. Integrating the organ into the recipient's self-schema.

D.W. Winnicott's transitional model described the psychological process in childhood where the child adopts a transitional object for comfort when a parent is absent. Recipients sometimes idealize the donor as a protective parental or god-like rescuing figure, identify with or project onto the donor as in a twin-ship relationship (good or evil twin), or may view the donor as a persecutor if the patient has had conflictual relationships with family members. Patients may communicate with the donor through magical thinking via thought transference as a defense against fears. Goetzmann theorized if the recipient continues to use the donor or organ as transitional objects, this may delay social and professional reintegration [91].

The first partial FT recipient in France confirmed some of these ideas in interviews, indicating that incorporating the face of her donor was challenging. She grieved both the death of her donor and the loss of her former appearance. She stated, "I used to think of her every day and 'talk' to her." She noted the differences between her original face and her donor's face. She thought if she could watch the film of the donor's face being removed and grafted onto her own face, then she could say goodbye to her donor. She expressed identification with the donor as well, calling her "a twin sister" since her donor had committed suicide. She had expected to look more like she did before her injury. She felt guilty that she was given so much after having done a "stupid thing." She also observed after being kissed on the cheeks by a clerk who recognized her that she was no longer thought of "as a victim of the plague." [93]

What was not anticipated was that the adjustment for those with facial injuries from their normal visage to a disfigured face is a much greater adjustment than adjusting to a new face after transplantation. For those with congenital differences such as neurofibromatosis, this also appears to be true, as the FT allows them to pass unnoticed in society. As stated in a recent article, FT is "unlikely to make people 'beautiful'; rather it will make them look normal and forgettable." [94]

Tools for Psychological Assessment and Psychological Outcomes in Face Transplant Candidates

Many FT teams have not quantitatively investigated body image, mood changes, perception of teasing, QOL, self-esteem, or social reintegration. There is a significant void in rating scales and instruments specific for psychiatric assessment and applicability to FT. Several rating scales were modified specifically for FT, such as the Perception of Teasing-FACES and the Physical Appearance State and Trait Anxiety Scale (PASTAS).

In view of the etiologies of facial disfigurement, including ballistic injuries, burns, congenital issues, and cancer and the many facial surgeries done prior to FT evaluation, the incidence of PTSD disorder may be high in FT candidates. In anticipation of future candidates, a review of PTSD instruments may prove useful. Generally a trade-off must be made between the best instrument and the most practical and time-efficient instrument clinically.

For initial screening for the presence of PTSD, the 10-item Trauma Screening Questionnaire may be superior to several other screening measures, including the PTSD Checklist [95], the Posttraumatic Stress Diagnostic Scale [96], the Davidson Trauma Scale [97], the 4-item SPAN [98], and the BPTSD-6 [99].

For screening purposes, documenting severity of symptoms and tracking all the DSM-IV-based criteria in an efficient way, the self-rated Posttraumatic Stress Diagnostic Scale (PDS) may suffice. This 49-item scale can be administered in 10–15 minutes, correlates with the Beck Depression Inventory (BDI) and State-Trait Anxiety Inventory, and has good reliability and validity [96].

Another measure that assesses DSM-IV criteria for PTSD that can be used for tracking changes in symptom severity is the Davidson Trauma Scale, containing 17 items. This rating scale has good test-retest reliability, shows a high correlation with other PTSD measures, and is not confounded by extroversion/introversion personality traits [97].

The Clinician-Administered PTSD Scale (CAPS-1) takes about 45 min to administer, provides a multidimensional view of the severity of PTSD, corresponds to established DSM-IV diagnostic criteria, delineates both current and lifetime diagnostic time frames for those with history of multiple traumatic events, has high sensitivity and specificity, and is a reliable and valid instrument [100].

Other instruments frequently used with PTSD patients include the Impact of Event Scale, the Mississippi Scale, and the Minnesota Multiphasic Personality Inventory PTSD Scale (MMPI-PTSD) – all of which may be used for screening for baseline symptoms, but none are diagnostic measures or useful for measuring treatment outcomes.

A recent review of quality of life after FT by Aycart et al. indicated that 11 of the 17 articles were descriptive, and only 4 centers reported data, with 1 study of 8 patients using prospective, systematic assessments with validated instruments [101]. The measures used to evaluate QOL and psychological variables greatly varied between the studies. Overall, of the 39 FT recipients, the quality of life outcomes have been published on only 14 patients in peer-reviewed literature. Considering that increasing the number of quality of life years is the rationale for FT, gathering more reliable quantitative data may be essential to determine the risk-benefit ratio for FT recipients [101].

Lantieri et al. published results of a prospective open study for six FT recipients, demonstrating that SF-36 scores were improved for all patients when comparing pre-transplant QOL to 2.5–8 years post-transplant for both physical and mental components [49]. However, patients with self-inflicted GSW reported less improvement than those with neurofibromatosis type 1. Lantieri et al. showed improvement in three patients on the Derriford Appearance Scale-59 and general improvement for these three patients on the University of Washington Head and Neck Disease-Specific questionnaire and Performance Status Scale for Head and Neck Cancer. Of the first five patients, data was omitted for two, as one died and the other decided to opt out of FT. One patient committed suicide by GSW at year 4 after FT [49]. This experience led the team to reconsider offering FT to patients with self-inflicted GSW.

Of note, although many surgeons may subscribe to the idea that all patients with self-inflicted GSW to the face will ultimately take their life in this way, evidence disputes this myth. Runeson et al. reviewed 48,649 patients treated for attempted suicide to see how many later successfully completed suicide and whether they used the same method [102]. Those who attempted via hanging were the most likely to commit suicide later by that method, 53.9% of men and 56.6% of women. Those who attempted suicide via firearm or explosive were less likely to complete suicide with that method later, 34.5% of men and 7.5% of women. Overall, only 11.8% of those that attempted suicide later completed suicide over 21–31 years follow-up [102].

To explore and demonstrate an example of the patient's psychological course post-FT, Coffman et al. did assessments every 3 months for 3 years, then every 6 months thereafter on the first FT recipient in Cleveland in 2008 [103]. The SF-36,

Rosenberg Self-Esteem Scale and Spielberger State-Trait Anxiety Inventory did not show much change over time for the first FT recipient. Her scores on Psychosocial Adjustment to Illness Scale-self-rated showed steady improvement after transplant in social integration and psychological distress for the first 3 years. The FACES-Perception of Teasing Scale, a single-center-derived instrument based on the original Perception of Teasing Scale, showed that verbal abuse in public diminished to nearly nonexistent over the first 3 years and that she was less bothered by the reactions she received in public. The Physical Appearance State, Trait Anxiety Scale, and Facial Anxiety Scale-State showed an increase in concern over weight gain in the first 3 months due to steroids and less anxiety about the face.

The patient's BDI score declined from 16 to 6 by 3 months post-FT while on escitalopram [103]. At the end of 2009, the BDI score was 14, reflecting CMV infection and challenges at home. However, in 3 months, the patient did not report any symptoms of depression on escitalopram 40 mg daily. On the PAIS-SR, the patient rated changes in her appearance that made her less attractive before transplant as "extremely," while after transplant she rated this as "a little bit." PAIS-SR psychological distress rose at 3 months post-transplant, then fell markedly over the next 4 months, until CMV infection caused extreme fatigue. Once she received a new medication and fatigue lifted, the psychological distress improved again. Although the SF-36 and WHOQOL-BREF were utilized, the PAIS-SR was more useful in reflecting social reintegration and psychological distress and other domains such as sexual functioning and attitudes toward health care [103].

Chang and Pomahac assessed three FT recipients at baseline, 3 and 6 months post-transplant, noting that physical QOL declined during the first 3 months, then improved on the Short Form-12 [104]. Mental health of all three patients also improved on SF-12 at 6 months. Two patients reported high scores on EuroQoL five-dimension scale [EuroQoL-5D] physical function during the time period, but the third patient's physical functioning declined during the 6 months after FT. Two patients showed an improvement in their romantic relationships on the Dyadic Adjustment Scale, while the other was not in a partnered relationship [104].

For the two groups that used The Facial Disability Index, there was no preoperative data. Diaz-Siso reported steady improvement in scores over 2–3 years post-transplant, and Fischer had only one score at a single time point for one patient at 1 year, three patients at 2.5 years, and one patient at 5 years [105, 106].

Lemmens et al. used many rating scales and showed that the patient's health-related QOL improved after FT but then declined more than mental QOL at 15 months. The Mini-International Neuropsychiatric Interview at 15 months showed lifetime depressive disorder as before the FT and no current depressive symptoms. This decline in physical QOL was attributed to medical complications that resulted from his medications. He showed improvement in resilience, affective responsiveness, and disease benefits, but his marital support and depth of the partnership bond decreased at 15 months [107].

Conclusions

Face transplantation offers a last resort intervention for patients with severe facial disfigurement. FT is not a life-saving but life-enhancing procedure, aimed at improving QOL and functionality. FT appears to decrease depression and verbal abuse patients experience in public and improve QOL and societal reintegration, though it may not alter anxiety, self-esteem, or sexual functioning. In terms of psychological monitoring, the PAIS-SR may have advantages over the SF-36 and WHOQOL-BREF rating scales for measuring psychological distress and social reintegration in this patient population. At present, UNOS is trying to collect SF-36 data from pre- and post-transplant on FT recipients to demonstrate QOL outcomes for this surgery motivated by improvement in quality of life. More systematic data should be collected to further examine whether the long-term physical and psychological outcomes of facial transplantation outweigh the risks of ongoing immunosuppression.

References

1. Dubernard JM, Lengelé B, Morelon E, Testelin S, Badet L, Moure C, et al. Outcomes 18 months after the first human partial face transplantation. N Engl J Med. 2007;357(24):2451–560.
2. Siemionow M, Sonmez E. Face as an organ. Ann Plast Surg. 2008;61:345–52.
3. Furr LA, Wiggins O, Cunningham M, Cunningham M, Vasilic D, Brown CS, et al. Psychosocial implications of disfigurement and the future of human face transplantation. Plast Reconstr Surg. 2007;120:559–65.
4. Siemionow M, Agaoglu G. The issue of "facial appearance and identity transfer" after mock transplantation: a cadaver study in preparation for facial allograft transplantation in humans. J Reconstr Microsurg. 2006;22:329–34.
5. Pomahac B, Aflaki P, Nelson C, Balas B. Evaluation of appearance transfer and persistence in central face transplantation: a computer simulation analysis. J Plast Reconstr Aesthet Surg. 2010;63:733–8.
6. Valente SM. Visual disfigurement and depression. Plast Surg Nurs. 2004;24:140–6.
7. Faces C. Facing disfigurement with confidence. London: Changing Faces; 2001.
8. Thompson A, Kent G. Adjusting to disfigurement: process involved in dealing with being visibly different. Clin Psychol Rev. 2001;21(5):663–92.
9. Rumsey N, Harcourt D. Body Image and disfigurement: issues and interventions. Body Image. 2004;1:83–97.
10. Furness P, Garrud P, Faulder A, Swift J. Coming to terms: a grounded theory of adaptation to facial surgery in adulthood. J Health Psychol. 2006;11:454–66.
11. Glynn SM. The psychosocial characteristics and needs of patients presenting with orofacial injury. Oral Maxillofac Surg Clin North Am. 2010;22:209–15.
12. Glynn SM, Shetty V, Elliot-Brown K, Leathers R, Belin TR, Wang J. Chronic posttraumatic stress disorder after facial injury: a 1-year prospective cohort study. J Trauma. 2007;62:410–8.
13. Bisson JI, Shepherd JP, Dhutia M. Psychological sequela of facial trauma. J Trauma. 1997;43:496–500.
14. Furness PJ. Exploring supportive care needs and experiences of facial surgery patients. Br J Nurs. 2005;14:641–5.
15. Brown B, Roberts J, Browne G, Byrne C, Love B, Streiner D. Gender differences in variables associated with psychosocial adjustment to burn injury. Res Nurs Health. 1988;11:23–30.
16. Katz MR, Irish JC, Devins GM, Rodin GM, Gullane PJ. Psychosocial adjustment in head and neck cancer: the impact of disfigurement, gender and social support. Head Neck. 2003;25:103–12.
17. Vickery LE, Latchford G, Hewison J, Bellew M, Feber T. The impact of head and neck cancer and facial disfigurement on the quality of life of patients and their partners. Head Neck. 2003;25:289–96.
18. Dropkin MJ. Coping with disfigurement and dysfunction after head and neck cancer surgery: a conceptual framework. Semin Oncol Nurs. 1989;5:213–9.
19. Dropkin MJ. Body image and quality of life after head and neck cancer surgery. Cancer Pract. 1999;7:309–13.
20. Newell R, Marks I. Phobic nature of social difficulty in facially disfigured people. Br J Psychiatry. 2000;176:177–81.
21. Rumsey N, Clarke A, Musa M. Altered body image: the psychological needs of patients. Br J Comm Nurs. 2002;7:563–6.
22. Levine E, Degutis L, Pruzinsky T, Shin J, Persing JA. Quality of life and facial trauma: psychological and body image effects. Ann Plast Surg. 2005;54:502–10.
23. Rumsey N. Body image and congenital conditions with visible differences. In: Cash TF, Pruzinsky T, editors. Body image: A handbook of theory, research, and clinical practice. New York: Guilford Press; 2002. p. 226–33.
24. Rumsey N. Body image in disfiguring congenital conditions. In: Cash TF, Pruzinsky T, editors. Body image: a handbook of theory, research, and clinical practice. New York: Guilford Press; 2002. p. 431–9.
25. Bradbury E. Counselling people with disfigurement. Leicester: British Psychological Society; 1996.
26. Malt U, Ugland O. A long-term psychosocial follow-up study of burned adults: review of the literature. Burns. 1980;6:190–7.
27. Desousa A. Psychological issues in oral and maxillofacial reconstructive surgery. Br J Oral Maxillofac Surg. 2008;46:661–4.
28. Walters E. Problems faced by children and families living with visible differences. In: Lansdown R, Rumey N, Bradbury E, Carr T, Partridge J, editors. Visible difference: coping with disfigurement. Oxford: Butterworth-Heinemann; 1997. p. 112–20.
29. Speltz M, Endriga M, Mason C. Early predictors of attachment in infants with cleft lip and/or palate. Child Dev. 1997;68:12–25.
30. Richman LC. Behavior and achievement of cleft palate children. Cleft Palate J. 1976;13:4–10.
31. Robinson E, Rumsey M, Partridge J. An evaluation of the impact of social interaction skills training for facially disfigured people. Br J Plast Surg. 1996;49:281–9.
32. Williams BJ, Paradise LP. Educational, occupational, and marital status of cleft palate adults. Cleft Palate J. 1973;10:223–9.
33. Ramstad T, Ottem E, Shaw WC. Psychosocial adjustment in Norwegian adults who had undergone standardised treatment of complete cleft lip and palate. II. Self-reported problems and concerns with appearance. Scand J Plast Reconstr Surg Hand Surg. 1995;29:329–36.

34. Rumsey N, Clarke A, White P, Wyn-Williams M, Garlick W. Altered body image: appearance-related concerns of people with visible disfigurement. J Adv Nurs. 2004;48:443–53.

35. Sarwer DB, Bartlett SP, Whitaker LA, Paige KT, Pertschuk MJ, Wadden TA. Adult psychological functioning of individuals born with craniofacial anomalies. Plast Reconstr Surg. 1999;103:412–8.

36. Pope AW, Ward J. Factors associated with peer social competence in preadolescents with craniofacial anomalies. J Pediatr Psychol. 1997;22:455–69.

37. Bradbury E. Understanding the problems. In: Lansdown R, Rumsey N, Bradbury E, Carr A, Partridge J, editors. Visibly different: coping with disfigurement. Oxford: Butterworth-Heinemann; 1997. p. 180–93.

38. Grant FC, Norcross NC. Repair of cranial defects by cranioplasty. Ann Surg. 1939;110:488–512.

39. Sedney C, Dillen W, Julien T. Clinical spectrum and radiographic features of the syndrome of the trephined. J Neurosci Rural Pract. 2015;6:438–41.

40. Gottlob I, Simonsz-Toth B, Heilbronner R. Midbrain syndrome with eye movement disorder: dramatic improvement after cranioplasty. Strabismus. 2002;10:271–7.

41. Bijlenga P, Zumofen D, Yilmaz H, Creisson E, De Tribolet N. Orthostatic mesodiancephalic dysfunction after decompressive craniectomy. J Neurol Neurosurg Psychiatry. 2007;78:430–3.

42. Ashayeri K, Jackson EM, Huang J, Brem H, Gordon CR. Syndrome of the trephined: a systematic review. Neurosurgery. 2016;79:525–33.

43. Yamaura A, Makino H. Neurological deficits in the presence of the sinking skin flap following decompressive craniectomy. Neurol Med Chir. 1977;17:43–53.

44. Honeybul S. Neurological susceptibility to a skull defect. Surg Neurol Int. 2014;5:83.

45. Schuind F, Abramowicz D, Schneeberger S. Hand transplantation: the state of the art. J Hand Surg. 2007;32E:2–17.

46. Gordon CR, Siemionow M, Papay F, Pryor L, Gatherwright J, Kodish E, et al. The world's experience with facial transplantation: what have we learned thus far? Ann Plast Surg. 2009;63:572–8.

47. Renshaw A, Clarke A, Diver AJ, Ashcroft RE, Butler PE. Informed consent for facial transplantation. Transpl Int. 2006;19:861–7.

48. Krakowczyk T, Maciejewski A, Szymczyk C, Oles K, Póltorak S. Face transplant in an advanced neurofibromatosis type I patient. Ann Transplant. 2017;22:53–7.

49. Lantieri L, Grimbert P, Ortonne N, Suberbielle C, Bories D, Gil-Vernet S, et al. Face transplant: long-term follow-up and results of a prospective open study. Lancet. 2016;388:1398–407.

50. Brown CS, Gander B, Cunningham M, Furr A, Vasilic D, Wiggins O, et al. Ethical considerations in face transplantation. Int J Surg. 2007;5:353–64.

51. Siemionow M, Bramstedt K, Kodish E. Ethical issues in face transplantation. Curr Opin Organ Transplant. 2007;12:193–7.

52. Coffman KL, Siemionow MZ. Ethics of facial transplantation revisited. Curr Opin Organ Transplant. 2014;19:181–7.

53. Aycart MA, Alhefzi M, Keuckelhaus M, Krezdorn N, Bueno EM, Caterson EJ, et al. A retrospective analysis of secondary revisions after face transplantation: assessment of outcomes, safety, and feasibility. Plast Reconstr Surg. 2016;138:690e–701e.

54. Sosin M, Rodriguez ED. The face transplantation update: 2016. Plast Reconstr Surg. 2016;137:1841–50.

55. Russo JE, Genden EM. Facial transplantation. Facial Plast Surg Clin North Am. 2016;24:367–77.

56. Smeets R, Rendenbach C, Birkelbach M, Al-Dam A, Gröbe A, Hanken H, et al. Face transplantation: on the verge of becoming clinical routine? Biomed Res Int. 2014;2014:907272. https://doi.org/10.1155/2014/907272. Epub 2014 Jun 9

57. Ozkan O. Facial transplantation: the Antalya, Turkey clinical experience. Paper presented at AO North America State of the Art: face reconstruction and transplantation biennial course. New York; 2015.

58. Vasilic D, Alloway RR, Barker JH, Furr A, Ashcroft R, Banis JC, et al. Risk assessment of immunosuppressive therapy in facial transplantation. Plast Reconstr Surg. 2007;120:657–68.

59. Guo S, Han Y, Zhang X, Lu B, Yi C, Zhang H, et al. Human facial allotransplantation: a 2-year follow-up study. Lancet. 2008;372:631–8.

60. Infante-Cossio P, Barerra-Pulido F, Gomez-Cia T, Faci Sicilia-Castro D, Garcia-Perla-Garcia A, Gacto-Sanchez P, et al. Facial transplantation: a concise update. Med Oral Patol Oral Cir Bucal. 2013;18:e263–27.

61. Morelon E, Petruzzo P, Kanitakis J, Dakpé S, Thaunat O, Dubois V, et al. Face transplantation: partial graft loss of the first case 10 years later. Am J Transplant. 2017; https://doi.org/10.1111/ajt.14218. [Epub ahead of print]

62. Cavadas P. Speed-update on world experience with clinic VCA. ASRT 3rd biennial meeting. Chicago; 2012.

63. Morris P, Bradley A, Doyal L, Earley M, Hagen P, Milling M, et al. Face transplantation: a review of the technical, immunological, psychological and clinical issues with recommendations for good practice. Transplantation. 2007;83:109–28.

64. Torres-Madriz G, Boucher HW. Immunocompromised hosts: perspectives in the treatment and prophylaxis of cytomegalovirus disease in solid-organ transplant recipients. Clin Infect Dis. 2008;47:702–11.

65. First MR, Peddi VR. Malignancies complicating organ transplantation. Transplant Proc. 1998;30:2768–70.

66. Penn I. Posttransplant malignancies. Transplant Proc. 1999;31:1260–2.

67. Carty MG, Bueno EM, Lehmann LS, Pomahac B. A position paper in support of face transplantation in the blind. Plast Reconstr Surg. 2012;130:319–24.

68. Bramstedt KA, Plock JA. Looking the world in the face: the benefits and challenges of facial transplantation for blind patients. Prog Transplant. 2016;27(1):79–83. pii: 152692481 [Epub ahead of print]

69. Sivak WN, Davidson EH, Komatsu C, Li Y, Miller MR, Schuman JS, et al. Ethical considerations of whole-eye transplantation. J Clin Ethics. 2016;27:64–7.

70. Davidson EH, Wang EW, Yu JY, Fernandez-Miranda JC, Wang DJ, Richards N, et al. Total human eye allotransplantation: developing surgical protocols for donor and recipient procedures. Plast Reconstr Surg. 2016;136:1297–308.

71. Bourne R, Li Y, Komatsu C, Miller MR, Davidson EH, He L, et al. Whole-eye transplantation: a look into the past and vision for the future. Eye. 2017;31:179–84.

72. Gordon CR, Siemionow M, Coffman K, Alam D, Eghtesad B, Zins JE, et al. The Cleveland Clinic FACES score: a preliminary assessment tool for identifying the optimal face transplant candidate. J Craniofac Surg. 2009;20:1969–74.

73. Clarke A, Butler PEM. Patient selection for facial transplantation II: psychological consideration. Int J Surg. 2004;2:116–8.

74. Coffman KL, Gordon CR, Siemionow MZ. Chapter 13, "Psychological aspects of face transplantation". In: Siemionow MZ, editor. The know-how of face transplantation. London: Springer; 2011. p. 143.

75. Farrer R. Psychological considerations in face transplantation. Int J Surg. 2004;2:77–8.

76. Schiller D, Freeman JB, Mitchell JP, Uleman JS, Phelps EA. A neural mechanism of first impressions. Nat Neurosci. 2009;12:508–14.

77. Lazarus R. Coping theory and research: past, present and future. Psychosom Med. 1993;55:234–47.

78. Horowitz MJ. Stress-response syndromes: a review of posttraumatic and adjustment disorders. Hosp Community Psychiatry. 1986;37:241–9.

79. Calahan C. Facial disfigurement and sense of self in head and neck cancer. Soc Work Health Care. 2004;40:73–87.
80. Girotto JA, MacKenzie E, Fowler C, Redett R, Robertson B, Manson PN. Long-term physical impairment and functional outcomes after complex facial fractures. Plast Reconstr Surg. 2001;108:312–27.
81. Scheller EL, Krebsbach PH. Gene therapy: design and prospects for craniofacial regeneration. J Dent Res. 2009;88:585–96.
82. Houston V, Bull R. Do people avoid sitting next to someone who is facially disfigured? Eur J Soc Psychol. 1994;24:279–84.
83. Macgregor FC. Facial disfigurement: problems and management of social interaction and implications for mental health. Aesthet Plast Surg. 1990;14:249–57.
84. Lansdown R, Rumsey N, Bradbury E, Carr T, Partridge J. Visibly different: coping with disfigurement. Oxford: Butterworth Heinemann; 1997.
85. Kiwanuka H, Aycart MA, Bueno EM, Patie Alhefzi M, Krezdorn N, Pomahac B. Patient recruitment and referral patterns in face transplantation: a single Center's experience. Plast Reconstr Surg. 2016;138:224–31.
86. Marchac A, Kuschner T, Paris J, Picard A, Vazquez MP, Lantieri L. Ethical issues in pediatric face transplantation: should we perform face transplantation in children? Plast Reconstr Surg. 2016;138:449–54.
87. Mäkitie AA, Salmi M, Lindford A, Tuomi J, Lassus P. Three-dimensional printing for restoration of the donor face: a new digital technique tested and used in the first facial allotransplantation patient in Finland. J Plast Reconstr Aesthet Surg. 2016;69:1648–52.
88. Attar. Looking for your own face. In: Washington P, editor. Persian poetry. New York/Toronto: AA Knopf, Inc; 2000. p. 59.
89. Cunningham M, Barbee A, Philhower C. Dimensions of facial physical attractiveness: the intersection of biology and culture. In: Rhodes G, Zebrowitz L, editors. Advances in visual cognition, vol. 1. Stamford: JAI/Ablex; 2002.
90. Cash TF. Body image and plastic surgery. In: Sarwer DB, Pruzinsky T, Cash TF, et al., editors. Psychological aspects of reconstructive and cosmetic surgery: clinical, empirical, and ethical perspective. Philadelphia: Lippincott Williams &Wilkins; 2006. p. 37–59.
91. Goetzmann L. "Is it me, or isn't it?"-transplanted organs and their donors as transitional objects. Am J Psychoanal. 2004;64(3):279–89.
92. http://www.telegraph.co.uk/news/worldnews/europe/france/3367041/Face-transplant-woman-struggles-with-identity.html
93. Times Online From The Sunday Times January 17, 2010 www.timesonline.co.uk/tol/life_and_style/.../article6987682.ece
94. [No authors listed]. 'Social anonymity': the ethics of facial transplantation. Br Dent J. 2016;221:126.
95. Blanchard EB, Jones-Alexander J, Buckley TC, Forneris CA. Psychometric properties of the PTSD checklist (PCL). Behav Res Ther. 1996;34:669–73.
96. Foa EB, Cashman L, Jaycox L, Perry K. The validation of a self-report measure of posttraumatic stress disorder: the posttraumatic diagnostic scale. Psychol Assess. 1997;9:445–51.
97. Davidson JR, Book SW, Colket JT, Tupler LA, Roth D, David D, et al. Assessment of a new self-rating scale for post-traumatic stress disorder. Psychol Med. 1997;27:153–60.
98. Meltzer-Brody S, Churchill E, Davison JRT. Derivation of the SPAN, a brief diagnostic screening test for post-traumatic stress disorder. Psychiatr Res. 1999;88:63–70.
99. Fullerton CS, Ursano RJ, Epstein RS, Crowley B, Vance KL, Craig J. Measurement of posttraumatic stress disorder in community samples. Nord J Psychiatry. 2000;54:5–12.
100. Dudley DB, Weathers FW, Nagy LM, Kaloupek DG, Gusman FD, Charney DS, et al. The development of a clinician-administered PTSD scale. J Trauma Stress. 1995;8:75–91.
101. Aycart MA, Kiwanuka H, Krezdorn N, Alhefzi M, Bueno EM, Pomahac B, et al. Quality of life after face transplantation: outcomes, assessment tools, and future directions. Plast Reconstr Surg. 2017;139:194–203.
102. Runeson B, Tidemalm D, Dahlin M, Lichtenstein P, Långström N. Method of attempted suicide as a predictor of subsequent successful suicide: national long term cohort study. BMJ. 2010;341:c3222–35.
103. Coffman KL, Siemionow MZ. Face transplantation: psychological outcomes at three-year follow-up. Psychosomatics. 2013;54:372–8.
104. Chang G, Pomahac B. Psychosocial changes 6 months after face transplantation. Psychosomatics. 2013;54:367–71.
105. Diaz-Siso JR, Parker M, Bueno EM, Sisk GC, Pribaz JJ, Eriksson E, et al. Facial allotransplantation: a 3–year follow-up report. J Plast Reconstr Aesthet Surg. 2013;66:1458–68.
106. Fischer S, Keuckelhaus M, Pauzenberger R, Bueno EM, Pomahac B. Functional outcomes of face transplantation. Am J Transplant. 2015;15:220–33.
107. Lemmens MD, Poppe C, Hendrickx H, Roche N, Peeters P, Vermeersch HF, et al. Facial transplantation in a blind patient: psychologic, marital, and family outcomes at 15 months follow-up. Psychosomatics. 2015;56:362–70.

Psychological and Psychosocial Aspects of Limb Transplantation

35

Martin Kumnig and Sheila G. Jowsey-Gregoire

Introduction

Vascularized Composite Allotransplantation Versus Solid Organ Transplantation

Solid organ transplantation (SOT) and vascularized composite allotransplantation (VCA) share a common history related to the combination of surgical and microsurgical challenges and a complex multidisciplinary care model [1, 2]. However, the technical demands of and psychosocial issues unique to VCA make VCA different from SOT [3]. The most notable difference between these two fields of transplantation is the visible nature of the VCA allograft [4, 5], which impacts the patients' self-image, ideas regarding the allograft, and psychological reaction to the allograft [6]. In addition to the challenge of accepting the allograft(s), VCA patients have had to cope with likely traumatic reactions to limb loss [3, 7, 8].

This chapter will focus on the psychosocial challenges in limb transplantation, including the psychosocial domains of the comprehensive pre- and post-transplant psychosocial evaluation of limb transplant patients, including the factors important in determining patients' eligibility for transplantation [9, 10]. Patient's motivation for limb transplantation can emerge from a variety of concerns, including functional and occupational limitations, body image concerns, the desire to have the sensation of touch, and restoration of bodily integrity. Thus, assessing motivation is a complex task in patients who are not medically ill and not requiring transplantation for life-saving purposes [3]. Several psychosocial and medical risk factors place limb transplant patients at higher risk for nonadherence and negative medical and/or psychological outcomes (e.g., developing depressive symptoms, post-traumatic stress disorder (PTSD), etc.) [11]. The most important development for the field is an emerging recognition that the pre- and post-transplantation psychosocial evaluation and treatment are an integral part of any transplant VCA program and that the identification of at-risk patients and those requiring ongoing counseling is a primary focus of the psychological evaluation [5].

Restorative Options for Patients with Limb Loss

The developments over the past 70 years in the fields of surgery and rehabilitation have enabled two different options for patients who have suffered limb loss: limb transplantation and prosthetic limbs [12]. Patients typically require limb transplantation due to traumatic injuries that occur in occupation settings, military engagements, motor vehicle, and other accidents. Some patients present with limb loss in the setting of sepsis or vascular malformations. The level of limb loss is significant for the recovery process, because nerve regeneration typically occurs at a rate of one inch per month resulting in particularly lengthy rehabilitation. Limb transplantation has the unique potential to not only restore motor skills but also to allow the return of sensation and restoration of bodily integrity [13]. Nevertheless, the impact of lifelong immunosuppression cannot be overstated, requiring medical teams and the patient to carefully weigh the potential benefits and risks [14–17]. Conversely, prostheses offer the potential to restore hand function without the risk of immunosuppression [18]. Myoelectric prostheses have increasingly advanced ergonomic and functional features [12]. Because there is no additional surgery needed and patients can return to near normal life, prosthetic fitting with myoelectric devices is the standard of care in below-elbow amputees [18]. Despite these advantages, abandonment of

M. Kumnig
Department of Medical Psychology,
Center for Advanced Psychology in Plastic and Transplant Surgery,
Innsbruck Medical University, Innsbruck, Austria
e-mail: Martin.Kumnig@i-med.ac.at

S. G. Jowsey-Gregoire (✉)
Department of Psychiatry and Psychology and Department of Surgery, Mayo Graduate School of Medicine,
Mayo Clinic Rochester, Rochester, MN, USA
e-mail: Jowsey-Gregoire.Sheila@mayo.edu

© Springer International Publishing AG, part of Springer Nature 2019
Y. Sher, J. R. Maldonado (eds.), *Psychosocial Care of End-Stage Organ Disease and Transplant Patients*,
https://doi.org/10.1007/978-3-319-94914-7_35

the prosthetic device occurs in about 20% of patients due to the inherent challenges of prosthetic use, including discomfort at the stump region, lack of functional benefit, excessive weight, lack of sensory feedback, and the need for the prosthesis to be serviced regularly [19].

Although the need for studies to analyze the functional and psychosocial differences between limb transplantation and prosthetic limbs has been noted [20–24], to date there is only one multicenter cohort study comparing the functional and quality of life (QOL) outcomes of patients who have undergone limb transplantation or prosthetic fitting [18]. While previous reports noted that limb transplants were superior to prostheses without adequately directly comparing the functional or psychosocial outcomes of both methods, this study showed that there were no significant differences when only motor function was considered. For most activities of daily living (ADL), both limb transplantation and prosthetic fitting provide reliable and sufficient hand function [18]. The functional results seem to be sustained with regular therapy to maintain the achieved capacities [25, 26]. However, in assessing the sensory capacity of the hand and perceived QOL, transplanted hands were far superior compared to prosthesis.

Research clearly shows that, given the lower risks associated with a prosthesis, the use of a prosthesis should remain the standard treatment for upper limp amputees, especially in unilateral cases [12, 18]. Additionally, the cost of each reconstructive procedure must be considered in the decision-making process. Cost-utility analyses that considered different financial factors, including surgical costs, inpatient treatment, hand therapy, outpatient visits, immunosuppression, and time-out of employment, have shown that prosthetic devices provide a reliable but less expensive treatment [27–29].

Limb transplantation and prosthetic fitting will continue to evolve. Interesting developments include possible induction of donor-specific tolerance for VCA versus new pattern-recognition control algorithms for prosthesis providing sensation and tactile feedback. Further research will be needed to reassess the advantages and disadvantages of both treatment options, including direct comparisons of specific amputation levels and potential functional, sensory, and esthetic advantages for each option [18].

Brief History and Medical Course

The concept of limb transplantation has evolved over time with attempts to transplant a limb occurring over a thousand years ago [2, 30, 31]. *The Legend of the Black Leg (Leggenda Aurea)* describes twins Cosmos and Damian, who transplanted the leg of a man with another man's limb in 348 AD

[32] (also see Chap. 8). Gaspare Tagliacozzi transplanted a nose from a slave to his master [33]. Other descriptions of tissue transplants were periodically reported including Bunger [34] transplanting a sheepskin and Carrel [35] who described attachment of an artery from a father to the leg of his infant suffering from intestinal bleeding [36]. Guthrie [37] experimented with dogs to transplant the head from one dog onto another. None of these efforts could surmount the challenges of rejection despite some degree of surgical innovation [38]. Medawar and colleagues [39] ultimately established the causes of rejection which led to the development of modern transplant immunology [30, 40]. Earle E. Peacock [41, 42] created the term composite tissue allograft in 1957, and the first limb transplant was performed in 1964 by Robert Gilbert [43] in Ecuador. Unfortunately, the graft had to be amputated 3 weeks later due to acute rejection. With this first early failure of limb transplantation, the field of VCA received no further substantive scientific efforts for most of the next three decades. Meanwhile immunosuppressive drug therapy innovations facilitated the success of SOT [2, 30].

Limb transplantation entered the current era in 1998 with pioneering work by Jean-Michel Dubernard [44–46] in Lyon, in 1999 Warren Breidenbach [47] in Louisville, and in 2000 Raimund Margreiter in Innsbruck [48], who performed successful limb transplants [31]. From 1998 to 2015, a total of 73 limb have been transplanted with 23 unilateral and 25 bilateral transplants, in a total of 48 patients [17]. VCA continues to grow as a field, although funding for this complex form of transplantation continues to be a barrier to the large-scale adoption of VCA. A number of transplant centers globally have created specific VCA programs [49]. Limited psychosocial research exists despite the years of experience with limb transplant [3].

Selection of Limb Transplant Candidates

VCA is a surgical procedure with the goals to regain limited or lost limb function and to improve patients' QOL, psychological well-being, and ADLs. The visible nature of the graft strikingly changes the transplant experience for limb transplant patients [4, 49]. Because limb loss is not a life-threatening illness, psychosocial factors become more important in the patients' motivation for improved functional outcomes, occupational attainment, improved body image and restoration of touch, and balanced against the risks of immunosuppression [3, 5, 15, 50]. The assessment of the patients' desire for limb transplantation is a psychologically complex process and warrants a VCA specific psychosocial evaluation protocol fully addressing these issues [16].

Psychosocial Domains of the Evaluation

Standardized evaluation guidelines and a shared research approach have not been developed yet [3–5, 13, 15, 16, 45, 47–67]. Recent efforts to attempt to address this deficiency are noted in the literature [49]. Although a variety of psychosocial evaluation protocols are used by transplant centers worldwide, specific psychosocial domains have emerged as important and predictive [3, 68–75]. As with any clinical psychological assessment in transplantation medicine, the assessment of limb transplant candidates has to include an understanding of the patient's prior psychiatric history (e.g., DSM-V diagnoses, associated prior treatments), substance use/abuse, health behaviors, prior history of coping and stress management, and mental status examination [5].

Adherence

Because of the need for lifelong adherence to immunosuppression and physical rehabilitation therapy [76], the patients' history of adherence is an important domain in pretransplant screening, and adherence will need to be addressed in post-transplant follow-up visits [3, 15, 49, 50]. Nonadherence postoperatively is predicted by pre-transplant nonadherence [77]. According to the theory of planned behavior, premorbid psychiatric status, current psychological state (e.g., high anxiety/depression), level of social support, and substance use history may be helpful in predicting pre- and post-transplant adherence [78, 79]. The International Registry on Hand and Composite Tissue Transplantation (IRHCTT) has reported that nonadherence has consistently been associated with rejection episodes, graft loss, and death [17]. These data highlight the need for careful patient selection to ensure that proper adherence to medication and treatment regimens occurs [3, 80].

Understanding of Motivation and Expectations

One of the major consequences of VCA is post-transplant immunosuppression as well as long-term physical rehabilitation therapy, necessitating the need to assess the patients' decision-making process to elicit their understanding of these requirements [81]. Decision-making can be especially stressful for patients when the surgical outcome is uncertain and when alternative treatment options are available [82]. Patients have different risk thresholds which contribute to their decision-making about how much risk they are willing to accept for improved function or esthetic restoration [83–88]. Thus, the evaluator must address all relevant psychosocial aspects of limb transplantation, including the assessment of patients' decision-making abilities [89].

The psychosocial evaluation should clarify if the patients have realistic expectations about the potential post-transplant functional and esthetic outcomes [3, 5, 15, 49, 50]. Otherwise, this could lead to a mismatch between patients' and surgical team's expectation about the outcome [82]. Similarly, although a patient might perceive an improvement of a particular body feature following the surgery, this may not have a corresponding impact on overall perception of body image (e.g., the allograft is perceived as foreign body with missing integration in the patients' self–/body concept) [90]. Therefore, the preparation for limb transplantation involves the careful assessment of patients' expectations, potential hand fantasies (e.g., about the donor and the actions have been performed by the deceased donor, etc.), and challenging unrealistic expectations (e.g., playing the piano as the patient used before traumatic hand loss, working in a horse breeding farm, being able to repair all parts of a motorcycle, etc.) [5].

Patients suffering from hand loss struggle with a variety of impairments in their daily living. Similar to chronically ill patients, their life is dominated by the medical experience, and their ADLs are limited [91]. Family/social support is essential to assist patients in their ADLs, which helps to normalize their life. Diverse psychosocial stressors such as loss of self-concept and self-esteem, and a feeling of uncertainty about the future [92], negatively affect patients' social, financial, and psychological well-being [93–95]. Most patients, especially those with bilateral limb transplantation, report their limited independence with ADLs as their primary motive for elective surgery [3]. Patients hope to significantly improve their QOL and ability to perform higher level of ADLs after limb transplantation, and most patients demonstrate a high degree of satisfaction with their postoperative outcome [13]. Overall health improvement, including improved QOL, has been reported after successful limb transplantation [92, 96–98], while post-transplant side effects and complications have been noted to respond to treatment protocols [99, 100]. In most cases, the patients' decision to undergo limb transplantation or prosthetic fitting depends more on how the treatment will fit into the patients' life, rather than on clinical indicators [101–104]. Thus, the successful outcome of limb transplantation appears to be highly dependent on the motivation and reasonable expectations of the patients [102].

Social Support

The transplant psychosocial assessment should determine family/social support before and after limb transplantation. The evaluation protocol should address the presence or absence of conflicted family relationships and also anticipate stress for the family that may come from intrusive media attention which has been reported in a number of cases [5]. Consideration of potential negative developments in the course of transplantation as well as improvements in QOL and ADLs will impact close family members.

Patients typically will experience an initial decrease in function, and caregivers will need to prepare for increased caregiver demands to assist with instrumental tasks of daily living while potentially also carrying a heavier burden of caring for children and maintaining employment [3]. During the ongoing post-transplant physical and occupational rehabilitation, family/social support is especially important [105, 106].

Body Image Issues

Additionally, limb transplantation, even when technically successful, is not a treatment to resolve long-standing body image disorders [81]. Visible grafts could adversely affect the patients' sense of themselves as an integrated whole, leading to rejection of the graft as undesirable [4, 7, 49, 107]. Psychological and social well-being will be influenced by disturbed body image due to limb loss that may associate with a range of concealing behaviors (e.g., neglect of personal hygiene such as cutting nails, etc.) in response to negative self-evaluation [79, 108–110]. Several cases have demonstrated the importance of the successful psychological integration of the allograft for post-transplant outcomes. Notably, patients must accept a new graft while adapting their loss of a part of their body that was unique to them [8]. This requires alterations in their sense of who they are, how the graft fits in with their body, and ultimately acceptance of the allograft as part of themselves [6]. Hence, body image issues need to be addressed and can provide information regarding the patients' self−/body concept and help to determine if successful integration of the graft can be expected [111]. Assessment of the families' expectations about limb transplantation (e.g., "Will I be able to accept my husband touching me with his new hands?") will be critical also. Ultimately, if the pre-transplant psychosocial assessment reveals a disordered body image or significant body image issues related to limb transplantation, proactive psychosocial interventions should be considered to assist the patients with their self-concept or body image processing [51].

Psychological Reactions

Another important area to assess is the patient's potential reaction to the initial traumatic event leading to disfigurement, loss of function, or in most cases to the loss of the limb (amputation) [4, 112–115]. The pre- and post-transplant psychosocial assessment should evaluate for PTSD resulting from the traumatic hand loss or after limb transplantation [3, 5, 15, 50]. Additionally, it is widely accepted that several psychosocial and medical risk factors, including exposure to immunosuppressive agents and lengthy recoveries leading to disruption of usual routines and employment, place transplant patients at higher risk for the development of depressive symptoms, anxiety, or regression [11].

Psychosocial Contraindications

Neuroplasticity, the human brain's ability to recognize itself by forming new neural connections throughout life, allows most VCA patients to adapt to major changes in their body and lives. Absolute psychosocial barriers are relatively uncommon in limb transplantation. Instead, we should focus on relative contraindications that require comprehensive evaluation. Furthermore, the psychosocial evaluation should identify potential vulnerabilities stemming from the patients' psychosocial risks that will necessitate supportive treatment. A number of modifiable risk factors for potential poor outcome can be treated prior to transplant and produce a meaningful remission of symptoms (e.g., anxiety or affective disorder). Chronic psychiatric conditions (e.g., schizophrenia, personality disorders, substance use disorders, etc.) may be more challenging, but careful evaluation and intensification of treatment may lead to well-selected patients achieving good outcomes. A one-time evaluation may be insufficient to assess severe chronic conditions. Decisions should be based on a comprehensive interdisciplinary evidence-based evaluation. In general, decisions for rejecting or accepting a limb candidate should be made on a "case-by-case basis" (e.g., evaluation of the individual psychosocial history, with collateral history from the spouse or significant other). Use of psychometric instruments may be helpful, but they do not predict outcomes. Another way to assess psychological contraindications is to consider the following questions:

- *Is the limb transplant patient sufficiently emotionally stable to cope with stresses which may come up before, during, and after transplantation?*
- *What is the potential for the development of somatization symptoms that could result in high medical resource utilization, prolonged disability, chronic pain, attention seeking, or other secondary gain as a result of undergoing an elective surgery?*
- *What is the motivation for undergoing limb transplantation, and are the patient's functional and esthetic expectations realistic?*
- *Is the patient prepared to handle the medical complications that she/he might experience?*

Pain Related to Amputation and Phantom Limb Pain

Assessment for chronic pain issues and exposure to opioid medications are important since a number of these patients may have phantom limb pain which may persist after transplantation. Fortunately, only a small number of patients are suffering from post-transplant phantom pain. Somatosensory cortical reorganization helps to immediately recognize the transplanted limb [116]. Consideration of pain rehabilitation approaches and non-opioid strategies is important since the patients could be at risk of opioid dependence which would complicate their recovery due to rebound pain, drug-seeking behavior, and possible cognitive effects.

Risk-Benefit Considerations

The risk-benefit ratio for limb transplantation is quite different than SOT, where the risks are offset by the life-saving nature of the procedure [3, 49, 67]. Limb transplant patients may overestimate the benefits of the procedure while not fully acknowledging the surgical risk, the demanding post-transplant medication regimen, and long-term rehabilitation [3, 83–85, 88, 91]. The lengthy rehabilitation with little initial functional or sensory improvement and consequences of nonspecific immunosuppression [88, 117] may lead to demoralization and nonadherence resulting in compromised outcomes [118]. In addition, subjective QOL outcomes must be weighed against the surgical procedure with medical risks [67, 86]. Thus, relevant QOL factors, including functional improvement, sense of identity, and risk tolerance for a non-life-saving procedure [88], contribute to risk-versus-benefit decisions which need to be grounded in a personal frame of reference [83–87].

Although immunoregulatory protocols continue to be developed with reduced toxicity [119], limb transplant patients face potential episodes of acute rejection [120] and immunosuppression-related complications. According to the data of the IRHCTT, the rejection rates of limb and face transplantations are about 85% in the first post-transplant year, and three recipients have died [17, 121]. Seven hand grafts were lost due to rejection in China [17, 122], and a similar number have been lost to rejection and other complications in European and American experience [17, 121–124]. Although rejection was often detected and treated without loss of graft, chronic allograft rejection is still the primary cause of long-term allograft failure [17, 120–122].

Immunosuppression-related complications are frequent but often reversed with proper medical treatment [121, 122]. Long-term side effects of immunosuppressive treatment include infection, metabolic derangements [9, 99, 125, 126], toxicity [99, 100, 127, 128], and cancer [9, 99, 100, 127–129]. The psychological status of limb transplant patients may be influenced by long-term side effects of immunosuppression. Effects of rejection episodes and delayed function or difficulties with the rehabilitation may cause anxiety and depression that can impact patients' adherence and require supportive treatment.

In summary, patients have different risk thresholds which contribute to their decision-making about how much risk they are willing to accept for improved function [83–87]

and QOL [88]. The risk versus benefit decisions have to be judged on wider criteria that must include all relevant psychosocial aspects of limb transplantation [89], necessitating rigorous patient selection and ongoing adherence assessment [80].

Tools for the Psychosocial Evaluation

Psychometric Screening

An overview of the different psychometric screening protocols in limb transplantation by Kumnig et al. [49] summarizes the various protocols and associated instruments previously reported. Practitioners may employ a variety of psychometric instruments to complement their clinical evaluation, and the use of psychometric instruments has been reported in about half of the published cases with variability in instruments used [49]. The weight which the instruments carry in their clinical decision-making is also variable. There is no international consensus on which instruments to use [49, 51].

The Chauvet research group, a multidisciplinary, international group focusing on VCA psychosocial evaluation and research, has convened two meetings to explore standardization of the VCA assessment and follow-up care [3]. Creating a screening instrument customized for these patients is a goal for the field [49, 130]. This collaborative approach is just a starting place for better understanding VCA patients, and this initiative hopefully will advance with the participation from multiple centers culminating in VCA-specific instruments not currently in existence [51].

In addition, the Chauvet research group compiled a list of validated psychometric instruments used by transplant centers to assess the following psychosocial domains [16] (see Table 35.1).

Interview Guidelines and Qualitative Assessment Procedures

International consensus exists for the primary importance of the clinical interview in the psychosocial assessment of limb transplant patients [15, 16]. A structured clinical interview ensures the evaluation of key psychosocial domains in limb transplantation [5] and identification of patients who most likely will comply with the rigorous pre- and post-transplant course [5]. It also facilitates the investigation of psychosocial factors in limb transplantation [156, 157].

Kumnig and colleagues [49] review the different interview protocols and qualitative research strategies used in assessing patients undergoing limb transplantation. In this report, a diagnostic clinical interview was part of the psychosocial assessment in 11 published papers. Additionally, other papers describe the use of the diagnostic interview and complementary psychometric testing as part of the psychosocial

Table 35.1 The most common tests used as psychometric instruments of psychosocial evaluation before and after limb transplantation

Psychosocial domain	Psychometric instruments
Depression	PHQ-9 by [131] Self-report depression scale for research in the general population (CES-D) by [132] BDI-II by [133]
Anxiety	GAD-7 by [134] BAI by [135] HADS by [136]
Quality of life	SF-36/SF-12 health survey by [137, 138] SWLS by [139] Q-LES-Q by [140]
Personality	MMPI by [141] NEO-PI-R by [142] PAI by [143] STAI by [144] SCID-II by [145] GSES by [146] PCS by [147]
Body image	RSES by [148] SSES by [149] MCSD by [150] MBA by [151] DAS-59 by [152] BES by [153]
Traumatic reactions	PSS-SR by [154] COPE inventory by [155]

PHQ-9 patient health questionnaire, *BDI-II* beck depression inventory, *GAD-7* generalized anxiety disorder questionnaire, *BAI* beck anxiety inventory, *HADS* hospital anxiety and depression scale, *SWLS* satisfaction with life scale, *Q-LES-Q* quality of life enjoyment and satisfaction questionnaire, *MMPI* minnesota multiphasic personality inventory, *NEO-PI-R* NEO personality inventory-revised, *PAI* personality assessment inventory, *STAI* state-trait anxiety inventory, *SCID-II* structured clinical interview for DSM-IV, *GSES* generalized self-efficacy scale, *PCS* perceived competence scale, *MCSD* multicultural social desirability, *GSES* generalized self-efficacy scale, *PCS* perceived competence scale, *RSES* rosenberg self-esteem scale, *SSES* self-esteem scale, *MBA* measure of body apperception, *DAS-59* derriford appearance scale, *BES* body esteem scale, *PSS-SR* PTSD symptom scale

assessment [158, 159]. A limited number of transplant centers use projective testing, including the Rorschach and the Thematic Apperception Test or the Draw-A-Person test [160]. Overall, most pre-transplant assessments and post-transplant progress are primarily evaluated by clinical observations and interviews [49].

Technical/Anatomic Issues

Unilateral Versus Bilateral

In addition to psychosocial factors that motivate patients to undergo limb transplantation, technical/anatomic issues, including bilateral or unilateral impairment and native or accidental loss of limb, may influence patients' decision-making process [5]. Patients with unilateral limb loss generally report difficulties with coping and psychological burden as a primary motivation for transplantation, as opposed to

bilateral amputees who are motivated by the need for increased function. Additionally, unilateral amputees are more risk-adverse group possibly because they must balance the transplant risks against the more limited functional benefits to be derived from an additional transplanted hand [87]. The risk threshold changes substantially in cases of bilateral hand amputees who experience significantly greater functional limitations and may be willing to accept the risk of rejection which is offset by the potential for significantly enhanced independence [3, 87]. Post-transplant, recipients of unilateral limb transplant report more difficulties with coping and psychosocial issues, compared to bilateral amputees. In cases of bilateral amputees, all sensory feedback has been lost for these patients, so it may not be sufficient to replace motor skills with a prosthesis; thus the benefit of restoring sensation and functional improvement may outweigh the risk of lifelong immunosuppression [18].

The transplant team needs to be attuned to the significance of the loss of function and expectations for improvement to offset risks from the transplant regimen [119, 122]. In addition, peer education between transplantation candidates and patients who have already undergone unilateral versus bilateral limb transplantation is important to help the candidates in their decision-making process [5, 161, 162].

Recent Injury Versus Chronic Impairment

When assessing patients for limb transplantation, several issues are unique, for example, differentiating between patients with recent injury and limb loss versus patients with chronic impairment (congenital hand loss or those who may be many years post injury) and have a high level of physical and psychological adaptation [3, 5, 51, 81]. Patients disfigured from birth report less disturbance in body image and better psychosocial adjustment than those disfigured from recent accidental injury [163]. The psychological adaptation process to the limb loss is demonstrated by the patients with congenital deformation who have incorporated their anomaly into their body image, typically habituated to social reactions, and have developed effective coping strategies to manage ADLs [164]. The psychological adaptation for patients who acquire disfigurement later in life often is more challenging, as they have to deal with reactions to the circumstances surrounding the onset (e.g., trauma, disease, accident), the loss of function, and appearance and body image [165].

Informed Consent

Informed consent for VCA recipients is a detailed process focusing on esthetic, functional, surgical, and post-transplant complications (including immunosuppressive effects and psychiatric disorders) [166–168]. Donor family informed consent also must occur with countries which have an "opt-out" system with implications for how families may experience the donor-related experience. Donor families need to be assured of the dignity that will be afforded to the donor and provided with the opportunity to decide if they wish to meet the recipient or remain anonymous [168].

The transplant center must have all appropriate staff and facilities to provide the care and ensure informed consent and anonymity for deceased donors families and limb transplant recipients [50].

Bioethical Considerations

Bioethical issues are myriad, and collaborating with biomedical ethics experts helps guide the technical and psychosocial challenges in modern limb transplant programs [3, 88]. The ethical principle of non-maleficence supports limited risk to patients and is balanced by the principle of patient autonomy [86, 167]. It would appear that beneficence and justice are less problematic ethical factors in this population [67]. Furthermore, three important ethical considerations in the ethical guidance process are related to ensuring appropriate patient selection, patient advocacy, and informed consent [166].

Bioethical issues in limb transplantation are quite complex [88] and may have an impact on patients' post-transplant motivation to go on with long-term rehabilitation and immunosuppressive treatment [169, 170]. The biomedical ethics consultation should be available on a case-by-case basis [67].

Financial Support

For VCA transplantation to be successful, the patient and his family must have sufficient financial resources to manage time off work, travel to the transplant center, housing, and post-transplant immunosuppressive medication. In addition, access to transportation is key to be able to attend therapy appointments and post-transplant visits to monitor for rejection and other complications. Family support in problem-solving related to financial issues and logistical support is an important aspect of addressing these concerns.

Ability to Tolerate Loss of Function

Following upper extremity transplantation, patients will have a lengthy recovery and initially experience decreased function due to the lack of nerve regeneration in the transplanted limb. The recovery process is gradual, and patients must be able to tolerate an initial loss of function while undergoing an intensive rehabilitation process. Family support during this time is essential, and the patient's innate psychological resilience will support their ability to tolerate this period of time. Coping characteristics such as optimism, problem-solving, flexibility, humor, and acceptance are of great benefit. The ability to develop a strong working relationship with the physical and occupational therapy teams is essential, and the mental health providers may need to interact with and support the physical therapy team during this process.

Media Interest

Upper extremity transplantation is a relatively recent and highly visual form of transplantation which has resulted in significant media interest. Maintaining patient confidentiality is challenging because friends and acquaintances of the recipients will become aware of the transplant. In the age of social media, the story can be quickly circulated beyond the transplant center. Teams should prepare the patient for the possibility of media awareness of the transplant and develop a plan for managing this which respects the patient's desires for privacy while providing support for a well-crafted media plan that decreases the possibility for intrusive media attention.

Donor Family Contact

Contact with the donor family is a highly personal decision between the donor and recipient. As in solid organ transplantation, some donor families wish to remain anonymous as do recipients. Utilizing knowledgeable social work staff who have experience with this interaction from their work with the solid organ population can be invaluable. Identifiers such as tattoos may increase the risk of the donor being identifiable, and as yet no clear guidelines exist about how best to address donor family privacy concerns in this setting. All parties will need to have realistic expectations about the possibility that the media or others may be able to identify both the donor and recipient due to the highly visible nature of upper extremity transplantation.

Conclusions

Hand and upper extremity transplantation has proven to be an option for the restoration of functional, sensory, and esthetic modalities following limb loss. Patients need to carefully weigh potential benefits against the risks imposed by a lifetime commitment to immunosuppressive medications. Patients with bilateral amputation may gain more functionally from upper extremity transplantation and additionally benefit from the restoration of sensation, compared to recipients of unilateral transplantation. VCA-related quality of life and psychosocial scales have yet to be developed, but utilizing experience gained with SOT and modifying existing semi-structured interviews to capture the unique facets of VCA allow for a reasonable, comprehensive evaluation process. Multicenter, collaborative research protocols will allow for adequate enrollment of subjects to advance our understanding of the important predictors of optimal outcomes following hand and upper extremity VCA.

References

1. Dubernard JM. Hand and face allografts: myth, dream, and reality. Proc Am Philos Soc. 2011;155:13–22.
2. Foroohar A, Elliott RM, Kim TW, Breidenbach W, Shaked A, Levin LS. The history and evolution of hand transplantation. Hand Clin. 2011;27:405–9.
3. Kumnig M, Jowsey SG, DiMartini A. Psychological aspects of hand transplantation. Curr Opin Organ Transplant. 2014;19(2):188–95.
4. Klapheke MM, Marcell C, Taliaferro G, Creamer B. Psychiatric assessment of candidates for hand transplantation. Microsurgery. 2000;20:453–7.
5. Kumnig M, Jowsey SG, Rumpold G, Weissenbacher A, Hautz T, Engelhardt TO, et al. The psychological assessment of candidates for reconstructive hand transplantation. Transpl Int. 2012;25:573–85.
6. Cherkassky L. A fair trial? Assessment of liver transplant candidates with psychiatric illnesses. J Med Ethics. 2011;37:739–42.
7. Carosella ED, Pradeu T. Transplantation and identity: a dangerous split? The Lancet. 2006;368:183–4.
8. Streisand RM, Rodrigue JR, Sears SF Jr, Perri MG, Davis GL, Banko CG. A psychometric normative database for pre-liver transplantation evaluations: the Florida cohort 1991–1996. Psychosomatics. 1999;40:479–85.
9. Petit F, Minns AB, Dubernard JM, Hettiaratchy S, Lee WP. Composite tissue allotransplantation and reconstructive surgery: first clinical applications. Ann Plast Surg. 2003;237:19–25.
10. Hettiaratchy S, Randolph MA, Andrew Lee WP. Long-term consideration of hand transplantation. Transplantation. [Letter to the Editor]. 2003;75:1605.
11. Dobbels F, Vanhaecke J, Dupont L, Nevens F, Verleden G, Pirenne J, et al. Pretransplant predictors of posttransplant adherence and clinical outcome: an evidence base for pretransplant psychosocial screening. Transplantation. 2009;87:1497–504.
12. Salminger S, Roche AD, Sturma A, Mayer JA, Aszmann OC. Hand transplantation versus hand prosthetics: Pros and Cons. Curr Surg Rep. 2016;4:8.
13. Hautz T, Engelhardt TO, Weissenbacher A, Kumnig M, Zelger B, Rieger M, et al. World experience after more than a decade of clinical hand transplantation: update on the Innsbruck program. Hand Clin. 2011;27:423–31.
14. Hettiaratchy S, Butler PEM. Extending the boundaries of transplantation. BMJ (Clinical research ed). 2003;326:1226–7.
15. Jowsey-Gregoire S, Kumnig M. Standardizing psychosocial assessment for vascularized composite allotransplantation. Curr Opin Organ Transpl. 2016;21(5):530–5.
16. Jowsey-Gregoire S, Kumnig M, Morelon E, Moreno E, Petruzzo P, Seulin C. The Chauvet 2014 meeting report: psychiatric and psychosocial evaluation and outcomes of upper extremity grafted patients. Transplantation. 2016;100(7):1453–9.
17. Petruzzo P, Lanzetta M, Dubernard JM. The international registry on hand and composite tissue transplantation (IRHCTT). Transplantation. 2015;99(Suppl):6S–2.
18. Salminger S, Sturma A, Roche AD, Hruby LA, Paternostro-Sluga T, Kumnig M, et al. Functional and psychosocial outcomes of hand transplantation compared with prosthetic fitting in below-elbow amputees: a multicenter cohort study. PLoS One. 2016;2(11):e0162507.
19. Biddiss EA, Chau TT. Upper limp prosthesis use and abandonment: a survey of the last 25 years. Prosthetics Orthot Int. 2007;31:236–57.
20. Agnew SP, Ko J, De La Garza M, Kuiken T, Dumanian G. Limb transplantation and targeted reinnervation: a practical comparison. J Reconstr Microsurg. 2012;28:63–8.
21. Jablecki J, Kaczmarzyk L, Patrzalek D, Domanasiewicz A, Chelmonski A. A detailed comparison of the functional outcome after mideforearm replantation versus mideforearm transplantation. Transplant Proc. 2009;41:513–6.
22. Graham B, Adkins P, Tsai TM, Firrell J, Breidenbach WC. Major transplantation versus revision amputation and prosthetic fitting in the upper extremity: a late functional outcomes study. J Hand Surg Am. 1998;23:783–9.
23. Peacock K, Tsai TM. Comparison of functional results of replantation versus prosthesis in a patient with bilateral arm amputation. Clin Orthop Relat Res. 1987;214:153–9.
24. Kay S, Wilks D. Invited comment: vascularized composite allotransplantation: an update on medical and surgical progess and remaining challanges. J Plast Reconstr Aesthet Surg. 2013;66:1456–7.
25. Bernardon L, Gazarian A, Petruzzo P, Packham T, Guillot M, Guigal V. Bilateral hand transplantation: functional benefits assessment in five patients with a mean follow-up of 7.6 years (range 4-13 years). J Plast Reconstr Aesthet Surg. 2015;68:1171–83.
26. Weissenbacher A, Hautz T, Pierer G, Ninkovic M, Zelger BG, Zelger B. Hand transplantation in its fourteenth year: the Innsbruck experience. Vasc Compos Allotransplant. 2014;1:11–21.
27. Chung KC, Oda T, Saddawi-Konefka D, Shauver MJ. An economic analysis of hand transplantation in the United States. Plast Reconstr Surg. 2010;125:589–98.
28. Chang J, Mathes DW. Ethical, financial, and policy considerations in hand transplantation. Hand Clin. 2011;27:553–60.
29. Brügger U. Should hand transplantation be reimbursed by a public payer? An up-to-date of a Swiss HTA for decision making in health care. HTAi conference, Seoul; 2013.
30. Tobin GR, Breidenbach WC, Ildstad ST, Marvin MM, Buell JF, Ravindra KV. The history of human composite tissue allotransplantation. Transplant Proc. 2009;41:466–71.
31. Gander B, Brown CS, Vasilic D, Furr A, Banis JCJ, Cunningham M, et al. Composite tissues allotransplantation of the hand and face: a new frontier in transplant and reconstructive surgery. Transpl Int. 2006;19:868–80.
32. Da Varagine J. Leggenda aurea. Florence: Libreria Editrice Fiorentina; 1952.
33. Barker CF, Markmann JF. Historical overview of transplantation. Cold Spring Harb Perspect Med. 2013;3:a014977.
34. Bunger C. Gelungener Versuch einer Nasenbildung aus einem völlig getrennten Hautstuck aus dem Beine. J Chir Augenheilk. 1823;4:569.
35. Carrel A. Landmark article, Nov 14, 1908: results of the transplantation of blood vessels, organs and limbs. JAMA. 1983;250:944–53.
36. Toledo-Pereyra LH. Classics of modern surgery: the unknown man of Alexis carrel– father of transplantation. J Invet Surg. 2003;16:243–6.
37. Guthrie CC. Blood-vessel surgery and its applications. New York: Longman Green; 1912.

38. Whitaker IS, Duggan EM, Alloway RR, Brown C, McGuire S, Woodle ES, et al. Composite tissue allotransplantation: a review of relevant immunological issues for plastic surgeons. J Plast Reconstr Aesthet Surg. 2008;61:481–92.

39. Billingham RE, Brent L, Medawar PB. 'Actively acquired tolerance' of foreign cells. Nat Clin Pract Nephrol. 1953;172:603–6.

40. Starzl TE. Peter Brian Medawar: father of Transplanation. J Am Coll Surg. 1995;180:332–6.

41. Peacock EE. Homologous composite tissue grafts of the digital flexor mechanism in human beings. Transplant Bull. 1960;7:418–21.

42. Peacock EE, Madden JW. Human composite flexor tendon allografts. Ann Surg. 1967;166:624–9.

43. Gilbert R. Transplant is successful with a cadaver forearm. Med Trib Med News. 1964;5:20–3.

44. Dubernard JM, Owen E, Herzberg G. The first transplantation of a hand in humans: early results. Chirurgie. 1999;124:358–65. discussion 65-67

45. Dubernard JM, Owen E, Herzberg G, Lanzetta M, Martin X, Kapila H, et al. Human hand allograft: report on first 6 months. Lancet. 1999;353:1315–20.

46. Dubernard JM, Owen E, Lefrancois N, Petruzzo P, Martin X, Dawahra M, et al. First human hand transplantation. Am J Transplant. 2000;13:S521–S4.

47. Jones JW, Gruber SA, Barker JH, Breidenbach WC, Team FtLHT. Successful hand transplantation: one-year follow-up. N Engl J Med. 2000;343:468–73.

48. Margreiter R, Brandacher G, Ninkovic M, Steurer W, Kreczy A, Schneeberger S. A double-hand transplant can be worth the effort! Transplantation. 2002;74:85–90.

49. Kumnig M, Jowsey SG, Moreno E, Brandacher G, Azari K, Rumpold G. An overview of psychosocial assessment procedures in reconstructive hand transplantation: the past, present, and future in psychosocial assessment of patients undergoing reconstructive hand transplantation. Transpl Int. 2014.; Article first published online: 14 November, 2013.

50. Kumnig M, Jowsey-Gregoire S. Key psychosocial challenges in vascularized composite allotransplantation. World J Transplant. 2014;27(5):417–27.

51. Kumnig M, Jowsey SG. Preoperative psychological evaluation of transplant patients: challenges and solutions. Transplant Res Risk Manag. 2015;7:35–43.

52. Breidenbach WC, Gonzales NR, Kaufman CL, Klapheke M, Tobin GR, Gorantla VS. Outcomes of the first 2 American hand transplants at 8 and 6 years posttransplant. J Hand Surg. 2008;33:1039–47.

53. Breidenbach WC, Tobin GR, Gorantla VS, Gonzalez RN, Granger DK. A position statement in support of hand transplantation. J Hand Surg. 2002;27:760–70.

54. Carta I, Convertino O, Cornaggia CM. Psychological investigation protocol of candidates for hand transplantation. Transplant Proc. 2001;33:621–2.

55. Dubernard JM, Petruzzo P, Lanzetta M, Parmentier H, Martin X, Dawahra M, et al. Functional results of the first humand double-hand transplantation. Ann Surg. 2003;238:128–36.

56. Jablecki J. World experience after more than a decade of clinical hand transplantation: update on the polish program. Hand Clin. 2011;27:433–42.

57. Landin L, Cavadas PC, Nthumba P, Munoz G, Gallego R, Belloch V, et al. Morphological and functional evaluation of visual disturbances in a bilateral hand allograft recipient. J Plast Reconstr Aesthet Surg. 2010;63:700–4.

58. Schuind F, Van Holder C, Mouraux D, Robert C, Meyer A, Salvia P, et al. Le premier cas belge de transplantation de main: Résultat á neuf ans. [The first Belgian hand transplantation case: nine years follow-up.]. Rev Med Brux. 2011;32:S66–70.

59. Schuind F, Van Holder C, Mouraux D, Robert C, Meyer A, Salvia P, et al. The first Belgian hand transplantation – 37 month term results. J Hand Surg. 2006;31:371–6.

60. Zhu L, Pei G, Gu L, Hong J. Psychological consequences derived during process of human hand allograft. Chin Med J. 2002;115:1660–3.

61. Cavadas PC, Landin L, Thione A, Rodríguez-Pérez JC, Garcia-Bello MA, Ibañez J, et al. The Spanish experience with hand, forearm, and arm transplantation. Hand Clin. 2011;27:443–53.

62. Cavadas P, Landin L, Ibanez J. Bilateral hand transplantation: results at 20 months. J Hand Surg. 2009;34E:434–43.

63. Kaufman CL, Blair B, Murphy E, Breidenbach WC. A new option for amputees: transplantation of the hand. J Rehabil Res Dev. 2009;46:395–404.

64. Petruzzo P, Dubernard JM. World experience after more than a decade of clinical transplantation: update on the French program. Hand Clin. 2011;27:411–6.

65. Petruzzo P, Badet L, Gazarian A, Lanzetta M, Parmentier H, Kanitakis J, et al. Bilateral hand transplantation: six years after the first case. Am J Transplant. 2006;6:1718–24.

66. Ravindra KV, Buell JF, Kaufman CL, Blair B, Marvin M, Nagubandi R, et al. Hand transplantation in the United States: experience with 3 patients. Surgery. 2008;144:638–44.

67. Tobin GR, Breidenbach WC, Klapheke MM, Bentley FR, Pidwell DJ, Simmons PD. Ethical considerations in the early composite tissue allograft experience: a review of the Louisville ethics program. Transplant Proc. 2005;37:1392–5.

68. Day E, Best D, Sweeting R, Russell R, Webb K, Georgiou G, et al. Predictors of psychological morbidity in liver transplant assessment candidates: is alcohol abuse or dependence a factor? Transpl Int. 2009;22:606–14.

69. Feurer ID, Russell RT, Pinson CW. Incorporating quality of life and patient satisfaction measures into a transplant outcomes assessment program: technical and practical considerations. Prog Transplant. 2007;17:121–8.

70. Fukunishi I, Sugawara Y, Takayama T, Makuuchi M, Kawarasaki H, Surman OS. Association between pretransplant psychological assessments and posttransplant psychiatric disorders in living-related transplantation. Psychosomatics. 2002;43:49–54.

71. Mascoloni SE, Marquez MF, Diez M, Berlolotti AM, Favaloro RR. Pretransplant psychological risk evaluation strongly predicts mortality after cardiac transplantation. J Heart Lung Transplant. 2006;25:S153–S.

72. Owen JE, Bonds CL, Wellisch DK. Psychiatric evaluations of heart transplant candidates: predicting post-transplant hospitalizations, rejection episodes, and survival. Psychosomatics. 2006;47:213–22.

73. Pascher A, Sauer IM, Walter M, Lopez-Haeninnen E, Theruvath T, Spinelli A, et al. Donor evaluation, donor risks, donor outcome, and donor quality of life in adult-to-adult living donor liver transplantation. Liver Transpl. 2002;8:829–37.

74. Sainz-Barriga M, Baccarani U, Scudeller L, Risaliti A, Toniutto PL, Costa MG, et al. Quality-of-life assessment before and after liver transplantation. Transplant Proc. 2005;37:2601–4.

75. von Steinbuchel N, Limm H, Leopold C, Carr D. Assessment of health-related quality-of-life in patients after heart transplantation under therapy with tacrolimus or cyclosporine. Transpl Int. 2000;13(Suppl 1):S609–14.

76. Ziegelmann JP, Griva K, Hankins M, Harrison M, Davenport A, Thompson D, et al. The Transplant Effects Questionnaire (TxEQ): the development of a ques-tionnaire for assessing the multidimensional outcome of organ transplantation – example of end stage renal diseases (ESRD). Br J Health Psychol. 2002;7:393–408.

77. Bunzel B, Laederach-Hofman K. Solid organ transplantation: are there predictors for post-transplant noncompliance? A literature review. Transplantation. 2000;70:711–6.

78. Goetzman L, Scheuer E, Naef R. Psychosocial situation and physical health in 50 patients > 1 year after lung transplantation. Chest. 2005;127:166–70.

79. Schwartzer R. Self-efficacy in the adoption and maintenance of health behaviours: theoretical approaches and a new model. In: Schwartzer R, editor. Self-efficacy: thought control of action. Washington, DC: Hemisphere; 1992. p. 217–43.

80. Schneeberger S, Landin L, Jableki J, Butler P, Hoehnke C, Brandacher G, et al. Achievements and challenges in composite tissue allotransplantation. Transpl Int. 2011;24:760–9.

81. Clarke A, Butler PEM. Face transplantation: psychological assessment and preparation for surgery. Psychol Health Med. 2004;9(3):315–26.

82. Rumsey N, Harcourt D. Body image and disfigurement: issues and interventions. Body Image. 2004;1:83–97.

83. Barker JH, Allen F, Cunningham M, Basappa PS, Wiggins O, Banis JC, et al. Risk assessment and management in hand and facial tissue transplantation. Eur J Trauma. 2011;37:469–76.

84. Brouha P, Naidu D, Cunningham M, Furr A, Majzoub R, Grossi FV, et al. Risk acceptance in composite-tissue allotransplantation reconstructive procedures. Microsurgery. 2006;26:144–50.

85. Cunningham M, Majzoub R, Brouha PCR, Laurentin-Perez LA, Naidu DK, Maldonado C, et al. Risk acceptance in composite tissue allotransplantation reconstructive procedures: instrument design and validation. Eur J Trauma. 2004;30:12–6.

86. Lanzetta M, Nolli R, Borgonovo A, Owen ER, Dubernard JM, Kapila H, et al. Hand transplantation: ethics, immunosuppression and indications. J Hand Surg. 2001;26:511–6.

87. Majzoub RK, Cunningham M, Grossi F, Maldonado C, Banis JC, Barker JH. Investigation of risk acceptance in hand transplantation. J Hand Surg Am. 2006;31A:295–302.

88. Simmons PD. Ethical considerations in composite tissue allotransplantation. Microsurgery. 2000;20:458–65.

89. Balasubramanian G, McKitty K, Fan SLS. Comparing automated peritoneal dialysis with continuous ambulatory peritoneal dialysis: survival and quality of life differences? Nephrol Dial Transplant. 2011;26:1702–8.

90. Sawer DB. Cosmetic surgery and changes in body image. In: Cash TF, Pruzinsky T, editors. Body image: a handbook of theory, research, and clinical practice. New York: Guilford; 2002. p. 422–30.

91. Sicard D. Ethical aspects of non-life-saving allografts with special regard to the hand. In: Lanzetta M, Dubernard JM, Petruzzo P, editors. Hand transplantation. Milan: Springer; 2011. p. 107–9.

92. Timmers L, Thong M, Dekker FW, Boeschoten EW, Heijmans M, Rijken M, et al. Illness perceptions in dialysis patients and their association with quality of life. Psychol Health. 2008;23(6):679–90.

93. Ginieri-Coccosso M, Theofilou P, Synodinou C, Tomaras V, Soldatos C. Quality of life, mental health and health beliefs in haemodialysis and peritoneal dialysis patients: investigating differences in early and later years of current treatment. BMC Nephrol. 2008;9:14–22.

94. Christensen A, Ehlers S. Psychological factors in end-stage renal disease: an emerging context for behavioral medicine research. J Consult Clin Psychol. 2002;70:712–24.

95. Griffin KW, editor. Comparison of quality of life in haemodialysis and peritoneal dialysis patients. Toronto: Peritoneal Dialysis Publications; 1994.

96. Fiebiger W, Mitterbauer C, Oberbauer R. Health-related quality of life outcomes after kidney transplantation. Health Qual Life Outcomes. 2004;2:2.

97. Neipp M, Karavul B, Jackobs S, Meyer zu Vilsendorf A, Richter N, Becker T. Quality of life in adult transplant recipients more than 15 years after kidney transplantation. Transplantation. 2006;81:1640–4.

98. Perlman RL, Finkelstein FO, Liu L, Roys E, Kiser M, Eisele G, et al. Quality of life in chronic kidney disease (CKD): a cross-sectional analysis in the renal research Institute-CKD study. Am J Kidney Dis. 2005;45:658–66.

99. Hautz T, Brandacher G, Zelger B, Gorantla VS, Lee AWP, Pratschke J, et al. Immunologic aspects and rejection in solid organ versus reconstructive transplantation. Transplant Proc. 2010;42:3347–53.

100. Ravindra K, Wu S, McKinney M, Xu H, Ildstad ST. Composite tissue allotransplantation: current challenges. Transplant Proc. 2009;41:3519–28.

101. NICE. Peritoneal dialysis: peritoneal dialysis in the treatment of stage 5 chronic kidney disease. London: Centre for Clinical Practice at NICE; 2011. [February 24, 2014]; Available from: www.nice.org.uk/guidance/CG125

102. Tong A, Hanson CS, Chapman JR, Halleck F, Budde K, Papachristou C, et al. The preferences and perspectives of nephrologists on patients' access to kidney transplantation: a systematic review. Transplantation. 2014;15:682–91.

103. Kimmel P. Psychosocial factors in dialysis patients. Kidney Int. 2001;59:1599–613.

104. Kutner NG, Johansen KL, Kaysen GA, Pederson S, Chen S, Agodoa LY, et al. The comprehensive dialysis study (CDS): a USRDS special study. Clin J Am Soc Nephrol. 2009;4:645–50.

105. Dew MA, Switzer GE, DiMartini A, Myaskovsky L, Crowley-Matoka M. Psychosocial aspects of living organ donation. In: Tan HP, Marcos A, Shapiro R, editors. Living donor transplantation. New York: Informa Healthcare; 2007. p. 7–26.

106. Lukasczik M, Neuderth S, Köhn D, Faller H. Psychologische Aspekte der Lebendnierenspende und -transplantation: Ein Überblick zum aktuellen Forschungsstand. Z Med Psychol. 2008;17:107–23.

107. Klapheke MM. Transplantation of the human hand: psychiatric considerations. Bull Menn Clin. 1999 Spr;63(2):159–173.

108. Bradbury E. The psychological and social impact of disfigurement to the hand in children and adolescents. Dev Neurorehabil. 2007;10:143–8.

109. Rumsey N. Body image and congenital conditions with visible differences. In: Cash TF, Pruzinsky T, editors. Body image: a handbook of theory, research, and clinical practice. New York: Guilford; 2002. p. 226–33.

110. Rumsey N. Optimizing body image in disfiguring congenital conditions. In: Cash TF, Pruzinsky T, editors. Body image: a handbook of theory, research, and clinical practice. New York: Guilford; 2002. p. 431–9.

111. De Pasquale C, Pistorio ML, Sorbello M, Parrinello L, Corona D, Gagliano M, et al. Body image in kidney transplantation. Transplant Proc. 2010;42:1123–6.

112. Schley MT, Wilms P, Toepfner S, Schaller HP, Schmelz M, Konrad CJ, et al. Painful and nonpainful phantom and stump sensations in acute traumatic amputees. J Trauma. 2008;65:858–64.

113. Meyer TM. Psychological aspects of mutilating hand injuries. Hand Clin. 2003;19:41–9.

114. Zeiler K. Ethics and organ transfer: a Merleau-Pontean perspective. Health Care Anal. 2009;17:110–22.

115. Lanzetta M, Petruzzo P, Vitale G, Lucchina S, Owen ER, Dubernard JM, et al. Human hand transplantation: what have we learned? Transplant Proc. 2004;36:664–8.

116. Frey S, Bogdanov S, Smith JC, Watrous S, Breidenbach WC. Chronically deafferented sensory cortex recovers a grossly typical organization after allogenic hand transplantation. Curr Biol. 2008;18:1530–4.

117. Kalluri HV, Hardinger KL. Current state of renal transplant immunosuppression: present and future. World J Transplant. 2012;24:51–68.

118. Baylis F. A face is not just like a hand: pace barker. Am J Bioeth. 2004;4:30–2.

119. Shores JT, Imbriglia JE, Lee WPA. The current state of hand transplantation. J Hand Surg. 2011;36:1862–7.

120. Brenner MJ, Tung TH, Jensen JN, Mackinnon SE. The spectrum of complications of immunosuppression: is the time right for hand transplantation? J Bone Joint Surg Am. 2002;84:1861–70.

121. IRHCTT. International registry on hand composite tissue transplantation. 2013 [November 27, 2013]; Available from: http://www.handregistry.com/.

122. Petruzzo P, Lanzetta M, Dubernard JM, Margreiter R, Schuind F, Breidenbach WC, et al. The international registry on hand and composite tissue transplantation. Transplantation. 2010;90:1590–4.

123. Kanitakis J, Jullien D, Petruzzo P, Hakim N, Claudy A, Revillard JP, et al. Clinicopathologic features of graft rejection of the first human hand allograft. Transplantation. 2003;76:688.

124. Landin L, Cavadas PC, Ibanez J, Roger I. Malignant skin tumor in a composite tissue (bilateral hand) allograft recipient. Plast Reconstr Surg. 2010;125:20e–1e.

125. Lanzetta M, Petruzzo P, Margreiter R, Dubernard JM, Schuind F, Breidenbach WC, et al. The international registry on hand and composite tissue transplantation. Transplantation. 2005;79:1210–4.

126. Lanzetta M, Petruzzo P, Dubernard JM, Margreiter R, Schuind F, Breidenbach WC, et al. Second report (1998-2006) of the international registry of hand and composite tissue transplantation. Transpl Immunol. 2007;18:1–6.

127. Wu S, Xu H, Ravindra K, Ildstad ST. Composite tissue allotransplantation: past, present and future-the history and expanding applications of CTA as a new frontier in transplantation. Transplant Proc. 2009;41:463–5.

128. Hettiaratchy S, Randolph MA, Petit F, Lee AWP, Butler PEM. Composite tissue allotransplantation: a new era in plastic surgery? Br Assoc Plast Surg. 2004;57:381–91.

129. Thaunat O, Badet L, El-Jaafari A, Kanitakis J, Dubernard JM, Morelon E. Composite tissue allograft extends a helping hand to transplant immunologists. Am J Transplant. 2006;6:2238–42.

130. Papachristu P. Strategies for psychiatric-psychosomatic evaluation of organ donors and recipients: the European experience. J Psychosom Res. 2013;74:555.

131. Spitzer RL, Kroenke K, Williams JB. Validation and utility of a self-report version of PRIME-MD: the PHQ primary care study. Primary care evaluation of mental disorders. Patient health questionnaire. JAMA. 1999;282:1737–44.

132. Radloff LS, Radloff LS. The CES-D scale: a self report depression scale for research in the general population. Appl Psychol Meas. 1977;1:385–401.

133. Beck AT, Steer RA, Brown GK. Manual for the beck depression inventory-II. San Antonio: Psychological Corporation; 1996.

134. Spitzer RL, Kroenke K, Williams JB. A brief measure for assessing generalized anxiety disorder: the GAD-7. Arch Intern Med. 2006;166:1092–7.

135. Beck AT, Steer RA. Beck anxiety inventory manual. San Antonio: Harcourt Brace and Company; 1993.

136. Zigmond AS, Snaith RP. The hospital anxiety and depression scale. Acta Psychiatr Scan. 1983;67:631–370.

137. Ware JE, Kosinski M, Keller SD. A 12-item short-form health survey: construction of scales and preliminary tests of reliability and validity. Med Care. 1996;34:220–33.

138. Ware JE, Sherbourne CD. The MOS 36-item short-form health survey (SF-36). I. Conceptual framework and item selection. Med Care. 1992;30:473–83.

139. Diener E, Emmons RA, Larsen RJ, Griffin S. The satisfaction with life scale. J Pers Assess. 1985;49:71–5.

140. Endicott J, Nee J, Harrison W, Blumenthal R. Quality of life enjoyment and satisfaction questionnaire: a new measure. Psychopharmacol Bull. 1993;29:321–6.

141. Hathaway SR, McKinley JC. The Minnesota multiphasic personality inventory. Minneapolis: University of Minnesota Press; 1943.

142. Costa PTJ, McCrae RR. Domains and facets: hierarchical personality assessment using the revised NEO personality inventory. J Pers Assess. 1995;64:21–50.

143. Morey LC. The personality assessment inventory professional manual. Lutz: Psychological Assessment Resources; 2007.

144. Spielberger CD, Gorsuch RL, Lushene R, Vagg PR, Jacobs GA. Manual for the state-trait anxiety inventory. Palo Alto: Consulting Psychologists Press; 1983.

145. First MB, Gibbon M, Spitzer RL, Williams JBW, Benjamin LS. Structured clinical interview for DSM-IV axis II personality disorders, (SCID-II). Washington, DC: American Psychiatric Press Inc; 1997.

146. Schwarzer R, Jerusalem M. Generalized self-efficacy scale. In: Weinman J, Wright S, Johnston M, editors. Measures in health psychology: a user's portfolio causal and control beliefs. Windsor: Nfer-Nelson; 1995. p. 35–7.

147. Williams GC, Deci EL. Internalization of biopsychosocial values by medical students: a test of self-determination theory. J Pers Soc Psychol. 1996;70:767–79.

148. Rosenberg M. Society and the adolescent self-image. Princeton: Princeton University Press; 1995.

149. Heatherton TF, Polivy J. Development and validation of a scale for measuring state self-esteem. J Pers Soc Psychol. 1991;60:895–910.

150. Constantine MG, Ladany N. Self-report multicultural counseling competence scales: their relation to social desirability attitudes and multicultural case conceptualizationability. J Couns Psychol. 2000;47:155–64.

151. Carver CS, Pozo-Kaderman C, Price AA, Noriega V, Harris SD, Derhagopian RP, et al. Concern about aspects of body image and adjustment to early stage breast cancer. Psychosom Med. 1998;60:168–74.

152. Carr T, Harris D, James C. The Derriford Appearance Scale (DAS-59): a new scale to measure individual responses to living with problems of appearance. Br J Health Psychol. 2000;5:201–15.

153. Franzoi SL, Shields SA. The body-esteem scale: multidimensional structure and sex differences in a college population. J Pers Assess. 1984;48:173–8.

154. Foa EB, Cashman L, Jaycox L. The validation of a self-report measure of posttraumatic stress disorder: the posttraumatic diagnostic scale. Psychol Assess. 1997;9:445–51.

155. Carver CS, Scheier MF, Weintraub JK. Assessing coping strategies: a theoretically based approach. J Pers Soc Psychol. 1989;56:267–83.

156. Mori DL, Klein W, Gallagher P. Validity of the MMPI-2 and Beck depression inventory for making decisions of organ allocation in renal transplantation. Psychol Rep. 1999;84:114–6.

157. Twillman RK, Manetto C, Wellisch DK, Wolcott DL. The transplant evaluation rating scale: a revision of the psychosocial levels system for evaluating organ transplant candidates. Psychosomatics. 1993;34:144–53.

158. Hautz T, Brandacher G, Engelhardt TO, Pierer G, Lee WPA, Pratschke J, et al. How reconstructive transplantation is different from organ transplantation – and how it is not. Transplant Proc. 2011;43:3504–11.

159. Gordon CR, Siemionow M. Requirements for the development of a hand transplantation program. Ann Plast Surg. 2009;63:262–73.

160. Goodenough F. Measurement of intelligence by drawings. New York: World Book Co; 1926.

161. Brunier G, Graydon J, Rothman B, Sherman C, Liadsky R. The psychological Well-being of renal peer support volunteers. J Adv Nurs. 2002;38:40–9.

162. Petrie K. Psychological well-being and psychiatric disturbance in dialysis and renal transplant patients. Br J Med Psychol. 1989;62:91–6.

163. Newell R. Body image and disfigurement care. London: Routledge; 2000a.

164. Newell R, Marks M. Evaluation of self-help leaflet in treatment of social difficulties following facial disfigurement. Int J Nurs Stud. 2000b;37:381–8.

165. Bradbury E. Understanding the problems. In: Lansdown R, Rumsey N, Bradburry E, Carr T, Partridge J, editors. Visibly different: coping with disfigurement. Oxford: Butter-worth-Heinemann; 1997. p. 180–93.

166. Bramstedt KA. Informed consent for facial transplantation. In: Siemionow M, editor. The know how of facial transplantation. London: Springer; 2011. p. 255–60.

167. Siemionow M, Coffman KL. Ethics of facial transplantation revisited. Curr Opin Organ Transpl. 2014;19:181–7.

168. Dickenson H. Ethical issues in limb transplants. Postgrad Med J. 1999;75:513–5.

169. Siegler M. Ethical issues in innovative surgery: should we attempt a cadaveric hand transplantation in a human subject? Transplant Proc. 1998;30:2779–82.

170. Moore FD. Three ethical revolutions ancient assumptions remodeled under pressure of transplantation. Transplant Proc. 1988;20:1061–7.

Psychological and Psychosocial Aspects of Uterine and Penile Transplantation

36

Andrea Ament and Sheila G. Jowsey-Gregoire

Introduction

The first successful organ transplant occurred in 1954: a kidney transplanted from a living donor. The 1960s brought a number of other successful organ transplants, including the liver, heart, and pancreas. Successful lung and intestine transplants occurred in the 1980s [1]. As advances in immunosuppression have decreased the rates of organ rejection, the opportunity to transplant non-vital organs has expanded; these non-vital organ transplants include hand, face, lower extremity, uterine, and penile, collectively known as vascularized composite allotransplantation (VCA).

History of Uterine Transplantation

Efforts to address female infertility have been a source of research for decades. For women who are unable to conceive or birth a child with current fertility treatments (i.e., hormonal therapies, intrauterine insemination, and in vitro fertilization), available options for child-rearing include gestational surrogate carrier, adoption, and fostering. Absolute uterine factor infertility (AUFI) affects 1/500 women worldwide [2], and for these women who wish to have children, only adoption and surrogacy are available. For women who are unable or prefer not to utilize these options, uterine transplant has become an emerging reality (see Table 36.1). Research into the viability of uterine trans-

Table 36.1 Uterine transplantation indications

The desire to carry and give birth to a child when unable to for the following indications
Hysterectomy
Postpartum hemorrhage
Multiple myomas
Cervical/uterine cancer
Multiple fibroids
Severe adenomyosis
Fibrous adhesions
Prior radiotherapy
Uterine malformation
Uterine agenesis (Mayer-Rokitansky-Küster-Hauser syndrome) 1/4500 women
Uterine hypoplasia
Countries where surrogacy and/or adoption are heavily restricted/prohibited
Sweden, Japan, Turkey, and Egypt, for example
Gestational surrogacy legal in only six European countries and illegal in five US states
Russia, Vietnam, and African countries restricting international adoption
Future theoretical considerations
Male-to-female transgender reassignment surgery

plantation in rats and nonhuman primates has been documented since the 1960s, with the first described rat pregnancy after allogenic uterus transplantation published in 2010 [3]. Report of the first successful human uterus transplantation was published in 2002, a case which involved a 26-year-old female recipient who lost her uterus to postpartum hemorrhage and a 46-year-old donor; the recipient developed acute vascular thrombosis 3 months after surgery, requiring hysterectomy [4]. The second case came in 2013, which also included the first clinical pregnancy via embryo transfer, 18 months after a 23-year-old female with Rokitansky syndrome (i.e., genetic disorder with underdevelopment or absence of vagina and uterus) was transplanted with a deceased donor uterus [5]. This pregnancy miscarried at 6 weeks gestation.

A Swedish group, led by Mats Brännström, published the first clinical trial of uterine transplantation in 2014, which

A. Ament (✉)
Department of Psychiatry and Behavioral Sciences, Stanford University, Stanford, CA, USA
e-mail: aament@stanford.edu

S. G. Jowsey-Gregoire
Mayo Graduate School of Medicine, Department of Psychiatry and Psychology and Department of Surgery, Mayo Clinic Rochester, Rochester, MN, USA
e-mail: Jowsey-Gregoire.Sheila@mayo.edu

© Springer International Publishing AG, part of Springer Nature 2019
Y. Sher, J. R. Maldonado (eds.), *Psychosocial Care of End-Stage Organ Disease and Transplant Patients*,
https://doi.org/10.1007/978-3-319-94914-7_36

included nine women who received uteri from live donors [6]. Two women required hysterectomy within the first few months, while seven women were able to achieve regular menstruation during the first year, with occasional subclinical rejection that was effectively treated with immunosuppressant therapy. In 2015, the same group published the landmark case of the first live birth after uterus transplant, in which a 35-year-old woman with Rokitansky syndrome received a uterus from a living 61-year-old two-parous donor who was a close family friend of the recipient. The recipient underwent in vitro fertilization with single-embryo transfer 1 year after transplantation, which resulted in a viable pregnancy. She continued immunosuppression while pregnant, and a course of corticosteroids for an episode of rejection while pregnant. The pregnancy ultimately resulted in the birth of a male baby with normal APGAR scores at 31 weeks gestation after caesarian section due to preeclampsia and abnormal cardiotocography [2]. The first uterine transplant in the United States was at the Cleveland Clinic in 2016, with a 26-year-old receiving a deceased donor uterus – the uterus had to be removed within a month after the transplant due to a Candidal infection. As of March 2018, 26 women have received a uterine transplantation, with 7 documented live births. The two most recent live births resulting from uterine transplantation have occurred in November 2017 and February 2018 at Baylor University Medical Center – both were from living donors, one of whom was nondirected.

Differences Between VCA and Solid Organ Transplantation

Different from solid organ transplantation, VCA involves transplantation with tissues of composite organs, including the skin, muscle, bone, vessels, and nerves, which make them immunologically complex [7]. The other fundamental difference between solid organ transplantation and VCA (including uterine and penile transplantation) is that the purpose of VCA is to enhance function and/or quality of life; the procedure is *not* required to save life, as in the case of solid organ transplantation. As such, implications of risk-benefit for VCA are different than for solid organ transplants. Both VCA and solid organ transplants require long-term immunosuppression for the survival of the graft – a treatment that comes with potentially significant adverse effects: this calls into question the ethical balance of proceeding with these procedures which are *life-enhancing*, rather than life-saving. Notably however, uterine transplant is the only transplant that is considered temporary, resulting in temporary exposure to immunosuppressants for the period of time that the recipient wishes to be childbearing.

Unique Factors Driving Needs for Uterine Transplantation

Absolute uterine factor infertility (AUFI) – characterized by any condition that causes congenital/iatrogenic absence or nonfunction of the uterus – affects 1/500 women of childbearing age, which corresponds to 1.5 million women worldwide [2]. Uterine transplantation is the first treatment available for AUFI, causes of which include congenital absence of the uterus (Rokitansky syndrome, aka Mayer-Rokitansky-Küster-Hauser syndrome) which affects 1/4500 women, previous hysterectomy, or severe intrauterine adhesions (see Table 36.1). It is also the first described organ transplant in which the graft is intended to be temporary and thus requires not one but two guaranteed surgeries [2]. Many factors are then involved in the timing of when to remove the organ, from how many pregnancies are desired, to risks and side effects of continued immunosuppression, to the decision-making autonomy of the recipient who is now the recipient of the new organ versus the medical team about eventual removal of the transplanted uterus.

Features of those expressing interest in becoming uterine transplant recipients and donors have been explored by two groups in the United States [8, 9]. Each group had significant interest (>250 potential recipients and 80 potential donors contacted the programs). Of the interested recipients, mean age was around 30-years-old, with about one-third having congenital absence of the uterus (mean age 28) and two-thirds having previous hysterectomy (mean age 33). In both studies, a subset of interested recipients already had one child (17% and 47%, respectively), and >93% of women were married or in a stable relationship. Religion did not appear to be a primary driving factor of interest. In one study, five candidates were male-to-female transgender, and one applicant had an intersex diagnosis. Of the donor candidates, 74% were altruistic/nondirected, mean age was 40, 90% had delivered at least one child, all had completed their own family, and 31% had undergone permanent pregnancy prevention. A study on the public attitudes toward transplantation in the United States showed 74% of 736 women were willing to donate their uterus [10]; a study in the United Kingdom showed that 94% of 528 healthcare professionals supported uterine transplantation [11], and a study in Sweden demonstrated that uterine transplant was felt to be more acceptable than surrogacy [12].

Psychosocial Assessment of Uterine Transplant Recipients

Psychosocial assessment for organ transplantation, though with little formal guidance from UNOS, has become more standardized at transplant centers, with four published psychosocial assessment tools: the Psychosocial Assessment for Candidates of Transplantation (PACT) [13], the Psychosocial Levels System (PLS) [14], the Transplant Evaluation Rating Scale (TERS) [15], and the Stanford Integrated Psychosocial Assessment for Transplantation (SIPAT) [16]. Please see Chap. 3 for the detailed description of psychosocial evaluation of solid organ transplant candidates. Ample evidence exists which demonstrates that psychosocial risk factors have a significant effect on graft outcomes; for example, psychiatric problems after transplantation lead to higher risk of infection, hospital readmissions, and higher medical costs; overall psychosocial risk is associated with number of rejection episodes [16, 17] and post-transplant mortality [18, 19].

A standardized evaluation for organ donors has also been established, called the Live Donor Assessment Tool (LDAT) [20] (See Chap. 4 for more details). As described above, evaluation of both recipients and donors for uterine transplantation adds a unique element to the risk-benefit analysis: both parties undergo substantial risk for procedures that are not required for the life of the recipient. For example, uterine donation from a deceased donor would reduce overall risks and complexity of the surgical procedure; however, thus far only uterine transplants from living donors have been able to result in a live birth. As live birth is the desired outcome driving uterine transplantation, the success rates of live vs deceased donors is an important consideration.

A particularly unique aspect to psychosocial considerations for uterine transplantation is the number of steps required for a "successful" outcome: (1) Identification of a donor, (2) successful transplantation, (3) lack of rejection, (4) successful embryo implantation by in vitro fertilization, (5) pregnancy without miscarriage, and (6) healthy live birth delivery. Additionally, uterine transplantation directly affects four individuals – recipient, donor, partner of recipient, and possible future child [21]. Careful psychosocial assessment of the recipient, her partner, and the donor is therefore imperative. Uterus recipient evaluation should include the same domains as any other organ transplantation. The psychosocial domains of interest include: psychiatric and substance use disorder history, family support, history of adherence, knowledge about transplantation, and health behaviors and factors measured by the above tools, all of which have been shown to predict medical and psychosocial outcomes, including rejection episodes, hospitalizations, infection rates, psychiatric decompensation, and support system failure [16, 17, 22].

Importantly, recipient evaluation for uterine transplant includes unique considerations that are not typical issues in other organ transplants. Motivations, attitude, and feelings around transplantation, pregnancy, childbearing, and potential success or failure of the procedure should be assessed. The recipient should also be assessed for other pregnancy options explored, relationship to donor, understanding of the

risks of immunosuppressives and pregnancy, acceptance of future hysterectomy, sexual function, partner support of transplantation, quality of life (including fertility), social desirability, self-esteem, body image, and coping [23]. In the most comprehensive study to date, nine uterine transplant recipients were assessed for quality of life, mood, relationship, and fertility quality of life. The study demonstrated decreases in physical function, and increases in bodily pain scores 3 months post-transplant, which subsequently normalized [24].

Health literacy related to immunosuppressive risks to the fetus needs to be assessed in the recipients, and as has been noted, cyclosporine, tacrolimus, and azathioprine have been associated with low birth weight and preterm labor [25]. Mycophenalate is contraindicated in pregnancy due to congenital malformations and miscarriage [25]. Steroids have no evidence of teratogenicity, and calcineurin inhibitors do not have an increased birth defect rate above the general population [26] (Table 36.2).

Obtaining collateral history from partners and exploring the partner's support and understanding of uterine transplant including the risks to the recipient and fetus are important. Issues related to the recipient's body image and concerns about sexuality should be addressed. Ensuring that the couple shares the same strong desire for having children would be reasonable, in addition to assessing the partner's expectations of positive or negative outcomes.

The groups who have completed or are undergoing uterine transplant clinical trials have documented that they perform extensive psychosocial evaluations for the potential

Table 36.2 Immunosuppressive risk to fetus in pregnant patients [25]

	FDA classification	Observations
Steroids	B – No evidence of risk in humans	No evidence of teratogenicity
Tacrolimus	C – Risks cannot be ruled out	Preterm birth, transient hyperkalemia, renal impairment observed
		No increased congenital malformations
Cyclosporine	C – Risks cannot be ruled out	Low birth weight associated
		No increased congenital malformations
Everolimus/ sirolimus	C – Risks cannot be ruled out	Limited data; contraindicated
Azathioprine	D – Positive evidence of risk	Prematurity, low birth weight
		Neonatal immunological problems (resolved within 1 year)
Mycophenolate mofetil	D – Positive evidence of risk	*Strictly contraindicated –* Miscarriage, several possible fetal malformations

recipients. One group's psychological evaluation included an in-depth interview and multiple standardized questionnaires, including Fertility Quality of Life Questionnaire, Millon Behavioral Medicine Diagnostic, Hospital Anxiety and Depression Scale, Posttraumatic Stress Disorder Checklist, Brief Coping Orientation to Problems Experienced Questionnaire, Connor-Davidson Resilience Scale 10, Drug Use Questionnaire, and Dyadic Adjustment Scale [9]. The other group performed semi-structured interviews assessing the following domains: psychological well-being, relationship, managing childlessness, knowledge about the project, and risk and relation with donor; these recipients additionally filled out standardized questionnaires regarding mood, quality of life, relationship, and fertility quality of life [21].

Psychosocial Assessment of Uterine Donors

The donor assessment should include motivators (both internal and external), knowledge of the donation process, risks of donation, relationship to recipient, evidence of coercion, financial gain or indecision, psychiatric issues, psychosocial stability, and substance use. Additional unique considerations include relationship to recipient (many recorded live donors have been family members) and donor's inability to pursue future pregnancies. In cases where mothers donate to daughters, the possibility of psychological coercion must be assessed, as well as a maternal donor's internal sense of guilt, self-blame, or obligation if her daughter was born with congenital absence of the uterus [27]. The donor surgery is more complex and lengthy than a typical hysterectomy and involves the typical risks of anesthesia, in addition to the more specific risk of ureteral injury. The evolution of robotic surgical strategies may improve the surgical strategies leading to decreased length of surgery for the donor. There is one initial observational study which explored the medical and psychological follow-up of nine live uterus donors. Donors were found to have higher baseline scores on the Psychological General Well-Being Index and the Dyadic Adjustment Scale; two donors had an increase in Hospital Anxiety and Depression Scale scores in the study period [28]. Donor complications have included one case of ureteric-vaginal fistula. The donors generally were related to the recipients, and most were postmenopausal [28] (Table 36.3).

Ethical Considerations

Ethical analysis of uterine transplantation has been described and emphasizes the importance of assessing the recipients' ability to provide informed consent, completing a thorough

Table 36.3 Unique considerations for psychosocial evaluation in uterus transplant

Recipient	Partner of recipient	Donor
Motivation for childbearing and pregnancy	Desire for child	Relationship to recipient
Prior pregnancies, children, and reproductive experiences	Understanding of risks for partner and fetus	Motivation (internal and external), in light of "non-life-saving transplant"
Other childbearing options explored	Relationship to donor	Prior experiences with pregnancy and childbearing, if any
Expectations of success or failure of the transplant, IVF, pregnancy, and live birth	Expectations of success or failure of the transplant, IVF, pregnancy, and live birth	Understanding around loss of childbearing ability, if still able
Relationship to donor and feelings around this	Impact on the sexual relationship with partner/recipient	Trauma, sexual history, and sexual function
Understanding of risks of immunosuppressants during pregnancy		Partner input, if applicable
Understanding of eventual hysterectomy		
Sexual function and expectations		
Partner support or lack thereof		
Quality of life regarding recovery from surgery, fertility treatments, future surgery		
Self-esteem and body image		

psychological evaluation of the recipient (and her partner), decreasing the possible exploitation of vulnerable women who currently serve as surrogates, and considering the possible risks to living donors (see Table 36.4) [29]. Uterine transplant allows women the opportunity for pregnancy (and generation of life), which for some individuals may be a central part of one's identity as woman and mother; as such, this type of transplant is life-enhancing but non-vital. Therefore, beneficence and autonomy need to carefully balance against the possible risks to the recipient, donor, and fetus. Bioethicists have opined that due to these risks, only deceased donations would be ethical [29], and in 2009 the International Federation of Obstetrics and Gynecology Committee reported it was unethical to remove a uterus for the purpose of transplantation [7]. However, given the risks of surrogacy, hysterectomy for the purpose of donation may be a less risky option, and the planned subsequent removal of the transplanted uterus may help decrease the risks of

Table 36.4 Elements of recipient informed consent for uterine transplantation [29]

1. Surgery lasts for 5 or more hours.
2. Possible complications due to anesthesia including pneumonia and deep vein thrombosis.
3. Risks of hemorrhages which may require transfusion.
4. Risks of infections which may require hysterectomy.
5. In vitro fertilization required to achieve pregnancy, which may fail.
6. Complications during pregnancy cannot be excluded; miscarriage may occur.
7. Possible risks to fetus from new vascular supply, altered uterine fixation.
8. Organ rejection can occur.
9. Organ rejection during pregnancy may warrant consideration of terminating pregnancy.
10. Risk of premature birth, along with short- and long-term risks of prematurity.
11. Long-term risk to fetus of immunosuppressant use during pregnancy is unknown.

longstanding immunosuppressive medication for the recipients. With the experience in solid organ transplantation of generally reasonable outcomes for offspring of pregnant recipients, the question of risk to the fetus is also more favorable than might be initially thought – risk of congenital malformations when using immunosuppressive drugs approved by the FDA during pregnancy is comparable to risk in normal pregnancy [21]. In an era of decreasing availability of adoptable infants and increasing scrutiny of surrogacy, women with absolute uterine factor infertility require ethical strategies to address their understandable desire for reproductive options.

Other ethical questions that have been raised regarding uterine transplantation include whether vulnerable populations could be financially coerced into donation. In the more distant future, innovations related to reconstructive transplantation, such as 3D printing of organs, may obviate the need for uterine transplantation. Uterine transplantation for non-genetic females is also of interest but poses unique physiologic challenges that will require further research. In addition, there has been a study looking at the attitudes regarding uterus donation of female-to-male transgender patients who were undergoing elective gender reassignment hysterectomy; of the 31 patients, 84% reported willingness to volunteer for donation after receiving detailed information about the procedure [30].

While the initial outcomes of the uterine transplant program in Sweden have been encouraging, other centers have not yet replicated this degree of success. How to best support the recipients who fail to become pregnant and when to consider explanting the uterus for these individuals are unknown. Managing recipients who have had graft failure or graft loss due to complications is also not described in detail in the literature. Not only will these events impact the recipients,

but they may also have implications for donors and spouses. Integrating mental health providers into the team to support and monitor for emerging symptoms of anxiety and distress in the event of adverse recipient or donor outcomes would be prudent.

Penile Transplantation

In contrast to uterine transplantation, penile transplantation has only been attempted few times with little thus far reported about the experience of the patients or the psychosocial assessment of these patients. Reasons for penile transplantation would be an attempt to restore urinary, reproductive, sexual, and aesthetic function, all of which may result in psychological consequences. Penile injuries are being seen more commonly in combat veterans exposed to improvised explosive devices, in addition to urotrauma due to cancer or motor vehicle accidents [31]. There are also reports of complications from ritual circumcision in South Africa, leading to severe penile injuries. The first penile transplant was performed in China in 2006, but the graft was removed apparently due to dissatisfaction by the patient and his wife [31]. The second transplant occurred in South Africa in a 21-year-old man whose penis had been damaged during a circumcision [31]. The first in the United States penile transplant occurred in Boston in a 64-year-old following surgery for a penile carcinoma [32]. In April 2018, the New York Times reported the transplant of a penis, scrotum, and a portion of the abdominal wall from a deceased donor to a recipient who was a veteran maimed by an improvised explosive device [33].

Many psychosocial factors are likely to be important in this transplant population, including the perception of the recipient and his partner about the transplant, body image concerns, sexuality, urinary issues, and consideration of a prosthesis or reconstructive surgery. Penile injury in particular has implications on physical intimacy, sexual identity, masculinity, fears of infertility, and suicidality [34]. In the case of the 21-year-old South African transplant recipient, careful psychological screening and follow-up was emphasized, and at a 24-month follow-up, he had achieved sexual function with a subsequent pregnancy of his partner, reported acceptance of his new organ, and had increased quality of life scores [35]. In the case of the 64-year-old Boston transplant recipient, at 6 months postoperatively, the patient regained normal appearance of the penis, full urinary function, and partial sensory and erectile function; furthermore, he reported improved health satisfaction, self-image, and optimism for the future [32]. In the most recent 2018 US case of the veteran who received a penile transplant, he reported having had thought about suicide before the possibility of a transplant gave him hope; at post-transplant he was quoted as "feeling whole again." In addition, this was the first case to transplant not just the penis but surrounding tissue including the scrotum. For ethical reasons, the donor testes were removed to eliminate the possibility that the recipient could produce children that were not genetically his own [33].

Public attitudes around penile donation and transplantation have not been studied. Societal acceptance of this form of transplantation also needs to occur in order for donor families to consider permitting this form of donation [36]. There are no formal guidelines for the psychosocial evaluation or ethical conduct of penile transplantation [22]. As with any form of transplantation, an assessment of psychiatric disorders including screening for posttraumatic stress disorder (PTSD) in the cases of trauma, family support, history of adherence, and knowledge about transplantation, including the need for lifelong immunosuppressive medication, is needed. Specific to penile transplant should be the increased focus on wishes regarding sexual activity, partner attitude/expectations, support system attitudes, ability to cope with possible stigma, scorn and failure of transplant, and tolerance for media publicity [31]. In the South African experience, screening for suicidality was especially important since the population identified has evidenced significant distress due to the catastrophic sequelae of the circumcision experience [37]. Informed consent should involve complete discussion about expectations of results around aesthetics, urinary, sexual, and reproductive function. As the three prior penile transplant cases received considerable attention from the media, the ability to cope and tolerate this would also potentially be an important factor to be considered for these patients, and careful discussion about the patient' desire for privacy would be a priority for the transplant team.

Conclusions

VCA involving reproductive organs is emerging as a solution for women with absolute uterine infertility and for men following penectomy or penile loss due to trauma. The benefits for these patient populations may be significant, but much needs to be learned about the medical and psychological implications of these forms of transplantation. Transplant teams will require experienced social workers, psychologists, and psychiatrists to assess and support the ongoing needs of these patients. As more centers develop programs, sharing information and developing shared research projects will yield valuable insights into how best to assess and manage emerging psychiatric disorders that may occur. Forums, such as the Chauvet Workshop which brings together key stakeholders in the psychosocial assessment of VCA patients, provide a useful platform for supporting collaboration [38].

References

1. https://www.unos.org/transplantation/history. Available from: https://www.unos.org/transplantation/history.
2. Brännström M, Johannesson L, Bokström H, Kvarnström N, Mölne J, Dahm-Kähler P, et al. Livebirth after uterus transplantation. Lancet. 2015;385(9968):607–16.
3. Diaz-Garcia C, Akhi S, Wallin A, Pellicer A, Brannstrom M. First report on fertility after allogenic uterus transplantation. Acta Obstet Gynecol Scand. 2010;89(11):1491–4.
4. Fegeeh W, Raffa H, Jabbad H, Marzouki A. Transplantation of the human uterus. Int J Gynecol Obstet. 2002;76(3):245–51.
5. Erman Akar M, Ozkan O, Aydinuraz B, Dirican K, Cincik M, Mendilcioglu I, et al. Clinical pregnancy after uterus transplantation. Fertil Steril. 2013;100:1358–63.
6. Brännström M, Johannesson L, Dahm-Kähler P, Enskog A, Mölne J, Kvarnström N, et al. First clinical uterus transplantation trial: a six-month report. Fertil Steril. 2014;101(5):1228–36.
7. Milliez J. Uterine transplantation FIGO committee for the ethical aspects of human reproduction and women's health. Int J Gynaecol Obstet. 2009;106(3):270.
8. Arian SE, Flyckt RL, Farrell RM, Falcone T, Tzakis AG. Characterizing women with interest in uterine transplant clinical trials in the United States: who seeks information on this experimental treatment? Am J Obstet Gynecol. 2017;216(2):190–1.
9. Johannesson L, Wallis K, Koon EC, McKenna GJ, Anthony T, Leffingwell SG, et al. Living uterus donation and transplantation: experience of interest and screening in a single center in the United States. Am J Obstet Gynecol. 2018;218(3):331e1–7.
10. Rodrigue JR, Tomich D, Fleishman A, Glazier AK. Vascularized composite allograft donation and transplantation: a survey of public attitudes in the United States. Am J Transplant. 2017;17(10):2687–95.
11. Saso S, Clarke A, Bracewell-Milnes T, Al-Memar M, Hamed AH, Thum MY, et al. Survey of perceptions of health care professionals in the United Kingdom toward uterine transplant. Prog Transplant. 2015;25(1):56–63.
12. Wennberg AL, Rodriguez-Wallberg KA, Milsom I, Brannstrom M. Attitudes towards new assisted reproductive technologies in Sweden: a survey in women 30-39 years of age. Acta Obstet Gynecol Scand. 2016;95(1):38–44.
13. Olbrisch M, Levenson J, Hamer R. The PACT: a rating scale for the study of clinic decision-making in psychosocial screening of organ transplant candidates. Clin Transpl. 1989;3:164–9.
14. Futterman A, Wellisch D, Bond G, Carr C. The psychosocial levels system. A new rating scale to identify and assess emotional difficulties during bone marrow transplantation. Psychosomatics. 1991;32(2):177–86.
15. Twillman R, Manetto C, Wellisch D, Wolcott D. The transplant evaluation rating scale. A revision of the psychosocial levels system for evaluating organ transplant candidates. Psychosomatics. 1993;34(2):144–53.
16. Maldonado J, Dubois H, David E, Sher Y, Lolak S, Dyal J, et al. The Stanford Integrated Psychosocial Assessment for Transplantation (SIPAT): a new tool for the psychosocial evaluation of pretransplant candidates. Psychosomatics. 2012;53(2):123–32.
17. Goetzmann L, Ruegg L, Stamm M, Ambühl P, Boehler A, Halter J, et al. Psychosocial profiles after transplantation: a 24-month follow-up of heart, lung, liver, kidney and allogeneic bone-marrow patients. Transplantation. 2008;86(5):662–8.
18. Owen J, Bonds C, Wellisch D. Psychiatric evaluations of heart transplant candidates: predicting post-transplant hospitalizations, rejection episodes, and survival. Psychosomatics. 2006;47(3):213–22.
19. Shapiro P, Williams D, Foray A, Gelman I, Wukich N, Sciacca R. Psychosocial evaluation and prediction of compliance problems and morbidity after heart transplantation. Transplantation. 1995;60(12):1462–6.

20. Iacoviello B, Shenoy A, Braoude J, Jennings T, Vaidya S, Brouwer J, et al. The live donor assessment tool: a psychosocial assessment tool for live organ donors. Psychosomatics. 2015;56(3):254–61.
21. Johannesson L, Jarvholm S. Uterus transplantation: current progress and future prospects. Int J Womens Health. 2016;8:43–51.
22. Hitschfeld M, Schneekloth T, Kennedy C, Rummans T, Niazi S, Vasquez A, et al. The psychosocial assessment of candidates for transplantation: a cohort study of its association with survival among lung transplant recipients. Psychosomatics. 2016;57(5):489–97.
23. Jowsey-Gregoire S, Kumnig M. Standardizing psychosocial assessment for vascularized composite allotransplantation. 2016;21(5). Available from: www.co-transplantation.com
24. Järvholm S, Johannesson L, Clarke A, Brännström M. Uterus transplantation trial: psychological evaluation of recipients and partners during the post-transplantation year. Fertil Steril. 2015;104(4):1010–5.
25. Ejzenberg D, Mendes L, Haddad L, Baracat E, D'Albuquerque L, Andraus W. Uterine transplantation: a systematic review. Clinics. 2016;71(11):679–83.
26. Blume C, Pischke S, von Versen-Hoynck F, Gunter HH, Gross MM. Pregnancies in liver and kidney transplant recipients: a review of the current literature and recommendation. Best Pract Res Clin Obstet Gynaecol. 2014;28(8):1123–36.
27. Lavoue V, Vigneau C, Duros S, Boudjema K, Leveque J, Piver P, et al. Which donor for uterus transplants: brain-dead donor or living donor? A systematic review. Transplantation. 2017;101(2):267–73.
28. Kvarnström N, Järvholm S, Johannesson L, Dahm-Kähler P, Olausson M, Brännström M. Live donors of the initial observational study of uterus transplantation—psychological and medical follow-up until 1 year after surgery in the 9 cases. Transplantation. 2017;101(3):664–70.
29. Petrini C, Gainotti S, Morresi A, Costa A. Ethical issues in uterine transplantation: psychological implications and informed consent. Transplant Proc. 2017;49:707–10.
30. Api M, Boza A, Ceyhan M. Could the female-to-male transgender population be donor candidates for uterus transplantation? Turkish J Obstet Gynecol. 2017;14(4):233–7.
31. Schol I, Ko D, Cetrulo CJ. Genitourinary vascularized composite allotransplantation. Curr Opin Organ Transplant. 2017;22(5):484–9. Epub ahead of print
32. Cetrulo CL Jr, Li K, Salinas HM, Treiser MD, Schol I, Barrisford GW, et al. Penis transplantation: first US experience. Ann Surg. 2018;267(5):983–8.
33. Grady D. 'Whole again': A vet maimed by an I.E.D. receives a transplanted penis. New York Times [serial on the Internet]. 2018 Available from: https://www.nytimes.com/2018/04/23/health/soldier-penis-transplant-ied.html
34. Lucas PA, Page PR, Phillip RD, Bennett AN. The impact of genital trauma on wounded servicemen: qualitative study. Injury. 2014;45(5):825–9.
35. van der Merwe A, Graewe F, Zuhlke A, Barsdorf NW, Zarrabi AD, Viljoen JT, et al. Penile allotransplantation for penis amputation following ritual circumcision: a case report with 24 months of follow-up. Lancet. 2017;390(10099):1038–47.
36. Caplan A, Kimberly L, Parent B, Sosin M, Rodriguez E. The ethics of penile transplantation: preliminary recommendations. Transplantation. 2017;101:1200–5.
37. Rasper A, Terlecki R. Ushering in the era of penile transplantation. Transl Androl Urol. 2017;6(2):216–21.
38. Kumnig M, Jowsey-Gregoire S. Key psychosocial challenges in vascularized composite allotransplantation. World J Transplant. 2016;6(1):91–102.

Bone Marrow Malignancies and Indications for Hematopoietic Cell Transplantation

37

Laura Johnston

Introduction

Hematopoietic cell transplantation (HCT), also known as blood and marrow transplantation (BMT), is an essential curative therapy for malignant and nonmalignant diseases. There are two forms of HCT: autologous and allogeneic. Autologous HCT utilizes the patient's own hematopoietic stem cells, while allogeneic HCT utilizes a healthy donor's hematopoietic stem cells. The hematopoietic graft or cells may be collected from the bone marrow, the peripheral blood, or the umbilical cord. Since the inception over 50 years ago, HCT's use has grown tremendously, with the millionth HCT reported in 2012 [1]. Soon after this report, the Worldwide Network for Blood and Marrow Transplantation published an observational study on the global development of HCT occurring from 1957 to 2012 [2]. Figure 37.1 demonstrates the steady rise of transplants, reaching 50,000 by 1991, to 500,000 by 2005, and 1,000,000 by 2012. At the time of this report, there was no evidence of saturation in the number of worldwide allogeneic HCTs.

Steady research and technologic advancements have allowed the increase in HCT, with a broader and older population receiving autologous and allogeneic HCT more safely and effectively. The Seattle group identified a reduction in non-relapse mortality (NRM) and improved overall survival (OS) from 1993–1997 to 2003–2007 in their allogeneic HCT recipients, identifying a reduction in organ damage, infection, and severe graft versus host disease (GVHD) responsible for the improved outcomes [3]. Extending the donor options to include not only the matched sibling donor (MSD), but the matched or minimally mismatched unrelated (URD), haploidentical related, and minimally mismatched umbilical

cord blood (UCB) donors offers a feasible donor for more than 80% of patients 20 years of age or older and for almost all pediatric patients based on a population-based genetic model from the US National Marrow Donor Program and UCB registries [4]. The trend in donor sources in the USA is illustrated in Fig. 37.2 [5]. As of 2006, the number of URDs exceeded MSDs, not only in the USA, but worldwide with over 22,000,000 registered donors from 57 countries and well over 600,000 UCB products HLA-typed and cryopreserved from 36 countries in 2015 [2]. The use of haploidentical donors has experienced the greatest rise in use with a 167% increase over 10 years noted from the Worldwide Network of BMT [6]. The increased use of these donor alternatives is legitimate due to similar outcomes seen regardless of donor source [7–12].

The trends in age for autologous and allogeneic HCT in the USA reported to the Center for International Blood and Marrow Transplant Research (CIBMTR) are shown in Fig. 37.3. The percent of patients greater than 60 years of age continues to increase, comprising greater than 50% of patients receiving autologous HCT for lymphoma and myeloma and approximately 25% of patients receiving allogeneic HCT. The ability to deliver allogeneic HCT with less morbidity and mortality via reduced intensity regimens has spurred the increase in the allogeneic HCT recipient's age, with a 2014 European Blood and Marrow Transplantation (EBMT) survey reporting 41% of the nearly 17,000 allogeneic HCTs utilizing a reduced intensity regimen [13, 14]. The majority of HCTs occur in the adult population with approximately four times the number of HCTs occurring in adults (7000 in 2015) than children (1600 in 2015) in the USA [5]. The diseases transplanted also vary between the pediatric and adult populations with a rare indication for HCT in nonmalignant disease in an adult, whereas this is a more common indication in a child.

As one can appreciate from the accompanying CIBMTR data on trends in HCT over time, age alone is not a determinant for HCT eligibility. There is an ever-increasing body of literature describing excellent outcomes in select elderly

L. Johnston
Division of Blood and Marrow Transplantation,
Department of Medicine, Stanford University School of Medicine,
Stanford, CA, USA
e-mail: korb@stanford.edu

© Springer International Publishing AG, part of Springer Nature 2019
Y. Sher, J. R. Maldonado (eds.), *Psychosocial Care of End-Stage Organ Disease and Transplant Patients*,
https://doi.org/10.1007/978-3-319-94914-7_37

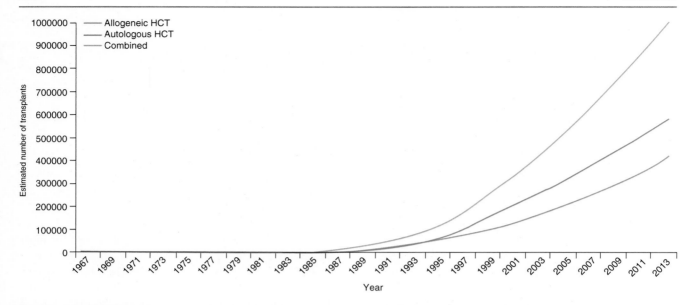

Fig. 37.1 Global development of hematopoietic cell transplantation by donor type from 1957 to 2012. The one millionth HCT was estimated to have been done by the end of 2012. (Fig. 37.1a [2])

Fig. 37.2 Estimated frequency of total number of transplants according to donor type done in the USA reported to the Center for International Blood Marrow Transplant Research prior to 2015. Slide 4 [5]

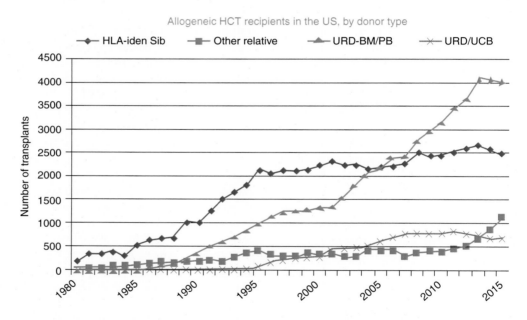

patients receiving autologous as well as allogeneic HCT regimens [15–17]. Predictors having a greater impact on outcomes include functional status, Karnofsky Performance Status, HCT-comorbidity index score, EBMT risk score, and pre-transplantation assessment of mortality risk score [16–22].

Patient Evaluation and Preparation for HCT

Patients considered for HCT are typically referred to a transplantation program by their primary hematologist or oncologist. The initial evaluation begins with a thorough review of the patient's medical and psychosocial history as well as the

current medical and psychosocial conditions, including assessment of the patient's financial and psychosocial support. The evaluation team often includes a BMT physician, a BMT nurse coordinator, a BMT social worker, a financial coordinator, and additional specialists dependent on patient-specific indications. Prior to HCT, in addition to assessing a patient's disease status with the appropriate disease-specific studies, the patient must also undergo a complete assessment of infectious disease and organ function, including routine laboratory data as well as cardiac and pulmonary function testing. Patients considered for allogeneic HCT must also undergo histocompatibility (HLA) testing and assessment of possible donors, which may include evaluating their healthy relatives. Patients are counseled and required to abstain from

Fig. 37.3 Trends in HCT for malignant diseases in the USA by recipient age reported to the CIBMTR prior to 2015. (**a**) Autologous HCT for non-Hodgkin lymphoma (NHL), Hodgkin lymphoma (HL), and multiple myeloma (MM). Slide 11 [5]; (**b**) Allogeneic HCT for acute myelogenous leukemia, acute lymphoblastic leukemia, NHL, HL, and MM. Slide 12 [5]

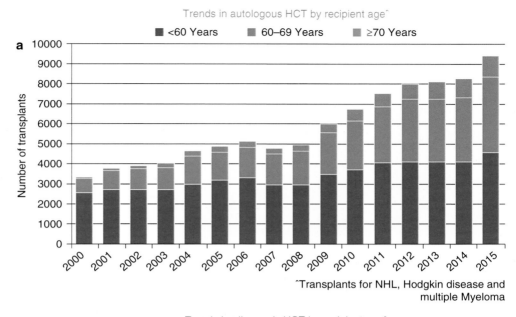

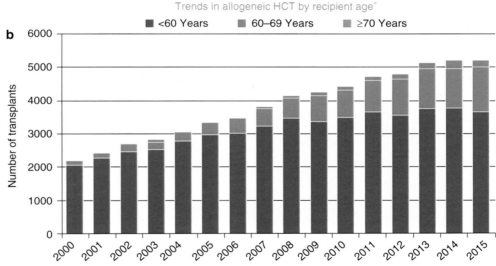

alcohol, tobacco, and all illicit drug use prior to HCT to minimize the risks associated with HCT.

HCT requires "preparation" of the patient, termed the preparative regimen. The preparative regimen serves two purposes: (1) to ensure adequate control of the disease and (2) to ensure adequate immunosuppression to allow successful engraftment of the donor cells. Traditionally, preparative regimens have utilized myeloablative or high-dose chemotherapy with or without radiation. Autologous HCT requires a high-dose regimen to ensure disease eradication, while allogeneic HCT also relies on the donor alloimmunity as a mode of disease control with lower dose or reduced intensity regimens occasionally employed in this setting. Myeloablative HCT begins with an approximate 4–7 days of preparative regimen, followed by a 2–3-week bone marrow

recovery period. During this time, patients are monitored as an inpatient or on a daily basis as an outpatient while they experience the side effects and toxicities of the regimen which include absolute neutropenia, anemia, thrombocytopenia requiring red blood cell and platelet transfusions, and increased risk of infections. Many patients experience gastrointestinal side effects of nausea, vomiting, diarrhea, and mouth sores that may limit oral nutrition and require pain medication. The autologous HCT patient is usually discharged to the care of their primary hematologist or oncologist within 1–2 months of their HCT. However, patients undergoing allogeneic HCT may receive a myeloablative or reduced intensity regimen, and thus due to the unique risks associated with allogeneic HCT, such as GVHD and infection, the allogeneic HCT recipient remains under the close observation of the transplant center until 80–100 days after HCT, regardless of the intensity of the regimen. Dependent on the transplant center, the allogeneic HCT recipient often continues with relatively frequent follow-up with their transplant center up to 1 year or more after HCT, dependent on the post-HCT clinical issues.

The indications for HCT in the USA are illustrated in Fig. 37.4 summarizing CIBMTR data from 2014 and Fig. 37.5

Fig. 37.4 Indications for HCT in the USA in 2014 as reported to the CIBMTR. Slide 13 [5]

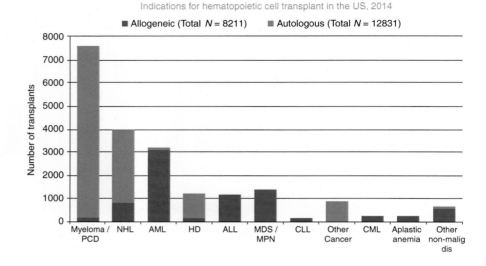

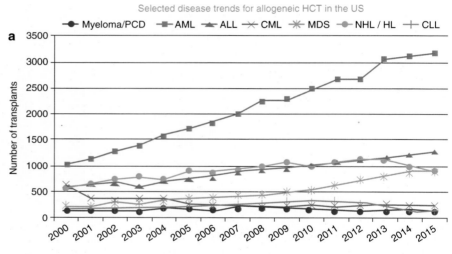

Fig. 37.5 Selected disease trends for HCT in the USA as reported to the CIBMTR from 2000 to 2015. (**a**) Allogeneic HCT, Slide 14 [5]; (**b**) Autologous HCT, Slide 15 [5]. PCD plasma cell dyscrasia, AML acute myelogenous leukemia, ALL acute lymphoblastic leukemia, CML chronic myeloid leukemia, MDS myelodysplasia, NHL/HL non-Hodgkin lymphoma/ Hodgkin lymphoma, CLL chronic lymphocytic leukemia

showing the trends by type of HCT and disease over time. The indications in the USA are similar to the indications reported from a 2014 EBMT survey [5, 13]. The most common indications for HCT in the USA in 2014 were multiple myeloma and lymphoma, accounting for 56% of all HCTs. Acute leukemias (acute myelogenous leukemia (AML), acute lymphoblastic leukemia (ALL), and myelodysplasia (MDS), combined with myeloproliferative neoplasms (MPN)) were the next most common, comprising approximately one third of HCTs and 70% of allogeneic HCTs. The European and US data from 2014 showed the allogeneic transplant activity increased in AML and MPN/MDS with a decrease in chronic lymphocytic leukemia (CLL). Autologous transplant activity showed the greatest increase in plasma cell disorders (PCD) including multiple myeloma (MM) and amyloidosis. The following section will review the most common indications for HCT in the adult population reflecting the published guidelines from the EBMT and the American Society of Blood and Marrow Transplantation (ASBMT), including respective outcomes based on the specific disease entities [23, 24].

Disease Specific Indications for HCT

Acute Myelogenous Leukemia

Acute myelogenous leukemia is the most common acute leukemia in adults with the median age of onset approximately 65 years of age with an estimated 21,000 new cases diagnosed in the USA in 2017 [25]. AML includes a heterogeneous group of blood cell cancers arising from clonal expansion of malignant hematopoietic precursor cells. The aberrant cells proliferate in the bone marrow and interfere with production of normal blood cells. Patients present with symptoms of anemia, such as fatigue, weakness, shortness of breath, dyspnea on exertion, infection, and excessive bruising and bleeding. Laboratory analyses reveal decreased red blood cells, platelets, and mature neutrophils. AML is generally rapidly lethal unless treated with intensive chemotherapy and/or targeted therapies together with supportive care [26].

Although AML is a relatively rare disease, it is the most common indication for allogeneic HCT with approximately 3200 patients receiving allogeneic HCT for AML in the USA in 2015 (see Fig. 37.5) [5]. AML is categorized into good-, intermediate-, and poor-risk disease based on cytogenetic and molecular markers identified at diagnosis (see Table 37.1) [27]. These disease-risk categories are important in determining indication for transplantation.

Allogeneic HCT with the best available donor (MSD, URD, haploidentical, and UCB) is standard of care for all intermediate- and poor-risk AML patients in first or subsequent complete remission (CR) and occasionally considered for patients not in CR [23, 24]. Favorable-risk AML patients are

Table 37.1 Risk status based on validated cytogenetics and molecular abnormalities[a] [27]

Risk status	Cytogenetics	Molecular abnormalities
Favorable risk	Core binding factor: inv(16)[b,c,d] or t(16;16)[b,c,d] or t(8;21)[b,d] or t(15;17)[d]	Normal cytogenetics: NPM1 mutation in the absence of FLT3-ITD or isolated biallelic (double) CEBPA mutation
Intermediate risk	Normal cytogenetics +8 alone t(9;11) Other nondefined	Core binding factor with KIT mutation[b]
Poor risk	Complex (≥3 clonal chromosomal abnormalities) Monosomal karyotype -5, 5q-, -7, 7q- 11q23-non t(9;11) inv(3), t(3;3) t(6;9) t(9;22)[e]	Normal cytogenetics: with FLT3-ITD mutation[f] TP53 mutation

[a]The molecular abnormalities included in this table reflect those for which validated assays are available in standardized commercial laboratories. Given the rapidly evolving field, risk stratification should be modified based on continuous evaluation of research data. Other novel genetic mutations have been identified that may have prognostic significance

[b]Emerging data indicate that the presence of KIT mutations in patients with t(8;21), and to a lesser extent inv(16), confers a higher risk of relapse. These patients are considered intermediate risk and should be considered for HCT or clinical trials, if available. Recent data suggest that certain KIT mutations may be more or less adverse in prognosis. *See Discussion*

[c]Paschka et al. [68]

[d]Other cytogenetic abnormalities in addition to these findings do not alter better risk status

[e]For Philadelphia+ AML t(9;22), manage as myeloid blast crisis in CML, with addition of tyrosine kinase inhibitors

[f]FLT3-ITD mutations are considered to confer a significantly poorer outcome in patients with normal karyotype, and these patients should be considered for clinical trials where available. There is controversy as to whether FLT3-TKD mutations carry an equally poor prognosis

recommended for allogeneic HCT with the best available donor if they are slow to achieve a first CR or if in second or subsequent CR. HCT in favorable-risk patients in first CR (CR1) is not routinely considered; however, the EBMT recommends consideration of HCT based on EBMT report results [28]. This EBMT report showed similar survival after autologous and allogeneic HCT for first CR patients with good-risk AML [28]. In addition, a meta-analysis demonstrated improved disease-free survival and a trend for improved OS in patients receiving autologous or MSD allogeneic HCT compared with standard chemotherapy [28, 29]. Autologous HCT may be considered for patients in CR, ideally if in a molecular remission. The OS in AML patients undergoing MSD and URD HCT from the CIBMTR from 2004 to 2014 is shown in Fig. 37.6, with results divided by disease phase at time of transplant [5]. The 3-year OS after an MSD HCT was

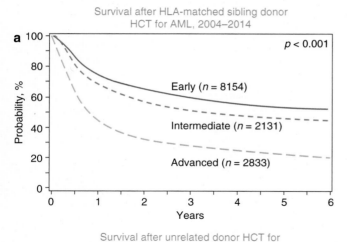

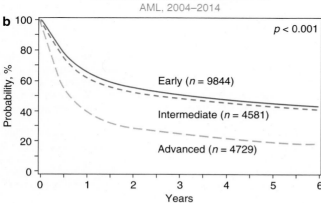

Fig. 37.6 Overall survival after HCT for acute myelogenous leukemia patients reported to the Center for International Blood Marrow Transplant Research from 2004 to 2014. (**a**) Matched sibling donor, Slide 20 [5]; (**b**) Unrelated donor, Slide 21 [5]. Early disease defined as first complete remission (CR), intermediate disease as second or subsequent CR, and advanced disease as primary induction failure or active disease. Comparisons across survival curves are univariate and do not adjust for all potentially important factors; consequently, results should be interpreted cautiously

59% ± 1% for patients with early AML, 51% ± 1% with intermediate AML and 27% ± 1% with advanced AML. The 3-year OS after a URD HCT was 51% ± 1% for patients with early, 48% ± 1% with intermediate, and 25% ± 1% with advanced AML. Although the comparisons across survival curves were univariate and did not control for multiple factors, disease status at time of HCT was an important predictor of survival with early disease defined as first CR, intermediate disease as second or subsequent CR, and advanced disease as primary induction failure or active disease.

Acute Lymphoblastic Leukemia

Acute lymphoblastic leukemia is a rare malignant disorder, estimated to be diagnosed in just under 6000 people in the USA in 2017, more commonly seen in childhood than adults

with the median age in adults of 39 years [25]. ALL originates from a B- or T-lymphocyte progenitor [26]. The proliferation and expansion of the clonal blast cells in the bone marrow lead to disruption of hematopoiesis resulting in anemia, neutropenia, and thrombocytopenia as well as occasional extramedullary expansion involving the lymph nodes, thymus, gonads, meninges, liver, and spleen. The laboratory findings may include anemia, neutropenia, and thrombocytopenia as well as circulating lymphoblasts in the peripheral blood and in the cerebrospinal fluid. The presenting symptoms of ALL are often related to the degree of bone marrow failure and site of extramedullary disease. Weakness and fatigue are common in addition to fevers that may or may not be related to anemia or infection. Bone pain and arthralgias are also relatively common, although more often in children. Contemporary ALL chemotherapy offers cure to nearly 90% of children and 40% of adults. These outcomes are due to the introduction of more aggressive pediatric chemotherapy regimens in the adolescent and young adult population leading to improved prognosis for patients younger than 35 years of age. Given these encouraging results, the indication for HCT is more controversial in adult ALL than AML with a reduced need for allogeneic HCT in this younger adult population [5, 30, 31].

Indication for HCT in the adult population is typically based on disease characteristics at the time of diagnosis. The high-risk features include age less than 1 year or over 35 years, white blood count of >30,000/ul for B-cell and >100,000/ul for T-cell phenotype, and high-risk cytogenetics (see Table 37.2) [32]. The ASBMT and EBMT agree on the recommendation of allogeneic HCT with the best donor available for patients with standard and high-risk ALL in CR2 and to "consider" HCT in patients with relapsed or refractory disease [23, 24]. The ASBMT and EBMT differ in their recommendations for patients in first CR. The ASBMT recommends allogeneic HCT as standard of care for standard- and high-risk patients. The EBMT limits its recommendation to a MSD or URD HCT in first CR patients with high-risk disease, only if persistent, or recurrent minimal residual disease (MRD) [33] and only in first CR patients

Table 37.2 Cytogenetic risk groups for B-ALL [32]

Risk groups	Cytogenetics
Good risk	Hyperdiploidy (51–65 chromosomes; cases with trisomy of chromosomes 4,10, and 17 appear to have the most favorable outcome); t(12;21)(p13;q22): ETV6-RUNX1
Poor risk	Hypodiploidy (<44 chromosomes); t(v;11q23):t(4;11) and other KMT2A rearranged t(-;11q23); t(9;22) (q34;q11.2): BCR-ABL1 (defined as high risk in the pre-TKI era); complex karyotype (5 or more chromosomal abnormalities); Ph-like ALL; intrachromosomal amplification of chromosome 21 (iAMP21)

with standard-risk disease if they are enrolled in a clinical trial. Although autologous HCT is not routinely considered for patients with ALL, the advent of monitoring MRD and promising results with autologous HCT in the setting of MRD negativity has led the EBMT to consider autologous HCT in patients with MRD negativity or molecular remission in the setting of Philadelphia chromosome-positive disease and the use of tyrosine kinase inhibitors [23, 34]. Figure 37.7 shows the OS for adult ALL patients receiving a MSD or URD HCT reported to the CIBMTR from 2004 to 2014 [5]. The outcomes among the nearly 10,000 adult patients receiving MSD and URD HCT were very similar. The 3-year OS after MSD in early ALL was 59% ± 1%, intermediate was 38% ± 2%, and advanced was 27% ± 2%. The corresponding 3-year OS after URD HCT in early ALL was 57% ± 1%, intermediate was 37% ± 1%, and advanced

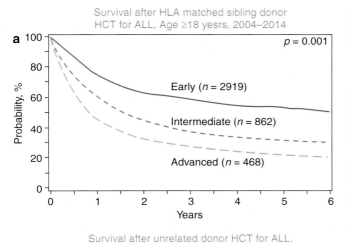

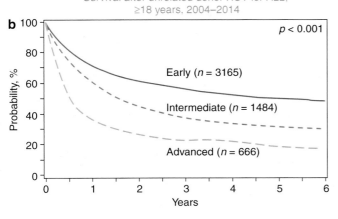

Fig. 37.7 Overall survival after HCT for adult acute lymphoblastic leukemia patients reported to the Center for International Blood Marrow Transplant Research from 2004 to 2014. (**a**) Matched sibling donor, Slide 29 [5]; (**b**) Unrelated donor, Slide 30 [5]. Early disease defined as first complete remission (CR), intermediate disease as second or subsequent CR, and advanced disease as primary induction failure or active disease. Comparisons across survival curves are univariate and do not adjust for all potentially important factors; consequently, results should be interpreted cautiously

was 24% ± 2%. As with AML, early disease was defined as first CR, intermediate disease as second or subsequent CR, and advanced disease as primary induction failure or active disease.

Myelodysplastic Syndromes

Myelodysplastic syndromes (MDS) are a heterogeneous group of clonal hematopoietic cell (HC) neoplasms identified by dysmorphic morphology, one or more HC cytopenias, and risk of clonal evolution to AML [26]. The estimated incidence is greater than 10,000 cases per year in the USA with a median age of onset >70 years of age and increasing incidence with age [35]. Patients may be asymptomatic or present with signs of anemia such as pallor, weakness, and dyspnea on exertion. Often patients present with fatigue that does not correlate with the degree of anemia. Less frequently, patients may present with infections related to severe neutropenia or neutrophil dysfunction as well as bleeding due to severe thrombocytopenia or platelet dysfunction. Laboratory findings include anemia, neutropenia, thrombocytopenia, and evidence of dysmorphic blood cell features on the peripheral blood smear as well as the bone marrow. The prognosis of the patient with MDS is dependent on various prognostic markers as depicted in the International Prognostic Scoring System (IPSS) [36, 37]. The IPSS determines a prognostic risk group for patients at the time of diagnosis as low, intermediate-1, intermediate-2, and high risk, based on percentage of leukemic blasts in the bone marrow, cytogenetic abnormalities, and number of peripheral blood cytopenias. Although patients' prognoses vary based on these features with OS ranging from months to many years, the only curative therapy for MDS is allogeneic HCT. The appropriate time to proceed to HCT remains somewhat controversial with a useful decision model developed to determine the benefit of proceeding to HCT at the time of diagnosis utilizing the IPSS [36, 38]. The decision model was designed to determine if transplant at diagnosis, after delay by several years, or at time of AML transformation was the optimal strategy. The decision model determined that proceeding to HCT at diagnosis in patients with Int-2- or high-risk disease was optimal, but awaiting evidence of AML transformation was optimal for patients with low and Int-1-risk disease. Since this decision model was proposed, there have been updated MDS prognostic scoring systems that refine expected survival and risk of AML, including the Revised IPSS and the World Health Organization Prognostic Scoring System (WPSS) [37, 39]. The R-IPSS and WPSS incorporate the degree of cytopenias and the need for transfusion support, both which predict outcomes at diagnosis and throughout the disease in patients proceeding or not proceeding to HCT. As expected, the disease-risk group

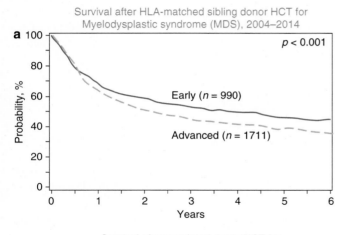

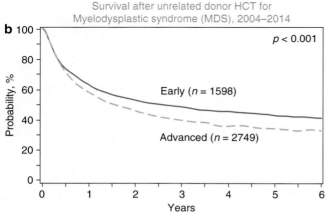

Fig. 37.8 Overall survival after HCT for myelodysplasia patients reported to the Center for International Blood Marrow Transplant Research from 2004 to 2014. (**a**) Matched sibling donor, Slide 23 [5]; (**b**) Unrelated donor, Slide 24 [5]. Early disease defined as refractory anemia or refractory anemia with ringed sideroblasts and advanced as refractory anemia with excess of blasts. Comparisons across survival curves are univariate and do not adjust for all potentially important factors; consequently, results should be interpreted cautiously

correlates with the outcome of HCT. Figure 37.8 shows the survival curves from patients receiving MSD and URD HCT reported to the CIBMTR from 2004 to 2014 [5]. As with AML and ALL, the 3-year OS is relatively similar between MSD and URD within each disease-risk group, 53% ± 2% and 49% ± 1% for recipients of sibling and unrelated donor transplants for early (refractory anemia or refractory anemia with ringed sideroblasts) or advanced (refractory anemia with excess of blasts) MDS, respectively, and 45% ± 1% and 40% ± 1% for recipients with advanced (Int-2, high) MDS.

Multiple Myeloma

Multiple myeloma accounts for approximately 10% of all hematologic malignancies with an incidence of 30,000 cases per year in the USA and a median age of onset of 66 years [40]. It is a hematologic disorder arising from the proliferation of clonal malignant plasma cells that produce an abnormal immunoglobulin protein [26]. The laboratory and clinical findings result from plasma cell proliferation and immunoglobulin overproduction leading to bone marrow suppression causing cytopenias; bone destruction causing fractures, bone pain, and hypercalcemia; and immunosuppression leading to infections and renal failure. Patients may be asymptomatic, with an incidental finding of anemia, or present with an unprovoked skeletal fracture or bone pain. Other symptoms may be related to hypercalcemia or renal failure including fatigue, altered mental status, weight loss, and failure to thrive. A patient's clinical course can vary from an indolent to highly aggressive course with survival ranging from over a decade to over 5 years.

Although MM is an uncommon disease, it is by far the greatest indication for autologous HCT worldwide and has the highest autologous transplant activity as evidenced in the US and European registries (see Figs. 37.4 and 37.5) [5, 13]. Unlike other indications for HCT, autologous HCT is not pursued as a curative therapy, but as a consolidative treatment after conventional therapy with the goal of prolonging progression free (PFS) and OS. The most recently published phase III trials comparing autologous HCT to "current-day" chemotherapy in patients in first remission continue to show prolonged PFS and improved or similar OS with autologous HCT [41–43]; hence, it remains standard of care to offer autologous HCT in first remission or sensitive relapse, typically up to the age of 70–75 years [23, 24]. Allogeneic HCT has been investigated in a tandem fashion with autologous HCT followed by a nonmyeloablative regimens without consistent benefit in PFS or OS and with associated greater morbidity and mortality [44]; hence, allogeneic HCT is not pursued outside of a clinical trial. Figure 37.9 illustrates the positive trend in survival of MM patients receiving autologous HCT reported to the CIBMTR from 2001 to 2014 with the 3-year overall survival increasing from 70% in 2001–2004 to 78% in 2013–2014 [5]. The overall outlook of MM continues to improve with the most recent induction therapies reaching responses similarly to those seen with autologous HCT; hence, the future benefit of autologous HCT remains to be determined [45].

Lymphoma

Lymphoma is comprised of multiple subsets of lymphomas characterized by their clinical, pathological, and genetic/molecular features via the World Health Organization Classification [46]. The most common indications for HCT in lymphomas will be reviewed here.

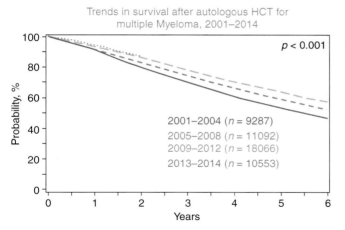

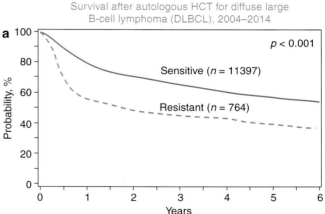

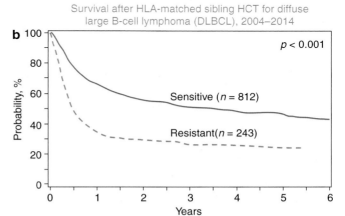

Fig. 37.9 Trends in overall survival after autologous HCT for patients with multiple myeloma reported to the Center for International Blood Marrow Transplant Research from 2001 to 2014. Slide 43 [5]. Comparisons across survival curves are univariate and do not adjust for all potentially important factors; consequently, results should be interpreted cautiously

Diffuse Large B-Cell Lymphoma

Diffuse large B-cell lymphoma (DLBCL) is one of the most common types of lymphoma, comprising approximately 25% of all non-Hodgkin lymphomas (NHL) [47]. The incidence is approximately 7 cases per 100,000 in the USA with a median age of 64 years. DLBCL is an aggressive malignancy of large, transformed B lymphocytes that leads to diffuse effacement of the normal lymph node or lymphatic organ. Patients present with symptoms related to rapid growth of lymph node masses. A third of patients have associated systemic or B symptoms of weight loss, fevers, and drenching night sweats. Patients with DLBCL in first remission after conventional chemoimmunotherapy are likely to enjoy long-term disease-free survival, with the consideration of HCT only in the setting of incomplete response or relapse of disease [48]. In this latter setting, DLBCL is the second most common indication for HCT following MM (see Fig. 37.4). The majority of HCTs for DLBCL are autologous with the standard indication in the setting of chemotherapy-sensitive relapsed disease [23, 24, 49]. The benefit of consolidative autologous HCT compared to standard salvage therapy was initially demonstrated via the PARMA trial in 1995, and it continues to be standard of care with PFS ranging from 30 to 70% compared to 10 to 15% without HCT [50, 51]. Allogeneic HCT is considered in patients with poorly responsive disease, either at initial presentation or upon relapse, and hence are typically patients with higher-risk disease compared to patients receiving autologous HCT. Allogeneic HCT is also considered an appropriate therapy in the setting of relapse after autologous HCT with multiple reports of prolonged survival following reduced intensity/nonmyeloablative allogeneic HCT [52].

Fig. 37.10 Overall survival after HCT for patients with diffuse large cell lymphoma reported to the Center for International Blood Marrow Transplant Research from 2004 to 2014. (**a**) Autologous HCT, Slide 39 [5]; (**b**) Allogeneic HCT, Slide 40 [5]. Comparisons across survival curves are univariate and do not adjust for all potentially important factors; consequently, results should be interpreted cautiously

Figure 37.10 shows the CIBMTR data of patients receiving autologous or MSD HCT for DLBCL from 2004 to 2014. The 3-year OS after autologous transplant was 65% ± 1% and 45% ± 2% for patients with chemosensitive and chemoresistant disease, respectively. The 3-year OS for patients receiving allogeneic HCT was 51% ± 2% and 27% ± 3% for patients with chemosensitive and chemoresistant disease, respectively.

Follicular Lymphoma

Follicular lymphoma is the second most common NHL, comprising approximately 20% of NHLs with an estimated incidence of 3 cases per 100,000 people in the USA [47]. FL is also the most common indolent lymphoma defined by survival measured in years if untreated. The median age of onset is 65 years with the average life span greater than 15 years. FL is a malignancy of B lymphocytes that causes lymph node effacement leading to diffuse lymphadenopathy and

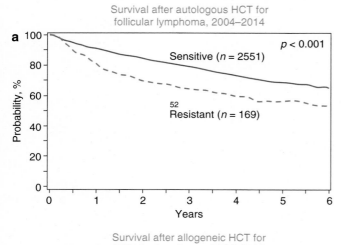

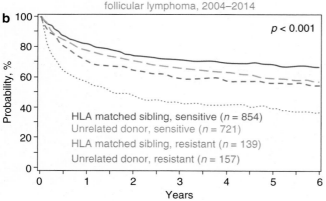

Fig. 37.11 Overall survival after HCT for patients with follicular lymphoma reported to the Center for International Blood Marrow Transplant Research from 2004 to 2014. (**a**) Autologous HCT, Slide 37 [5]; (**b**) Allogeneic HCT, Slide 38 [5]. Comparisons across survival curves are univariate and do not adjust for all potentially important factors; consequently, results should be interpreted cautiously

commonly associated with bone marrow infiltration. Patients are often asymptomatic at diagnosis with eventual need for treatment due to progressive lymphadenopathy and occasional cytopenias due to the bone marrow infiltration [26]. Indication for HCT is beyond the first or second remission, in the setting of relapsed or refractory disease [23, 24]. As with MM, autologous HCT is not likely curative and is approached with the goal of prolonging PFS and OS and maintaining quality of life. Autologous HCT is considered for patients with chemotherapy-sensitive first or second relapse without a clear benefit in patients having failed three or more prior therapies [53, 54]. A somewhat unique situation in which autologous HCT may be utilized earlier in the treatment of FL is in the setting of transformation to a more aggressive histology, an event occurring at a predicted 3% risk per year from FL diagnosis [55]. Autologous HCT may offer long-term control of the more aggressive histology,

however, with a more likely risk of persistent or recurrent, indolent FL histology in the future. Allogeneic HCT, however, does offer curative potential in FL and is an ideal indication for reduced intensity regimens, harnessing the immunologic benefits of the graft versus lymphoma effect without the morbidity and mortality of more aggressive HCT regimens [53, 56, 57]. One of the most promising reports comes from the MD Anderson experience reporting an 11-year PFS of 78% in patients with recurrent and refractory FL, including patients having failed autologous HCT [56]. Figure 37.11 shows the survival curves for FL patients reported to the CIBMTR treated with autologous and allogeneic HCT from 2004 to 2014 [5]. The progressive decline in the survival curves in the autologous HCT group illustrates the lack of curative potential despite encouraging 3-year OS of 79% ± 1% and 65% ± 0.4% for patients with chemosensitive and chemoresistant disease, respectively. On the other hand, the allogeneic HCT curves demonstrate plateaus and possible curative endpoints with 3-year OS ranging from 43% to 72% for MSD and URD HCT in patients with chemosensitive and chemoresistant disease.

Mantle Cell Lymphoma

Mantle cell lymphoma (MCL) is a relatively rare type of lymphoma with four to eight cases per million people, comprising approximately 7% of NHLs and a median age at diagnosis of 68 years [58]. MCL is also a B-cell neoplasm with a pathognomonic chromosomal abnormality of t(11;14) [26]. MCL most often presents with disseminated lymphadenopathy, occasional visceral organ involvement, such as the gastrointestinal tract, as well as the bone marrow. Patients may present without symptoms other than painless, swollen lymph nodes or an incidental pathologic finding on a routine colonoscopy. Others may have systemic complaints such as weight loss, fevers, and night sweats or rarely with a leukemic phase noted on a peripheral blood smear. Although MCL is much less common than FL, the CIBMTR reports a similar number of patients undergoing HCT for MCL as FL in the USA [5]. Dissimilar to FL, MCL has a more aggressive course in the majority of patients, and if left untreated, patients may die of their disease within a few years of diagnosis [59]. Autologous HCT is the standard approach for transplant eligible patients (typically less than 60–65 years) in first CR [23, 24, 60], and similarly to FL, a lack of plateau in the OS curve depicts the likely noncurative potential of autologous HCT albeit with a 3-year OS of 79% (see Fig. 37.12) [5]. Allogeneic HCT is indicated for patients with relapse after intensive induction, refractory to intensive induction, or failure of autologous HCT with 3-year OS of 53%. The possibility of curative potential is evidenced by the plateau in the survival curve, again similar to FL undergoing allogeneic HCT [5].

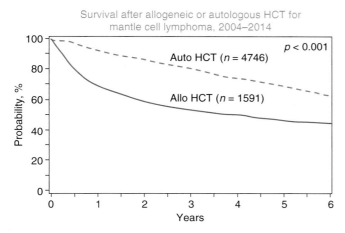

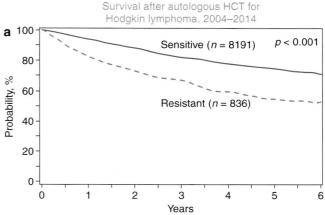

Fig. 37.12 Overall survival after HCT for patients with mantle cell lymphoma reported to the Center for International Blood Marrow Transplant Research from 2004 to 2014. Slide 41 [5]. Comparisons across survival curves are univariate and do not adjust for all potentially important factors; consequently, results should be interpreted cautiously

Hodgkin Lymphoma

Classical Hodgkin lymphoma (HL) is a distinct entity from NHL comprising 10% of all lymphomas and with an estimated 8300 new cases in 2017 [25]. It is derived from a mature B lymphocyte with loss of most of the B-cell-specific expression profile. As with other lymphomas, HL disease manifests with lymph node replacement and occasional involvement of extra-nodal sites [26]. Classical HL refers to four subgroups with the most common being nodular sclerosing HL, 70% of all classical HL in the USA and Europe [61]. Classical HL has two peak median ages of onset, at approximately 20 years and 65 years. The most common presenting symptom is painless swelling above the diaphragm corresponding to the area of lymphadenopathy. Less frequently patients may have fevers, weight loss, or drenching night sweats. Somewhat unique to HL is unexplained diffuse pruritus as well as a rare association of pain in an affected lymph node after ingestion of alcohol. By far the majority of patients will be cured with their initial conventional therapy. Autologous HCT is pursued with cura-tive intent and indicated for patients with first relapse or pri-mary refractory HL [24, 46] with the outcome dependent on pre-transplant characteristics. The CIBMTR identified four adverse prognostic factors (Karnofsky performance score <90, chemotherapy resistance at time of HCT, number of prior che-motherapy regimens, and extranodal disease at time of HCT) that defined three risk groups with 4-year PFS ranging from 42% to 71% [62]. Allogeneic HCT is indicated for patients with refractory disease as well as for patients with relapse post-autologous HCT, also with curative intent [23, 24]. Figure 37.13 illustrates the outcomes of HL patients receiving autologous and allogeneic HCT reported to the CIBMTR from 2004 to 2014 [5].

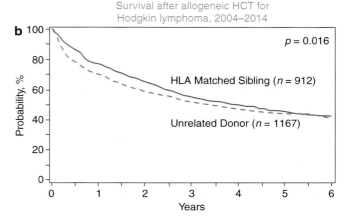

Fig. 37.13 Overall survival after HCT for patients with Hodgkin lym-phoma reported to the Center for International Blood Marrow Transplant Research from 2004 to 2014. (**a**) Autologous HCT, Slide 35 [5]; (**b**) Allogeneic HCT, Slide 36 [5]. Comparisons across survival curves are univariate and do not adjust for all potentially important factors; conse-quently, results should be interpreted cautiously

Aplastic Anemia

Aplastic anemia (AA) is a life-threatening form of bone mar-row failure and, if untreated, leads to death within 1 year [63]. Severe AA is characterized by absence of red blood cells, neu-trophils, monocytes, and platelets and their respective precur-sors in the bone marrow. Laboratory data identify profound anemia, neutropenia, and thrombocytopenia with a bone mar-row devoid of hematopoietic elements. Patients present with symptoms of anemia including fatigue, weakness, dizziness; symptoms of thrombocytopenia with gum and nose bleeding, easy bruising, and rash (petechiae); and infections. The major-ity of AA cases present without a precipitating cause; however, AA may occur following a viral illness, exposure to toxic chemicals, medications, or an associated autoimmune or con-nective tissue disorder. As a rare disease, with an incidence of two per million per year, it is a relatively uncommon indication for allogeneic HCT and never an indication for autologous

L. Johnston

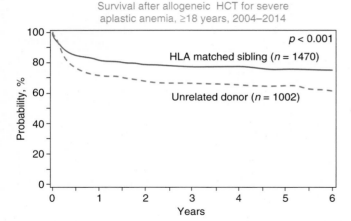

Fig. 37.14 Overall survival after allogeneic HCT for adult patients with severe aplastic anemia reported to the Center for International Blood Marrow Transplant Research from 2004 to 2014. Slide 14 [5]. Comparisons across survival curves are univariate and do not adjust for all potentially important factors; consequently, results should be interpreted cautiously

HCT. However, severe AA is one of the few, if not only, diseases, in which allogeneic HCT is the standard of care at the time of diagnosis for an individual <40–50 years of age with a MSD or MURD [23, 24, 64]. Age impacts outcome of HCT with review of over 1300 patients transplanted between 1991 and 2004 reported by the CIBMTR showing 5-year survival of 82% if younger than 20 years of age, 72% for those 20–40 years of age, and approximately 50% for those older than 40 years with a MSD [65]. The EBMT reported similar outcomes for patients 30–40 years and 40–50 years of age with MSDs, however, with need to carefully consider comorbidities as well as the preparative regimen utilized to minimize the regimen-related toxicities [66]. The EBMT has also reported similar outcomes for adults receiving MSD versus MURD in the more recent era; hence, it is the standard of care to consider URD BMT as a first-line therapy for the younger patients including younger adults [67]. For patients greater than 40–50 years of age or without a MSD or MURD, allogeneic HCT is indicated as a second-line therapy, after failure of standard immunosuppressive therapy [23, 24, 64]; however, outcomes of HCT in these clinical settings are also improving with consideration for HCT earlier in diagnosis likely becoming more frequent in the near future. The CIBMTR data for AA adult patients transplanted from 2004 to 2014 are shown in Fig. 37.14 supporting the excellent outcomes for recipients of a MSD or an URD with 3-year OS of 78% ± 1% and 67% ± 2%, respectively [5].

Conclusions

The indications for HCT reviewed above comprise approximately 75% and nearly 90% of adult patients receiving allogeneic and autologous HCT, respectively [5, 13]. We are now well beyond the millionth HCT worldwide with the population of patients considered for HCT continuing

to expand. The extension of donor sources, reduction in regimen-related toxicities, and improvements in pre-transplant risk assessment allow us to offer the curative potential of HCT to the patient population of greatest likelihood to have these diagnoses.

References

1. Program NMD. National marrow donor program: media fact sheet: 1 million blood stem cell transplants Worldwide; 2012.
2. Gratwohl A, Pasquini MC, Aljurf M, Atsuta Y, Baldomero H, Foeken L, et al. One million haemopoietic stem-cell transplants: a retrospective observational study. Lancet Haematol. 2015;2(3):e91–100.
3. Gooley TA, Chien JW, Pergam SA, Hingorani S, Sorror ML, Boeckh M, et al. Reduced mortality after allogeneic hematopoietic-cell transplantation. N Engl J Med. 2010;363(22):2091–101.
4. Gragert L, Eapen M, Williams E, Freeman J, Spellman S, Baitty R, et al. HLA match likelihoods for hematopoietic stem-cell grafts in the U.S. registry. N Engl J Med. 2014;371(4):339–48.
5. D'Souza APM, Zhu X. Current use and outcome of hematopoietic stem cell transplantation: CIBMTR summary slides, 2016. http://www.cibmtr.org2016.
6. Niederwieser D, Baldomero H, Szer J, Gratwohl M, Aljurf M, Atsuta Y, et al. Hematopoietic stem cell transplantation activity worldwide in 2012 and a SWOT analysis of the worldwide network for blood and marrow transplantation group including the global survey. Bone Marrow Transplant. 2016;51(6):778–85.
7. Saber W, Cutler CS, Nakamura R, Zhang MJ, Atallah E, Rizzo JD, et al. Impact of donor source on hematopoietic cell transplantation outcomes for patients with myelodysplastic syndromes (MDS). Blood. 2013;122(11):1974–82.
8. Saber W, Opie S, Rizzo JD, Zhang MJ, Horowitz MM, Schriber J. Outcomes after matched unrelated donor versus identical sibling hematopoietic cell transplantation in adults with acute myelogenous leukemia. Blood. 2012;119(17):3908–16.
9. Marks DI, Woo KA, Zhong X, Appelbaum FR, Bachanova V, Barker JN, et al. Unrelated umbilical cord blood transplant for adult acute lymphoblastic leukemia in first and second complete remission: a comparison with allografts from adult unrelated donors. Haematologica. 2014;99(2):322–8.
10. Brunstein CG, Fuchs EJ, Carter SL, Karanes C, Costa LJ, Wu J, et al. Alternative donor transplantation after reduced intensity conditioning: results of parallel phase 2 trials using partially HLA-mismatched related bone marrow or unrelated double umbilical cord blood grafts. Blood. 2011;118(2):282–8.
11. Bashey A, Zhang X, Sizemore CA, Manion K, Brown S, Holland HK, et al. T-cell-replete HLA-haploidentical hematopoietic transplantation for hematologic malignancies using post-transplantation cyclophosphamide results in outcomes equivalent to those of contemporaneous HLA-matched related and unrelated donor transplantation. J Clin Oncol. 2013;31(10):1310–6.
12. Zhang H, Chen J, Que W. A meta-analysis of unrelated donor umbilical cord blood transplantation versus unrelated donor bone marrow transplantation in acute leukemia patients. Biol Blood Marrow Transplant. 2012;18(8):1164–73.
13. Passweg JR, Baldomero H, Bader P, Bonini C, Cesaro S, Dreger P, et al. Hematopoietic stem cell transplantation in Europe 2014: more than 40 000 transplants annually. Bone Marrow Transplant. 2016;51(6):786–92.
14. McClune BL, Weisdorf DJ. Reduced-intensity conditioning allogeneic stem cell transplantation for older adults: is it the standard of care? Curr Opin Hematol. 2010;17(2):133–8.

15. Muffly L, Pasquini MC, Martens M, Brazauskas R, Zhu X, Adekola K, et al. Increasing use of allogeneic hematopoietic cell transplantation in patients aged 70 years and older in the United States. Blood. 2017;130(9):1156–64.

16. Michaelis LC, Hamadani M, Hari PN. Hematopoietic stem cell transplantation in older persons: respecting the heterogeneity of age. Expert Rev Hematol. 2014;7(3):321–4.

17. Wildes TM, Stirewalt DL, Medeiros B, Hurria A. Hematopoietic stem cell transplantation for hematologic malignancies in older adults: geriatric principles in the transplant clinic. J Natl Compr Cancer Netw. 2014;12(1):128–36.

18. Muffly LS, Kocherginsky M, Stock W, Chu Q, Bishop MR, Godley LA, et al. Geriatric assessment to predict survival in older allogeneic hematopoietic cell transplantation recipients. Haematologica. 2014;99(8):1373–9.

19. Sorror ML, Logan BR, Zhu X, Rizzo JD, Cooke KR, McCarthy PL, et al. Prospective validation of the predictive power of the hematopoietic cell transplantation comorbidity index: a Center for International Blood and Marrow Transplant Research Study. Biol Blood Marrow Transplant. 2015;21(8):1479–87.

20. Gratwohl A, Stern M, Brand R, Apperley J, Baldomero H, de Witte T, et al. Risk score for outcome after allogeneic hematopoietic stem cell transplantation: a retrospective analysis. Cancer. 2009;115(20):4715–26.

21. Parimon T, Au DH, Martin PJ, Chien JW. A risk score for mortality after allogeneic hematopoietic cell transplantation. Ann Intern Med. 2006;144(6):407–14.

22. Sorror M, Storer B, Sandmaier BM, Maloney DG, Chauncey TR, Langston A, et al. Hematopoietic cell transplantation-comorbidity index and Karnofsky performance status are independent predictors of morbidity and mortality after allogeneic nonmyeloablative hematopoietic cell transplantation. Cancer. 2008;112(9):1992–2001.

23. Sureda A, Bader P, Cesaro S, Dreger P, Duarte RF, Dufour C, et al. Indications for Allo- and auto-SCT for haematological diseases, solid tumours and immune disorders: current practice in Europe, 2015. Bone Marrow Transplant. 2015;50(8):1037–56.

24. Majhail NS, Farnia SH, Carpenter PA, Champlin RE, Crawford S, Marks DI, et al. Indications for autologous and allogeneic hematopoietic cell transplantation: guidelines from the American Society for Blood and Marrow Transplantation. Biol Blood Marrow Transplant. 2015;21(11):1863–9.

25. Siegel RL, Miller KD, Jemal A. Cancer statistics, 2017. CA Cancer J Clin. 2017;67(1):7–30.

26. Kaushansky K, Lichtman MA, Prchal J, Levi M, Press O, Burns L, et al., editors. Williams Hematology. 9th ed. New York: McGraw-Hill Education; 2016.

27. NCCN Guidelines: Acute Myeloid Leukemia 2017 June 6, 2017 Contract No.: Version 3.2017.

28. Gorin NC, Labopin M, Frassoni F, Milpied N, Attal M, Blaise D, et al. Identical outcome after autologous or allogeneic genoidentical hematopoietic stem-cell transplantation in first remission of acute myelocytic leukemia carrying inversion 16 or t(8;21): a retrospective study from the European cooperative Group for Blood and Marrow Transplantation. J Clin Oncol. 2008;26(19):3183–8.

29. Schlenk RF, Taskesen E, van Norden Y, Krauter J, Ganser A, Bullinger L, et al. The value of allogeneic and autologous hematopoietic stem cell transplantation in prognostically favorable acute myeloid leukemia with double mutant CEBPA. Blood. 2013;122(9):1576–82.

30. Boissel N. How should we treat the AYA patient with newly diagnosed ALL? Best Pract Res Clin Haematol. 2017;30(3):175–83.

31. Stock L, Advani, Geyer, Harvey, Mullighan, Willman, et al. Favorable outcomes for older adolescents and young adults (AYA) with acute lymphoblastic leukemia (ALL): early results of U.S. Intergroup Trial C10403. Blood. [abstract]. 2013;124:796.

32. NCCN Guidelines: Acute Lymphoblastic Leukemia 2017 October 27, 2017 Contract No.: Version 5.2017.

33. Chen X, Wood BL. How do we measure MRD in ALL and how should measurements affect decisions. Re: treatment and prognosis? Best Pract Res Clin Haematol. 2017;30(3):237–48.

34. Giebel S, Labopin M, Gorin NC, Caillot D, Leguay T, Schaap N, et al. Improving results of autologous stem cell transplantation for Philadelphia-positive acute lymphoblastic leukaemia in the era of tyrosine kinase inhibitors: a report from the acute Leukaemia working Party of the European Group for blood and marrow transplantation. Eur J Cancer. 2014;50(2):411–7.

35. Ma X, Does M, Raza A, Mayne ST. Myelodysplastic syndromes: incidence and survival in the United States. Cancer. 2007;109(8):1536–42.

36. Greenberg P, Cox C, LeBeau MM, Fenaux P, Morel P, Sanz G, et al. International scoring system for evaluating prognosis in myelodysplastic syndromes. Blood. 1997;89(6):2079–88.

37. Greenberg PL, Tuechler H, Schanz J, Sanz G, Garcia-Manero G, Sole F, et al. Revised international prognostic scoring system for myelodysplastic syndromes. Blood. 2012;120(12):2454–65.

38. Cutler CS, Lee SJ, Greenberg P, Deeg HJ, Perez WS, Anasetti C, et al. A decision analysis of allogeneic bone marrow transplantation for the myelodysplastic syndromes: delayed transplantation for low-risk myelodysplasia is associated with improved outcome. Blood. 2004;104(2):579–85.

39. Malcovati L, Germing U, Kuendgen A, Della Porta MG, Pascutto C, Invernizzi R, et al. Time-dependent prognostic scoring system for predicting survival and leukemic evolution in myelodysplastic syndromes. J Clin Oncol. 2007;25(23):3503–10.

40. Kyle RA, Gertz MA, Witzig TE, Lust JA, Lacy MQ, Dispenzieri A, et al. Review of 1027 patients with newly diagnosed multiple myeloma. Mayo Clin Proc. 2003;78(1):21–33.

41. Gay F, Oliva S, Petrucci MT, Conticello C, Catalano L, Corradini P, et al. Chemotherapy plus lenalidomide versus autologous transplantation, followed by lenalidomide plus prednisone versus lenalidomide maintenance, in patients with multiple myeloma: a randomised, multicentre, phase 3 trial. Lancet Oncol. 2015;16(16):1617–29.

42. Palumbo A, Cavallo F, Gay F, Di Raimondo F, Ben Yehuda D, Petrucci MT, et al. Autologous transplantation and maintenance therapy in multiple myeloma. N Engl J Med. 2014;371(10):895–905.

43. Attal M, Lauwers-Cances V, Hulin C, Leleu X, Caillot D, Escoffre M, et al. Lenalidomide, Bortezomib, and dexamethasone with transplantation for myeloma. N Engl J Med. 2017;376(14):1311–20.

44. Armeson KE, Hill EG, Costa LJ. Tandem autologous vs autologous plus reduced intensity allogeneic transplantation in the upfront management of multiple myeloma: meta-analysis of trials with biological assignment. Bone Marrow Transplant. 2013;48(4):562–7.

45. Kumar SK, Dispenzieri A, Lacy MQ, Gertz MA, Buadi FK, Pandey S, et al. Continued improvement in survival in multiple myeloma: changes in early mortality and outcomes in older patients. Leukemia. 2014;28(5):1122–8.

46. Swerdlow SH, Campo E, Pileri SA, Harris NL, Stein H, Siebert R, et al. The 2016 revision of the World Health Organization classification of lymphoid neoplasms. Blood. 2016;127(20):2375–90.

47. Morton LM, Wang SS, Devesa SS, Hartge P, Weisenburger DD, Linet MS. Lymphoma incidence patterns by WHO subtype in the United States, 1992-2001. Blood. 2006;107(1):265–76.

48. Zhou Z, Sehn LH, Rademaker AW, Gordon LI, Lacasce AS, Crosby-Thompson A, et al. An enhanced international prognostic index (NCCN-IPI) for patients with diffuse large B-cell lymphoma treated in the rituximab era. Blood. 2014;123(6):837–42.

49. Oliansky DM, Czuczman M, Fisher RI, Irwin FD, Lazarus HM, Omel J, et al. The role of cytotoxic therapy with hematopoietic stem cell transplantation in the treatment of diffuse large B cell lymphoma: update of the 2001 evidence-based review. Biol Blood Marrow Transplant. 2011;17(1):20–47 e30.

50. Hamlin PA, Zelenetz AD, Kewalramani T, Qin J, Satagopan JM, Verbel D, et al. Age-adjusted international prognostic

index predicts autologous stem cell transplantation outcome for patients with relapsed or primary refractory diffuse large B-cell lymphoma. Blood. 2003;102(6):1989–96.

51. Philip T, Guglielmi C, Hagenbeek A, Somers R, Van der Lelie H, Bron D, et al. Autologous bone marrow transplantation as compared with salvage chemotherapy in relapses of chemotherapy-sensitive non-Hodgkin's lymphoma. N Engl J Med. 1995;333(23):1540–5.

52. Rezvani AR, Kanate AS, Efron B, Chhabra S, Kohrt HE, Shizuru JA, et al. Allogeneic hematopoietic cell transplantation after failed autologous transplant for lymphoma using TLI and anti-thymocyte globulin conditioning. Bone Marrow Transplant. 2015;50(10):1286–92.

53. Oliansky DM, Gordon LI, King J, Laport G, Leonard JP, McLaughlin P, et al. The role of cytotoxic therapy with hematopoietic stem cell transplantation in the treatment of follicular lymphoma: an evidence-based review. Biol Blood Marrow Transplant. 2010;16(4):443–68.

54. Cao TM, Horning S, Negrin RS, Hu WW, Johnston LJ, Taylor TL, et al. High-dose therapy and autologous hematopoietic-cell transplantation for follicular lymphoma beyond first remission: the Stanford University experience. Biol Blood Marrow Transplant. 2001;7(5):294–301.

55. Lossos IS, Gascoyne RD. Transformation of follicular lymphoma. Best Pract Res Clin Haematol. 2011;24(2):147–63.

56. Khouri IF, Saliba RM, Erwin WD, Samuels BI, Korbling M, Medeiros LJ, et al. Nonmyeloablative allogeneic transplantation with or without 90yttrium ibritumomab tiuxetan is potentially curative for relapsed follicular lymphoma: 12-year results. Blood. 2012;119(26):6373–8.

57. Rezvani AR, Storer B, Maris M, Sorror ML, Agura E, Maziarz RT, et al. Nonmyeloablative allogeneic hematopoietic cell transplantation in relapsed, refractory, and transformed indolent non-Hodgkin's lymphoma. J Clin Oncol. 2008;26(2):211–7.

58. Zhou Y, Wang H, Fang W, Romaguer JE, Zhang Y, Delasalle KB, et al. Incidence trends of mantle cell lymphoma in the United States between 1992 and 2004. Cancer. 2008;113(4):791–8.

59. Cheah CY, Seymour JF, Wang ML. Mantle cell lymphoma. J Clin Oncol. 2016;34(11):1256–69.

60. Robinson S, Dreger P, Caballero D, Corradini P, Geisler C, Ghielmini M, et al. The EBMT/EMCL consensus project on the role of autologous and allogeneic stem cell transplantation in mantle cell lymphoma. Leukemia. 2015;29(2):464–73.

61. Loscher W, Nau H, Wahnschaffe U, Honack D, Rundfeldt C, Wittfoht W, et al. Effects of valproate and E-2-en-valproate on functional and morphological parameters of rat liver. II. Influence of phenobarbital comedication. Epilepsy Res. 1993;15(2):113–31.

62. Hahn T, McCarthy PL, Carreras J, Zhang MJ, Lazarus HM, Laport GG, et al. Simplified validated prognostic model for progression-free survival after autologous transplantation for hodgkin lymphoma. Biol Blood Marrow Transplant. 2013;19(12):1740–4.

63. Young NS. Aplastic anaemia. Lancet. 1995;346(8969):228–32.

64. Bacigalupo A. How I treat acquired aplastic anemia. Blood. 2017;129(11):1428–36.

65. Gupta V, Eapen M, Brazauskas R, Carreras J, Aljurf M, Gale RP, et al. Impact of age on outcomes after bone marrow transplantation for acquired aplastic anemia using HLA-matched sibling donors. Haematologica. 2010;95(12):2119–25.

66. Bacigalupo A, Socie G, Schrezenmeier H, Tichelli A, Locasciulli A, Fuehrer M, et al. Bone marrow versus peripheral blood as the stem cell source for sibling transplants in acquired aplastic anemia: survival advantage for bone marrow in all age groups. Haematologica. 2012;97(8):1142–8.

67. Bacigalupo A, Socie G, Hamladji RM, Aljurf M, Maschan A, Kyrcz-Krzemien S, et al. Current outcome of HLA identical sibling versus unrelated donor transplants in severe aplastic anemia: an EBMT analysis. Haematologica. 2015;100(5):696–702.

68. Paschka P, et al. Secondary genetic lesions in acute myeloid leukemia with inv(16) or t(16;16): a study of the German-Austrian AML study group (AMLSG). Blood. 2013;121:170–7.

Mental Health Prior to Hematopoietic Cell Transplantation

38

Sheila Lahijani

Introduction

The estimated annual combined incidence of leukemia, lymphoma, and multiple myeloma in the United States (US) is about 173,000, which is approximately 10% of all cancers [1]. Myelodysplastic syndrome (MDS) consists of stem cell disorders characterized by ineffective hematopoiesis with cytopenias and progression to leukemia in one third of cases; MDS is diagnosed annually in about 10,000 people in the United States [2, 3]. These blood dyscrasias may affect children, young adults, and those older than 65 years of age. Over time, cure rates have increased as has prolonged survival due to novel treatment regimens that can accompany hematopoietic cell transplant (HCT). HCT, which is discussed in Chaps. 37 and 40, is a potentially curative treatment involving the transplantation of stem cells from a donor (allogeneic) or from the patient (autologous). Approximately 20,000 HCTs are performed each year in the United States. The annual number of allogeneic transplant recipients has surpassed 8000 per year in the United States since 2013; the number of autologous transplant recipients has increased at a faster rate due to transplants being performed with reduced intensity regimens for plasma cell and lymphoproliferative disorders in older adults [4, 5]. Psychosocial distress and comorbid psychiatric symptoms and/or disorders in individuals with blood dyscrasias are common and may be greater in severity than the general population without cancer. Distress is a term used to describe the array of psychiatric symptoms and psychosocial issues that transplant recipients experience specific to the disease and transplant. Symptoms of distress are assessed to be the most intense before transplantation and over time can improve or resolve [6]. Adjustment, depressive, and anxiety disorders are most common in patients with cancer [7]. Of

notable concern is worsening of psychiatric symptoms in individuals with preexisting psychiatric disorders who develop hematologic malignancies and need to undergo HCT. In this patient population, there is particular consideration for medication nonadherence, drug-drug interactions, and drug-disease interactions [8].

Individuals with psychiatric issues are at risk for worse health outcomes, longer hospitalizations, and increased mortality [9, 10]. In patients undergoing HCT, mental health stability is of paramount importance given the associated physical and psychological factors associated with HCT and post-transplant sequelae, such as infection and graft versus host disease (GVHD). Psychological distress and alterations in thinking are common in these patient population who are often in isolation in the hospitalized setting [11]. Patients experience additional disruptions to their lives when being separated from their support systems, experiencing financial problems, having housing concerns, and dealing with other life stressors in the setting of illness. Among psychosocial risk factors, those associated with negative outcomes following transplantation include limited social support, history of poor adherence, comorbid untreated psychiatric disorder, use of avoidance-based coping, and active substance use [12]. Therefore, given the wide range of distress with which individuals may present, the screening, diagnosis, treatment of psychiatric symptoms, and disorders should be routinely provided to this patient population by a cross-disciplinary collaborative approach.

Psychiatric Symptoms and Disorders

Anxiety

While anxiety disorders in the DSM-5 include their own diagnostic criteria, the shared feature is heightened distress related to a threat and efforts to avoid or flee from the perceived danger [13]. The prevalence of anxiety in patients with cancer varies from approximately 10–30% given variable assessment

S. Lahijani
Department of Psychiatry and Behavioral Sciences, Stanford University School of Medicine, Palo Alto, CA, USA
e-mail: lahijani@stanford.edu

© Springer International Publishing AG, part of Springer Nature 2019
Y. Sher, J. R. Maldonado (eds.), *Psychosocial Care of End-Stage Organ Disease and Transplant Patients*,
https://doi.org/10.1007/978-3-319-94914-7_38

methods [14]. People may experience anxiety symptoms from the onset of diagnosis and throughout the illness experience with shifts in roles, changes in functioning, financial stressors, and existential inquires. Anxiety may present as new symptom in these transitions or be reactivated from the past with the diagnosis of cancer [15]. Furthermore, patients with cancer may experience many factors related to the disease and associated with the treatment. In addition, medications, such as corticosteroids and antiemetics, as well as comorbid medical problems, such as a pulmonary embolism, may present as anxiety. Irrespective of the etiology, the presence of anxiety, especially in the form of a disorder, may negatively impact patients' quality of life (QOL) and treatment outcomes (Fig. 38.1). Thus, the screening, assessment, and treatment of anxiety disorders in patients with hematological malignancy is critical to comprehensive cancer care both for hospitalized patients and those undergoing outpatient evaluations for HCT. In a large 3-year prospective study of hospitalized patients undergoing HCT using the Hospital Anxiety and Depression Scale (HADS), anxiety was found to be the highest at the beginning of the hospitalization. This was related to the uncertainty and the fear undergoing the HCT, an aggressive medical therapy [16]. Guidelines from the American Society of Clinical Oncology recommend periodic screening for anxiety in patients with cancer with the use of screening tools and referral to mental health providers as clinically indicated [17] (Table 38.1).

Depression

In a survey by the World Health Organization (WHO), 9.3–23% of participants with one or more chronic medical problem also had comorbid depression; depression had the largest impact on worsening mean health scores and increasing disability compared with other chronic conditions [18]. In a meta-analysis of 94 studies, the prevalence of depression in the cancer setting was 38% [14]. Depression in cancer is associated with greater physical, social, and existential distress and with measurable reductions in QOL [19]. Furthermore, depression in patients with advanced cancer may be associated with higher symptom burden [20].

Many factors may contribute to depression in patients with hematological malignancies. These include poor symptom control (e.g., mucositis), comorbid neurological disorders (e.g., cognitive impairment), and metabolic disorders (e.g., thyroid dysfunction). Cytotoxic therapies, disruptions in the hypothalamic pituitary adrenal axis, increases in pro-inflammatory cytokines, and paraneoplastic syndromes may also contribute to depressive symptoms in this patient population. Thus, it is important to note that comorbid medical disorders and/or treatments or symptoms associated with hematological malignancies (e.g., weakness, fatigue) can make it difficult to diagnose depressive disorders. Therefore, identifying risk factors for depressive disorders in this patient population is important for prevention and early diagnosis

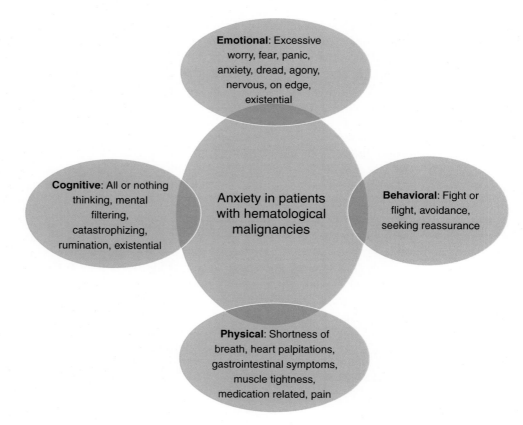

Fig. 38.1 Domains of Anxiety in Patients with Hematological Malignancies

Table 38.1 Categories of anxiety disorders in patients with hematological malignancies

Anxiety disorders in hematological malignancies	
Primary psychiatric disorders	Generalized anxiety disorder Panic disorder Agoraphobia and other phobias Social anxiety disorder Obsessive-compulsive disorder Acute stress disorder Post-traumatic stress disorder Adjustment disorder with anxiety
Substance-induced anxiety disorder	Corticosteroids Antiemetics Stimulants Anticholinergics Withdrawal from nicotine, alcohol, benzodiazepines
Anxiety disorders due to medical condition	Somatic symptoms: Nausea, vomiting, pain Thyroid dysfunction Electrolyte derangements (e.g., hypercalcemia) Pulmonary embolism Pulmonary effusions

and treatment of depression. Additional contributory factors can be categorized into two groups: (1) general predisposing factors for depression and (2) psychosocial and personality factors. Past history of depression, family history of depression, and poor social support are among general predisposing factors for depressions. These have been associated with inflammatory responses in the brain. Personality factors also have been studied; Type D personality, characterized by negative affectivity and social inhibition, has been associated with worse mental health. However, studies have shown variable association between these biological and nonbiological factors [21]. In a recent multicenter study, a diagnosis of pre-HCT depression was associated with lower overall survival, higher risk of acute GVHD, and less days spent alive and out of the hospital during the first 100 days after HCT. These findings highlight the impact of pre-HCT depression on post-HCT outcomes and further identify the need for psychosocial assessments of patients with hematological malignancies prior to undergoing HCT [22].

Demoralization

Demoralization is a term and concept introduced many years ago by Jerome Frank that recently has been described as a specific clinical entity in the oncology setting. Demoralization is characterized by existential despair, hopelessness, helplessness, and a subjective personal failure to achieve one's goals. It is associated with the loss of meaning and purpose in life. As a syndrome, it must persist for at least 2 weeks without the presence of a major psychiatric episode. Demoralization may be viewed as a spectrum that

encompasses disheartenment, despondency, despair, and fulminant demoralization syndrome, the last of which causes significant functional impairment [23–25]. There are two dominant measures of demoralization: a structured interview called the Diagnostic Criteria for Psychosomatic Research (DCPR) and the Demoralization Scale (DS), which is a self-report questionnaire [23.24]. Validation of the DS has allowed the estimation of demoralization among cancer patients to be 16% [26].

More recently, the Demoralization Scale-II was created as a self-report measure of demoralization consisting of 16 items and 2 subscales (meaning and purpose, distress and coping ability) [27]. Demoralization is clinically separate from depressive disorders, has a high prevalence in medical disorders, and, therefore, needs to be evaluated, measured, and treated during the course of the cancer illness experience. Differentiating between demoralization and depressive disorders is important for treatment planning and alignment of goals between providers and patients. Analyses of current measures of demoralization demonstrate that demoralization should be considered as a significant clinical entity in cancer settings to improve QOL [28]. In a longitudinal study of patients with acute leukemia evaluating physical and psychological well-being, depression, hopelessness, and demoralization were distinguished, and further investigation was recommended to evaluate, diagnose, and manage this distress in patients with leukemia [29]. With respect to demoralization in patients with cancer, a recent study showed an association with a significantly increased risk for suicidal ideation, further highlighting the importance of psychiatric evaluations of patients with hematologic malignancies [30].

Suicide

Compared to the general population, individuals with cancer are at higher risk of suicide [31]. In a retrospective cohort study, there was a two times higher incidence of suicide in those with cancer compared to those without cancer. Patients were 13 times more likely to commit suicide within 1 week of receiving a cancer diagnosis. Patients were three times more likely to commit suicide within 1 year of cancer diagnosis than the general population [32]. Studies including individuals with hematological malignancies also have reported an increased risk of suicide [31, 33]. The risk of attempted and completed suicide was evaluated in a large population-based Swedish cohort study of over 40,000 patients diagnosed with lymphoma, myeloma, and leukemia. Patients with a hematological malignancy had a two times higher risk of completed suicide compared to those without cancer. A history of severe mental illness and a history of attempted suicide before diagnosis were associated with higher risk, although the overall greater risk of suicide was not isolated to this group. The risk was highest within the first 3 months following diagnosis, and a 1.7-fold increase in risk of completed suicide remained after the first year of diagnosis. The findings of this study suggest an increase in suicidal intent in those with hematological malignancy [34].

In another large population-based study, patients with hematological malignancies were again found to be at increased risk for completed suicide and suicide attempt, particularly those with preexisting depressive disorders and alcohol use disorders [35]. Therefore, early identification of high-risk patients immediately after diagnosis and during follow-up is important as a preventative measure for suicide risk. These findings emphasize the need for multidisciplinary teams, psychiatric evaluations, and treatment to improve QOL measures and also to decrease the risk of suicide in patients with hematological malignancies.

Delirium

Delirium is a neurobehavioral syndrome characterized by alterations in awareness, attention, cognition, language, and perception that is an abrupt change from the person's baseline due to a variety of endocrinologic, immunologic, neuroinflammatory, neurologic, and/or metabolic effects [36]. It is associated with increased morbidity and mortality, longer length of hospitalization, higher health-care costs, and distress among patients and their families. Delirium is a very common neuropsychiatric presentation in patients with cancer. Despite a prevalence of 10–30%, delirium continues to be underdiagnosed and untreated in patients hospitalized with cancer [37].

In patients with hematological malignancies, several pretransplantation risk factors for delirium have been identified. These include lower pre-transplant renal, hepatic and cognitive functioning, acute leukemia, total body irradiation, and prior substance use. Additionally, chemotherapy-related hormonal changes in females and hypermagnesemia have been associated with a higher delirium risk. The diagnosis and treatment of delirium prior to HCT may reduce the risk and severity of delirium after HCT [38]. In a study by Fann, et al., potentially modifiable pre-transplantation risk factors were liver dysfunction, dehydration, and renal dysfunction. Pain control and judicious use of opioid medications were associated with lower risk of delirium. Identifying risk factors for delirium symptom severity is important in decreasing the morbidity from delirium before, during, and after HCT [39].

Somatic Symptoms

Pain

In cancer, pain is a multidimensional experience of physical symptoms, personality factors, cognition, and social and behavioral relations. The experience of pain may change over the course of the cancer illness experience. A patient with cancer who has pain can be best treated when all of the different aspects of the pain are considered and addressed [40]. In patients with hematological malignancies, oral mucositis is among the most debilitating side effects of myeloablative therapy prior to HCT. Mucositis results from damage to mucosal epithelium of the mouth and throat with activation of proinflammatory cytokines in the submucosa, leading to oral ulceration. Oral mucositis can impact all aspects of QOL and interfere with daily activities, such as talking, eating, swallowing, and sleeping. The Oral Mucositis Daily Questionnaire (OMDQ) is a valid and reliable tool that can be used to measure mucositis severity. Treatment of mucositis includes basic oral care, anti-inflammatory agents, anesthetic agents, coating agents, and antimicrobials [41, 42]. Other types of pain in patients with blood dyscrasias include bone pain, paresthesias, treatment-related pain, infection-related pain, and skeletal lesions. Both preventative and interventional measures should be implemented to optimize the pain management of patients prior to undergoing HCT. Nonpharmacological and pharmacological treatments can be of particular benefit, and patient-related variables, such as performance status, comorbidities (including psychiatric illness), and concurrent medications should be considered when making clinical decisions about treatment [43, 44]. Research over the years has demonstrated that depression, anxiety, distress, and lower QOL are associated with greater levels of pain in patients with cancer. Using a biopsychosocial approach when evaluating pain can elicit such contributory factors and better delineate pain management options [45].

Fatigue

Fatigue in cancer is a persistent, subjective experience of physical, emotional, and/or cognitive tiredness or exhaustion related to cancer or cancer treatment which is disproportionate to activity and interferes with usual functioning. Fatigue is a highly distressing symptom of cancer and is associated with decreased QOL and significant psychological and functional morbidity [46]. Severe fatigue has been reported more frequently in patients with hematologic malignancies than in those with solid tumors. Fatigue may be a presenting symptom at time of diagnosis of a hematologic malignancy; "B" symptoms of lymphoma include fatigue. A major contributor to increased fatigue and diminished QOL is anemia related to both the disease state and treatments. Other mechanisms, such as endocrine changes, physical deconditioning, impaired sleep, and alterations in cytokines, also have been proposed [47]. Physical exercise has been studied and recommended as an intervention for patients who will undergo HCT to improve physical activity, performance status, and quality of life [48, 49]. Managing psychiatric symptoms, anemia, metabolic derangements, and any nutritional deficiencies can improve the severity of fatigue. Psychopharmacologic agents should be considered, particularly in cases where a patient's functional status is compromised prior to transplant [46, 50].

Sleep

Sleep disorders, such as difficulty falling asleep, difficulty maintaining sleep, early awakening, and daytime sleepiness, are prevalent among patients with cancer. Sleep in patients with cancer may be impacted by a number of factors, including anxiety, depression, pain, and fatigue and may be related to biochemical changes associated with cancer and antineoplastic treatment [51].

Reasons for sleep disorders include thinking, pain or discomfort, concerns about health, concerns about family or friends, cancer diagnosis, physical effects of cancer, and concerns about finances [52].

Sleep disturbances and insomnia co-occur in symptom clusters in patients with cancer. The presence of symptom comorbidity in cancer may be related to underlying inflammatory processes common to all of them. The maintenance of circadian rhythms and consistent sleep wake patterns can reduce depressive symptomatology, improve overall perception of quality of life, and potentially improve outcomes and survival. Individuals with insomnia demonstrate cognitive, physiological, and cortical hyperarousal, cognitive patterns, and attentional biases. Cognitive behavioral therapy for insomnia (CBT-I) is a multimodal intervention to address these contributory factors. CBT-I has five main components: sleep restriction, stimulus control, sleep hygiene, cognitive restructuring, and relaxation training. A review of the literature has showed that CBT-I is associated with statistically and clinically significant improvements in subjective sleep outcomes in patients with cancer. CBT-I also may improve mood, fatigue, and quality of life during and after cancer treatment [53]. Pharmacologic interventions for sleep have not been adequately studied in patients with cancer. While they should be offered when indicated, caution must be exercised when prescribing these agents due to the potential for increased sedation, drug-drug interactions, delirium, and/or dependency.

Evaluation and Diagnosis

Screening

Major depression, minor depression, anxiety disorders, and adjustment disorders are among the most common psychiatric presentations in patients with cancer. A clinically significant mood disorder can be predicted in four in ten patients early in their disease course [14]. Many patients also experience emotional difficulty after a cancer diagnosis but do not meet criteria for a DSM-V disorder. The concept of distress has garnered popularity as the sixth vital sign, following

temperature, blood pressure, pulse, respiratory rate, and pain. The National Comprehensive Cancer Network (NCCN) has established distress management guidelines and defined distress as the "multifactorial unpleasant emotional experience of a psychological (cognitive, behavioral, emotional), social, and/or spiritual nature that may interfere with the ability to cope effectively with cancer, its physical symptoms and its treatment" [54, 55]. NCCN and other national guidelines promote the need for integrated psychosocial care and the use of psychometric assessments to help clinicians identify emotional problems in patients with cancers. Psychometric assessment would contribute to ruling out patients who do not need professional help (screening) and confirming the presence of a treatment psychiatric disorder (case finding). Psychometric assessment also would help quantify the severity of the disorder while monitoring for response to treatment [56].

The American College of Surgeons has established the Commission on Cancer's Cancer Program Standards which includes a process to integrate and monitor psychosocial distress screening and referral for the provision of psychosocial care. The standards require that all cancer patients be screened for distress a minimum of one time at a pivotal medical visit as determined by the program. The method of screening must utilize the expertise of physicians who can administer and interpret the screening tool. The tool used to screen should be a standardized, validated instrument. The distress screening then is to be discussed with the patient at the medical visit which may prompt a referral to a mental health provider [57].

Using the distress thermometer or asking a patient "are you worried?" or "are you depressed?" is a simple way to assess distress or anxiety [58, 59]. Screening for psychiatric symptoms and disorders in patients with cancer may include the use of a reliable, validated screening questionnaire or tool, of which there are many. The Generalized Anxiety Disorder-7 scale (GAD-7) and the Patient Health Questionnaire-9 (PHQ-9) are widely validated and used measures in medical populations [60, 61]. The Hospital Anxiety and Depression Scale (HADS) is the most extensively validated scale for screening emotional distress in patients with cancer. The thresholds for clinical decision-making vary widely, however, across studies [62]. A systematic review of assessment instruments to measure emotional distress in patients with cancer demonstrated the utility of both the HADS and the Center for Epidemiologic Studies Depression Scale (CES-D). The reviewers emphasized the importance of using short tools for screening of patients who undergo strenuous treatments, such as those with hematologic malignancies. Shorter tools may be better implemented in the setting of hospitalization prior to HCT [63]. While there are ongoing efforts to improve psychometric assessments for patients with cancer, such as the National Institute of Health project Patient-Reported Outcomes Measurement

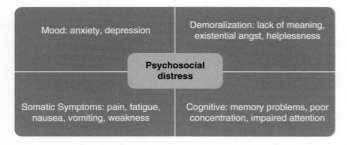

Fig. 38.2 Examples and sources of psychosocial distress

Information System network, the standard for psychosocial evaluation of patients with cancer continues to be structured clinical interviews (Fig. 38.2).

Psychiatric Interview and Exam

Once a patient with a hematologic malignancy is determined by having signs of emotional distress, depression, anxiety, or another psychiatric symptom, a psychiatric assessment is considered the next step. Many dimensions of a person's psychological symptoms may be explored further with a clinical interview. The aim of a standard psychiatric interview and exam would be to establish whether or not there is a psychiatric disorder or another condition requiring clinical psychiatric and/or psychosocial attention. During the exam, clinical data is collected to support a differential diagnosis and a comprehensive formulation. The formulation may include the clinical diagnosis which can be derived from the DSM-V. There also may be a discussion about other variables in the patient's presentation, including coping and attachment, vulnerabilities, strengths, history of life events, and social support. Factors affecting the individual with cancer distinct from the clinical diagnosis may describe further the individual's psychosocial suffering [64].

Quality of Life

Several domains of health-related QOL have been studied in patients treated with auto-HCT and allo-HCT. These include biomedical functioning (symptoms, disease, treatment), physical functioning (activities of daily living, sleep, fatigue), psychological functioning (cognitive, emotional, psychiatric symptoms), social functioning (social relations, support, education, socioeconomic status, work), and sexual functioning. Low social support and psychological distress prior to HCT have been identified to be predictors of diminished health-related QOL following HCT. Therefore, identifying factors that predict health-related QOL following HCT is important in understanding the ways patients may adapt to the consequences of the disease and treatment, such as resulting GVHD [65]. QOL assessments completed by patients before HCT have shown a strong association with

post-transplant physical and psychological functioning and also shown to be a strong independent predictor of post-HCT self-reported recovery through the first year [66]. Associations among psychosocial distress, coping responses, and QOL indicate that poor psychosocial functioning pre-HCT increases the likelihood of impaired QOL across the illness experience. Therefore, those who are more vulnerable should be identified and offered interventions earlier to help influence post-HCT outcomes [67]. A longitudinal study of QOL and physical and psychological symptoms experienced by patients with hematologic malignancies hospitalized for HCT and also their caregivers demonstrated the importance of addressing pre-HCT QOL, anxiety, depression, and fatigue in patients and offering psychiatric interventions where indicated. Additionally, the distress experienced by patients' caregivers was highlighted as another opportunity for supportive care interventions [68].

Social Support

The role of social support on the impact of illness has been extensively studied. Social support is believed to affect health in three ways: (1) regulating thoughts, feelings, and behaviors to promote health, (2) fostering an individual's sense of meaning in life, and (3) facilitating health-promoting behaviors. Supportive relationships have been identified in the literature as an important component in the adjustment and psychosocial functioning of patients with cancer. In patients who undergo HCT, social support has been associated with significantly better psychosocial adjustment [69]. The use of the Psychosocial Assessment of Candidates for Transplantation (PACT) scale has been studied in patients with hematological malignancies undergoing allo-HCT. "Family or support system availability" was identified as an important subscale and associated with a decreased risk of mortality [70]. Social support, self-efficacy, and optimism before HCT have been associated with health-related QOL after HCT. Prior to HCT, patients may be offered a list of support groups, educational resources, and online support and also be encouraged to identify family, friends, and existing members of their community for support [71].

Caregivers for patients with hematologic malignancies are expected to provide extensive support throughout the illness and transplant. Caregivers and patients may experience changes in employment, housing, and shifts in roles. Caregivers are tasked with a variety of responsibilities related to providing medical support (e.g., monitoring and administering medications) and navigating logistical challenges (e.g., transportation). A review of the literature demonstrated that psychosocial distress among HCT caregivers is highest pre-HCT and decreases over time. Factors associated with this distress include being a female caregiver, higher levels of subjective burden, and higher symptom distress in the patient. Caregivers for patients undergoing HCT experience uncertainty while adapting to changing roles and needing to balance their own needs with the patients' needs [72].

Studies suggest that rates of distress for caregivers following HCT may be the same as or greater than that of the patients in the immediate post-HCT period. Offering educational interventions and problem-solving therapy has demonstrated benefit in reducing caregiver distress and dyadic distress between the patient and his/her caregiver [73]. In a multicenter longitudinal study, the dyadic coping of patients with hematologic malignancies and their partners was investigated using the SF-12 questionnaire for QOL and the Dyadic Coping Inventory (DCI). Baseline QOL was the strongest predictor of physical and mental QOL for patients and their partners. Analyses of the DCI suggested the importance of incorporating patients' partners in a systematic way to help improve understanding of illness, improve compliance, and strengthen psychosocial adjustment [74].

Financial Burden

The national cost of cancer care is expected to increase due to adoption of more expensive targeted treatments as standard of care. Additionally, as the population ages, the impact on cancer prevalence may exceed the impact of declining cancer incidence rates for some cancers. This will result in an increase in both the number of cancer survivors and cancer expenditures [75]. As the number of patients with cancer in the United States increases, the numbers of patients with cancer who are treated with chemotherapy and diagnosed with neutropenia are also expected to rise. In patients with hematologic malignancies, patients face hospitalizations for cancer-related neutropenia and associated infections. Hospitalizations related to neutropenic complications result in significant medical costs, longer lengths of hospital stay, morbidity, and mortality [76].

The term "financial toxicity" is used to describe the financial hardship as a result of cancer diagnosis and treatment. Financial toxicity encompasses adverse economic consequences due to medical treatment that may result in nonadherence and lifestyle changes for patients, impacting their QOL and increasing the morbidity and mortality of treatments. Higher costs of newer treatment, more out of pocket costs, barriers in communication about costs, and medical comorbidities are cited as sources of increased financial toxicity in patients with hematological malignancies. One area of intervention, therefore, may be increasing communication between providers and patients to influence shared decision-making, health behaviors, and health outcomes [77].

Unmet Psychosocial Needs

A particular area of importance in patients with hematologic malignancies is unmet psychosocial needs. Psychosocial needs relate to a desire or requirement for support or help that underlies a patient's emotional or psychological welfare.

Examples include maintaining a sense of identity, body image, spirituality, relationships, social support, or practical issues related to a patient's illness experience. These needs are underreported to clinicians and may be left unacknowledged. In patients with hematological malignancies, the manner and setting in which treatment is received can differ from those diagnosed with solid tumors. Treatment is intensive, carries a high burden of illness, and can impact a patient's social, occupational, and family functioning. Data shows that fear of recurrence, needs relating to information, psychological needs, and fertility issues are unmet psychosocial needs in patients with hematological malignancies [78]. Currently, there is a lack of randomized trials of psychosocial interventions to address unmet psychosocial needs of these patients. Challenges are related to underutilized screening guidelines and tools in addition to lack of time allocated for managing these unmet needs. Increased efforts to screen for unmet needs in this population of patients would contribute to developing evidence-based interventions [79].

Special Considerations

Sexuality and Fertility

Patients with hematologic malignancies undergo treatments that affect body image, sexual function, hormone levels, and reproductivity. Myeloablative regimens cause loss of ovarian function and sexual dysfunction. High-dose conditioning regimens of HCT cause gonadal and hormonal dysfunction [73]. The deterioration in fertility potential may be temporary or permanent. Fertility issues and difficulties related to sexuality span the illness experience and thus may impact the mental welfare of patients who are pre-HCT. Biological factors (e.g., treatment related), behavioral factors (e.g., medical prohibitions on sexual activity), relational issues (e.g., partner response to sexual changes), and psychological factors (e.g., sexual esteem) all contribute to compromised sexuality. The review of literature demonstrates that those who will receive HCT may experience long-term sexual problems, including decreased libido, decreased sexual activity, genital changes, erectile and/or ejaculatory dysfunction, and altered sexual appearance. Measures should be considered for sexual health counseling and fertility preservation in patients with hematological malignancies [80–82].

Substance Use Disorders

All aspects of the cancer illness experience can be impacted by the use of substances and substance use disorders (SUD). Illicit drug or alcohol use disorders can cause nonadherence to potentially life-saving treatments. SUD can affect pain management and increase morbidity and mortality. It has remained a challenge to diagnose SUDs in patients with cancer partly due to underdiagnosis. Patients with cancer with historic or current SUD may participate in aberrant drug-taking behavior which may prompt a treatment team to consult a psycho-oncologist. Prescription drug abuse, including opioids, may complicate pain management and compromise both medical and psychiatric stability. Tobacco use disorders have been shown to impact HCT outcomes, thus inferring the need for tobacco use cessation. A multidisciplinary approach for pain and symptom management is recommended in patients with cancer who have SUD [83–85].

Decision-Making Capacity

Patients with cancer may have comorbid cognitive difficulties, dementia, or delirium related to a premorbid history of neuropsychiatric problems or as a consequence of the cancer and associated treatment. While screening measures and assessment tools are available, a diagnostic evaluation by a trained expert, such as a psychiatrist, would facilitate clinical decision-making, particularly in cases where decision-making capacity is of concern. Decision-making capacity consists of the patient's ability to understand relevant information, appreciate the situation and its consequences, manipulate information rationally, and communicate choices. Decision-making capacity can fluctuate with changes in patients' underlying medical or psychiatric problems, fatigue, or medication-related effects. Therefore, there may be a need to evaluate decision-making capacity more than once. In patients being evaluated for HCT, consideration of the aforementioned factors is important when assessing decision-making capacity to assent to or to refuse a proposed treatment or intervention [86].

Treatment

Psychopharmacologic

Psychotropic medications are frequently used in this patient population to treat psychiatric symptoms and disorders, as well as to manage nonpsychiatric conditions, such as fatigue, delirium, suppressed appetite, neuropathic pain, as well as nausea and vomiting. Optimal treatment of contributory medical problems, such as insomnia, with medications should be tried as a means to improve psychosocial health. While there is a spectrum of indications for psychopharmacologic agents, many agents may also increase the risk for hematopoietic dysfunction. Caution should be exercised to minimize adding to the burden of neutropenia, agranulocytosis, abnormal bleeding, and platelet dysfunction. Psychopharmacologic agents may interact with anticancer therapies, causing worsening gastrointestinal side effects, anticholinergic effects, and increased sedation. Psychotropic agents should be utilized as indicated, among other appropriate interventions, to improve the medical and psychiatric health of patients with hematologic malignancies prior to HCT, while monitoring for tolerance and side effects [73, 87]. See Table 38.2.

Non-Psychopharmacologic

Different modalities of psychotherapy have demonstrated efficacy for managing mood symptoms in patients with cancer [88]. These include cognitive behavioral therapy,

Table 38.2 Psychopharmacologic agents commonly used in patients with hematological malignancies

Medication class	Uses	Risks	Interactions	Hematologic effects
Antidepressants	SSRIs and SNRIs: Depression, anxiety, panic Mirtazapine: Sleep, appetite, nausea Bupropion: Fatigue	SSRIs: GI disturbances, headache SNRIs: GI disturbances, headache, hypertension Mirtazapine: Rare risk of agranulocytosis Bupropion: Seizures	MAOI interaction (e.g., procarbazine) CYP450 2D6 and 3A4 interactions (e.g., fluoxetine, paroxetine)	Cytopenias, platelet, impaired platelet aggregation
Anxiolytics: Benzodiazepines	Anxiety	Sedation, delirium, fatigue, respiratory depression, misuse	Narcotics, other sedative hypnotics	Cytopenias, platelet, impaired platelet aggregation
Antipsychotics	Anxiety, delirium, sleep Olanzapine: Nausea	Orthostatic hypotension, akathisia, EPS	QT prolongation with other agents, higher risk of EPS with antiemetics	Cytopenias, eosinophilia (clozapine)
Mood stabilizers, Anticonvulsants	Anxiety, irritability, delirium Gabapentin: Neuropathic pain	Sedation, weight gain Valproic acid: Transaminitis, decreased platelet aggregation, hair loss	Possible additive one marrow suppression with cytotoxic therapy	Cytopenia, anemia
Psychostimulants	Fatigue, concentration, depression	Anxiety, headache	Increased stimulation with corticosteroids	Not available

SSRIs selective serotonin reuptake inhibitors, *SNRIs* serotonin norepinephrine reuptake inhibitors, *MAOI* monoamine oxidase inhibitor, *EPS* extrapyramidal symptoms

problem-solving therapy, interpersonal therapies, group intervention, and behavioral activation. Relaxation therapy, mindfulness-based therapy, meaning-centered therapy, and dignity therapy are other approaches with principles that may be used to manage different causes of emotional distress. Other therapies, such as existential and psychodynamic, may be helpful in the setting of advanced disease. These many therapeutic approaches may be applied as indicated to patients with hematological malignancies before, during, and after HCT [73]. Please refer to Chap. 43 for further psychotherapeutic interventions.

Conclusions

The American Society for Blood and Marrow Transplantation HCT guidelines for clinical centers include a psychiatric/psychosocial assessment as part of the medical evaluation for all HCT candidates [89]. Improving a treating team's knowledge of a patient's psychosocial distress, psychiatric history, social support, and other important psychosocial factors can influence medical outcomes before, during, and after HCT. Standardized approaches, such as the PACT, have been developed in identifying psychosocial concerns before HCT. Associations have been shown between psychosocial health and QOL with adherence to treatment, length of hospital stay, morbidity, and mortality. Screening measures to complement clinical interviews and exams can offer valuable opportunities to intervene and improve psychosocial variables in patients with hematologic malignancies. While there are many future directions for research, the psychosocial assessment of this patient population remains of paramount importance in assessing the risks for HCT, which may be the only treatment option. Therefore, a multidisciplinary, collaborative approach to meet the psychosocial needs of patients with hematological malignancies can contribute to better HCT outcomes.

References

1. American Cancer Society. Cancer facts and figures 2017. Atlanta: American Cancer Society; 2013.
2. Adès L, Itzykson R, Fenaux P. Myelodysplastic syndromes. Lancet. 2014;383(9936):2239–52.
3. Sekeres MA. Epidemiology, natural history, and practice patterns of patients with myelodysplastic syndromes in 2010. J Natl Compr Cancer Netw. 2011;9(1):57–63.
4. D'Souza A, Zhu X. Current uses and outcomes of hematopoietic cell transplantation (HCT): CIBMTR summary slides; 2017.
5. Majhail NS, Farnia SH, Carpenter PA, Champlin RE, Crawford S, Marks DI, et al. Indications for autologous and allogeneic hematopoietic cell transplantation: guidelines from the American Society for Blood and Marrow Transplantation. Biol Blood Marrow Transplant. 2015;21(11):1863–9.
6. Syrjala KL, Langer SL, Abrams JR, Storer B, Sanders JE, Flowers ME, et al. Recovery and long-term function after hematopoietic cell transplantation for leukemia or lymphoma. JAMA. 2004;291(19):2335–43.
7. Mehnert A, Brähler E, Faller H, Härter M, Keller M, Schulz H, et al. Four-week prevalence of mental disorders in patients with cancer across major tumor entities. J Clin Oncol. 2014;32(31):3540–6.
8. Akaho R, Sasaki T, Yoshino M, Hagiya K, Akiyama H, Sakamaki H. Bone marrow transplantation in subjects with mental disorders. Psychiatry Clin Neurosci. 2003;57(3):311–5.
9. Pinquart M, Duberstein PR. Depression and cancer mortality: a meta-analysis. Psychol Med. 2010;40(11):1797–810.
10. Prina AM, Cosco TD, Dening T, Beekman A, Brayne C, Huisman M. The association between depressive symptoms in the community, non-psychiatric hospital admission and hospital outcomes: a systematic review. J Psychosom Res. 2015;78(1):25–33.
11. Sasaki T, Akaho R, Sakamaki H, Akiyama H, Yoshino M, Hagiya K, et al. Mental disturbances during isolation in bone marrow transplant patients with leukemia. Bone Marrow Transplant. 2000;25(3):315.
12. Jowsey SG, Taylor ML, Schneekloth TD, Clark MM. Psychosocial challenges in transplantation. J Psychiatr Pract®. 2001;7(6):404–14.
13. American Psychiatric Association. Diagnostic and statistical manual of mental disorders (DSM-5®): American Psychiatric Pub; Washington, DC; 2013.
14. Mitchell AJ, et al. Prevalence of depression, anxiety, and adjustment disorder in oncological, haematological, and palliative-care settings: a meta-analysis of 94 interview-based studies. Lancet Oncol. 2011;12(2):160–74.
15. Kangas M, Henry JL, Bryant RA. The course of psychological disorders in the 1st year after cancer diagnosis. J Consult Clin Psychol. 2005;73(4):763.
16. Prieto JM, Atala J, Blanch J, Carreras E, Rovira M, Cirera E, et al. Patient-rated emotional and physical functioning among hematologic cancer patients during hospitalization for stem-cell transplantation. Bone Marrow Transplant. 2005;35(3):307–14.
17. Andersen BL, DeRubeis RJ, Berman BS, Gruman J, Champion VL, Massie MJ, et al. Screening, assessment, and care of anxiety and depressive symptoms in adults with cancer: an American Society of Clinical Oncology guideline adaptation. J Clin Oncol. 2014;32(15):1605–19.
18. Moussavi S, Chatterji S, Verdes E, Tandon A, Patel V, Ustun B. Depression, chronic diseases, and decrements in health: results from the world health surveys. Lancet. 2007;370(9590):851–8.
19. Wilson KG, Chochinov HM, Skirko MG, Allard P, Chary S, Gagnon PR, et al. Depression and anxiety disorders in palliative cancer care. J Pain Symptom Manag. 2007;33(2):118–29.
20. Grotmol KS, Lie HC, Loge JH, Aass N, Haugen DF, Stone PC, et al. Patients with advanced cancer and depression report a significantly higher symptom burden than non-depressed patients. Palliat Support Care. 2018;10:1–7.
21. Caruso R, Nanni MG, Riba M, Sabato S, Mitchell AJ, Croce E, et al. Depressive spectrum disorders in cancer: prevalence, risk factors and screening for depression: a critical review. Acta Oncol. 2017;56(2):146–55.
22. El-Jawahri A, Chen YB, Brazauskas R, He N, Lee SJ, Knight JM, et al. Impact of pre-transplant depression on outcomes of allogeneic and autologous hematopoietic stem cell transplantation. Cancer. 2017;123(10):1828–38.
23. Kissane DW, Clarke DM, Street AF. Demoralization syndrome-a relevant psychiatric diagnosis for palliative care. J Palliat Care. 2001;17(1):12.
24. Clarke DM, Kissane DW. Demoralization: its phenomenology and importance. Aust N Z J Psychiatry. 2002;36(6):733–42.
25. Robinson S, Kissane DW, Brooker J, Burney S. A systematic review of the demoralization syndrome in individuals with progressive disease and cancer: a decade of research. J Pain Symptom Manag. 2015;49(3):595–610.

26. Mehnert A, Vehling S, Höcker A, Lehmann C, Koch U. Demoralization and depression in patients with advanced cancer: validation of the German version of the demoralization scale. J Pain Symptom Manag. 2011;42(5):768–76.

27. Robinson S, Kissane DW, Brooker J, Hempton C, Michael N, Fischer J, et al. Refinement and revalidation of the demoralization scale: the DS-II—external validity. Cancer. 2016;122(14):2260–7.

28. Grassi L, Nanni MG. Demoralization syndrome: new insights in psychosocial cancer care. Cancer. 2016;122(14):2130–3.

29. Gheihman G, Zimmermann C, Deckert A, Fitzgerald P, Mischitelle A, Rydall A, et al. Depression and hopelessness in patients with acute leukemia: the psychological impact of an acute and life-threatening disorder. Psycho-Oncology. 2016;25(8):979–89.

30. Vehling S, Kissane DW, Lo C, Glaesmer H, Hartung TJ, Rodin G, et al. The association of demoralization with mental disorders and suicidal ideation in patients with cancer. Cancer. 2017;123(17):3394–401.

31. Hem E, Loge JH, Haldorsen T, Ekeberg Ø. Suicide risk in cancer patients from 1960 to 1999. J Clin Oncol. 2004;22(20):4209–16.

32. Fang F, Fall K, Mittleman MA, Sparén P, Ye W, Adami HO, et al. Suicide and cardiovascular death after a cancer diagnosis. N Engl J Med. 2012;366(14):1310–8.

33. Misono S, Weiss NS, Fann JR, Redman M, Yueh B. Incidence of suicide in persons with cancer. J Clin Oncol. 2008;26(29):4731–8.

34. Mohammadi M, Moradi T, Bottai M, Reutfors J, Cao Y, Smedby KE. Risk and predictors of attempted and completed suicide in patients with hematological malignancies. Psycho-Oncology. 2014;23(11):1276–82.

35. Hultcrantz M, Svensson T, Derolf ÅR, Kristinsson SY, Lindqvist EK, Ekbom A, et al. Incidence and risk factors for suicide and attempted suicide following a diagnosis of hematological malignancy. Cancer Med. 2015;4(1):147–54.

36. Maldonado JR. Neuropathogenesis of delirium: review of current etiologic theories and common pathways. Am J Geriatr Psychiatry. 2013;21(12):1190–222.

37. Breitbart W, Alici Y. Evidence-based treatment of delirium in patients with cancer. J Clin Oncol. 2012;30(11):1206–14.

38. Fann JR, Roth-Roemer S, Burington BE, Katon WJ, Syrjala KL. Delirium in patients undergoing hematopoietic stem cell transplantation. Cancer. 2002;95(9):1971–81.

39. Fann JR, Hubbard RA, Alfano CM, Roth-Roemer S, Katon WJ, Syrjala KL. Pre-and post-transplantation risk factors for delirium onset and severity in patients undergoing hematopoietic stem-cell transplantation. J Clin Oncol. 2011;29(7):895–901.

40. Stiefel F. Psychosocial aspects of cancer pain. Support Care Cancer. 1993;1(3):130–4.

41. Stiff PJ, Erder H, Bensinger WI, Emmanouilides C, Gentile T, Isitt J, et al. Reliability and validity of a patient self-administered daily questionnaire to assess impact of oral mucositis (OM) on pain and daily functioning in patients undergoing autologous hematopoietic stem cell transplantation (HSCT). Bone Marrow Transplant. 2006;37(4):393.

42. Lalla RV, Bowen J, Barasch A, Elting L, Epstein J, Keefe DM, et al. MASCC/ISOO clinical practice guidelines for the management of mucositis secondary to cancer therapy. Cancer. 2014;120(10):1453–61.

43. Niscola P, Romani C, Scaramucci L, Dentamaro T, Cupelli L, Tendas A, et al. Pain syndromes in the setting of haematopoietic stem cell transplantation for haematological malignancies. Bone Marrow Transplant. 2008;41(9):757.

44. Niscola P, Tendas A, Scaramucci L, Giovannini M, De Sanctis V. Pain in blood cancers. Indian J Palliat Care. 2011;17(3):175.

45. Novy DM, Aigner CJ. The biopsychosocial model in cancer pain. Curr Opin Support Palliat Care. 2014;8(2):117–23.

46. Berger AM, Mooney K, Alvarez-Perez A, Breitbart WS, Carpenter KM, Cella D, et al. Cancer-related fatigue, version 2.2015. J Natl Compr Cancer Netw. 2015;13(8):1012–39.

47. Wang XS, Giralt SA, Mendoza TR, Engstrom MC, Johnson BA, Peterson N, et al. Clinical factors associated with cancer-related fatigue in patients being treated for leukemia and non-Hodgkin's lymphoma. J Clin Oncol. 2002;20(5):1319–28.

48. Wiskemann J, Huber G. Physical exercise as adjuvant therapy for patients undergoing hematopoietic stem cell transplantation. Bone Marrow Transplant. 2008;41(4):321.

49. Wiskemann J, Dreger P, Schwerdtfeger R, Bondong A, Huber G, Kleindienst N, et al. Effects of a partly self-administered exercise program before, during, and after allogeneic stem cell transplantation. Blood. 2011;117(9):2604–13.

50. Dimeo F, Schmittel A, Fietz T, Schwartz S, Köhler P, Böning D, et al. Physical performance, depression, immune status and fatigue in patients with hematological malignancies after treatment. Ann Oncol. 2004;15(8):1237–42.

51. Roscoe JA, Kaufman ME, Matteson-Rusby SE, Palesh OG, Ryan JL, Kohli S, et al. Cancer-related fatigue and sleep disorders. Oncologist. 2007;12(Supplement 1):35–42.

52. Davidson JR, MacLean AW, Brundage MD, Schulze K. Sleep disturbance in cancer patients. Soc Sci Med. 2002;54(9):1309–21.

53. Garland SN, Johnson JA, Savard J, Gehrman P, Perlis M, Carlson L, et al. Sleeping well with cancer: a systematic review of cognitive behavioral therapy for insomnia in cancer patients. Neuropsychiatr Dis Treat. 2014;10:1113.

54. Holland JC, Bultz BD. The NCCN guideline for distress management: a case for making distress the sixth vital sign. J Natl Compr Cancer Netw. 2007;5(1):3–7.

55. Holland JC, Andersen B, Breitbart WS, Buchmann LO, Compas B, Deshields TL, et al. Distress management. J Natl Compr Cancer Netw. 2013;11(2):190–209.

56. Mitchell AJ. Screening and assessment for distress. In: Holland JC, et al., editors. Psycho-oncology. 3rd ed. New York: Oxford University Press; 2015. p. 384–95.

57. American College of Surgeons. Cancer Program Standards (CPS) 2016. [Online] https://www.facs.org/quality-programs/cancer/coc/standards. Accessed 1 Feb 2018.

58. Roth AJ, Kornblith AB, Batel-Copel L, Peabody E, Scher HI, Holland JC. Rapid screening for psychologic distress in men with prostate carcinoma. Cancer. 1998;82(10):1904–8.

59. Chochinov HM, Wilson KG, Enns M, Lander S. "Are you depressed?" screening for depression in the terminally ill. Am J Psychiatr. 1997;154:674–6.

60. Spitzer RL, Kroenke K, Williams JB, Löwe B. A brief measure for assessing generalized anxiety disorder: the GAD-7. Arch Intern Med. 2006;166(10):1092–7.

61. Kroenke K, Spitzer RL, Williams JB. The PHQ-9: validity of a brief depression severity measure. J Gen Intern Med. 2001;16:606–13.

62. Vodermaier A, Millman RD. Accuracy of the hospital anxiety and depression scale as a screening tool in cancer patients: a systematic review and meta-analysis. Support Care Cancer. 2011;19(12):1899.

63. Vodermaier A, Linden W, Siu C. Screening for emotional distress in cancer patients: a systematic review of assessment instruments. J Natl Cancer Inst. 2009;101(21):1464–88.

64. Grassi L, Caruso R, Sabato S, Massarenti S, Nanni MG. Psychosocial screening and assessment in oncology and palliative care settings. Front Psychol. 2015;5:1485.

65. Braamse AM, Gerrits MM, van Meijel B, Visser O, van Oppen P, Boenink AD, et al. Predictors of health-related quality of life in patients treated with auto-and Allo-SCT for hematological malignancies. Bone Marrow Transplant. 2012;47(6):757.

66. Andorsky DJ, Loberiza FR Jr, Lee SJ. Pre-transplantation physical and mental functioning is strongly associated with self-reported recovery from stem cell transplantation. Bone Marrow Transplant. 2006;37(9):889.

67. Pillay B, Lee SJ, Katona L, Burney S, Avery S. Psychosocial factors associated with quality of life in allogeneic stem cell transplant patients prior to transplant. Psycho-Oncology. 2014;23(6):642–9.

68. El-Jawahri AR, Traeger LN, Kuzmuk K, Eusebio JR, Vandusen HB, Shin JA, et al. Quality of life and mood of patients and family caregivers during hospitalization for hematopoietic stem cell transplantation. Cancer. 2015;121(6):951–9.
69. Molassiotis A, Van Den Akker OB, Boughton BJ. Perceived social support, family environment and psychosocial recovery in bone marrow transplant long-term survivors. Soc Sci Med. 1997;44(3):317–25.
70. Foster LW, McLellan L, Rybicki L, Dabney J, Visnosky M, Bolwell B. Utility of the psychosocial assessment of candidates for transplantation (PACT) scale in allogeneic BMT. Bone Marrow Transplant. 2009;44(6):375.
71. Hochhausen N, Altmaier EM, McQuellon R, Davies SM, Papadopolous E, Carter S, et al. Social support, optimism, and self-efficacy predict physical and emotional Well-being after bone marrow transplantation. J Psychosoc Oncol. 2007;25(1):87–101.
72. Beattie S, Lebel S. The experience of caregivers of hematological cancer patients undergoing a hematopoietic stem cell transplant: a comprehensive literature review. Psycho-Oncology. 2011;20(11):1137–50.
73. Fann JR, Levy M. Hematopoietic Dyscrasias and stem cell transplantation. In: Holland JC, editor. Psycho-oncology. New York: Oxford University Press; 2015. p. 148.
74. Ernst J, Hinz A, Niederwieser D, Döhner H, Hönig K, Vogelhuber M, et al. Dyadic coping of patients with hematologic malignancies and their partners and its relation to quality of life–a longitudinal study. Leuk Lymphoma. 2017;58(3):655–65.
75. Mariotto AB, Robin Yabroff K, Shao Y, Feuer EJ, Brown ML. Projections of the cost of cancer care in the United States: 2010–2020. J Natl Cancer Inst. 2011;103(2):117–28.
76. Tai E, Guy GP, Dunbar A, Richardson LC. Cost of cancer-related neutropenia or fever hospitalizations, United States, 2012. J Oncol Pract. 2017;13(6):e552–61.
77. McNulty J, Khera N. Financial hardship—an unwanted consequence of cancer treatment. Curr Hematol Malig Rep. 2015;10(3):205–12.
78. Swash B, Hulbert-Williams N, Bramwell R. Unmet psychosocial needs in haematological cancer: a systematic review. Support Care Cancer. 2014;22(4):1131–41.
79. Barata A, Wood WA, Choi SW, Jim HS. Unmet needs for psychosocial care in hematologic malignancies and hematopoietic cell transplant. Curr Hematol Malig Rep. 2016;11(4):280–7.
80. Agarwal A, Said TM. Fertility issues in hematologic malignancies. In: Sekeres MA, editor. Clinical malignant hematology. New York: McGraw-Hill Professional; 2006. p. 1171–8.
81. Thygesen KH, Schjødt I, Jarden M. The impact of hematopoietic stem cell transplantation on sexuality: a systematic review of the literature. Bone Marrow Transplant. 2012;47(5):716.
82. Jean CY, Syrjala KL. Sexuality after hematopoietic stem cell transplantation. Cancer J (Sudbury, Mass.). 2009;15(1):57.
83. Kirsh KL, Rzetelny, Passik SD. Substance use disorders. In: Holland JC, editor. Psycho-oncology. New York: Oxford University Press; 2015. p. 148.
84. Ehlers SL, Gastineau DA, Patten CA, Decker PA, Rausch SM, Cerhan JR, et al. The impact of smoking on outcomes among patients undergoing hematopoietic SCT for the treatment of acute leukemia. Bone Marrow Transplant. 2011;46(2):285.
85. Chang G, John Orav E, McNamara T, Tong MY, Antin JH. Depression, cigarette smoking, and hematopoietic stem cell transplantation outcome. Cancer. 2004;101(4):782–9.
86. Appelbaum PS, Grisso T. Assessing patients' capacities to consent to treatment. N Engl J Med. 1988;319(25):1635–8.
87. Leigh H. Chap. 27. In: Leigh H, editor. Handbook of consultation-liaison psychiatry: Springer; Hoboken, NJ; 2016. p. 389–91.
88. Watson M, Kissane DW, editors. Handbook of psychotherapy in cancer care: Wiley; Hoboken, NJ; 2011.
89. American Society for Blood and Marrow Transplantation (ASBMT) HSCT guidelines. 2016. [Online] http://asbmt.org/practice-resources/practice-guidelines. Accessed 1 Feb 2018.

History of Hematopoietic Cell Transplantation

39

Jaroslava Salman, Kimberly Shapiro,
and Stephen J. Forman

Early Discoveries

In 1868, Ernst Neumann (former Prussia) and Giulio Bizzozero (Italy), both contemporaries of William Osler, the father of modern medicine, independently made the initial observations leading to the recognition of the marrow as the origin of blood formation in mammals [1]. Mature blood cells exit the bone marrow cavity through small blood vessels penetrating the bone cortex. Based on this discovery, physicians tried to employ various "treatments" for leukemia, e.g., instructing patients to swallow fresh bone marrow from young cattle [2]. However, it was not until the 1940s when the immunologic basis for tumor transplants was established through experiments in mice leading to the recognition of the histocompatibility transplant antigen system [3].

The explosion of two atomic bombs at the end of World War II and the effects of radiation on the bone marrow function of survivors of the nuclear exposure rekindled the scientific interest in bone marrow transplantation. Discovery of the immunologic basis for graft rejection and tolerance in mice by Sir Peter Brian Medawar (a British biologist, born in Brazil), who was considered to be the father of transplantation, helped to propel this pursuit further [4].

Number of experiments in mice revealed that they can survive lethal irradiation exposure if their spleens were shielded by lead foils [5]. At the time, it was unclear whether this recovery can be attributed to humoral or cellular factors, but subsequent experiments in the early 1950s by Egon Lorenz (biophysicist at NCI Bethesda) and colleagues, as well as D.W.H. Barnes and J.F. Loutit (both at Medical Research Council in Berkshire, England) indicated that the recovery conferred by spleen and marrow infusion might be due to living

cells, supporting the cellular hypothesis. Final proof for the cellular hypothesis came in 1956 when Ford and colleagues (Medical Research Council in Berkshire, England) showed that the marrow of transplanted mice displayed the cytogenetic characteristics of the donor. In the same year, Barnes and colleagues reported on the treatment of murine leukemia with high-dose irradiation followed by marrow graft infusion [2].

Early Experiments with HCT in Humans

The first experiments with hematopoietic cell transplantation (HCT) in humans were reported by Thomas and colleagues (University of Washington, Fred Hutchinson Cancer Research Center) in 1957 when they infused bone marrow to patients after they received radiation and chemotherapy [6].

That same year, several laboratory workers were treated with human bone marrow transplant after exposure to radiation due to the Vinca nuclear research reactor accident in the former Yugoslavia. Although recovery of hematopoietic function did occur, it was unclear if long-lasting benefit is sustainable. These early experiences led to the use of HCT to promote recovery of hematopoietic function after myeloablative chemotherapy and radiation [7].

In 1958, European scientists Jean Dausset (French immunologist) [8] and Jon van Rood (Dutch immunologist) [9] described the human leukocyte antigen-1(HLA) groups that were soon recognized as crucial genetic factors for donor selection in both experimental and clinical medicine. Subsequently, in 1968, 100 years after Neumann and Bizzozero's discoveries, the first curative and successful bone marrow transplants were performed in several infants with immunodeficiency disorders who received a transplant from their HLA-matched siblings. However, marrow transplantation from sibling donors for patients with advanced leukemia or bone marrow failure conditions proved considerably more challenging than transplantation for immunodeficiency disease.

In parallel discoveries, the concept of storing autologous hematopoietic cells while patients are exposed to high dose

J. Salman (✉) · K. Shapiro
Department of Psychiatry and Psychology, City of Hope, Duarte, CA, USA
e-mail: jsalman@coh.org

S. J. Forman
Department of Hematology and Hematopoietic Cell Transplantation, City of Hope, Duarte, CA, USA

© Springer International Publishing AG, part of Springer Nature 2019
Y. Sher, J. R. Maldonado (eds.), *Psychosocial Care of End-Stage Organ Disease and Transplant Patients*,
https://doi.org/10.1007/978-3-319-94914-7_39

of irradiation and/or high-dose cancer drugs with subsequent cell reinfusion was developed in the 1960s [2].

Building on the HLA system discoveries, allogeneic sibling donors of stem cells were used. However, the initial results were disappointing, and there was a sense that the transplantation barrier from one individual to another could not be overcome. This caused many researchers to abandon the idea that bone marrow transplantation could be used to treat hematological malignancies [5].

The use of autologous transplantation was also disappointing due to contamination with tumor cells. Fortunately, preclinical and clinical research continued despite the skepticism, and areas of histocompatibility, conditioning regimens, and prevention and treatment of graft-versus-host disease (GVHD) held the interest of scientists.

Further Advancements of the 1970s

With the advent of immunosuppressive drugs, improvements in conditioning regimens, and antibiotic treatments of the 1970s, interest in HCT was revived, and overall survival (6 months) rates rose to 70%. In their seminal report, Seattle transplant team of Thomas and colleagues described the first 100 patients treated with bone marrow transplant (73 for advanced leukemia and 27 for aplastic anemia) [10].

The Center for International Blood and Marrow Transplant Research (CIBMTR) was initiated in 1972 to collect and analyze data from transplant centers across the world. Currently, more than 390 transplant centers participate in submitting data to the CIBMTR for the purpose of analyzing outcomes of allogeneic and autologous transplants. It also serves as a resource for trends related to the use of HCT for treatment of different diseases and includes data related to type of transplant, use of various preparative regimens, and patient-related demographic data.

The Era of 1980s–1990s

The first transplants for thalassemia major and for sickle cell disease were performed in Seattle, opening the field for successful treatment of severe nonmalignant hematologic disorders. New approaches for the prevention of GVHD were developed. The potent combination of cyclosporine with methotrexate was introduced and became a new standard [2]. In 1980, ganciclovir was discovered by Kevin Ogilvie from Canada [11]. This new antiviral drug made it possible to control and reverse infections with cytomegalovirus (CMV), a serious complication which had previously caused fatal post-transplant infection in about 15% of HCT patients. In addition, new and powerful molecular tests were developed which were based on the polymerase chain reaction principle, originally invented by Kary Mullis (American biochemist) [12], that allowed the rapid and noninvasive monitoring of CMV presence and progression in patients post-transplant [2].

General interest in HCT continued to grow, and by 1986, approximately 5000 transplants were performed each year at more than 200 transplant centers [13]. In clinical practice, multiple criteria were taken into consideration in evaluating the patient's candidacy for transplant, including disease status, type of transplant, and patient risk factors. Chemotherapy-based preparative regimens, such as busulfan and cyclophosphamide, replaced the use of total body irradiation.

Interest in the use of the stem cell collected from the peripheral blood was introduced in the mid- to late 1980s. Stem cells were found to circulate in the peripheral blood following the administration of colony-stimulating factors with or without chemotherapy. Advances in cryopreservation and storage of stem cells allowed further growth in the use of autologous stem cell transplant which became common for treatment of a variety of hematologic diseases as well as solid tumors [7].

In 1986, the National Bone Marrow Transplant Donor Registry, known as the National Marrow Donor Program (NMDP), was formed in the United States. By managing a worldwide network of affiliated organizations, the agency coordinates the collection of hematopoietic cells for patients who lack a suitably matched donor in their family.

Be The Match is the organization operated by the NMDP. Since the organization began operations in 1987, it has facilitated a total of 68,000 transplants, including nearly 6300 transplants in 2014 alone, for patients in need of a cure (www.bethematch.org).

In the 1990s the use of both autologous and allogeneic stem cell transplants continued to expand. Improved understanding of HLA typing allowed the rising use of the unrelated donor as a source of stem cells for transplantation, and a number of conditioning regimens were developed to treat a variety of specific diseases. Furthermore, non-myeloablative stem cell transplant was introduced as an alternative treatment option. Using less toxic conditioning regimens helped to minimize treatment-related non-hematologic and hematologic toxicities, such as neutropenia, anemia, and thrombocytopenia. Since conditioning regimens were better tolerated by elderly patients, they opened the door for increased transplantation in this vulnerable population [7]. During this period of time, umbilical cord blood (UCB) attracted the interest as a potential source of stem cells for transplantation. The UCB is a rich source of stem cells that can be used for allogeneic or autologous stem cell transplant. The stem cells can be infused fresh or collected and stored for later use [14].

The Autologous Bone Marrow Transplant Registry was formed in 1990 to support international data collection related to autologous transplantation.

Twenty-First-Century Developments

The use of HCT for the treatment of a variety of malignant and nonmalignant hematologic diseases and autoimmune conditions continued to grow, and various reduced intensity regimens have been introduced over the past decade. Some contain low-dose total body irradiation and chemotherapy, while others consist of combinations of various drugs [2]. The lower toxicity and decreased morbidity and mortality of these regimens extend this treatment modality to patients who would previously not be considered suitable for transplant. Age is no longer considered an impediment to successful stem cell transplant [15]. There have been ongoing efforts to improve the prevention and treatment of GVHD, a significant cause of morbidity and mortality associated with HCT. A National Institute of Health Consensus Development Project developed criteria for the diagnosis, management, and clinical trials of chronic GVHD [16]. The possibility of induction of tolerance for solid organ transplants by the administration of donor hematopoietic cells has been one of the exciting new ways of stem cell transplant application [17].

Conclusions

The idea that the bone marrow could be used to treat hematologic disorders has been around for over a century. However, it wasn't until World War II that the bone marrow research took off in the wake of the atomic bomb explosions. The initial research worldwide was conducted using laboratory animals. First human trials of bone marrow transplantation were unsuccessful and almost led to abandonment of future explorations. Fortunately, subsequent critical scientific discoveries in the field of immunology, genetics, and pharmacology helped to propel the research forward.

Contemporary application of HCT includes young and elderly patients with a wide variety of hematological disorders. The ongoing and progressive research by numerous transplant teams throughout the world will allow continued progress toward developing novel, improved treatment modalities and an even a wider application of the use of hematopoietic stem cell transplantation [5].

Timeline

1868 – Neumann and Bizzozero, two experimental pathologists, reported their observations that blood cells of mammals are produced inside the bone marrow.

1945 – Atomic bomb explosions revealed the effects of radiation on the bone marrow function of the survivors.

1948 – Histocompatibility complex in mice (H-2) introduced by George Snell.

1949 – Jacobson and colleagues demonstrated that mice could survive lethal irradiation exposure *by shielding the spleen with lead foil.*

1954 – Barnes and Loutit's experiments supported the cellular hypothesis of the bone marrow recovery.

1956 – Barnes and colleagues reported on the treatment of murine leukemia with high-dose irradiation followed by marrow graft infusion.

1957 – Thomas and colleagues conducted first attempts to treat patients with total body irradiation and chemotherapy with subsequent marrow grafting.

1958 – Dausset and van Rood describe the HLA (human leukocyte antigen) groups.

1968 – Successful marrow transplant from HLA-matched sibling to infants with congenital immunodeficiency disorders took place.

1975 – Seattle transplant team of Thomas and colleagues described the first 100 patients treated with bone marrow transplant (73 for advanced leukemia and 27 for plastic anemia).

1976 – Immunosuppressive activity of cyclosporine is discovered.

1979 – Favorable outcomes were reported with matched sibling donors.

1980s – Successful transplants in treatment of nonmalignant hematologic disorders took place. New approaches for prevention of GVHD were discovered.

1980 – Ganciclovir was discovered by Ogilvie.

1985 – PCR was discovered.

1987 – The National Marrow Donor Program was founded.

1989–1999 – Ganciclovir to treat CMV infections in transplant patients was introduced; cord blood registries were developed.

2000–present – Reduced intensity regimens allowing transplantation of elderly, and medically vulnerable patients are discovered. Induction of tolerance for solid organ transplants by giving donor hematopoietic cells and new applications of HCT are discovered.

Glossary of Terms

Autologous Cells derived from the same individual.

Allogeneic Cells obtained from a genetically distinct individual of the same species.

Cellular Factor Aspect of the immune response related to white blood cells, rather than circulating antibodies.

CMV (Cytomegalovirus) A herpes virus that becomes latent after primary infection and causes few symptoms in the general population. However, it can reactivate in immunosuppressed transplant patients and is a significant cause of morbidity and mortality due to infection of multiple organs including the lungs, gastrointestinal tract, and central nervous system.

CSF (Colony-Stimulating Factors) Proteins that bind to receptors on the surface of hematopoietic stem cells, activating them to proliferate and differentiate into a specific kind of blood cell.

Conditioning Regimen Treatments used to prepare a patient for stem cell transplant. May involve chemotherapy, monoclonal antibody therapy, and radiation treatments of the entire body.

Cryopreservation A process of cooling cells to very low temperatures to preserve structure and function.

Cytogenetics Branch of genetics concerned with the structure and function of chromosomes.

HCT (Hematopoietic Cell Transplantation) Also referred to as a bone marrow transplant, HCT is a procedure that infuses healthy blood stem cells into the body to replace diseased or damaged bone marrow.

Hematopoietic The formation of blood.

HLA (Human Leukocyte Antigen) A protein marker found on most cells in the body used to determine a match for bone marrow.

Humoral Factor Immune responses involving antibodies in body fluids.

Murine Affecting mice or related rodents.

Myeloablative Chemotherapy High-dose chemotherapy that kills cells in the bone marrow, including cancer cells and normal blood-forming cells in the marrow. It is usually followed by a bone marrow transplant.

PCR (Polymerase Chain Reaction) A technique used in molecular biology to amplify a single copy or a few copies of a piece of DNA. This can generate up to millions of copies of a particular DNA sequence for further study.

References

1. Cooper B. The origins of bone marrow as the seedbed of our blood: from antiquity to the time of Osler. PRO. 2011;24(2):115–8.
2. Blume KG, Thomas ED. A history of allogeneic and autologous hematopoietic cell transplantation. In: Thomas' hematopoietic cell transplantation. 5th ed. San Francisco: Wiley Blackwell; 2016. p. 1–11.
3. Snell GD. Methods for the study of histocompatibility genes. J Genet. 1948;49(2):87–108.
4. Medawar PB. The immunology of transplantation. Harvey Lect. 1956;(Series 52):144–76.
5. Little MT, Storb R. History of haematopoietic stem-cell transplantation. Nat Rev Cancer. [Review]. 2002;2(3):231–8.
6. Thomas ED, Lochte HL Jr, Lu WC, Ferrebee JW. Intravenous infusion of bone marrow in patients receiving radiation and chemotherapy. N Engl J Med. 1957;257(11):491–6.
7. Ezzone SA. History of hematopoietic stem cell transplantation. Semin Oncol Nurs. [Article]. 2009;25(2):95–9.
8. Dausset J. Iso-leuko-antibodies. Acta Haematol. 1958;20(1–4): 156–66.
9. Van Rood JJ, Eernisse JG, Van Leeuwen A. Leucocyte antibodies in sera from pregnant women. Nature. 1958;181(4625):1735–6.
10. Thomas E, Storb R, Clift RA, Fefer A, Johnson FL, Neiman PE, et al. Bone-marrow transplantation (first of two parts). N Engl J Med. 1975;292(16):832–43.
11. Smith KO, Galloway KS, Kennell WL, Ogilvie KK, Radatus BK. A new nucleoside analog, 9-[[2-hydroxy-1-(hydroxymethyl)ethoxyl] methyl]guanine, highly active in vitro against herpes simplex virus types 1 and 2. Antimicrob Agents Chemother. 1982;22(1):55–61.
12. Mullis K, Faloona F, Scharf S, Saiki R, Horn G, Erlich H. Specific enzymatic amplification of DNA in vitro: the polymerase chain reaction. Cold Spring Harb Symp Quant Biol. 1986;51(Pt 1):263–73.
13. Bortin MM, Horowitz MM, Gale RP. Current status of bone marrow transplantation in humans: report from the international bone marrow transplant registry. Nat Immun Cell Growth Regul. 1988;7(5–6):334–50.
14. Ballen KK. New trends in umbilical cord blood transplantation. Blood. 2005;105(10):3786–92.
15. Sorror ML, Sandmaier BM, Storer BE, Franke GN, Laport GG, Chauncey TR, et al. Long-term outcomes among older patients following nonmyeloablative conditioning and allogeneic hematopoietic cell transplantation for advanced hematologic malignancies. JAMA. 2011;306(17):1874–83.
16. Filipovich AH, Weisdorf D, Pavletic S, Socie G, Wingard JR, Lee SJ, et al. National Institutes of Health consensus development project on criteria for clinical trials in chronic graft-versus-host disease: I. Diagnosis and staging working group report. Biol Blood Marrow Transplant J Am Soc Blood Marrow Transpl. 2005;11(12):945–56.
17. Storb R, Gyurkocza B, Storer BE, Sorror ML, Blume K, Niederwieser D, et al. Graft-versus-host disease and graft-versus-tumor effects after allogeneic hematopoietic cell transplantation. J Clin Oncol Off J Am Soc Clin Oncol. 2013;31(12):1530–8.

Additional References

www.bethematch.org.
www.cibmtr.org.

Medical Course and Complications After Hematopoietic Cell Transplantation

40

Janice (Wes) Brown and Judith A. Shizuru

Introduction

The field of hematopoietic cell transplantation (HCT) is constantly evolving. Many elements of the transplant procedure are optimized for the specific patient, their comorbidities, the type of conditioning regimen, available donors, and the disease entity for which they are undergoing transplantation. Each of these variables can significantly impact the incidence and severity of medical complications; however, an understanding of the most common medical complications can facilitate the overall care of the patient.

The first one hundred days post-transplant are designated as the peri-transplant period. Events are typically classified as *early,* which includes the preparative regimen through day (D) +100, or *late* which refers to events that occur after D+100. Although complications are recognized to occur as a continuum, the nomenclature is still helpful and will be used here. Serious medical complications can arise as early as during conditioning or as late as several years post-transplant.

Conditioning/Preparative Regimen

Conditioning/preparative regimens are aimed at both preparing patients to accept donor allografts and, when applicable, to eradicate malignancies. These regimens are either radiation- and/or chemotherapy-based. High-dose, myeloablative total body irradiation (TBI) in combination with chemotherapy has been used for decades to condition patients for HCT. More recently, attenuated (non-myeloablative) doses of TBI have been used and are preferred for elderly and more frail patients. Regimens of chemotherapy alone are also used. The most common chemotherapeutic agents include

busulfan, cyclophosphamide, melphalan, fludarabine, and etoposide [1]. The toxicities of these chemotherapy agents and their management have been well described [1–6].

The effects of myeloablative TBI warrant special mention. Myeloablative TBI is most commonly given in 8–12 fractions over 4 days for a total dose of 12–15 Gray (Gy). In addition to the well-recognized toxicities of substantially increased risk for mucositis, nausea, emesis, fatigue, and headaches, TBI has been associated with long-term deleterious effects on musculoskeletal system and growth in children as well as fertility, nephritis, and pneumonitis in adults. Increased risks of secondary malignancies, neurocognitive disorders, and endocrinologic disturbances have also been well recognized in adults and children [7–13].

Mucositis is one of the most impactful complications of HCT that occurs during the acute peri-transplant period as it results in pain, disruption of sleep, impairment of nutritional maintenance and medication compliance, and increased risk for infection and may be so severe as to require invasive support for airway protection [11, 14]. Mucosal injury often involves the entire gastrointestinal (GI) tract with resulting abdominal discomfort with or without diarrhea. The risk of mucositis can be anticipated by the intensity of the conditioning regimen. The combination of chemotherapy with intensive radiation is associated with the highest risk and the greatest severity. The resolution of mucositis is temporally associated with the recovery of peripheral neutropenia for reasons that have not been well understood.

Intravenous opioid are almost invariably required for pain control, and programmable patient-controlled analgesia delivery systems, with or without a basal delivery rate, are often highly successful. Intravenous nutritional supplementation can be delivered when nutritional status is poor and the patient can safely tolerate parenteral nutrition. Mucositis is also associated with a markedly increased risk for bloodstream infections due to bacteria and/or candida, with or without sepsis.

Some comfort and potentially attenuation of severity and infectious risk may be achieved by frequent daily rinses with

J. W. Brown (✉) · J. A. Shizuru
Division of Blood and Marrow Transplantation,
Department of Medicine, Stanford University School of Medicine,
Stanford, CA, USA
e-mail: wesbrown@stanford.edu; Jshizuru@stanford.edu

© Springer International Publishing AG, part of Springer Nature 2019
Y. Sher, J. R. Maldonado (eds.), *Psychosocial Care of End-Stage Organ Disease and Transplant Patients*,
https://doi.org/10.1007/978-3-319-94914-7_40

saline, antimicrobial preparations, and/or topical anaesthetics. Of note, toxic levels of anesthetic are possible (via lidocaine absorption), although rare.

In the presence of active bleeding and ulcerations, gentle oral care and platelet transfusions may help. The removal of sloughed tissue should be approached with great care by an experienced care provider. Palifermin, a truncated human recombinant keratinocyte growth factor, is currently the only agent with FDA approval for the prevention and attenuation of mucositis associated with chemotherapy [15].

Other commonly used conditioning modalities that warrant special mention are anti-thymocyte globulin (ATG) and the monoclonal anti-CD52 antibody alemtuzumab. ATG or alemtuzumab have been included in a number of conditioning regimens with goal of improving engraftment by depletion of host T cells [16–20]. Although the specific indications and intermediate and long-term effects of the two agents may differ, they share the risk for infusion-related hypotension, fever, chills, hypoxemia, and rash, which frequently prompt empiric antimicrobial therapy [21, 22]. These antibodies can remain in the serum for an extended period after the donor graft is infused and thus modify donor cell activity, including impairment of immune reconstitution [20, 23, 24].

Infectious Complications

The increased risk for infections is anticipated by the patient; however, the duration and nature of this increased susceptibility is often underappreciated [25]. Patient and care teams are often appropriately vigilant for risks for exogenous exposure to infections; however, the vast majority of infections result from organisms that are endogenous to that patient and present prior to the HCT procedure. Members of the herpesvirus family are ubiquitous and establish latency after acute infection. Reactivation of these DNA viruses causes the greatest morbidity and mortality post-transplantation. Therefore, serologies of herpes simplex 1 and 2 (HSV-1, HSV-2), varicella zoster virus (VZV), Epstein-Barr virus (EBV), and cytomegalovirus (CMV) should be documented and readily available to the care teams. Other pre-transplant tests should include hepatitis B surface antigen, hepatitis B surface antibody, hepatitis C antibody, hepatitis C RNA, human T-cell lymphotropic viruses 1 and 2 (HTLV-1/−2) serology, human immunodeficiency virus (HIV) serology, toxoplasma serology, and syphilis screening [26]. Mandated donor testing often includes West Nile virus using a test for nucleic acid.

Individual risk assessment should include a detailed history of past infections, dental problems, places of residence and/or travel, the use of complementary treatments including herbal medications, smoking, occupational and vocational activities, and exposure to animals. Consultation with an infectious disease specialty service is recommended regarding specific screening testing based on exposures such as endemic fungi, *Schistosoma*, and *Mycobacterium tuberculosis* [27–29].

Special Situations that May Require Additional Pre-transplant Evaluation

History of Infection with or Isolation of Antibiotic-Resistant Organisms

Any history of infection and/or colonization with bacteria harboring antimicrobial resistance, such as methicillin-resistant *Staphylococcus aureus* (MRSA), vancomycin-resistant *Enterococcus* (VRE), or multidrug-resistant or carbapenem-resistant gram-negative rods, should be noted and documented to take into consideration when choosing empiric antimicrobials for fever [30, 31].

Oral Health

The status of a patient's dentition should be assessed, with any recommended radiographs performed, prior to transplantation by a dentist/oral surgeon. Poor dentition and gingivitis are associated with an increased risk for severe mucositis as well as the risk of local and systemic infection [32, 33]. Collaborative staging of any procedures is ideal in determining optimal timing relative to transplant.

Preexisting Fungal Infections

There are no definitive, data-based recommendations regarding the need for and timing of radiographic studies in the setting of a suspected or proven fungal infection. However, confirmation of stabilization and/or improvement in areas of suspected involvement (e.g., chest CT) is generally recommended prior to proceeding to transplantation. Similarly, if a patient is being treated with a mold-active azole, it is reasonable to document a baseline trough serum levels as one factor that may be used in interpreting post-transplant clinical deterioration.

Clostridium difficile (*C. difficile*)

There are no data to suggest that a single episode of *C. difficile* infection which is responsive to treatment requires any special prophylaxis. However, in the setting of recurrent or protracted *C. difficile* infection, recurrent colitis becomes a significant risk [34, 35]. Commonly recommended practices include avoidance of antibiotics, especially quinolones, and consideration of prophylaxis, especially if the patient is documented to be a carrier of *C. difficile* (i.e., the organism is detected in the patient's stool even in the absence of symptoms). The choice of prophylaxis should be influenced by history of response to specific agents. Fidaxomicin is licensed for recurrent *C. difficile* although not specifically studied in HCT patients. Activity of rifaximin against *C. difficile* has not been proven although a number of case reports have been published [34, 35].

Overall Timing of Infections

Early in the history of transplantation, a specific temporal sequence of the two most apparent medical complications – infections and graft-versus-host disease (GVHD) – was observed. Moreover, a variety of factors may influence the timing, frequency, and severity of these complications [36, 37]. Familiarity with the medical complications of a myeloablative preparative regimen followed by transplantation of a bone marrow graft from a HLA-matched, related donor provides a framework to understand the impact of these factors.

Grafts of mobilized peripheral blood (MPB) are comprised of a greater percentage and absolute number of myeloid progenitors which contribute to the marked shortening of the neutropenic period, although the incidence of fever is not substantially different. Nonmyeloablative and reduced intensity preparative regimens do result in marked reduction in neutropenia and associated fever.

Fever During Neutropenia: Bacterial Infections

The well-established approach to fever during neutropenia, as outlined by consensus panels, is recommended [38, 39]. Patients with severe mucositis are at higher risk for documented bacteremia, candidemia, and sepsis [6]. *Streptococcal mitis* warrants special mention as this organism is associated with severe sepsis in 5–15% of cases with a high mortality rate despite appropriate antibiotic treatment [40]. At this time, the vast majority of isolates in the United States are susceptible to cefepime; however, an increasing percentage of isolates from an increasing number of other countries are resistant to penicillin [41]. As most HCT patients have received antibiotics for previous episodes of infection, they are at potential risk for drug-resistant organisms, and the selection of antimicrobials for patients with severe sepsis syndrome should reflect this risk [42–44].

Invasive Fungal Infections

Candida

Prior to the widespread use of low-dose amphotericin and/or fluconazole prophylaxis, candidemia was nearly as common as proven bacteremia and carried a higher mortality rate. A number of studies demonstrated that 400 mg of fluconazole daily significantly reduced candidemia and all-cause mortality. One study noted an increased incidence of aspergillosis in the group treated with fluconazole compared to no prophylaxis; it was postulated that overall increase in survival resulted in more patients at risk for other infectious complications [45, 46].

Invasive Mold Infections and Emerging Fungal Pathogens

During the past 20 years, there has been an explosion of mold-active antifungal agents which have vastly improved the survivability of a fungal infection post-HCT with less toxicity than was seen with Amphotericin B. In addition to two lipid formulations of the polyene Amphotericin B, which offer markedly reduced risk of nephrotoxicity, the other two main classes of antifungals are echinocandins (caspofungin) and triazoles (itraconazole, voriconazole, posaconazole, and isavuconazole) [47–51]. The shorter period of neutropenia after MPB than after BM grafts has also modestly decreased the incidence of fungal infection. In a randomized, double-blind trial in patients with GVHD, 5.3% and 9% of the posaconazole group developed proven or probable invasive aspergillosis (IA), respectively, as compared to fluconazole (2.3% and 7%, $p = 0.006$) [52]. Another randomized, double-blind, placebo-controlled trial of voriconazole versus fluconazole failed to demonstrate a similar magnitude of protection; however, in the former study, the *Aspergillus* galactomannan assay was an important criteria. The sensitivity of this assay is significantly decreased by mold-active agents (e.g., posaconazole) which may have affected the number of patients with "probable" IA.

Education regarding reducing exposures and wearing of fitted HEPA-filtered masks are two strategies employed by some centers. Unfortunately, fungal infections still represent a significant cause of morbidity and mortality with the several weeks-to-months long treatment associated with a psychosocial, physical, and financial burden on the patient. Prompt administration of antifungal treatment, while actively working to identify pathogen, holds the best promise to improve survivability. The increasing reports of resistance to various licensed antifungal and emerging fungal species have been reported [50, 53].

Viruses

HTLV-1, HTLV-2

Serologic testing for HTLV-1 and HTLV-2 is routine for both patients and their donors. These viruses have higher prevalence in certain areas of the world including Japan, Africa, and the Caribbean [54]. A very small minority of patients with HTLV may develop a spastic myelopathy, hyperinfection with *Strongyloides*, or T-cell leukemia/other T-cell malignancies. Due to the very low prevalence in the United States and unclear route of transmission, available literature regarding the significance of either donor or patient being seropositive for HTLV is still not well characterized. The general consensus at this time is that patient should be presented with the possibility of increased risk of HTLV-related complications. Limited data and exploratory studies are underway to determine which agents may have efficacy in reducing transmission and/or disease sequelae [55–57]. Of note, an HTLV-positive individual should be notified and offered to discuss potential risk with partner who can then be evaluated by their personal physician.

Herpesviruses

HSV-1, HSV-2, and VZV

In addition to their classification as alpha-herpesviruses, HSV-1, HSV-2, and VZV are grouped together for discussion since acyclovir (ACV) and valacyclovir (VCV) have been shown to prevent clinically significant reactivations. Diseases due to HSV have ranged from the classic oral or genital mucosal ulcerations to life-threatening visceral or central nervous system (CNS) disease. ACV prophylaxis during the early post-HCT period substantially reduced the incidence of HSV disease. However, because the median time to VZV reactivation is approximately D+ 90, the duration of prophylaxis was not immediately clear. In the ensuing decades, protracted ACV or VCV has been shown to decrease the average severity and, if administered for a duration of greater than approximately 1 year post-transplant, decreased the incidence of zoster. The use of immunomodulatory agents such as bortezomib-based therapies for myeloma is associated with increased VZV reactivation, and continued anti-VZV prophylaxis is recommended [58–61]. VZV reactivation after HCT is more likely than in other patients to be disseminated, involve viscera, and be without skin lesions (*zoster sine herpete*) posing challenges to diagnosis. One classic manifestation within the visceral involvement is reactivation in the celiac plexus which can present as syndrome of severe abdominal pain, possibly with ileus mimicking pseudo-obstruction, and hyponatremia. Although no randomized control trials exist, most investigators recommend continuation of HSV/VZV prophylaxis throughout treatment with immunosuppressive agents [55, 59–66].

Of note, there has not been a randomized, controlled trial to compare doses of ACV and/or VCV. Of note, in non-HCT patients, a lower dose is usually favored, whereas in recipients of HCT, higher dosing is often, but not invariably used. Sporadic reports often fuel the higher-dose practice based on the concern regarding selection for resistance by administering lower doses of antivirals in a situation where antiviral immune reconstitution is suboptimal [67–69].

Cytomegalovirus (CMV)

CMV can establish latency in a wide variety of cells, including hematopoietic progenitor cells, and has been shown to reactivate even in healthy patients. However, the risk for clinically apparent disease due to CMV is determined by the degree of immune dysfunction resulting from allogeneic transplant and increased in the setting of grafts that have various degrees of HLA mismatch, from unrelated donors or alternative sources, and/or in the setting of GVHD. T-cell depletion, whether resulting from antibody treatment of the patient or ex vivo depletion of the graft itself, independently and substantially increases risk for CMV viremia as well as disease [70].

Until the development of treatment strategies based on early detection of viremia, CMV was the leading infectious cause of death following HCT. These strategies are referred to as preemptive [66, 71]. Boeckh et al. demonstrated that a prophylactic strategy did reduce the incidence of proven tissue disease when compared to a preemptive strategy defined as starting antiviral therapy based on the immunohistochemistry-based detection of antigenemia prior to any clinically apparent disease; however, overall mortality was not different between the groups due to the toxicity of ganciclovir. Currently, most centers employ preemptive strategies to reduce CMV disease based on the regular screening of CMV by PCR in plasma or, less likely, CMV antigenemia testing [72–75].

Until late 2017, medications licensed for CMV treatment included the nucleoside analogue ganciclovir, inorganic phosphate derivative foscarnet, and cidofovir. The toxicity profile of each of these drugs has been well documented [73]. In 2017, a randomized, double-blind, placebo-controlled trial demonstrated efficacy of letermovir and led to its licensing, preventing CMV viremia in allogeneic transplant patients without marrow, renal, or hepatic toxicity [76].

Post-transplant, the timing, magnitude, incidence of disease, and response of CMV viremia to therapy are some of the most sensitive indicators of the reconstituting immunologic response. A detailed discussion of each transplant scenario is beyond the scope of this chapter; however, any factor that delays or stunts reconstitution, most notably T and possibly NK lineages, can be associated with an increased impact of CMV. For example, a graft comprised of umbilical cord blood, GVHD, and any condition that requires intermediate–/high-dose steroids all substantially increase risk of CMV disease. Under some, but not all, circumstances, a CMV seropositive patient receiving a graft from a seronegative donor may have a higher risk for reactivation requiring treatment and resulting in increased risk of serious CMV infection until the naive graft has generated an appropriate immune response.

Post-transplant Lymphoproliferative Disorder (PTLD)

PTLD most commonly represents the monoclonal or polyclonal expansion of lymphocytes and, in the vast majority of cases, B-cell expansion that is driven by EBV oncogenes [77]. However, lymphoproliferative disorders may be related to causes other than EBV and should be suspected in any patient with unexplained syndromes. To varying degrees, both viral replication and impaired immune surveillance contribute to risk of developing PTLD. Although cases have been reported even following autologous HCT, T-cell depletion of graft and addition of T-cell-specific antibodies increase the risk with an incidence reported from 1–5%. Prior to the availability of anti-CD19+ 20+ antibodies, (i.e., rituximab), approaches to treatment were centered around reducing immunosuppression and instituting conventional chemotherapy if disease progressed [78–81]. The treatment of viral-mediated diseases, such as PTLD, using adoptive transfer of virus-specific effector cells is an active area of investigation [82].

Early diagnosis of PTLD requires a certain degree of clinical vigilance as patients have few or no complaints. The most common symptoms are fever and nonspecific constitutional symptoms, such as malaise. Any lymphoid tissue may be involved; however, lung, GI, and CNS disease are notoriously difficult to diagnose and can be mistaken for other disorders prior to tissue sampling. Quantitative EBV PCR of the plasma may help in identifying patients at risk, although there is no consensus about the precise relationship of viral load and risk [83, 84]. Some investigators advocate prophylaxis or preemptive treatment of high-risk patients with rituximab [85–87]. Consensus recommendations include assessing extent of disease with a PET and/or CT scan as well as a biopsy of involved tissue whenever possible and inclusion of rituximab for suspected or proven disease.

Human Herpesvirus-6 (HHV6)

Of the herpesviruses commonly recognized to be associated with disease, the significance of HHV6 viremia is the most dependent on the clinical scenario [65, 88, 89]. HHV6 may be the most ubiquitous of herpesviruses. Both retrospective and prospective large case series of HCT patients at single centers note the high frequency of symptomatic detection of HHV6 in plasma during the early post-transplant period [90, 91]. In addition, a variety of smaller case series reveal that symptomatic HHV6 may be associated with fever and rash and overlap with the occurrence of acute GVHD during the peri-engraftment period [88, 89, 92, 93]. HHV6 may be associated with delayed engraftment, neurologic disorders, and, less likely, pulmonary disease [88, 89, 92, 93]. In some patients and/or their donors, HHV6 may be integrated into their cellular genome, and viral "load" may be very high as

determined by quantitative PCR testing. Whether or not patients with HHV6 integration can develop HHV6 disease from reactivated virus post-HCT is an area of controversy; however, the issue may be moot as HHV-6 may be transmitted in the donor graft [94].

Even in the absence of HHV6 genomic integration, there are no clinical data to support benefit from treatment of isolated, asymptomatic HHV6 viremia [88, 89]. Patients with viremia who may benefit from empiric or preemptive treatment include (1) the recipients of UCB, haploidentical, and/or T-cell-depleted grafts, (2) patient with a history of anti-T-lymphocyte antibody treatments such as alemtuzumab or ATG, and/or (3) patients who have delayed engraftment or graft loss. Isolation of the virus from the symptomatically affected organ system (e.g., cerebrospinal fluid in the setting of neuropathy) supports the treatment for HHV6-related disease [89, 90, 95].

Adenovirus

Adenovirus, a double-stranded DNA virus, was once thought to only result from an exogenous exposure. Our current understanding of adenovirus is far from complete. To add to the complexity, the significance of adenovirus and response to therapy differ greatly between adult and pediatric patients. Since the development of commercially available PCR-based assays of blood and tissue to detect virus, high-grade adenovirus viremia has been associated with increased all-cause mortality [96, 97]. The pathophysiology and optimal approaches to adenovirus are currently an active area of study.

Respiratory Viruses

HCT patients have significantly increased morbidity and mortality due to respiratory viruses even when compared to other patients undergoing treatments for malignancy [98–102]. Symptoms at presentation do not parallel those seen in healthy patients. Although the period of increased susceptibility is not yet known, patients with even seemingly minor respiratory symptoms in the peri-transplant period and/or who have GVHD should be tested. Specific risk factors are associated with lower respiratory tract disease and death due to respiratory virus infection, including the pre- and peri-engraftment period, GVHD, neutropenia, or lymphopenia (absolute lymphocyte count reported as <100) [103–106]. Patients with protracted delays in T-cell reconstitution, including recipients of T-cell depleted or UCB grafts or T-cell depleting therapies, also appear to be at significantly increased risk [107].

Influenza viruses, respiratory syncytial virus (RSV), human metapneumovirus (hMPV), parainfluenza viruses (PIV), and adenovirus are included in most multiplex PCR diagnostic panels. These four viruses can be diagnosed at the stage of upper respiratory infection or involvement of the lower tract disease and are collectively associated with the highest morbidity and mortality.

Treatment for respiratory viruses is determined by the specific virus and/or the clinical findings. Furthermore, treatment duration cannot be extrapolated from studies of healthy patients and should be individualized based on patient's response. Prompt treatment for influenza is universally recommended regardless of the duration of symptoms prior to diagnosis [102]. Treatment for RSV is generally recommended for patients in the higher-risk category. Many studies support the use of ribavirin administered orally for patients without lower tract disease; however, aerosolized ribavirin may be indicated for patients with hypoxemia and infiltrates consistent with lower respiratory tract disease [105, 106, 108]. Adjunctive therapy with IVIG is generally supported in RSV infection. The approach to hMPV and PIV is still a topic of debate.

Specific Infections and Considerations

Although the list of emerging infectious diseases will continue to evolve, certain infections warrant special mention due to either their relative frequency, challenges in diagnoses, and/or presentation that may easily be mistaken for more common opportunistic infections.

Nocardia

Infections due to *Nocardia* spp. are often diagnosed late, in large part due to the limitations in diagnostic testing and its most common presentation of a pulmonary nodule and/or infiltrate that has no specific characteristics differentiating it from the more common fungal and bacterial infections [109]. Furthermore, *Nocardia*, with or without pulmonary involvement, can present with bacteremia and direct inoculation due to trauma and has the propensity to involve the CNS. The bacteria of the genus *Nocardia* are found in soil and may be commensal oral organisms that stain weakly positive with gram stains and acid-fast stains. As with fungal infections, presentation may vary widely with respect to symptoms and signs. Most premortem diagnoses are confirmed by detecting acid-fast bacilli (AFB)-positive organisms by staining and culture of respiratory secretions, blood, and/or biopsy tissue. Newer real-time PCR test has just been recently released (Viracor, Eurofins Diagnostics), and results of molecular diagnostic testing have demonstrated utility [110]. The most active agents against *Nocardia.*, defined by percentage of isolates tested, include sulfamethoxazole/trimethoprim, linezolid, and carbapenems [109, 111, 112]. However, susceptibility testing should be performed to guide therapy.

Post-transplant Vaccination

With the exponential growth and improved survival post-transplant, studies are ongoing regarding whether a patient achieves functional reconstitution of protective memory against historically encountered pathogens and/or vaccines. Guidelines have been developed to provide a reasonable framework for revaccination post-HCT. The goal is for patients to be started on a revaccination schedule 6–12 months post-HCT. They should be (re)vaccinated with nonlive vaccines against childhood illnesses, tetanus toxoid, hepatitis B, *Haemophilus influenzae* B, and pneumococcus [113–116]. Although there is no data yet regarding immunogenicity studies in HCT patients of the newly licensed VZV subunit vaccine, Shingrix (GSK), there does not appear to be a contraindication, and it does not carry the theoretical risk of disease resulting from the live-attenuated VZV vaccine, Zostavax (Merck) [117].

Changes in Fecal Microbiota

Study of the fecal microbiota is currently an area of active research. Investigators are seeking to understand the impact of the fecal microbiota on transplant outcomes, including the incidence of GVHD and, reciprocally, how is the microbiota modified by the complexities of care post-HCT. At this time, few conclusions can be made, but data from large consortia studies are expected in the near future [118–121].

Noninfectious Complications/Organ Injury

Renal

Renal injury remains a common complication of HCT with reported incidence ranging from 10% to 70% with lower risks reported after autologous HCT. In addition to the peri-transplant period, patients may have a lifetime increased risk for renal disease [122–142]. As with many complications of HCT, acute (AKI) and chronic renal injury (CKI) are defined as significant increase in serum creatinine (SCR) that occurs prior to and after D+100, respectively. Comorbidity assessment at the time of HCT includes multiple measurements of organ function including SCR. Patients with increased risk for death associated with the number and severity of comorbid conditions also have an increased risk for renal injury, due to factors such as toxicities of the preparative regimen, exposure to nephrotoxic drugs, development of complications such as hepatic sinusoidal obstruction syndrome or thrombotic microangiopathy, and GVHD [122]. Multiple criteria to define renal injury are used; however, a doubling of SCR is one generally accepted indicator, with the median onset of AKI in the range of 33–38 days. Risk for mortality parallels the degree of AKI with >50% reported in patients requiring dialysis. The reported incidence of CKI post-HCT varies from 7% to 48%; however, data continues to evolve with an ever-increasing number of survivors, especially as the onset of CKI may be several years post-HCT [122, 123, 125–127].

To what extent AKI or CKI may result from an inflammatory process is an area of active study and some debate [122, 125, 128, 129]. There is no substantial clinical data based on histologic changes, except of limited reports of inflammation in various renal structures including glomeruli, capillaries, and tubules. As discussed previously, the diagnosis of GVHD is not wholly reliant on specific criteria, nor do such criteria exist for the kidney injury. In rodent models of GVHD, endothelial injury appears to result from inflammatory processes including increased enhanced expression of adhesion molecules (e.g., MCP-1) that are apparently mediated by CD3+ T cells. Specific attention has been paid to an endogenous serine protease inhibitor, known as elafin. Elevation of urinary elafin is associated with AKI and CKI, which is notable given a previously reported association between elafin and skin GVHD [122, 123].

Thrombotic microangiopathy (TMA) which, by definition, is thrombosis of small vessels (arterioles and capillaries) occurs in a variety of syndromes largely defined by clinical presentation and suspected trigger [130–132]. As a well-recognized complication of HCT, TMA deserves separate mention as a risk factor for renal injury. The initial common precipitating event is believed to be endothelial injury resulting in a cascade of increase in local prostaglandin and prostacyclin production, thrombin formation, and increased leukocyte adhesion. Although TMA is often labelled as idiopathic, various forms of TMA have been associated with drugs, including calcineurin inhibitors, antifungal and antiviral agents, infectious triggers, and immunomodulatory and immunotoxic therapies, and GVHD [123].

Hepatic Veno-occlusive Disease/Sinusoidal Obstruction Syndrome (VOD/SOS)

During the first 3 weeks post-transplant, hepatic endothelial injury may result from the preparative regimen for HCT leading to a syndrome known as VOD/SOS, typically defined as a triad of increase in abdominal girth and increase in body weight due to ascites, hepatomegaly with or without pain, and hyperbilirubinemia. However, updated criteria have been proposed, at least in part due to differences between the syndrome observed in adults versus pediatric patients [133]. For example, in children, there is no time limit to the onset of the syndrome, and unexplained consumptive, refractory thrombocytopenia may be seen. For adults, later onset (past D+21) VOD/SOS has been reported. Unpredictable in its occurrence, patients with VOD/SOS may develop multi-organ failure with mortality exceeding 80% [134, 135]. Ultrasonography with Doppler studies reveals a reversal of sinusoidal venous flow resulting from a cascade of events leading to extraluminal compression, thrombosis within the central veins and sinusoidal tracts, and portal hypertension [136]. In certain cases, liver biopsy and measurement of transhepatic venous pressure gradients are helpful in confirming the diagnosis. Factors associated with increased risk include age, history of certain chemotherapy regimens and/or radiation to the abdomen, and iron overload [134, 136]. Although the rarity of the event limited study design, defibrotide reportedly restores thrombolytic balance and is the only licensed agent in the United States and EU to treat severe VOD/SOS after HCT for patients >1 month of age [135]. The long-term effects of VOD/SOS have not been well characterized, although one long-term sequela is a significantly increased risk for chronic renal injury [123].

Immunologic Sequelae of HCT

Graft-Versus-Host Disease

Although patients may perceive that increased susceptibility to infection is the greatest hurdle post-HCT, GVHD has the greatest impact on overall morbidity and mortality, risk of infection, and quality of life [137–142]. GVHD occurs when the donor-derived immune cells (graft) mount an immunologic attack on allogeneic molecules present on patient's cells (host) which they continue to view as foreign. Two comprehensive reviews of the pathophysiology and clinical spectrum of GVHD have been published recently [137, 143]. Clinical familiarity with the diagnosis, treatment, and sequelae of GVHD is necessary to optimize the care of the HCT patient.

In addition to choice donor selection and preparative regimen, current commonly used approaches to reduce the incidence of GVHD result in increased risk for infection. The major approaches involve T-cell depletion of the graft; prophylactic calcineurin inhibitors, mTOR inhibitors, corticosteroids, and methotrexate; post-transplant cyclophosphamide to reduce alloreactive cells; and peri-transplant immunomodulatory/antibody therapy. These approaches all result in a potential increase in infectious complications, although this risk may be attenuated. For example, anti-thymocyte globulin has been used in HCT for decades and has been shown to decrease the graft rejection and acute GVHD; however, the potential for clinically significant deleterious effects on immune reconstitution is highly dependent on ATG pharmacodynamics, especially in the setting of UCB HCT [18, 20, 87, 144–146].

The NIH consensus classification system in 2005 and its revision in 2014 defines "acute" GVHD (aGVHD) as syndromes that are typical for GVHD that occur prior to D+100 and "recurrent" or "late, acute" GVHD as similar syndromes that occur after D+100 [147]. "Chronic" GVHD (cGVHD) occurs after D+100 and without features of aGVHD. In 2005, syndromes with features typical for both aGVHD and cGVHD were designated as "overlap"; however, the revised statement recommends elimination of the "overlap" category, classifying patients as aGVHD versus cGVHD and then documenting all manifestations whether typical or not [147–149].

Regardless of severity, both aGVHD and cGVHD are associated with a significantly increased risk for infection and infection-related mortality [36, 70, 99, 150–153]. This compromise of protection against bacterial, viral, and fungal pathogens results from both a direct and deleterious effect on functional immune reconstitution and the administration of immunosuppressive therapies. The prophylactic administration of antimicrobials against the following pathogens is recommended at least for the duration of immunosuppressive therapy for aGVHD and cGVHD: *Pneumocystis jiroveci, HSV-1, HSV-2, and VZV.* Antiviral prophylaxis for VZV is often continued for 1 year post-allogeneic transplant as this duration has been shown to reduce incidence and severity of reactivation.

The increased risk for disease due to CMV associated with GVHD has been well-recognized [70, 142, 154]. To complicate matters, plasma PCR is not highly sensitive for gastrointestinal disease. However, until recently the toxicity profile of the licensed anti-CMV antivirals precluded prophylaxis. The newly licensed antiviral letermovir may serve as a candidate for prophylaxis as Phase 3 studies in allo-BMT patients demonstrated efficacy in the absence of myelo- or nephrotoxicity.

GVHD is also associated with a significantly increased risk for invasive fungal infections; however, center-specific practices vary regarding infection control practices, surveillance, and prophylaxis with mold-active agents versus fluconazole [37, 50, 98, 151, 155, 156]. A high risk for infection due to encapsulated bacterial organisms is a hallmark of cGVHD which prompts indefinite prophylaxis with agents such as penicillin or trimethoprim-sulfamethoxazole.

Hypogammaglobulinemia is common during the peri-HCT period and in the setting of GVHD. Regular measurement of total IgG level is a common practice with intravenous immunoglobulin administration if the level is <400 mg/dl [157–160].

Optimizing survival in HCT is dependent on a continued awareness of risk for infection, thorough evaluation with a lowered threshold for empiric antimicrobial therapy with any substantive or unexplained change in clinical status, and appropriate prophylaxis. Although patients with GVHD may have suboptimal responses, guidelines have been established for vaccination of all patients post-HCT.

Although there is some degree of overlap, the risk factors for and clinical syndromes associated with aGVHD differ from cGVHD. Disparity in HLA encoded by the major histocompatibility complex (MHC), female donor for male patient, and increased age of donor and/or patient are associated with increased risk for aGVHD [138, 143, 161]. Many studies report that aGVHD risk may parallel the content of alloreactive T cells in the graft resulting in a higher rate associated with transplantation of MPB and a lower rate associated with UCB when compared to BM [121, 138, 143]. However, a growing body of data including preclinical models, genetic analyses of the role of minor histocompatibility antigens, a recent randomized trial of MPB versus BMT, and other studies of UCB transplant demonstrate how much still remains to be understood.

Acute GVHD

Typical syndromes associated with aGVHD include involvement of the skin, gastrointestinal tract, and liver. Each system is assessed based on an established grading system of Grade 1, 2, 3, or 4 representing increasing severity [147]. A single organ system or any combination of organ systems may be involved. Even when multiple organ systems are involved, the severity and timing of involvement may differ greatly. Moreover, aGVHD organ systems may demonstrate different degrees of responsiveness to therapy.

The most common organ system targeted is the skin. Manifestations of aGVHD can range from an eruption, most commonly maculopapular, but can evolve to life-threatening desquamation of the entire dermal surface [122, 143, 161]. Skin biopsies reveal varying degrees of inflammation of the epidermal and dermal layers, particularly perivascular or adjacent to dyskeratotic keratinocytes, and apoptosis in the basal layer of the epidermis [162]. Any portion of the gastrointestinal tract can be involved in GVHD. Esophago-gastro-duodenal disease may present as nausea, vomiting, abdominal pain, and/or anorexia. Small bowel and colonic disease may also present with abdominal pain, often described as cramping, and varying degrees of diarrhea which may be watery and/or bloody. Endoscopic examination ranges from normal-appearing mucosa to shallow ulcerations to severe mucosal denudation. Similar to histologic findings in skin, lymphocytic inflammation may be seen although apoptosis, especially at crypt bases, is highly supportive of the diagnosis of GVHD [163–165]. Hepatic aGVHD results from lymphocytic inflammation surrounding portal vein and/or bile ducts (pericholangitis) with subsequent destruction and presents as jaundice without pain or with mild RUQ pain. Liver biopsy, typically via a transjugular approach, is the most useful diagnostic modality [166]. Corticosteroids are the first-line therapy for aGVHD, and steroid-resistant disease is associated with a high mortality rate [143].

Chronic GVHD

The potentially devastating impact of cGVHD cannot be overstated. In spite of calcineurin inhibitor and antimetabolite therapy as prophylaxis, 30–70% of recipients of HCT will develop cGVHD which can result in profound debilitation, poor quality of life, and significant increase in mortality [137, 141, 148, 167]. Risk factors for cGVHD overlap with those for aGVHD and include peripheral blood as the source of the graft, female donor for a male recipient, and HLA-mismatched graft from an unrelated donor. History of Grade 3 or 4 aGVHD and donor lymphocyte infusions post-HCT have also been identified as risk factors for cGVHD. The pathophysiology of cGVHD involves inflammation that ultimately facilitates a fibrotic tissue response. Most recent work has supported a multiphase process which may be triggered by inflammatory response to exposure to a microbe, such as translocated organisms through the gastrointestinal mucosa. The ensuing dysfunction of cellular and humoral immunity then facilitates a fibrosis-inducing cascade [137]. Although the NIH consensus criteria provide a framework for the severity of disease in eight key organ systems (i.e., the skin, mouth, eye, liver, lungs, genitalia, and musculoskeletal), any system can be involved. Specific symptoms and findings are graded individually and assigned a score after which the clinician assigns an overall score. This system has facilitated studies of GVHD and potential therapies [147, 168, 169].

A substantial increase in transplant-related mortality is consistently reported in association with cGVHD in the following conditions: (1) platelet count less than 100 K/ul at the time of diagnosis, (2) progressive as opposed to quiescent disease, (3) severe disease, and (4) involvement of the liver, lungs, or gastrointestinal tract. Although cGVHD is also consistently associated with a decrease in relapse in patients with acute leukemia, this potential salutary effect is not reflected in an improvement in overall survival [137].

Cutaneous Manifestations

The most common manifestations of cGVHD are maculopapular rash and/or erythema. Eruption may have features that are lichen planus-like, sclerosis-like, papulosquamous lesions or ichthyosis, and/or keratosis pilaris-like eruptions. Changes in pigmentation are not uncommon [162, 170]. Most commonly, patients present with pain, pruritus, and progressively symptomatic fasciitis with or without sclerodermatous changes. The percentage of body surface area involved determines severity with Grade 4 defined as >50% involvement. Depending on the specific tissues involved and the extent of disease, cGVHD may lead to chronic pain, loss of range of motion, disfigurement, and impairment in ADLs including simple ambulation.

An increased incidence of skin cancer, especially squamous cell carcinoma, has long been recognized, and close surveillance by experienced specialist in dermatology and timely resection of suspicious lesions are recommended. Patients are also at significantly increased risk for infection which is exacerbated by poor wound healing [162, 170].

General consensus recommendations include minimizing damage resulting from ultraviolet rays A and B by repeated topical application of sunscreens with sun protection factor of 30 or greater. Avoidance of sun exposure during peak hours is also recommended. Diligent skin cancer surveillance should be performed regularly. Use of drugs known to increase photosensitivity, such as trimethoprim-sulfamethoxazole, should be balanced against risk. Voriconazole, a triazole antifungal medication, has been reported by some to increase risk for dermal injury, squamous cell carcinoma, and other cutaneous malignancies [171–174].

Once thought to be a rare complication, cGVHD of the musculoskeletal system is being diagnosed with increasing frequency with manifestations which are as varied as those seen in non-transplant autoimmune rheumatologic diseases. Polyserositis can involve musculoskeletal structures in addition to the serosal surfaces of the viscera [170]. Early and continued involvement of specialists in kinesiology and rehabilitation medicine is recommended.

Oral

Oral GVHD is the most common manifestation that provides the most common impetus for the addition of a second- or third-line immunosuppressive agent [149, 175–180]. Increasing severity is scored based on the physical findings, symptoms, and limitations on oral intake. Patients report significant discomfort due to dryness, alterations in taste, difficulty with swallowing, and pain. In addition to the impact of chronic discomfort, oral GVHD can also profoundly reduce quality of life by altering enjoyment of food and ability to eat which can lead to significant malnutrition. Decreased saliva production can disrupt taste and the ability to eat. If severe and prolonged, the loss of dental and gingival protection can lead to rapid progression of caries and tooth loss [137, 149].

Much has been published about the incidence and impact of mucositis and more detailed aspects of the oral health, such as gingivitis, caries, and ulcerations. In a recent notable study, Doss et al. presented their findings of a prospective, longitudinal study of dental plaque, gingivitis, and mucositis in 19 pediatric patients (5.1–12.8 years old) undergoing HCT [33, 181–184]. Using standardized indices they determined that plaque accumulation, gingival inflammation, mucositis, and oral ulcerations were seen in 85%, 85%, 68%, and 58%, respectively. Of note, the median severity gingivitis and ulcerations peaked at D+7, whereas coating of the mucosa and overall dental hygiene continued to deteriorate through D+28 [181, 183]. Patients who received myeloablative preparative regimens had more severe gingivitis and ulcerations but similar changes in dental hygiene and mucosal coating which were comparable to those in patients who received reduced intensity conditioning. Studies such as these are crucial in the beginning to understand pathophysiology, and they underscore the increased need for improvements in oral hygiene [182, 184]. Ongoing collaboration with a specialized maxillofacial/dental specialist is encouraged.

Ophthalmologic

In an excellent review, Tung notes that despite reported rates from 30% to 85%, ocular GVHD is likely underreported in part due to imprecision in disease classification [185]. Risk factors for ocular GVHD include a history of aGVHD of other organ systems including the skin and/or oropharyngeal, older age, female donor of graft for a male patient, and MPB graft. Ocular GVHD may be acute or chronic with the latter typically less severe in presentation. Hyperacute ocular GVHD often occurs as part of systemic process occurring during the peri-engraftment period for which corticosteroids are the first-line therapy. Ocular aGVHD may present as excessive tearing and/or dryness of the eye and discomfort including itching, burning, photophobia, or changes in visual acuity [180, 185, 186].

Examination most commonly reveals nonspecific membranous conjunctivitis due to inflammation likely due to infiltration with donor T and NK cells with a notable depletion of the specialized epithelial goblet cells which are responsible for tear stability. Sloughing of corneal cells, cellular debris, and infectious and noninfectious keratitis may also be noted. There might also be eyelid involvement with lichenoid changes with histologic examination revealing inflammation, apoptosis, and necrosis. The onset of ocular cGVHD is most commonly reported to be between 7 and 10 months post-HCT when the patient presents with lacrimal gland dysfunction manifested as excessive tearing and/or dryness, ultimately resulting in keratoconjunctival sicca, injection, scarring of the conjunctiva, and nasolacrimal duct obstruction. cGVHD of the eyelid structures may result in entropion which may, in turn, result in corneal damage and require surgical intervention. When the posterior structures of the eye are involved, discomfort and visual changes may be more prominent [186, 187].

The most common ocular complaints are related to disruption of tear production and stability. Lymphocytic infiltration can ultimately lead to obstruction due to severe scarring of the lacrimal glands. Attentive therapy with regular examination by an ophthalmologist is recommended; treatments include lubrication, anti-inflammatory agents, scleral lenses, and surgical intervention. Infection and inflammation can further compromise the ocular physiology [188–190].

Gastrointestinal

As with other organ involvement, the diagnosis of gastrointestinal cGVHD is based on clinical signs and symptoms which may be supported by, but not dependent on, additional studies. Any portion of the GI tract can be involved with focal findings of esophageal webbing or strictures and symptoms such as nausea, emesis, diarrhea, and wasting. New onset pancreatic exocrine insufficiency is a well-recognized manifestation of cGVHD. The Pathology Working Group Report of the NIH Consensus Development Project outlined minimal histologic criteria which, interestingly, do not differ between aGVHD and cGVHD [163, 164, 191–193]. The hallmark of GVHD is epithelial cell apoptosis, which is more marked in the intestines than in the stomach, and predominantly seen in the regenerative compartment of the crypt. In more advanced GVHD, inflammation, crypt abscesses, epithelial destruction, and cytoplasmic granular debris may be seen. Apoptosis not due to GVHD has been reported early (earlier than D+20) post-transplant likely secondary to myeloablative conditioning regimen, infections, and drugs including proton-pump inhibitors and mycophenolate mofetil (MMF) [164, 194].

MMF can cause colitis that is histologically difficult to distinguish from GVHD. CMV is also associated with epithelial apoptosis, although even if immunohistochemical or molecular studies confirm the presence of CMV, this does not rule out GVHD. The presence and density of eosinophils in the infiltrate has been described as a correlative finding but may be more common in aGVHD [195].

For a variety of reasons, small bowel involvement can be more difficult to diagnose and may result from a different pathophysiology. Although not consistently described, pericapillary hemorrhage and rupture of capillary basement membrane are associated with severe small bowel disease [137, 164].

Debate exists regarding the optimal site for biopsy; furthermore, in these patients at high risk for concomitant processes, a site optimal for GVHD may not be optimal for diagnosing infection [163, 193, 196, 197].

Hepatic

Elevations of hepatic transaminases and/or bilirubin are common post-HCT. Unlike other organ syndromes seen in cGVHD, hepatic involvement commonly is presumed when liver test abnormalities persist without other explanation.

Hepatic cGVHD typically parallels involvement and response to therapy of other system(s) [136, 141, 166]. However, many factors confound interpretation of hepatic abnormalities in this population, including drug hepatotoxicity and high risk for iron overload. There are no pathognomonic ultrasonographic or other radiographic findings, although MRI may be helpful in assessing the degree of iron overload. A growing number of PCR-based assays may help diagnose or rule out infectious causes such as hepatitis viruses, CMV, and adenovirus. Transjugular liver biopsy may be important to perform microbiologic and molecular studies [136, 166].

Pulmonary

The impact of the increasing survivorship of HCT patients is arguably most evident in the rapidly evolving understanding of the pulmonary manifestations of cGVHD [51, 198, 199]. The presentation of pulmonary disease is often confounded by conditions common in the post-HCT patient, including deconditioning and infection. As most patients will present with a nonspecific mild shortness of breath that may steadily worsen and/or persistent cough, the possibility of pulmonary cGVHD should be considered, especially in the setting of other organ involvement with cGVHD. The best characterized manifestation is narrowing of the terminal airways by a peribronchiolar and intraluminal fibrosis process referred to as bronchiolitis obliterans syndrome (BOS) which was first described in HCT patients in 1984 [198–200]. Since that time, new-onset airflow obstruction due to BOS has been included in the diagnostic criteria for cGVHD. Diagnosis of post-HCT BOS is not based on lung biopsy but primarily on results of spirometric testing including one of the following if the patient has extrapulmonary cGVHD: (1) a ratio of forced expiratory volume in 1 second (FEV1) to forced vital capacity (FVC) on less than 0.7, (2) FEV1 less than 75% of predicted value, (3) and evidence of air trapping with residual volume > 120% of predicted. High-resolution CT scan demonstrating bronchiolitis is also a diagnostic finding. Reduced FVC has been correlated with increased mortality in one series, and recent reports of survival at 2 years after diagnosis have improved possibly due to earlier recognition and treatment. Finally, the patient should not have an active pulmonary infection at the time the diagnosis of pulmonary cGVHD. Using the initial criteria established in 2005, 14% of patients with extrapulmonary cGVHD and 5% of all allogeneic patients were felt to have pulmonary cGVHD [168, 199, 202].

High-dose systemic corticosteroids are the first-line treatment for pulmonary cGVHD. Adjunctive treatment with fluticasone (anti-inflammatory), azithromycin (immunomodulatory), and montelukast (antifibrotic) resulted in sustained stability of FEV1 in a prospective, multicenter, single-arm trial [203]. Extracorporeal photophoresis has also been demonstrated to be of potential benefit but has largely been used in patients with steroid-refractory disease and/or as an attempt to reduce steroid exposure [180]. With the exception of two randomized, double-blinded placebo-controlled trials, data about adjunctive and/or secondary therapies are limited to reports and/or small series. In the first trial, azithromycin alone failed to demonstrate benefit [203]. In the second of these trials, budesonide/formoterol treatment resulted in a 12% FEV1 improvement [199]. A broad number of immunomodulatory therapies are actively being studied in large, well-designed trials [180]. At this time, there is not sufficient data to demonstrate approaches that can prevent pulmonary cGVHD.

Reports of a respiratory infection prior to the development of BOS are common and support the hypothesis that a trigger may result in an aberrant alloreactivity reaction. It is interesting to note that BOS is not felt to occur in recipients of a T-cell depleted graft. As with other studies of cGVHD, B cells appear to play a role in development of this inflammatory response, although limited studies of CD20 depletion have not demonstrated consistent benefit.

Other pulmonary pathologies have been described following HCT [198, 200, 201, 204]. Parenchymal involvement consistent with interstitial lung disease (ILD) is frequently observed in patients with pulmonary cGVHD. The most common presentation of ILD includes fever, cough, and shortness of breath, and 70% who are eventually diagnosed with ILD have GVHD. Given the marked increased susceptibility to infection resulting from cGVHD, it is not yet possible in the acute setting to distinguish infection with or without ILD or ILD alone. Moreover, the ability to diagnose infections even from bronchoscopic specimens remains highly limited. Diagnosis is typically confirmed by the patient's clinical and radiographic course. Additional pulmonary syndromes that have been reported include the following: organizing pneumonia resulting from intraluminal granulation tissue, largely comprised of fibroblasts and macrophages in distal airspaces; pleuroparenchymal fibroelastosis; diffuse alveolar damage; and other organizing pneumonias that have been described post-HCT. These and other potential manifestations of alloreactive disease warrant additional studies.

Genitalia

Early detection of vulvovaginal cGVHD has been shown to decrease need for surgical intervention. Establishing the diagnosis is highly dependent on patient awareness and timely examination by a knowledgeable clinician. Vulvovaginal cGVHD does not typically happen in isolation, and it should be considered in all women with other involvement [170–174].

Patients most commonly present with vaginal dryness and/or discharge, dyspareunia, and vulvar pain. These symptoms overlap with estrogen deficiency and may improve with estrogen treatment; however, in collaboration with the HCT team, treatment directed against cGVHD should be given to minimize severe sequelae. Vulvar changes can range from erythema, lichen planus-like and/or sclerosis-like features, ulcerations, fissures, fusion of labia, and scarring and fibrosis of the vagina that can lead to complete stenosis. A high degree of vigilance regarding infections should be maintained given the increased susceptibility to infection associated with all forms of cGVHD [205, 206, 208, 209].

Genital cGVHD in men is believed to be at least as under-recognized as it is in women. In two recent studies of men who had received an allogeneic HCT, 4–13% were felt to have features consistent with genital cGVHD [168, 207, 210]. Men most commonly present with dyspareunia, urinary complaints, and/or sexual dysfunction. Skin changes parallel those seen in women. Other findings include inflammation of the glans penis; changes may lead to difficulty in retracting foreskin, lichenoid lesions, sclerotic lesions, and/or urethral stenosis/strictures.

Cardiovascular Disease (CVD) and the Metabolic Syndrome

Clinically significant late (>1 year post-HCT) CVD is a now a well-recognized complication of HCT and is more common following allogeneic HCT [211–216]. The Bone Marrow Transplant Survivor Study found that the risk for CVD-related deaths was 2.3-fold higher than the risk for the general population. This result was echoed by Chow and colleagues who noted a >three-fold risk of significant CVD-related morbidity and mortality.

In retrospective analysis of pre- and post-HCT factors, Saro et al. found that patients who developed clinically evident CVD had a significantly lower OS rate (52.4%) compared to HCT patients who did not develop CVD (80.6%) [212]. As with non-HCT recipients, comorbidities such as obesity; hypertension; diabetes, especially due to insulin resistance; and dyslipidemia are associated with increased risk. They noted that if patients had two or more of the four identified cardiovascular risk factors, they had a fivefold increased risk of CVD and even higher risk for cerebrovascular complications. Perhaps the most important observation made by Saro et al. is that the increased risk was associated with the development of these comorbidities post-transplant. This finding supports the potential benefit of avoidance and/or management of these comorbidities.

A constellation of characteristics known as metabolic syndrome (MetS) has been shown to be closely associated with premature CVD risk in the general population and has a reported prevalence of 31–40% in post-HCT patients [217–219]. As of 2009, MetS is defined by the International Diabetes Federation and American Heart Association as ≥3 of the following risk factors: abdominal obesity, elevated triglycerides (≥150 mg/dl or > −1.7 mm/L), low high-density lipoprotein cholesterol (<40 mg/dL or 1.0 mmol/L for men and <50 mg/dL for women), blood pressure ≥130/≥85 mmHg; and/or fasting glucose ≥100 mg/dl (≥5.6 mmol/L). Treatment for dyslipidemias, hypertension, and/or hyperglycemia also meets the individual criteria. In the general population, MetS increases the risk for CVD, DM, and stroke.

Although MetS has not yet been demonstrated to have a direct impact on CVD post-HCT, the CIBMTR Late Effects and Quality of Life Working Committee and the EBMT Complications and Quality of Life Working Party published their recommendations for screening and preventative practice of MetS in a reasonable attempt to mitigate any CVD risk factors [217, 218, 220, 221].

Interestingly, pre-HCT chest radiation exposure was also associated with a ninefold increase in coronary artery disease compared to patients without a history of radiation exposure. These data are consistent with previous reports that radiation induces vascular injury with endothelial, intimal, and medial scarring. Inflammatory responses may also contribute, although little is known about the relative contribution of a GVHD-like effect. Radiation of the head and/or neck was not associated with increased cerebrovascular disease in contrast to the increased risk reportedly seen in patients who received radiation in the treatment of head and neck cancers [212–214]. Of drugs commonly used for conditioning, high-dose cyclophosphamide has long been recognized to be cardiotoxic, although it is not clear if there is any association with subsequent atherosclerosis [214].

Endocrine/Metabolic

Bone Metabolism and Vitamin D

As would be predicted by the decrease in physical activity, gonadal failure, significant corticosteroid and calcineurin inhibitor exposure, and deficiencies in calcium and/or vitamin D that are common in HCT patients, decreased bone mineral density (BMD) is now recognized as a serious potential complication, especially in long-term survivors [222–226]. Rapid resorption with resulting loss in BMD can be detected as early as 1–2 years post-HCT. A retrospective analysis revealed that 5% of >3500 allo-HCT patients had a pathologic fracture which occurred at a median of 85 months post-transplant [223]. In addition to the classic risk factors listed above, immune-mediated processes detrimental to the homeostasis of bone have been proposed, including derangements in the receptor activator of nuclear factor kappa-B ligand which increases osteoclast activity and osteoprotegerin which inhibits osteoclast activity [223, 227]. The NIH cGVHD Consensus Project Ancillary and Supportive Care Guidelines has recommended annual BMD measurements. In recent study, 258 patients (145 males, 113 females) with a median age of 48 years and moderate to severe cGVHD following allo-HCT (84% PB graft, 86% with an HLA-matched donor, and 62% with a related donor) underwent a 1-week comprehensive evaluation including dual-energy X-ray absorptiometry (DEXA) to determine BMD at the femoral neck, lumbar spine, and total hip [228]. Patients were also evaluated using standardized scores of assessment of osteoporosis, nutrition, and physical activity. In the univariate analysis, lower body weight and malnutrition were associated with osteoporosis at all three sites; however, a variety of characteristics were related to risks at one or two other sites. For example, higher current glucocorticoid dose was associated with osteoporosis in the total hip. Interestingly, vitamin D deficiency was not associated with osteoporosis in this study, although it is noted that a high percentage of patients were on replacement therapy. With the rapidly increasing number and age of HCT patients, further study will be crucial. Current recommendations include close collaboration with endocrinology specialists to begin monitoring for osteoporosis post-HCT regardless of age, optimization of vitamin D level, minimization of inactivity and steroid exposure, limited course of sex hormone therapy replacement, and bisphosphonates for patients on steroids for greater than 2 months [229].

Thyroid

Disruption of thyroid gland dysfunction is one of the most common endocrine complications of transplantation and has been best characterized in children and after allogeneic transplantation [12, 230–234]. At one large center where pre- and post-transplantation serum thyroid function testing was routine, 259 adult patients who did not have pre-existing thyroid disease and who had survived ≥2 years after allogeneic transplant were analyzed. Of all patients, 30.5% developed thyroid dysfunction, and 11% of these patients had clinically apparent disease (8% with hypothyroidism and 3% with hyperthyroidism). The median time to thyroid dysfunction was 3.03 years, and high-dose TBI was identified as a risk factor (68%). In contrast, other case series have revealed an association between TBI, TBI dose, increased age, and GVHD [9, 233, 235, 236]. It is likely that studies of longer duration with detailed analysis of immunosuppressive duration may be needed to understand the true incidence of thyroid dysfunction. Some data has

indicated that the risk for thyroid carcinoma is higher in HCT patients. In one such study with an extended period of follow-up of 791 pediatric patients, thyroid masses were detected at a median of 9.9 years post-transplant and occurred in 0.02% of patients [237]. In this report, over two-thirds of the masses were papillary carcinomas, and the remainders were benign [237].

Reproduction/Fertility

Although limited, the majority of reports regarding the impact of HCT on gonadal function have focused on ovarian failure due to the toxicity of the conditioning regimen, reported to be 44–100% with correspondingly lower pregnancy rates [5, 13, 238–241]. Jadoul and Donnez provided an informative review of published data [13]. TBI is associated with the highest risk of ovarian failure, decreased potential for recovery of function, and the lowest subsequent pregnancy rates [13]. Risk from TBI increases if the female is older than 10 years old and/or is postpuberty. A total dose of 10 cGy appears to result in nearly universal ovarian failure. Myeloablative doses of chemotherapy, most commonly cyclophosphamide, busulfan, or melphalan, are also associated with rates of ovarian failures as high as 70–100%, with risk also associated with age and melphalan being possibly less gonadotoxic than busulfan. The decreased risk for irreversible ovarian failure resulting from the conditioning regimen in younger females is believed to be, in part, due to an increased number of nongrowing follicles in younger girls. However, complex effects on the vasculature of the ovary and uterus are not fully understood.

True impact on fertility can only be determined by analysis of spontaneous pregnancy rates and live births in large population of post-BMT patients with adequate follow-up and sufficient homogenicity regarding factors such as age at time of transplant, prior and pre-transplant gonadotoxic therapies, and hormonal therapies. There is no definitive laboratory test to determine ovarian function [241]; however, follicle-stimulating hormone and anti-Mullerian hormone are potentially useful.

Approaches to facilitate future reproductive potential include gamete preservation by ovarian fragment, oocyte, or sperm banking, reducing ovarian gonadotoxic therapy, and attempts to protect the ovaries by administration of gonadotropin-releasing hormone. Timely referral to a specialist in reproductive endocrinology as part of transplant preparation may maximize future fertility and/or options for reproduction [204, 242]. Reduced intensity and/or non-myeloablative preparative regimens may also result in reduced gonadal toxicity and is currently under study.

Immunomodulatory Therapies: Lessons from Rituximab and Checkpoint Inhibitors

The use of therapeutic immunomodulatory antibodies in the treatment of cancer continues to expand. Rituximab, an engineered chimeric antibody against the CD20 surface protein on B cells, was licensed in 2006 for treatment of non-Hodgkin's lymphoma but is now widely used for a wide range of malignancies and autoimmune disorders and is being studied as an adjunctive treatment for GVHD. Although rituximab treatment results in a prolonged and profound depletion of B cells, there has been a paucity of infectious complications even in HCT patients possibly due to the fact that plasma cells do not express CD20. Infectious complications reported include progressive multifocal leukoencephalopathy due to JC virus, hepatitis B reactivation, and impaired immunoglobulin response to influenza vaccine immunization. To date, no increase in infection-related mortality has been reported in HCT patients who received rituximab [243, 244].

Antibodies against regulators of peripheral immune tolerance, such as the protein receptors CTLA-4 (cytotoxic T-lymphocyte-associated protein 4) and PD-1 (programmed cell death 1), result in the "immune checkpoint blockade." Interestingly, adverse effects of these therapies mirror genetic autoimmune polyendocrinopathies (e.g., colitis, thyroiditis, hypophysitis, type-1 diabetes, and adrenal insufficiency) and are reported in over 10% of recipients [245, 246]. The use of checkpoint inhibitors to reduce relapse after autologous HCT is an area of active study. The utility of these drugs after allogeneic HCT is being approached with caution given preclinical mouse models demonstrating augmentation of alloreactive T-cell proliferation and GVHD. A retrospective analysis of 39 patients with lymphoma who had received a PD-1 inhibitor median of 62 days prior to allogeneic HCT was found to have significant reductions in both PD-1+ T cells and ratios of Treg cells to CD4+ or CD8+ cells; however, conclusions cannot yet be made regarding impact of prior treatment on GVHD [243].

Sleep Disorders

Information regarding disruptions in sleep in HCT recipients is frequently captured by questionnaire studies regarding quality of life with limited data regarding short- versus long-term effects [247–250]. Studies by Bevan et al. and Rischer et al. report that as many as 77% of HCT patients experience sleep disturbances, most notably during the peri-transplant period. However, there is limited published data regarding sleep using standard tools of assessment [249, 251]. Nelson et al. recently reported the prevalence and severity of sleep disruptions as measured by actigraphic data from 7 consecutive 24-hour periods and accepted self-report scales in 84 patients who had undergone autologous transplant 6–18 months prior to enrollment [252]. The demographics of their patients was notable for a median age of 60 years and 45%, 4.8%, and 11% self-identified as female, Hispanic, and nonwhite, respectively. In their study, 41% of patients reported significant sleep disruption which correlated with a decrease in objectively calculated total sleep time, but no other measures of sleep disruption. Interestingly, both younger and Hispanic patients took longer to fall asleep (sleep latency). In all groups, longer sleep latency correlated with increase in fear of cancer recurrence. Hispanic patients were more likely to have worse quality of sleep than non-Hispanic patients. As has been previously reported, sleep disruption decreased with increased time since transplantation. Average sleep efficiency was below the lower level of recommended sleep quality. Interestingly, subjective reports were considered to be the more clinically relevant outcome, but did not correlate well with objective data from actigraphy. Collectively, data supports increased awareness of the profound consequences and need for interventions for sleep disruptions in HCT patients [247, 249, 251–253]. Additional studies, especially longitudinal, with attention to factors such as age, cancer status, and ethnicity are needed.

Conclusions

Post-HCT patients may experience a variety of infectious and noninfectious complications. Patients are susceptible to a variety of viruses, bacteria, and fungi. Noninfectious complications can involve any organ and include GVHD, which can severely decrease quality of life, lead to multiple other comorbidities, and decrease survival. Knowledge of such complications can help physicians, patients, and caregivers plan accordingly, anticipate vigilantly, and treat promptly.

References

1. Bruserud O, Reikvam H, Kittang AO, Ahmed AB, Tvedt TH, Sjo M, et al. High-dose etoposide in allogeneic stem cell transplantation. Cancer Chemother Pharmacol. 2012;70:765–82.
2. Hill BT, Rybicki L, Carlstrom KD, Jagadeesh D, Gerds A, Hamilton B, et al. Daily weight-based busulfan with cyclophosphamide and etoposide produces comparable outcomes to four-times-daily busulfan dosing for lymphoma patients undergoing autologous stem cell transplantation. Biol Blood Marrow Transplant. 2016;22:1588–95.
3. Ben-Barouch S, Cohen O, Vidal L, Avivi I, Ram R. Busulfan fludarabine vs busulfan cyclophosphamide as a preparative regimen before allogeneic hematopoietic cell transplantation: systematic review and meta-analysis. Bone Marrow Transplant. 2016;51:232–40.
4. Krivoy N, Hoffer E, Lurie Y, Bentur Y, Rowe JM. Busulfan use in hematopoietic stem cell transplantation: pharmacology, dose

adjustment, safety and efficacy in adults and children. Curr Drug Saf. 2008;3:60–6.

5. Even-Or E, Ben-Haroush A, Yahel A, Yaniv I, Stein J. Fertility after treatment with high dose Melphalan in women with acute myelogenous leukemia. Pediatr Blood Cancer. 2016;63:334–6.

6. Chaudhry HM, Bruce AJ, Wolf RC, Litzow MR, Hogan WJ, Patnaik MS, et al. The incidence and severity of oral mucositis among allogeneic hematopoietic stem cell transplantation patients: a systematic review. Biol Blood Marrow Transplant. 2016;22:605–16.

7. Danylesko I, Shimoni A. Second malignancies after hematopoietic stem cell transplantation. Curr Treat Options in Oncol. 2018; https://doi.org/10.1007/s11864-018-0528-y.

8. Jackson TJ, Mostoufi-Moab S, Hill-Kayser C, Balamuth NJ, Arkader A. Musculoskeletal complications following total body irradiation in hematopoietic stem cell transplant patients. Pediatr Blood Cancer. 2018;65(4) https://doi.org/10.1002/pbc.26905.

9. Slatter MA, Gennery AR, Cheetham TD, Bhattacharya A, Crooks BN, Flood TJ, et al. Thyroid dysfunction after bone marrow transplantation for primary immunodeficiency without the use of total body irradiation in conditioning. Bone Marrow Transplant. 2004;33

10. Oya N, Sasai K, Tachiiri S, Sakamoto T, Nagata Y, Okada T, et al. Influence of radiation dose rate and lung dose on interstitial pneumonitis after fractionated total body irradiation: acute parotitis may predict interstitial pneumonitis. Int J Hematol. 2006;83:86–91.

11. Bowen JM, Wardill HR. Advances in the understanding and management of mucositis during stem cell transplantation. Curr Opin Support Palliat Care. 2017;11:341–6.

12. Farhadfar N, Stan MN, Shah P, Sonawane V, Hefazi MT, Murthy HS, et al. Thyroid dysfunction in adult hematopoietic cell transplant survivors: risks and outcomes. Bone Marrow Transplant. 2018;1 https://doi.org/10.1038/s41409-018-0109-5.

13. Jadoul P, Donnez J. How does bone marrow transplantation affect ovarian function and fertility? Curr Opin Obstet Gynecol. 2012;24(3):164–71. https://doi.org/10.1097/GCO.0b013e328353bb57.

14. Riley P, Glenny AM, Worthington HV, Littlewood A, Fernandez Mauleffinch LM, Clarkson JE, et al. Interventions for preventing oral mucositis in patients with cancer receiving treatment: cytokines and growth factors. Cochrane Database Syst Rev. 2017;11:CD011990.

15. Schmidt V, Niederwieser D, Schenk T, Behre G, Klink A, Pfrepper C, et al. Efficacy and safety of keratinocyte growth factor (palifermin) for prevention of oral mucositis in TBI-based allogeneic hematopoietic stem cell transplantation. Bone Marrow Transplant. 2018; https://doi.org/10.1038/s41409-018-0135-3.

16. Giralt S. The role of Alemtuzumab in Nonmyeloablative hematopoietic transplantation. Semin Oncol. 2006;33:36–43.

17. Kharfan-Dabaja MA, Nishihori T, Otrock ZK, Haidar N, Mohty M, Hamadani M. Monoclonal antibodies in conditioning regimens for hematopoietic cell transplantation. Biol Blood Marrow Transplant. 2013;19:1288–300.

18. Kröger N, Solano C, Wolschke C, Bandini G, Patriarca F, Pini M, et al. Antilymphocyte globulin for prevention of chronic graft-versus-host disease. N Engl J Med. 2016; https://doi.org/10.1056/NEJMoa1506002.

19. Arai Y, Jo T, Matsui H, Kondo T, Takaori-Kondo A. Efficacy of antithymocyte globulin for allogeneic hematopoietic cell transplantation: a systematic review and meta-analysis. Leuk Lymphoma. 2017;58:1840–8.

20. de Koning C, Admiraal R, Nierkens S, Boelens JJ. Immune reconstitution and outcomes after conditioning with anti-thymocyte-globulin in unrelated cord blood transplantation; the good, the bad, and the ugly. Stem Cell Investig. 2017;4:38. https://doi.org/10.21037/sci.2017.05.02.

21. Yañez San Segundo L, et al. Differences of antithymocyte globulin (ATG) side effects during allogeneic stem cell transplantation. Blood. 2015;126

22. Österborg A, Karlsson C, Lundin J, Kimby E, Mellstedt H. Strategies in the management of alemtuzumab-related side effects. Semin Oncol. 2006;33:29–35.

23. McCune JS, Bemer MJ, Long-Boyle J. Pharmacokinetics, pharmacodynamics, and pharmacogenomics of immunosuppressants in allogeneic hematopoietic cell transplantation: part II. Clin Pharmacokinet. 2016;55:551–93.

24. Nikolousis E, Nagra S, Pearce R, Perry J, Kirkland K, Byrne J, et al. Impact of pre-transplant co-morbidities on outcome after alemtuzumab-based reduced intensity conditioning Allo-SCT in elderly patients: a British Society of Blood and Marrow Transplantation study. Bone Marrow Transplant. 2015;50:82–6.

25. Mehta RS, Rezvani K. Immune reconstitution post allogeneic transplant and the impact of immune recovery on the risk of infection. Virulence. 2016;7:901–16.

26. Gajurel K, Dhakal R, Montoya JG. Toxoplasma prophylaxis in haematopoietic cell transplant recipients: a review of the literature and recommendations. Curr Opin Infect Dis. 2015;28:283–92.

27. Kauffman CA, Freifeld AG, Andes DR, Baddley JW, Herwaldt L, Walker RC, et al. Endemic fungal infections in solid organ and hematopoietic cell transplant recipients enrolled in the Transplant-Associated Infection Surveillance Network (TRANSNET). Transpl Infect Dis. 2014; https://doi.org/10.1111/tid.12186.

28. Patel SS, Rybicki LA, Corrigan D, Bolwell B, Dean R, Liu H, et al. Prognostic factors for mortality among day +100 survivors after allogeneic hematopoietic cell transplantation. Biol Blood Marrow Transplant. 2018; https://doi.org/10.1016/j.bbmt.2018.01.016.

29. Muñoz L, Santin M. Prevention and management of tuberculosis in transplant recipients: from guidelines to clinical practice. Transplantation. 2016;100(9):1840–52. https://doi.org/10.1097/TP.0000000000001224.

30. Scheich A, Lindner S, Koenig R, Reinheimer C, Wichelhaus TA, Hogardt M, et al. Clinical impact of colonization with multidrug-resistant organisms on outcome after allogeneic stem cell transplantation in patients with acute myeloid leukemia. Cancer. 2018;124:286–96.

31. Hefazi M, Damlaj M, Alkhateeb HB, Partain DK, Patel R, Razonable RR, et al. Vancomycin-resistant Enterococcus colonization and bloodstream infection: prevalence, risk factors, and the impact on early outcomes after allogeneic hematopoietic cell transplantation in patients with acute myeloid leukemia. Transpl Infect Dis. 2016;18:913–20.

32. Sultan AS, Zimering Y, Petruzziello G, Alyea E III, Antin JH, Soiffer RJ, et al. Oral health status and risk of bacteremia following allogeneic hematopoietic cell transplantation. Oral Surg Oral Med Oral Pathol Oral Radiol. 2017;124:253–60.

33. Bogusławska-Kapała A, Hałaburda K, Rusyan E, Gołąbek H, Strużycka I. Oral health of adult patients undergoing hematopoietic cell transplantation. Pre-transplant assessment and care. Ann Hematol. 2017;96:1135–45.

34. Boyle NM, Magaret A, Stednick Z, Morrison A, Butler-Wu S, Zerr D, et al. Evaluating risk factors for Clostridium difficile infection in adult and pediatric hematopoietic cell transplant recipients. Antimicrob Resist Infect Control. 2015;4(41)

35. Dubberke ER, Reske KA, Olsen MA, Bommarito KM, Seiler S, Silveira FP, et al. Risk for Clostridium difficile infection after allogeneic hematopoietic cell transplant remains elevated in the postengraftment period. Transplant Direct. 2017;3(e145)

36. Hiemenz JW. Management of infections complicating allogeneic hematopoietic stem cell transplantation. Semin Hematol. 2009; https://doi.org/10.1053/j.seminhematol.2009.03.005.

37. Miller HK, Braun TM, Stillwell T, Harris AC, Choi S, Connelly J, et al. Infectious risk after allogeneic hematopoietic cell transplantation complicated by acute graft-versus-host disease. Biol Blood Marrow Transplant. 2017;23:522–8.

38. Freifeld AG, Bow EJ, Sepkowitz KA, Boeckh MJ, Ito JI, Mullen CA, et al. Clinical practice guideline for the use of antimicrobial agents in neutropenic patients with cancer: 2010 update by the infectious diseases society of America. Clin Infect Dis. 2011;52:e56–93.

39. Taplitz RA, Kennedy EB, Flowers CR. Outpatient management of fever and neutropenia in adults treated for malignancy: American Society of Clinical Oncology and Infectious Diseases Society of America Clinical Practice Guideline Update. J Clin Oncol. 2018;36(14):1443–53. https://doi.org/10.1200/JCO.2017.77.6211.

40. Shelburne SA, Sahasrabhojane P, Saldana M, Yao H, Su X, Horstmann N, et al. Streptococcus mitis strains causing severe clinical disease in cancer patients. Emerg Infect Dis. 2014;20:762–71.

41. Doern, G. V, Ferraro, M. J., Brueggemann, A. B. & Ruoff, K. L. Emergence of high rates of antimicrobial resistance among viridans group streptococci in the United States. Antimicrob Agents Chemother 40, 891–894 (1996).

42. Engelhard D, Akova M, Boeckh MJ, Freifeld A, Sepkowitz K, Viscoli C, et al. Bacterial infection prevention after hematopoietic cell transplantation. Bone Marrow Transplant. 2009;44:467–70.

43. Alp S, Akova M. Management of febrile neutropenia in the era of bacterial resistance. Ther Adv Infect Dis. 2013;1:37–43.

44. Cohen SA, Woodfield MC, Boyle N, Stednick Z, Boeckh M, Pergam SA, et al. Incidence and outcomes of bloodstream infections among hematopoietic cell transplant recipients from species commonly reported to be in over-the-counter probiotic formulations. Transpl Infect Dis. 2016;18:699–705.

45. van Burik JH, Leisenring W, Myerson D, Hackman RC, Shulman HM, Sale GE, et al. The effect of prophylactic fluconazole on the clinical spectrum of fungal diseases in bone marrow transplant recipients with special attention to hepatic candidiasis. An autopsy study of 355 patients. Medicine (Baltimore). 1998;77:246–54.

46. Marr KA, Seidel K, Slavin MA, Bowden RA, Schoch HG, Flowers ME, et al. Prolonged fluconazole prophylaxis is associated with persistent protection against candidiasis-related death in allogeneic marrow transplant recipients: long-term follow-up of a randomized, placebo-controlled trial. Blood. 2000;96:2055–61.

47. Cortegiani A, Russotto V, Maggiore A, Attanasio M, Naro AR, Raineri SM, et al. Antifungal agents for preventing fungal infections in non-neutropenic critically ill patients. Cochrane Database Syst Rev. 2016; https://doi.org/10.1002/14651858.CD004920.pub3.

48. Segal BH, Almyroudis NG, Battiwalla M, Herbrecht R, Perfect JR, Walsh TJ, et al. Prevention and early treatment of invasive fungal infection in patients with cancer and neutropenia and in stem cell transplant recipients in the era of newer broad-spectrum antifungal agents and diagnostic adjuncts. Clin Infect Dis. 2007;44(3):402–9.

49. Garcia-Vidal C, Viasus D, Carratalà J. Pathogenesis of invasive fungal infections. Curr Opin Infect Dis. 2013;26(3):270–6. https://doi.org/10.1097/QCO.0b013e32835fb920.

50. Choi JK, Cho SY, Yoon SS, Moon JH, Kim SH, Lee JH, et al. Epidemiology and risk factors for invasive fungal diseases among allogeneic hematopoietic stem cell transplant recipients in Korea: results of "RISK" study. Biol Blood Marrow Transplant. 2017;23:1773–9.

51. Roychowdhury M, Pambuccian SE, Aslan DL, Jessurun J, Rose AG, Manivel JC, et al. Pulmonary complications after bone marrow transplantation: an autopsy study from a large transplantation center. Arch Pathol Lab Med. 2005;129:366–71.

52. Ullmann AJ, Lipton JH, Vesole DH, Chandrasekar P, Langston A, Tarantolo SR, et al. Posaconazole or fluconazole for prophylaxis in severe graft-versus-host disease. N Engl J Med. 2007;356:335–47.

53. Busca A, Tortorano AM, Pagano L. Reviewing the importance and evolution of fungal infections and potential antifungal resistance in haematological patients. J Glob Antimicrob Resist. 2015; https://doi.org/10.1016/j.jgar.2015.09.002.

54. Willems L, Hasegawa H, Accolla R, Bangham C, Bazarbachi A, Bertazzoni U, et al. Reducing the global burden of HTLV-1 infection: an agenda for research and action. Antivir Res. 2017; https://doi.org/10.1016/j.antiviral.2016.10.015.

55. Eisen D, Essell J, Broun ER, Sigmund D, DeVoe M. Clinical utility of oral valacyclovir compared with oral acyclovir for the prevention of herpes simplex virus mucositis following autologous bone marrow transplantation or stem cell rescue therapy. Bone Marrow Transplant. 2003;31:51–5.

56. Macchi B, Balestrieri E, Frezza C, Grelli S, Valletta E, Marçais A, et al. Quantification of HTLV-1 reverse transcriptase activity in ATL patients treated with zidovudine and interferon-α. Blood Adv. 2017;1:748–52.

57. Moreno-Ajona D, Yuste JR, Martín P, Gállego Pérez-Larraya J. HTLV-1 myelopathy after renal transplant and antiviral prophylaxis: the need for screening. J Neurovirol. 2018; https://doi.org/10.1007/s13365-018-0627-3.

58. Morfin F, Bilger K, Boucher A, Thiebaut A, Najioullah F, Bleyzac N, et al. HSV excretion after bone marrow transplantation: a 4-year survey. J Clin Virol. 2004;30:341–5.

59. Dignani MC, Mykietiuk A, Michelet M, Intile D, Mammana L, Desmery P, et al. Valacyclovir prophylaxis for the prevention of Herpes simplex virus reactivation in recipients of progenitor cells transplantation. Bone Marrow Transplant. 2002;29:263–7.

60. Ljungman P, Wilczek H, Gahrton G, Gustavsson A, Lundgren G, Lönnqvist B, et al. Long-term acyclovir prophylaxis in bone marrow transplant recipients and lymphocyte proliferation responses to herpes virus antigens in vitro. Bone Marrow Transplant. 1986;1:185–92.

61. Ong DSY, Bonten MJM, Spitoni C, Verduyn Lunel FM, Frencken JF, Horn J, et al. Molecular diagnosis and risk stratification of sepsis consortium. Clinical infectious diseases epidemiology of multiple herpes viremia in previously immunocompetent patients with septic shock. Clin Infect Dis. 2017;64:1204–10.

62. Lipsitch M, Bacon TH, Leary JJ, Antia R, Levin BR. Effects of antiviral usage on transmission dynamics of herpes simplex virus type 1 and on antiviral resistance: predictions of mathematical models. Antimicrob Agents Chemother. 2000;44:2824–35.

63. Kanbayashi Y, Matsumoto Y, Kuroda J, Kobayashi T, Horiike S, Hosokawa TY, et al. Predicting risk factors for varicella zoster virus infection and postherpetic neuralgia after hematopoietic cell transplantation using ordered logistic regression analysis. Ann Hematol. 2017;96:311–5.

64. Klein A, Miller KB, Sprague K, DesJardin JA, Snydman DR. A randomized, double-blind, placebo-controlled trial of valacyclovir prophylaxis to prevent zoster recurrence from months 4 to 24 after BMT. Bone Marrow Transplant. 2011;46:294–9.

65. Brennan DC, Aguado JM, Potena L, Jardine AG, Legendre C, Säemann MD, et al. Effect of maintenance immunosuppressive drugs on virus pathobiology: evidence and potential mechanisms. Rev Med Virol. 2013; https://doi.org/10.1002/rmv.1733.

66. Green ML, Leisenring W, Stachel D, Pergam SA, Sandmaier BM, Wald A, et al. Efficacy of a viral load-based, risk-adapted, pre-emptive treatment strategy for prevention of cytomegalovirus disease after hematopoietic cell transplantation. Biol Blood Marrow Transplant. 2012; https://doi.org/10.1016/j.bbmt.2012.05.015.

67. Akahoshi Y, Kanda J, Ohno A, Komiya Y, Gomyo A, Hayakawa J, et al. Acyclovir-resistant herpes simplex virus 1 infection early

after allogeneic hematopoietic stem cell transplantation with T-cell depletion. J Infect Chemother. 2017;23:485–7.

68. Fujii H, Kakiuchi S, Tsuji M, Nishimura H, Yoshikawa T, Yamada S, et al. Application of next-generation sequencing to detect acyclovir-resistant herpes simplex virus type 1 variants at low frequency in thymidine kinase gene of the isolates recovered from patients with hematopoietic stem cell transplantation. J Virol Methods. 2018;251:123–8.

69. Ariza-Heredia EJ, Chemaly RF, Shahani LR, Jang Y, Champlin RE, Mulanovich VE. Delay of alternative antiviral therapy and poor outcomes of acyclovir-resistant herpes simplex virus infections in recipients of allogeneic stem cell transplant – a retrospective study. Transpl Int. 2018; https://doi.org/10.1111/tri.13142.

70. Cohen L, Yeshurun M, Shpilberg O, Ram R. Risk factors and prognostic scale for cytomegalovirus (CMV) infection in CMV-seropositive patients after allogeneic hematopoietic cell transplantation. Transpl Infect Dis. 2015;17:510–7.

71. Goodier MR, Jonjić S, Riley EM, Juranić Lisnić V. CMV and natural killer cells: shaping the response to vaccination. Eur J Immunol. 2018;48:50–65.

72. Krawczyk A, Ackermann J, Goitowski B, Trenschel R, Ditschkowski M, Timm J, et al. Assessing the risk of CMV reactivation and reconstitution of antiviral immune response post bone marrow transplantation by the QuantiFERON-CMV-assay and real time PCR. J Clin Virol. 2018;99–100:61–6.

73. El Chaer F, Shah DP, Chemaly RF. How I treat resistant cytomegalovirus infection in hematopoietic cell transplantation recipients. Blood. 2016;128:2624–36.

74. Nakamura R, La Rosa C, Longmate J, Drake J, Slape C, Zhou Q, et al. Viraemia, immunogenicity, and survival outcomes of cytomegalovirus chimeric epitope vaccine supplemented with PF03512676 (CMVPepVax) in allogeneic haemopoietic stem-cell transplantation: randomised phase 1b trial. Lancet Haematol. 2016;3:e87–98.

75. Boeckh M, Nichols WG, Chemaly RF, Papanicolaou GA, Wingard JR, Xie H, et al. Valganciclovir for the prevention of complications of late cytomegalovirus infection after allogeneic hematopoietic cell transplantation: a randomized trial. Ann Intern Med. 2015;162:1–10.

76. Marty FM, Ljungman P, Chemaly RF, Maertens J, Dadwal SS, Duarte RF, et al. A phase III randomized, double-blind, placebo-controlled trial of letermovir for prevention of cytomegalovirus infection in adult CMV-seropositive recipients of allogeneic hematopoietic cell transplantation. N Engl J Med. 2017;377(25):2433–44.

77. Meij P, van Esser JW, Niesters HG, van Baarle D, Miedema F, Blake N, et al. Impaired recovery of Epstein-Barr virus (EBV)-specific CD8+ T lymphocytes after partially T-depleted allogeneic stem cell transplantation may identify patients at very high risk for progressive EBV reactivation and lymphoproliferative disease. Blood. 2003; https://doi.org/10.1182/blood-2002-10-3001.

78. Klionsky DJ, Abdelmohsen K, Abe A, Abedin MJ, Abeliovich H, Acevedo Arozena A, et al. Guidelines for the use and interpretation of assays for monitoring autophagy (3rd edition). Autophagy. 2016;12:1–222.

79. Dumas PY, Ruggeri A, Robin M, Crotta A, Abraham J, Forcade E, et al. Incidence and risk factors of EBV reactivation after unrelated cord blood transplantation: a Eurocord and Société Française de Greffe de Moelle-Therapie Cellulaire collaborative study. Bone Marrow Transplant. 2012;48:253–6.

80. Furuya A, Ishida M, Hodohara K, Yoshii M, Okuno H, Horinouchi A, et al. Epstein-Barr virus-related post-transplant lymphoproliferative disorder occurring after bone marrow transplantation for aplastic anemia in Down's syndrome. Int J Clin Exp Pathol. 2014;7:438–42.

81. Lim WH, Russ GR, Coates PTH. Review of Epstein-Barr virus and post-transplant lymphoproliferative disorder post-solid organ transplantation. Nephrology. 2006; https://doi.org/10.1111/j.1440-1797.2006.00596.x.

82. Sutrave G, Blyth E, Gottlieb DJ. Cellular therapy for multiple pathogen infections after hematopoietic stem cell transplant. Cytotherapy. 2017;19:1284–301.

83. Chiereghin A, Bertuzzi C, Piccirilli G, Gabrielli L, Squarzoni D, Turello G, et al. Successful management of EBV-PTLD in allogeneic bone marrow transplant recipient by virological-immunological monitoring of EBV infection, prompt diagnosis and early treatment. Transpl Immunol. 2016;34:60–4.

84. Aguilera N, Gru AA. Reexamining post-transplant lymphoproliferative disorders: newly recognized and enigmatic types. Semin Diagn Pathol. 2018; https://doi.org/10.1053/j.semdp.2018.02.001.

85. Strippel C, Mönig C, Golombeck KS, Dik A, Bönte K, Kovac S, et al. Treating refractory post-herpetic anti-N-methyl-d-aspartate receptor encephalitis with rituximab. Oxf Med Case Rep 2017;2017(7):omx034.

86. Peric Z, Cahu X, Chevallier P, Brissot E, Malard F, Guillaume T, et al. Features of EBV reactivation after reduced intensity conditioning unrelated umbilical cord blood transplantation. Bone Marrow Transplant. 2011;47:251–7.

87. Hassan R, Stefanoff CG, Maradei S, Fernandes GA, Barros MH, Carestiato FN, et al. EBV-associated post transplant lymphoproliferative disorder of the 'loser' graft cell origin following double unrelated umbilical cord blood transplantation. Bone Marrow Transplant. 2009;44:193–5.

88. de Pagter PJ, Schuurman R, Meijer E, van Baarle D, Sanders EA, Boelens JJ, et al. Human herpesvirus type 6 reactivation after haematopoietic stem cell transplantation. J Clin Virol. 2008; https://doi.org/10.1016/j.jcv.2008.08.008.

89. Betts BC, Young JAH, Ustun C, Cao Q, Weisdorf DJ. Human herpesvirus 6 infection after hematopoietic cell transplantation: is routine surveillance necessary? Biol Blood Marrow Transplant. 2011; https://doi.org/10.1016/j.bbmt.2011.04.004.

90. Smith C, Khanna R. Immune regulation of human herpesviruses and its implications for human transplantation. Am J Transplant. 2013; https://doi.org/10.1111/ajt.12005.

91. de Pagter PJ, et al. Human herpesvirus type 6 reactivation after haematopoietic stem cell transplantation. J Clin Virol. 2008;43:361–6.

92. Mori Y, Miyamoto T, Nagafuji K, Kamezaki K, Yamamoto A, Saito N, et al. High incidence of human herpes virus 6-associated encephalitis/myelitis following a second unrelated cord blood transplantation. Biol Blood Marrow Transplant. 2010; https://doi.org/10.1016/j.bbmt.2010.05.009.

93. Mariotte E, Schnell D, Scieux C, Agbalika F, Legoff J, Ribaud P, et al. Significance of herpesvirus 6 in BAL fluid of hematology patients with acute respiratory failure. Infection. 2011; https://doi.org/10.1007/s15010-011-0114-8.

94. Pantry S, Medveczky P. Latency, integration, and reactivation of human Herpesvirus-6. Viruses. 2017;9:194.

95. Papadopoulou A, Gerdemann U, Katari UL, Tzannou I, Liu H, Martinez C, et al. Activity of broad-spectrum T cells as treatment for AdV, EBV, CMV, BKV, and HHV6 infections after HSCT. Sci Transl Med. 2014;6:242ra83.

96. Lion T. Adenovirus infections in immunocompetent and immunocompromised patients. Clin Microbiol Rev. 2014; https://doi.org/10.1128/CMR.00116-13.

97. Cupit-Link MC, Nageswara Rao A, Warad DM, Rodriguez V, Khan S. EBV-PTLD, adenovirus, and CMV in pediatric allogeneic transplants with alemtuzumab as part of pretransplant conditioning: a retrospective single center study. J Pediatr Hematol Oncol. 2018;1 https://doi.org/10.1097/MPH.0000000000001138.

98. Safdar A, Rodriguez GH, Mihu CN, Mora-Ramos L, Mulanovich V, Chemaly RF, et al. Infections in non-myeloablative hematopoietic stem cell transplantation patients with lymphoid malignancies: spectrum of infections, predictors of outcome and proposed guidelines for fungal infection prevention. Bone Marrow Transplant. 2009;45:339–47.

99. Ustun C, Slabý J, Shanley RM, Vydra J, Smith AR, Wagner JE, et al. Human parainfluenza virus infection after hematopoietic stem cell transplantation: risk factors, management, mortality, and changes over time. Biol Blood Marrow Transplant. 2012; https://doi.org/10.1016/j.bbmt.2012.04.012.

100. Raanani P, Gafter-Gvili A, Paul M, Ben-Bassat I, Leibovici L, Shpilberg O, et al. Immunoglobulin prophylaxis in hematopoietic stem cell transplantation: systematic review and meta-analysis. J Clin Oncol. 2009; https://doi.org/10.1200/JCO.2008.16.8450.

101. Campbell AP, Guthrie KA, Englund JA, Farney RM, Minerich EL, Kuypers J, et al. Clinical outcomes associated with respiratory virus detection before allogeneic hematopoietic stem cell transplant. Clin Infect Dis. 2015;61:192–202.

102. Kmeid J, Vanichanan J, Shah DP, El Chaer F, Azzi J, Ariza-Heredia EJ, et al. Outcomes of influenza infections in hematopoietic cell transplant recipients: application of an immunodeficiency scoring index. Biol Blood Marrow Transplant. 2016;22:542–8.

103. Shah DP, Shah PK, Azzi JM, Chemaly RF. Parainfluenza virus infections in hematopoietic cell transplant recipients and hematologic malignancy patients: a systematic review. Cancer Lett. 2016;370:358–64.

104. Sidwell RW, Barnard DL. Respiratory syncytial virus infections: recent prospects for control. Antivir Res. 2006; https://doi.org/10.1016/j.antiviral.2006.05.014.

105. Chemaly RF, Shah DP, Boeckh MJ. Management of respiratory viral infections in hematopoietic cell transplant recipients and patients with hematologic malignancies. Clin Infect Dis. 2014; https://doi.org/10.1093/cid/ciu623.

106. Gilbert BE, et al. Further studies with short duration ribavirin aerosol for the treatment of influenza virus infection in mice and respiratory syncytial virus infection in cotton rats. Antivir Res. 1992;172

107. Hutspardol S, et al. Significant transplantation-related mortality from respiratory virus infections within the first one hundred days in children after hematopoietic stem cell transplantation. Biol Blood Marrow Transplant. 2015;21:1802–7.

108. Gilbert BE, Wyde PR, Wilson SZ, Robins RK. Aerosol and intraperitoneal administration of ribavirin and ribavirin triacetate: pharmacokinetics and protection of mice against intracerebral infection with influenza A/WSN virus. Antimicrob Agents Chemother. 1991; https://doi.org/10.1128/AAC.35.7.1448.

109. Molina A, Winston DJ, Pan D, Schiller GJ. Increased incidence of nocardial infections in an era of atovaquone prophylaxis in allogeneic hematopoietic stem cell transplant recipients. Biol Blood Marrow Transplant. 2018; https://doi.org/10.1016/j.bbmt.2018.03.010.

110. Rouzaud, C. et al. Clinical assessment of a *Nocardia* spp. polymerase chain reaction (PCR)-based assay for the diagnosis of nocardiosis. J Clin Microbiol. 2018;JCM.00002–18. doi:https://doi.org/10.1128/JCM.00002-18.

111. Welsh O, Vera-Cabrera L, Salinas-Carmona MC. Current treatment for nocardia infections. Expert Opin Pharmacother. 2013;14:2387–98.

112. Shannon K, Pasikhova Y, Ibekweh Q, Ludlow S, Baluch A. Nocardiosis following hematopoietic stem cell transplantation. Transpl Infect Dis. 2016;18:169–75.

113. Small TN, Cowan MJ. Immunization of hematopoietic stem cell transplant recipients against vaccine-preventable diseases. Expert Rev Clin Immunol. 2011;7:193–203.

114. Verolet CM, Posfay-Barbe KM. Live virus vaccines in transplantation: friend or foe? Curr Infect Dis Rep. 2015;17:472.

115. Lee D-G. Vaccination of hematopoietic stem cell transplantation recipients: perspective in Korea. Infect Chemother. 2013;45:272–82.

116. Palazzo M, et al. Revaccination after autologous hematopoietic stem cell transplantation is safe and effective in patients with multiple myeloma receiving lenalidomide maintenance. Biol Blood Marrow Transplant. 2017; https://doi.org/10.1016/j.bbmt.2017.12.795.

117. Cunningham AL, et al. Efficacy of the herpes zoster subunit vaccine in adults 70 years of age or older. N Engl J Med. 2016;375:1019–32.

118. Weber D, et al. Microbiota disruption induced by early use of broad-spectrum antibiotics is an independent risk factor of outcome after allogeneic stem cell transplantation. Biol Blood Marrow Transplant. 2017; https://doi.org/10.1016/j.bbmt.2017.02.006.

119. Shono Y, van den Brink MRM. Gut microbiota injury in allogeneic haematopoietic stem cell transplantation. Nat Rev Cancer. 2018; https://doi.org/10.1038/nrc.2018.10.

120. Vossen JM, et al. Complete suppression of the gut microbiome prevents acute graft-versus-host disease following allogeneic bone marrow transplantation. PLoS One. 2014;9:e105706.

121. Zeiser R, Socié G, Blazar BR. Pathogenesis of acute graft-versus-host disease: from intestinal microbiota alterations to donor T cell activation. Br J Haematol. 2016; https://doi.org/10.1111/bjh.14295.

122. Hingorani S. Renal complications of hematopoietic-cell transplantation. N Engl J Med. 2016; https://doi.org/10.1056/NEJMra1404711.

123. Kemmner S, Verbeek M, Heemann U. Renal dysfunction following bone marrow transplantation. J Nephrol. 2017; https://doi.org/10.1007/s40620-016-0345-y.

124. Parikh CR, et al. Comparison of ARF after myeloablative and nonmyeloablative hematopoietic cell transplantation. Am J Kidney Dis. 2005; https://doi.org/10.1053/j.ajkd.2004.11.013.

125. Liu Y, et al. Acute kidney injury following haplo stem cell transplantation: incidence, risk factors and outcome. Bone Marrow Transplant. 2018;53(4):483–6. https://doi.org/10.1038/s41409-017-0030-3.

126. Piñana JL, et al. A time-to-event model for acute kidney injury after reduced-intensity conditioning stem cell transplantation using a tacrolimus- and sirolimus-based graft-versus-host disease prophylaxis. Biol Blood Marrow Transplant. 2017; https://doi.org/10.1016/j.bbmt.2017.03.035.

127. Parikh CR, et al. Impact of acute kidney injury on long-term mortality after nonmyeloablative hematopoietic cell transplantation. Biol Blood Marrow Transplant. 2008;14(3):309–15. https://doi.org/10.1016/j.bbmt.2007.12.492.

128. Girsberger M, Halter JP, Hopfer H, Dickenmann M, Menter T. Kidney pathology after hematologic cell transplantation-a single-center observation study of indication biopsies and autopsies. Biol Blood Marrow Transplant. 2018;24:571–80.

129. Yango AF, et al. West Nile virus infection in kidney and pancreas transplant recipients in the Dallas-Fort Worth Metroplex during the 2012 Texas epidemic. Transplantation. 2014;97(9):953–7. https://doi.org/10.1097/01.TP.0000438621.81686.ab.

130. Stavrou E, Lazarus HM. Thrombotic microangiopathy in haematopoietic cell transplantation: an update. Mediterr J Hematol Infect Dis. 2010;2:2010033.

131. Gavriilaki E, Sakellari I, Anagnostopoulos A, Brodsky RA. Transplant-associated thrombotic microangiopathy: opening Pandora's box. Bone Marrow Transplant. 2017;52:1355–60.

132. Epperla N, Hemauer K, Hamadani M, Friedman KD, Kreuziger LB. Impact of treatment and outcomes for patients with posttransplant drug-associated thrombotic microangiopathy. Transfusion. 2017;57:2775–81.

133. Cowan J, Cameron DW, Knoll G, Tay J. Protocol for updating a systematic review of randomised controlled trials on the prophylactic use of intravenous immunoglobulin for patients undergoing haematopoietic stem cell transplantation. BMJ Open. 2015;5(8):e008316. https://doi.org/10.1136/bmjopen-2015-008316.

134. Khattry N, Shah M, Jeevangi NK, Joshi A. Late-onset hepatic veno-occlusive disease post autologous peripheral stem cell transplantation successfully treated with oral defibrotide. J Cancer Res Ther. 2009;5:312.

135. Richardson PG, et al. Defibrotide sodium for the treatment of hepatic veno-occlusive disease/sinusoidal obstruction syndrome. Expert Rev Clin Pharmacol. 2018; https://doi.org/10.1080/17512433.2018.1421943.

136. Mahgerefteh SY, et al. Radiologic imaging and intervention for gastrointestinal and hepatic complications of hematopoietic stem cell transplantation. Radiology. 2011; https://doi.org/10.1148/radiol.10100025.

137. Zeiser R, Blazar BR. Pathophysiology of chronic graft-versus-host disease and therapeutic targets. N Engl J Med. 2017; https://doi.org/10.1056/NEJMra1703472.

138. Teshima T, Reddy P, Zeiser R. Acute graft-versus-host disease: novel biological insights. Biol Blood Marrow Transplant. 2016;22:11–6.

139. Pidala J, et al. Patient-reported quality of life is associated with severity of chronic graft-versus-host disease as measured by NIH criteria: report on baseline data from the Chronic GVHD Consortium. Blood. 2011;117:4651–7.

140. Pallua S, et al. Impact of GvHD on quality of life in long-term survivors of haematopoietic transplantation. Bone Marrow Transplant. 2010;45:1534–9.

141. Cooke KR, et al. The biology of chronic graft-versus-host disease: a task force report from the National Institutes of Health Consensus Development Project on Criteria for Clinical Trials in Chronic Graft-versus-Host Disease. Biol Blood Marrow Transplant. 2017;23:211–34.

142. Wikstrom ME, et al. Acute GVHD results in a severe DC defect that prevents T-cell priming and leads to fulminant cytomegalovirus disease in mice. Blood. 2015;126:1503–14.

143. Zeiser R, Blazar BR. Acute graft-versus-host disease — biologic process, prevention, and therapy. N Engl J Med. 2017; https://doi.org/10.1056/NEJMra1609337.

144. Duinhouwer LE, et al. Impaired thymopoiesis predicts for a high risk of severe infections after reduced intensity conditioning without anti-thymocyte globulin in double umbilical cord blood transplantation. Bone Marrow Transplant. 2018; https://doi.org/10.1038/s41409-018-0103-y.

145. Schaenman JM, et al. Early CMV viremia is associated with impaired viral control following nonmyeloablative hematopoietic cell transplantation with a total lymphoid irradiation and antithymocyte globulin preparative regimen. Biol Blood Marrow Transplant. 2011; https://doi.org/10.1016/j.bbmt.2010.08.010.

146. Kalra A, et al. Risk factors for post-transplant lymphoproliferative disorder after thymoglobulin-conditioned hematopoietic cell transplantation. Clin Transpl. 2018;32:e13150.

147. Shulman HM, et al. NIH consensus development project on criteria for clinical trials in chronic graft-versus-host disease: II. The 2014 Pathology Working Group Report. Biol Blood Marrow Transplant. 2015;21(4):589–603. https://doi.org/10.1016/j.bbmt.2014.12.031.

148. Carpenter PA, et al. National Institutes of Health Consensus Development Project on criteria for clinical trials in chronic graft-versus-host disease: V. The 2014 Ancillary Therapy and Supportive Care Working Group Report. Biol Blood Marrow Transplant. 2015;21(7):1167–87. https://doi.org/10.1016/j.bbmt.2015.03.024.

149. Treister NS, et al. Oral chronic graft-versus-host disease scoring using the NIH consensus criteria. Biol Blood Marrow Transplant. 2010;16:108–14.

150. Torelli GF, et al. The immune reconstitution after an allogeneic stem cell transplant correlates with the risk of graft-versus-host disease and cytomegalovirus infection. Leuk Res. 2011; https://doi.org/10.1016/j.leukres.2011.03.009.

151. Miceli MH, Churay T, Braun T, Kauffman CA, Couriel DR. Risk factors and outcomes of invasive fungal infections in allogeneic hematopoietic cell transplant recipients. Mycopathologia. 2017;182:495–504.

152. Bunting MD, et al. GVHD prevents NK-cell-dependent leukemia and virus-specific innate immunity. Blood. 2017;129:630–42.

153. Riches ML, et al. Risk factors and impact of non-Aspergillus mold infections following allogeneic HCT: a CIBMTR infection and immune reconstitution analysis. Bone Marrow Transplant. 2016;51:277–82.

154. Boeckh M, et al. Late cytomegalovirus disease and mortality in recipients of allogeneic hematopoietic stem cell transplants: importance of viral load and T-cell immunity. Blood. 2003; https://doi.org/10.1182/blood-2002-03-0993.

155. Girmenia C, et al. Incidence and outcome of invasive fungal diseases after allogeneic stem cell transplantation: a prospective study of the gruppo italiano trapianto midollo osseo (GITMO). Biol Blood Marrow Transplant. 2014; https://doi.org/10.1016/j.bbmt.2014.03.004.

156. Matsumura-Kimoto Y, et al. Association of cumulative steroid dose with risk of infection after treatment for severe acute graft-versus-host disease. Biol Blood Marrow Transplant. 2016; https://doi.org/10.1016/j.bbmt.2016.02.020.

157. Howell JE, Gulbis AM, Champlin RE, Qazilbash MH. Retrospective analysis of weekly intravenous immunoglobulin prophylaxis versus intravenous immunoglobulin by IgG level monitoring in hematopoietic stem cell transplant recipients. Am J Hematol. 2012; https://doi.org/10.1002/ajh.22229.

158. Wehr C, et al. Multicenter experience in hematopoietic stem cell transplantation for serious complications of common variable immunodeficiency. J Allergy Clin Immunol. 2015;135:988–97.e6.

159. Parikh SA, et al. Hypogammaglobulinemia in newly diagnosed chronic lymphocytic leukemia: natural history, clinical correlates, and outcomes. Cancer. 2015; https://doi.org/10.1002/cncr.29438.

160. Wahn V. From immune substitution to immunomodulation. Semin Hematol. 2016; https://doi.org/10.1053/j.seminhematol.2016.04.003.

161. Lee C, et al. Prediction of absolute risk of acute graft-versus-host disease following hematopoietic cell transplantation. PLoS One. 2018;13(1):e0190610. https://doi.org/10.1371/journal.pone.0190610.

162. Strong Rodrigues K, Oliveira-Ribeiro C, de Abreu Fiuza Gomes S, Knobler R. Cutaneous graft-versus-host disease: diagnosis and treatment. Am J Clin Dermatol. 2018;19(1):33–50. https://doi.org/10.1007/s40257-017-0306-9.

163. Mehta RS, Cao Q, Holtan S, Macmillan ML, Weisdorf DJ. Upper GI GVHD: similar outcomes to other grade II graft-versus-host disease. Bone Marrow Transplant. 2017; https://doi.org/10.1038/bmt.2017.90.

164. Washington K, Jagasia M. Pathology of graft-versus-host disease in the gastrointestinal tract. Hum Pathol. 2009; https://doi.org/10.1016/j.humpath.2009.04.001.

165. Ferrara JLM, Smith CM, Sheets J, Reddy P, Serody JS. Altered homeostatic regulation of innate and adaptive immunity in lower gastrointestinal tract GVHD pathogenesis. J Clin Investig. 2017; https://doi.org/10.1172/JCI90592.

166. Matsukuma KE, Wei D, Sun K, Ramsamooj R, Chen M. Diagnosis and differential diagnosis of hepatic graft versus host disease

(GVHD). J Gastrointest Oncol. 2016; https://doi.org/10.3978/j.issn.2078-6891.2015.036.

167. Hamilton BK, et al. Association of socioeconomic status with chronic graft-versus-host disease outcomes. Biol Blood Marrow Transplant. 2018;24:393–9.

168. Jagasia MH, et al. National Institutes of Health Consensus Development Project on criteria for clinical trials in chronic graft-versus-host disease: I. The 2014 Diagnosis and Staging Working Group Report. Biol Blood Marrow Transplant. 2015;21(3):389–401.e1. https://doi.org/10.1016/j.bbmt.2014.12.001.

169. Alexander BT, et al. Use of cytomegalovirus intravenous immune globulin for the adjunctive treatment of cytomegalovirus in hematopoietic stem cell transplant patients NIH public access. Pharmacotherapy. 2010;30:554–61.

170. Marks C, et al. German-Austrian-Swiss Consensus Conference on clinical practice in chronic graft-versus-host disease (GVHD): guidance for supportive therapy of chronic cutaneous and musculoskeletal GVHD. Br J Dermatol. 2011; https://doi.org/10.1111/j.1365-2133.2011.10360.x.

171. Belbasis L, Stefanaki I, Stratigos AJ, Evangelou E. Non-genetic risk factors for cutaneous melanoma and keratinocyte skin cancers: an umbrella review of meta-analyses. J Dermatol Sci. 2016;84:330–9.

172. Martens MC, Seebode C, Lehmann J, Emmert S. Photocarcinogenesis and skin Cancer prevention strategies: an update. Anticancer Res. 2018;38:1153–8.

173. Levine MT, Chandrasekar PH. Adverse effects of voriconazole: over a decade of use. Clin Transpl. 2016;30:1377–86.

174. Williams K, Mansh M, Chin-Hong P, Singer J, Arron ST. Voriconazole-associated cutaneous malignancy: a literature review on photocarcinogenesis in organ transplant recipients. Clin Infect Dis. 2014;58:997–1002.

175. Hull K, et al. Oral chronic graft-versus-host disease in Australia: clinical features and challenges in management. Intern Med J. 2015;45:702–10.

176. Chaudhry HM, et al. The incidence and severity of oral mucositis among allogeneic–hematopoietic stem cell transplantation patients: a systematic review. Biol Blood Marrow Transplant. 2016;22:605–16.

177. Alborghetti MR, et al. Late effects of chronic graft-vs.-host disease in minor salivary glands. J Oral Pathol Med. 2005;34:486–93.

178. Petti S, Polimeni A, Berloco PB, Scully C. Orofacial diseases in solid organ and hematopoietic stem cell transplant recipients. Oral Dis. 2013; https://doi.org/10.1111/j.1601-0825.2012.01925.x.

179. Lee SJ, et al. Success of immunosuppressive treatments in patients with chronic graft-versus-host disease. Biol Blood Marrow Transplant. 2017; https://doi.org/10.1016/j.bbmt.2017.10.042.

180. Yalniz FF, et al. Steroid refractory chronic graft-versus-host-disease: cost-effectiveness analysis. Biol Blood Marrow Transplant. 2018; https://doi.org/10.1016/j.bbmt.2018.03.008.

181. Doss LM, et al. Oral health and hematopoietic stem cell transplantation: a longitudinal evaluation of the first 28 days. Pediatr Blood Cancer. 2018;65:e26773.

182. Santos-Silva AR, Feio Pdo S, Vargas PA, Correa MEP, Lopes MA. cGVHD-related caries and its shared features with other 'dry-mouth'-related caries. Braz Dent J. 2015;26:435–40.

183. Barrach RH, de Souza MP, Da Silva DPC, Lopez PS, Montovani JC. Oral changes in individuals undergoing hematopoietic stem cell transplantation. Braz J Otorhinolaryngol. 2015; https://doi.org/10.1016/j.bjorl.2014.04.004.

184. Guenther A, et al. Dental status does not predict infection during stem cell transplantation: a single-center survey. Bone Marrow Transplant. 2017;52:1041–3.

185. Tung CI. Graft versus host disease: what should the oculoplastic surgeon know? Curr Opin Ophthalmol. 2017; https://doi.org/10.1097/ICU.0000000000000400.

186. Gama I, Rodrigues W, Franco J, Almeida L, Monteiro-Grillo M. Chronic ocular graft vs host disease as a serious complication of allogeneic hematopoietic stem cell transplantation: case report. Transplant Proc. 2015;47(4):1059–62. https://doi.org/10.1016/j.transproceed.2015.03.038.

187. Zinkernagel MS, Petitjean C, Wikstrom ME, Degli-Esposti MA. Kinetics of ocular and systemic antigen-specific T-cell responses elicited during murine cytomegalovirus retinitis. Immunol Cell Biol. 2012;90:330–6.

188. Ogawa Y, Kuwana M. Dry eye as a major complication associated with chronic graft-versus-host disease after hematopoietic stem cell transplantation. Cornea. 2003;22:S19–27.

189. Ivanir Y, Shimoni A, Ezra-Nimni O, Barequet IS. Prevalence of dry eye syndrome after allogeneic hematopoietic stem cell transplantation. Cornea. 2013;32:e97–e101.

190. Pathak M, et al. Ocular findings and ocular graft-versus-host disease after allogeneic stem cell transplantation without total body irradiation. Bone Marrow Transplant. 2018;1 10.1038/s41409-018-0090-z

191. Bassim CW, et al. Malnutrition in patients with chronic GVHD. Bone Marrow Transplant. 2014; https://doi.org/10.1038/bmt.2014.145.

192. Naymagon S, et al. Acute graft-versus-host disease of the gut: considerations for the gastroenterologist. Nat Rev Gastroenterol Hepatol. 2017; https://doi.org/10.1038/nrgastro.2017.126.

193. Cloutier J, Wall DA, Paulsen K, Bernstein CN. Upper versus lower endoscopy in the diagnosis of graft-versus-host disease. J Clin Gastroenterol. 2017; https://doi.org/10.1097/MCG.0000000000000609.

194. Sung AD, et al. Late gastrointestinal complications of allogeneic hematopoietic stem cell transplantation in adults. Biol Blood Marrow Transplant. 2018;24:734–40.

195. Meijs L, Zusterzeel R, Wellens HJ, Gorgels AP. The Maastricht??? Duke bridge: an era of mentoring in clinical research??? A model for mentoring in clinical research – a tribute to Dr. Galen Wagner. J Electrocardiol. 2017; https://doi.org/10.1016/j.jelectrocard.2016.10.009.

196. Westerhoff M, Lamps LW. Mucosal biopsy after bone marrow transplantation. Surg Pathol Clin. 2017; https://doi.org/10.1016/j.path.2017.07.006.

197. Liu A, Meyer E, Johnston L, Brown J, Gerson LB. Prevalence of graft versus host disease and cytomegalovirus infection in patients post-haematopoietic cell transplantation presenting with gastrointestinal symptoms. Aliment Pharmacol Ther. 2013; https://doi.org/10.1111/apt.12468.

198. Bergeron A, Cheng GS. Bronchiolitis obliterans syndrome and other late pulmonary complications after allogeneic hematopoietic stem cell transplantation. Clin Chest Med. 2017; https://doi.org/10.1016/j.ccm.2017.07.003.

199. Gazourian L, et al. Pulmonary clinicopathological correlation after allogeneic hematopoietic stem cell transplantation: an autopsy series. Biol Blood Marrow Transplant. 2017; https://doi.org/10.1016/j.bbmt.2017.06.009.

200. Jain NA, et al. Repair of impaired pulmonary function is possible in very-long-term allogeneic stem cell transplantation survivors. Biol Blood Marrow Transplant. 2014;20:209–13.

201. Sharma S, et al. Pulmonary complications in adult blood and marrow transplant recipients: autopsy findings. Chest. 2005;128:1385–92.

202. Grube M, et al. Risk factors and outcome of chronic graft-versus-host disease after allogeneic stem cell transplantation—results from a single-center observational study. Biol Blood Marrow Transplant. 2016; https://doi.org/10.1016/j.bbmt.2016.06.020.

203. Hildebrandt GC, et al. Diagnosis and treatment of pulmonary chronic GVHD: report from the consensus conference on

clinical practice in chronic GVHD. Bone Marrow Transplant. 2011;46:1283–95.

204. Fujikura Y, et al. Pleuroparenchymal fibroelastosis as a series of airway complications associated with chronic graft-versus-host disease following allogeneic bone marrow transplantation. Intern Med. 2014;53:43–6.

205. Kornik RI, Rustagi AS. Vulvovaginal graft-versus-host disease. Obstet Gynecol Clin N Am. 2017; https://doi.org/10.1016/j.ogc.2017.05.007.

206. Chung CP, Sargent RE, Chung NT, Lacey JV, Wakabayashi MT. Graft-versus-host disease-associated vulvovaginal symptoms after bone marrow transplantation. Biol Blood Marrow Transplant. 2016;22:378–9.

207. Hamilton BK, Goje O, Savani BN, Majhail NS, Stratton P. Clinical management of genital chronic GvHD. Bone Marrow Transplant. 2017; https://doi.org/10.1038/bmt.2016.315.

208. Li Z, et al. Sexual health in hematopoietic stem cell transplant recipients. Cancer. 2015; https://doi.org/10.1002/cncr.29675.

209. Spinelli S, et al. Female genital tract graft-versus-host disease following allogeneic bone marrow transplantation. Haematologica. 2003;88:1163–8.

210. Dyer G, et al. A survey of fertility and sexual health following allogeneic haematopoietic stem cell transplantation in New South Wales, Australia. Br J Haematol. 2016;172:592–601.

211. Pophali PA, et al. Male survivors of allogeneic hematopoietic stem cell transplantation have a long term persisting risk of cardiovascular events. Exp Hematol. 2014; https://doi.org/10.1016/j.exphem.2013.07.003.

212. Armenian SH, et al. Predictors of late cardiovascular complications in survivors of hematopoietic cell transplantation. Biol Blood Marrow Transplant. 2010; https://doi.org/10.1016/j.bbmt.2010.02.021.

213. Chow EJ, et al. Late cardiovascular complications after hematopoietic cell transplantation. Biol Blood Marrow Transplant. 2014; https://doi.org/10.1016/j.bbmt.2014.02.012.

214. Borchert-Mörlins B, et al. Cardiovascular risk factors and subclinical organ damage after hematopoietic stem cell transplantation in pediatric age. Bone Marrow Transplant. 2018; https://doi.org/10.1038/s41409-018-0104-x.

215. Shah GL, et al. Impact of toxicity on survival for older adult patients after CD34+selected allogeneic hematopoietic stem cell transplantation. Biol Blood Marrow Transplant. 2018; https://doi.org/10.1016/j.bbmt.2017.08.040.

216. Pang A, et al. Corin is down-regulated and exerts cardioprotective action via activating pro-atrial natriuretic peptide pathway in diabetic cardiomyopathy. Cardiovasc Diabetol. 2015;14:134.

217. Shalitin S, et al. Endocrine dysfunction and parameters of the metabolic syndrome after bone marrow transplantation during childhood and adolescence. Bone Marrow Transplant. 2006;37:1109–17.

218. Shalitin S, et al. Endocrine and metabolic disturbances in survivors of hematopoietic stem cell transplantation in childhood and adolescence. Horm Res Paediatr. 2018; https://doi.org/10.1159/000486034.

219. Oudin C, et al. Metabolic syndrome in adults who received hematopoietic stem cell transplantation for acute childhood leukemia: an LEA study. Bone Marrow Transplant. 2015;50:1438–44.

220. DeFilipp Z, et al. Metabolic syndrome and cardiovascular disease following hematopoietic cell transplantation: screening and preventive practice recommendations from CIBMTR and EBMT. Bone Marrow Transplant. 2017;52:173–82.

221. Bourdieu A, et al. Steady state peripheral blood provides cells with functional and metabolic characteristics of real hematopoietic stem cells. J Cell Physiol. 2018;233:338–49.

222. Bechard LJ, Gordon C, Feldman HA, Venick R, Gura K, Guinan EC, et al. Bone loss and vitamin D deficiency in children under-

going hematopoietic cell transplantation. Pediatr Blood Cancer. 2015;62:687–92.

223. McClune BL, Polgreen LE, Burmeister LA, Blaes AH, Mulrooney DA, Burns LJ, et al. Screening, prevention and management of osteoporosis and bone loss in adult and pediatric hematopoietic cell transplant recipients. Bone Marrow Transplant. 2011;46:1–9.

224. Ebeling PR, et al. Mechanisms of bone loss following allogeneic and autologous hemopoietic stem cell transplantation. J Bone Miner Res. 1999;14:342–50.

225. Petryk A, et al. Bone mineral density in children with fanconi anemia after hematopoietic cell transplantation. Biol Blood Marrow Transplant. 2015;21:894–9.

226. Polgreen LE, et al. Changes in biomarkers of bone resorption over the first six months after pediatric hematopoietic cell transplantation. Pediatr Transplant. 2012;16:852–7.

227. McClune BL, Majhail NS. Osteoporosis after stem cell transplantation. Curr Osteoporos Rep. 2013; https://doi.org/10.1007/s11914-013-0180-1.

228. Pirsl F, Curtis LM, Steinberg SM, Tella SH, Katić M, Dobbin M, et al. Characterization and risk factor analysis of osteoporosis in a large cohort of patients with chronic graft-versus-host disease. Biol Blood Marrow Transplant. 2016;22:1517–24.

229. Weilbaecher KN. Mechanisms of osteoporosis after hematopoietic cell transplantation. Biol Blood Marrow Transplant. 2000;6:165–74.

230. Boulad F, Bromley M, Black P, Heller G, Sarafoglou K, Gillio A, Papadopoulos E, et al. Thyroid dysfunction following bone marrow transplantation using hyperfractionated radiation. Bone Marrow Transplant. 1995;15

231. Al-Fiar FZ, Colwill R, Lipton JH, Fyles G, Spaner D, Messner H. Abnormal thyroid stimulating hormone (TSH) levels in adults following allogeneic bone marrow transplants. Bone Marrow Transplant. 1997;19

232. Isshiki Y, Ono K, Shono K, Onoda M, Yokota A. Autoimmune thyroid dysfunction after allogeneic hematopoietic stem cell transplant. Leuk Lymphoma. 2016;57

233. Savani BN, Koklanaris EK, Le Q, Shenoy A, Goodman S, Barrett AJ. Prolonged chronic graft-versus-host disease is a risk factor for thyroid failure in long-term survivors after matched sibling donor stem cell transplantation for hematologic malignancies. Biol Blood Marrow Transplant. 2009;15

234. Gunasekaran U, Agarwal N, Jagasia MH, Jagasia SM. Endocrine complications in long-term survivors after allogeneic stem cell transplant. Semin Hematol. 2012;49:66–72.

235. Al-Hazzouri A, Cao Q, Burns LJ, Weisdorf DJ, Majhail NS. Similar risks for hypothyroidism after allogeneic hematopoietic cell transplantation using TBI-based myeloablative and reduced-intensity conditioning regimens. Bone Marrow Transplant. 2009;43

236. Li X, et al. Avascular necrosis of bone after allogeneic hematopoietic cell transplantation in children and adolescents. Biol Blood Marrow Transplant. 2014;20:587–92.

237. Cohen A, et al. Risk for secondary thyroid carcinoma after hematopoietic stem-cell transplantation: an EBMT Late Effects Working Party Study. J Clin Oncol. 2007;25

238. Guida M, et al. Reproductive issues in patients undergoing hematopoietic stem cell transplantation: an update. J Ovarian Res. 2016;9:72.

239. Roberts SC, et al. Validity of self-reported fertility-threatening cancer treatments in female young adult cancer survivors. J Cancer Surviv. 2017;11:517–23.

240. Snarski E, et al. Onset and outcome of pregnancy after autologous haematopoietic SCT (AHSCT) for autoimmune diseases: a retrospective study of the EBMT autoimmune diseases working party (ADWP). Bone Marrow Transplant. 2015;50:216–20.

241. Scanlon M, et al. Patient satisfaction with physician discussions of treatment impact on fertility, menopause and sexual health among pre-menopausal women with Cancer. J Cancer. 2012;3:217–25.

242. Nahata L, Cohen LE, Lehmann LE, Yu RN. Semen analysis in adolescent cancer patients prior to bone marrow transplantation: when is it too late for fertility preservation? Pediatr Blood Cancer. 2013;60:129–32.

243. Soiffer RJ, Davids MS, Chen Y-B. Tyrosine kinase inhibitors and immune checkpoint blockade in allogeneic hematopoietic cell transplantation. Blood. 2018; https://doi.org/10.1182/blood-2017-10-752154.

244. Schneider S, Potthast S, Komminoth P, Schwegler G, Böhm S. PD-1 checkpoint inhibitor associated autoimmune encephalitis. Case Rep Oncol. 2017;10:473–8.

245. Baris S, et al. Clinical heterogeneity of immunodysregulation, polyendocrinopathy, enteropathy, X-linked: pulmonary involvement as a non-classical disease manifestation. J Clin Immunol. 2014;34:601–6.

246. Husebye ES, Anderson MS, Kämpe O. Autoimmune polyendocrine syndromes. N Engl J Med. 2018;378(12):1132–41. https://doi.org/10.1056/NEJMra1713301.

247. Nelson AM, et al. Sleep disruption among cancer patients following autologous hematopoietic cell transplantation. Bone Marrow Transplant. 2017; https://doi.org/10.1038/s41409-017-0022-3.

248. Jim HSL, et al. Sleep disruption in hematopoietic cell transplantation recipients: prevalence, severity, and clinical management. Biol Blood Marrow Transplant. 2014;20:1465–84.

249. Rischer J, Scherwath A, Zander AR, Koch U, Schulz-Kindermann F. Sleep disturbances and emotional distress in the acute course of hematopoietic stem cell transplantation. Bone Marrow Transplant. 2009;44:121–8.

250. Andrykowski M, et al. Energy level and sleep quality following bone marrow transplantation. Bone Marrow Transplant. 1997;20:669–79.

251. Ross A, Yang L, Klagholz SD, Wehrlen L, Bevans MF. The relationship of health behaviors with sleep and fatigue in transplant caregivers. Psychooncology. 2016;25:506–12.

252. Nelson AM, et al. Sleep quality following hematopoietic stem cell transplantation: longitudinal trajectories and biobehavioral correlates. Bone Marrow Transplant. 2014;49:1405–11.

253. Graef DM, et al. Sleepiness, fatigue, behavioral functioning, and quality of life in survivors of childhood hematopoietic stem cell transplant. J Pediatr Psychol. 2016;41:600–9.

Post-transplant Psychosocial and Mental Health Care of Hematopoietic Cell Transplant Recipients

Renee Garcia

Introduction

Receiving the diagnosis of a hematopoietic malignancy is a terrifying experience, often leading to a hematopoietic stem cell transplant (HCT) as a potentially life-saving intervention. While physicians recognize the magnitude of the HCT process and oncologists make all efforts to communicate the challenging nature of HCT experience, most patients would agree that they still did not realize how multidimensional and all-encompassing the HCT process can be. In the time leading up to the post-HCT period, patients have already endured so much that they are emotionally and physically depleted heading into the post-HCT period.

Impact of HCT Hospitalization

Regardless of HCT type, the pre-HCT period and hospitalization is marked by invasive medical procedures. Studies have shown that this can leave a lasting impact beyond the expected physical pain and distress, including changes in one's body image and loss of a sense of personal control [1]. Many prospective studies have followed the development of anxiety, depression, and emotional distress during their hospitalization. One longitudinal prospective study followed anxiety and depression rates from the time of admission to day 28 and beyond post-engraftment [2]. The study found that 10% of patients already have the presence of anxiety and depressive symptoms on admission [2]. Anxiety remained present throughout hospitalization unresolved and with unchanged prevalence rates. Depressive symptoms on the other hand increased during the hospitalization from 10% on admission to a peak depression incidence of 22% at 2 weeks [2]. Patients most vulnerable to developing depression were females, those with introverted personality traits, and patients with higher anxiety and poor performance on admission [2].

The emotional state and level of distress have been an area of interest for many studies, but variations in methods of quantifying and classifying this distress impede head-to-head comparison. Prospective research does demonstrate that approximately 40% of HCT patients will develop a clinically significant psychiatric disorder, mostly adjustments disorders, depression, anxiety, and delirium [1, 3, 4]. As one would expect with patients undergoing HCT, there are many medical variables that contribute to the likelihood of emotional distress, including steroid use, higher regimen-related toxicity, acute graft-versus-host disease (GVHD), and type of HCT performed. These variables are often statistically controlled for when attempting to assess the impact of psychiatric morbidity on post-HCT outcomes. Studies identified several independent predictors for the development of emotional distress, such as low personal control, high pre-transplant anxiety or depression, and past psychiatric history [1, 5–7]. These predictors or risk factors should be considered and included in pre-transplant psychiatric screening as a way of identifying high-risk patients who may benefit from additional psychosocial support. The types of support while patients are hospitalized can range from visits from loved ones, chaplain/spiritual care, to brief focused psychotherapy or psychoeducational interventions with social work or psychiatry consultants [8, 9].

Post-HCT Psychiatric Sequelae

There is a certain relief that comes when an HCT patient achieves a state of medical stability to the point of being able to leave the acute care setting. The completion of another phase of treatment and transitioning into the survivorship phase is bittersweet for many HCT recipients. Many patients will go on to experience long-term physical effects from the

R. Garcia
Department of Psychiatry and Behavioral Sciences, Stanford University School of Medicine, Stanford, CA, USA

Hoag Presbyterian Memorial Hospital, Newport Beach, CA, USA
e-mail: Rgarcia7@stanford.edu

© Springer International Publishing AG, part of Springer Nature 2019
Y. Sher, J. R. Maldonado (eds.), *Psychosocial Care of End-Stage Organ Disease and Transplant Patients*,
https://doi.org/10.1007/978-3-319-94914-7_41

toxicity and immunosuppression involved in HCT treatment itself (please see Chap. 40), not to mention psychological and emotional distress inherent in such a taxing experience.

In fact, many clinical studies have examined the impact on HCT survivors' quality of life (QOL) and their psychological and emotional well-being. Challenges in synthesizing the available literature on the subject include lack of structured clinical interviews limiting knowledge of psychiatric diagnoses, complex interplay between physical aspects of HCT treatment and mood disturbance, use of self-report measures with limited applicability to HCT or cancer population, and difficulty identifying predictors due to variations in measures used and diverse medical histories [10].

Despite limitations, all healthcare providers understand that some form or variation of *psychosocial distress* is inevitable. The National Comprehensive Cancer Network (NCCN) created guidelines in 2018 for the recognition, evaluation, and treatment of cancer-related distress [10]. The term distress is broadly defined as "a multifactorial unpleasant experience of a psychological (i.e., cognitive, behavioral, emotional), social, spiritual, and/or physical nature that may interfere with the ability to cope with cancer treatment, and its physical symptoms" which "extends along a continuum, from common normal anxiety, panic, social isolation, and existential and spiritual crisis [10]."

Depression

The development of sadness while undergoing, for most, the most daunting, terrifying experience of their lives is expected to some degree. However, when sadness transitions to point of impacting a patient's ability to function, it translates to lack of participation in medical care, heightened somatic symptoms, prolonged hospital stays, and nonadherence. In fact, depression is the most well-studied psychiatric diagnosis in the HCT literature. The rates of depression in HCT survivors vary depending on time point in HCT process from time of hospital admission to 10-year post-HCT, but it is estimated that 15–20% of HCT patients will develop major depressive disorder (MDD) at some point [12].

Despite the robust quantity of literature examining psychiatric symptoms in HCT patients, most studies have utilized brief self-report measures that are not always based on the diagnostic *Diagnosis and Statistical Manual* (DSM) criteria, thus only suggesting presence of a disorder [13]. In fact, psychiatric symptomatology is often embedded within other psychological health or QOL measures. In recent years, more research studies are attempting to include structured clinical interviews so that psychiatric prevalence data can be collected and utilized for purposes of developing treatment interventions.

Diagnosing depression in an HCT population must take into account the significant overlay between the expected physical effects from treatment toxicity and the classic neurovegetative symptoms of major depression. Psychiatrists working with the medically ill patients have long performed psychiatric assessments recognizing the significant overlap between physical symptoms associated with medical illness and classic neurovegetative symptoms of depression [14]. Consultation-liaison psychiatrists commonly focus more on the depressive nature of their cognitions when diagnosing a depressive disorder and less so on the physical effects. Depressive cognitions include negative feelings or thoughts of self, feeling like a burden, thinking that people "would be better off without me," helplessness, and hopelessness or despair. This is not to say that the physical effects of depression are not present in depressed HCT patients but that they are less reliable indicators and symptoms when assessing severity of depressive symptoms [12–14].

Prevalence rates of depression vary depending on time point of patient in HCT process. Many studies have found that depression rates are highest when patients are hospitalized, as high as 31–38% [5], and in the midst of physical, emotional, and psychological stress, but then gradually decline over the course of the first post-transplant year [14–16]. Length of the longitudinal studies varies with many focusing on the first few years post-transplant. Other studies that have evaluated depression as far as ten years post-transplantation find that risk of psychological distress and depression gradually declines with time from HCT; and, in some, rates of anxiety and depression are comparable to population norms [17, 18]. Long-term survivorship depression rates are estimated to be approximately 11% in HCT population [17, 19].

Depression carries significant implications for HCT patients' long-term medical outcomes and has been associated with increased hospital length of stay and nonadherence to post-HCT regimen [2, 5, 19, 20]. There is currently a mixed evidence base regarding depression's impact on mortality. Some studies have found a positive correlation with higher mortality, while others have not replicated or supported this relationship [16, 21, 22]. Many have wondered if depression is merely a surrogate marker for illness severity or whether it impacts survival directly, but currently the relationship between psychiatric morbidity/depression and mortality/survival remains unclear in HCT population [21].

Several studies have been conducted with the goal of identifying which patients are at highest risk for depression, so that appropriate interventions can be developed and implemented. Many different sociodemographic or various clinical factors have been evaluated, with mixed results for some factors. The most consistent risk factors for the development of depression were younger age, lower socioeconomic status, chronic pain, and the presence of GVHD [19] (See Table 41.1). Those with moderate to severe depression have been found to have worse QOL and reduced social functioning; however, depression did not impact return to work rates [23, 24].

Table 41.1 Risk factors associated with various psychiatric disorders

Depression	Anxiety	PTSD	Delirium
Younger ages	Low income	Negative appraisal of HCT experience	Post-HCT:
Chronic pain	Poor self-reported health status		Higher opioid requirements
Female gender			Current/prior pain
Severity of cGVHD	Exposure to prednisone	Use of avoidance-based coping strategies	Impaired renal function (higher BUN/CR, lower CrCl)
Pre-HCT distress		Lower levels of social support	
Low self-reported emotional functioning		Greater social constraint	Lower oxygen saturation
High physical symptom burden pre-HCT		Prior exposure to negative life events	Lower hemoglobin
		Poorer physical functioning	Lower albumin
		Presence of pre-HCT distress	

References: [2, 5–7, 12, 18, 19, 29, 31, 32, 38, 40, 47, 51]

The most worrisome symptom of depression is suicidality, representing the continuum of suicidal ideation, intent, self-injurious behavior, attempts, and completed suicide [25]. Little epidemiologic data is known about suicidality in the HCT population; however, few studies have included suicidal ideation in secondary measures. One comparison study found that suicidal ideation was 13 times more likely to occur in depressed HCT patients than nondepressed HCT patients [19]. A prospective study found that 6.7% HCT survivors reported suicidal thoughts, but when rates were adjusted for household income, it eliminated the difference between the HCT survivor and their sibling comparison group [18]. Interestingly, there was no association between suicidality and the presence of multiple medical problems; however, negative patients' perceptions of their health status were associated with an increased likelihood of reporting suicidal ideation. This association highlights the impact that a patient's perception can have on their medical care [18].

Lastly, many have hypothesized that there is a genetic vulnerability to the development of depression or emotional/psychological stress. The diathesis-stress model was first proposed in the setting of understanding the origins of schizophrenia and then later applied to depression. The diathesis-stress model essentially proposes that "there is a synergism between the diathesis and stress that yields an effect beyond their combined separate effects into depressive symptomatology and thus, the effects of stress on the depression risk are dependent on the diathesis [26]." One retrospective study of 107 HCT patients evaluated the relationship between genetic factors and psychological distress [27].

While there was no association found with most genetic factors (i.e., 5HTTLPR, STin2, FKBP5, CRHR1 TAT haplotype), the single nucleotide polymorphism of brain-derived neurotropic factor (BDNF) Val66Met demonstrated a non-statistically significant association with depression development, possibly due to small sample size. However, this may indicate a genetic vulnerability toward the development of psychological distress or depression [27].

Anxiety

Anxiety is a feeling of worry, nervousness, or unease, typically about an imminent event or something with an uncertain outcome. In the setting of an HCT, a sense of uncertainty is inevitable given the inability to predict whose HCT will be curative or potentially lead to their death. Additionally, there is significant amount of anticipatory anxiety related to the expectation of the high-dose chemotherapy or body irradiation, high-risk period of heightened vulnerability to infections, HCT infusions, prolonged hospitalization, and neutropenic medical isolation [13, 28, 29].

Anxiety can take on many forms and presentations, but it can be helpful to categorize anxiety manifestations into physical and psychological symptoms. The physical components of anxiety include the hyperactivity, restlessness, and inability to relax or sit still. These can be side effects of the treatment itself, such as steroids, opioids, hormonal blockers, and antiemetics and thus can often be ameliorated by a medication change or dose adjustment.

The psychological aspects of anxiety are not as straightforward or easy to treat. Many patients with cancer and HCT struggle with health, family, and personal fears that, to some degree, are expected and appropriate. However, for a significant minority of patients, anxiety symptoms can be disabling and detrimental to quality of life. Commonly experienced fears include that of death, recurrence, physical pain, or discomfort (see Table 41.2). One study found that 23–29% of HCT patients experience a significant fear of illness progression [28]. It also appears that younger age is associated with this fear of progression in the post-allogeneic HCT population [29]. In one study, 27% of patients had moderate to severe anxiety symptoms, 29% had fear of progression, and 15% were with significant posttraumatic stress disorder (PTSD) symptoms [29].

While there are no direct comparison investigations, one study found rates of psychological distress to be similar among a predominantly autologous population and mixed autologous/allogeneic populations [29]. With the higher transplant-related mortality risk with allogeneic HCT, most would assume that allogeneic HCT would also be associated with a higher rate of distress. However, if rates of psychological distress are similar between HCT types, it may indicate a

Table 41.2 Most commonly experienced biopsychosocial effects

Biopsychosocial implications for HCT patients		
Biologic	Psychologic	Social
Pain	Loss of independence	Financial uncertainty/insecurity
Fatigue	Changes in body image	Career stunting
Poor sleep	Fear of recurrence/death	Relationship changes
Poor appetite	Intrusive recollections	Disruption of personal goals
Poor concentration	Sense of isolation/stigmatization	Inability to engage in social activities
Oral symptoms: Mucositis, sores	Uncertainty regarding future	
Skin changes	Concerns about illness, treatments, and side effects	
Sexual dysfunction		
Infertility		
Low functionality		

References: [1, 2, 6, 8, 10, 17, 29, 30]

stronger influence of the patient's perception of danger and fear on their distress levels as compared to the actual evidence-based risk [29].

Posttraumatic Stress Disorder

Undergoing either an autologous or allogeneic HCT provides the unfortunate perfect milieu of triggers to induce trauma-based disorders, including acute stress disorder (ASD) and PTSD. While HCT is a well-established treatment and provides hope for a cure for many with hematologic malignancies, it also carries with it high levels of uncertainty, morbidity, and mortality [30]. This sense of uncertainty and psychological distress is overlaid on extreme conditions, including high rate of medical complications, tentative chances of survival, and prolonged periods of medical isolation in hospital [32]. It is not a surprise then that HCT patients go on to develop ASD, posttraumatic stress symptoms (PTSS), and PTSD at a higher rate than the general population. In fact, studies estimate PTSD rates between 15–28% in HCT patients [29–32].

Many studies suggest that the rates of psychological distress, depression, and anxiety are high in the phase leading up to transplant and remain elevated up to 2 weeks after transplantation [33–35]. Psychological distress then proceeds to drop off with decreases noted at 3 months, 12 months, and 2-year post-transplant [34, 36, 37]. One prospective study found that HCT patients who experienced a decrease in QOL and an increase in depressive symptoms during their hospitalization (admission to week 2) had higher rates of PTSD symptoms and lower QOL 6 months post-HCT [32]. Prevalence of PTSD or PTSS seem to peak around the 6-month mark as one study found rate of 28% at 6 months post-HCT [32] and, unfortunately, PTSD or PTSS symptoms can persist in up to 41% of patients for up to 10 years post-HCT [38, 39].

Many studies have been conducted to identify which HCT patients are most vulnerable to the development of PTSD. The

identified psychological and psychosocial risk factors include negative appraisals of the transplant experience, use of avoidance-based coping strategies, lower levels of social support, greater social constraints, greater number of negative life events, history of psychological disturbances, current psychological distress, and reduced physical functioning [9, 38, 40].

There have been a few novel approaches taken to target PTSD symptoms in the HCT population. Cognitive behavioral therapy (CBT) interventions have been shown to decrease emotional distress. In fact, one study showed that a ten-session telephone-based cognitive behavioral (T-CBT) intervention with HCT survivors can decrease PTSD symptoms, general distress, and depressive symptoms even up to 12 months post-intervention [41]. However, an internet-based coping intervention in HCT patients did not demonstrate any effect on psychological functioning or distress [42]. It was postulated that the internet-based approach impeded the development of a therapeutic relationship or alliance. However, another T-CBT intervention with HCT survivors found that higher therapeutic alliance prospectively predicted reductions in depressive symptomatology; higher task scores predicted decreased overall distress, reexperiencing, avoidance, and depressive symptoms; and higher bond scores predicted decreased reexperiencing and depressive symptoms [43, 44].

Delirium and Neurocognitive Effects

Delirium is the most common psychiatric disorder diagnosed in the acute care setting [45]. Up to 50% of HCT recipients will experience a delirious episode at some point during the first 4 weeks post-HCT [46, 47, 54]. Delirium has been associated with many acute and long-term negative outcomes, including prolonged hospital stays and increased morbidity and mortality [46–52]. Unfortunately, approximately 50% of delirium cases in advanced cancer patients go unrecognized missing an opportunity for an intervention [46, 53].

Few studies have investigated the risk factors associated with the development of delirium pre- and post-HCT transplant. The identified post-HCT risk factors for delirium include higher opioid requirements, current/prior pain, renal dysfunction, lower oxygen saturation, lower hemoglobin, and lower albumin [46, 47].

In one study, HCT patients who experienced a delirious episode during the first 4 weeks after transplantation were compared to HCT patients without delirium [56]. At 6 months, those with delirium had significantly more distress, fatigue, worse physical health, higher cognitive impairments (memory, executive functioning, attention, processing speed), decreased health-related QOL (HRQOL), and subjective neurocognitive dysfunction [56]. At 1 year, all effects remained persistent with the addition of worse depressive and PTSD symptoms [51, 52].

Many patients subjectively identify cognitive difficulties often referred to as "chemo-brain." It may be difficult to disentangle which effects are primary versus secondary to the malignancy and/or due to other comorbid medical problems [55]. However, studies have identified that HCT patients who had received cranial irradiation or intrathecal chemotherapy as part of the initial treatment or preparation for HCT were at a higher risk for development of neurocognitive impairments [55, 57]. One study specifically examined the effects of total body irradiation in HCT patients and found that 60% of patients had mild to moderate cognitive impairments up to 82 months post-HCT [58].

The most common impairments were in areas of selective attention, executive function, information processing speed, psychomotor coordination, verbal learning, and verbal/visual memory [56, 58]. Some studies support that some cognitive functioning can be restored up to 1 year post-HCT [57–59]. One longitudinal study noted significant recovery of cognitive functioning in HCT recipients from the transplant to up to 5 years in all domains, except verbal recall and motor dexterity; however, 41.5% of patients still maintained mild to greater global deficit scores compared to 19.7% of controls [59].

Somatic Symptoms

The most frequently reported somatic symptoms by HCT patients include fatigue, general weakness, oral sores or pain, nausea, diarrhea, insomnia, and sexual dysfunction [57, 60–62]. This section will highlight a few key somatic symptoms that have implications in the diagnosis of psychiatric disorders or sequelae, including fatigue, insomnia, and effects of GVHD.

Fatigue is the most frequently reported somatic symptoms post-HCT. Fatigue has been shown to affect transplant-related distress and impair physical functioning and QOL for at least 5 years post-HCT [63]. Studies have shown rates of severe fatigue to be 30–42% in post-HCT patients, but the longitudinal course of fatigue severity is not fully clear [62, 64]. The data suggests that there is potential for fatigue improvements in the 3–4 years post-HCT, but for approximately 25% of patients, severe fatigue symptoms persist beyond the 10–15-year mark [11, 63, 64]. Risk factors for the development of fatigue post-HCT include female sex, current chronic pain, current severity of chronic graft-versus-host disease (cGVHD), and younger age [65].

Sleep disturbances are common amongst post-HCT patients with prevalence of 50% pre-transplant, up to 82% during hospitalization, and up to 43% post-HCT [65, 66]. One study found that sleep worsened during the first 4 weeks post-HCT transplant but improved by the end of first 100 days [67–69]. The survivorship guidelines recommend screening for sleep disruption at regular time points citing fact that insomnia has been associated with decreased daytime functioning, worse QOL, and distress [68]. An interesting relationship between the quality of sleep and inflammation in cancer patients has been evaluated with specific associations found with IL-6, IL-1RA, and TNF-α [70]. This relationship has not been well-studied in the HCT population in particular, but one study in HCT patients demonstrated that poorer sleep quality was associated with higher levels of IL-6 and greater burden of depression and anxiety [66].

GVHD is a complication associated with allogeneic HCT where the newly transplanted cells attack the recipient's body. The presence of acute or chronic GVHD has been associated with decline in physical functioning, QOL, emotional well-being, general health, and role functioning [12, 14, 57, 71, 72]. Chronic GVHD has been also shown to impact HCT survivors' likelihood of returning to work, but there is potential for improved QOL over time despite cGVHD [17, 35, 57, 71, 72].

Quality of life is defined as "satisfaction with psychological, cognitive, physical, and social aspects of functioning [73]." QOL reductions have been found to be associated with transplant-related distress, higher somatic complaints or symptom burden, presence of GVHD, lower physical functioning, and lower levels of social support [35, 74]. In the post-HCT period, the most prevalent concerns for survivors were management of physical symptoms, maintaining health status, maintaining employment, changes in appearance, and lack of sexual interest/satisfaction, which suggests that QOL interventions should address those aspects post-HCT [63].

Treatment Recommendations and Areas of Future Development for HCT Survivors

Multiple studies in HCT patients have found that the most common unmet needs are psychiatric in nature, including depression, anxiety, fear of recurrence, and cognitive deficits

[75–77]. These unmet psychiatric needs may be a manifestation of underdiagnosis or underrecognition of psychiatric symptomatology, thus leading to overall undertreatment of these disorders [29]. It is estimated that only 39% of HCT patients endorsing distress were prescribed any psychotropic medications and only 22% were engaged in some form of psychotherapy [29]. See Table 41.3 on important psychotropic medication class considerations in HCT patients.

The NCCN publishes guidelines for a comprehensive approach to the management of cancer-related distress [10]. These guidelines are updated at regular intervals with the most recent release at beginning of 2018. They detail the assessment of distress from point of screening with their validated NCCN Distress Thermometer Screening Tool all

the way to the identification and diagnosis of psychiatric disorders [10]. Each psychiatric disorder class has its own set of specific treatment guidelines highlighting appropriate evaluation, treatment, and follow-up. All NCCN guidelines can be found on www.nccn.org. See Fig. 41.1. Algorithm for the Management of Cancer-Related Distress and Psychiatric treatment.

An important aspect of addressing cancer-related distress is recognizing that unrelieved physical symptoms must first be managed in an effort to mitigate their impact on, or confound, psychiatric symptomatology assessments [10]. Additionally, receiving a diagnosis of a hematopoietic malignancy is expected to be distressing, and it is considered within the range of normal to experience symptoms of fear,

Table 41.3 Psychotropic medication considerations in HCT patients

Medication class		Medication names	Indications	Important considerations
Antidepressants	SSRI	Fluoxetine Escitalopram Sertraline Citalopram Paroxetine	Depression Anxiety PTSD Dementia-related agitation	Increased risk of bruising and bleeding due to decreased platelet aggregation. SSRI most associated with abnormal bleeding – Fluoxetine, paroxetine, sertraline – Given high serotonergic effects.
	SNRI	Venlafaxine Desvenlafaxine Duloxetine Levomilnacipran		Avoid use with other medications potentiating bleeding risk: NSAIDs, aspirin Varying CYP450 profiles with – Fluoxetine, paroxetine, duloxetine – With most interactions SNRI medications have the added benefit of assisting with chronic neuropathic pain.
	DNRI	Bupropion	Depression Fatigue ADHD	Can induce CNS stimulation – Restlessness, anxiety, insomnia Risk of appetite suppression Reduces seizure threshold and has been associated with seizures in setting of electrolyte imbalances
	Tetracyclic	Mirtazapine	Depression Anxiety Insomnia Appetite stimulation Nausea	Agranulocytosis occurs in ~1/1000 (similar to other antidepressants), which can occur early and late into treatment. Often used purely for sleep and/or appetite stimulation Risk of sedation given anti-histamine properties and long half-life May confer mild antiemetic properties via 5HT3 antagonism
	TCAs	Amitriptyline Nortriptyline Desipramine Clomipramine	Depression Anxiety Insomnia Neuropathic pain	Risk for cardiotoxicity and should be avoided in heart disease patients (i.e., orthostasis, conduction abnormalities, arrhythmias) Anticholinergic properties can lead to blurry vision, dry mouth, constipation, urinary retention, and confusion/delirium Risk for daytime sedation via anti-histamine properties
	MAOIs	Selegiline Phenelzine Tranylcypromine	Depression Anxiety	Should not be used in the medically ill and avoided if possible Selegiline comes in transdermal patch only to be considered in select patients with inability to tolerate oral medications

Table 41.3 (continued)

Medication class		Medication names	Indications	Important considerations
Anxiolytics	Benzodiazepine	Lorazepam Clonazepam Diazepam Alprazolam	Acute anxiety Chronic anxiety (less preferred)	Effective for the short-term management of acute anxiety Should be avoided in long-term treatment due to risk of tolerance, dependency and cognitive impairment Proven deliriogenic properties that is dose dependent Discontinued/tapered if delirium arises Plan should be in place to taper and discontinue use when used for >2 weeks Risk of sedation, falls and respiratory depression (especially with opioids) Should be avoided purely for indication of sleep
	Non-benzodiazepine	Hydroxyzine Gabapentin Guanfacine	Acute anxiety	Hydroxyzine: Risk of sedation, dry mouth, constipation Gabapentin: Avoid in significant renal impairment; risk of sedation, myoclonus, confusion/neurotoxicity Guanfacine: Ideal for physiologically driven anxiety of racing heart, restlessness, tension; risk of hypotension, bradycardia
		SSRI, SNRI, TCA, MAOI classes	Chronic, long-term anxiety	
Antipsychotics	1st generation (typical)	Haloperidol Chlorpromazine Fluphenazine Loxapine	Delirium Dementia related agitation Severe anxiety Depression augmentation Schizophrenia Schizoaffective disorder	Risk of parkinsonism, bradykinesia, tremor, cogwheeling, rigidity, akathisia Varying sedative properties depending on neurotransmitter receptor profile Risk of QTc prolongation, avoid use of other QTc prolonging medications Agranulocytosis occurs in ~1/1000 in this class Neuroleptic malignant syndrome (NMS) risk is higher than with atypicals
	2nd generation (atypical)	Risperidone Ziprasidone Olanzapine Aripiprazole Quetiapine Paliperidone Lurasidone Clozapine	Bipolar disorder Steroid-induced mood or psychotic disorders	Neutropenia occurs in ~4% with risperidone, 2% with quetiapine or paliperidone, and ~1% in atypicals as class Cases of severe neutropenia or agranulocytosis reported but are rare. Risk for orthostasis, sedation, urinary retention, dry mouth, parkinsonism (less than typicals) Risk of NMS and can contribute to risk of serotonin toxicity Risk of thrombocytopenia with quetiapine Avoid clozapine due to additive risk of myelosuppression Olanzapine has evidence for improved chemotherapy-induced nausea/vomiting control when combined with standard antiemetics
Mood stabilizers	Anti-epileptic drugs (AEDs)	Valproic acid Carbamazepine Oxcarbamazepine Topiramate	Bipolar disorder Schizoaffective disorder Delirium Impulsivity Steroid-induced mood disorders	Thrombocytopenia and hemolytic anemia associated with AED use. Valproate associated with thrombocytopenia (5–40%), neutropenia (5–26%), pancreatitis Carbamazepine has 0.5% risk of neutropenia Risk of sedation, cognitive slowing/blunting, weight gain
	Non-AED	Lithium		Lithium can induce thrombocytosis and leukocytosis Contraindicated in patients with renal dysfunction, cardiovascular disease Multiple drug interactions with anti-HTN meds (ACEI, diuretics) Level is sensitive to renal function and salt and water balance with narrow therapeutic index

(continued)

Table 41.3 (continued)

Medication class		Medication names	Indications	Important considerations
Psychostimulants	Amphetamine based	Methylphenidate Dextroamphetamine Dextroamphetamine Amphetamine Lisdexamfetamine	Depression Fatigue ADHD Delirium	Commonly used to treat the classic neurovegetative symptoms of depression or fatigue/inattention in medically ill Used to improve level of arousal/alertness in hypoactive delirium Amphetamine-based meds can function as inotropes and thus can increase blood pressure, heart rate. Risk of insomnia, hyperactivity, anxiety, psychosis/hallucinations, agitation, appetite suppression Amantadine dose requires adjustment in renal impairments
	Non-amphetamine based	Modafinil Armodafinil Amantadine Atomoxetine		

References: [57, 78, 79, 84–86]

DNRI dopamine/norepinephrine reuptake inhibitor, *MAOI* monoamine oxygenase inhibitor, *TCA* tricyclic antidepressant, *SNRI* serotonin/norepi *ACEI* angiotensin-converting enzyme inhibitor, *ADHD* attention deficit hyperactivity disorder, *CNS* central nervous system nephrine reuptake inhibitor, *SSRI* selective serotonin reuptake inhibitor

worry, and sadness [8, 10, 18, 28, 29]. Hence, being aware of the expected distress symptoms and first-line supportive interventions is crucial to reducing risk of distress escalating to point of developing a psychiatric disorder.

When a psychiatric disorder does develop, or is present pre-HCT, management should be based on an individualized combination of psychotherapy and psychopharmacology. Many psychotherapeutic interventions have an evidence based in a cancer population, including educational-behavioral interventions to improve adherence, group psychotherapy, individual psychotherapy, and mindfulness meditation [10]. Psychotropic medications are commonly used in HCT patients despite the fact that there are no current randomized controlled trials specifically evaluating efficacy, tolerability, common adverse reactions, or special considerations in this population [57]. Additionally, the decision to initiate a psychotropic medication in medically complex HCT patients requires thoughtful consideration of the patient's current medical status, other medical comorbidities, onset of action, route of administration, potential for drug interactions, common adverse effects, and somatic symptom profile [78].

The principle of "start low and go slow" applies to this population given propensity for complex, multidrug medication regimens and significant risk of drug-drug interactions [78]. The treating psychiatrist absolutely requires an up-to-date medication list and should be notified of any new medications or discontinued medications as it can lead to alterations in drug levels via cytochrome P450 (CYP450) interactions [79]. CYP450 interactions can potentially lead to toxicity symptoms via enzymatic inhibition of drug metabolism, or reduce effectiveness of a medication by induction effects [78, 79]. Collaboration with the primary oncologist regarding expected treatments, chemotherapy, and immunosuppressants can facilitate well-informed psy-

chotropic medication choices early and reduce likelihood of having to later make a medication switch to avoid pharmacokinetic or pharmacodynamics interactions [57, 78, 79].

Psychotropic medications are well known for their propensity for adverse effects, which often negatively impacts primary oncologist's comfort level managing psychiatric disorders. See Table 41.3 for review of relevant target symptoms, adverse effects, and beneficial secondary effects of certain medications.

For those with premorbid psychiatric disorders, long-term administration of psychotropic medications may be required and should be thoroughly discussed between the patient and treating psychiatrist. HCT patients who developed psychiatric disorders in midst of the grueling HCT process may not require long-term psychotropic medication treatment. The decision to continue or to discontinue should be based on patient's preferences, severity of psychopathology, psychiatric symptom remission status, tolerability, and current level of functioning [10]. When deciding to discontinue psychotropic medications, it is recommended that the dose be downtitrated under supervision of a psychiatrist or mental health provider.

Conclusions

HCT survivors would greatly benefit from having access to and receiving appropriate psychiatric and psychological treatments. Given the pattern of especially heightened psychological distress during the peri-transplant period and ongoing psychosocial needs, supportive services should be incorporated at all stages of the HCT process: pre-transplant, during the transplant process, and years into the post-transplant period [80]. Important post-transplant interventions include normalizing frequent somatic complaints and experiences, low threshold for proactive symptom management with palliative care consultation, and

Fig. 41.1 NCCN adapted guidelines for management of distress and psychiatric treatment

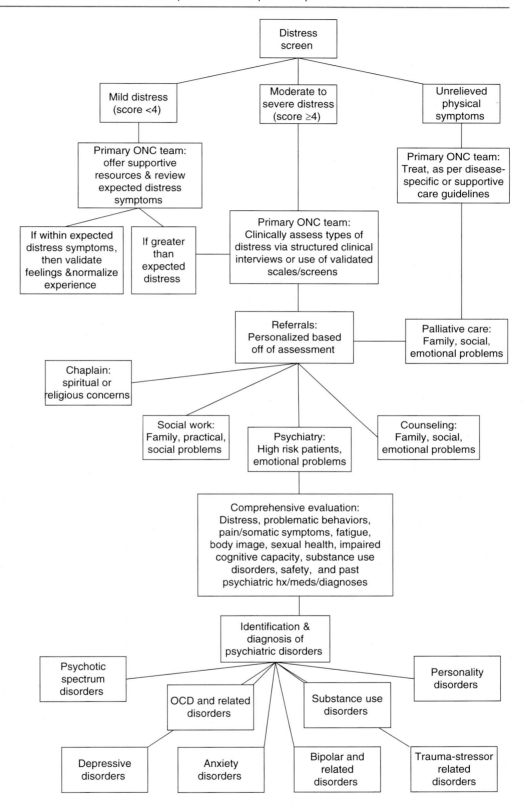

facilitating the development of realistic and appropriate short- and long-term expectations regarding the transplant process as a whole and the prolonged recovery period. Finally, there are many complementary and alternative medicine approaches or interventions that can provide additional layer of support and comfort to HCT patients, including the use of healing survivorship narratives, music, and exercise interventions [81–83].

References

1. Fife BL, Huster GA, Cornetta KG, Kennedy VN, Akard LP, Broun ER. Longitudinal study of adaptation to the stress of bone marrow transplantation. J Clin Oncol. 2000;18:1539–49.

2. Tecchio C, Bonetto C, Bertani M, Cristofalo D, Lasalvia A, Nichele I, et al. Predictors of anxiety and depression in hematopoietic stem cell transplant patients during protective isolation. Psycho-Oncology. 2013;22:1790–7.

3. Sasaki T, Akaho R, Sakamaki H, Sasaki T, Akaho R, Sakamaki H, et al. Mental disturbances during isolation in bone marrow transplant patients with leukemia. Bone marrow transplant 2000 mental disturbances during isolation in bone marrow transplant patients with leukemia. Bone Marrow Transplant. 2000;25:315–8.

4. Prieto JM, Blanch J, Atala J, Carreras E, Rovira M, Cirera E, et al. Psychiatric morbidity and impact on hospital length of stay among hematologic cancer patients receiving stem-cell transplantation. J Clin Oncol. 2002;1:1907–17.

5. Schulz-Kindermann F, Hennings U, Ramm G, Zander AR, Hasenbring M. The role of biomedical and psychosocial factors for the prediction of pain and distress in patients undergoing high-dose therapy and BMT/ PBSCT. Bone Marrow Transplant. 2002;29:341–51.

6. Prieto JM, Blanch J, Atala J, Carreras E, Rovira M, Cirera E, et al. Stem cell transplantation: risk factors for psychiatric morbidity. Eur J Cancer. 2006;42:514–20.

7. Trask PC, Paterson A, Riba M, Brines B, Griffith K, Parker P, et al. Assessment of psychological distress in prospective bone marrow transplant patients. Bone Marrow Transplant. 2002;29:917–25.

8. Block SD. Diagnosis and treatment of depression in patients with advanced illness. Epidemiol Psychiatr Soc. 2010;19:103–9.

9. Mosher CE, Redd WH, Rini CM, Burkhalter JE, DuHamel KN. Physical, psychological, and social sequelae following hematopoietic stem cell transplantation: a review of the literature. Psycho-Oncology. 2009;18:113–27.

10. Holland JC, Deshields TL, Anderson B, Braun I, Breitbart WS, Buchmann LO, et al. NCCN clinical practice guidelines in oncology for distress management. National Comprehensive Cancer Network. January 2018. https://www.nccn.org/professionals/physician_gls/default.aspx#distress.

11. Jim HS, Sutton SK, Jacobsen PB, Martin PJ, Flowers ME, Lee SJ. Risk factors for depression and fatigue among survivors of hematopoietic cell transplantation. Cancer. 2016;122:1290–7.

12. Hoodin F, Zhao L, Carey J, Levine JE, Kitko C, et al. Impact of psychological screening on routine outpatient care of hematopoietic cell transplantation survivors. Biol Blood Marrow Transplant. 2013;19:1493–7.

13. Weiner M, Lovitt R. Conservation withdrawal vs depression in medically ill patients: Rorchach case. J Pers Assess. 1980;44:5.

14. Syrjala KL, Chapko MK, Vitaliano PP, Cummings C, Sullivan KM. Recovery after allogeneic marrow transplantation: prospective study of predictors of long-term physical and psychosocial functioning. Bone Marrow Transplant. 1993;11(4):319–27.

15. Meyers CA, Weitzner M, Byrne K, Valentine A, Champlin RE, Przepiorka D. Evaluation of the neurobehavioral functioning of patients before, during, and after bone marrow transplantation. J Clin Oncol. 1994;12(4):820–6.

16. Prieto JM, Atala J, Blanch J, Carreras E, Rovira M, Cirera E, et al. Role of depression as a predictor of mortality among cancer patients after stem-cell transplantation. J Clin Oncol. 2005;23(25):6063–71.

17. Hjermstad MJ, Loge JH, Evensen SA, Kvaloy SO, Fayers PM, Kaasa S. The course of anxiety and depression during the first year after allogeneic or autologous stem cell transplantation. Bone Marrow Transplant. 1999;24(11):1219–28.

18. Sun CL, Francisco L, Baker KS, Weisdorf DJ, Forman SJ, Bhatia S. Adverse psychological outcomes in long-term survivors of hematopoietic cell transplantation: a report from the Bone Marrow Trans-plant Survivor Study (BMTSS). Blood. 2011;118:4723–31.

19. Artherholt SB, Hong F, Berry DL, Fann JR. Risk factors for depression in patients undergoing hematopoietic cell transplantation. Biol Blood Marrow Transplant. 2014;20:946–950.3.

20. Mumby PB, Hurley C, Samsi M, Thilges S, Parthasarathy M, Stiff PJ. Predictors of non-compliance in autologous hematopoietic SCT patients undergoing out-patient transplants. Bone Marrow Transplant. 2012;47:556–61.

21. Pillay B, Lee SJ, Katona L, Burney S, Avery S. Psychosocial factors predicting survival after allogeneic stem cell transplant. Support Care Cancer. 2014;22(9):2547–55.

22. Loberiza FR, Rizzo JD, Bredeson CN, Antin JH, Horowitz MM, Weeks JC, et al. Association of depressive syndrome and early deaths among patients after stem-cell transplantation for malignant diseases. J Clin Oncol. 2002;20:2118–26.

23. Pulgar A, Alcala A, Reyes Del Paso GA. Psychosocial predictors of quality of life in hematological cancer. Behav Med. 2015;41:1–8.

24. Horsboel TA, Bültmann U, Nielsen CV, Nielsen B, Andersen NT, de Thurah A. Are fatigue, depression and anxiety associated with labour market participation among patients diagnosed with haematological malignancies? A prospective study. Psychooncology. 2015;24:408–15.

25. Meyer RE, Salzman C, Youngstrom EA, Clayton PJ, Goodwin FK, Mann J, et al. Suicidality and risk of suicide--definition, drug safety concerns, and a necessary target for drug development: a consensus statement. J Clin Psychiatr. 2010;71(8):1–21.

26. Colodro-Conde L, Couvy-Duchesne B, Zhu G, Coventry WL, Byrne EM, Gordon S, et al. A direct test of the Diathesis-Stress model for depression. Mol Psychiatry. 2017 July 11 [Epub ahead of print].

27. Romanowicz M, Ehlers S, Walker D, Decker P, Rundell J, Shinozaki G, et al. Testing a diathesis-stress model: potential genetic risk factors for development of distress in context of acute leukemia diagnosis and transplant. Psychosomatics. 2012;53:456–62.

28. Sarkar S, Scherwath A, Schirmer L, Schulz-Kindermann F, Neumann K, Kruse M, et al. Fear of recurrence and its impact on quality of life in patients with hematological cancers in the course of allogeneic hematopoietic SCT. Bone Marrow Transplant. 2014;49:1217–22.

29. Hefner J, Kapp M, Drebinger K, Dannenmann A, Einsele H, Grigoleit GU, et al. High prevalence of distress in patients after allogeneic hematopoietic SCT: fear of progression is associated with a younger age. Bone Marrow Transplant. 2014;49:581–4.

30. Fife BL, Fausel CA. Hematopoietic Dyscrasias and stem cell/bone marrow transplantation. In: Holland JC, editor. Psycho-oncology. 2nd ed. New York: Oxford University Press; 2010. p. 191–5.

31. Kuba K, Esser P, Scherwath A, Schirmer L, Schulz-Kindermann F, Dinkel A, et al. Cancer-and-treatment-specific distress and its impact on post-traumatic stress in patients undergoing allogeneic hematopoietic stem cell transplantation (HSCT). Psycho-Oncology. 2017;26:1164–71.

32. El-Jawahri AR, Vandusen HB, Traeger LN, Fishbein JN, Keenan T, Gallagher ER, et al. Quality of life and mood predict posttrau-

matic stress disorder after hematopoietic stem cell transplantation. Cancer. 2016;122:806–12.

33. Prieto JM, Atala J, Blanch J, Carreras E, Rovira M, Cirera E, et al. Patient-rated emotional and physical functioning among hematologic cancer patients during hospitalization for stem-cell transplantation. Bone Marrow Transplant. 2005;35:307–14.

34. Syrjala KL, Langer SL, Abrams JR, Storer B, Sanders JE, Flowers ME, et al. Recovery and long-term function after hematopoietic cell transplantation for leukemia or lymphoma. JAMA. 2004;291:2335–43.

35. Hjermstad MJ, Knobel H, Brinch L, Fayers PM, Loge JH, Holte H, et al. A prospective study of health related quality of life, fatigue, anxiety and depression 3-5 years after stem cell transplantation. Bone Marrow Transplant. 2004;34:257–66.

36. Schulz-Kindermann F, Zander AR, Mehnert A, Scherwath A, Schirmer L. Cognitive functions and treatment-related distress in the course of high-dose therapy and allogeneic stem-cell transplantation: results of a prospective study in patients with hematological malignancies. Bone Marrow Transplant. 2006;15:402–3.

37. Gruber U, Fegg M, Buchmann M, Kolb H, Hiddemann W. The long-term psychosocial effects of haematopoetic stem cell transplantation. Eur J Cancer Care. 2003;12:249.

38. Jacobsen PB, Sadler IJ, Booth Jones M, Soety E, Weitzner M, Fields KK. Predictors of posttraumatic stress disorder symptomatology following bone marrow transplantation for cancer. J Consult Clin Psychol. 2002;70:235–40.

39. Rusiewicz A, Duhamel KN, Burkhalter J, Ostroff J, Winkel G, Scigliano E, et al. Psychological distress in long-term survivors of hematopoietic stem cell transplantation. Psychooncology. 2008;17:329–37.

40. Widows MR, Jacobsen PB, Fields KK. Relation of psychological vulnerability factors to posttraumatic stress disorder symptomatology in bone marrow transplant recipients. Psychosom Med. 2000;62:873–82.

41. DuHamel KN, Mosher CE, Winkel G, Labay LE, Rini C, Meschian YM, et al. Randomized clinical trial of telephone-administered cognitive-behavioral therapy to reduce post-traumatic stress disorder and distress symptoms after hematopoietic stem-cell transplantation. J Clin Oncol. 2010;28(23):3754–61.

42. David N, Schlenker P, Prudlo U, Larbig W. Internet-based program for coping with cancer: a randomized controlled trial with hematologic cancer patients. Psychooncology. 2013;22:1064–72.

43. Munder T, Wilmers F, Leonhart R, Linster HW, Barth J. Working alliance inventory-short revised (WAI-SR): psychometric properties in outpatients and inpatients. Clin Psychol Psychother. 2010;17(3):231–9.

44. Applebaum AJ, DuHamel KN, Winkel G, Rini C, Greene PB, Mosher CE, et al. Therapeutic alliance in telephone administered cognitive-behavioral therapy for hematopoietic stem cell transplant survivors. J Consult Clin Psychol. 2012;80:811–6.

45. Maldonado JR. Delirium in the acute care setting: characteristics, diagnosis and treatment. Crit Care Clin. 2008;24(4):657–722.

46. Beglinger LJ, Duff K, Van Der Heiden S, Parrott K, Langbehn D, Gingrich R. Incidence of delirium and associated mortality in hematopoietic stem cell transplantation patients. Biol Blood Marrow Transplant. 2006;12:928–35.

47. Fann JR, Roth-Roemer S, Burington BE, Katon WJ, Syrjala KL. Delirium in patients undergoing hematopoietic stem cell transplantation. Cancer. 2002;95:1971–81.

48. Bruera E, Bush SH, Willey J, Paraskevopoulos T, Li Z, Palmer JL, et al. Impact of delirium and recall on the level of distress in patients with advanced cancer and their family caregivers. Cancer. 2009;115(9):2004–12.

49. Siddiqi N, House AO, Holmes JD. Occurrence and outcome of delirium in medical in-patients: a systematic literature review. Age Ageing. 2006;35(4):350–64.

50. Fong TG, Jones RN, Shi P, Marcantonio ER, Yap L, Rudolph JL, et al. Delirium accelerates cognitive decline in Alzheimer disease. Neurology. 2009;72(18):1570–5.

51. Fann JR, Alfano CM, Roth-Roemer S, Katon WJ, Syrjala KL. Impact of delirium on cognition, distress, and health-related quality of life after hematopoietic stem-cell transplantation. J Clin Oncol. 2007;25(10):1223–31.

52. Fann JR, Alfano CM, Roth-Roemer S, Katon WJ, Syrjala KL. Impact of delirium on distress, health-related quality of life, and cognition 6 months and 1 year after hematopoietic cell transplant. Biol Blood Marrow Transplant. 2010;16:824–31.

53. Wada T, Wada M, Onishi H. Characteristics, interventions, and outcomes of misdiagnosed delirium in cancer patients. Palliat Support Care. 2010;8(2):125–31.

54. Caraceni A, Nanni O, Maltoni M, Piva L, Indelli M, Arnoldi E, et al. Impact of delirium on the short term prognosis of advanced cancer patients. Italian multicenter study group on palliative care. Cancer. 2000;89:1145–9.

55. Levy MR, Fann JR. The neuropsychiatry of hematopoietic stem cell transplantation. Eur J Psychiatr. 2006;20:107–28.

56. Schulz-Kindermann F, Mehnert A, Scherwath A, Schirmer L, Schleimer B, Zander AR, et al. Cognitive function in the acute course of allogeneic hematopoietic stem cell transplantation for hematological malignancies. Bone Marrow Transplant. 2007;39:789–99.

57. Rueda-Lara M, Lopez-Patton MR. Psychiatric and psychosocial challenges in patients undergoing haematopoietic stem cell transplants. Int Rev Psychiatry. 2014;26(1):74–86.

58. Harder H, Cornelissen JJ, Van Gool AR, , Duivenvoorden HJ, Eijkenboom WM, van den Bent MJ. Cognitive functioning and quality of life in long term adult survivors of bone marrow transplantation . Cancer, 2002, 95 , 183–192 .

59. Syrjala KL, Artherholt SB, Kurland BF, Langer SL, Roth-Roemer S, Elrod JB, et al. Prospective neurocognitive function over 5 years after allogeneic hematopoietic cell transplantation for cancer survivors compared with matched controls at 5 years. J Clin Oncol. 2011;29:2397–404.

60. Bevans MF, Mitchell SA, Marden S. The symptom experience in the first 100 days following allogeneic hematopoietic stem cell transplantation (HSCT). Support Care Cancer. 2008;16:1243–54.

61. Le RQ, Bevans M, Savani BN, Mitchell SA, Stringaris K, Koklanaris E, et al. Favorable outcomes in patients surviving 5 or more years after allogeneic hematopoietic stem cell transplantation for hematologic malignancies. Biol Blood Marrow Transplant. 2010;16:1162–70.

62. Lee SJ, Fairclough D, Parsons SK, Soiffer RJ, Fisher DC, Schlossman RL, et al. Recovery after stem-cell transplantation for hematologic diseases. J Clin Oncol. 2001;19:242–52.

63. Mosher CE, DuHamel KN, Rini C, Corner G, Lam J, Redd WH. Quality of life concerns and depression among hematopoietic stem cell transplant survivors. Support Care Cancer. 2011;19:1357–65.

64. Gielissen MF, Schattenberg AV, Verhagen CA, Rinkes MJ, Bremmers ME, Bleijenberg G. Experience of severe fatigue in long-term survivors of stem cell transplantation. Bone Marrow Transplant. 2007;39:595–603.

65. Jim HS, Evans B, Jeong JM, Gonzalez BD, Johnston L, Nelson AM, et al. Sleep disruption in hematopoietic cell transplantation recipients: prevalence, severity, and clinical management. Biol Blood Marrow Transplant. 2014;20:1465–84.

66. Nelson AM, Coe CL, Juckett MB, Rumble ME, Rathouz PJ, Hematti P, et al. Sleep quality following hematopoietic stem cell transplantation: longitudinal trajectories and biobehavioral correlates. Bone Marrow Transplant. 2014;49:1405–11.

67. Rischer J, Scherwath A, Zander AR, Koch U, Schulz-Kindermann F. Sleep disturbances and emotional distress in the acute course of

hematopoietic stem cell transplantation. Bone Marrow Transplant. 2009;44:121–8.

68. National Comprehensive Cancer Network. Clinical practice guidelines in oncology survivorship version 2013. http://www.nccn.org/professionals/physician_gls/pdf/survivorship.pdf.

69. Boonstra L, Harden K, Jarvis S, Palmer S, Kavanaugh-Carveth P, Barnett J, et al. Sleep disturbance in hospitalized recipients of stem cell transplantation. Clin J Oncol Nurs. 2011;15:271–6.

70. Liu L, Mills PJ, Rissling M, Fiorentino L, Natarajan L, Dimsdale JE, et al. Fatigue and sleep quality are associated with changes in inflammatory markers in breast cancer patients undergoing chemotherapy. Brain Behav Immun. 2012;26:706–13.

71. Couriel D, Carpenter PA, Cutler C, Bolaños-Meade J, Treister NS, Gea-Banacloche J, et al. Ancillary therapy and supportive care of chronic graft-versus-host disease: National Institutes of Health consensus development project on criteria for clinical trials in chronic graft-versus-host disease. Ancillary therapy and supportive care working group report. Biol Blood Marrow Transplant. 2006;12:375–96.

72. Bush NE, Donaldson GW, Haberman MH, Dacanay R, Sullivan KM. Conditional and unconditional estimation of multidimensional quality of life after hematopoietic stem cell transplantation: a longitudinal follow-up of 415 patients. Biol Blood Marrow Transplant. 2000;6:576–91.

73. Pidala J, Anasetti C, Jim H. Quality of life after allogeneic hematopoietic cell transplantation. Blood. 2009;114:7–19.

74. Andrykowski MA, Bishop MM, Hahn EA, Cella DF, Beaumont JL, Brady MJ, et al. Long-term health related quality of life, growth, and spiritual Well-being after hematopoietic stem-cell transplantation. J Clin Oncol. 2005;23:599–608.

75. Boyes AW, , Clinton-McHarg T, Waller AE, Steele A, D'Este CA, Sanson-Fisher RW. Prevalence and correlates of the unmet supportive care needs of individuals diagnosed with a haematological malignancy. Acta Oncol 2015;54:507–514.

76. Hall A, D'Este C, Tzelepis F, Lynagh M, Sanson-Fisher R. Factors associated with haematological cancer survivors experiencing a high level of unmet need across multiple items of supportive care: a cross-sectional survey study. Support Care Cancer. 2014;22:2899–909.

77. Lobb EA, Joske D, Butow P, Kristjanson LJ, Cannell P, Cull G, et al. When the safety net of treatment has been removed: patients' unmet needs at the completion of treatment for haematological malignancies. Patient Educ Couns. 2009;77:103.

78. Marcangelo M, Heinrich TW. Psychiatric issues in solid organ transplantation. Harv Rev Psychiatry. 2009;17:398.

79. Yap KY, Tay WL, Chui WK, Chan A. Clinically Relevant Drug Interactions between Anticancer drugs and psychotropic agents. Eur J Cancer Care. 2011;20:6–32.

80. McQuellon RP, Russell GB, Rambo TD, Craven BL, Radford J, Perry JJ, et al. Quality of life and psychological distress of bone marrow transplant recipients: the time trajectory to recover over the first year. Bone Marrow Transplant. 1998;21:477–86.

81. Mishra SI, Scherer RW, Snyder C, Geigle PM, Berlanstein DR, Topaloglu O. Exercise interventions on health-related quality of life for people with cancer during active treatment. Cochrane Database Syst Rev. 2012;(8):CD008465. https://doi.org/10.1002/14651858.CD008465.pub2.

82. Benish-Weisman M, Wu LM, Weinberger-Litman SL, Redd WH, Duhamel KN, Rini C. Healing stories: narrative characteristics in cancer survivorship narratives and psychological health among hematopoietic stem cell transplant survivors. Palliat Support Care. 2014;12:261–7.

83. Bradt J, Dileo C, Magill L, Teague A. Music interventions for improving psychological and physical outcomes in cancer patients. Cochrane Database Syst Rev. 2016;(8):CD006911. https://doi.org/10.1002/14651858.CD006911.pub3.

84. Schwartz A, Ward M. Challenges in pharmacologic management of the hospitalized patient with psychiatric comorbidity. J Hosp Med. 2013;8(9):523.

85. Manitpisitkul W, McCann E, Lee S, Weir MR. Drug interactions in transplant patients: what everyone should know. Curr Opin Nephrol Hypertens. 2009;18:404–11.

86. Lahijani S, Harris K. Medical complications of psychiatric treatment. Crit Care Clin. 2017;33:713–34.

Part X

General Considerations in the Treatment of Transplant Patients

Psychopharmacology in Transplant Patients

42

Martha C. Gamboa and Stephen J. Ferrando

Introduction

The journey of a patient suffering from end-stage organ failure is usually full of pathophysiological alterations and psychosocial challenges. The perspective of organ transplantation brings about its own host of trials. Rates of anxiety and depressive disorders in this population are equal or higher than those in patients with other chronic medical conditions [1, 2]. If not identified and treated appropriately pre- or post-transplant, anxiety and depressive disorders may negatively impact graft and patients' morbidity and mortality outcomes [3]. Neurocognitive disorders are common pre- and post-transplant [4–7]. These disorders can be exacerbated by exogenous substances as well as by other comorbidities and need to be recognized and appropriately treated in order to increase adherence to treatment, optimize quality of life, and improve graft and patient survival [3].

As with any other medically ill patient requiring psychopharmacological interventions, medication choices derive from a careful and comprehensive psychiatric and medical history, a complete mental status examination, collection of collateral information whenever possible, review of pertinent tests, and arrival to a psychiatric diagnosis and differential. In transplant patients, given the severity of their organ failure as well as the possibility of multiple comorbidities, the pharmacological management of psychiatric disorders requires special considerations, including pharmacokinetic, pharmacodynamic, drug-drug interactions and attention to specific medical issues.

M. C. Gamboa (✉) · S. J. Ferrando
Department of Psychiatry and Behavioral Sciences,
New York Medical College, Valhalla, NY, USA
e-mail: Martha.gamboa@wmchealth.org

Basic Pharmacological Concepts

Pharmacokinetics

Pharmacokinetics describes the processes and transformations medications undergo in the human body, including absorption, distribution, metabolism and elimination of the drugs and their metabolites.

Absorption

Drug *absorption* refers to the rate at which a pharmacological compound leaves the site of administration and reaches the systemic circulation. *Bioavailability* refers to the percentage of the drug that successfully arrived to the systemic circulation compared to the initial given dose. It depends not only on the drug preparation but on the multiple factors that interfere with absorption in each individual situation. Absorption of a drug requires its pass through cell membranes. Lipid soluble and non-ionized drugs are more easily absorbed than hydrophilic and ionized compounds. The oral route is the most common, inexpensive, and convenient means of drug administration. Most drug absorption from the gastrointestinal (GI) tract occurs by passive diffusion. An orally administered drug reaches the portal vein circulation after crossing the gastric or duodenal enterocyte and the endothelium of the capillary portal vein. The portal vein will carry the drug to the liver. However, the drug may undergo biotransformation at the intestine and the liver prior to reaching the systemic circulation. This process known as the *first pass* decreases drug bioavailability. Other routes of administration, such as the intravenous and sublingual, obviate the process of absorption, hence avoiding hepatic and intestinal first-pass elimination. Drugs that undergo extensive first-pass metabolism require a higher dose when given orally compared to intravenous administration. Factors that alter drug absorption include the surface area for absorption, the physical state of the drug (solid, solution, suspension), its water solubility, the drug concentration at the absorption site,

© Springer International Publishing AG, part of Springer Nature 2019
Y. Sher, J. R. Maldonado (eds.), *Psychosocial Care of End-Stage Organ Disease and Transplant Patients*,
https://doi.org/10.1007/978-3-319-94914-7_42

the presence of food, the presence of other drugs, gastric pH changes, vitamin D deficiency, changes in gastric emptying and intestinal motility, vomiting, intestinal flora, splanchnic blood flow, and the presence of intestinal edema. Additionally, the activity of enterocyte and hepatocyte membrane-embedded transporters such as the ATP-binding cassette (ABC) transporters can block the entrance of substrate drugs into the intestinal wall or into the hepatocyte, thus decreasing drug absorption.

Drug Distribution

Once a drug reaches the systemic circulation, it is distributed throughout the body and its compartments. Factors that alter drug concentration and distribution to tissues and fluids include blood flow, nutritional state, membrane permeability, as well as drug characteristics such as lipophilicity or hydrophilicity, drug pH, and protein-binding capacity. The term *volume of distribution* refers to the relationship between the total amount of drug in the body and the concentration of drug measured in a biological fluid. The volume of distribution seems larger for lipophilic drugs (most psychotropics) as these drugs are sequestered into lipid compartments, rendering low serum levels. The opposite takes place for hydrophilic drugs as they have high serum concentrations, hence, lower volumes of distribution. However, if edema is present, this causes expansion of the extracellular volume and may increase the volume of distribution of hydrophilic drugs, leading to lower serum concentrations.

Drug Metabolism

Drug metabolism refers to the biotransformation of drug compounds into more polar, water-soluble, and inactive molecules that could then be eliminated via urine, bile, or stool. This biotransformation is accomplished by the metabolic enzyme systems largely found in the liver and the intestinal wall, particularly in the smooth endoplasmic reticulum of enterocytes and hepatocytes but also in the intestinal lumen and intestinal microbiota. Metabolic reactions are organized in phases 1 and 2. *Phase 1* reactions are catabolic and involve oxidation, reduction, and hydrolysis processes. The cytochrome P450 (CYP450) mono-oxidase system contributes to the large majority of phase 1 reactions. Some benzodiazepines, such as lorazepam, oxazepam, and temazepam, do not undergo phase 1 metabolic reactions. *Phase 2* reactions are anabolic and involve conjugation reactions, in which water-soluble molecules are added to a drug or metabolite, leading to inactive and polar products easily excreted in the urine. They include glucuronidation, sulfation, and methylation [8]. The activity of phase 1 and 2 enzymes can be induced or inhibited by co-administration of other substances, including drugs, foods, and smoking. Enzyme induction or inhibition can result in lower or higher than desired drug or metabolite levels, potentially causing serious clinical consequences.

Additionally, intestinal microorganisms, which include anaerobic bacteria and yeasts, coexist in the human intestine and participate in non-oxidative drug biotransformation reactions such as reduction, hydrolysis, decarboxylation, dehydroxylation, dealkylation, dehalogenation, and deamination. Medications that alter the equilibrium of the gut microbiota can in turn alter the metabolism of co-administered drugs substrates of microorganism enzymes [9, 10]. Other factors that affect drug metabolism include the presence of portosystemic shunts, the quality of the splanchnic blood flow, as well as individual enzyme variations. Recent attention has been given to alterations in the function of CYP450 enzymes by the presence of chronic kidney disease via direct uremic toxins or via inhibition of their expression [11–13].

Elimination

Most drugs and their metabolites are eliminated as polar hydrophilic compounds in the urine. A smaller portion of drugs are eliminated via the hepatobiliary system in the feces. Membrane-embedded transporter systems have an important role in drug elimination. These transporters are present in the intestinal cells, in the hepatocytes, in the renal tubule cells, in the capillary endothelial cells of the blood-brain barrier, as well as in other tissues. Membrane transporters are divided in two superfamilies: solute-linked carrier (SLC) transporters and ATP-linked cassette (ABC) transporters. P-glycoprotein (P-gp) belongs to the later family and is also known as ABCB1 for ATP-binding cassette B1 [14]. When substrate drugs arrive to the intestinal lumen, ABC efflux transporters located in the apical brush border can expel them back to the intestinal lumen. In the enterocyte, substrate drugs undergo phase 1 and 2 metabolism and are subsequently transferred to the portal capillary system. Portal blood carries drugs or their metabolites to the liver. At the hepatocyte level, drugs and their metabolites are transferred by influx (mostly SLC) transporters from the basolateral border to the cytoplasm where the drug undergoes phase 1 and 2 metabolic reactions. The drug metabolites are then transferred mostly via ABC transporters to the bile through the apical border of the cell and then delivered to the duodenum. In the small intestine, drugs can be reactivated by microbiota enzymes and then reabsorbed (enterohepatic circulation) or eliminated in the feces. For example, lorazepam is conjugated in the liver to its inactive metabolite, lorazepam glucuronide. This compound may be excreted in the bile to the intestine, where β-glucuronidase breaks the ester linkage and converts it back to lorazepam, which in turn can be reabsorbed to the portal circulation or eliminated in feces.

The elimination of drugs or their metabolites through the kidney takes place through glomerular filtration, active tubular secretion, and passive tubular reabsorption. Factors limiting glomerular filtration of drugs include molecular size and albumin binding. Only unbound drugs pass freely from plasma in the glomerular capillary to the glomerular filtrate. Membrane transporters located in the proximal tubule including SLC transporters and ABC transporters including P-glycoprotein secrete drugs into the filtrate. In the proximal and distal renal tubules the non-ionized fraction of the weak acids or bases is passively reabsorbed. The ionized fraction of the drug remains in the filtrate and is excreted in the urine. Additionally, some drugs undergo active reabsorption to the main circulation via membrane transporters located in the distal tubular lumen.

Pharmacodynamics

Pharmacodynamic processes refer to the drug effects on the organism, including the intended and therapeutic, as well as the side effects. Drug effects derive from the interaction between the drug and its receptors and can be altered by the presence of other drugs and medical conditions. Psychiatric medications usually act on multiple receptors; hence potentiation of the effects of other nonpsychiatric drugs is common. For example, amitriptyline is a tricyclic antidepressant which increases the synaptic concentration of serotonin and norepinephrine in the central nervous system by inhibition of their reuptake at the presynaptic neuronal level. However, amitriptyline also has anticholinergic effects, and its concurrent use with diphenhydramine, a histamine H1 antagonist, can increase the risk for side effects, including drowsiness, xerostomia, blurry vision, constipation, and delirium.

Post-transplant Psychopharmacological Issues

The administration of psychiatric medications following organ transplantation should derive from careful review of the patient's overall medical status, the graft function, the level of functioning of the absorbing, metabolizing and eliminating organs, as well as the potential drug-drug interactions, particularly with immunosuppressant agents. Unfortunately, some post-transplant patients suffer primary graft failure requiring early re-transplantation, while others may suffer delayed graft functioning, requiring close monitoring and medication dose adjustments. Once the transplanted organ assumes normal physiological functioning, and proper absorption, metabolism, and elimination are established, medications could be prescribed at their regular doses. Acute rejection occurs in approximately 20% of liver transplant patients in the first 6 months after surgery [15], in 10% of intestinal transplant recipients within the first month [16, 17], in up to 60% of kidney transplant patients in the first 6 months, and in up to 50% of heart transplant patients within the first year [16]. Acute graft rejection usually requires more aggressive management

with immunosuppressant agents [18], including high-dose steroids, which themselves can cause a wide variety of neuropsychiatric symptoms.

Initial postoperative psychopharmacological interventions usually focus on management of delirium and neuropsychiatric side effects from immunosuppressants, as well as treatment of anxiety related to perceived traumatic perioperative events such as intense uncontrolled pain, intubation, inability to communicate, and the use of restraints. Following the acute recovery phase, additional indications for psychopharmacological interventions include the presence of anxiety and/or depressive symptoms interfering with recovery, adjustment to medications side effects, decreased appetite, and insomnia. Long-term, post-transplant patients have to deal with the fear of rejection, body image issues, acceptance of role changes, financial concerns, hospital bills, cravings for smoking, alcohol or other substances, as well as re-hospitalizations in the context of organ rejection or immunosuppression-related complications. These include neurocognitive impairments, serious infections, increased cancer risk, and compromise of kidney function in some cases leading to initiation of renal replacement therapy. Mental health professionals caring for transplant patients need to be alert to patients' post-transplant biopsychosocial changes and adaptations. Additionally, it is important to understand basic aspects of immunosuppressants commonly used in post-transplant patients in order to confidently recognize their psychoactive side effects, as well as recommend and prescribe psychiatric medications when needed.

Immunosuppressants

Important nonspecific immunosuppressant side effects include weight gain, hypertension, diabetes, and dyslipidemias [19, 20]. These comorbidities are important to consider when deciding on the addition of a psychopharmacological agent, given that many psychotropics are associated with weight gain and metabolic syndrome.

Corticosteroids
Steroids play an important role in transplantation at various stages, including induction, maintenance, and management of rejection. Steroids bind to glucocorticoid-responsive elements in DNA preventing the transcription of cytokine genes and receptors. They also decrease cell-mediated immunity and T-cell activation. Methylprednisolone, prednisolone, and prednisone are substrates of CYP3A4. At high doses glucocorticoids inhibit and at low doses induce CYP3A4. Several psychiatric drugs are either inducers or inhibitors of CYP3A4; therefore, drug-drug interactions are expected when used concurrently [20]. Common neuropsychiatric side effects of glucocorticoids include agitation, anxiety,

cognitive impairments, delusions, delirium, euphoria, hallucinations, as well as personality changes [21]. The most validated risk factor for these side effects is the dose, particularly doses higher than 40 mg per day [21]. Other risk factors include blood-brain barrier damage, hypoalbuminemia and co-administration of CYP 3A4 inhibitors [21]. On the other hand, depressed mood, fatigue, mania, and delirium can occur upon withdrawal of steroids [21–23].

It is important to educate patients and caregivers regarding the possibility of steroid-induced neuropsychiatric adverse effects including changes in mood and cognitive abilities. A history of mood disorders as well as previous neuropsychiatric adverse reactions to steroids alerts the clinician about the need to consider prophylactic interventions. Unfortunately, there is a paucity of well-powered randomized controlled trials informing on the efficacy and safety of specific agents for this purpose. Similarly, the literature on the treatment of steroid-induced neuropsychiatric disorders is based on multiple case reports and small trials. For steroid-induced mania in the transplant population, the reduction and discontinuation of the steroid dose are not always possible, and the temporary addition of a neuroleptic such as olanzapine could be considered a first step [21, 24, 25]. In this case, the monitoring of glucose control should be emphasized. The use of lithium is second choice due to nephrotoxicity concerns in the presence of calcineurin inhibitors and potential co-administration of diuretics. Antiepileptics can also be used, including valproic acid and gabapentin [24, 26]. Benzodiazepines can also be helpful, particularly clonazepam [27].

Calcineurin Inhibitors (CNIs)

Tacrolimus and cyclosporine are the cornerstone drugs in solid organ transplantation [19]. Although they are not chemically related to each other, they have similar mechanisms of action since they both bind to cytoplasmic isomerases that are abundant in all tissues. Cyclosporine binds to cyclophilin and tacrolimus binds to the immunophilin FK-binding protein (FKBP) forming complexes that inhibit calcineurin. Calcineurin is a cytoplasmic phosphatase necessary for the activation of a T-cell-specific transcription factor involved in the synthesis of interleukins by activated T cells. CNIs are highly lipophilic and undergo extensive first-pass metabolism. They are substrates for the cytochrome CYP3A4, CYP3A5, as well as the P-glycoprotein transporter.

Since these medications have pharmacokinetic and pharmacodynamic variability, therapeutic drug monitoring is routine. Low blood levels increase risk of rejection, while high levels increase risk of adverse effects, including neurotoxicity, nephrotoxicity, infection, and neoplasias. Due to individual variability, rejection as well as toxicities can occur within therapeutic drug levels. The mechanism underlying CNIs' neurotoxic effects is not yet well understood, but it

may be related to the role of calcineurin in neuronal cell functioning [28]. Tacrolimus and cyclosporine may cause similar neuropsychiatric side effects, including agitation, anxiety, cognitive impairment, depression, dysarthria, fatigue, hallucinations, insomnia, lethargy, neuropathy, and seizures [19, 29]. Both agents have also been associated with the development of posterior reversible encephalopathy syndrome (PRES), a rare neurologic condition presenting in approximately 0.5–5% of solid organ transplant patients [30–32]. The characteristic clinical symptoms in post-transplant PRES include seizures, headache, acute encephalopathy syndrome, autonomic instability, and visual symptoms, while magnetic resonance imaging (MRI) findings consist of an abnormal and reversible increased signal in the fluid-attenuated inversion recovery (FLAIR) images, with characteristic distribution in the parietal and occipital lobes, and less frequently in the posterior frontal, temporal lobe, cerebellum, brainstem, thalamus, and basal ganglia [33, 34]. Early diagnosis is important, although there is no clear consensus regarding immunosuppressant management in this context. Some studies recommend a decrease and even a complete discontinuation of CNI and switching to other immunosuppressant agents [35].

Long-term neuropsychiatric side effects of CNIs include cognitive impairment and tremors [19].

In addition, the long-term use of CNIs can lead to nephrotoxicity [19]. This emphasizes the need to monitor renal function particularly when medications that do not undergo liver metabolism and that are fully or almost fully eliminated by the kidney are co-administered (i.e., gabapentin, amantadine, lithium).

Cyclosporine

This agent is available for oral and intravenous administration. The oral absorption of cyclosporine is erratic and incomplete and depends on the presence of food, bile acids, and gastrointestinal motility [36]. Cyclosporine is extensively metabolized in the liver via CYP3A4, forming many metabolites, and it undergoes extensive first-pass effect following oral administration. In plasma, cyclosporine is both a substrate and an inhibitor of CYP3A4 and P-glycoprotein. Given that many psychiatric drugs are metabolized by CYP3A4, there are multiple possibilities for significant drug-drug interactions [29]. Psychiatric drugs that inhibit CYP3A4, such as fluvoxamine, nefazodone, and fluoxetine, can increase cyclosporine levels and risk of toxicity. On the other hand, CYP3A4 inducers, such as carbamazepine, phenobarbital, and modafinil, can decrease cyclosporine levels risking transplant rejection. Furthermore, since cyclosporine itself is an inhibitor of CYP3A4, it can increase the levels of buspirone, most benzodiazepines, iloperidone, quetiapine, and ziprasidone. Additionally, P-glycoprotein inducers, such as *Hypericum perforatum* (i.e., St. John's wort), can also induce

CYP3A4 [37] and thus reduce cyclosporine levels, increasing risk of rejection. Since cyclosporine inhibits P-glycoprotein, it can increase the bioavailability of several psychiatric medications including carbamazepine, lamotrigine, olanzapine, phenytoin, paroxetine, quetiapine, risperidone, and venlafaxine, among others. Cyclosporine can cause hyperkalemia by decreasing potassium tubular excretion. This may be a mechanism underlying its association with increased cardiac arrhythmia risk [38]. Therefore, concurrent use of cyclosporine and potentially arrhythmogenic psychiatric drugs needs to be executed under careful monitoring.

Tacrolimus

Tacrolimus is available for intravenous and oral administration. Its oral absorption is incomplete and variable and also reduced in the presence of food. Tacrolimus is highly protein bound to plasma proteins: 99% is primarily bound to albumin and alpha1 acid glycoprotein. This CNI is metabolized extensively in the liver via CYP3A4 to several metabolites. Tacrolimus is a substrate of P-glycoprotein. It is also a substrate and inhibitor of uridine 5'-diphosphate glucuronosyltransferase (UGT). Tacrolimus use can be associated with QT prolongation [39, 40]. Given that many psychotropic agents can prolong the QT interval [41] and that they often are substrates and/or inhibitors of CYP3A4, caution is advised when they are co-administered with tacrolimus. Close monitoring of the electrocardiogram, tacrolimus levels, as well as serum electrolytes including sodium, potassium, and calcium is advised. Drug dosage reduction may be necessary.

Mechanistic Target of Rapamycin (mTOR) Inhibitors

Sirolimus and everolimus exert their principal immunosuppressive effects by inhibiting the ability of the cytoplasmic enzyme complex mTOR to regulate the growth, proliferation, and survival of lymphocytes and other immunocompetent cells. Sirolimus and everolimus are metabolized in the liver and intestinal wall by CYP3A4 and CYP3A5 and, to a minor extent, by CYP2C8. They are both substrates of ABCB1, while everolimus has inhibitory action on CYP3A4 and ABCB. Its metabolites are excreted primarily in feces. Neuropsychiatric side effects include tremor, insomnia, headache, and pain [42].

Polyclonal and Monoclonal Antibodies

Antithymocyte globulin (ATG) is a purified gamma globulin obtained by immunizing rabbits (thymoglobulin) or horses (Atgam) with human thymocytes [43, 44]. ATG induces lymphocyte depletion in the periphery by complement-dependent cell lysis. Premedication with steroids, acetaminophen, and/or antihistamine approximately 1 h prior to infusion is recommended to minimize the antithymocyte globulin-induced cytokine release syndrome, characterized

by fever, chills, and rigors, but can also include dyspnea, nausea/vomiting, diarrhea, hypotension, hypertension, malaise, rash, and headache The metabolism and elimination of this drug is unknown. The principal neuropsychiatric side effects of thymoglobulin include chills, pain, headache, malaise, and anxiety [43, 44].

Basiliximab is a monoclonal antibody that blocks the T-cell IL-2 receptor preventing IL-2-induced T-cell activation [45]. Basiliximab is a powerful induction agent, but it is not used to treat acute rejection, as it does not cause lymphocyte depletion. Common neuropsychiatric adverse effects include insomnia, fatigue, pain, headache, tremor, agitation, anxiety, and depression [45].

Alemtuzumab is a monoclonal antibody that has profound lymphocyte-depleting effects [46, 47]. It causes cell death by complement-mediated cytolysis, antibody-mediated cytotoxicity, and apoptosis. Alemtuzumab causes a long-lasting T-cell depletion, which prolongs infection and lymphoproliferative disorder risks. Psychiatric adverse effects include insomnia, anxiety, and suicidal ideation [46, 47].

Rituximab is a monoclonal antibody that binds specifically to a B-lymphocyte differentiation antigen on pre-B- and mature B-lymphocytes [48]. Neuropsychiatric side effects include anxiety, chills, delirium, depression, dizziness, fatigue, insomnia, migraine, myalgias, neuropathy, paresthesias, and pain [48].

Inhibitors of Purine Synthesis
Mycophenolate Mofetil

The active drug mycophenolic acid inhibits inosine-5'-monophosphate dehydrogenase (IMPDH), a rate-limiting enzyme in the purine synthesis. Mycophenolic acid suppresses the proliferation of T- and B-lymphocytes. Common neuropsychiatric side effects include pain, headache, dizziness, tremor, insomnia, and anxiety [49].

Azathioprine

Azathioprine is metabolized to 6-mercaptopurine (6-MP). 6-MP substitutes the purine base guanine in RNA. Mercaptopurine ribonucleotides are incorporated into RNA and halt DNA synthesis. The immunosuppressive activity of azathioprine is due to its ability to inhibit delayed hypersensitivity reactions and cellular cytotoxic activity. Neuropsychiatric side effects include malaise and myalgias [50].

Others

Belatacept is a selective T-cell costimulation blocker. This medication is indicated for rejection prophylaxis in adults receiving kidney transplant. Neuropsychiatric side effects include anxiety, dizziness, headache, insomnia, pain, tremor, and Guillain-Barre syndrome, and it has been implicated in post-transplant lymphoproliferative disorder (PTLD) [51].

Psychiatric Medications

Antidepressants

Antidepressants are commonly used in the transplant population to assist in the management of various psychiatric syndromes, including depression, anxiety, insomnia, pain, and appetite stimulation.

Selective Serotonin Reuptake Inhibitors (SSRIs)

Among transplant patients, most SSRI studies have taken place in patients with end-stage heart or kidney disease [13, 52–54]. As a family, SSRIs share some side effects.

SSRIs increase bleeding risk as they inhibit platelet activation and thus may increase bleeding time [55, 56]. This can be particularly problematic in end-stage liver disease, since patients with cirrhosis are prone to bleeding in the context of coagulopathy, thrombocytopenia, and variceal formation. Additionally, platelet dysfunction can also be present in patients with kidney failure. Many end-stage organ disease patients are managed with anticoagulants and/or aspirin, and special caution needs to be taken when co-administration of an antidepressant is needed.

All SSRIs can potentially prolong QT interval; therefore, caution is needed in the context of predisposing medical conditions and co-administration with other QT prolonging drugs [41]. Of note, of the SSRI agents, citalopram is associated with the most QT prolongation [41]. In addition, SSRIs have been associated with hyponatremia [57, 58]. The use of SSRI agents has been associated with bone metabolism dysfunction; thus they may increase the risk for fractures. Therefore, caution is required when use in the context of chronic corticosteroid therapy [59]. Despite of these potential issues, SSRIs remain the first-line treatment for the treatment of depression in transplant patients due to their superior safety profile and less drug-drug interactions when compared to other antidepressants [60].

Sertraline

Sertraline is well absorbed after oral administration. It is 98% protein bound and is metabolized by CYP3A4 to desmethylsertraline [61]. At low doses the parent drug and its metabolite cause weak inhibition of CYP2D6, which can become clinically relevant at high doses [62, 63]. Sertraline does not inhibit CYP3A4 in vivo [64], which is favorable for patients taking immunosuppressant agents. However, at least one study found an association of sertraline and increased cyclosporine levels [65]. Sertraline elimination half-life increases in the context of liver failure. Sertraline has been helpful in decreasing pruritus in cholestatic jaundice patients, which constitutes an added benefit in this clinical scenario [66]. It has been shown to be helpful for sensation of dyspnea in patients with chronic obstructive pulmonary disease [67]. In addition, sertraline has been helpful in reducing dialysis-related hypotension which makes this medication appealing in patients with difficulty tolerating dialysis [68]. Dose adjustment is not recommended in kidney failure. However in mild liver failure, it is advised to decrease the dose to half of the usual. Furthermore, in moderate to advanced liver failure, sertraline is not recommended [69].

Citalopram

Citalopram is composed of S and R enantiomers. The S enantiomer (escitalopram) is pharmacologically active. Citalopram is absorbed rapidly following oral administration and is metabolized by CYP3A4 and CYP2C19 [61]. Citalopram is a weak inhibitor of 2D6, and concurrent administration with metoprolol leads to increased levels of the beta-blocker [70]. Citalopram has the Food and Drung Administration (FDA) warning regarding its potential to prolong QT [41]. Citalopram is also the only agent that carries specific recommendations, including a maximum daily dose of 20 mg/day in patients suffering with hepatic impairment or in those older than 60 years and a maximum 40 mg dose/day in young and healthier patients [71], although the merit of this warning has been debated [72].

Escitalopram

The S enantiomer of citalopram is rapidly absorbed following oral administration. Escitalopram is 56% protein bound [61]. It is metabolized by CYP2D6, 2C19, and 3A4 and weakly inhibits CYP2D6 [61]. Dose adjustment is recommended in hepatic and severe renal impairment [69]. QT can still be prolonged by escitalopram, although to a lesser degree compared to citalopram [41].

Paroxetine

Paroxetine is metabolized by CYP2D6, strongly inhibits CYP2D6, and has a mild inhibitory effect of CYP2C9 and CYP2C19 [61]. Paroxetine has significant anticholinergic properties, which can contribute to many side effects, including delirium and cognitive impairment. It has a relatively short half-life, which may be associated with severe serotonin withdrawal, upon abrupt discontinuation. In addition, its use is associated with significant weight gain, as compared to other SSRIs. In severe renal (creatinine clearance <30%) and hepatic impairment, the manufacturer recommends slower titration and lower maximum daily dosages.

Fluoxetine

Fluoxetine is metabolized by CYP2D6 and CYP2C9 [61]. Fluoxetine and its active metabolite, norfluoxetine, inhibit CYP2D6, CYP2C9, CYP2C19, and CYP3A4 [61]. Fluoxetine has the longest half-life of all the SSRIs (i.e., 7 days) [69]. In patients with severe impaired renal function, additional accumulation of fluoxetine and norfluoxetine may occur. Patients with liver cirrhosis require lower than usual doses or less frequent administration intervals.

Fluvoxamine

Fluvoxamine is metabolized primarily by deamination and acetylation. Fluvoxamine is a substrate of CYP1A2 and CYP2D6 [61]. This drug is a potent inhibitor of CYP1A2 and exerts less inhibition of CYP2C19, CYP2C9, and CYP3A4. There is limited information regarding its safety in kidney and liver impairment. Due to its significant potential for interactions, it is usually avoided in the transplant population.

Serotonin Norepinephrine Reuptake Inhibitors (SNRIs)

SNRIs are chemically unrelated to each other. As in the case of tricyclic antidepressants (TCAs), SNRIs inhibit serotonin and norepinephrine reuptake [61]. However, in contrast to TCAs, SNRIs do not have much affinity for other receptors. In addition to their use in major depression, SNRIs may be useful in the treatment of pain disorders. SNRIs are associated with increases in blood pressure and heart rate; therefore, caution is recommended in patients with hypertension, cerebrovascular disease, and cardiac disease.

Venlafaxine

Venlafaxine is a potent inhibitor of neuronal serotonin and norepinephrine reuptake and weak inhibitor of dopamine reuptake [61]. Venlafaxine functions like an SSRI in low doses and as a dual mechanism agent affecting both serotonin and norepinephrine at doses above 225 mg per day. Venlafaxine has a short half-life and is associated with increased risk of serotonin withdrawal. Venlafaxine is metabolized by CYP2D6. Two cases of serotonin toxicity have been reported in patients receiving venlafaxine and CNIs, likely due to CNI-inhibitory effect of P-glycoprotein [73]. Dose reduction of venlafaxine is indicated in kidney and liver impairment.

Desvenlafaxine

Desvenlafaxine is the major active metabolite of venlafaxine [61]. Desvenlafaxine undergoes hepatic metabolism primarily by conjugation and in less proportion by oxidation via CYP3A4. Desvenlafaxine is a weak inhibitor of CYP2D6 and a weak inductor of CYP3A4; however, clinical studies have not found clinically relevant interactions when this medication is co-administered with CYP2D6 and CYP3A4 substrates, at doses up to 100 mg/day. Desvenlafaxine dosing needs to be adjusted in the setting of renal and hepatic impairment [74].

Duloxetine

Duloxetine is metabolized by the liver, via CYP1A2 and CYP2D6 into multiple inactive metabolites [61]. Duloxetine is associated with increased risk of idiopathic hepatic failure [75, 76]. Duloxetine use should be avoided in hepatic impairment and in cases of kidney failure with creatinine clearance lower than 30 mL/min.

Milnacipran

Milnacipran is a SNRI that has been used in the treatment of depression in Europe for many years but only approved in the USA for the treatment of fibromyalgia. Milnacipran undergoes hepatic metabolism and should be used with caution in kidney and liver impairment. Its dosage should be reduced if the creatinine clearance is lower than 30 mL/minute and its use is not recommended in end-stage renal disease. However, the manufacturer does not recommend dose adjustment in case of hepatic impairment.

Levomilnacipran

Levomilnacipran is an enantiomer of racemic milnacipran. Levomilnacipran is metabolized in the liver primarily by CYP3A4 to inactive metabolites. Levomilnacipran is a weak substrate of P-glycoprotein. More than half of the dose of levomilnacipran is excreted by the kidney. Dosage adjustment is needed in the context of renal impairment with creatinine clearance lower than 30 mL/min.

Other Antidepressants
Mirtazapine

Mirtazapine has central presynaptic alpha$_2$-adrenergic antagonist effects, leading to increased release of norepinephrine and serotonin [61]. Additionally it is a potent antagonist of 5-HT$_2$ and 5-HT$_3$ serotonin receptors and H$_1$ histamine receptors and a moderate antagonist at peripheral alpha$_1$-adrenergic and muscarinic receptors. Mirtazapine is metabolized by CYP2D6, CYP1A2, CYP3A4, and CYP2C9 [61]. This medication has been associated with rare potentially life-threatening agranulocytosis [77]; therefore, caution is necessary when given concurrently with immunosuppressant agents and in patients before and after hematopoietic cell transplantation. Common side effects include sedation, increased appetite, and weight gain, which are desirable effects in patients who need to increase oral intake and improve sleep, particularly pre-transplant. Mirtazapine does not inhibit CYP enzymes. By blocking 5-HT2A receptors, mirtazapine potentially blocks JC virus from entering into glial cells, and for this reason, it has been used in the treatment of progressive multifocal leukoencephalopathy (PML), a condition that can occur in immunosuppressed patients. However, data on transplant patients treated with mirtazapine for PML is scarce, and the level of evidence supporting mirtazapine use in this scenario is low so far [78]. Mirtazapine clearance is decreased in the context of kidney and liver impairment.

Vilazodone

Vilazodone inhibits the reuptake of serotonin and is a 5-HT1A receptor partial agonist. It is metabolized mainly by CYP3A4; thus caution should be used when combined with immunosuppressant agents. Vilazodone is metabolized in less degree by 2C19 and 2D6 [79]. No dose adjustments are reportedly needed in renal or hepatic impairment based on small studies.

Nefazodone

Nefazodone inhibits neuronal reuptake of serotonin and nor-epinephrine and also blocks 5-HT and alpha1 receptors [61]. Nefazodone is rapidly absorbed following oral administration. Nefazodone is metabolized by CYP3A4 and CYP2D6, and it is an inhibitor of CYP3A4. It also exerts weak inhibition of CYP2D6 [80]. It undergoes extensive first pass, with a bioavailability of 20%. It is 99% protein bound. Nefazodone has been associated with rare cases of acute liver failure, leading to liver transplantation and death in few, and its product label has a black box warning to this respect [81]. For this and its potential for drug-drug interactions, nefazodone is not recommended in transplant patients.

Trazodone

Trazodone inhibits the reuptake of serotonin and acts as a 5-HT2a receptor antagonist [61]. Additionally, trazodone blocks H_1 histamine and alpha1-adrenergic receptors, mechanisms involved in its sedative effect. Trazodone is rapidly absorbed after oral administration. Its concentration peaks at 1 hour. It is 90% protein bound and its bioavailability is 80%. It is metabolized by CYP3A4 and CYP2D6 and it does not seem to inhibit or induce CYP enzymes. It is associated with orthostatic hypotension due to its alpha1-adrenergic effects. Trazodone should be used with caution in patients with kidney and/or liver impairment due to the possibility of accumulation, reduction in its excretion, and increased risk of side effects.

Vortioxetine

Vortioxetine inhibits the reuptake of serotonin and has agonist activity at the 5-HT$_{1A}$ receptor and antagonist activity at the 5-HT$_3$ receptor. Vortioxetine is metabolized by CYP2D6 isoenzyme. Its use in severe hepatic impairment is not recommended. Dosage adjustment is recommended for CYP2D6 poor metabolizers and when given concurrently with strong CYP2D6 inhibitors.

Bupropion

Bupropion is a relatively weak inhibitor of the neuronal uptake of norepinephrine and dopamine, and does not inhibit monoamine oxidase or the reuptake of serotonin [61]. Bupropion is a substrate of CYP2B6 and a strong inhibitor of CYP2D6 [61]. Dose needs to be adjusted in end-stage liver disease. Bupropion lacks sedative side effects; hence it is an alternative for patients suffering from decreased energy. It is also used for smoking cessation [61]. It can cause tachycardia and increased blood pressure [61]. It can decrease seizure threshold, especially in patients with electrolyte abnormalities or structural brain abnormalities.

Monoamine Oxidase Inhibitors (MAOIs)

By inhibiting the monoamine oxidase enzyme, MAOIs (tranylcypromine, phenelzine, isocarboxazid, selegiline) increase monoamine concentrations in the presynaptic neuron [61]. These monoamines include dopamine, tyramine, serotonin, norepinephrine, epinephrine, and phenylethylamine. There are two monoamine oxidase isoenzymes: A and B. MAO-A is found primarily in the brain, liver, gut, and placenta; its primary substrates are norepinephrine, epinephrine, and serotonin. MAO-B is found in the brain, liver, and platelets; its main substrates are dopamine, phenylethylamine, histamine, and tyramine. Some MAOIs inhibit both isoenzymes (A and B) and are irreversible inhibitors, while others are selective for one or the other and are mostly reversible inhibitors. Most MAOIs produce a nonspecific reduction in the activity of hepatic drug-metabolizing enzymes. MAOIs inhibit MAO in the gut which can lead to life-threatening tyramine pressor effects. Due to drug-drug and food-drug potential interactions, MAOIs are not considered as first line in the treatment of depression in patients with medical comorbidities, including transplant candidates and recipients [69, 82].

Tricyclic Antidepressants (TCAs)

TCAs' tolerability and lethality in overdose have placed them as second choice in the management of depression, behind SSRIs. By virtue of their involvement in the blockade of several receptors, including acetylcholine muscarinic, alpha1, and histamine receptors, the use of TCA increases the risk of arrhythmias, QTc prolongation, intraventricular conduction delays, orthostatic hypotension, weight gain, as well as lipid changes. Use of TCAs in the transplant population requires careful follow-up [69]. TCAs are metabolized by the CYP system. Secondary amines such as desipramine, nortriptyline, and protriptyline are primarily substrates of CYP2D6, while tertiary amines such as imipramine, clomipramine, and amitriptyline are substrates for CYP1A2 and CYP2C19. Dose adjustment is necessary in kidney and liver impairment.

Herbal Supplements

Patients might be using herbal supplements; thus it is important to inquire about this use and properly counsel patients. For example, St. John's wort, an herbal known for its antidepressant actions, extracted from the plant *Hypericum perforatum*, is actually an inducer of 3A4 and P-glycoprotein [83]. In fact, concurrent use of St. John's wort and cyclosporine has caused graft rejections [83–85].

Stimulants

Besides attention deficit and hyperactivity disorders, psychostimulants can be used in the treatment of apathy and depression, when faster effect is needed [86]. In 2006, the FDA requested that all manufacturers of stimulant medications include a class label change that sudden death has been reported in pediatric patients with structural cardiac abnormalities receiving stimulants [87]. Prior to initiation of stimulants, patients need to be evaluated for possible heart conditions including physical examination, electrocardiogram, and family history of cardiac illness.

Methylphenidate

Methylphenidate blocks dopamine uptake in central adrenergic neurons by blocking dopamine transport proteins. This causes increase of the sympathomimetic activity in the central nervous system. Methylphenidate is available for oral and transdermal administration. Methylphenidate is not metabolized by the CYP system, and it does not seem to be an inhibitor of CYP isozymes. Instead, methylphenidate is metabolized via de-esterification to its main metabolite, ritalinic acid, which is inactive and is eliminated by the kidney. This drug has not been studied in renal or hepatic impairment.

A small retrospective study in liver transplant patients targeting psychomotor and cognitive slowing, lack of motivation for recovery, poor rehabilitation effort, social withdrawal, and apathy found positive effect from methylphenidate [88]. A recent meta-analysis also provided further support for efficacy of methylphenidate in treatment of fatigue in patients with cancer and those undergoing hematopoietic cell transplantation [89]. Patients need to be monitored for risk of developing tachyarrhythmias and hypertension. A case report described the successful use of methylphenidate in a patient with heart transplant and depression who developed catatonic symptoms after initiation of sertraline [90]. However, a recent publication also reported a case of a 12-year-old child who developed liver failure, requiring liver transplantation, presumed to be associated with methylphenidate hepatotoxicity [91].

Dextroamphetamine

Dextroamphetamine is the D-isomer of amphetamine and is twice as potent as racemic amphetamine. Escalating doses of dextroamphetamine produce the progressive release of norepinephrine, dopamine, and serotonin from storage sites in the nerve terminal. Dextroamphetamine is available in oral presentation. Its metabolism is hepatic, via CYP monooxygenase and glucuronidation, with renal elimination. Renal and hepatic impairment may lead to decreased elimination and prolonged exposure; therefore, doses should be titrated carefully [92].

Modafinil

Modafinil mechanism of action is not fully understood. It appears that modafinil induces alertness by activating wakefulness-related systems such as hypocretin, histamine, α-adrenergic, glutamate, and dopamine, likely by blocking the activity of the dopamine transporter and modulating norepinephrine and serotonin transporters [93]. Dose reduction is recommended in patients with severe hepatic impairment. Elimination half-life is around 15 hours. Modafinil is metabolized by and weakly induces CYP3A4; thus it can hypothetically lead to decreased blood levels of immunosuppressants also metabolized by CYP3A4. Elimination is mostly hepatic, with kidney excretion of inactive metabolites.

Benzodiazepines

Benzodiazepines produce central nervous system depression including sedation, skeletal muscle relaxation, anticonvulsant activity, and coma by interacting with gamma aminobutyric acid A (GABA-A) receptors. Potentiation of GABA effects increases the inhibition of the ascending reticular activating system. The use of benzodiazepines in patients with end-stage organ disease requires vigilance due to the potential to cause excessive sedation, respiratory depression (worsened by co-administration of opioids), increased risk of falls, and worsened cognition. Some benzodiazepines such as diazepam, lorazepam, and midazolam are available for parenteral use. In liver disease, oxazepam, temazepam, and lorazepam are preferred as they do not undergo phase 1 metabolism (i.e., oxidation), but only phase 2 by glucuronidation. Benzodiazepines act within few minutes of administration, which makes them very appealing for rapid anxiety relief. Due to their potential for tolerance and cognitive decline in the longer term, prolonged use of benzodiazepines should be avoided. Their use pre- and post-transplant can also increase risk of delirium. Cigarette smoking may increase clearance of alprazolam, lorazepam, oxazepam, diazepam, and demethyldiazepam [94].

Lorazepam

Its availability for oral, intravenous, and intramuscular use makes lorazepam a very appealing medication in many settings. Lorazepam elimination half-life is 12–15 hours and protein binding is around 90%. Its metabolite, lorazepam glucuronide, is inactive and excreted in urine. Use in severe renal impairment is not recommended. Use in severe hepatic impairment requires caution and dose adjustment.

Clonazepam

Clonazepam is orally administered. It undergoes extensive hepatic metabolism including involvement of the CYP system as well as conjugation reactions. Its metabolites are inactive and undergo renal excretion. Clonazepam is 85% bound to proteins. Its half-life eliminations is 17–60 hours in adults. In renal and hepatic impairment, clonazepam should be used with caution due to risk of accumulation.

Alprazolam

Alprazolam is available for oral use. Extended release presentations are available. Alprazolam undergoes metabolism via CYP3A4 to active and inactive metabolites, which do not appear to be clinically significant. Protein binding is around 80–90%. Elimination of immediate release formulations is between 6 and 16 hours. Dose adjustment in advanced hepatic impairment is necessary. Pharmacokinetic studies in special populations such as in patients with liver or kidney impairment are lacking for the extended release formulation.

Other

Buspirone

Buspirone is a non-benzodiazepine anxiolytic used in the treatment of generalized anxiety disorder. Its mechanism of action is not well understood, but it is likely through suppression of serotonergic activity and enhancement of noradrenergic and dopaminergic cell firing [95]. Its main action seems to be a partial agonism of 5-HT1A receptors. Buspirone undergoes extensive first-pass effect, and it is metabolized via hepatic oxidation, primarily via CYP3A4 to active and inactive metabolites. Buspirone elimination half-life is 1–10 hours. Anxiolytic activity starts around 4 weeks into the initiation. Use in patients with pulmonary pathology may be advantageous given its lack of respiratory depression. Half-life elimination is prolonged in renal and hepatic impairment. The administration of buspirone in advanced kidney and liver disease is not recommended.

Antipsychotics

Typical and atypical antipsychotics are used in the transplant population for treatment of preexisting and new onset psychosis and mood disorders, delirium, and refractory anxiety. Antipsychotic use in the post-transplant patients brings about concerns related to QTc prolongation [41], particularly when co-administered with tacrolimus which can also prolong the QT and/or cyclosporine which could increase the risk of arrhythmia.

Typical Antipsychotics

Haloperidol

Haloperidol is a high-potency typical antipsychotic. The therapeutic effect in the treatment of positive psychotic symptoms is thought to result from the central postsynaptic dopamine-2 receptor blockade in the mesolimbic pathway [96]. Haloperidol is available for oral and parenteral (i.e., IM and IV) administration. Intravenous use of haloperidol is not approved by the FDA; however, it is frequently used in the intensive care setting where cardiac monitoring is continuous and for the management of postoperative agitation and/or delirium or immunosuppressant-induced psychotic symptoms. Haloperidol is metabolized by glucuronidation and via CYP2D6 and CYP3A4 isozymes, to inactive metabolites. Haloperidol is 90% protein bound. No dose adjustment is needed in renal or hepatic impairment. Frequent monitoring of QTc for potential prolongation is recommended. Pseudoparkinsonism and other extrapyramidal symptoms can result from dopamine blockade in the nigrostriatal pathway; therefore, this is an additional aspect that requires close monitoring, taking into account that calcineurin inhibitors can cause myoclonus and tremors. Slow CYP2D6 metabolizers may be at increased risk for haloperidol side effects.

Atypical Antipsychotics

Atypical antipsychotics can increase risk of dyslipidemias, obesity, glucose intolerance, and hypertension [96]. In the transplant setting, this side effect profile represents an added concern given the similarities with that of the immunosuppressant agents.

Aripiprazole

Aripiprazole is available in oral and intramuscular extended release forms. The oral forms include tablet, disintegrated tablet, and solution. The mechanism of action of aripiprazole is unique among antipsychotics due to its partial agonism of dopaminergic D-2 receptors. It is also a partial agonist of 5-HT1A receptors and an antagonist of 5-HT2A receptors. This medication seems to be one of the least QTc prolonging among the antipsychotics [41]. Aripiprazole is metabolized by CYP3A4 and CYP2D6 to an active metabolite, dehydroaripiprazole. No dose adjustment is needed in hepatic or renal impairment. The elimination half-life of immediate release aripiprazole is 75 hours and 94 hours for dehydroaripiprazole. For poor CYP2D6 metabolizers, half-life elimination of aripiprazole is 146 hours [97].

Olanzapine

Olanzapine can be administered by mouth in the forms of regular tablet form and orally disintegrated tablet. Olanzapine is also available for intramuscular administration in immediate and extended release injections. Olanzapine is a potent antagonist of serotonin 5-HT2A and 5-HT2C, dopamine D 1–4, histamine H1, and alpha1-adrenergic receptors [96]. Olanzapine has moderate antagonism of 5-HT3 and muscarinic M1–5 receptors. Olanzapine is metabolized by direct glucuronidation and oxidation via CYP1A2 and CYP2D6. Cigarette smoking may alter its metabolism via CYP1A2 induction. Olanzapine dose does not need to be adjusted in renal impairment and is not dialyzable. Olanzapine dose does not require adjustment in liver impairment except when given in combination with fluoxetine. In that case the manufacturer recommends that the initial olanzapine dose should be limited to 2.5 to 5 mg daily [98].

Quetiapine

Quetiapine is available in immediate and extended release oral forms. Quetiapine is an antagonist of serotonin 5-HT1A and 5-HT2, dopamine D1 and D2, histamine H1, and adrenergic alpha1- and alpha2 receptors. It is metabolized by CYP3A4 to active and inactive compounds. In the setting of hepatic impairment, there is a 30% reduction in the medication clearance. Half-life of quetiapine in patients with normal hepatic function is roughly 6 hours. Patients with creatinine clearance between 10 and 30 mL/min have a decrease in the clearance of the drug of approximately 25% [99]. Due to its alpha1-antagonist effect, it can cause significant hypotension, which can be an issue in fragile postoperative patients.

Risperidone

Risperidone is available for oral administration in the forms of tablet, orally disintegrated tablet, and oral solution. Risperidone can also be administered intramuscularly in the form of reconstituted suspension. Risperidone has a high 5-HT2 and dopamine D2 receptor antagonist activity. It also antagonizes alpha1, alpha2-adrenergic, and histaminergic receptors. Risperidone has low to moderate affinity for 5-HT1C, 5-HT1D, and 5-HT1A receptors. Risperidone is metabolized mainly by CYP2D6 to 9-hydroxyrisperidone. N-dealkylation is a second minor pathway. Risperidone dose needs to be adjusted in renal and hepatic impairment [100].

Lurasidone

Lurasidone is an atypical antipsychotic with mixed serotonin-dopamine antagonist activity. Lurasidone exhibits high affinity for D2, 5-HT2A, and 5-HT7 receptors and moderate affinity for alpha2C-adrenergic receptors and is a partial agonist for 5-HT1A receptors. Lurasidone is available in tablet form. The absorption of lurasidone is increased in the fed state. Lurasidone is metabolized via CYP3A4. It requires dose adjustment in moderate kidney and hepatic impairment. Lurasidone seems to have a minimal impact on QTc prolongation [101].

Antiepileptic Drugs (AEDs)

Gabapentin

Although gabapentin is structurally similar to the neurotransmitter GABA, it does not bind to $GABA_A$ or $GABA_B$ receptors, and it does not appear to influence synthesis or uptake of GABA [102]. High-affinity gabapentin binding sites have been located throughout the brain; these sites correspond to the presence of voltage-gated calcium channels specifically possessing the alpha2-delta-1 subunit [102]. This channel appears to be located presynaptically and may modulate the release of excitatory neurotransmitters which participate in epileptogenesis and nociception. Gabapentin is not metabolized by the liver. It is only 3% protein bound and it lacks significant drug interactions. It was developed as an anticonvulsant, and it has been used as adjunct in the treatment of partial seizures. It has also been used in the treatment of spasticity in multiple sclerosis, amyotrophic lateral sclerosis, postherpetic neuralgia, and moderate to severe primary restless legs syndrome. Gabapentin has also been used in the setting of alcohol withdrawal and dependence, with positive results for decreased cravings and anxiety and improved sleep [103–105]. In addition, it is used for acute and neuropathic pain and can be helpful for treatment of social phobia [106]. Gabapentin is also used for treatment of anxiety [102] and has been suggested for such use in transplant populations, especially when benzodiazepines are to be avoided [69]. However, further studies specific to transplant populations are needed. Due to its renal excretion, gabapentin dose needs adjustment based on creatinine clearance. Additionally, after a 4-hour hemodialysis, a small supplemental dose may be necessary. Side effects include sedation and myoclonus.

Valproic Acid

Valproic acid is approved for the treatment of different seizure types, prophylaxis for migraine, and management of mania associated with bipolar disorder. It has also been used for delirium management [107]. Valproic acid undergoes extensive hepatic metabolism mainly via glucuronide conjugation, mitochondrial beta-oxidation, and in lesser extent oxidation by CYP2C9, CYP2C19, and CYP2A6 [108]. Protein binding is 80–90% and dependent on drug concentration. Half-life elimination is 9–19 hours in adults [108]. Valproic acid does not need dose adjustment in renal impairment; however, monitoring of free fraction of the drug instead of the total fraction is more appropriate, given that in kidney disease protein binding decreases. The use of valproic acid is not recommended in patients with liver impairment due to decreased clearance and the risk of hepatotoxicity. Hepatic disease is also associated with decreased albumin concentrations and increase in the free drug fraction. Free instead of total concentrations of valproic acid should be monitored in liver impairment, if the medication is indeed used in this setting [109]. Other conditions that lead to increased free fraction of the drug are cachexia and elevated free fatty acids. Elevated free fraction increases risk of lethargy and cognitive slowing. Of note, valproic acid is decreased by 80% when combined with carbapenems [108]. Other undesirable side effects for the transplant patients include thrombocytopenia and platelet dysfunction; hence, close monitoring is needed [110]. Moreover, valproic acid carries a black box warning against life-threatening pancreatitis. It is contraindicated in pregnancy due to significant risk of congenital malformations, such as neural tube defects, and decreased intelligence quotient (IQ) scores in offspring.

Carbamazepine

Carbamazepine has multiple properties including anticonvulsant, anticholinergic, antineuralgic, antidiuretic, muscle relaxant, mood stabilizing, and antiarrhythmic. Carbamazepine is metabolized via CYP3A4 to an active metabolite. Carbamazepine is considered a potent inducer of CYP3A4 (autoinduction). Given that immunosuppressants are for the most part metabolized by this isozyme, the concurrent use of carbamazepine will likely reduce their levels risking rejection. As carbamazepine is an autoinductor, its half-life is variable for the first 3–5 weeks after initiation of a fixed carbamazepine dose. In addition to drug-drug interactions with immunosuppressants, another problematic aspect of carbamazepine use in transplant patients is the risk for leukopenia and blood dyscrasias, such as aplastic anemia and agranulocytosis [110]. Carbamazepine can alter bone metabolism and vitamin D levels. Carbamazepine should be used with caution in hepatic impairment, and it may require discontinuation if liver function worsens or dysfunction becomes apparent. It requires dose adjustment in renal impairment.

Oxcarbazepine

Compared to carbamazepine, oxcarbazepine is not associated with blood dyscrasias. It is a weak inducer of CYP3A4 but can still decrease immunosuppressant levels. It has also been associated with decreased vitamin D levels. Autoinduction has not been observed. Oxcarbazepine is metabolized in the liver to an active compound. Oxcarbazepine is a dose-dependent CYP2C19 inhibitor. Hyponatremia is a common side effect. Oxcarbazepine has not been studied in severe hepatic impairment. In renal impairment the clearance of the active metabolite changes from approximately 9 hours to 19 hours.

Topiramate

Besides its uses in the treatment of several types of seizures and migraine prophylaxis, topiramate continues to be studied as adjunctive therapy for bipolar disorder. It also has emerging evidence for treatment of alcohol dependence [111]. Topiramate is not extensively metabolized, with nearly 70% of the dose being eliminated by the kidney unchanged. Topiramate requires adjustment for renal impairment and an added post-dialysis dose. It should be used with caution in hepatic impairment given that its clearance can be reduced. Overall, due to its side effects, including cognitive dysfunction, topiramate is not desirable in patients receiving potentially neurotoxic medications such as CNIs.

Lithium

Lithium is available in oral form. Lithium is approved for the treatment of manic episodes and as maintenance treatment for bipolar I disorder. Lithium is also effective as an adjunct for refractory depression and for reducing the risk of suicide in patients with mood disorders [96]. Lithium is not metabolized by liver and is eliminated solely by the kidney [96]. It has minimal protein binding of 15%. Dose needs to be adjusted according to creatinine clearance and dialysis status. Its half-life elimination in adults is 18–36 hours. Lithium clearance is affected by kidney function as well as by hyponatremia, hypernatremia, diuretic use, and dehydration [112]. Potential electrolyte changes and fluid shifts in transplant patients and the potential concurrent use with sodium-depleting diuretics, especially thiazides and angiotensin-converting enzyme inhibitors, make the safe use of lithium challenging in the post-transplant patient, particularly early after surgery. Lithium can cause adverse effects in the heart, believed to be related to intracellular hypokalemia and extracellular hyperkalemia imbalance that can give rise to cardiac arrest. It can also cause nephrotoxicity, tremors, weight gain, and cognitive slowing, all potential side effects of commonly used immunosuppressants. Therefore, the use of lithium in the late post-transplant patient needs to be carefully considered using the best clinical judgment and individualized approach based on the patient's history.

Medications Used in the Treatment of Substance Use Disorders

Acamprosate

Acamprosate appears to increase the activity of the GABA-ergic system, and decreases activity of glutamate within the CNS, including a decrease in activity at N-methyl D-aspartate (NMDA) receptors. Acamprosate may affect CNS calcium channels. Acamprosate does not undergo hepatic metabolism and is eliminated unchanged via the kidneys. It requires dose adjustment in renal impairment, and it is contraindicated when creatinine clearance is lower than 30% [113].

Disulfiram

Disulfiram interferes with the hepatic oxidation of acetaldehyde, which leads to its accumulation and unpleasant symptoms if the patient ingests ethanol. Symptoms include throbbing headache and neck, dyspnea, vomiting, diaphoresis, thirst, chest pain, palpitations, hypotension, blurred vision, vertigo, weakness, anxiety, syncope, and confusion. Cardiac collapse and deaths have been reported [114, 115]. Disulfiram has also been associated with rare cases of fulminant hepatic failure, and liver transplantation in such a patient has been reported [116]. Due to multiple potential interactions with other drugs, disulfiram is not recommended in transplant patients.

Naltrexone

Naltrexone is an opioid antagonist used to help maintain an opioid-free state in patients with opioid use disorders and in the management of patients with alcohol use disorder, decreasing the cravings, alcohol use, and alcohol relapse. Naltrexone is associated with increased risk for hepatotoxicity [117]. The CYP system is not involved in the metabolism of naltrexone. Dose adjustment may be necessary in hepatic and renal impairment. Naltrexone needs to be discontinued when pain control requires opioid agonists, such as prior or after surgical procedures.

Methadone

Methadone is an opioid agonist used in the maintenance of opioid use disorder [118, 119]. It undergoes hepatic metabolism via CYP3A4, CYP2D6, CYP2B6, CYP2C19, and CYP2C9 and is a substrate of P-glycoprotein [119]. It requires dose adjustment in severe renal impairment and caution is needed in hepatic impairment. Methadone can prolong QTc, and thus monitoring is required [118]. Methadone half-life varies between 8 hours and 59 hours in adults. Management of pain postoperatively can be accomplished by continuing the pre-transplant methadone dose and adding another opioid temporarily or increasing the pre-transplant methadone dose. With chronic use, methadone can autoinduce its metabolism. Please see Chap. 45 on further discussion of methadone in transplant patients.

Buprenorphine

Buprenorphine is a semisynthetic mixed opioid agonist-antagonist. It has a ceiling effect which may make it comparatively safer than full opioid agonists [119]. It is metabolized by CYP3A4. See Chap. 45 on further discussion of buprenorphine in transplant patients.

Alpha2 Agonists

Dexmedetomidine

Dexmedetomidine is a selective alpha$_2$-adrenoceptor agonist with sympatholytic, sedative, and analgesic effects, similar to clonidine. Intravenous dexmedetomidine drips are used in intensive care settings for the management of sedation in patients requiring ventilatory support or periprocedurally. It has been shown to decrease risk of delirium in ICU populations, as compared to other sedative drips, such as propofol or benzodiazepines [120, 121].

Protective neurocognitive effects in orthotopic liver transplantation are being studied with encouraging results; however, further research is needed [122]. Dexmedetomidine

undergoes hepatic metabolism via N-glucuronidation, N-methylation, and CYP2A6. Its elimination half-life is 2 hours. Although no dose adjustment is recommended in kidney impairment, dose reduction should be considered in hepatic impairment as the clearance is reduced in varying degrees based on the level of impairment. Dexmedetomidine can cause bradycardia and lower blood pressure.

Conclusions

Transplant recipients are at increased risk for cognitive, anxiety, and mood disorders; thus they may require treatment with a variety of psychopharmacological agents. Clinicians should be aware of neuropsychiatric side effects of medications used in transplant recipients, pharmacodynamics and pharmacokinetics of psychotropic agents in patients with end-stage organ disease and post-transplant, and drug-drug interactions. Some general guidelines are summarized below:

- Most immunosuppressant agents are substrates of CYP3A4; hence, attention needs to be given to the multiple potential interactions with psychiatric medications.
- In general, start psychiatric medications at a low dose and titrate slowly while monitoring for potential side effects and drug-drug interactions.
- Monitor for recent changes of concurrent medications, as additions or discontinuations may alter the metabolism of the remaining medications, and adjust accordingly.
- CNIs are nephrotoxic, and mTOR inhibitors can cause kidney function alterations; hence, close monitoring and adjustment of psychiatric medications such as lithium and gabapentin may become necessary.
- Discontinue medications when they are no longer needed and caution patients and team members of the potential consequences of introduced changes as well as the signs and symptoms that need to be monitored.
- Inquire about all medications the patient is taking, including herbal supplements.
- Avoid starting new medications in a long-acting form if possible. This will allow rapid withdrawal of the medication in case of intolerable side effects.

References

1. Dew MA, DiMartini AF, DeVito Dabbs AJ, Fox KR, Myaskovsky L, Posluszny DM, et al. Onset and risk factors for anxiety and depression during the first 2 years after lung transplantation. Gen Hosp Psychiatry. 2012;34(2):127–38.
2. Dew MA, Kormos RL, DiMartini AF, Switzer GE, Schulberg HC, Roth LH, et al. Prevalence and risk of depression and anxiety-

related disorders during the first three years after heart transplantation. Psychosomatics. 2001;42(4):300–13.

3. Dew MA, Rosenberger EM, Myaskovsky L, DiMartini AF, DeVito Dabbs AJ, Posluszny DM, et al. Depression and anxiety as risk factors for morbidity and mortality after organ transplantation: a systematic review and meta-analysis. Transplantation. 2015;100(5):988–1003.

4. Smith PJ, Rivelli S, Waters A, Reynolds J, Hoyle A, Flowers M, et al. Neurocognitive changes after lung transplantation. Ann Am Thorac Soc. 2014;11(10):1520–7.

5. Smith PJ, Rivelli SK, Waters AM, Hoyle A, Durheim MT, Reynolds JM, et al. Delirium affects length of hospital stay after lung transplantation. J Crit Care. 2015;30(1):126–9.

6. Basinski JR, Alfano CM, Katon WJ, Syrjala KL, Fann JR. Impact of delirium on distress, health-related quality of life, and cognition 6 months and 1 year after hematopoietic cell transplant. Biol Blood Marrow Transplant J Am Soc Blood Marrow Transplant. [Clinical Trial Research Support, N.I.H., Extramural Research Support, Non-U.S. Gov't]. 2010;16(6):824–31.

7. DiMartini A, Crone C, Fireman M, Dew MA. Psychiatric aspects of organ transplantation in critical care. Crit care Clin. [Research Support, N.I.H., Extramural Review]. 2008;24(4):949–81, x.

8. Rang H, Ritter R, Flower RJ, Rang GH. Drug metabolism and elimination. Rang and Dale's pharmacology. Livingstone: Elsevier Churchill; 2016. p. 116–24.

9. Enright EF, Gahan CG, Joyce SA, Griffin BT. The Impact of the Gut Microbiota on Drug Metabolism and Clinical Outcome. Yale J Biol Med. [Review Research Support, Non-U.S. Gov't]. 2016;89(3):375–82.

10. Klaassen CD, Cui JY. Review: mechanisms of how the intestinal microbiota alters the effects of drugs and bile acids. Drug Metab Dispos Biol Fate Chem. [Research Support, N.I.H., Extramural Review]. 2015;43(10):1505–21.

11. Dreisbach AW, Lertora JJ. The effect of chronic renal failure on hepatic drug metabolism and drug disposition. Semin Dial. [Research Support, Non-U.S. Gov't Research Support, U.S. Gov't, P.H.S. Review]. 2003;16(1):45–50.

12. Holford NG. Pharmacokinetics & pharmacodynamics: rational dosing & the time course of drug action. In: Katzung BG, Trevor AJ, editors. Basic and clinical pharmacology. 13th ed. New York: McGraw-Hill; 2015.

13. Lake DF, Briggs AD. Immunopharmacology. In: Katzung BG, Trevor AJ, editors. Basic and clinical pharmacology. 13th ed. New York: McGraw-Hill; 2015.

14. Muller J, Keiser M, Drozdzik M, Oswald S. Expression, regulation and function of intestinal drug transporters: an update. Biol Chem. [Review Research Support, Non-U.S. Gov't]. 2017;398(2):175–92.

15. Levitsky J, Goldberg D, Smith AR, Mansfield SA, Gillespie BW, Merion RM, et al. Acute rejection increases risk of graft failure and death in recent liver transplant recipients. Clin Gastroenterol Hepatol Off Clin Pract J Am Gastroenterol Assoc. [Observational Study]. 2017;15(4):584–93e2.

16. Fireman M, DiMartini A, Crone C. Organ transplantation. In: Ferrando S, Levenson JL, Owen JA, editors. Clinical manual of psychopharmacology in medically ill. Arlington: American Psychiatric Publishing; 2010. p. 597–631.

17. Wu GS, Cruz RJ Jr, Cai JC. Acute antibody-mediated rejection after intestinal transplantation. World J Transplant. 2016;6(4):719–28.

18. Lake J. Liver transplantation. In: Friedman S, editor. Current diagnosis and treatmetn in gastroenterology. New York: McGraw-Hill; 2003. p. 813–34.

19. Fireman M, DiMartini AF, Armstrong SC, Cozza KL. Immunosuppressants. Psychosomatics. [Review]. 2004;45(4):354–60.

20. Wynn G. Transplant surgery and rheumatology. Immunosuppressants. In: Wynn G, Oesterheld J, Gozza K, Armstrong S, editors. Clinical manual of drug interaction principles for medical practice. Washingon, DC: American Psychiatric Publishing, Inc.; 2009. p. 461–72.

21. Dubovsky AN, Arvikar S, Stern TA, Axelrod L. The neuropsychiatric complications of glucocorticoid use: steroid psychosis revisited. Psychosomatics. [Review]. 2012;53(2):103–15.

22. Wolkowitz OM. Long-lasting behavioral changes following prednisone withdrawal. JAMA. [Case Reports Letter]. 1989;261(12):1731–2.

23. Fardet L, Nazareth I, Whitaker HJ, Petersen I. Severe neuropsychiatric outcomes following discontinuation of long-term glucocorticoid therapy: a cohort study. J Clin Psychiatry. 2013;74(4):e281–6.

24. West S, Kenedi C. Strategies to prevent the neuropsychiatric side-effects of corticosteroids: a case report and review of the literature. Curr Opin Organ Transplant.. [Case Reports Review]. 2014;19(2):201–8.

25. Goldman LS, Goveas J. Olanzapine treatment of corticosteroid-induced mood disorders. Psychosomatics. [Case Reports]. 2002;43(6):495–7.

26. Roxanas MG, Hunt GE. Rapid reversal of corticosteroid-induced mania with sodium valproate: a case series of 20 patients. Psychosomatics. 2012;53(6):575–81.

27. Viswanathan R, Glickman L. Clonazepam in the treatment of steroid-induced mania in a patient after renal transplantation. N Engl J Med.. [Case Reports Letter]. 1989;320(5):319–20.

28. Sun X, Wu Y, Chen B, Zhang Z, Zhou W, Tong Y, et al. Regulator of calcineurin 1 (RCAN1) facilitates neuronal apoptosis through caspase-3 activation. J Biol Chem. [Research Support, Non-U.S. Gov't]. 2011;286(11):9049–62.

29. Trzepacz PT, DiMartini A, Tringali R. Psychopharmacologic issues in organ transplantation. Part I: Pharmacokinetics in organ failure and psychiatric aspects of immunosuppressants and anti-infectious agents. Psychosomatics. [Review]. 1993;34(3):199–207.

30. Song T, Rao Z, Tan Q, Qiu Y, Liu J, Huang Z, et al. Calcineurin inhibitors associated posterior reversible encephalopathy syndrome in solid organ transplantation: report of 2 cases and literature review. Medicine. [Case Reports Research Support, Non-U.S. Gov't Review]. 2016;95(14):e3173.

31. Rosso L, Nosotti M, Mendogni P, Palleschi A, Tosi D, Montoli M, et al. Lung transplantation and posterior reversible encephalopathy syndrome: a case series. Transplant Proc. 2012;44(7):2022–5.

32. Smith PJ, Stonerock GL, Ingle KK, Saulino CK, Hoffman B, Wasserman B, et al. Neurological sequelae and clinical outcomes after lung transplantation. Transplant Direct. 2018;4(4):e353.

33. Chen S, Hu J, Xu L, Brandon D, Yu J, Zhang J. Posterior reversible encephalopathy syndrome after transplantation: a review. Mol Neurobiol. [Review]. 2016;53(10):6897–909.

34. Schusse CM, Peterson AL, Caplan JP. Posterior reversible encephalopathy syndrome. Psychosomatics. [Case Reports Review]. 2013;54(3):205–11.

35. Hayes D Jr, Adler B, Turner TL, Mansour HM. Alternative tacrolimus and sirolimus regimen associated with rapid resolution of posterior reversible encephalopathy syndrome after lung transplantation. Pediatr Neurol. [Case Reports]. 2014;50(3):272–5.

36. Curtis JJ, Jones P, Barbeito R. Large within-day variation in cyclosporine absorption: circadian variation or food effect? Clin J Am Soc Nephrol CJASN. [Research Support, Non-U.S. Gov't]. 2006;1(3):462–6.

37. Aronson J. Meyler's side effects of herbal medicines. Amsterdam: Elsevier Science; 2008.

38. Finsterer J, Ohnsorge P. Influence of mitochondrion-toxic agents on the cardiovascular system. Regul Toxicol Pharmacol RTP [Review]. 2013;67(3):434–45.

39. Hodak SP, Moubarak JB, Rodriguez I, Gelfand MC, Alijani MR, Tracy CM. QT prolongation and near fatal cardiac arrhythmia after intravenous tacrolimus administration: a case report. Transplantation. [Case Reports Research Support, Non-U.S. Gov't]. 1998;66(4):535–7.

40. Ikitimur B, Cosansu K, Karadag B, Cakmak HA, Avci BK, Erturk E, et al. Long-term impact of different immunosuppressive drugs on QT and PR intervals in renal transplant patients. Ann Noninvasive Electrocardiol Off J Int Soc Holter Noninvasive Electrocardiol Inc. 2015;20(5):426–32.

41. Beach SR, Celano CM, Noseworthy PA, Januzzi JL, Huffman JC. QTc prolongation, torsades de pointes, and psychotropic medications. Psychosomatics. [Review]. 2013;54(1):1–13.

42. Bradley J, Watson C. mTOR inhibitors: Sirolimus and everolimus. In: Morris P, Knechtle S, editors. Kidney transplantation: principles and practice. London: Elsevier Health Sciences; 2014. p. 267–86.

43. Atgam (lymphocyte immune globulin, antithymocyte globulin [equine]) [prescribing information]. New York: Pfizer, Inc; 2015.

44. Thymoglobulin (antithymocyte glbolung [rabbit] package insert. Cambridge, MA: Genzyme Corportaion; 2016.

45. Simulect (basiliximab) package insert. East Hanover: Novartis Pharmaceuticals Corporation; 2005.

46. Campath (alemtuzumab) package insert. Cambridge, MA: Genzyme Corporation; 2014.

47. Lemtrada (alemtuzumab) injection package insert. Camridge, MA: Genzyme Corporation; 2017.

48. Rituxan (rituximab) package insert. South San Francisco: Genentech, Inc.; 2013.

49. Myfortic (mycophenolate sodium) [prescribing information]. East Hanover: Novartis Pharmaceuticals Corporation; 2015.

50. Azathioprine.Lexicomp Online®, Lexi-Drugs. Hudson: Lexi-Comp, Inc.; 2017.

51. Gruessner A, Jie T, Papas K, Porubsky M, Rana A, Smith M, et al. Transplantation. In: Bruncardi F, Andersen D, Billiar T, Dunn D, Hunter J, Matthews J, et al., editors. Schwartz's principles of surgery. New York: McGraw-Hill; 2015.

52. O'Connor CM, Jiang W, Kuchibhatla M, Silva SG, Cuffe MS, Callwood DD, et al. Safety and efficacy of sertraline for depression in patients with heart failure: results of the SADHART-CHF (Sertraline against depression and heart disease in chronic heart failure) trial. J Am Coll Cardiol. [Randomized Controlled Trial Research Support, N.I.H., Extramural]. 2010;56(9):692–9.

53. Kalender B, Ozdemir AC, Yalug I, Dervisoglu E. Antidepressant treatment increases quality of life in patients with chronic renal failure. Ren Fail. 2007;29(7):817–22.

54. Gottlieb SS, Kop WJ, Thomas SA, Katzen S, Vesely MR, Greenberg N, et al. A double-blind placebo-controlled pilot study of controlled-release paroxetine on depression and quality of life in chronic heart failure. Am Heart J. [Randomized Controlled Trial Research Support, Non-U.S. Gov't Research Support, U.S. Gov't, Non-P.H.S.]. 2007;153(5):868–73.

55. Jeong BO, Kim SW, Kim SY, Kim JM, Shin IS, Yoon JS. Use of serotonergic antidepressants and bleeding risk in patients undergoing surgery. Psychosomatics. [Review]. 2014;55(3):213–20.

56. Eckersley MJ, Sepehripour AH, Casula R, Punjabi P, Athanasiou T. Do selective serotonin reuptake inhibitors increase the risk of bleeding or mortality following coronary artery bypass graft surgery? A meta-analysis of observational studies. Perfusion. 2018;1:267659118765933.

57. Varela Pinon M, Adan-Manes J. Selective Serotonin reuptake inhibitor-induced hyponatremia: clinical implications and therapeutic alternatives. Clin Neuropharmacol. [Case Reports]. 2017;40(4):177–9.

58. De Picker L, Van Den Eede F, Dumont G, Moorkens G, Sabbe BG. Antidepressants and the risk of hyponatremia: a class-by-class review of literature. Psychosomatics. [Review]. 2014;55(6):536–47.

59. Tsapakis EM, Gamie Z, Tran GT, Adshead S, Lampard A, Mantalaris A, et al. The adverse skeletal effects of selective serotonin reuptake inhibitors. Eur Psychiatry J Assoc Eur Psychiatr. [Review]. 2012;27(3):156–69.

60. Sher Y, Zimbrean P. Psychiatric aspects of organ transplantation in critical care: an update. Crit Care Clin. [Review]. 2017;33(3):659–79.

61. DeBattista C. Antidepressant agents. In: Katzung B, Trevor A, editors. Basic and clinical pharmacology. New York: McGraw-Hill; 2015.

62. Crewe HK, Lennard MS, Tucker GT, Woods FR, Haddock RE. The effect of selective serotonin re-uptake inhibitors on cytochrome P4502D6 (CYP2D6) activity in human liver microsomes. Br J Clin Pharmacol. [Comparative Study]. 1992;34(3):262–5.

63. Ozdemir V, Naranjo CA, Herrmann N, Shulman RW, Sellers EM, Reed K, et al. The extent and determinants of changes in CYP2D6 and CYP1A2 activities with therapeutic doses of sertraline. J ClinPsychopharmacol. [Comparative Study Research Support, Non-U.S. Gov't]. 1998;18(1):55–61.

64. Preskorn SH, Alderman J, Greenblatt DJ, Horst WD. Sertraline does not inhibit cytochrome P450 3A-mediated drug metabolism in vivo. Psychopharmacol Bull [Comparative Study]. 1997;33(4):659–65.

65. Lill J, Bauer LA, Horn JR, Hansten PD. Cyclosporine-drug interactions and the influence of patient age. Am J Health Syst Pharm AJHP Off J Am Soc Health Syst Pharm. [Research Support, Non-U.S. Gov't]. 2000;57(17):1579–84.

66. Mayo MJ, Handem I, Saldana S, Jacobe H, Getachew Y, Rush AJ. Sertraline as a first-line treatment for cholestatic pruritus. Hepatology. [Randomized Controlled Trial Research Support, N.I.H., Extramural Research Support, Non-U.S. Gov't]. 2007;45(3):666–74.

67. Smoller JW, Pollack MH, Systrom D, Kradin RL. Sertraline effects on dyspnea in patients with obstructive airways disease. Psychosomatics. [Case Reports]. 1998;39(1):24–9.

68. Yalcin AU, Sahin G, Erol M, Bal C. Sertraline hydrochloride treatment for patients with hemodialysis hypotension. Blood Purif. [Clinical Trial]. 2002;20(2):150–3.

69. Crone CC, Gabriel GM. Treatment of anxiety and depression in transplant patients: pharmacokinetic considerations. Clin Pharmacokinet. [Comparative Study Review]. 2004;43(6):361–94.

70. Sandson NB, Armstrong SC, Cozza KL. An overview of psychotropic drug-drug interactions. Psychosomatics. [Review]. 2005;46(5):464–94.

71. FDA Drug Safety Communication: revised recommendations for Celexa (citalopram hydrobromide) related to a potential risk of abnormal heart rhythms with high doses. U.S. Food and Drug Administration; 2012 [cited 2018 5/14/2018]; Available from: https://www.fda.gov/Drugs/DrugSafety/ucm297391.htm.

72. Gerlach LB, Kales HC, Maust DT, Chiang C, Stano C, Choe HM, et al. Unintended consequences of adjusting citalopram prescriptions following the 2011 FDA warning. Am J Geriatr Psychiatry Off J Am Assoc Geriatr Psychiatry. 2017;25(4):407–14.

73. Newey CR, Khawam E, Coffman K. Two cases of serotonin syndrome with venlafaxine and calcineurin inhibitors. Psychosomatics. [Case Reports]. 2011;52(3):286–90.

74. Desvenlafaxine. Lexicomp® Online, Lexi-Drugs. Hudson: Lexi-Comp, Inc; [cited 2017 28 Dec]; Available from: https://online.lexi.com.

75. Voican CS, Corruble E, Naveau S, Perlemuter G. Antidepressant-induced liver injury: a review for clinicians. Am J Psychiatry. [Review]. 2014;171(4):404–15.

76. Wernicke J, Pangallo B, Wang F, Murray I, Henck JW, Knadler MP, et al. Hepatic effects of duloxetine-I: non-clinical and clinical

trial data. Curr Drug Saf. [Research Support, Non-U.S. Gov't Review]. 2008;3(2):132–42.

77. Hartmann PM. Mirtazapine: a newer antidepressant. Am Fam Physician. [Review]. 1999;59(1):159–61.

78. Jamilloux Y, Kerever S, Ferry T, Broussolle C, Honnorat J, Seve P. Treatment of progressive multifocal Leukoencephalopathy With Mirtazapine. Clin Drug Investig. [Review]. 2016;36(10):783–9.

79. Boinpally R, Alcorn H, Adams MH, Longstreth J, Edwards J. Pharmacokinetics of vilazodone in patients with mild or moderate renal impairment. Clin Drug Investig. [Clinical Trial, Phase I Research Support, Non-U.S. Gov't]. 2013;33(3):199–206.

80. Owen JR, Nemeroff CB. New antidepressants and the cytochrome P450 system: focus on venlafaxine, nefazodone, and mirtazapine. Depress Anxiety. [Research Support, U.S. Gov't, P.H.S. Review]. 1998;7(Suppl 1):24–32.

81. Nefazodone hydrochloride tablet package insert. Jacksonville: Ranbaxy Pharmaceutical Inc.; 2008.

82. Livingston MG, Livingston HM. Monoamine oxidase inhibitors. An update on drug interactions. Drug Saf. [Review]. 1996;14(4):219–27.

83. Borrelli F, Izzo AA. Herb-drug interactions with St John's wort (Hypericum perforatum): an update on clinical observations. AAPS J. [Review]. 2009;11(4):710–27.

84. Moschella C, Jaber BL. Interaction between cyclosporine and Hypericum perforatum (St. John's wort) after organ transplantation. Am J kidney Dis Off J Natl Kidney Found. [Case Reports]. 2001;38(5):1105–7.

85. Turton-Weeks SM, Barone GW, Gurley BJ, Ketel BL, Lightfoot ML, Abul-Ezz SR. St John's wort: a hidden risk for transplant patients. Prog Transplant. [Case Reports]. 2001;11(2):116–20.

86. Hardy SE. Methylphenidate for the treatment of depressive symptoms, including fatigue and apathy, in medically ill older adults and terminally ill adults. Am J Geriatr Pharmacother. [Research Support, N.I.H., Extramural Research Support, Non-U.S. Gov't Review]. 2009;7(1):34–59.

87. FDA Drug Safety Communication: safety review update of medications used to treat attention-deficit/hyperactivity disorder (ADHD) in children and young adults. U.S. Food & Drug Administration2011 [cited 2018 May 13]; Available from: https://www.fda.gov/Drugs/DrugSafety/ucm277770.htm.

88. Plutchik L, Snyder S, Drooker M, Chodoff L, Sheiner P. Methylphenidate in post liver transplant patients. Psychosomatics. [Case Reports]. 1998;39(2):118–23.

89. Tomlinson D, Robinson PD, Oberoi S, Cataudella D, Culos-Reed N, Davis H, et al. Pharmacologic interventions for fatigue in cancer and transplantation: a meta-analysis. Curr Oncol. [Review]. 2018;25(2):e152–e67.

90. Corchs F, Teng CT. Amphetamine, catatonic depression, and heart transplant: a case report. Revista Bras Psiquiatr. [Case Reports Letter]. 2010;32(3):324–6.

91. Tong HY, Diaz C, Collantes E, Medrano N, Borobia AM, Jara P, et al. Liver transplant in a patient under methylphenidate therapy: a case report and review of the literature. Case Rep Pediatr. 2015;2015:437298.

92. Dextroamphetamine. Clinical Key [cited 2018 Jan 4]; Available from: http://www.clinicalkey.com.

93. Murillo-Rodriguez E, Barciela Veras A, Barbosa Rocha N, Budde H, Machado S. An overview of the clinical uses, pharmacology, and safety of Modafinil. ACS Chem Neurosci. [Research Support, Non-U.S. Gov't]. 2018;9(2):151–8.

94. Desai HD, Seabolt J, Jann MW. Smoking in patients receiving psychotropic medications: a pharmacokinetic perspective. CNS Drugs. [Review]. 2001;15(6):469–94.

95. Eison AS, Temple DL, Jr. Buspirone: review of its pharmacology and current perspectives on its mechanism of action. Am J Med. [Review]. 1986;80(3B):1–9.

96. Meltzer H. Antipsychotic agents & lithium. In: Katzung B, Trevor A, editors. Basic and clinical pharmacology. New York: McGraw-Hill; 2015.

97. de Bartolomeis A, Tomasetti C, Iasevoli F. Update on the Mechanism of Action of Aripiprazole: Translational Insights into Antipsychotic Strategies Beyond Dopamine Receptor Antagonism. CNS Drugs. [Research Support, Non-U.S. Gov't Review]. 2015;29(9):773–99.

98. Zyprexa (olanzapine, all formulations) package insert. Indianapolis: Eli Lilly and company; 2017.

99. Quetiapine. [cited 2018 Jan 5]; Available from: http://clinicalkey.com.

100. Risperidone. Lexicomp Online ®. Lexi-drugs®. Hudson: Lexicomp, Inc; [cited 2018 Jan 5].

101. Citrome L. A review of the pharmacology, efficacy and tolerability of recently approved and upcoming oral antipsychotics: an evidence-based medicine approach. CNS Drugs. [Review]. 2013;27(11):879–911.

102. Greenblatt HK, Greenblatt DJ. Gabapentin and pregabalin for the treatment of anxiety disorders. Clinical Pharmacol Drug Dev. [Editorial]. 2018;7(3):228–32.

103. Leung JG, Hall-Flavin D, Nelson S, Schmidt KA, Schak KM. The role of gabapentin in the management of alcohol withdrawal and dependence. Ann Pharmacother. [Review]. 2015;49(8):897–906.

104. Leung JG, Rakocevic DB, Allen ND, Handler EM, Perossa BA, Borreggine KL, et al. Use of a gabapentin protocol for the Management of Alcohol Withdrawal: a preliminary experience expanding from the consultation-liaison psychiatry service. Psychosomatics. 2018;21

105. Maldonado JR. Novel Algorithms for the Prophylaxis and Management of Alcohol Withdrawal Syndromes-Beyond Benzodiazepines. Criti Care Clin. [Review]. 2017;33(3):559–99.

106. Pande AC, Davidson JR, Jefferson JW, Janney CA, Katzelnick DJ, Weisler RH, et al. Treatment of social phobia with gabapentin: a placebo-controlled study. J Clin Psychopharmacol. [Clinical Trial Multicenter Study Randomized Controlled Trial Research Support, Non-U.S. Gov't]. 1999;19(4):341–8.

107. Sher Y, Miller AC, Lolak S, Ament A, Maldonado JR. Adjunctive valproic acid in management-refractory hyperactive delirium: a case series and rationale. J Neuropsychiatr Clin Neurosci. 2015:appineuropsych14080190.

108. Sher Y, Miller Cramer AC, Ament A, Lolak S, Maldonado JR. Valproic acid for treatment of hyperactive or mixed delirium: rationale and literature review. Psychosomatics. [Review]. 2015;56(6):615–25.

109. Haroldson JA, Kramer LE, Wolff DL, Lake KD. Elevated free fractions of valproic acid in a heart transplant patient with hypoalbuminemia. Ann Pharmacother. [Case Reports]. 2000;34(2):183–7.

110. Verrotti A, Scaparrotta A, Grosso S, Chiarelli F, Coppola G. Anticonvulsant drugs and hematological disease. Neurol Sci Off J Ital Neurol Soc Ital Soc Clin Neurophysiol. [Review]. 2014;35(7):983–93.

111. Guglielmo R, Martinotti G, Quatrale M, Ioime L, Kadilli I, Di Nicola M, et al. Topiramate in alcohol use disorders: review and update. CNS Drugs. [Review]. 2015;29(5):383–95.

112. DasGupta K, Jefferson JW. The use of lithium in the medically ill. Gen Hosp Psychiatry. [Review]. 1990;12(2):83–97.

113. Acamprosate [prescribing information]. Morgantown: Mylan Pharmaceuticals Inc; 2015.

114. Moreels S, Neyrinck A, Desmet W. Intractable hypotension and myocardial ischaemia induced by co-ingestion of ethanol and disulfiram. Acta Cardiol. [Case Reports]. 2012;67(4):491–3.

115. Jeronimo A, Meira C, Amaro A, Campello GC, Granja C. Cardiogenic shock caused by disulfiram. Arq Bras Cardiol. [Case Reports]. 2009;92(3):e16–8.

116. Mohanty SR, LaBrecque DR, Mitros FA, Layden TJ. Liver transplantation for disulfiram-induced fulminant hepatic failure. J Clin Gastroenterol. [Case Reports Review]. 2004;38(3):292–5.

117. Garbutt JC. Efficacy and tolerability of naltrexone in the management of alcohol dependence. Curr Pharm Des [Review]. 2010;16(19):2091–7.

118. Westermeyer J, Adabag S, Anand V, Thuras P, Yoon G, Batres YCT. Methadone maintenance dose/weight ratio, long QTc, and EKG screening. Am J Addict. 2016;25(6):499–507.

119. Schumacher M, Basbaum A, Way W. Opioid analgesics & antagonists. In: Katzung B, Trevor A, editors. Basic and clinical pharmacology. New Yok: McGraw-Hill; 2015.

120. Xia ZQ, Chen SQ, Yao X, Xie CB, Wen SH, Liu KX. Clinical benefits of dexmedetomidine versus propofol in adult intensive care unit patients: a meta-analysis of randomized clinical trials. J Surg Res. [Comparative Study Meta-Analysis Research Support, Non-U.S. Gov't Review]. 2013;185(2):833–43.

121. Maldonado JR, Wysong A, van der Starre PJ, Block T, Miller C, Reitz BA. Dexmedetomidine and the reduction of postoperative delirium after cardiac surgery. Psychosomatics. 2009;50(3):206–17.

122. Xu G, Li LL, Sun ZT, Zhang W, Han XP. Effects of Dexmedetomidine on postoperative cognitive dysfunction and serum levels of b-amyloid and neuronal microtubule-associated protein in orthotopic liver transplantation patients. Ann transplant. [Randomized Controlled Trial]. 2016;21:508–15.

Psychotherapy in Transplant Patients

43

Mariana Schmajuk, Earl DeGuzman, and Nicole Allen

Introduction

Patients living with organ dysfunction and transplants face a complex array of stressors and challenges. Managing complex chronic health problems is emotionally demanding and time-intensive, and it is not surprising that anxiety, depression, and insomnia are prevalent in the transplant population. Even patients who have fully successful transplants must cope with adverse side effects of medications and potentially new complications. As discussed throughout this textbook, these stressors may overwhelm psychological functioning and lead to distress and suffering. Poor psychological functioning may present in a variety of ways: lower quality of life, increased nonadherence, and poor engagement in medical care.

Interventions to reduce symptoms of stress and improve quality of life after transplantation are necessary and, at times, drug-free strategies may be preferred due to the complexity of transplant medication regimens or as an adjunctive treatment.

At its heart, psychotherapy is aimed at mitigating the distress of the life cycle of transplantation from organ dysfunction to the post-transplantation period. Ultimately, through treatment with a mental health professional, patients can gain new techniques to cope with ongoing life stressors.

M. Schmajuk (✉)
Department of Psychiatry and Behavioral Sciences, Stanford University School of Medicine, Stanford, CA, USA
e-mail: m.schmajuk@stanford.edu

E. DeGuzman
Traditions Behavioral Health, Napa, CA, USA

N. Allen
Department of Psychiatry, Lenox Hill Hospital/Northwell Health, New York, NY, USA

Department of Psychiatry, Donald and Barbara Zucker School of Medicine at Hofstra/Northwell, Hempstead, NY, USA

Department of Psychiatry, SUNY Downstate School of Medicine, Brooklyn, NY, USA

Goals may include enhancing coping strategies, facilitating adjustment to living with a new organ, increasing social supports, or simply improving a patient's sense of purpose and self-esteem. Additional goals may include improving adherence to risk reduction and medical care.

Supportive and Problem-Solving Approaches

Adjusting to illness and the long-term challenges of transplantation can affect the patient's quality of life and mood. Healthcare professionals play a key role in assisting with a patient's adjustment. Supportive psychotherapy is founded in transitional psychoanalysis and is based heavily on a positive relationship between clinician and patient. It is particularly useful in two groups of patients: (1) previously well-functioning patients who are psychologically destabilized by one or more life events or (2) patients with a chronic or recurrent disability. The aim of treatment is to support the patient's more mature or adaptive defenses. The clinician aims to optimize the patient's competence in coping with current circumstances. Therapy may be complemented with psychopharmacology and education. For example, a clinician may be able to alleviate fear and uncertainty by providing clear information and education on their disease process [1].

Literature on supportive psychotherapy specifically in transplant patients is limited. One small observational study noted that almost half of all patients listed for heart transplantation, on a ventricular assist device (VAD), or successfully bridged from VAD to transplant, utilized psychological services when offered. The study suggests that this patient population experiences enough emotional distress to warrant access to and benefit from psychotherapeutic support [2].

Generally supportive therapy should focus on empowering the patient and helping them feel less vulnerable. Supportive therapy may include a substantial amount of psychoeducation and education on their medical problems in a

© Springer International Publishing AG, part of Springer Nature 2019
Y. Sher, J. R. Maldonado (eds.), *Psychosocial Care of End-Stage Organ Disease and Transplant Patients*,
https://doi.org/10.1007/978-3-319-94914-7_43

jargon-free manner. Thus, the mental health clinician's familiarity with medical processes, prognosis, complications, and medication side effects is helpful to offer the utmost support to the patient.

Relational Therapies

Psychodynamic psychotherapy (PDT) is a briefer form of psychoanalytically based treatment, involving analyzing and interpreting psychological mechanisms held outside of the patient's awareness so as to resolve unconscious conflicts and achieve resolution of physical and psychological symptoms. Treatment sessions often occur one to two times per week, lasting a few weeks to a few years [3]. Whereas past research has focused on addressing specific psychodynamic components of onset of disease, patients' reactions to disease, and transference-countertransference issues [4], others have discussed the focus on affect expression, attempts to avoid distressing thoughts and feelings, identification of recurrent themes, past experiences, interpersonal relations, and fantasy life [3, 5]. For the medically ill, especially those with end-stage organ disease with need for transplantation, PDT may be beneficial due to patient concerns about fears of death, abandonment, physical incapacity, or demoralization when placed in the sick role within the foreign and depersonalized hospital milieu [6].

While past research has examined the role of PDT among cancer patients [7, 8], the overarching commonality of PDT among both cancer and transplant disease models point to the importance of addressing perceived psychosocial burden in the context of resilience factors [9]: favorable coping skills, self-efficacy, sense of coherence, optimism, and social support. This is particularly relevant as 50% of transplant patients were found to have a need for psychological care, especially for affective and anxiety disorders [10]. Poor transplant outcomes have been associated with weak or absent support systems, history of nonadherence, active psychiatric pathology, significant cognitive impairment, and personality disorders with impulsivity [11]. Studies among the transplant population have sought to address these issues. In fact, an intensive psychodynamically oriented interview was found to be a useful approach for bone marrow transplant candidates [12], whereas a psychodynamically based dreamwork was helpful in aiding transplant patients adjust to their new organ [13].

Medically ill patients experience a wide array of core emotions: anger, anxiety, guilt, fright, shame, sadness, happiness, envy, relief, and hope [14]. Moreover, patients may express these emotions in different ways to cope with stress and illness, depending on one's temperament, attachment, developmental experiences, and personality style. Seven personality styles were historically identified in the medical set-

ting [15]: (1) dependent with fears of abandonment and need for care, (2) obsessive and detail-oriented, (3) narcissistic with feelings of superiority and need to feel invulnerable, (4) masochistic with worthlessness and help-rejecting, (5) paranoid and distrustful, (6) histrionic with over dramatization and need for attention, and (7) schizoid with loneliness and avoidance of care. Understanding the different personality styles is crucial in helping patients cope with stress and fostering the patient-doctor therapeutic alliance. For instance, a transplant patient with perceived lack of symptom improvement may engage in help-rejecting behaviors to fulfill an unconscious need to assume the sick role and to avoid fear of abandonment. The physician who recognizes this personality style may improve the therapeutic alliance through setting realistic treatment expectations and emphasizing continued medical care beyond the hospital encounter.

In addition to the multitude of physical, psychological, affective, behavioral, and cognitive challenges involved in the transplant process, patients suffering from end-organ failure are faced with the prospect of a limited life expectancy, wherein fear of death, inner conflicts, and the ambiguity of a timely and successful transplant come to the fore in one's quality of life [9]. Thus, the goals of PDT may extend beyond symptom remission, facilitating an open exploration of one's fears, desires, dreams, and fantasies, all of which influence how the patient views the self and others, interprets or makes sense of experience, avoids aspects of experience, or interferes with the potential capacity of finding joy and meaning in life [3].

When faced with the onset and progression of illness, transplant patients may find it additionally difficult to face stressors akin to what Strain and Grossman describe as types of stress hospitalized patients experience [16]:

1) Threat to narcissistic integrity. By accepting the "sick role," the patient may experience a narcissistic injury when faced with pain and suffering that may occur before and after transplantation. A diminution of function, vitality, and locus of control may be heightened by complications of post-transplant delirium, increased hospital length of stay, neurotoxicity of immunosuppressive medications, graft rejection, retransplantation, or death [9, 10, 17].

2) Fear of strangers. The hospital environment is often stressful for patients, particularly when one's well-being is dependent on the care of others. There are often changes in hospital staff day-to-day which can be quite stressful. There are multiple members on physician teams and these teams change. Frequently, patients find multiple hospital staff walk into their rooms at all times of day: multiple physicians from primary and consulting teams, social workers, dieticians, nurses, assistants, radiology technicians, and others. For those with history of trauma

or paranoia, patients may find it difficult to trust others whose actions may in fact be benign and beneficial [18]. Ego-supportive therapy may be helpful in further providing support, reassurance, and encouragement with the goal of both achieving symptom alleviation and fostering a positive transference [7].

3) Separation anxiety. Patients might experience separation anxiety, given the new and often changing environment of the hospital setting, which can instill unfamiliarity, disruption, and lack of structure. While in the hospital, patients are separated from their homes and extended families, their routines, and daily structures. Some are required to move closer to the transplant center to await the surgery and for an extended time after the transplantation. Some patients might need to go to rehabilitation or skilled nursing facilities after the immediate transplant hospitalization, and it might not be apparent when they are safe to return home. Patients may develop anxiety when their capacity to adapt to change is tested, which may be further complicated by post-transplant delirium and cognitive deficits.

4) Fear of loss of love and approval. Physical changes and adaptation of the sick role can sometimes instill within patients feelings of disapproval and loss of love from their physicians, nurses, and family members. Transplant patients may develop chronic worries about retransplantation, serious comorbidities, and death [19]. These feelings may be even more distressing when one feels ongoing suffering along with limited perception of recovery, exposing underlying fantasies of past failed attachments and dependency conflicts.

5) Fear of loss of control of developmentally achieved functions. Given the multitude of physical changes and expectations for recovery within the post-transplant period, patients may find it challenging and frustrating to regain these physical and mental functions that were once under one's control. From difficulties in regaining abilities to breathe on their own after a ventilator, to speak and vocalize on one's behalf, to urinate and defecate, to adhering to one's complex medication regimen and new lifestyle recommendations, or to returning to work or other meaningful activities—all these may threaten self-esteem and ability to tolerate loss of control [18].

6) Fear of loss or injury to body parts. This fear can be analogous to castration anxiety, or the fear of not only losing one's body part, but also to one's ability to function in society. Moreover both occupational and sexual function deficits persist after transplantation [20] which may be threatening to one's physical vulnerability, symbolic sense of empowerment, and basic safety needs [18].

7) Reactivation of feelings of guilt and shame and fears of retaliation for previous transgressions. Patients may question their illness or even their decision to pursue transplantation in the first place. The experience of guilt toward the donor, for instance, after one has accepted a new organ, may arise and increase stress and nonadherence with treatment and recovery. This phenomenon occurs in the context of the psychodynamic conceptualization of organ integration or the psychological process of experiencing the transplanted organ as part of the patient's self and not as part of the donor or as a foreign, external object [21]. The transplantation process may evoke strong doubts of one's identity and meaning of life. This is especially the case when guilt is unconsciously enacted as a masochistic punishment for accepting and failing to successfully integrate an organ from a deceased donor; rather, instead of viewing the new organ as part of one's identity, it is viewed as "foreign" [21].

Related to personality attributes and coping styles utilized in the context of illness is the theory of attachment, or the history of lifelong patterns of responding to threats in the environment that are learned in the interaction between infant and caregiver, especially during the first two years of life. Attachment insecurity may affect stress regulation, resulting in altered use of external regulators of affect (e.g., substance abuse, eating and sexual behaviors) or protective factors (e.g., treatment adherence, symptom reporting) [22]. For instance, in *secure* attachment, there is an internalized sense of worth, effectiveness in eliciting care when required, and self-efficacy in dealing with most stressors. Other patients may be in a *preoccupied* attachment, wherein they are likely to be excessively care-seeking, anxious, and dependent. In *dismissing* attachment, patients may be overly self-sufficient and avoidant of care when provided to them, which often leads to stress when confronted with being in the hospital during the transplant process. And lastly, *fearful* attachment characterizes those who are self-conscious, doubting, and suspicious [22, 23].

Furthermore, psychodynamic factors are inherent in the interactions between physicians and patients. Countertransference describes both the physician's unconscious and conscious total emotional reaction to a patient [24] with certain physician characteristics identified as most susceptible: those with senses of perfectionism, exaggerated sense of responsibility, and fantasies of rescue and omnipotence [25, 26]. These may subsequently lead to feelings of frustration, anger, helplessness, and behavioral enactments of avoidance and abandonment of both the patient and the environment, particularly if certain patient characteristics evoke these countertransference reactions: the "whining self-pitier," the suicidal patient [27], or the "hateful patient" [28].

Groves [28] identifies four styles of patients and qualities of dependent interactions with medical professionals: "dependent clingers" who might request constant support, "entitle demanders" who use intimidation and guilt induction to obtain reassurance, "manipulative help rejectors" who exhaust medical providers by returning again and again with the perception that medical interventions have failed, and "self-destructive deniers" who frequently display behaviors that are contraindicated for their medical conditions (i.e., the recent cardiac transplant patient who is shoveling snow). From a practical point of view, physician awareness of these subtypes is helpful especially for those who service patients with end-stage organ disease and transplantation as these patients require frequent medical care that is both overwhelming and demanding. Staff and physicians may feel inundated by the requests that patients make and may themselves become exhausted by the care of these patients.

Through the process of exploring a patient's overall attachment history, personality style, coping mechanisms, intrapsychic conflicts and transference reactions, as one journeys through the stages of transplantation, a life narrative can conceptualize and subsequently inform the patient-doctor relationship about the psychodynamic underpinnings of one's experience with anger, despair, and anxiety in the face of chronic medical illness within the hospital and clinic setting. With the help of the clinician, the patient can begin to understand the role and meaning of illness in the overall context of one's life narrative.

Existential Therapies

Existential Psychotherapy

Existential therapy derives from existentialism or the philosophical examination of the basic struggles of human existence. From Friedrich Nietzsche's *the will to power* [29] to Viktor Frankl's *self-transcendence* [30] – the individual, by virtue of one's existence, or what Martin Heidegger referred to as *being-in-the-world* [31], seeks to satiate biological, psychological, and social needs to achieve the capacity to symbolize, imagine, and create personal meaning. Here, the individual's existence is negotiated within one's relationship to the self and others, both within the finite boundaries of life and death [32–34].

Within the transplant setting, patients may experience increasing and persistent stress, particularly when faced with the immediacy of disease onset and progression that may ultimately develop into an existential crisis, of which the extreme possibility is death [35]. For example, in hematological cell transplantation (HCT), over 90% of survivors experience at least one serious physical complication, with chronic graft-versus-host disease (cGVHD) representing one significant factor in quality of life [36]. Complex physical, emotional, and social challenges are faced, which may all continue well into the post-transplant recovery phase [37, 38]. For both the patient and one's spouse or significant other, this period may represent a "dynamic interaction" during which the transplant couple may face unpredictability as they put their "life on hold" [39]. Although family relationships return to "normal" [40] sometime after transplantation, these relationships may experience prolonged anxiety, decreased perceived quality of life, changes in role function, and marital distress [41–43]. Thus, clinicians may help patients and their family navigate through the transplant process by finding meaning in suffering, especially as this process can often generate unrelenting anxiety, lack of freedom, isolation, guilt, and hopelessness in the midst of physical pain, emotional angst, prospect of death, and the uncertainty of end of life [32, 44].

Existential psychotherapy provides an opportunity for patients to address questions about their existence and to understand and ease anxiety when facing questions about one's mortality. Several philosophical principles underlie existential therapy: (a) humans need to find meaning and purpose in their lives; (b) humans have the capacity to freely choose and change values; (c) humans will face challenges in their life and function best when tackling these challenges; (d) all emotions (negative and positive) are essential to being human and are an opportunity for therapeutic work; and (e) relationships and interactions with one's environment are fundamental to the human experience [45, 46].

The concept of organ transplantation, for instance, illustrates the founding ground of Heidegger's *being-in-the-world*, particularly when a patient suffering from a failing organ undergoes the alien experience of feeling hurt, tired, and nauseated—sensations that may heighten not only anxiety at the prospect of a malfunctioning organ that may entail receiving a new organ but also obtrusive feelings of mortality and death [33]. For instance, candidates for heart transplant have been found to have high levels of psychological distress related to the possibility of an unavailable heart and the potential of life-threatening heart failure [47]. The finitude that a patient may experience when confronted with these possibilities embodies the limitations associated with the physicality of the body, all the while striving for self-transcendence in finding meaning in one's life beyond physical and emotional suffering [47, 48].

Existential therapy can be valuable for transplant patients who are able to access emotional experiences or to overcome barriers that preclude a patient's ability to cope with the transplantation process. As a "fellow traveler" through this process, the clinician supports the patient to confront anxiety in the setting of death, isolation, freedom, and emptiness inherent in one's suffering [34]. The clinician then can elicit personal choices and encourage the patient to focus on responsibility in making one's own decisions and to continually derive personal meaning [32, 34].

Dignity Therapy

Dignity therapy is a psychotherapeutic approach to patients who are nearing death that focuses on the production of a "generativity document" and aims to maximize the dignity conserving practices and perspectives of the patient. Dignity therapy was created by Dr. Harvey Max Chochinov based upon his work with patients with end-stage cancer. He was inspired to consider the impact and meaning of dignity at the end of life by the Dutch study on euthanasia and other medical decisions to end life (MDEL) published in 1991. This study found that "loss of dignity" was the most common reason given by physicians who had participated in hastening the death of their patient, cited in 57% of cases [49]. The intended targeted patients of dignity therapy are those facing a life-threatening illness or life-limiting circumstances. Many of the patients who have taken part in dignity therapy are patients with cancer diagnoses; the therapy has also been utilized for patients with other terminal diagnoses such as neurodegenerative disorders, end-stage renal disease, end-stage chronic obstructive pulmonary disease (COPD), and the frail elderly.

Traditionally, dignity therapy takes place over four sessions and is comprised of two main tasks: an interview with the patient in which she speaks about her life and the experiences that have been most important to her, and the creation of a "generativity document" which is an edited transcript of the interview. Dr. Chochinov suggests a question protocol that can be used to guide the interview, but generally the interviewer should allow and help the patient to speak about what is meaningful to her. The document can then be given to the patient's family if she so desires. This process allows the patient approaching death to consider who she is and what she has felt throughout her life and to leave behind an enduring legacy for others.

The efficacy of dignity therapy has been studied numerous times, both by Dr. Chochinov's group and by others around the world. Dignity therapy has been found to improve quality of life and spiritual well-being and lessen sadness and depression. Dignity therapy has also been found helpful for the families of patients with terminal illnesses [50]. The efficacy of dignity therapy in different patient populations continues to be actively studied; at least seven studies were published in 2017 related to dignity therapy, including studies on its efficacy in patients with Huntington's disease, as used by nursing staff, for loved ones, and in newly diagnosed cancer patients [51–53].

Given that dignity therapy is primarily intended for patients facing death, its use in a transplant population would be most efficacious and appropriate for those patients in potentially terminal situations, e.g., a patient in liver failure awaiting transplant but with little hope of making it off the waiting list, a patient following lung transplant with progressive bronchiolitis obliterans, or a patient with end-stage organ disease who decided not to pursue transplant or was declined by the team. Generally patients should be more than 2 weeks away from death in order to have time to complete the process, and although insight into their prognosis is not necessary, it can be helpful to maximize the impact of the therapy. No literature has yet been published applying dignity therapy to transplant patients in particular.

Meaning-Centered Psychotherapy

Meaning-centered psychotherapy was developed by Dr. William Breitbart at Memorial Sloan Kettering Cancer Center in response to the need for an intervention for advanced cancer patients struggling with despair, hopelessness, and desire for hastened death, but not necessarily depressed [54]. The intervention was originally developed as a group therapy; later an individual form of the therapy was developed to address the difficulties of coordinating groups of very medically ill people. Meaning-centered psychotherapy was largely inspired by the work of Victor Frankl who wrote the book *Man's Search for Meaning* in 1946 based on his experiences in a concentration camp during World War II [39].

This therapy is designed specifically for demoralized patients with a limited prognosis. The therapy aims to bring meaning to patients' lives through encouraging them to consider their choice of attitudes toward life and death; their connection with life through love, art, humor, nature, and relationships; their engagement with life through creative pursuits; and their understanding of their own identity and legacy. Group meaning-centered psychotherapy takes place over eight sessions, and individual meaning-centered psychotherapy over seven sessions, with each session focusing on a slightly different aspect of meaning. Each session consists of some didactic instruction and some experiential exercises.

The efficacy of both group and individual meaning-centered psychotherapy has been studied extensively. In the first randomized controlled trial, patients with advanced cancer who participated in group meaning-centered psychotherapy were found to report significantly improved "meaning/peace" and "faith" and show a significant decrease in anxiety and desire for death as compared to patients who participated in supportive psychotherapy [55]. The first randomized controlled trial of individual meaning-centered psychotherapy in patients with cancer showed an improvement in spiritual well-being and overall quality of life, as well as a decrease in physical symptom distress, but the same decrease in anxiety and desire for death was not found.

There is no literature currently on the use of meaning-centered psychotherapy in transplant patients. Although meaning-centered psychotherapy was designed for and has been studied in patients with cancer with a limited prognosis, its use to mitigate demoralization in patients with end-stage organ disease, facing transplant, or post-transplant could be significant. For example, one session of meaning-centered psychotherapy focuses on exploring the patient's identity before and after cancer; this exercise could easily be adapted for a patient with an illness requiring transplant or who is living with a transplanted organ.

Structured Therapies

Cognitive-Behavioral Therapy

Originally developed by Aaron Beck for depression, cognitive-behavioral therapy (CBT) has now been demonstrated to be an effective treatment for many psychiatric conditions. CBT relies on a cognitive model of psychological distress. CBT is based on the theory that emotion, behavior, and cognition are interconnected and psychological distress is due to problematic thinking patterns. Specific CBT approaches vary in emphasis but share the common underlying features of being problem-focused, goal-directed, and time-limited. With the help of a practitioner, patients learn to challenge and modify dysfunctional beliefs so that their distress can be alleviated [56].

Sensky [57] has described in detail how CBT has been adapted for use in people with physical illnesses. In the medical setting, an ideal starting point for cognitive therapy is to understand the patient's perception of his medical problems and explore any links between the physical and emotional states. An individual's thoughts and perceptions of their illness or their body sensations and how these thoughts influence their behaviors, physiology, and emotions are central to the cognitive model. For example, if even benign bodily sensations are regarded as being symptoms of disease, several consequences ensue: (1) the patient may become emotionally distressed, which may increase bodily sensations; (2) the patient will pay more attention to these symptoms and worry will increase; (3) the patient employs coping strategies that may exacerbate symptoms instead of relieving them; and (4) caretakers, including doctors, may respond to the patient in a way that intensifies the patient's concerns, attention to bodily sensations, and dysfunctional coping. Working closely with the patient and having the patient actively collaborate with their physician can restore a patient's sense of mastery or control over his illness. Overall, the aim is to help the patient examine the beliefs underlying his illness and understand how they affect his behavior.

Despite extensive empirical evidence of CBT utility in a vast number of medical problems such as HIV, cardiovascular diseases, insomnia, and renal failure [58–66], there are no studies to examine its effect on quality of life or depression in patients with or awaiting transplantation. Given its proven efficacy for depression and anxiety, one might imagine that CBT is a very helpful non-pharmacological approach to psychotherapy in patients who are pre- or post-transplant.

Acceptance and Commitment Therapy

Similar to cognitive-behavioral therapy, acceptance and commitment therapy (ACT) focuses on increasing psychological flexibility by using acceptance and mindfulness strategies. Developed by Steven Hayes in 1982, ACT is founded on the idea that suffering is normal but can be made manageable through the development of cognitive flexibility. This is achieved through the three pillars of ACT: (1) being *present* in the moment and maintaining awareness of what one is feeling, (2) observing and being open to emotions as they evolve, and (3) clarification of a patient's personal values and what is meaningful to his life. With these three pillars in mind, practitioners and patients are able to create an action plan to more effectively handle painful thoughts and feelings. Over time, patients gain mastery in tolerating and accepting negative feelings. Further, they are able to create action plans that help them engage in behaviors that align best with their value systems [67].

ACT has been empirically tested and demonstrated promise for the treatment of depression and anxiety, as well as chronic medical conditions [68, 69]. ACT has also become popular in behavioral medicine for a variety of chronic illnesses and conditions that require changes in health behaviors, such as diabetes and smoking cessation [70, 71]. ACT has been shown to reduce distress and improve functioning among people living with chronic medical conditions such as patients with cancer, migraines, and chronic pain [70, 72, 73].

In patients with transplant and organ dysfunction, ACT may be particularly well-suited as it offers a model of healthy adaptation to patients' often challenging medical and psychosocial realities and encourages patients to be present in the moment, open, and focused on what matters to them. While no empirical studies have analyzed the efficacy of ACT for people with organ dysfunction and transplant, the foundations of ACT and effectiveness in other chronic medical conditions suggest that ACT would likely be helpful in patients undergoing transplant.

Mindfulness-Based Cognitive Therapy and Mindfulness-Based Stress Reduction

Mindfulness training is a method for self-regulation of attention. Mindfulness increases awareness of inner thoughts, emotions, and bodily sensations while fostering an attitude of acceptance. Using breathing meditation and yoga stretches, it helps participants become more aware of the present moment and be aware of changes in the body and mind [74].

Programs that rely on the tradition of meditation are mindfulness-based stress reduction (MBSR) and mindfulness-based cognitive therapy (MBCT). Both are highly structured, educational, patient-focused interventions with formal training in mindfulness meditation. MBSR was developed by Jon Kabat-Zinn and aims to help patients manage physical and emotional pain [75]. MBSR programs generally consist of 60–90 min sessions over 7–10 weekly group sessions. Mindfulness-based cognitive therapy (MBCT) has been adapted from mindfulness-based stress reduction approaches as a treatment for depression [76]. While both rely on the tradition of meditation, MBCT also includes several techniques from cognitive therapy focusing on the links between thinking and feeling and participants to effectively respond when depression threatens to overwhelm them.

With training patients learn to perceive emotional and physical states as they are and let thoughts come and go in awareness with no attempts to change, suppress, or elaborate on them. MBSR was developed to help individuals with chronic health conditions cope with difficult physical symptoms not improving with standard medical care, with the early work focusing on chronic pain [75]. MCBT encourages participants to "let go" of thoughts in order to interrupt the link between low mood and negative thoughts. With this skill, patients are able to tolerate distressing thoughts, moods, and bodily sensations. They are encouraged to stay in the present moment and not focus on the past or future.

The practice of mindfulness is associated with distinct physiological effects including an increase in parasympathetic nervous system activation [77], which may lead to the reduction of distressing physical symptoms. MBSR has been demonstrated to help patients with a variety of illnesses adjust and improve their quality of life [62, 63, 78]. For example, cancer patients practicing mindfulness experience reduced stress, pain, and fatigue, as well as improved sleep [79, 80]. The benefits of mindfulness practice with MBSR may contribute to the overall improvement in parasympathetic nervous system activation, such as reduced sinus arrhythmia [77, 81] and long-term decreased cortisol, proinflammatory cytokines, and blood pressure in cancer patients.

Transplant patients often have to live with difficult physical symptoms and medication side effects. Even with excellent function of the transplanted organs, immunosuppressive medications generate adverse effects and cause new complications.

In the first randomized control trial of MBSR in patients with solid organ transplant, it was found that patients who had 8 weeks of MSBR training had lower depression rating scores and better sleep. At 1 year, anxiety, depression, qual-

ity of life, and sleep remained improved from baseline in those who received MSBR compared to those with only psychoeducation [82].

Therapies Aimed at Adherence

A significant part of a patient's candidacy for organ transplantation is medication adherence, which has been associated with improved outcomes among solid organ transplant candidates [83]. Individuals with chronic kidney disease, for example, experience complex and dynamic physical and emotional lifestyle changes, all of which may affect patients' motivation to manage their illness [84]. Nonadherence, varying in incidence from 19% to 25% per year, with vital and lifelong post-transplant immunosuppressants, has been associated with significant complications, including graft rejection, increased health-care costs, lower quality of life, and mortality [85, 86]. For transplant recipients, the ability to follow recommended treatment may be complicated by not only the complex medication regimens, but also by the burden of experiencing cognitive barriers (e.g., forgetfulness), need to attend frequent medical visits, undergoing laboratory tests, and adjusting to lifestyle modifications [87]. This may result in diminished motivation and disengagement of patients from their clinicians.

Originally developed within the field of addiction as an alternative to the confrontational approach of treating substance use disorders, motivational interviewing (MI) is a collaborative, goal-oriented approach that builds intrinsic personal motivation and growth as a result of the exploration of a patient's conflict between ambivalence and need to change [88]. Although few have tested MI among the transplant population, Dobbels and colleagues have shown that MI, in addition to other multicomponent behavioral interventions based on social cognitive theory, increased adherence to tacrolimus among post-transplant heart, liver, and lung recipients, sustainable even at 5 years post-intervention [89, 90]. MI has been an effective method of encouraging patients with chronic kidney disease in self-managing their care [91]. For instance, among a randomized sample of 793 patients with chronic kidney disease in 9 different Dutch hospitals, those patients who were coached MI by a nurse practitioner had increased adherence rates with improvement in self-management over the course of 5 years and corresponding decrease of cardiovascular comorbidity and mortality, all-cause mortality, renal function, vascular damage, and improvement of quality of life [92].

Although MI is typically thought of as a brief intervention, it can also be conceptualized as a communication style to enhance intrinsic motivation to change while exploring and resolving ambivalence. Four principles underlie this collaborative approach [93]:

Engaging The process of establishing a helpful connection and working relationship inherent in the therapeutic alliance between the patient and clinician.

Focusing The process by which a patient develops and maintains a direction in the conversation about change and the movement toward a specific goal.

Evoking The process of eliciting the patient's own motivations for change, which represents the heart of MI, rather than from a solely paternalistic approach or "righting reflex." This may be problematic if advice put forth by the clinician is incongruent with the patient's own personal values.

Planning The process that encompasses the patient both developing commitment to change and formulating a concrete plan of action, all the while promoting patient autonomy in decision-making and eliciting change talk.

Related to these four principles are core interviewing skills that are flexibly utilized in order to invite change talk and to explore resistance to change [93]:

Open-Ended Questions Encourage the patient to reflect and elaborate on motivations for change.

Affirmations The clinician comments on the patient's strengths, abilities, good intentions, and efforts as a way to promote acceptance and support of the patient as well as self-efficacy.

Reflective Listening The process by which the clinician restates empathetically one's understanding of what the patient had said and to encourage the patient to discuss more about one's ambivalence and motivation for change.

Summarizing A clinician's best understanding of the patient's experience with ambivalence and motivation for change, while further collecting change talk statements and linking discrepancies underlying resistance to change. This allows the clinician to paint a "whole picture" for the patient to negotiate ambivalence with one's desire, ability, reason, need, and commitment to change behavior.

MI is an effective and empirically based intervention and communication style that cuts across several disciplines to address behavioral problems wherein ambivalence and motivation to change are salient. For the transplant patient, treatment nonadherence, especially with immunosuppressants (and the risks associated with rejection and graft loss), highlights the importance of MI as a behavioral intervention that informs the way in which the clinician collaboratively works with the patient to strengthen one's own motivation and commitment to change and sustain a good quality of life.

Caregiver Support

Transplantation is a family affair. The whole family is necessary to support the patient through the evaluation, waiting list, and actual transplantation process. It is no surprise that family members play a key role in providing support and as a result have increased distress, anxiety, and depressive symptoms themselves. The rates of depression and anxiety-related disorders in caregivers for transplant patients exceed those found in other caregiver populations. In one study with 3-year follow-up, the rates of psychiatric disorders in transplant recipient caregivers were major depressive disorder (MDD), 31.6%; adjustment disorders, 35.4% (29.4% with anxious mood); post-traumatic stress disorder related to the transplant (PTSD-T), 22.5%; generalized anxiety disorder, 7.3%; and any assessed disorder, 56.3%. Thus, focus on caregiver support is essential when caring for a patient who is considering and undergoing transplant.

In small studies of caregivers of transplant recipients, MBSR led to lower scores of perceived stress and anxiety [94]. Caregivers can also benefit from stress reduction techniques.

Group Therapy

Transplant patients have many shared experiences and concerns. Transplant patients face special issues: lack of community knowledge regarding transplant, concerns about source of their donor, lifelong needs for immunosuppression and resultant risks of infection, and changes in physical appearance [95]. Given this shared experience, one might conjecture that patients can benefit from hearing from others' experiences. In a brief open group therapy program for renal transplant patients, Buchanan noted that patients benefited from learning to cope by observing others in the group. Further, by spending time together, patients developed a sense of community and develop realistic expectations of the future [96]. Structured programs that address both pre-transplant and post-transplant experiences have been outlined and have the potential to be effective in alleviating patients' and families' concerns in a resource-efficient manner [95].

Conclusions

The psychological needs of transplant and end-stage organ disease patients are complex and require a multidisciplinary approach. Improving patients' access to resources is essential in developing more structured and evidence-based treatments. While more research needs to be done in the field of psychotherapy and non-pharmacological interventions for mood disorders in transplant patients, we might extrapolate the benefits of these interventions from other chronically ill patient populations.

Despite the limitations in evidence and research, there is support that a variety of treatment modalities are useful non-pharmacological options for this vulnerable population. Supportive and psychodynamic psychotherapies are effective in bolstering the patient's preexisting resilient or adaptive coping mechanisms. Existential and meaning-centered psychotherapy can be helpful in patients questioning meaning in the face of challenges related to organ transplantation. CBT and ACT may help patients with distorted perceptions of their illness or those who are particularly struggling with physical symptoms. Dignity therapy is useful for patients nearing the end of life, and motivational interviewing is helpful for patients struggling with adherence to treatment recommendations. In addition, caregivers for transplant patients require support and would also likely benefit from interventions such as dignity therapy.

Further research is required to assist providers identifying characteristics of patients that might be most suited for particular interventions. For now, we depend on the skill of mental health providers and patient's principal caretakers to identify interventions that may alleviate a patient's distress and improve their quality of life.

Resources for therapy	
Supportive and problem-solving approaches	*Textbook of Psychotherapeutic Treatments* Edited by Glen O. Gabbard [24].
Psychodynamic psychotherapy	*Brief Psychotherapy at the Bedside: Countering Demoralization from Medical Illness* by James Griffith and Lynne Gaby [97] *Existential Psychotherapy* by Irvin Yalom [34]
Cognitive-behavioral therapy	*Coping with Chronic Illness: A Cognitive-Behavioral Therapy Approach for Adherence and Depression* by Steven Safren, Jeffrey Gonzalez, Nafisseh Soroudi [98]
Acceptance and commitment therapy	*Acceptance and Change: Content and Context in Psychotherapy* by Steven Hayes [99]
Mindfulness-based cognitive-behavioral therapy	*Full Catastrophe Living: Using the Wisdom of Your Body and Mind to Face Stress, Pain, and Illness* by Jon Kabat-Zinn [100]
Dignity therapy	*Dignity Therapy: Final Words for Final Days* by Harvey Chochinov [101]
Meaning-centered psychotherapy	*Meaning-Centered Group Psychotherapy for Patients with Advanced Cancer: A Treatment Manual* by Breitbart, William Poppito, Shannon R [102].
Motivational interviewing	*Motivational Interviewing: Helping People Change* by William miller and Stephen Rollnick [93]

References

1. Bloch S. An introduction to the psychotherapies. 4th ed. Oxford. New York: Oxford University Press; 2006.
2. Heilmann C, Kuijpers N, Beyersdorf F, Berchtold-Herz M, Trummer G, Stroh AL, et al. Supportive psychotherapy for patients with heart transplantation or ventricular assist devices. Eur J Cardiothorac Surg. 2011 Apr;39(4):e44–50.
3. Shedler J. The efficacy of psychodynamic psychotherapy. Am Psychol. 2010 Feb-Mar;65(2):98–109.
4. Blumenfield M. The place of psychodynamic psychiatry in consultation-liaison psychiatry with special emphasis on countertransference. J Am Acad Psychoanal Dyn Psychiatry. 2006 Spring;34(1):83–92.
5. Nash SS, Kent LK, Muskin PR. Psychodynamics in medically ill patients. Harv Rev Psychiatry. 2009;17(6):389–97.
6. Wahl CW. The physician's treatment of the dying patient. Ann N Y Acad Sci. 1969 Dec 19;164(3):759–75.
7. Straker N. Psychodynamic psychotherapy for cancer patients. J Psychother Pract Res. 1997 Winter;7(1):1–9.
8. Postone N. Psychotherapy with cancer patients. Am J Psychother. 1998 Fall;52(4):412–24.
9. Schulz KHKS. Psychosocial challenges before and after organ transplantation. Transplant Research and Risk Management. 2015;7(1):45–8.
10. DiMartini A, Crone C, Fireman M, Dew MA. Psychiatric aspects of organ transplantation in critical care. Crit Care Clin 2008 Oct;24(4):949–81, x.
11. Jowsey SG, Taylor ML, Schneekloth TD, Clark MM. Psychosocial challenges in transplantation. J Psychiatr Pract. 2001 Nov;7(6):404–14.
12. Hoffman LH, Szkrumelak N, Sullivan AK. Psychiatric assessment of candidates for bone marrow transplantation: a psychodynamically-oriented approach. Int J Psychiatry Med. 1999;29(1):13–28.
13. Barrett D. Trauma and dreams. Cambridge: Harvard University Press; 1996.
14. Lazarus RDFS. Stress, appraisal and coping. New York, NY: Springer; 1984.
15. Kahana RJBG. Personality types in medical management. In: Zingberg N, editor. Psychiatry and medical practice in a general hospital. New York, NY: International University Press; 1964.
16. Strain JJ, Grossman S. Psychological care of the medically ill : a primer in liaison psychiatry. New York: Appleton-Century-Crofts; 1975.
17. Sher Y, Mooney J, Dhillon G, Lee R, Maldonado JR. Delirium after lung transplantation: association with recipient characteristics, hospital resource utilization, and mortality. Clin Transpl. 2017;31(5)
18. Schwartz HJ, Bleiberg E, Weissman SH. Psychodynamic concepts in general psychiatry. Washington, DC: American Psychiatric Press; 1995.
19. Goetzmann L, Irani S, Schwegler K, Stamm M, Spindler A, Bricman R, et al. Lung function, sociodemographic characteristics, and psychological reaction to transplant associated with chronic stress among lung recipients. Anxiety Stress Coping. 2010;23(2):213–33.
20. Goetzmann L, Irani S, Moser KS, Schwegler K, Stamm M, Spindler A, et al. Psychological processing of transplantation in lung recipients: a quantitative study of organ integration and the relationship to the donor. Br J Health Psychol. 2009 Nov;14(Pt 4):667–80.

21. Neukom M, Corti V, Boothe B, Boehler A, Goetzmann L. Fantasized recipient-donor relationships following lung transplantations: a qualitative case analysis based on patient narratives. Int J Psychoanal. 2012 Feb;93(1):117–37.
22. Maunder RG, Hunter JJ. Attachment and psychosomatic medicine: developmental contributions to stress and disease. Psychosom Med. 2001 Jul-Aug;63(4):556–67.
23. Bartholomew K, Horowitz LM. Attachment styles among young adults: a test of a four-category model. J Pers Soc Psychol. 1991 Aug;61(2):226–44.
24. Gabbard GO. Long-term psychodynamic psychotherapy: a basic text. 2nd ed. Arlington: American Psychiatric Association; 2010.
25. Gabbard GO. The big chill : the transition from residency to managed care nightmare. Acad Psychiatry. 1992 Sep;16(3):119–26.
26. Schwab JJ. Handbook of psychiatric consultation. New York: Appleton-Century-Crofts; 1968.
27. Maltsberger JT, Buie DH. Countertransference hate in the treatment of suicidal patients. Arch Gen Psychiatry. 1974 May;30(5):625–33.
28. Groves JE. Taking care of the hateful patient. N Engl J Med. 1978 Apr 20;298(16):883–7.
29. Nietzche F. The will to power. Kaufman W, editor. New York: Vintage Books; 1967.
30. Frankl VE. Man's search for meaning. Young readers edition. Ed. Boston: Beacon Press; 2017.
31. Heidegger M. Being and Time. London: S.C.M Press; 1962.
32. Breitbart W, Gibson C, Poppito SR, Berg A. Psychotherapeutic interventions at the end of life: a focus on meaning and spirituality. Can J Psychiatr. 2004 Jun;49(6):366–72.
33. Svenaeus F. What is an organ? Heidegger and the phenomenology of organ transplantation. Theor Med Bioeth. 2010 Jun;31(3):179–96.
34. Yalom ID. Existential psychotherapy. New York: Basic Books; 1980.
35. Dunn E, Arber A, Gallagher A. The immediacy of illness and existential crisis: Patients' lived experience of under-going allogeneic stem cell transplantation for haematological malignancy. A phenomenological study. Eur J Oncol Nurs. 2016 Apr;21:90–6.
36. Cant AJGA, Jackson G. Why hematopoietic stem cell transplantation and for whom? In: Cant AJCC, Skinner R, editors. Practical hematopoietic stem cell transplantation. Oxford: Blackwell Publishing Ltd; 2007.
37. Andrykowski MA, Bishop MM, Hahn EA, Cella DF, Beaumont JL, Brady MJ, et al. Long-term health-related quality of life, growth, and spiritual well-being after hematopoietic stem-cell transplantation. J Clin Oncol. 2005 Jan 20;23(3):599–608.
38. Cooke L, Gemmill R, Kravits K, Grant M. Psychological issues of stem cell transplant. Semin Oncol Nurs. 2009 May;25(2):139–50.
39. Williams M. Life on hold: A theory of spouse response to the waiting period prior to heart transplantation. Unpublished doctoral dissertation. Unpublished doctoral dissertation, University of Arizona.
40. Hwang HF. Patient and family adjustment to heart transplantation. Prog Cardiovasc Nurs 1996 Spring;11(2):16–8, 39.
41. McCurry AH, Thomas SP. Spouses' experiences in heart transplantation. West J Nurs Res. 2002 Mar;24(2):180–94.
42. McSweeney JCRR, Innerarity SA, et al. What about me? Spouses' quality of life after heart transplantation. J Transpl Coord. 1995;5(2):59–94.
43. Mishel MH, Murdaugh CL. Family adjustment to heart transplantation: redesigning the dream. Nurs Res. 1987 Nov-Dec;36(6):332–8.
44. Frankl VE. Man's search for meaning : an introduction to logotherapy. Boston: Beacon Press; 1963.
45. Corey G. Theory and practice of counseling and psychotherapy. 2nd ed. Monterey: Brooks/Cole Pub. Co.; 1982.
46. Vos J, Craig M, Cooper M. Existential therapies: a meta-analysis of their effects on psychological outcomes. J Consult Clin Psychol. 2015 Feb;83(1):115–28.
47. Kop WJ. Role of psychological factors in the clinical course of heart transplant patients. J Heart Lung Transplant. 2010 Mar;29(3):257–60.
48. Hiatt JF. Spirituality, medicine, and healing. South Med J. 1986 Jun;79(6):736–43.
49. Van Der Maas PJ, Van Delden JJ, Pijnenborg L, Looman CW. Euthanasia and other medical decisions concerning the end of life. Lancet. 1991 Sep 14;338(8768):669–74.
50. Chochinov HM, Kristjanson LJ, Breitbart W, McClement S, Hack TF, Hassard T, et al. Effect of dignity therapy on distress and end-of-life experience in terminally ill patients: a randomised controlled trial. Lancet Oncol. 2011 Aug;12(8):753–62.
51. Moskowitz CB, Rao AK. Making a measurable difference in advanced Huntington disease care. Handb Clin Neurol. 2017;144:183–96.
52. Dose AM, Hubbard JM, Mansfield AS, McCabe PJ, Krecke CA, Sloan JA. Feasibility and acceptability of a dignity therapy/life plan intervention for patients with advanced Cancer. Oncol Nurs Forum. 2017 Sep 1;44(5):E194–202.
53. Juliao M. The efficacy of dignity therapy on the psychological well-being in loved ones of terminally ill patients. J Palliat Med. 2017 Nov;20(11):1182–3.
54. Breitbart W, Rosenfeld B, Pessin H, Kaim M, Funesti-Esch J, Galietta M, et al. Depression, hopelessness, and desire for hastened death in terminally ill patients with cancer. JAMA. 2000 Dec 13;284(22):2907–11.
55. Breitbart W, Rosenfeld B, Gibson C, Pessin H, Poppito S, Nelson C, et al. Meaning-centered group psychotherapy for patients with advanced cancer: a pilot randomized controlled trial. Psychooncology. 2010 Jan;19(1):21–8.
56. Beck AT. Cognitive therapy and the emotional disorders. New York: International Universities Press; 1976.
57. Sensky T. Cognitive therapy with patients with chronic physical illness. Psychother Psychosom. 1989;52(1–3):26–32.
58. Church J. The application of cognitive-behavioural therapy for depression to people with human immunodeficiency virus (HIV) and acquired immune deficiency syndrome (AIDS). Psychooncology. 1998 Mar-Apr;7(2):78–88.
59. Johnston DW. Cognitive behaviour therapy for cardiovascular diseases. Z Kardiol. 2000;89(Suppl 9):IX/78–81.
60. Smith MT, Huang MI, Manber R. Cognitive behavior therapy for chronic insomnia occurring within the context of medical and psychiatric disorders. Clin Psychol Rev. 2005 Jul;25(5):559–92.
61. Cukor D. Use of CBT to treat depression among patients on hemodialysis. Psychiatr Serv. 2007 May;58(5):711–2.
62. McElhiney MC, Rabkin JG, Rabkin R, Nunes EV. Provigil (modafinil) plus cognitive behavioral therapy for methamphetamine use in HIV+ gay men: a pilot study. Am J Drug Alcohol Abuse. 2009;35(1):34–7.
63. Cully JA, Stanley MA, Deswal A, Hanania NA, Phillips LL, Kunik ME. Cognitive-behavioral therapy for chronic cardiopulmonary conditions: preliminary outcomes from an open trial. Prim Care Companion J Clin Psychiatry. 2010;12(4).
64. Greer JA, Park ER, Prigerson HG, Safren SA. Tailoring cognitive-behavioral therapy to treat anxiety comorbid with advanced Cancer. J Cogn Psychother. 2010 Jan 1;24(4):294–313.
65. Garland SN, Carlson LE, Stephens AJ, Antle MC, Samuels C, Campbell TS. Mindfulness-based stress reduction compared with cognitive behavioral therapy for the treatment of insomnia comorbid with cancer: a randomized, partially blinded, noninferiority trial. J Clin Oncol. 2014 Feb 10;32(5):449–57.
66. Hudson JL, Moss-Morris R, Game D, Carroll A, Chilcot J. Improving Distress in Dialysis (iDiD): a tailored CBT self-

management treatment for patients undergoing dialysis. J Ren Care. 2016 Dec;42(4):223–38.

67. Hayes SC, Strosahl K, Wilson KG. Acceptance and commitment therapy : an experiential approach to behavior change. New York: Guilford Press; 1999.

68. Twohig MP, Levin ME. Acceptance and commitment therapy as a treatment for anxiety and depression: a review. Psychiatr Clin North Am. 2017 Dec;40(4):751–70.

69. Powers MB. Zum Vorde Sive Vording MB, Emmelkamp PM. Acceptance and commitment therapy: a meta-analytic review. Psychother Psychosom. 2009;78(2):73–80.

70. Gregg JA, Callaghan GM, Hayes SC, Glenn-Lawson JL. Improving diabetes self-management through acceptance, mindfulness, and values: a randomized controlled trial. J Consult Clin Psychol. 2007 Apr;75(2):336–43.

71. Bricker J, Wyszynski C, Comstock B, Heffner JL. Pilot randomized controlled trial of web-based acceptance and commitment therapy for smoking cessation. Nicotine Tob Res. 2013 Oct;15(10):1756–64.

72. McCracken LM, Sato A, Wainwright D, House W, Taylor GJ. A feasibility study of brief group-based acceptance and commitment therapy for chronic pain in general practice: recruitment, attendance, and patient views. Prim Health Care Res Dev. 2014 Jul;15(3):312–23.

73. Dindo L. One-day acceptance and commitment training workshops in medical populations. Curr Opin Psychol. 2015 Apr 1;2:38–42.

74. Shennan C, Payne S, Fenlon D. What is the evidence for the use of mindfulness-based interventions in cancer care? A review Psychooncology. 2011 Jul;20(7):681–97.

75. Kabat-Zinn J. An outpatient program in behavioral medicine for chronic pain patients based on the practice of mindfulness meditation: theoretical considerations and preliminary results. Gen Hosp Psychiatry. 1982 Apr;4(1):33–47.

76. Segal Z, Vincent P, Levitt A. Efficacy of combined, sequential and crossover psychotherapy and pharmacotherapy in improving outcomes in depression. J Psychiatry Neurosci. 2002 Jul;27(4):281–90.

77. Azam MA, Katz J, Mohabir V, Ritvo P. Individuals with tension and migraine headaches exhibit increased heart rate variability during post-stress mindfulness meditation practice but a decrease during a post-stress control condition – a randomized, controlled experiment. Int J Psychophysiol. 2016 Dec;110:66–74.

78. Kim BJ, Cho IS, Cho KI. Impact of mindfulness based stress reduction therapy on myocardial function and endothelial dysfunction in female patients with microvascular angina. J Cardiovasc Ultrasound. 2017 Dec;25(4):118–23.

79. Carlson LE, Garland SN. Impact of mindfulness-based stress reduction (MBSR) on sleep, mood, stress and fatigue symptoms in cancer outpatients. Int J Behav Med. 2005;12(4):278–85.

80. Tacon AM. Mindfulness: existential, loss, and grief factors in women with breast cancer. J Psychosoc Oncol. 2011;29(6):643–56.

81. Ditto B, Eclache M, Goldman N. Short-term autonomic and cardiovascular effects of mindfulness body scan meditation. Ann Behav Med. 2006 Dec;32(3):227–34.

82. Gross CR, Kreitzer MJ, Thomas W, Reilly-Spong M, Cramer-Bornemann M, Nyman JA, et al. Mindfulness-based stress reduction for solid organ transplant recipients: a randomized controlled trial. Altern Ther Health Med. 2010 Sep-Oct;16(5):30–8.

83. Castleberry AW, Bishawi M, Worni M, Erhunmwunsee L, Speicher PJ, Osho AA, et al. Medication nonadherence after lung transplantation in adult recipients. Ann Thorac Surg. 2017 Jan;103(1):274–80.

84. Martino S. Motivational interviewing to engage patients in chronic kidney disease management. Blood Purif. 2011;31(1–3):77–81.

85. Dew MA, Dimartini AF, De Vito Dabbs A, Zomak R, De Geest S, Dobbels F, et al. Adherence to the medical regimen during the first two years after lung transplantation. Transplantation. [Comparative StudyResearch Support, N.I.H., Extramural]. 2008 Jan 27;85(2):193–202.

86. Vlaminck H, Maes B, Evers G, Verbeke G, Lerut E, Van Damme B, et al. Prospective study on late consequences of subclinical non-compliance with immunosuppressive therapy in renal transplant patients. Am J Transplant. 2004 Sep;4(9):1509–13.

87. Patzer RESM, Reese PP, Przytula K, Koval R, Ladner DP, Levitsky JM, et al. Medication understanding, non-adherence, and clinical outcomes among adult kidney transplant recipients. Clin Transpl. 2016;30(10):1294–305.

88. Rollnick S, Miller WR. Stephan. Motivational interviewing: preparing people for change. New York: Guildford Press; 2002.

89. De Bleser LMM, Dobbels F, Russell C, De Geest S. Interventions to improve medication-adherence after transplantation: a systematic review. Transpl Int. 2009;22(8):780–97.

90. Dobbels FDBL, Berben L, Kristanto P, Dupont L, Nevens F, Vanhaecke J, et al. Efficacy of a medication adherence enhancing intervention in transplantation: the MAESTRO-Tx trial. J Heart Lung Transplant. 2017;36(5):499–508.

91. McCarley P. Patient empowerment and motivational interviewing: engaging patients to self-manage their own care. Nephrol Nurs J. 2009;36(4):409–13.

92. Van Zuilen AD, Wetzels JF, Bots ML, Van Blankestijn PJ, MASTERPLAN Study Group. MASTERPLAN: study of the role of nurse practitioners in a multifactorial intervention to reduce cardiovascular risk in chronic kidney disease patients. J Nephrol. 2008;21(3):261–7.

93. Miller WRS. Motivational interviewing: helping people change. 3rd ed. New York, NY: Guildford Press; 2013.

94. Haines J, Spadaro KC, Choi J, Hoffman LA, Blazeck AM. Reducing stress and anxiety in caregivers of lung transplant patients: benefits of mindfulness meditation. Int J Organ Transplant Med. 2014;5(2):50–6.

95. Abbey S, Farrow S. Group therapy and organ transplantation. Int J Group Psychother. 1998 Apr;48(2):163–85.

96. Buchanan DC. Group therapy for kidney transplant patients. Int J Psychiatry Med. 1975;6(4):523–31.

97. Griffith J, Gaby L. Brief psychotherapy at the bedside: countering demoralization from medical illness. Psychosomatics. 2005;46(2):109–16.

98. Safren S, Gonzalez J, Soroudi N. Coping with chronic illness: a cognitive-behavioral therapy approach for adherence and depression. New York: Oxford University Press; 2008.

99. Hayes SC. Acceptance and change : content and context in psychotherapy. Reno, NV: Context Press; 1994.

100. Kabat-Zinn J. Full catastrophe living: using the wisdom of your body and mind to face stress, pain, and illness. New York: Bantam Books; 2013.

101. Chochinov HM. Dignity therapy : final words for final days. Oxford/New York: Oxford University Press; 2012.

102. Breitbart W, Poppito SR. Individual meaning-centered psychotherapy for patients with advanced cancer : a treatment manual. Oxford: Oxford University Press; 2014.

Social Work Interventions in End-Stage Organ Disease and Transplant Patients

44

Caitlin J. West and Kelsey Winnike

Introduction

Social workers play an integral role in the transplantation process for patients, their families and caregivers, and the medical teams. The focus of the practice in solid organ transplant social work involves psychosocial evaluation, addressing identified areas of psychosocial vulnerability or risk factors, and working as part of a multidisciplinary team to best support patients and their families during this complex and challenging process. While the transplant social work practices and evaluation tools may vary between transplant centers and across organ groups, the Centers for Medicare and Medicaid Services (CMS) have created mandates for all transplant centers. These mandates are aimed at standardizing care, guiding best practices, ensuring equal access to care, and ultimately protecting the health and safety of solid organ transplant patients (see Table 44.1).

Psychosocial Evaluation

Social workers are frequently among the first transplant team members to have in-depth interactions with patients. This often begins with a thorough psychosocial evaluation.

For the purpose of this chapter, we will not cover the distinct differences in the evaluation process and unique ethical considerations that occur in the psychosocial evaluation of and work with living donors (see Chap. 4). However, it is important to acknowledge this unique area of organ transplantation in social work practice.

The psychosocial evaluation includes the patient and ideally his or her identified support persons/caregivers. This

Table 44.1 CMS mandates for the solid organ transplant programs [1]

CMS regulation reference	Regulation
Regulation X092	A social worker must be part of the solid organ transplant team. "Transplant centers must make social services available, furnished by qualified social workers to transplant patients, living donors and their families" [1]
Regulation X053	A psychosocial evaluation must be conducted for potential transplant candidates. "In nearly all cases, the transplant program must conduct and document the psychosocial evaluation conducted on a prospective transplant candidate before his/her placement on the waitlist. With exception to emergency situations" [1]
Regulation X093	A qualified professional is "an individual who meets licensing requirements in the state in which he or she practices; and (1) Completed a course of study with specialization in clinical practice and holds a master's degrees from a graduate school of social work accredited by the Council on Social Work Education; or (2) Worked as a social worker in a transplant center as of June 28, 2007 and has served for at least 2 years as a social worker, 1 year of which was in a transplantation program and has established a consulting relationship with a qualified social worker" [1] (e.g., Masters of Social Work (MSW), Licensed Clinical Social Worker(LCSW))

process helps the multidisciplinary transplant team identify patients' strengths and protective factors that will assist the patient in navigating the complex transplant process as well as possible risk factors that can lead to negative outcomes. The detailed psychosocial evaluation aims to optimize physical, emotional, and mental well-being of patients post-transplantation [2]. Please refer to Chap. 3 for full review of the psychosocial evaluation process for potential candidates at Stanford Health Care. The identified risk factors allow transplant social workers to develop targeted interventions to minimize risks and assist patients in optimizing their transplant candidacy and post-transplant physical and emotional outcomes. As part of their intervention, social workers refer

C. J. West
Department of Social Work,
University of Colorado Hospital, Aurora, CO, USA

K. Winnike (✉)
Department of Social Work and Case Management, Stanford Health Care, Stanford, CA, USA
e-mail: KWinnike@stanfordhealthcare.org

© Springer International Publishing AG, part of Springer Nature 2019
Y. Sher, J. R. Maldonado (eds.), *Psychosocial Care of End-Stage Organ Disease and Transplant Patients*,
https://doi.org/10.1007/978-3-319-94914-7_44

patients to transplant psychiatrists for further evaluation of areas of concern and/or for treatment. Any concerns identified by transplant social workers that might interfere with successful management of a transplant are brought to the attention and discussed during the multidisciplinary transplant committee meeting [3].

Pre-transplant, psychosocial updates are completed, at minimum, annually after the initial evaluation and psychosocial needs are reassessed frequently and across the continuum of transplantation. Patient's psychosocial status might change while awaiting transplant or postoperatively (e.g., caregiver plan or mental health changes), and social workers are on the frontline to identify changes and intervene, as needed, to optimize outcomes.

Psychoeducation

A thorough assessment of patients and caregivers' health literacy is a key component of the initial psychosocial evaluation and can help the medical team to adapt education. Social workers have an obligation to ensure that patients and families have a realistic overview of the solid organ transplant process. In fact, CMS mandates that patients are informed of both medical and psychosocial risks [1]. More specifically, CMS outlines that the potential risks of depression, post-traumatic

stress disorder (PTSD), generalized anxiety disorder, anxiety regarding dependence on others, and feelings of guilt should be discussed with transplant candidates [1]. It is essential for patients to understand that solid organ transplant is not a cure and that they will be trading one disease for another condition requiring a lifetime of medical treatment. Furthermore, CMS requires that discussion of psychosocial risks takes place early in the evaluation process and is repeated whenever any major change in medical or psychosocial status occurs [1].

A multidisciplinary approach to patient education in the patient's primary language through individual or group education sessions, videos, and handouts can improve patients' understanding of the complex transplant process. Incorporating psychoeducation into the initial psychosocial evaluation can also enhance patients and families' understanding of the transplant process and reinforce information that has already been reviewed or might follow this evaluation.

Financial Preparedness

Undergoing transplantation can significantly impact financial stability. In preparing for transplant, it is essential for social workers to provide education around the significant costs of transplantation to patients and families (see Table 44.2) [4]. Both medical and nonmedical expenses are

Table 44.2 Estimated US average 2017 billed charges per transplant

Transplant	30 days pre-transplant	Procurement	Hospital transplant admission	Physician during transplant admission	180 days post-transplant discharge	Outpatient immuno-suppressants & other prescriptions	Total
Single Organ/Tissue							
Bone Marrow -Allogenic	$60,200	$72,200	$465,200	$22,600	$249,800	$22,700	$892,700
Bone Marrow -Autologous	61,500	15,300	226,300	10,700	81,300	14,500	409,600
Cornea	NA	NA	21,900	8,300	NA	NA	30,200
Heart	43,300	102,100	887,400	92,300	222,800	34,500	1,382,400
Intestine	28,400	106,100	669,600	60,000	260,600	22,600	1,147,300
Kidney	30,100	96,800	159,400	24,900	75,000	28,600	414,800
Liver	41,400	94,100	463,200	56,100	126,900	30,800	812,500
Lung - Single	27,900	106,100	475,000	49,600	163.200	39,900	861,700
Lung - Double	38,800	127,600	679,100	68,900	226,500	49,800	1.190.700
Pancreas	13,400	97,900	131,400	19,600	62,600	22,100	347,000
Multiple Organ							
Heart-Lung	93,100	155,900	1,731,900	162,800	373,600	46,700	2,564,000
Intestine with Other Organs	69,000	260,700	803,200	96,600	313,000	42,600	1,585,100
Kidney-Heart	136,300	126,700	1,582,100	163,900	450,200	71,700	2,530,900
Kidney-Pancreas	36,500	135,100	274,500	35,900	107,000	29,100	618,100
Liver-Kidney	77,000	160.100	648,900	81.700	216.900	45,100	1,229.700
Other Multi-Organ	85,500	188,400	1,078,900	122,700	327,500	52,400	1,855,400

Reprinted with permission from Bentley, TS, Phillips, SJ. 2017. U.S. organ and tissue transplant cost estimates and discussion. In: Milliman Research Report. 2017.

important to consider in financially preparing for transplant. Anticipated medical expenses include, but are not limited to, insurance deductibles, co-pays, and post-transplant medications. Nonmedical costs include, but are not limited to, pre-transplant travel; lodging and food; medical flight for transplant; pending distance from transplant center; post-transplant temporary relocation, if indicated; and loss of wages by patients and caregivers.

Social workers can support patients and families by providing education regarding fundraising. While there is a plethora of existing fundraising organizations available, a select few are transplant specific. The National Foundation for Transplants, Children's Organ Transplant Association, and Help Hope Live are all 501(c)(3) nonprofit organizations that provide one-on-one guidance to patients and families throughout the fundraising process. The above organizations will manage funds raised and patients can submit bills for direct billing or receipts for reimbursement. Funds collected with the help of these particular organizations are not taxable due to nonprofit status and will not impact patient's eligibility for or jeopardize assistance programs, such as Medicaid or Supplemental Security Income (SSI).

Documentation and Discharge Planning

Transplant social workers are responsible for participating in and maintaining appropriate and supporting documentation on patients throughout the transplant continuum, starting with the psychosocial evaluation. In addition, it is mandated that social workers are actively involved throughout the initial hospitalization for transplantation [1]. Social workers must partner with members of the transplant multidisciplinary team to develop comprehensive safe discharge plans to optimize outcomes after patients leave the hospital.

Discharge planning for transplant is an important topic that is first discussed during the initial psychosocial evaluation, with ongoing discussions across the transplant continuum. Social workers facilitate discussions around caregiver plans, access to medications, relocation, temporary lodging arrangements, and financial preparedness in an effort to proactively plan for discharge post-transplant. At Stanford Health Care, social workers are responsible for facilitating post-transplant lodging and ensuring that there is a safe and adequate lodging plan in place.

Available temporary lodging arrangements and resources will vary across transplant centers. In fact, at Stanford Health Care post-transplantation relocation policies vary significantly even across organ groups. For example, Stanford's lung transplant team requires their patients to reside within a 45-min radius of the hospital, including time spent in traffic. In contrast, Stanford's kidney transplant team determines whether patients are medically required to relocate on a case

by case basis. If available, patients are provided with psychoeducation regarding lodging benefits through their insurance. Patients are strongly encouraged to financially prepare for relocation expenses through saving and fundraising. See financial preparedness section for further details. In the event of an ongoing financial hardship, a financial screening can be completed to assess for potential subsidies.

Lastly, education plays a significant role in the discharge planning process. Patients and their caregivers are required to participate in education with various members of the multidisciplinary team. This typically includes the post-transplant nurse coordinator, registered dietician, and pharmacist. Social workers are actively involved throughout the transplant process, but take on a critical role during the final stages of discharge planning, in addition to case managers, to ensure patients and their caregivers feel confident to leave the hospital and successfully manage care on their own.

Therapeutic Interventions

Adjustment to illness can vary widely across the disease spectrum and may depend on the acute versus chronic nature of the condition. De Ridder et al. defines chronic illnesses as disorders that persist for a protracted period and impact a person's ability to function [5]. Consequently, chronic illnesses can provoke significant changes in lifestyle that may negatively impact a person's overall well-being and quality of life [6].

With a multitude of potential losses in mind, it is not surprising that some individuals with chronic illness have more difficulty adjusting than others. There are unique challenges related to the uncertain and erratic nature of the disease course [7]. Loss of control frequently pervades all aspects of a chronic illness [8]. In addition, fears regarding loss of self-image, dependency, stigma of illness, abandonment, expression of anger, isolation, and death can overtake patients with chronic illness [9]. Potential responses to chronic illness include increased anxiety, depression, alienation, abandonment, emotional ambivalence, hopelessness, powerlessness, and withdrawal from relationships [7, 10, 11]. Many of these responses occur in transplant recipients. In fact, Goetzmann et al. found that 41% of transplant recipients experienced psychosocial hardship after transplant, including depression and anxiety, psychological stress, and lower quality of life [12].

Psychosocial interventions to reduce symptoms of distress with non-pharmacological approaches may facilitate improved quality of life and more adaptive coping among post-transplant recipients [13]. Transplant social workers are at the forefront of interfacing with transplant patients and are able to evaluate their emotional states and ideally intervene with non-pharmacological measures. There are a variety of psychotherapeutic techniques available (see Chap. 43 for further details). One intervention that can be easily employed or recommended by transplant social workers is mindfulness training or mindfulness-based stress reduction (MBSR). In the first randomized controlled trial of MBSR in transplant recipients, Gross et al. found that MBSR reduced symptoms of distress and improved mental health and vitality in recipients of solid organ transplant [13]. Social workers may consider exploring MBSR training and/or recommending a MBSR program to transplant recipients.

It is also important for transplant social workers to liaise with transplant and/or community psychiatrists and therapists to refer patients for further evaluation and treatment when needed. In particular, community mental health-care providers with experience and expertise in dealing with adjustment to chronic illness can provide invaluable support and therapeutic interventions for transplant patients.

Post-Transplant Interventions

After a patient is discharged from the hospital, social workers follow patients for the life of the organ. Social workers use outpatient clinic as an opportunity to provide ongoing assessment and psychosocial support around adjustment to life post-transplant. Having a strong social work presence in clinic can help facilitate timely interventions to optimize patients' psychosocial outcomes. During the post-transplant period, it is common for social workers to assist with a variety of issues, such as medication access, motivation and adherence, mental health concerns, caregiver support, and barriers to care such as changes in insurance, transportation issues, financial strain, and support related to end of life issues.

Peer Support and Internet Resources

It is broadly recognized that peer support is valuable to transplant patients, but the subject is underresearched [13]. Wright found that heart transplant patients enrolled in a formal mentorship program appreciated the information and support to help them cope [14]. Interestingly, Wright further found that medical topics were among the most frequently discussed topics during such meetings, indicating that although patients had received information from their medical teams, it was essential for them to process this information with their peers who had a similar experience. In a study of liver transplant patients, the support group intervention demonstrated improved physiological, psychological, and social adaptation of liver transplant recipients [15]. In a systematic literature review of volunteer-delivered peer support programs in oncology, Campbell et al. observed that several studies found wide ranging benefits of peer support, including reassurance,

reduction in isolation, increased information sharing, improved coping skills, an enhanced understanding of the experience, and a sense of normalcy [16]. Social workers can promote these valuable peer connections by developing transplant-specific peer mentorship programs and support groups.

Patients may benefit from one-to-one connections with peers who have shared experiences. Augmenting patient care through support and education from a peer perspective is the primary goal of peer mentorship programs [17]. At Stanford, the Peer-to-Peer Mentor Program is another valuable resource for patients awaiting transplant. Patients are paired with peer mentors and the two connect by email, phone, or in-person, based on personal preference and geographical proximity. The transplant social workers often assist in identifying appropriate mentors and provide them with linkage to the Peer-to-Peer Mentor Program. In addition, social workers can identify transplant candidates who may benefit from a one-to-one peer connection and provide psychoeducation about the program and benefits of peer mentorship.

Many transplant centers offer traditional in-person support groups for patients and caregivers [17]. At Stanford, Health Care, solid organ transplant support groups are generally conducted on a monthly or every other month basis lasting an hour to an hour and a half. Pre- and post-transplant patients and their caregivers are invited to attend. Social workers organize and facilitate these meetings.

Many of the Stanford transplant support groups utilize a psychoeducational framework. Social workers collaborate with the transplant multidisciplinary team to coordinate psychoeducation sessions regarding each team member's area of expertise to further support patients and their caregivers across the transplant continuum. For example, pharmacists discuss strategies for managing complex post-transplant medications, psychiatry presents on psychological care in all phases of transplantation, and transplant nurse practitioners and coordinators cover what to expect in post-transplant clinic and how to stay well post-transplant. Dieticians review the importance of nutrition, and physical therapists review the importance of staying active and strong throughout transplantation. Support groups also serve as a vehicle for physicians and transplant leadership to maintain open communication and build rapport with patients and families. Physician and transplant leadership can offer organ-specific programmatic updates while also presenting a unique opportunity for patients and caregivers to openly ask questions of the physicians and the programs. Social work will liase with local donor networks to arrange having a donor family present to the group. The donor family presentation provides a unique opportunity for patients and families to hear a donor family's perspective and the powerful impact that transplantation has on both parties.

While these in-person connections are immensely valuable, they can also be inconvenient for some patients due to geographic proximity, space, time, and patient mobility [18, 19]. Furthermore, individual and group dynamics may impact a person's willingness to contribute his or her own experiences due to concerns around privacy, confidentiality, and fear of embarrassment [18, 19]. The Internet offers individuals additional opportunities to communicate with one another anytime and remain anonymous in doing so, if preferred [18]. It allows patients and caregivers the opportunity to connect with a wide array of individuals with shared health interests worldwide [20], such as organ-specific transplantation.

Transplant recipients are now able to access organ-specific social media sites to broaden their support network [18]. Grumme and Gordon described that transplant recipients found a sanctuary in an international transplant community support group online, where recipients were able to share their unique feelings and experiences post-transplant in a safe environment [18]. Transplant recipients' postings reveal a willingness to share experiences and a sense of community for members to support each other.

Online resources might also be especially useful for younger transplant patients. For example, a pilot study on an innovative Internet program *Teens Taking Charge: Managing My Transplant Online* provided teens with solid organ transplants with relevant transplant information, self-management and transition skills, as well as opportunities for peer support [21]. Initial findings found positive regard and engagement from teens, with more interventions and studies planned by the research group [21]. Social workers can recognize such opportunities for their patient populations, bringing a variety of adapted interventions to clinics.

Caregivers

It is widely known that the availability of one or more dedicated caregivers is a fundamental aspect of a patient's post-transplant success [22–24]. Caregivers have multifaceted roles throughout the pre-, peri-, and postoperative phases of transplant. Pre-transplant, caregivers are often required to accompany patients to medical appointments, including the pre-transplant evaluation [25]. During the perioperative phase, caregivers await surgery updates, provide bedside support, and consult with providers for medical decision-making [25]. Post-transplant, caregivers participate in bedside discharge teaching, assist in managing a complex medication regimen, provide transportation and accompany patients to follow-up appointments, assist with practical needs (e.g., meal preparation, refilling prescriptions, cleaning, laundry), provide emotional support, and potentially relocate, if indicated.

While caregiver requirements vary across transplant centers and organ groups, reviewing programmatic expectations in detail with patients and identified caregivers is essential during the psychosocial evaluation. Social workers at Stanford Health Care provide psychoeducation about the program's caregiver requirements and assess identified caregivers' ability to serve in that capacity. Caregivers should not only be available but fully functional and able to assist with a myriad of tasks post-transplant. They must be well known to transplant candidates and demonstrate full commitment to patients' post-transplant recovery. In addition, caregivers must be able to drive and have access to reliable transportation to accompany patients to their outpatient visits. Furthermore, the caregivers' physical or mental health conditions should not interfere with their ability to provide care for patients post-transplant. Alcohol, tobacco, and substance use disorders are also important considerations to assess in potential caregivers as these may impact their ability to effectively serve in that capacity. Identified caregivers must be able to take leave from work and/or other household responsibilities for the time required to serve in this role. The financial implications of taking leave from work are important to consider in assessing caregivers' ability to commit to the role. While caregivers may be eligible for unpaid job protection of up to 12 weeks annually under the Family and Medical Leave Act [26], some states, albeit quite limited, offer paid family leave programs, which can help alleviate the financial burden of caring for a loved one. Social workers can assist in determining if a caregiver meets criteria for a state paid family leave program. They can also help facilitate coordination of leave forms and documentation needed to support the caregiver's efforts to take an extended leave from their job.

Caring for patients with chronic illnesses is stressful and taxing [27]. Vitaliano et al. found that caregivers reported higher levels of somatic complaints and affective distress than non-caregivers [28]. Multiple studies have indicated that distressed caregivers often report feeling resentful, depressed, anxious, overwhelmed, and exhausted [29–31]. Caregivers often prioritize patient needs before their own during the pre-, peri-, and post-transplant periods [25]. Parekh et al. found that caregivers were more susceptible to burnout and experienced higher levels of burden when their own needs were disregarded [32]. Relationships between patients and caregivers often evolve during the transplant process with changing roles and responsibilities that can strain the relationship. Ongoing assessment of caregiver support is needed to bolster such strained relationships [33]. How caregivers cope with stress has implications for their own mental and physical health and impacts their ability to effectively meet the caregiver responsibilities [25]. Mollberg et al. suggested that caregivers may impact recipients' long-term outcomes by affecting adherence to the daily post-transplant treatment regimen [34]. With this in mind, it is essential that caregivers are well supported throughout the transplant process.

Early detection of caregiver distress and adjustment challenges affords social work clinicians a critical opportunity to provide additional support and referrals to mental health services [25], as indicated. Goetzinger et al. further emphasize the importance of a secondary caregiver plan, which offers the primary caregiver relief and respite to attend to their own needs [25]. Social workers can provide psychoeducation regarding the importance of developing a secondary caregiver plan prior to listing for transplant. Social workers can further assist distressed caregivers in developing more adaptive coping mechanisms, which can promote self-efficacy, confidence, and personal control [25].

Conclusions

In conclusion, social workers are essential members of the multidisciplinary transplantation teams. Social workers serve a critical role providing valuable assessment, psychoeducation, treatment strategies, and interventions aimed at optimizing a patient's candidacy pre-transplant and optimizing outcomes post-transplant. Although the primary focus is often directed toward the patient, supporting the caregivers during this complex process is paramount to the success and well-being of the patient/caregiver system. More research is needed on behalf and by transplant social workers regarding a variety of multimodal interventions to further advance transplant social work practice and support patients and caregivers in having a successful transplant journey.

References

1. Department of Health and Human Services, Centers for Medicare & Medicaid Services, Center for Clinical Standards and Quality/Survey & Certification Group. Interpretive guidelines for organ transplant conditions of participation. 2016. https://www.cms.gov/Medicare/Provider-Enrollment-and-Certification/SurveyCertificationGenInfo/Downloads/Survey-and-Cert-Letter-16-10.pdf. Accessed 14 Dec 2017.
2. Wise T. Update on consultation–liaison psychiatry (psychosomatic medicine). Curr Opin Psychiatry. 2008;21(2):196–200.
3. Kuntz K, Weinland S, Butt Z. Psychosocial challenges in solid organ transplantation. J Clin Psychol Med Settings. 2015;22(2–3):122–35.
4. Bentley TS, Phillips SJ. 2017 U.S. organ and tissue transplant cost estimates and discussion. In: Milliman Research Report. 2017. http://www.milliman.com/uploadedFiles/insight/2017/2017-Transplant-Report.pdf. Accessed 19 Nov 2017.
5. De Ridder D, Geenen R, Kuijer R, van Middendorp H. Psychological adjustment to chronic disease. Lancet. 2008;372:246–55.
6. Sprangers M, de Regt E, Andries F, et al. Which chronic conditions are associated with better or poorer quality of life? J Clin Epidemiol. 2000;53:895–907.
7. Sidell N. Adult adjustment to chronic illness: a review of the literature. Health Soc Work. 1997;22(1):5–11. Available from: Academic Search Premier
8. Miller J. Coping with chronic illness: overcoming powerlessness. Philadelphia: F.A. Davis; 1983.
9. Pollin I. Taking charge: overcoming the challenge of long-term illness. New York: Random House; 1994.
10. Lapham E, Ehrhart L. Young adulthood: establishing intimacy. In: Lapham E, Shevlin K, editors. The impact of chronic illness on psychosocial stages of human development. Washington, DC: National Center for Education in Maternal and Child Health; 1986. p. 91–104.
11. McLaughlin T, Aupont O, Bambauer K, Stone P, Mullan M, Colagiovanni J, et al. Improving psychological adjustment to chronic illness in cardiac patients: the role of depression and anxiety. J Gen Intern Med. 2005;20:1084–90.
12. Goetzmann L, Ruegg L, Stamm M, Ambuhl P, Boehler A, Halter J, et al. Psychosocial profiles after transplantation: a 24-month follow-up of heart, lung, liver, kidney and allogeneic bone-marrow patients. Transplantation. 2008;86(5):662–8.
13. Gross CR, Kreitzer MJ, Thomas W, Reilly-Spong M, Cramer-Bornemann M, Nyman JA, et al. Mindfulness-based stress reduction for solid organ transplant recipients: a randomized controlled trial. Alternative Therapies. 2010;16(5):30–7.
14. Wright L, Pennington J, Abbey S, Young E, Haines J, Ross H. Evaluation of a mentorship program for heart transplant patients. J Heart Lung Transplant. 2001;20(9):1030–3.
15. Ordin YS, Yarayurt O. Effects of a support group intervention on physical, psychological, and social adaptation of liver transplant recipients. Exp Clin Transplant. 2016;14(3):329–37.
16. Campbell HS, Phaneuf MR, Deane K. Cancer peer support programs—do they work? Patient Educ Couns. 2004;55:3–15.
17. Wright L. Mentorship programs for transplant patients. Prog Transplant. 2000;10:267–72.
18. Grumme V, Gordon S. Social media use by transplant recipients for support and healing. CIN. 2016;34(12):570–7.
19. Walther J, Boyd S. Attraction to computer-mediated social support. In: Lin C, Atkin D, editors. Communication technology and society: audience adoption and uses. Creskill, NJ: Hampton Press; 2002. p. 153–88.
20. Eysenbach G. The impact of the internet on cancer outcomes. CA Cancer J Clin. 2003;53(6):356–71. https://doi.org/10.3322/canjclin.53.6.356.
21. Korus M, Crunchley E, Stinson JN, Gold A, Anthony SJ. Usability testing of the internet program: "teens taking charge: managing my transplant online.". Pediatr Transplant. 2015;19:107–19.
22. Christiansen AJ, Turner CW, Slaughter JM, Holman JM. Perceived family support as a moderator psychological Well-being in end-stage renal disease. J Behav Med. 1989;12:249.
23. Moran PJ, Christensen AJ, Ehlers SL, Bertolatus JA. Family environment, intrusive ideation, and adjustment among renal transplant candidates. Ann Behav Med. 1999;21:311.
24. Levenson JL, Olbrish ME. Shortage of donor organs and long waits. Psychosomatics. 1987;28:399.
25. Goetzinger AM, Blumenthal JA, O'Hayer CA, Babyak MA, Hoffman BM, Ong L, et al. Stress and coping in caregivers of patients awaiting solid organ transplantation. Clin Transpl. 2012;26:97–104.

26. United States Department of Labor. Wage and hour division (WHD): family and medical leave act. https://www.dol.gov/whd/fmla/. Accessed 22 Feb 2018.
27. Pinquart M, Sorensen S. Differences between caregivers and non-caregivers in psychological health and physical health: a meta-analysis. Psychol Aging. 2003;18:250.
28. Vitaliano PP, Zhang J, Scanlan JM. Is caregiving hazardous to one's physical health? A Meta-Analysis Psychol Bull. 2003;129:946.
29. Billings DW, Folkman SF, Acree M, Moskowitz JT. Coping and physical health during caregiving: the roles of positive and negative affect. J Pers Soc Psychol. 2000;79:131.
30. Chappell N, Colin RR. Burden and Well-being among caregivers: examining the distinction. The Gerontologist. 2002;42:772.
31. Goode KT, Haley WE, Roth DL, Ford GR. Predicting longitudinal changes in caregiver physical and mental health: a stress process model. Health Psychol. 1998;17:190.
32. Parekh PI, Bluementhal JA, Babyak MA, et al. Psychiatric disorders and quality of life in patients awaiting lung transplantation. Chest. 2003;124:1682.
33. Berry OO, Kymissis C. Key role of social supports in cardiac transplant treatment team. J Psychiatr Pract. 2016;22(2):133–9.
34. Mollberg NM, Farjah F, Howell E, Ortiz J, Backhus L, Mulligan M. Impact of primary caregivers on long-term outcomes after lung transplantation. J Heart Lung Transplant. 2015;34(1):59–64.

Substance Use Disorders in Transplant Patients

45

Marian Fireman

Introduction

Evaluation of transplant candidates focuses on those who are most ill and those who will benefit the most from transplant. Selection of candidates seeks to identify those patients who will care for the transplanted organ, including not using substances that may negatively impact patient and graft survival. It is hoped that careful and appropriate selection of transplant candidates will lead to good post-transplant outcomes and long survival post-transplant.

Alcohol, tobacco, and other substance use disorders are common in the general population in the United States and globally. The lifetime prevalence of alcohol use disorders (AUDs) in the United States is approximately 29% [1]. Tobacco use has been declining in the United States. Current estimated lifetime prevalence of tobacco use disorders is 20–25%; it is estimated that approximately 15% of the general population are current smokers [2]. Substance use disorders (SUDs), excluding alcohol and tobacco, are also common; nearly 4% currently meet criteria for SUDs and lifetime prevalence of SUDs in the United States is nearly 10% [3]. Many more individuals use a variety of substances recreationally, but may not actually meet criteria for a disorder. Alcohol, tobacco, and drug use disorders are difficult to treat, relapse rates are high, and at any one time, only approximately 10% of those in need of treatment are actually receiving such treatment. Medical complications of these disorders cause significant morbidity and mortality. Currently, in the United States, alcohol, tobacco, illicit drug, and prescription drug use are identified as the primary factors in one out of every four deaths [4]. Alcohol, tobacco, and other drugs cause a wide range of health consequences, both those directly related to the drug use and indirect effects related to the method of use. Such problems include cardiovascular

disease, malignancy, hepatitis, HIV-related illness, and other infectious complications. These substances may have adverse effects on virtually every organ system. It is estimated that these substances cost the United States more than $740 billion yearly for health care, crime, and lost productivity [4]. Smoking decreases life expectancy by approximately 14 years, and excessive alcohol use decreases life expectancy by at least 10–12 years. Drug overdose deaths have skyrocketed and now are the leading cause of death of Americans under 50 years of age [5]. The medical complications of these disorders may cause and often do contribute to end-stage organ disease. Not unexpectedly, a large percentage of patients with end-stage organ disease will have a current or past history of alcohol, tobacco, and/or other substance use [6]. These findings are summarized in Fig. 45.1.

Concerns in Transplant

Addiction is a chronic illness with remissions and relapses. The etiology of addiction is complex with the illness disrupting the functioning of the brain and the ability of the individual to modulate and control social, emotional, and cognitive behavior. Relapse is a major concern when evaluating transplant candidates as recurrent use of alcohol, tobacco, and other substances may result in direct or indirect damage to the transplanted organ, rejection of the graft, and medical

Addiction Diagnoses and End-Stage Organ Disease

- Heart transplant candidates
  - ~30% alcohol use disorders
  - ~90% tobacco use disorder
- Lung transplant candidates
  - ~70% tobacco use disorder
- Liver transplant candidates
  - 25-75% alcohol use disorders
  - ~25% other substance use disorders

Fig. 45.1 Addiction diagnoses and end-stage organ disease

M. Fireman
Department of Psychiatry, Oregon Health and Science University, Portland, OR, USA
e-mail: firemanm@ohsu.edu

© Springer International Publishing AG, part of Springer Nature 2019
Y. Sher, J. R. Maldonado (eds.), *Psychosocial Care of End-Stage Organ Disease and Transplant Patients*,
https://doi.org/10.1007/978-3-319-94914-7_45

complications that are a direct result of the substance use, poor adherence, and difficult management issues for the transplant team. A large percentage of transplant candidates do have a history of alcohol, tobacco, and substance use disorder, and many may be only recently abstinent from these substances. As a result, much attention has been paid to risk of relapse in this group. Early identification of individuals with a history of alcohol, tobacco, and other SUDs is important as some of these individuals may benefit from assessment and ongoing treatment of these disorders. Appropriate treatment addressing the alcohol, tobacco, or other SUD may enhance adherence with care and transplant outcomes. In addition, is it important to identify individuals who may not be transplant candidates. These individuals may include those who are unable to stop alcohol or other substance use and individuals who are not able to be adequately adherent with medications and medical care [7].

Alcohol

Many studies address the issue of whether patients with alcohol use disorders (AUDs) should be transplanted and the risk of post-transplant alcohol use in these individuals. Despite a large number of studies, the risk of post-transplant alcohol relapse and the question as to whether relapse impacts transplant outcomes remains controversial. Unfortunately, despite the fact that this issue has been studied by many authors for over 25 years, there are no standard guidelines or even a consensus among centers with regard to a standardized approach to the evaluation of transplant candidates who consume alcohol. The issue is mainly addressed in the liver transplant literature. There are few studies related to other solid organ transplants. A number of factors may account for the wide variety of approaches seen at different transplant centers. Differences in resources, program size, availability of addiction experts with knowledge of organ transplant, and different approaches to the selection process are among the factors that have been proposed [8].

Starzl [9] described liver transplant as the "ultimate sobering experience" based on an early study in which only 2 of 35 patients who survived greater than 2 months post-transplant relapsed to the use of alcohol. Kumar [10], Bird [11], and Osorio [12] noted in several small studies that patients with a minimum of 6 months abstinence from alcohol prior to transplant had lower relapse rates and proposed a required period of 6 months of abstinence prior to liver transplantation. These studies were followed by many other studies describing relapse rates varying from approximately 5% to greater than 90%. Unfortunately, these studies were largely retrospective and used differing definitions of relapse, different periods of follow-up, and various patient populations [13]. When a definition of "any use" of

alcohol is used, greater than 70% of patients are noted to use alcohol when assessed at 10–13 years post-transplant. "Heavy use" is often defined as more than 2 standard drinks per day, 14 drinks per week, or 4 drinks per occasion. Ongoing "heavy" drinking would seem to be a more appropriate definition of relapse. When relapse is defined as "heavy drinking," approximately 20–40% of patients are noted to have relapsed when assessed at 10 years post-transplant. Approximately half of those patients (10–20%) have returned to continuous heavy drinking [13]. A provocative paper by Pageaux questions whether alcohol relapse post-transplant impacts patient or graft survival [14]. A number of studies have shown both good patient and graft survival post-transplant in patients who have relapsed and returned to heavy drinking. However, complications of heavy alcohol use include nonadherence, rejection, and increased rates of steatohepatitis. A number of deaths have been noted in these patients; however, overall patient survival is comparable or even better than those transplanted for other diseases [6, 15–17]. It has been noted that patients who do relapse to the use of alcohol have increased mortality from cardiovascular disease and de novo neoplasms. It has been proposed that this observation is likely due to concurrent relapse to tobacco use in these individuals. Thus, cessation of smoking should be an important goal for all transplant patients [15, 18–23].

Many risk factors for relapse to alcohol use post-transplant have been proposed and studied. These are summarized in Fig. 45.2. Many studies have assessed a variety of the proposed relapse risk factors and noted conflicting results. This is likely because of the retrospective nature of most studies, differing selection criteria for transplant, different definitions of relapse, and different patient populations. Most studies assess a variety of clinical and demographic variables. The most consistent predictors of alcohol relapse have been a diagnosis of AUD, comorbid psychiatric diagnoses, co-occurring other SUDs, poor social support, positive family history of AUD, and ongoing tobacco use. Severity of AUD, insight, motivation for sobriety, willingness to accept treatment, and cognitive impairment have also been associated with increased risk for relapse [6, 13, 15, 18, 19, 24–31]. A few studies have evaluated the efficacy of substance abuse treatment in the pre-transplant period [32, 33]. One study found fewer relapses in those patients who had ongoing treatment both pre- and post-transplant [34].

Many studies have focused on length of pre-transplant sobriety as the most important predictor of post-transplant abstinence. However, data in support of the so-called 6-month rule is weak, and the rule has increasingly been questioned as being arbitrary. A minimum of 6 months of sobriety prior to transplant was supported by some studies and refuted by others [13, 30, 35, 36]. DiMartini et al. in a prospective study noted that patients with shorter lengths of

Fig. 45.2 Proposed risk factors for alcohol and substance use post-transplant

Proposed Risk Factors for Alcohol and Substance Use Post-Transplant

- Younger age
- Male gender
- Shorter length of pre-transplant abstinence
- Polysubstance use
- Failed prior addiction treatment
- Lack of engagement in addiction treatment
- Lack of substitute activities
- Unstable home
- Lack of stable job
- Criminal activity
- Family history of addictive disease
- Noncompliance with medical treatment
- Cognitive impairment

- Higher quantity and/or frequency of use
- Longer duration of use
- Ongoing use despite severe medical and/or psychosocial consequences
- Co-morbid psychiatric illness
- Co-morbid personality disorder
- Tobacco use
- Denial of addiction diagnosis
- Continued association with people/places/things associated with substance use
- Lack of social support for sobriety
- Worse medical prognosis
- Earlier onset of substance use disorder
- Childhood abuse

Fig. 45.3 Abstinence prognostic factors in patients diagnosed with alcohol/substance use disorders

Abstinence Prognostic Factors in Patients Diagnosed with Alcohol/Substance Use Disorders

Positive Factors

- Activities to replace substance use
- Sources of hope/self-esteem
- Negative reinforcement for use
- Acceptance of diagnosis and treatment recommendations
- Relationships that promote sobriety
- Lack of co-morbid mental health or personality disorder
- Strong social support system

Negative Factors

- Poor social support system
- Lack of substitute activities and/or ongoing associations with activities associated with substance use
- Criminal activity
- Personality disorder
- Poor compliance
- Worse medical prognosis
- Polysubstance use

sobriety prior to transplant were at higher relapse risk, but there was no minimum length of sobriety that accurately predicted post-transplant abstinence [37]. Although data supporting the "6-month rule" remains inconclusive at best and is not a requirement recommended by UNOS, many programs still use this guideline. One group of patients thought to have increased rates of alcohol relapse and a poorer post-transplant prognosis are those who have a history of abusing multiple substances. It is thought that these patients differ in a number of ways from those with primary alcohol use disorders. These patients with polysubstance use often have a history of childhood abuse, alcohol and drug use in childhood or early adolescence, and comorbid personality disorders [8]. Proposed positive and negative prognostic factors are summarized in Fig. 45.3.

Beresford [38] proposed a careful evaluation of multiple factors in assessing risks of relapse. In this paper, he proposed applying the prognostic factors identified in Valliant's landmark studies on alcoholism. More recently, Beresford and Lucey have proposed a standardized approach of the evaluation of these patients. They state that a proper evaluation of the patient should include the following six factors. These are (1) clinical history, (2) cognitive assessment, (3) diagnostic assessment with regard to presence of alcohol and/or substance use disorder, (4) acceptance of the diagnosis of alcohol/substance use disorder, (5) evaluation of social stability, and (6) application of Valliant's factors that predict abstinence [8]. Valliant proposed four factors that were positive predictors of long-term sobriety. These included substitute activities that filled time previously spent drinking, relationships that supported ongoing sobriety, negative reinforcement for drinking behaviors, and sources that provided the person hope and improved self-esteem [8, 40]. Other authors and clinicians propose a thorough assessment of the patient, including a complete medical, psychiatric, psychosocial, and drug and alcohol history. In addition, a social support person who knows the patient well should be interviewed independently, if possible, to verify the history. All available records should be reviewed to corroborate the history, and random screening for use of alcohol and other drugs should be conducted. Assessment with regard to whether the patient is merely "abstinent" or truly "sober" should also be conducted. Abstinence is merely not using alcohol or other substances, while sobriety refers to engaging in a lifestyle that supports ongoing abstinence. Evidence of true sobriety could include structured time in productive activities; relationships that promote sobriety; avoidance of people, places, and things that might trigger relapse; and a comprehensive relapse prevention plan [39].

One of the emerging controversial topics is transplantation of patients with severe alcohol hepatitis who do not have time to establish long-term abstinence. Mortality among patients presenting with severe alcoholic hepatitis is high, and for those patients who are not responsive to medical management, proceeding to early liver transplantation is the only alternative treatment option. Mathurin et al. [41] first reported that early liver transplantation in this patient population improved survival and that carefully selected patients had low rates of relapse to the use of alcohol. Patients selected for early transplant were screened carefully and none had any psychiatric comorbidity. All had strong social support and committed to lifetime abstinence. On the basis of early studies, it is argued that early liver transplantation should be utilized in carefully selected individuals with refractory severe acute alcoholic hepatitis [42, 43]. Although relapse rates were low in this and similar studies, particularly compared to a non-transplant population, they are still in the 10–20% range at an average follow-up of just 2 years [44–49]. Further prospective studies of this patient population are needed, including the long-term relapse rates and effects on graft and patient survival. Factors, such as insight into their alcohol use disorder, influencing patients' risk of relapse, also need to be further elucidated. Consideration should also be given to methods to enhance supporting the sobriety of these patients post-transplant.

While most studies of post-transplant relapse are in liver transplant patients, several studies have addressed this issue in heart, kidney, and lung transplantation [6]. Approximately 80% of lung transplant patients in a US study endorsed low to moderate alcohol use pre-transplant. After transplant about 40% used alcohol, all at low or moderate levels [50]. Several studies have addressed this issue in kidney transplant patients. Use of alcohol, tobacco, or illicit drugs predicted a small but significant risk of graft loss in a US study; unfortunately, the study analyzed a large database which did not differentiate patients with alcohol use only from those with use of more than one substance [51]. Another study analyzed the association between a pre-transplant diagnosis of alcohol dependence and increased risk of graft loss as well as post-transplant mortality [52]. Several European studies noted that >50% of post-renal transplant patients used alcohol, but heavy alcohol use was rare [53, 54]. There are several small studies of heart transplant patients. These studies noted that pre-transplant substance use was associated with post-transplant nonadherence but had no effect on patient survival [55, 56].

Patients with alcohol use disorders can be successfully transplanted, and survival in this patient population is comparable to patients without alcohol use disorders. Patients with alcohol-related liver disease who undergo liver transplant have superior survival rates to other liver transplant patients, likely because the disease will not recur in the absence of alcohol relapse. Up to 40–50% of patients do relapse with 10–20% drinking at very harmful levels. Outcomes in these patients are still good; however, a small percentage do have complications including steatohepatitis in liver transplant recipients, nonadherence with medications, rejection, graft loss, and death. All patients presenting for organ transplant with alcohol use disorders need careful evaluation, but multiple studies report successful transplantation, excellent survival, and excellent outcomes in these patients. Relapse to ongoing heavy use of alcohol occurs at low rates but can lead to significant morbidity and mortality. Patients should be carefully assessed by the transplant team, and early interventions to treat the disorder are highly recommended. Many patients will need ongoing supports for sobriety both pre- and post-transplant. The issue of which "risk factors for relapse" are most important remains controversial and consensus is lacking. The most prudent approach may be the thorough evaluation of multiple factors in the context of a comprehensive clinical assessment.

Marijuana

Marijuana use among transplant candidates and recipients remains quite controversial. Currently marijuana is legal for recreational use in nine states and Washington, D.C. It is legal for medical use in 29 states [57]. Approximately 60% of the US population lives in a state where marijuana is legal in some form, making it likely that patients will have a current or past history of marijuana use. There is no consensus among transplant centers regarding whether marijuana use in transplant candidates is acceptable or not; some centers have excluded patients who use cannabis, while other centers routinely accept these patients as transplant candidates [58–60].

Public opinion in general supports allowing cannabis users to receive organ transplants [61, 62]. As of the writing of this chapter, eight states have passed legislation stating that patients cannot be denied transplant solely on the basis of marijuana use.

Medical concerns about marijuana use have included potential respiratory, cardiovascular, gastrointestinal, cognitive, and infectious complications. In addition, risk for malignancy may be increased and there is increasing evidence of marijuana-drug interactions [63–67]. Several case reports have highlighted infectious concerns regarding complications of marijuana use, such as disseminated aspergillosis and lupoid pneumonias [63, 68–70].

There has been at least one published case of tacrolimus toxicity caused by suspected cannabinoid inhibition of CYP3A4 and P-glycoprotein [71]. Several other studies of renal and liver transplant recipients did not show worse outcomes among marijuana users [72–74]. Virtually all the case reports and studies to date have addressed smoking of marijuana, while little is known about use of cannabis in other forms.

Patients may use marijuana or other cannabis products to treat medical conditions. Others may be occasional recreational users, while some have diagnosable cannabis use disorders and some are self-medicating a variety of psychiatric conditions. The last two categories are concerning for adverse outcomes. In these cases, patients should be referred for appropriate addiction and/or psychiatric evaluation, and any necessary treatment before the patient is considered an acceptable transplant candidate. Inhalation of products of combustion is associated with negative consequences, and thus benefits of smoked cannabis are likely outweighed by the negative effects.

In summary, risks associated with occasional marijuana use in transplant patients are low, but not completely known and not insignificant. Risk in those with marijuana use disorder is likely higher, but has not been systematically studied. It is recommended that marijuana use be considered as a risk factor, but not an absolute contraindication to transplant, and both patients and staff be educated regarding the risks and benefits of marijuana use in this population [58, 63, 69, 72].

Methadone and Buprenorphine

Methadone and buprenorphine are highly effective therapies for opioid use disorders. Many patients with histories of opioid use disorders are able to maintain abstinence and improve psychosocial functioning in the community with opioid substitution therapies. It is well-documented that a high percentage of patients on opioid substitution therapies relapse when methadone is tapered [75, 76]. Less is known about relapse after buprenorphine taper. The issue of whether to accept methadone and buprenorphine maintained individuals for organ transplantation remains controversial. Many centers have had a policy that these patients need to be tapered off methadone in order to be transplant candidates, a practice that unfortunately may actually cause relapse. There are four published reports regarding the use of methadone in organ transplantation; all studies were in liver transplant recipients. All four studies were limited by small sample sizes, but all noted that patient and graft survival were similar in methadone maintenance therapy (MMT) patients and the general transplant population [77–80]. It has been proposed [81] that MMT patients should not be automatically denied transplantation and should not be tapered off methadone prior to transplant. These patients should be comprehensively evaluated on an individual basis, applying similar criteria as used in other patients. Post-transplant, MMT patients should continue to receive a stable methadone dose; in addition, adequate medication for pain control should be prescribed. Short-acting opioids should be tapered as quickly as possible [81]. Although there are no studies of treatment of transplant patients with buprenorphine, Aldemir [82] reported two cases of successful post-transplant treatment of opioid-dependent patients with buprenorphine/naloxone. It is recommended that the approach to patients receiving buprenorphine or buprenorphine/naloxone be similar to those on MMT. Buprenorphine may be a safer long-term option in this patient population, as it has fewer potential drug-drug interactions with immunosuppressant and other post-transplant medications [83].

Tobacco

Smoking is recognized as a leading cause of morbidity and mortality in the general population. Smoking is a risk factor for a wide range of diseases including cardiovascular disease, respiratory illness, stroke, and malignancy. Smoking is also known to impair wound healing, increase risk for infection, accelerate the development of renal disease, and increase postsurgical complications. Post-transplant complications associated with smoking include increased vascular complications, increased graft loss, and increased all-cause mortality.

Although many smokers do successfully stop smoking prior to transplant, post-transplant relapse to use of tobacco is estimated to be at least 20% or higher [20]. For example, among LT recipients, up to 60% have lifetime history of tobacco use, 15% continue to smoke following their transplantation, and nearly 58% of those requiring transplantation for ALD return to smoking following a transplant [22, 84].

A number of studies have addressed the issue of complications related to post-transplant tobacco smoking. Post-transplant smoking has been linked with decreased post-transplant survival, renal dysfunction, and malignancy in heart transplant recipients [20]. In a study of heart transplant recipients followed for 13 years, 27% of patients tested positive for cotinine at least once during the follow-up and 15% tested positive on more than one occasion. Patients with post-transplant smoking had increased death from malignancy and graft coronary artery disease with median survival decreased from 16.3 to 11.9 years [85]. Of note, in a different study, heart transplant patients who were abstinent from tobacco for greater than 1 year prior to transplant had lower risk of tobacco relapse as compared to those who were abstinent for less than 1 year (8.4% versus 40%, P = 0.006) [86].

Decreased survival and chronic kidney disease have been observed in lung transplant recipients [87]. Lung transplant recipients who resumed tobacco after transplant have been reported to have increased rate of oncologic events, including lung cancer [88]. In a study of 276 lung transplant recipients, 11% self-reported smoking resumption post-transplant. Higher rates of post-transplant smoking at 23% were noted in patients with emphysema due to chronic obstructive pulmonary disease (COPD). Risk factors for tobacco resumption included shorter cessation period prior to transplantation, lower socioeconomic status, exposure to second-hand smoke, emphysema, and death of a spouse [89].

Rates of smoking in kidney transplant candidates range between 24% and 33%, while up to 90% of smokers continue to smoke postoperatively [20]. Smoking in renal transplant recipients is linked with graft loss, graft non-function, decreased survival, and malignancy [90, 91].

Smoking in liver transplant recipients is linked with decreased survival, vascular complications (including hepatic artery thrombosis), and biliary complications [18, 20–22, 92]. For example, in a single-center retrospective study of 1275 LT recipients, 22% were active smokers, 25% were previous smokers, and 53% were non-smokers at the time of LT listing. While 70% of previous and non-smokers survived at 10 years, only 55% of current smokers did so (P < 0.01) [93].

Tobacco use at the time of listing can also be associated with worse post-transplant outcomes. In one study of 316 patients newly listed for heart transplant at 17 hospitals, at 5-year follow-up, 14% of never-smoking patients died as compared to 18% of former smokers versus 42% of those who smoked at the time of wait listing. This mortality was also dependent on the amount of time that had passed since quit date: the longer patients were abstinent from tobacco use at the time of listing, the better was their survival post-transplant [94].

Late complications of smoking post-transplant include cardiovascular disease and malignancy. One study noted the absence of early complications in liver transplant that were attributable to tobacco use. The authors suggested that late complications were likely similar to the negative health effects of smoking in general, rather than a specific transplant complication related to tobacco use [95].

On the basis of the available studies, there is compelling evidence that post-transplant smoking results in poorer medical outcomes, increased graft loss, and decreased survival. Most transplant programs currently encourage smokers to cease tobacco use prior to consideration for transplantation, but there is considerable variation from organ to organ and program to program regarding this requirement. In general, lung transplant programs view smoking as an absolute contraindication and most heart transplant programs require smoking cessation. In fact, the International Society for Heart and Lung Transplantation (ISHLT), in their heart transplant listing guidelines, stated that "It is reasonable to consider active tobacco smoking as a relative contraindication to transplantation. Active tobacco smoking during the previous 6 months is a risk factor for poor outcomes after transplantation" [96]. They also stated that active substance abuse, including tobacco, should be an absolute contraindication against listing on the lung transplant waitlist [97]. An increasing number of liver and renal transplant programs now require smoking cessation prior to transplant listing. It is recommended patients with a history of tobacco use be offered counseling as well as medications for both smoking cessation and relapse prevention pre- and post-transplant [20].

One interesting topic is how tobacco use in organ donors influences transplant outcomes. In fact, several studies have looked at solid organ transplant outcomes with transplanted organs from donors with a smoking history. Recipients of hearts, lungs, and kidneys from donors with tobacco use histories tended to have decreased survival and increased morbidity [20, 98, 99]. In particular, lung transplant recipients receiving organs from donors who smoked have decreased rates of survival at 3 years post-transplant [20]. Similarly, one study of liver transplant recipients who received organs from donors that smoked shows an increased risk of death [100]. It is important to note that these results were not replicated in all studies and that declining these organs would likely result in patients dying on the waiting list [20].

Opioids

Opioid addiction is a serious global health problem, and misuse of prescription opioids in the United States has reached epidemic proportions [101]. Despite this, the issue of addiction to prescription opioids has received little attention in the transplant literature, and few studies have been published to date. The published studies address chronic prescription opioid use, but not opioid use disorders per se. In these studies, it is noted that those patients with the highest levels of prescription opioid use prior to transplant had increased post-transplant death and graft loss [102, 103]. Post-renal transplant patients with the highest levels of opioid use [102] had increased risk of ventricular arrhythmias, alcohol and other substance use, mental status changes, and accidents following transplant. Although, these patients were not diagnosed with opioid use disorders, the authors concluded that high levels of pre-transplant opioid use did predict an increased risk of post-renal transplant complications. A similar study of liver transplant recipients showed decreased survival and increased graft loss in patients receiving high levels of opioids while on the transplant waiting list and during the first year post-transplant [103]. Patients with pre-transplant chronic prescription opioid use should be evaluated carefully for the presence of an opioid use disorder. Patients with opioid use disorders should be referred for substance abuse treatment and consideration should be given to use of opioid maintenance therapies in these patients. Post-transplant, opioids for pain control should be used appropriately but chronic opioid use for nonmalignant pain should be avoided in all patients.

Other Drugs

The topic of other illicit drug use is often discussed by transplant professionals, but there are few published studies. It is accepted that patients with active injection drug use should not be transplanted, and a period of abstinence as well as substance abuse treatment is highly recommended. Few studies have addressed substance use other than alcohol, tobacco, marijuana, and methadone maintenance therapy, and a majority of studies address liver transplantation. A meta-analysis by Dew et al. showed low relapse to illicit drug use following liver transplantation [13]. Confounding factors that may have influenced these results include small sample sizes, limited studies mainly in liver recipients, variations in selection criteria, unclear definitions of substance use disorders, and differing definitions and methodologies of detecting relapse. It is thought that patients with pre-transplant SUDs are more likely to relapse post-transplant and have issues with nonadherence and poorer post-transplant outcomes, but systematic studies are lacking [6, 13, 19, 104–106].

Most studies in this patient population address "polysubstance use" rather than evaluating relapse to individual substances. One study showed that 17% of patients relapsed to polysubstance use after transplant. In this study pre-transplant, substance use disorder was the only factor that predicted relapse [107]. Another study showed a relapse rate of 27% and did not find any predictive factors or effect on post-transplant outcomes [108]. These studies are limited by small numbers, differing patient populations, differing definitions of relapse, and use of the term "polysubstance use" rather than addressing individual use of substances. Outside

of opioids, no studies of prescription drug misuse in organ transplant patients could be located in the literature. It is suggested that use of benzodiazepines, barbiturates, and other sedative-hypnotics be minimized in this patient population because of the risks of cognitive impairment, respiratory depression, and adverse drug interactions.

Evaluation of a Patient with a Substance Use Disorder and Treatment Interventions

Currently, there are no universally accepted national or international guidelines with regard to the approach to transplant patients with alcohol and other substance use disorders. The US Department of Health and Human Services' Organ Procurement and Transplantation Network has published ethical guidelines for allocation of human organs for transplant. These guidelines discuss in detail the principles of utility, justice, and respect for persons in the determination of organ allocation. In doing so, the guidelines imply that past behaviors should not exclude a patient from consideration for transplant. The principle of utility discusses the need to maximize benefit and minimize harm in determining which patients receive organs. Social considerations should not be factors in organ allocation; rather medical conditions that predict poorer outcome should be weighted heavily. The principle of justice states that organs should be allocated to those with medical need who will benefit the most. Respect for persons implies that individuals' autonomy is important and that patients have a choice with regard to accepting transplant or not. These principles also imply that all patients needing organs should be considered with equal respect and concern; recipients who will benefit from transplant and where there is a probability of a good outcome should receive priority and that extending life and relieving suffering should also be a guiding principle [109]. In applying these principles, patients with alcohol and other substance use disorders should be considered equally with other patients. Historically, these patients are known to be less likely to be referred for transplant and, if referred, may be referred when they are so ill that the likelihood of survival, even with transplant, is low.

The requirement for a minimum period of 6 months of abstinence prior to transplant (the "6-month rule") has increasingly fallen out of favor as a guideline, and multiple studies have questioned its validity on its own as a predictor of future abstinence. Instead, most experts currently propose a thorough evaluation of multiple factors in evaluating risk for relapse post-transplant. All patients with alcohol or other substance use disorders should receive a thorough evaluation including complete clinical history, thorough review of records, corroborating history from a third-party "social support person" (family member, friend, care provider), and cognitive assessment [8]. The clinical history should include a very complete history of alcohol, tobacco, and other substance use. Each substance should be discussed separately and attention should be given to the age of onset, quantity used, frequency of use, consequence of use, length of time since last use, and reasons for discontinuing use. Episodes of past substance abuse treatment should be explored including the nature of such treatment, reasons for attending treatment, what was learned, and whether treatment resulted in a period of abstinence or sobriety. The patient should be questioned as to their understanding of the contribution of substance use to their medical illness, if applicable, and relapse risk factors should be investigated. The presence of comorbid mental health or personality disorders should be determined. The patient should be questioned regarding whether or not they accept that they have an alcohol or substance use disorder and whether they are willing to accept treatment for the disorder, if that is recommended. Commitment to future abstinence and willingness to engage in activities to support abstinence must be determined. A thorough psychosocial assessment is important in determining the social stability of the patient. Factors that predict future abstinence such as substitute activities, relationships that hinge on sobriety, negative consequences for use, and sources of hope/self-esteem should be assessed. Ongoing random screening for alcohol tobacco, and other substance use should occur; the evaluators should be aware of the limitations and potential errors in such testing [110, 111]. Ongoing alcohol and/or other substance use, inability to commit to future abstinence, lack of insight and acceptance of the alcohol or substance use disorder diagnosis, lack of social stability, and multiple relapse risk factors are considered by many to be contraindications to transplant.

Patients with histories of alcohol and/or substance use disorders with verified long periods of pre-transplant sobriety (i.e., 5 years or more) may be securely abstinent and at low risk for future relapse. However, many patients with up to 2 years of pre-transplant sobriety may relapse post-transplant. Alcohol and substance abuse treatment should be recommended for these patients and required for those assessed at high risk for relapse. Psychosocial interventions are effective for the general population with alcohol and substance use disorders. Pharmacologic interventions may increase treatment success for those with alcohol, tobacco, and opioid use disorders. Several studies have shown that addiction treatment in the pre-transplant period may reduce post-transplant relapse [32, 33]. Some patients may be too ill or cognitively impaired to comply with pre-transplant treatment; post-transplant treatment is recommended for these individuals. Unfortunately, many patients do not comply with recommendations for ongoing post-transplant addiction treatment. Addolorato [33] noted that treatment provided by addiction specialists who were part of the transplant team yielded lower relapse rates and improved patient survival as compared to those patients receiving treatment in other settings.

Patients may relapse while on the transplant waiting list. Several studies have identified up to 20–25% of patients with alcohol relapse while on the waiting list [15, 112]. There is no consensus as to how to approach these patients. Some programs will permanently remove these patients from the transplant waiting list, and others will require addiction treatment, while other programs may increase monitoring.

In addition, in the United States, 3rd-party payors (i.e., insurance companies) may have additional requirements for organ transplant candidates. They may require a verified period of abstinence; documented negative drug, alcohol, and tobacco screens; or a period of addiction treatment that meets certain requirements.

The addiction specialist consulting to the transplant team has several important roles. In addition to comprehensive evaluation of the patient, they must advise the team objectively regarding the evaluation and treatment recommendations. Explicit recommendations should be made with regard to addiction treatment including the recommended setting (residential, outpatient, etc.) and the type of treatment. Recommendations should be tailored to the specific patient. The consultant and the team must keep in mind that abstinence and sobriety are not the same and that sobriety is the goal of treatment. The patient may need education and may lack motivation for treatment; motivational interviewing may need to be a component of the recommendations. The patient's adherence to recommendations must be monitored and clear expectations should be outlined. It is suggested that the patient be given a reasonable but not unlimited amount of time to comply with recommendations. Patients should have ongoing, random screening to document compliance with recommendations and ongoing abstinence. Early referrals to treatment are always recommended. Patients may be quite ill and the available time for treatment should be used wisely. Education of the transplant team is another important role of the consultant. The team must understand that addiction is a chronic illness with remissions and relapses and that abstinence and sobriety are not synonymous. In addition, length of sobriety prior to transplant on its own may not be helpful in predicting future abstinence. A thorough evaluation and accurate diagnosis is necessary and appropriate treatment may improve outcomes. Both the patient and the transplant team need support from the addictions consultant.

Conclusions

Alcohol, tobacco, and substance use disorders are common in patients being evaluated for organ transplantation. Most studies of alcohol and other substance use disorders in transplant patients have been in the liver transplant population. These studies indicate that carefully selected patients transplanted for ALD can do as well in terms of patient and graft survival as patients transplanted for other indications: however, patients can resume alcohol consumption and this can lead to heavy drinking. Relapse to use of tobacco is not uncommon and is associated with increased morbidity and mortality. Marijuana use in transplant patients should be evaluated on individual basis. Studies on other illicit substances are lacking in transplant populations. Multiple risk factors for relapse, graft loss, poor outcomes, decreased survival, and medical complications have been proposed, but there is still no consensus as to which factors are most important. The "6-month rule" for abstinence has been found to be arbitrary with multiple studies questioning its validity as a predictor of future abstinence. Instead, most experts currently propose a thorough evaluation of multiple factors in evaluating risk for relapse post-transplant. Transplant and addiction psychiatrists play an important role in patient evaluation and treatment pre- and post-transplant as well as transplant team education and support.

References

1. Grant BF, Goldstein RB, Saha TD, Chou SP, Jung J, Zhang H, et al. Epidemiology of DSM-5 alcohol use disorders: results from the national epidemiologic survey on alcohol and related conditions III. JAMA Psychiat. 2015;72:757–66.
2. Centers for Disease Control. Cigarette Smoking in the United States. 2017. htttps://www.cdc.gov/tobacco/campaign/tips/resources/data/cigarette-smoking-in-united-states.html. Accessed 9 Oct 2017.
3. Grant BF, Saha TD, Ruan WJ, Goldstein RB, Chou SP, Jung J, et al. Epidemiology of DSM-5 drug use disorder: results from the national epidemiologic survey on alcohol and related conditions III. JAMA Psychiat. 2016;73:39–47.
4. National Institutes of Health. Health consequences of Drug Misuse. 2017. https://www.drugabuse.gov/publications/health-consequences-drug-misuse. Accessed 9 Oct 2017.
5. American Society of Addiction Medicine. Opioid Addiction Disease Facts and Figures. 2016. https://www.asam.org/docs/default-source/advocacy/opioid-addiction-disease-facts-figures.pdf. Accessed 20 Jan 2018.
6. Parker R, Armstrong MJ, Corbett C, Day EJ, Neuberger JM. Alcohol and substance use in solid-organ transplant recipients. Transplantation. 2013;96:1015–24.
7. DiMartini AF, Sotelo JL, Dew MA. Organ transplantation. In: Levenson JL, editor. Textbook of psychosomatic medicine. Washington, DC: American Psychiatric Publishing; 2011. p. 725–58.
8. Beresford TP, Lucey ML. Towards standardizing the alcohol evaluation of potential liver transplant recipients. Alcohol Alcohol. 2017;104:1–10. https://doi.org/10.1093/alcalc/agx.
9. Starzl TE, Van Thiel D, Tzakis AG, Iwatsuki S, Todo S, Marsh JW, et.al. Orthotopic liver transplantation for alcoholic cirrhosis. JAMA 1988;260:2542-2544.
10. Kumar S, Stauber RE, Gavaler JS. Orthotopic liver transplantation for alcoholic liver disease. Hepatology. 1990;11:159–64.
11. Bird GLA, O'Grady JG, Harvey FAH, Caine RY, Williams R. Liver transplantation in patients with alcoholic cirrhosis: selection criteria and rates of survival and relapse. BMJ. 1990;301:15–7.
12. Osorio RW, Ascher NL, Avery M, Bacchetti P, Roberts JP, Lake JR. Predicting recidivism after orthotopic liver transplantation for alcoholic liver disease. Hepatology. 1994;20:105–10.
13. Dew MA, DiMartini AF, Steel J, De Vito DA, Myaskovsky L, Unruh M, Greenhouse J. Meta-analysis of the risk for relapse to substance use after transplantation of the liver or other solid organs. Liver Transpl. 2008;14:159–72.
14. Pageaux GP, Bismuth M, Perney P, Costes V, Jaber S, Possoz P, et al. Alcohol relapse after liver transplantation for alcoholic liver disease: does it matter? J Hepatol. 2003;38:629–34.
15. DiMartini AF, Crone C, Dew MA. Alcohol and substance abuse in liver transplant patients. Clin Liver Dis. 2011;15:727–51.
16. Testino G, Leone S. Alcohol and liver transplantation. Alcohol Alcohol. 2017;52:129.
17. Rice JP, Eickhoff J, Agni R, Ghufran A, Brahmbhatt R, Lucey MR. Abusive drinking after liver transplantation is associated with allograft loss and advanced allograft fibrosis. Liver Transpl. 19 2013;19: 1377–1386.
18. Lucey MR. Liver transplantation for alcoholic liver disease. Nat Rev – Gastroent Hepatol. 2014;11:300–7.
19. Lucey MR, Weinrieb RM. Alcohol and substance abuse. Semin Liver Dis. 2008;29:66–73.
20. Corbett C, Armstrong MJ, Neuberger J. Tobacco smoking and solid organ transplantation. Transplantation. 2012;94:979–87.
21. Oliveira CP, Stefano JT, Alvares-da-Silva MR. Cardiovascular risk, atherosclerosis and metabolic syndrome after liver transplantation: a mini review. Expert Rev Gastroenterol Hepatol. 2013;7:361–4.
22. Ursic-Bedoya J, Donnadieu-Rigole H, Faure S, Pageaux G. Alcohol use and smoking after liver transplantation: complications and prevention. Best Pract Res Clin Gastroenterol. 2017;31:181–5.
23. Iruzubieta P, Crespo J, Fabrega E. Long-term survival after liver transplantation for alcoholic cirrhosis. World J Gastroenterol. 2013;19:9198–208.
24. Heinrich TW, Marcangelo M. Psychiatric issues in solid organ transplantation. Harvard Rev Psychiatry. 2009;17:398–406.
25. Rodrigue JR, Hanto DW, Curry MP. The alcohol relapse risk assessment: a scoring system to predict the risk of relapse to any alcohol use after liver transplant. Prog Transplant. 2013;23: 310–8.
26. Marroni CA. Management of alcohol recurrence before and after liver transplantation. Clin Res Hepatol Gastroenterol. 2015;39:S109–14.
27. Dom G, Wojnar M, Crunelle CL, Thon N, Bobes J, Pruess UW, et al. Assessing and treating alcohol relapse in liver transplantation candidates. Alcohol Alcohol. 2015;50:164–72.
28. Lee MR, Leggio L. Management of alcohol use disorder in patients requiring liver transplant. Am J Psychiatry. 2015;172:1182–9.
29. Choudary NS, Kumar N, Saigal S, Rai R, Saraf N, Soin AS. Liver transplantation for alcohol related liver disease. J Clin Exp Hepatol. 2016;6:47–53.
30. Karim Z, Intaraprasong P, Scudamore C, Erb SR, Soos JG, Cheung E, et al. Predictors of significant alcohol drinking after liver transplantation. Can J Gastroenterol. 2010;24:245–50.
31. Rustad JK, Stern TS, Prabhakar M, Musselman D. Risk factors for alcohol relapse following orthotopic liver transplantation: a systemic review. Psychosomatics. 2015;56:21–35.
32. Weinrieb RM, Van Horn DHA, Lynch KG, Lucey MR. A randomized controlled study of treatment for alcohol dependence in patients awaiting liver transplantation. Liver Transpl. 17 2011;17: 539–547.
33. Addolorato G, Mirijello A, Leggio L, Ferrulli A, D'Angelo C, Vassallo G, et al. Liver transplantation in alcoholic patients: impact of an alcohol addiction unit within a liver transplant center. Alcohol Clin Exp Res. 2013;37:1601–8.
34. Rodrigue JR, Hanto DW, Curry MP. Substance abuse treatment and its association with relapse to alcohol use after liver transplantation. Liver Transpl. 2013;19:1387–95.

35. Rice JP, Lucey MR. Should length of sobriety be a major determinant in liver transplant selection? Curr Opin Organ Transplant. 2013;18:259–64.

36. DeGottardi A, Spahr L, Golez P, Morard I, Mentha G, Guilland O. A simple score for predicting alcohol relapse after liver transplantation. Arch Int Med. 2007;167:1183–8.

37. DiMartini AF, Dew MA, Day N, Fitzgerald MG, Jones BL, deVera M, Fontes P. Trajectories of alcohol consumption following liver transplantation. Am J Transplant. 2010;10:2305–12.

38. Beresford TP, Turcotte JG, Merion R, Burtch G, Blow FC, Campbell D, et al. A rational approach to liver transplantation for the alcoholic patient. Psychosomatics. 1990;31:241–54.

39. Anderson CF, personal communication.

40. Valliant GE. The natural history of alcoholism revisited. Cambridge: Harvard University Press; 1995.

41. Mathurin P, Moreno C, Samuel D, Dumortier J, Salleron J, Durand F, et al. Early liver transplantation for severe alcoholic hepatitis. NEJM. 2011;365:1790–800.

42. Busutill RW, DuBray BJ. Liver transplantation for alcoholic hepatitis. Ann Surg. 2017;265:30–1.

43. Jesudian AB, Brown RS. Acute alcoholic hepatitis as indication for liver transplantation. Curr Opin Organ Transplant. 2016;21:107–10.

44. Artu F, Louvet A, Mathurin P. Liver transplantation for patients with alcoholic hepatitis. Liver Int. 2017;37:337–9.

45. Im GY, Kim-Schluger L, Shenoy A, Schubert E, Goel A, Friedman SL, et al. Early liver transplantation for severe alcoholic hepatitis in the United States – a single center experience. Am J Transplant. 2016;16:841–9.

46. Lucey MR, Rice JP. Liver transplantation for severe alcoholic hepatitis crosses the Atlantic. Am J Transplant. 2016;16:1739–40.

47. Schneekloth TD, Niazi SK, Simonetto DA. Alcoholic hepatitis: appropriate indication for liver transplantation? Curr Opin Organ Transplant. 2017;22:578–83.

48. Stroh G, Rosell T, Dong F, Forster J. Early liver transplantation for patients with acute alcoholic hepatitis: public views and the effects on organ donation. Am J Transplant. 2015;15:1598–604.

49. Testino L, Burra P, Bonino F, Piani F, Sumberaz A, Peressutti R, et al. Acute alcoholic hepatitis, end stage alcoholic liver disease and liver transplantation: an Italian position statement. World J Gastroenterol. 2014;20:14642–51.

50. Evon DM, Burker EJ, Sedway JA, Cicale R, Davis K, Egan T. Tobacco and alcohol use in lung transplant candidates and recipients. Clin Transpl. 2005;19:207–14.

51. Sandhu GS, Khattak M, Woodward RS, Hanto DW, Pavlakis M, Dimitri N, Goldfarb-Rumyantzev AS. Impact of substance abuse on access to renal transplantation. Transplantation. 2011;91:86–93.

52. Gueye AS, Chelamcharla M, Baird BC, Nguyen C, Tang H, Barenbaum AL, et al. The association between recipient alcohol dependency and long-term graft and recipient survival. Nephrol Dial Transplant. 2007;22:891–8.

53. Zelle DM, Agarwal PK, Ramirez JLP, van der Heide JJ, Corpeleijn E, Gans RO, Navis G, Bakker SJ. Alcohol consumption, new onset diabetes after transplantation, and all-cause mortality in renal transplant recipients. Transplantation. 2011;92:203–8.

54. Fierz K, Steiger J, Denhaerynck K, Dobbels F, Bock A, De Geest S. Prevalence, severity and correlates of alcohol use in adult renal transplant recipients. Clin Transpl. 2006;20:171–8.

55. Hanrahan JS, Eberly C, Mohanty PK. Substance abuse in heart transplant recipients: a 10-year follow-up study. Prog Transplant. 2001;11:285–90.

56. Shapiro PA, Williams DL, Foray AT, Gelman IS, Wukich N, Sciacca R. Psychosocial evaluation and prediction of compliance problems and mortality after heart transplantation. Transplantation. 1995;60:1462–6.

57. Robinson M, Berke J, Gould S. Business insider- legal marijuana states 2018. January 23, 2018. http://www.businessinsider.com/legal-marijuana-states-2018-1. Accessed 1 Feb 2018.

58. Neyer J, Uberoi A, Hamilton M, Kobashigawa JA. Marijuana and listing for heart transplant: a survey of transplant providers. Circ Heart Fail. 2016;9:1–8.

59. Allen LA, Ambardekar AV. Hashing it out over cannabis: moving toward a standardized guideline on substance use for cardiac transplantation eligibility that includes marijuana. 2016.

60. Pondrom S. Transplantation and marijuana use. Am J Transplant. 2016;16:1–2.

61. Schwartz C. Medical marijuana patients in California are being denied organ transplants but that could change soon. 2015. http://www.huffingtonpost.com/2015/02/24/marijuana-organ-transplant_n_6736672.htm. Accessed 5 Feb 2018.

62. Miller, K. Marijuana user who lost place on transplant list asks lawmakers to change hospital policy. 2017. https://www.pressherald.com/2017/03/27/bill-would-prohibit-hospitals-from-rejecting-organ-recipients-who-use-medical-marijuana/. Accessed 5 Feb 2018.

63. Coffman KL. The debate about marijuana usage in transplant candidates: recent medical evidence on marijuana health effects. Curr Opin Organ Transplant. 2008;13:189–95.

64. Marijuana: Drug Facts. 2018. https://www.drugabuse.gov/publications/drugfacts/marijuana. Accessed 5 Feb 2018.

65. National Academies of Sciences, Engineering, and Medicine. The Health Effects of Cannabis and Cannabinoids: The Current State of Evidence and Recommendations for Research. Washington, DC: The National Academies Press. 2017. https://doi.org/10.17226/24625.

66. Fishman JA. Infection in solid-organ transplant recipients. NEJM. 2007;357:2601–14.

67. Huang JY, Zhang ZF, Tashkin DP, Feng B, Straif K, Hashibe M. An epidemiologic review of marijuana and cancer: an update. Cancer Epidemiol Biomark Prev. 2015;24:15–31.

68. Vethanayagam D, Pugsley S, Dunn EJ, Russell D, Kay JM, Allen C. Exogenous lipid pneumonia related to smoking weed oil following cadaveric renal transplantation. Can Respir J. 2000;7:338–42.

69. Marks WH, Florence L, Lieberman J, Chapman P, Howard D, Roberts P, et al. Successfully treated invasive pulmonary Aspergillosis associated with smoking marijuana in a renal transplant recipient. Transplantation. 1996;61:1771–4.

70. Hamadeh R, Ardehali A, Locksley RM, York MK. Fatal Aspergillosis associated with smoking contaminated marijuana in a bone marrow transplant recipient. Chest. 1988;94:423–33.

71. Hauser N, Sahai T, Richards R, Roberts T. High on cannabis and calcineurin inhibitors: a word of warning in the era of legalized marijuana. Case Rep Transplant. 2016; doi:https://doi.org/10.1155/2016/4028492.

72. Greenan G, Ahmad SB, Anders MG, Leeser A, Bromberg JS, Niederhaus SV. Recreational marijuana use is not associated with worse outcomes after renal transplantation. Clin Transpl. 2016;30:1340–6.

73. Ranney DN, Acker WB, Al-Holou SN, Ehrlichman L, Lee DS, Lewin SA, et al. Marijuana use in potential liver transplant candidates. Am J Transplant. 2009;9:280–5.

74. Rai HS, Winder GS. Marijuana use and organ transplantation: a review and implications for clinical practice. Current Psychiatry Rep. 2017;19:91.

75. Schuckit MA. Treatment of opioid use disorders. NEJM. 2016;375:357–68.

76. Renner JA, Knapp CM, Ciraulo DA, Epstein S. Opioids. In: Kranzler HR, Ciraulo DA, Zindel LR, editors. Clinical manual of addiction psychopharmacology. Washington, DC: American Psychiatric Publishing; 2014. p. 97–136.

77. Liu LU, Schiano TD, Lau N, O'Rourke M, Min AD, Sigal SH, et al. Survival and risk of recidivism in methadone dependent patients undergoing liver transplantation. Prog Transplant. 2001;11:50–7.

78. Hancock MM, Prosser CC, Ransibrahmanakul K, Lester L, Craemer E, Bourgeois JA, Rossario L. Liver transplant and hepatitis C in methadone maintenance therapy: a case report. Subst Abuse Treat Prev Policy. 2007;2:5.

79. Kanchana TP, Kaul V, Manzarbeitia C, Reich DJ, Hails KC, Munoz SJ, Rothstein KD. Liver transplantation for patients on methadone maintenance. Liver Transpl. 2002;8:778–82.

80. Weinrieb RM, Barnett R, Lynch KG, DePiano M, Atanda A, Olthoff KM. A matched comparison study of medical and psychiatric complications and anesthesia and analgesia requirements in methadone-maintained liver transplant recipients. Liver Transpl. 2004;10:97–106.

81. Jiao M, Greanya ED, Haque M, Yoshida EM, Soos JG. Methadone maintenance therapy in liver transplantation. Prog Transplant. 2010;20:209–14.

82. Aldemir E, Coskunul H, Kilic M, Sert I. Treatment of opioid dependence with buprenorphine/naloxone after liver transplantation:report of two cases. Transpl Proc. 2016;48:2769–72.

83. Fireman M, DiMartini AF, Crone CC. Organ transplantation. In: Ferrando SJ, Levenson JL, editors. Clinical manual of psychopharmacology in the medically ill. Washington, DC: American Psychiatric Association Publishing; 2017. p. 597–631.

84. Dulaney DT, Dokus KM, McIntosh S, Al-Judaibi B, Ramaraju GA, Tomiyama K, et al. Tobacco use is a modifiable risk factor for post-transplant biliary complications. J Gastrointest Surg. 2017;10:1643–9.

85. Botha P, Peaston R, White K, Forty J, Dark JH, Parry G. Smoking after cardiac transplantation. Am J Transplant. 2008;8:866–71.

86. Basile A, Bernazzali S, Diciolla F, Lenzini F, Lisi G, Maccherini M, et al. Risk factors for smoking abuse after heart transplantation. Transpl Proc. 2004;36:641–2.

87. Hellemons ME, Agarwal PK, van der Bij W, Verschuuren EA, Postmus D, Erasmus ME, et al. Former smoking is a risk factor for chronic kidney disease after lung transplantation. Am J Transplant. 2011;11:2490–8.

88. Ruttens D, Verleden S, Vos R, Vaneylen A, Vandermeulen E, Thomeer T, et al. The impact of smoking relapse on the outcome after lung transplantation. Eur Respir J. 2012;40:S56.

89. Vos R, De Vusser K, Schaevers V, Schoonis A, Lemaigre V, Dobbels F, et al. Smoking resumption after lung transplantion: a sobering truth. Eur Respir J. 2010;35:1411–3.

90. Nourbala MH, Nemati E, Rostami Z, Einollahi B. Impact of cigarette smoking on kidney transplant recipients: a systematic review. Iran J Kidney Dis. 2011;5:141–8.

91. Hurst FP, Altieri M, Patel PP, Jindal TR, Guy SR, Sidawy AN, Agodoa LY, et al. Effect of smoking on kidney transplant outcomes: analysis of the United States Renal Data System. Transplantation. 2011;92:1101–7.

92. DiMartini AF, Javed L, Russell S, Dew MA, Fitzgerald MG, Jain A, Fung J. Tobacco use following liver transplantation for alcoholic liver disease: an underestimated problem. Liver Transpl. 2005;11:679–83.

93. Mangus RS, Fridell JA, Kubal CA, Loeffler AL, Krause AA, Bell JA, et al. Worse long-term patient survival and higher cancer rates in liver transplant recipients with a history of smoking. Transplantation. 2015;99:1862–8.

94. Gali K, Spaderna H, Smits JM, Bramstedt KA, Weidner G. Smoking status at the time of listing for a heart transplant predicts mortality on the waiting list: a multicenter prospective observational study. Prog Transplant. 2016;26:117–21.

95. Li Q, Wang Y, Ma T, Liu X, Wang B, Zheng W, et al. Impact of cigarette smoking on early complications after liver transplantation: a single center experience and meta-analysis. PLoS One. 2017;12:1–15.

96. Mehra M, Canter CE, Hannan MM, Semigran MJ, Uber PA, Baran DA, et al. The 2016 International Society for Heart Lung Transplantation listing criteria for heart transplantation: a 10 year update. J Heart Lung Transplant. 2016;35:1–23.

97. Weill D, Benden C, Corris PA, Dark JH, Davis RD, Lederer DJ, et al. A consensus document for the selection of lung transplant candidates: 2014-an update from the pulmonary transplantation Council of the International Society for heart and lung transplantation. J Heart Lung Transplant. 2014;34:1–15.

98. Tsao CI, Chen RJ, Chou NK, Ko WJ, Chi NH, Yu HY, et al. The influence of donor characteristics on survival after heart transplantation. Transplant Proc. 2008;40:2636–7.

99. Bonser RS, Taylor R, Collett D, Thomas HL, Dark JH, Neuberger J, et al. Effect of donor smoking on survival after lung transplantation: a cohort study of a prospective registry. Lancet. 2012;380:747–55.

100. Fruhauf NR, Fischer-Frohlich CL, Kutschmann M, Schmidtmann I, Kirste G. Joint impact of donor and recipient parameters on the outcome of liver transplantation in Germany. Transplantation. 2011;92:1378–84.

101. National Institute of Drug Abuse. Trends and statistics. 2017. https://www.drugabuse.gov/related-topics/trends-statistics. Accessed 9 Oct 2017.

102. Lentine KL, Lam NN, Xiao H, Tuttle-Newhall JE, Axelrod D, Brennan DC, et al. Associations of pre-transplant prescription narcotic use with clinical complications after kidney transplantation. Am J Nephrol. 2015;41:165–76.

103. Randall HB, Alhamad T, Schnitzler M, Zhang Z, Ford-Glanton S, Axelrod DA, et al. Survival implications of opioid use before and after liver transplantation. Liver Transpl. 2017;23:305–14.

104. Donnadieu-Rigole H, Perney P, Ursic-Bedoya J, Faure S, Pageaux G. Addictive behaviors in liver transplant recipients: the real problem? World J Hepatol. 2017;9:953–8.

105. Tome S, Said A, Lucey MR. Addictive behavior after solid organ transplantation: what do we know already and what do we need to know? Liver Transpl. 2008;14:127–9.

106. Webb K, Shepherd L, Neuberger J. Illicit drug use and liver transplantation: is there a problem and what is the solution? Transpl Int. 2008;21:923–9.

107. Gedaly R, McHugh PP, Johnston TD, Jeon H, Koch A, Clifford TM, Ranjan D. Predictors of relapse to alcohol and illict drugs after liver transplantation for alcoholic liver disease. Transplantation. 2008;86:1090–5.

108. Nickels M, Jain A, Sharma R, Orloff M, Tsoulfas G, Kashyap R, Bozorgzadeh A. Polysubstance abuse in liver transplant patients and its impact on survival outcomes. Exp Clin Transplant. 2007;5:680–5.

109. Department of Health and Human Resources. Ethical Principles in the Allocation of Human Organs. 2015. https://optn.transplant.hrsa.gov/resources/ethics/ethical-principles-in-the-allocation-of-human-organs/. Accessed 24 Dec 2017.

110. American Society of Addiction Medicine. Drug Testing: A White Paper. 2013. https://www.asam.org/drug-testing-a-white-paper-by-asam.pdf. Accessed 20 Jan 2018.

111. Piano S, Marchioro L, Gola E, Rosi S, Morando F, Cavallin M, et al. Assessment of alcohol consumption in liver transplant candidates and recipients: the best combination of tools available. Liver Transpl. 2014;20:815–22.

112. Carbonneau M, Jensen LA, Bain VG, Kelly K, Meeberg G, Tandon P. Alcohol use while on the liver transplant waiting list: a single center experience. Liver Transpl. 2010;16:91–7.

Special Considerations in Pediatric Transplant Patients

Lauren M. Schneider, Catherine Naclerio, and Carol Conrad

Introduction

Pediatrics is defined by the American Academy of Pediatrics as the "specialty of medical science concerned with the physical, mental, and social health of children from birth to young adulthood…that deals with biological, social, and environmental influences on the developing child and with the impact of disease and dysfunction on development. Children differ from adults anatomically, physiologically, immunologically, psychologically, developmentally, and metabolically [1]." It is for these reasons and then some that children are more than simply little adults. By encompassing a broad range of developmental stages, pediatric transplant presents unique complexities and specific considerations that warrant attention when caring for these patients.

Pediatric solid organ transplant (SOT) began in the early 1950s with the first pediatric kidney transplant. Heart and liver transplants quickly followed in the 1960s [2]. The implementation of immunosuppressant medication in the 1980s to delay organ rejection guaranteed SOT as the gold standard treatment for pediatric patients in organ failure. In 1984, the United Network for Organ Sharing (UNOS) was created to oversee organ donation, procurement, and transplantation across transplant centers and to collect data on patients and outcomes [3]. Based on Organ Procurement Transplant Network (OPTN) data as of December 2017, there have been a total of 51,078 pediatric SOTs since 1988.

L. M. Schneider (✉)
Division of Child and Adolescent Psychiatry,
Department of Psychiatry and Behavioral Sciences,
Stanford University School of Medicine, Stanford, CA, USA
e-mail: lmikula@stanford.edu

C. Conrad
Division of Pulmonary Pediatrics, Department of Pediatrics,
Stanford University School of Medicine, Stanford, CA, USA

C. Naclerio
PGSP-Stanford Psy.D. Consortium, Palo Alto, CA, USA

In 2016, 1878 of the transplants were in youths ranging from less than 1 year old to 17 years old. The largest group of pediatric recipients fell between the ages of 11 and 17. With advances in medical care, pediatric SOT patients today benefit from better medical outcomes, but they also face distinct challenges as they navigate development with a transplant. Attention and support can be helpful both during the pretransplant period and following transplant.

Evaluation

Medical Aspects

The OPTN calls for pediatric and adult transplant teams to be good stewards of a valuable, limited resource. This obligation is balanced with the need to best serve one's patient. "Because donated organs are a severely limited resource the best potential recipients should be identified. The probability of a good outcome must be highly emphasized to achieve the maximum benefit for all transplants [4]." Therefore, a thorough medical evaluation is necessary to determine the need for transplant as well as listing status, with each organ type weighing specific considerations.

For example, the timing of lung transplantation is influenced most by the underlying allocation system. In 2005, the allocation of lungs in the United States was modified to apply to candidates over 12 years of age based on a combination of transplant benefit and medical urgency by means of a calculated score. All lung transplant candidates aged 12 years or older are listed on the Adult Lung Transplant Allocation List by means of a calculation, resulting in the lung allocation score (LAS) [5]. Each year, there are approximately 100 times more adults than children undergoing lung transplantation. Thus, older children and adolescents "compete" with adults for organs. Once evaluated, perhaps the most difficult decision for pediatric lung transplant physicians is determining the appropriate time to accept organs that will best secure a survival benefit. Donor availability is of issue, given size matching, as well as cultural issues, but the most difficult issue is predicting survival without transplant. Even in the case of cystic fibrosis (CF), for which the natural history of the disease process in children has been modeled [6, 7], many factors, including the improvement in care in recent years, have led to better quality of life (QOL) and survival to adulthood. Thus, the limited predictive data, variable course, and unique diagnoses lead most pediatric centers to carefully consider multiple factors, including waiting list survival estimates, growth and nutrition status, frequency of hospitalizations, and potential for improvement in overall QOL before committing a child to lung transplant.

With regard to heart transplant, the United Network for Organ Sharing (UNOS) developed a recipient priority system for candidates awaiting a heart transplant. Similar to the listing practices for adult candidates, Status 1A individuals have top priority and will be offered the heart first. They are severely ill, not expected to survive more than a month, and in intensive care or on advanced life support. Status 1B individuals are the next priority and are receiving intravenous medication and/or mechanical assistance to make their hearts work, either in the hospital or in their home. They are expected to survive longer than a month. Status 2 individuals are usually not hospitalized and not receiving intravenous medication or mechanical assistance.

The criteria for pediatric kidney transplant candidates involve determining the estimated post-transplant survival (EPTS) score. This score reflects several factors including age, time on dialysis, diabetes status, previous organ transplants, and sensitization status. It is a percentage score indicating length of time one candidate will need a donated kidney as compared to other candidates. In the kidney allocation system (KAS), the EPTS is considered against the kidney donor profile index (KDPI), a score describing the potential longevity of the donated kidney, in order to determine matches. Notably, pediatric patients are given priority in the KAS [8].

Alternatively, pediatric liver transplant candidates aged 12 to 17 years are assigned a PELD (pediatric end-stage liver disease) or MELD (model for end-stage liver disease) score. Children younger than 12 years of age are assigned a PELD score. The PELD is a disease severity scoring system for children, designed to improve the organ allocation in transplantation based on the severity of liver disease rather than time on the waiting list. The MELD/PELD ranges from 6 (less ill) to 40 (gravely ill). The urgency of liver transplantation for pediatric acute liver failure (ALF) is typically not reflected by their PELD/MELD score. Patients with ALF and in need of liver transplantation are given priority over those listed with a PELD/MELD score and are listed as Status 1A or 1B. Transplant rates were highest in 2014–2015 for candidates with MELD/PELD 35 or higher, compared to those with MELD/PELD less than 15 [9].

Psychosocial Aspects

The OPTN bylaws mention that a psychosocial evaluation for transplant candidacy should occur to identify good candidates. Just as is true for adult transplant, however, no specific requirements are provided with regard to what is to be included in the psychosocial evaluation, and OPTN encourages transplant centers to develop their own guidelines, examining each candidate individually [4]. The works of Annuziato and Lefkowitz have provided general guidelines that allow teams to utilize the psychosocial evaluation to identify both risk and protective factors present for the family. These works also advocate for the evaluation to include recommendations for mental health interventions that would address and hopefully mitigate the identified risk factors, which may result in medical morbidity or in some cases mortality [10, 11]. Specific risk or protective factors that are to be assessed often vary between transplant centers, as only suggestions or guidelines exist. Annuziato and colleagues reviewed the adult transplant literature and proposed that psychosocial evaluations should include the following content areas for children and adolescents: comprehension, expectations and outlook, mental health screening, cognitive assessment, family functioning, social support, and behavioral health. Similarly, recommended domains of assessment in Lefkowitz and colleagues' review include adherence, patient psychological and cognitive functioning, and family functioning.

Given that family issues are often out of the pediatric patient's control, children's behavior can be more dynamic, and that future behavior may be more challenging to predict, psychosocial factors as exclusions for transplant listing are less common than what one might see with adult programs [10, 11]. However, given the limited resources, teams are forced to consider the likelihood of success for a pediatric patient and their family. This need is counterbalanced with the difficulty that arises when considering declining a pediatric patient, given the unique and often emotionally charged factors that can be at play [11]. During the psychosocial evaluation, it is recommended that the patient and family's expectations for transplant be explored, so that true informed consent and assent can be obtained. Considerations for whether one believes transplant to be a cure; anticipation of expected treatment demands, including a lifetime of immunosuppressant medications; and understanding of the potential side effects of the treatments or medications should be assessed.

Furthermore, best practices for pediatric psychosocial evaluations encourage clinicians to specify at the outset what information will be collected and how it will be utilized; implement a standardized assessment process, while also varying assessment procedures based on age, developmental level, illness factors, and other pediatrics specific factors; and attend to and acknowledge the influence cultural factors have on health beliefs or health behavior [11]. Moreover, assessing all domains for all patients and families will improve standardization across centers [11].

Killian examined the relationship between physician reports of adherence with a number of familial risk factors in a pediatric transplant population. Association was established with the age of the child at the time of transplant, parental education levels, having a two-parent family, significant psychosocial problems, and the pre-transplant life support status of the patient. However, this was a retrospective study; unfortunately, as Lefkowitz et al. noted, there is scant prospective research examining the role of pre-transplant psychosocial risk and protective factors on post-transplant outcomes. Therefore, the effectiveness of interventions to mitigate pre-transplant risk factors also remains unknown. Taken together, these works conclude with the need to develop standardized and evidence-based pediatric pre-transplant psychosocial assessments, which include a focus on familial risk factors [12].

Due to the significant role that caregivers play in the pediatric transplant patient's overall life and specifically with the management of their medical care, pediatric clinicians need to ensure that they have assessed the functioning and readiness of the caregivers in addition to the patient. Taken one step further, one should evaluate the functioning of the family unit as a whole. Family functioning has been shown to impact behavioral symptoms, adjustment to the illness, and adherence to a medical regimen; strong family cohesion and support have been linked to better adherence, less behavioral symptoms, and better adjustment to the illness [13–15].

Moreover, pediatric practices cover a range of developmental categories, ranging from infancy to young adulthood, with each stage having its own unique set of exclusions or exceptions, further complicating evaluations. For instance, caregiver involvement should adapt to the patient's changing developmental needs, necessitating that one's evaluation or assessment can account for these nuances involving degree of caregiver participation. It is for these reasons that pediatric teams can't simply administer adult measures to a pediatric population. A pediatric-specific tool is needed, and attempts to create a standardized psychosocial evaluation tool have been made.

Fung and Shaw created the Pediatric Transplant Rating Instrument (P-TRI) [16]. They modeled the instrument on existing adult measures but adapted it for the pediatric population by incorporating a developmental perspective and evaluation of family factors. Following a literature review of the relevant pediatric risk factors, they designed a 17-item rating scale to identify and describe risk factors that may affect post-transplant outcomes. The P-TRI presented a standardized and systematic approach to pediatric transplantation, which was groundbreaking [16]. Unfortunately, the P-TRI had psychometric issues with interrater reliability, which prevented clinicians from implementing it in such a way that a meaningful cutoff score is obtained representing a level of risk [17]. Given that it is the only pediatric measure to date, a number of centers incorporate the questions from the P-TRI into a psychosocial evaluation, but don't present a cutoff score.

Continued interest remains within the pediatric transplant community to clarify the role that psychosocial factors play in medical outcomes as well as to develop a well-validated psychosocial screening tool that is valid, reliable, and easy to use. Schneider, Almond, and Shaw, investigators at Stanford University, have leveraged lessons learned from the P-TRI and in 2016 developed the Stanford Pediatric Psychosocial Optimization Tool (SPPOT) [18]. SPPOT is a self-report questionnaire that has two self-report versions for children and adolescents/young adults and four versions for parents of patients ranging in age from 0 to 30, corresponding with different developmental modules. The parent versions include an infant, toddler, school age, and adolescent/young adult versions. Domains include adherence, caregiver supervision, medical coping, psychiatric history (both patient and parent), cognitive, developmental and behavioral issues, family issues, social support, and relationship with the medical team [18]. Lastly, the SPPOT incorporates a screen of current psychiatric problems utilizing the Patient Health Questionnaires [19]. Efforts are underway to study its predictive validity vis-a-vis the relationship between baseline SPPOT scores and medical outcomes, including patterns of nonadherence and episodes of graft rejection and graft loss. The authors' goal is to develop a tool that can identify risks and then provide recommendations to minimize the risks, in a systematic way that can be applied to all participants and hopefully eventually allow for a fair and equitable evaluation process in child and adolescent transplant candidates (Table 46.1).

One area that deserves attention is the recognition of neurocognitive impairments in this patient population and ways to appropriately and ethically address this in the pre-transplant evaluation. Building from earlier findings [20–24], Reed Knight and colleagues found that pediatric kidney, liver, and heart patients' intellectual functioning at the time of the pre-transplant evaluation was within the average range overall; however, scores were significantly lower than the normal population across organs. Academic achievement scores were also significantly lower than the normal population, with means in the low average to average ranges [25].

Antonini and colleagues also found preschool-aged heart and liver transplant patients to have cognitive delays at the time of transplant evaluations, though, as is often the case, limitations due to a small sample size and variable scores are to be noted [26]. Given the rapid maturation that occurs during childhood with regard to neurological development, as discussed by Mohammed, identification of and early interventions targeting deficits are particularly important [26, 27]. It is, therefore, recommended that intellectual and academic functioning be evaluated at the time of the pre-transplant evaluation, so that appropriate accommodations or supports can be implemented. This will also help medical teams to set

Table 46.1 Components of a pediatric psychosocial evaluation from the Stanford Pediatric Psychosocial Optimization Tool [18]

	Self-report: school age	Self-report: adolescent/young adult	Parent report: infant	Parent report: young child	Parent report: school age	Parent report: adolescent/young adult
Demographic information	X	X	X	X	X	X
Concerns about transplant	X	X	X	X	X	X
Motivation for transplant	X	X	X	X	X	X
Adherence	X	X	X	X	X	X
Parental supervision			X	X	X	X
Medical coping	X	X		X	X	X
Relationship with the medical team	X	X	X	X	X	X
Patient social support	X	X				
Family support	X	X	X	X	X	X
Logistical issues			X	X	X	X
Parental social and logistical support			X	X	X	X
Externalizing problems	X	X		X	X	X
Cognitive/developmental issues			X	X	X	X
Trauma history	X	X				
Parent psychiatric history – Self-report			X	X	X	X
Patient psychiatric history – Parent report				X	X	X
Patient psychiatric history – Self-report (18yo+)		X				
Self-report rating of current psychiatric concerns		X	X	X	X	X

appropriate expectations for the role that patients or caregivers will have in the patient's disease management. For example, it may be helpful to increase adult supervision during medication administration times if a patient is unlikely to be able to manage the regimen independently or customize transplant education accordingly [11]. If over time the patient is able to increase their role in their self-care, expectations are to then be adjusted [11]. It is worth noting that identification of intellectual impairments or more specifically intellectual disability at the time of transplant is not to be done so as to in any way allow for discrimination of this patient group; rather, as mentioned in Dobbels' editorial, pre-transplant screening on a case-by-case basis, irrespective of intellectual disability, should occur [28].

While attention has been on the initial pre-transplant evaluation, it is considered best practice to reevaluate patients and families. Dew et al. demonstrate the need for ongoing evaluation, as fluctuations in caregiver and patient presentations occur with adult patients [29]. Perhaps ongoing reevaluations are of even greater importance in a pediatric population, with the ever-evolving and constant development of children and adolescents. Furthermore, Annunziato et al. discussed how reevaluation is of importance, given that new findings may be uncovered once a more trusting relationship

is established and also after one has had the opportunity to receive mental health interventions that were recommended at the initial pre-transplant evaluation to address identified risk factors [10].

Selection/Listing Process

Solid organ transplant first begins with consent. The consent process requires members of the medical team to ensure that both patients and parents/caregivers understand the risks and benefits of SOT in order to give informed consent, which is obtained for pediatric patients over the age of 18 and from parents or caregivers of patients under 18 [30]. In addition to gaining consent from parents, it is ethically responsible to also gain assent or agreement from the minor patient [31]. As with all types of candidates, assurance that the patient and support system can and will adhere to the rigorous therapeutic plan before and after the transplant must be obtained. Should the patient decline transplant, the medical team and caretakers must then weigh the benefits of respecting the patient's wishes while also balancing the need for an indicated and life-saving treatment [31].

Similar to adult transplant, following informed consent and a comprehensive pre-transplant evaluation, the medical team will present the patient and discuss the varied risks and benefits of transplant. Ethical issues regarding the scare medical resource are considered, including psychosocial concerns [30]. At the conclusion of the multidisciplinary team meeting a decision is provided regarding treatment planning, and if approved the patient is placed on the transplant wait list.

Wait List

Based on OPTN data as of December 2017, there were 1995 patients under the age of 18 waiting for an organ transplant. Wait times for organs can vary widely based on the organ type. The 2012 UNOS annual data report shared that 40% of pediatric renal transplant patients waited less than a year, and the remainder of patients waited between 1 and 4 years for a transplant [32]. Conversely, the majority of pediatric heart transplant patients are transplanted within a year of being listed active on the transplant list [32].

The demand for heart transplants continues to grow steadily, as heart transplant continues to afford advanced heart failure patients the best option for long-term survival. The number of heart transplant candidates who are listed and the number of heart transplants performed continue to increase. As found at the end of 2015, the number of active candidates on the heart transplant waiting list increased by 130% over the last decade. The number of heart transplants increased by 26.8% in the past decade and only by 5.2% between 2014 and 2015. It is apparent that the growth in the waiting list has exceeded the growth in the number of transplants. This may reflect the increase of effective employment of cardiac assist devices that allow patients to survive longer on the waiting list. At the end of 2015, 230 pediatric candidates remained actively listed, 34% of whom were 11–17 years of age, followed by ages younger than 1 year (25.8%), 1 to 5 years (24.2%), and 6 to 10 years (16.0%). Fifteen percent died on the wait list or were too sick to undergo transplant. However, 48 (7.6%) children were removed due to improved condition.

Similar to heart transplant, the ratio of wait list deaths to transplants in pediatric lung candidates is higher than that in adults. Despite the highest lung transplant rates in 2015 for both populations combined, the 2014–2015 overall mortality rate was 16.5 deaths per 100 wait list years compared with 8.6 in 2004–2005, and was highest for candidates aged 12 to 17 years, at 40.0 deaths per 100 wait list years likely due to the increasingly sick candidate pool [33]. The number of active candidates on the lung transplant waiting list at year-end has grown by 14.7% over the past decade, while the number of active and inactive new additions to the waiting

list has increased by 42.4% over the same time period [33]. Data from the Scientific Registry of Transplant Recipients (SRTR) report in 2016 measured a range of wait times for as brief as 30 days, to between 2 and 3 years.

According to OPTN data as of December 2017, there were 1051 pediatric patients awaiting kidney transplant with 566 of those patients being adolescent patients, aged 11 to 17 years old. The majority of pediatric kidney patients wait between 6 months and 2 years for transplant. In 2015, ten patients aged 1–17 died while waiting for transplant. Unique to kidney transplant is that patients can incorporate their time on dialysis prior to being listed as part of the overall wait time for transplant. With regard to liver transplant, in 2015, the number of new active candidates added to the pediatric liver transplant waiting list was 689, down from a peak of 826 in 2005. Waiting time has decreased slightly over time such that 52.7% of candidates waited for less than 1 year in 2015, compared with 36.4% in 2005.

Recipient characteristics, wait list mortality, and patient and transplant outcomes differ for intestine transplant and intestine-liver transplant. Over the past decade, the age distribution of candidates wait listed for intestine and intestine-liver transplant shifted from primarily pediatric to increasing proportions of adults. In 2015, a total of 141 intestine transplants were performed in both adults and children. Between 2006 and 2015, the number of intestine transplants declined by 19.4%, from 175 to 141. Numbers of intestine transplants without a liver increased from a low of 51 in 2013 to 70 in 2015. Intestine-liver transplants increased from a low of 44 in 2012 to 71 in 2015. Most of the listed candidates receive a graft within 1 year of listing. In 2015, transplant rates were highest for adult intestine-liver transplants, at 151.5 per 100 wait list years, and lowest for pediatric intestine transplant, at 18.8 per 100 wait list years.

The time waiting for transplant can be emotionally taxing for patients and their families as patients face the threat of dying before receiving an organ [34, 35]. This time is understandably marked by anxiety and uncertainty. Often patients and families are adjusting their lives to prepare for transplant. For example, families may be asked to temporarily relocate to be closer to their transplant center in case an organ becomes available. If the entire family moves or if only the patient and one parent move, disruptions to the family's life are guaranteed, with potential impacts on the schooling of the children, employment of the parents, and overall support of the community or extended family.

Concerns regarding the potential donor may also arise as the patient and family learn about the deceased donor process. Children and adolescents may have questions or worries both before and after transplant about their donor, their donor's family, and the circumstances around the donor's death. Alternatively, patients pursuing living donation must also process their own unique considerations, such as who will donate the organ and whether the patient is comfortable with a living donor donation. A major benefit to living donation is that it can be scheduled, which can alleviate the uncertainty of waiting. However, with living donation you must identify caregivers for both the pediatric patient and the donor. Oftentimes one parent would like to donate, which in turn strains the entire family system when two members are recovering from an invasive surgery. Similarly, siblings are sometimes asked to donate. Special attention should be given to ensure that the sibling does not feel coerced or pressured. Lastly, the patient will also require individual attention to assess for and discuss potential guilt or disinterest in living donation, which may be particularly relevant for older children, adolescents, and young adults, who are aware of and sensitive to these potential issues.

Transplant Outcomes

Medical Outcomes

Medical outcomes have generally improved over time and vary per organ group. Although survival after pediatric lung transplantation has improved over the past decade, long-term survival rates remain well below heart and other solid organ transplants. Lung transplantation is considered in children with end-stage or progressive lung disease or life-threatening pulmonary vascular disease, for which there is no other medical therapy. Regardless of the underlying diagnosis, all candidates have a clear diagnosis and trajectory of illness such that the child is at high risk of death, despite optimal medical therapy. Mortality after lung transplant is greatest in the first year, with approximately 15% of all recipients dying because of infection and graft failure [34]. Nonetheless, the overall survival rate has improved over the last 30 years. Survival is similar among pediatric recipients under the age of 12, including infants, but worst among adolescents, when conditional survival to 1 year is considered. Before 2000, median survival was 3.3 years among all children, but median survival improved substantially to 5.8 years after 2000, and, upon conditional analysis limited to survival to 1 year, pediatric median survival has increased to 8.7 years compared with 9.6 years in adults [36]. The ongoing challenges to better outcomes include optimization of patient selection and altering allocation policies to ensure that pediatric lung transplantation confers survival and/or QOL benefit.

Patient mortality following heart transplant has declined. Among pediatric patients who underwent heart transplant in 2014, the 1-year survival rate was greater than 90%. Overall, in 2015, 1-year and 5-year patient survival rates were 88.7% and 77.2%, respectively, among recipients who underwent transplant in 2003–2010. Five-year patient survival was 71.2% for recipients aged younger than 1 year, 78.4% for ages 1 to 5 years, 87.5% for ages 6 to 10 years, and 77.4% for ages 11 to 17 years.

Outcomes for pediatric renal transplant recipients are generally very good. Data from 2008–2015 showed that 1-year graft survival rates for renal patients were 95.2% for ages 1–5, 96.4% for ages 6–10, and 97.0% for ages 11–17. Survival rates decreased at the year 5 point, with ages 1–5 and ages 6–7 demonstrating 87.6% and 87.9% graft survival, respectively, and ages 11–17 showing 78.1% graft survival rate [35]. Notably, adolescent renal patients are considered to have the worst long-term outcomes compared to all other age groups, with the only exception being adults over the age of 65 [37]. Nonadherence to medications has been identified as a principle explanation for this pattern [38].

The 5-year graft survival within the adolescent-age group after liver transplant is slightly lower than for the 6–10-year-old age group (79% vs. 87%, respectively) but was 75.0% for recipients aged younger than 1 year and 78.2% for ages 1 to 5 years. For all ages combined, the 5-year survival averages 85% [9].

Demand for pancreas transplants overall has declined dramatically in the past decade, likely due to a combination of factors including improvements in noninvasive therapies for diabetes weighed against the difficulty and potential complications of the transplant surgery. Annually, the number of pediatric pancreas transplants appears to be stable at about 30–50 per year since 2008. The overall survival rate for recipients of a pancreas is high, at approximately greater than 97% at 5 years, but the survival of functioning grafts are reported in the range of 55–65% at 5 years after transplant [39].

The number of intestine transplants has remained low over the decades. Intestine and intestine-liver transplant remains important in the treatment of intestinal failure, despite decreased morbidity associated with parenteral nutrition. Intestine transplants may be performed in isolation, with a liver transplant, or as part of a multi-visceral transplant. Short gut syndrome (congenital and non-congenital) is the main cause of disease leading to intestine and to intestine-liver transplant. Intestine graft survival has improved since the early 1990s but has plateaued over the past decade. Patient survival was lowest for adult intestine-liver recipients (1- and 5-year survival 68.6% and 35.7%, respectively) and highest for pediatric intestine recipients (1- and 5-year survival 88.1% and 74.6%, respectively), though rates differ among age groups, with longest survival of both patient and graft occurring in the 6–10-year-old recipients and lower in the children aged either <1 year of age or adolescent age range [40].

Psychosocial Outcomes

Solid organ transplant is associated with complex treatment regimens, frequent doctors' appointments, and lifestyle restrictions [41, 42]. The majority of patients adaptively cope with the changes that come with transplant, but a significant subpopulation experiences difficulties with the transition to post-transplant care [43].

Health-related quality of life captures the domains of physical functioning, mental health, and general health perceptions [44]. QOL for the first 1 to 2 years following transplant is rated lower than expected and lower than patients with other chronic conditions; however, it has been found to increase over time [45]. Other studies have found that transplant patients generally report lower QOL compared to healthy peers but similar to other chronic illness groups [46, 47]. Parents of pediatric transplant patients tend to rate QOL as worse than the patients themselves [48]. Additionally, this pattern of lower-rated QOL has been found in both children and adolescents [37, 45, 49, 50]. Care needed post-transplant may disrupt social development such as playing sports and staying out late with friends and in turn impacts QOL [50]. Times of particular vulnerability may include transitioning home from the hospital; returning to previous routines, such as reintegration into school or readopting an exercise regimen; and reestablishing family functioning [45, 51].

Research has shown individual characteristics related to adherence (i.e., rescheduled clinic appointments or medication adherence) predicted lower QOL in adolescent transplant patients [44]. Similarly, the perception of adverse side effects from medications was significantly related to both physical and psychological well-being of the patient. Side effects from medications can include a decrease in energy, weight gain, and changes in facial appearance, all of which can impact an adolescent's sense of self [42]. Adolescents who perceived these side effects as worse reported a lower QOL [42]. Adolescents may then stop taking medications to avoid side effects, leading to issues with nonadherence. Similarly, transplant has been associated with a negative impact on biological aspects of development, which may contribute to lower perceived QOL [37, 52].

Family functioning following transplant is vulnerable to the impact of stress and burden that is associated with SOT [53]. Research has shown that factors such as parental income and family conflict can negatively impact QOL [44]. Taken in combination with the new medical requirements, financial obligations, increased monitoring of the patient, and lifestyle changes, families may experience more conflict and decreased functioning [53]. Furthermore, families with high levels of parental stress, worse child behavior, and more dysfunctional child-parent interactions were found to have worse medication adherence [54].

Based on the abovementioned research, it is not surprising that the development of distress and, in some cases, psychiatric disorders occurs after SOT [55–57]. Depression and anxiety related to illness uncertainty, organ rejection, medical procedures, and body image distortions commonly develop following transplant [58]. Furthermore, patients with a history of psychiatric illness prior to transplant are at increased risk of experiencing emotional difficulties [43, 56]. Adolescent renal transplant patients had a significantly higher incidence of depression in addition to anxiety and phobias compared to healthy peers [59]. Shaw et al. found that almost a third of their renal transplant sample carried a psychiatric diagnosis, with a statistically higher occurrence in adolescents compared to children [60]. Psychiatric diagnoses for the entire sample included major depression (50%), adjustment disorder (50%), psychological factors affecting other medical condition (20%), oppositional defiance disorder (10%), and substance use disorder (10%) [60]. DeMaso et al. found that approximately one fourth of their pediatric heart transplant sample exhibited emotional difficulties at some point in the first 5 years following transplant.

Posttraumatic stress symptoms may develop in both pediatric SOT patients and their parents or caregivers following transplant, as the process may qualify as medical trauma [61]. Understanding the development of posttraumatic stress in patients and families dealing with chronic illness is of particular importance as it relates to nonadherence [61]. Difficulties taking medication or attending required medical appointments may be a manifestation of avoidance symptoms [62]. Mintzer and colleagues found that approximately 16% of their sample of pediatric solid organ transplant patients met full criteria for posttraumatic stress disorder (PTSD) following transplant [63]. An additional 14% endorsed significant subthreshold symptoms and met criteria for two out of the three clusters of symptoms [63]. Furthermore, Young and colleagues have documented 50% of parents of transplant patients reported at least moderately severe PTSD symptoms, and 44.6% reported that the symptoms resulted in moderate to severe impairment in their functioning. Further, 27.1% of parents reported symptoms that met diagnostic criteria for PTSD [64]. Therefore, models such as those proposed by Kazak and colleagues that explain the development of posttraumatic stress symptoms in patients and families dealing with pediatric chronic illness deserve attention and possible modification to the transplant population [65, 66].

Quality of life and psychological problems are areas that warrant assessment post-transplant, given documented deficits. Similarly, assessment of neurocognitive functioning is equally important. In 2009, Alonso reviewed the available literature on neurodevelopmental outcomes in pediatric solid organ transplant recipients and found that in all cases neurologic comorbidities increased the risk of delay [67]. Given urges to assess this functioning at the time of the evaluation and then after transplant, it is hoped that more longitudinal data can be gathered to better understand these processes and the impact of transplant on pediatric patients.

Adherence

Treatment adherence has emerged as a critical issue for pediatric patients following SOT [38, 68, 69]. Adherence is a term used to describe a patient's ability to comply with a medical treatment plan [68, 70]. It is often defined behaviorally by how consistently a patient takes prescribed medication, attends regularly scheduled clinic appointments, and adapts to recommended lifestyle changes [68, 71]. Adherence to medications is heavily emphasized in SOT because of the large role it plays in graft survival [68, 70]. Failure to properly take immunosuppressant medications can lead to increased hospitalizations, organ rejection, organ failure, and in some cases death [46, 68–70, 72]. The complexity of the immunosuppressant medication regimen (e.g., doses per day, number of medications needed, and timed schedule) directly affects adherence rates [69]. For example, in pediatric kidney transplant patients, adherence decreased as number of medications increased [69].

Adolescent SOT patients have the highest occurrence of nonadherence compared to other age groups [60, 70, 72–77]. Approximately 30% of SOT patients are nonadherent, with adolescents demonstrating higher rates of nonadherence compared to children; approximately 42%–45% of adolescents have been documented as nonadherent compared to approximately 20% of younger children [60, 78]. Dew et al. (2009) conducted a meta-analysis to determine a prevalence rate of nonadherence in pediatric transplant patients and found that 12.9 cases per 100 patients per year were nonadherent to appointments and lab tests and that accounted for the largest occurrence of nonadherence in the pediatric sample. Additionally, 6 cases out of 100 patients were nonadherent to their immunosuppressant medications [38].

Several risk factors have been linked to nonadherence, including age, socioeconomic status, race, family functioning, and psychological status [38, 72, 76, 79–81]. Adolescence serves as a significant risk factor, as this stage of development is marked by impulsivity, increased risky behaviors, increased attention to body image, and increased emotionality [79, 80]. Psychiatric diagnoses have also been found to be related to nonadherence after transplant [55, 56, 60, 75, 82]. Patients experiencing higher levels of anxiety, depression, and posttraumatic stress endorsed more barriers to medication adherence and demonstrated poorer medication adher-

ence overall [83]. Notably, barriers to medication adherence remain stable over time [84].

Given that difficulties with adherence and psychosocial concerns have been well documented in the adolescent population, recent research has focused on identifying evidence-based treatments [74, 85]. However, small sample sizes, inconsistent and nonstandardized means of measuring adherence, and a lack of randomized clinical trials have made it difficult to identify best practices and determine appropriate interventions [86]. Tailoring interventions to the specific needs of particular populations may have the best chance to demonstrate efficacy [87, 88].

Multicomponent treatments employing a variety of interventions, such as psychoeducation, behavioral strategies, and cognitive tools, have proven effective with other groups and may benefit pediatric transplant patients [74]. Educational and instructional interventions on their own have been shown to have only a small effect on adherence in adolescent transplant patients [89, 90]. Interventions should incorporate the patient, the family, and the medical team [91]. Further, they should be skills-based and cover several domains, including education, emotional response, and social supports [91].

Research has shown promising results with regard to multicomponent interventions for pediatric SOT patients. Fennel et al. showed improvements in adherence to prednisone for renal transplant patients following a brief intervention that combined education and behavioral strategies [92]. Shemesh et al. found improvements in graft functioning after participation in an intervention that combined increased medical visits with behavior strategies to improve adherence [93]. Hashim, Vadnais, and Miller adapted dialectal behavioral therapy to address nonadherent adolescent renal transplant patients and found that the combination of multiple behavioral interventions improved adherence [94]. Lastly, Naclerio found that renal transplant patients were six times less likely to lose their graft after participation in a multicomponent therapy that addressed adherence and adjustment to transplant through behavioral strategies, problem solving, and cognitive processing [95]. Larger studies are needed to better understand mechanisms of change.

With society seeing rapid advancements in technology, the electronic delivery of psychosocial interventions has the potential to be a powerful tool. While some research has reported that the effect of technology on adherence has not yet been shown to be efficacious [90], others recognize the utility and developmental appropriateness of the technology when working with adolescents. Text messages have been used as behavioral interventions to improve adherence, such as reminders to take medications or attend laboratory appointments [52, 96]. Online portals have been used to deliver education, such as information on medications and adherence, as well as foster communities of peers to provide support, discuss common fears and worries, and process the transplant experience [97–99].

Transitioning

Transitioning refers to the process of graduating a patient from pediatric to adult medical teams [100, 101]. For some patients, this can be a vulnerable time period as they are expected to take on more responsibility in their medical care. Negative outcomes, such as nonadherence, rejection, and graft loss, are possible during this period [100]. Therefore, pediatric medical teams have begun to focus on readiness to transition by administering questionnaires that assess key components of self-management [100].

Mixed evidence has been found regarding the impact of transitioning to adult care on medication adherence [73, 102]. One study found that adherence was not significantly worsened when kidney transplant patients were transitioned to an adult care setting within the same institution [102]. Other researchers have argued that young adults, ages 18–24, experience similar difficulties as adolescents with regard to adherence and suffer from similar poor outcomes as they begin to transition from pediatric to adult medical care [73].

Transitioning to adult care impacts many levels of a system, including the patient, the family, the pediatric medical team, and the adult medical team. Barriers to a successful transition can include patient's developmental stage, family's ability to support increasing patient responsibility, pediatric team's bond with patient, and adult team's uncertainty of treating issues specific to adolescence/young adulthood [101]. Providing education on diagnoses, medications, and how to navigate the health-care system is recommended. It is also important to address concerns from the family and encourage that they support the adolescent or young adult to take on more responsibility in care. Medical teams can benefit from having team members specifically assigned to aiding in transition-related issues [103]. Evidence-based practice guidelines as well integrated psychosocial programs are now a focus of research in order to better address potential barriers to transitioning [101, 104].

Conclusions

With medical outcomes improving significantly in recent years, pediatric SOT patients are living longer than ever before and, in turn, are faced with unique challenges requiring further attention and research. QOL following transplant can be negatively impacted by increased medical appointments, hospitalizations, medication side effects, and changes in typical routines. Nonadherence to a new medical regimen is also not uncommon and is associated with a host of medical and psychological consequences. Taken in combination, pediatric SOT patients and their families juggle multiple demands leaving the entire family system taxed. Standardized, multidisciplinary evaluations aimed at identifying and addressing both medical and psychosocial factors that pose risk to

successful transplantation are recommended for comprehensive, patient-centered support. Moreover, understanding how to minimize the effects of transplantation and immunosuppression on these critical processes in children is paramount. Lastly, identifying the etiologies responsible for and addressing the poor outcomes in the adolescent population remain an important area for study.

References

1. Rimsza ME, Hotalin AJ, Keown ME, Marcin JP, Moskowitz WB, Sigrest TD, et al. Definition of a pediatrician. Pediatrics. 2015;135(4):780.
2. Azeka E, Saavedra LC, Fregni F. Clinical research in pediatric organ transplantation. Clinics. 2014;69(S1):73–5.
3. Sharing UN for O. History [Internet]. 2017 [cited 2017 Jan 1]. Available from: https://unos.org/transplantation/history/
4. Network OP and T. General Considerations in Assessment for Transplant Candidacy. 2015.
5. Egan TM, Edwards LB. Effect of the lung allocation score on lung transplantation in the United States. J Hear Lung Transplant [Internet]. Elsevier; 2016;35(4):433–439. Available from: http://linkinghub.elsevier.com/retrieve/pii/S1053249816000577
6. Liou TG, Adler FR, Huang D. Use of lung transplantation survival models to refine patient selection in cystic fibrosis. Am J Respir Crit Care Med. 2005;171(9):1053–9.
7. Belkin RA, Henig NR, Singer LG, Chaparro C, Rubenstein RC, Xie SX, et al. Risk factors for death of patients with cystic fibrosis awaiting lung transplantation. Am J Respir Crit Care Med. 2006;173(6):659–66.
8. Sharing UN for O. Kidney Allocation System [Internet]. 2017 [cited 2017. Jul 12]. Available from: https://optn.transplant.hrsa.gov/learn/professional-education/kidney-allocation-system/
9. Kim WR, Lake JR, Smith JM, Skeans MA, Schladt DP, Edwards EB, et al. OPTN/SRTR 2015 annual data report: liver. Am J Transplant [Internet]. 2017;17 Suppl 1:174–251. Available from: http://www.ncbi.nlm.nih.gov/pubmed/28052604
10. Annunziato RA, Fisher MK, Jerson B, Bochkanova A, Shaw RJ. Psychosocial assessment prior to pediatric transplantation: a review and summary of key considerations. Pediatr Transplant. 2010;14(5):565–74.
11. Lefkowitz DS, Fitzgerald CJ, Zelikovsky N, Barlow K, Wray J. Best practices in the pediatric pretransplant psychosocial evaluation. Pediatr Transplant. 2014;18(4):327–35.
12. Killian MO. Psychosocial predictors of medication adherence in pediatric heart and lung organ transplantation. Pediatr Transplant. 2017;21(4).
13. Drotar D. Relating parent and family functioning to the psychological adjustment of children with chronic health conditions: what have we learned? What do we need to know? J Pediatr Psychol [Internet] 1997 Apr 1;22(2):149–165. Available from: http://jpepsy.oxfordjournals.org/cgi/doi/10.1093/jpepsy/22.2.149
14. Wysocki T, Gavin L. Paternal involvement in the Management of Pediatric Chronic Diseases: associations with adherence, Quality of Life, and Health Status. J Pediatr Psychol. 2006;31(5):501–11.
15. DiMatteo MR. Social support and patient adherence to medical treatment: a meta-analysis. Health Psychol [Internet]. 2004 Mar [cited 2015 Jul 29];23(2):207–18. Available from: http://www.ncbi.nlm.nih.gov/pubmed/15008666
16. Fung E, Shaw RJ. Pediatric Transplant Rating Instrument – a scale for the pretransplant psychiatric evaluation of pediatric organ transplant recipients. Pediatr Transplant [Internet]. 2008 Mar

[cited 2015 Jul 29];12(1):57–66. Available from.: http://www.ncbi.nlm.nih.gov/pubmed/18186890

17. Fisher M, Storfer-Isser A, Shaw RJ, Bernard RS, Drury S, Ularntinon S, et al. Inter-rater reliability of the pediatric transplant rating instrument (P-TRI): challenges to reliably identifying adherence risk factors during pediatric pre-transplant evaluations. Pediatr Transplant. 2011;

18. Schneider LM, Almond CS, Shaw RJ. The stanford pediatric psychosocial optimization tool. In: Presentation to the Stanford Children's Health Transplant Leadership Meeting. 2016. p. (Unpublished).

19. Spitzer RL, Kroenke K, Williams JBW. Validation and utility of a self-report version of PRIME-MD the PHQ primary care study. J Am Med Assoc. 1999;282(18):1737–44.

20. Baum M, Freier MC, Freeman KR, Chinnock RE. Developmental outcomes and cognitive functioning in infant and child heart transplant recipients. Prog Pediatr Cardiol. 2000;11:159–63.

21. Chinnock RE, Freier MC, Ashwal S, Pivonka-Jones J, Shankel T, Cutler D, et al. Developmental outcomes after pediatric heart transplantation. J Hear Lung Transplant. 2008;27:1079–84.

22. Haavisto A, Korkman M, Holmberg C, Jalanko H, Qvist E. Neuropsychological profile of children with kidney transplants. Nephrol Dial Transplant. 2012;27:2594–601.

23. Sorensen LG, Neighbors K, Martz K, Zelko F, Bucuvalas JC, Alonso EM. Cognitive and academic outcomes after pediatric liver transplantation: functional outcomes group (FOG) results. Am J Transplant. 2011;11:303–11.

24. Uzark K, Spicer R, Beebe DW. Neurodevelopmental outcomes in pediatric heart transplant recipients. J Hear Lung Transplant. 2009;28(12):1306–11.

25. Reed-Knight B, Lee JL, Cousins LA, Mee LL. Intellectual and academic performance in children undergoing solid organ pre-transplant evaluation. Pediatr Transplant. 2015;19:229–34.

26. Antonini TN, Beer SS, Miloh T, Dreyer WJ, Caudle SE. Neuropsychological functioning in preschool-aged children undergoing evaluation for organ transplant. Clin Neuropsychol. 2017;31(2):352–70.

27. Mohammad S, Alonso EM. Approach to optimizing growth, rehabilitation, and neurodevelopmental outcomes in children after solid-organ transplantation. Pediatric Clinics of North America. 2010. pp. 539–57.

28. Dobbels F. Intellectual disability in pediatric transplantation: pitfalls and opportunities. Pediatr Transplant. 2014;18(7):658–60.

29. Dew MA, Goycoolea JM, Stukas AA, Switzer GE, Simmons RG, Roth LH, et al. Temporal profiles of physical health in family members of heart transplant recipients: predictors of health change during caregiving. Health Psychol. 1998;17(2):138–51.

30. Committe on Hospital Care, Section on Surgery and S on CC. Policy Statment-Pediatric Organ Donation and Transplantation. Am Acad Pediatr [Internet]. 2010;125(4):822–8. Available from: http://pediatrics.aappublications.org/cgi/doi/10.1542/peds.2010-0081

31. Kelly SL, Morris N, Mee L, Brosig C, Self MM. The role of pediatric psychologists in solid organ transplant candidacy decisions: ethical considerations. Clin Pract Pediatr Psychol [Internet] 2016;4(4):417–422. Available from: http://doi.apa.org/getdoi.cfm?doi=10.1037/cpp0000155

32. States U, Transplantation O. OPTN/SRTR 2012 Annual Data Report 2014.

33. Valapour M, Skeans MA, Smith JM, Edwards LB, Cherikh WS, Uccellini K, et al. OPTN/SRTR 2015 annual data report: lung. Am J Transplant [Internet]. 2017;17 Suppl 1:357–424. Available from: http://www.ncbi.nlm.nih.gov/pubmed/28052607

34. Almond CSD, Thiagarajan RR, Piercey GE, Gauvreau K, Blume ED, Bastardi HJ, et al. Waiting list mortality among children listed for heart transplantation in the United States. Circulation [Internet]. 2009 Mar. 10 [cited 2015 Jul 29];119(5):717–27. Available from: http://www.pubmedcentral.nih.gov/articlerender.fcgi?artid=4278666&tool=pmcentrez&rendertype=abstract

35. Department of Health and Human Services, Health Resources and Services Administration, Healthcare Systems Bureau, Division of Transplantation, Rockville, MD; United Network for Organ Sharing, Richmond, VA; University Renal Research and Education Associati M. 2015 Annual Report of the U.S. Organ Procurement and Transplantation Network and the Scientific Registry of Transplant Recipients: Transplant Data 2008–2015.

36. Goldfarb SB, Levvey BJ, Cherikh WS, Chambers DC, Khush K, Kucheryavaya AY, et al. Registry of the International Society for Heart and Lung Transplantation: Twentieth Pediatric Lung and Heart-Lung Transplantation Report – 2017; Focus Theme: Allograft ischemic time. J Hear Lung Transplant [Internet]. Elsevier Inc.; 2017;36(10):1070–9. Available from: https://doi.org/10.1016/j.healun.2017.07.017

37. Bartosh SM, Ryckman FC, Shaddy R, Michaels MG, Platt JL, Sweet SC. A national conference to determine research priorities in pediatric solid organ transplantation. Pediatr Transplant [Internet]. 2008 Mar [cited 2015 Jul 29];12(2):153–66. Available from: http://doi.wiley.com/10.1111/j.1399-3046.2007.00811.x

38. Dew MA, Dabbs AD, Myaskovsky L, Shyu S, Shellmer D a, DiMartini AF, et al. Meta-analysis of medical regimen adherence outcomes in pediatric solid organ transplantation. Transplantation [Internet]. 2009 Sep. 15 [cited 2015 Jul 29];88(5):736–46. Available from: http://www.pubmedcentral.nih.gov/articlerender.fcgi?artid=2769559&tool=pmcentrez&rendertype=abstract

39. Kandaswamy R, Stock PG, Gustafson SK, Skeans MA, Curry MA, Prentice MA, et al. OPTN/SRTR 2015 annual data report: pancreas. Am J Transplant. 2017;17:117–73.

40. Smith JM, Skeans MA, Horslen SP, Edwards EB, Harper AM, Snyder JJ, et al. OPTN/SRTR 2015 annual data report: intestine. Am J Transplant. 2017;17:252–85.

41. Hsu DT. Biological and psychological differences in the child and adolescent transplant recipient. Pediatr Transplant [Internet]. 2005 Jun [cited 2015 Jul 29];9(3):416–21. Available from: http://www.ncbi.nlm.nih.gov/pubmed/15910401

42. Simons LE, Anglin G, Warshaw BL, Mahle WT, Vincent RN, Blount RL. Understanding the pathway between the transplant experience and health-related quality of life outcomes in adolescents. Pediatr Transplant [Internet]. 2008 Mar [cited 2015 Jul 29];12(2):187–93. Available from: http://www.ncbi.nlm.nih.gov/pubmed/18307667

43. DeMaso DR, Douglas Kelley S, Bastardi H, O'Brien P, Blume ED. The longitudinal impact of psychological functioning, medical severity, and family functioning in pediatric heart transplantation. J Heart Lung Transplant [Internet]. 2004 Apr [cited 2015 Jul 29];23(4):473–80. Available from: http://www.ncbi.nlm.nih.gov/pubmed/15063408

44. Devine K a, Reed-Knight B, Loiselle K a, Simons LE, Mee LL, Blount RL. Predictors of long-term health-related quality of life in adolescent solid organ transplant recipients. J Pediatr Psychol [Internet]. 2011 Sep;36(8):891–901. Available from: http://www.pubmedcentral.nih.gov/articlerender.fcgi?artid=3935000&tool=pmcentrez&rendertype=abstract

45. Brosig C, Pai A, Fairey E, Krempien J, McBride M, Lefkowitz DS. Child and family adjustment following pediatric solid organ transplantation: factors to consider during the early years post-transplant. Pediatr Transplant [Internet]. 2014 Sep [cited 2015 Jun 26];18(6):559–67. Available from: http://www.ncbi.nlm.nih.gov/pubmed/24923434

46. Fredericks EM, Lopez MJ, Magee JC, Shieck V, Opipari-Arrigan L. Psychological functioning, nonadherence and health outcomes after pediatric liver transplantation. Am J Transplant [Internet]. 2007 Aug [cited 2015 Jul 29];7(8):1974–83. Available from: http://www.ncbi.nlm.nih.gov/pubmed/17617862

47. Kim J, Marks S. Long-term outcomes of children after solid organ transplantation. Clinics [Internet]. 2014 Jan. 15 [cited 2015 Jul 29];69(Suppl 1):28–38. Available from: http://clinics.org.br/article.php?id=1262

48. Reed-Knight B, Loiselle K a, Devine K a, Simons LE, Mee LL, Blount RL. Health-related quality of life and perceived need for mental health services in adolescent solid organ transplant recipients. J Clin Psychol Med Settings [Internet]. 2013 Mar [cited 2015 May 21];20(1):88–96. Available from: http://www.pubmedcentral.nih.gov/articlerender.fcgi?artid=3916010&tool=pmcentrez&rendertype=abstract

49. Alonso, Estella M; Neighbors, Katie; Barton; Franca B.; McDiarmid, Sue V.; Dunn, Stephen P.; Mazariegos, George V.; Landgraf, Jeanne M.; Bucuvalas JC, and the S of the PLTRG. Health-related quality of life and family functioning following pediatric liver transplantation. Liver Transplant. 2008;14:460–468.

50. Ratcliff MB, Blount RL, Mee LL. The relationship between adolescent renal transplant recipients' perceived adversity, coping, and medical adherence. J Clin Psychol Med Settings [Internet]. 2010 Jun [cited 2015 Jun 23];17(2):116–24. Available from: http://www.ncbi.nlm.nih.gov/pubmed/20386962

51. Lerret SM, Weiss ME. How ready are they? Parents of pediatric solid organ transplant recipients and the transition from hospital to home following transplant. Pediatr Transplant [Internet]. 2011 Sep [cited 2015 Jul 29];15(6):606–16. Available from: http://www.ncbi.nlm.nih.gov/pubmed/21736682

52. Miloh T, Annunziato R, Arnon R, Warshaw J, Parkar S, Suchy FJ, et al. Improved adherence and outcomes for pediatric liver transplant recipients by using text messaging. Pediatrics. 2009;124:e844–50.

53. Cousino MK, Rea KE, Schumacher KR, Magee JC, Fredericks EM. A systematic review of parent and family functioning in pediatric solid organ transplant populations. Pediatr Transplant. 2017;21(3):1–13.

54. Gerson a C, Furth SL, Neu a M, Fivush B a. Assessing associations between medication adherence and potentially modifiable psychosocial variables in pediatric kidney transplant recipients and their families. Pediatr Transplant [Internet]. 2004 Dec [cited 2015 Jul 29];8(6):543–50. Available from: http://www.ncbi.nlm.nih.gov/pubmed/15598321

55. Corbett C, Armstrong MJ, Parker R, Webb K, Neuberger JM. Mental health disorders and solid-organ transplant recipients. Transplantation [Internet]. 2013 Oct 15 [cited 2015 May 21];96(7):593–600. Available from: http://www.ncbi.nlm.nih.gov/pubmed/23743726

56. Heinrich TW, Marcangelo M. Psychiatric issues in solid organ transplantation. Harv Rev Psychiatry [Internet]. 2009 Jan [cited 2015 Jul 29];17(6):398–406. Available from.: http://www.ncbi.nlm.nih.gov/pubmed/19968454

57. Steele RG, Aylward BS, Jensen CD, Wu YP. Parent- and Youth-Reported Illness Uncertainty: Associations With Distress and Psychosocial Functioning Among Recipients of Liver and Kidney Transplantations. Child Heal Care [Internet]. 2009 Jul. 16 [cited 2015 Jul 29];38(3):185–99. Available from: http://www.tandfonline.com/doi/abs/10.1080/02739610903038768

58. Rainer JP, Thompson CH, Lambros H. Psychological and psychosocial aspects of the solid organ transplant experience--a practice review. Psychotherapy (Chic) [Internet]. 2010 Sep [cited 2015 Jul 29];47(3):403–12. Available from.: http://www.ncbi.nlm.nih.gov/pubmed/22402095

59. Berney-Martinet S, Key F, Bell L, Lépine S, Clermont M-J, Fombonne E. Psychological profile of adolescents with a kidney transplant. Pediatr Transplant [Internet]. 2009 Sep [cited 2015 Jul 29];13(6):701–10. Available from.: http://www.ncbi.nlm.nih.gov/pubmed/18992062

60. Shaw RJ, Palmer L, Blasey C, Sarwal M. A typology of nonadherence in pediatric renal transplant recipients. Pediatr Transplant. 2003;7(14):489–93.

61. Supelana C, Annuziato R, Kaplan D, Helcer J, Stuber M, Shemesh E. PTSD in solid organ transplant recipients: current understanding and future implications. Pediatr Transplant. 2016;20(1):23–33.

62. Shemesh E, Lurie S, Stuber ML, Emre S, Patel Y, Vohra P, et al. A pilot study of posttraumatic stress and nonadherence in pediatric liver transplant recipients. Pediatrics. 2000;105(2):E29.

63. Mintzer LL, Stuber ML, Seacord D, Castaneda M, Mesrkhani V, Glover D. Traumatic stress symptoms in adolescent organ transplant recipients. Pediatrics [Internet]. 2005 Jun [cited 2015 Aug 2];115(6):1640–4. Available from: http://www.ncbi.nlm.nih.gov/pubmed/15930227

64. Young GS, Mintzer LL, Seacord D, Castan M, Mesrkhani V, Stuber ML. Symptoms of posttraumatic stress disorder in parents of transplant recipients: recipients: incidence, severity, and related factors. Pediatrics. 2003;111(6):e725–31.

65. Kazak AE, Simms S, Alderfer MA, Rourke MT, Crump T, Mcclure K, et al. Feasibility and preliminary outcomes from a pilot study of a brief psychological intervention for families of children newly diagnosed with Cancer. J Pediatr Psychol. 2005;30(8):644–55.

66. Kazak AE, Rourke MT, Alderfer MA, Pai A, Reilly AF, Meadows AT. Evidence-based assessment, intervention and psychosocial Care in Pediatric Oncology: a blueprint for comprehensive services across treatment. J Pediatr Psychol. 2007;32(9):1099–110.

67. Alonso EM, Sorensen LG. Cognitive development following pediatric solid organ transplantation. Curr Opin Organ Transplant. 2009;15:522–5.

68. Chisholm M a. Issues of adherence to immunosuppressant therapy after solid-organ transplantation. Drugs [Internet]. 2002;62(4):567–75. Available from: http://link.springer.com/10.2165/00003495-200262040-00002

69. Nevins TE, Robiner WN, Thomas W. Predictive patterns of early medication adherence in renal transplantation. Transplantation [Internet]. 2014 Oct 27 [cited 2015 Jul 29];98(8):878–84. Available from.: http://www.ncbi.nlm.nih.gov/pubmed/24831921

70. Foster BJ, Pai ALH. Adherence in adolescent and young adult kidney transplant recipients. Open Urol Nephrol J [Internet] 2014 Dec 16;7(1):133–143. Available from: http://benthamopen.com/ABSTRACT/TOUNJ-7-133

71. McGrady ME, Hommel KA. Medication adherence and health care utilization in pediatric chronic illness: a systematic review. Pediatrics [Internet]. 2013 Oct [cited 2015 Jun 7];132(4):730–40. Available from: http://www.pubmedcentral.nih.gov/articlerender.fcgi?artid=3784296&tool=pmcentrez&rendertype=abstract

72. Connelly J, Pilch N, Oliver M, Jordan C, Fleming J, Meadows H, et al. Prediction of medication non-adherence and associated outcomes in pediatric kidney transplant recipients. Pediatr Transplant [Internet]. 2015 Aug. [cited 2015 Jul 29];19(5):555–62. Available from: http://www.ncbi.nlm.nih.gov/pubmed/25917112

73. Foster BJ. Heightened graft failure risk during emerging adulthood and transition to adult care. Pediatr Nephrol [Internet]. 2015 Apr. [cited 2015 Jul 16];30(4):567–76. Available from: http://www.ncbi.nlm.nih.gov/pubmed/24890339

74. Fredericks EM, Dore-Stites D. Adherence to immunosuppressants: how can it be improved in adolescent organ transplant recipients? Curr Opin Organ Transplant [Internet]. 2010 Oct [cited 2015 Jul 29];15(5):614–20. Available from: http://www.pubmedcentral.nih.gov/articlerender.fcgi?artid=3092530&tool=pmcentrez&rendertype=abstract

75. Kahana SY, Frazier TW, Drotar D. Preliminary quantitative investigation of predictors of treatment non-adherence in pediatric transplantation: A brief report. Pediatr Transplant [Internet]. 2008 Sep [cited 2015 Aug 2];12(6):656–60. Available from: http://doi.wiley.com/10.1111/j.1399-3046.2007.00864.x

76. Oliva M, Singh TP, Gauvreau K, Vanderpluym CJ, Bastardi HJ, Almond CS. Impact of medication non-adherence on survival after pediatric heart transplantation in the U.S.A. J Heart Lung Transplant [Internet]. Elsevier; 2013 Sep [cited 2015 Jul 29];32(9):881–8. Available from.: http://www.ncbi.nlm.nih.gov/pubmed/23755899

77. Takemoto SK, Pinsky BW, Schnitzler M A, Lentine KL, Willoughby LM, Burroughs TE, et al. A retrospective analysis of

immunosuppression compliance, dose reduction and discontinuation in kidney transplant recipients. Am J Transplant [Internet]. 2007 Dec [cited 2015 Jul 29];7(12):2704–11. Available from: http://www.ncbi.nlm.nih.gov/pubmed/17868065

78. Dobbels F, Ruppar T, De Geest S, Decorte A, Van Damme-Lombaerts R, Fine RN. Adherence to the immunosuppressive regimen in pediatric kidney transplant recipients: a systematic review. Pediatr Transplant [Internet]. 2010 Aug [cited 2015 Jul 29];14(5):603–13. Available from.: http://www.ncbi.nlm.nih.gov/pubmed/20214741

79. Bunzel B, Laederach-Hofmann K. Solid organ transplantation: are there predictors for Posttransplant noncompliance? A literature overview. Transplantation [Internet] 2000 Sep;70(5):711–716. Available from: http://content.wkhealth.com/linkback/openurl?sid=WKPTLP:landingpage&an=00007890-200009150-00001

80. Casey BJ, Jones RM, Hare TA. The adolescent brain. Ann New York Acad Sci. 2008;1124:111–26.

81. Jarzembowski T, John E, Panaro F, Heiliczer J, Kraft K, Bogetti D, et al. Impact of non-compliance on outcome after pediatric kidney transplantation: an analysis in racial subgroups. Pediatr Transplant [Internet]. 2004 Aug;8(4):367–71. Available from: http://www.ncbi.nlm.nih.gov/pubmed/15265164

82. Rosenberger EM, Dew MA, Crone C, DiMartini AF. Psychiatric disorders as risk factors for adverse medical outcomes after solid organ transplantation. Curr Opin Organ Transplant [Internet]. 2012 Apr [cited 2015 Jul 29];17(2):188–92. Available from: http://www.pubmedcentral.nih.gov/articlerender.fcgi?artid=4470498&tool=pmcentrez&rendertype=abstract

83. McCormick King ML, Mee LL, Gutiérrez-Colina AM, Eaton CK, Lee JL, Blount RL. Emotional functioning, barriers, and medication adherence in pediatric transplant recipients. J Pediatr Psychol [Internet]. 2014 Apr;39(3):283–93. Available from.: http://www.ncbi.nlm.nih.gov/pubmed/24080552

84. Lee JL, Eaton C, Gutie AM, Devine K, Simons LE, Mee L, et al. Longitudinal stability of specific barriers to medication adherence. J Pediatr Psychol. 2014;39(7):667–76.

85. Fredericks EM, Zelikovsky N, Aujoulat I, Hames A, Wray J. Post-transplant adjustment--the later years. Pediatr Transplant [Internet]. 2014 Nov. [cited 2015 Jul 29];18(7):675–88. Available from.: http://www.ncbi.nlm.nih.gov/pubmed/25220845

86. De Bleser L, Matteson M, Dobbels F, Russell C, De Geest S. Interventions to improve medication-adherence after transplantation: a systematic review. Transpl Int [Internet]. 2009 Aug [cited 2015 Jul 29];22(8):780–97. Available from: http://www.ncbi.nlm.nih.gov/pubmed/19386076

87. Goldbeck L, Fidika A, Herle M, Quittner A. Psychological interventions for individuals with cystic fibrosis and their families (Review). Cochrane Database Syst Rev. 2014;6:1–152.

88. Kazak AE. Evidence-based interventions for survivors of childhood Cancer and their families. J Pediatr Psychol. 2005;30(1):29–39.

89. Beck DE, Fennell RS, Yost RL, Robinson JD, Geary MB, Ch B, et al. Evaluation of an educational program on compliance with medication regimens in pediatric patients with renal transplants. J Pediatr. 1980;96(6):1094–7.

90. Kahana S, Drotar D, Frazier T. Meta-analysis of psychological interventions to promote adherence to treatment in pediatric chronic health conditions. J Pediatr Psychol. 2008;33(6):590–611.

91. Henry HKM, Schor EL. Supporting self-management of chronic health problems. Pediatrics [Internet]. 2015 May. [cited 2015 Jun 2];135(5):789–92. Available from.: http://www.ncbi.nlm.nih.gov/pubmed/25896841

92. Fennell R, Foulkes L, Boggs S. Family-based program to promote medication compliance in renal transplant children. Transpl Proc. 1994;26(1):102–3.

93. Shemesh E, Annunziato RA, Shneider BL, Dugan CA, Warshaw J, Kerkar N, et al. Improving adherence to medications in pediatric liver transplant recipients. Pediatr Transplant. 2008; 12(3):316–23.

94. Hashim BL, Vadnais M, Miller AL. Improving adherence in adolescent chronic kidney disease: a dialectical behavior therapy (DBT) feasibility trial. Clin Pract Pediatr Psychol [Internet]. 2013;1(4):369–79. Available from: http://hz9pj6fe4t.search.serialssolutions.com.proxy.cc.uic.edu/?ctx_ver=Z39.88-2004&ctx_enc=info:ofi/enc:UTF-8&rfr_id=info:sid/ProQ:psycinfo&rft_val_fmt=info:ofi/fmt:kev:mtx:journal&rft.genre=article&rft.jtitle=Clinical+Practice+in+Pediatric+Psychology&

95. Naclerio C. The impact of a brief, manualized therapy protocol on medication adherence in adolescent kidney transplant recipients: Palo Alto University; 2017.

96. McKenzie RB, Berquist WE, Foley MA. Park K, Windsheimer JE, Litt, Iris F. Text messaging improves participation in laboratory testing in adolescent liver transplant patients. J Particip Med. 2015;7:1–15.

97. Korus M, Cruchley E, Stinson JN, Gold A, Anthony SJ. Usability testing of the internet program: "teens taking charge: managing my transplant online". Pediatr Transplant [Internet]. 2015;19(1):107–17. Available from: http://ovidsp.ovid.com/ovidweb.cgi?T=JS&PAGE=reference&D=prem&NEWS=N&AN=25495484

98. Bers MU, Beals LM, Chau C, Satoh K, Blume ED, Demaso DR, et al. Use of a virtual community as a psychosocial support system in pediatric transplantation. Pediatr Transplant. 2010;14(2):261–7.

99. Freier C, Oldhafer M, Offner G, Dorfman S, Kugler C. Impact of computer-based patient education on illness-specific knowledge and renal function in adolescents after renal transplantation. Pediatr Transplant. 2010;14(5):596–602.

100. Kerkar N, Annunziato R. Transitional care in solid organ transplantation. Semin Pediatr Surg [Internet]. Elsevier. 2015;24(2):83–7. Available from: https://doi.org/10.1053/j.sempedsurg.2015.01.006

101. Annunziato R A, Freiberger D, Martin K, Helcer J, Fitzgerald C, Lefkowitz DS. An empirically based practice perspective on the transition to adulthood for solid organ transplant recipients. Pediatr Transplant [Internet]. 2014 Dec [cited 2015 Jul 29];18(8):794–802. Available from: http://www.ncbi.nlm.nih.gov/pubmed/25224273

102. Akchurin OM, Melamed ML, Hashim BL, Kaskel FJ, Del Rio M. Medication adherence in the transition of adolescent kidney transplant recipients to the adult care. Pediatr Transplant [Internet]. 2014 Aug. [cited 2015 Jul 29];18(5):538–48. Available from.: http://www.ncbi.nlm.nih.gov/pubmed/24820521

103. LaRosa C, Glah C, Baluarte HJ, Meyers KEC. Solid-organ transplantation in childhood: transitioning to adult health care. Pediatrics [Internet]. 2011;127(4):742–53. Available from: http://pediatrics.aappublications.org/cgi/doi/10.1542/peds.2010-1232

104. Annunziato R A, Emre S, Shneider BL, Dugan C A, Aytaman Y, McKay MM, et al. Transitioning health care responsibility from caregivers to patient: a pilot study aiming to facilitate medication adherence during this process. Pediatr Transplant [Internet]. 2008 May. [cited 2015 Jul 29];12(3):309–15. Available from.: http://www.ncbi.nlm.nih.gov/pubmed/18435606

Palliative Care in Transplant Patients

47

Anna Piotrowski and Susan Imamura

Introduction

Historically transplantation and palliative medicine have been seen on the opposite ends of the spectrum, with transplant medicine focusing on aggressive life prolongation and palliative care being equated with end-of-life care. However, recent trends show that these specialties are not mutually exclusive.

Due to advances in medicine and technology, many more people than ever before are living with chronic and end-stage illness and have the possibility of organ transplantation as a means of potential treatment. Patients with leukemia, multiple myeloma, and some types of lymphoma may now have the option of a bone marrow transplant. However, some patients evaluated for transplant might not be found appropriate candidates due to medical or psychosocial reasons or may pass while awaiting a transplant [1, 2]. Others may not survive the transplant or postoperative period or may have complications which limit their quality of life (QOL) or long-term survival [2]. In addition, patients undergoing transplantation trade one chronic illness for another, as all transplant recipients must take a complicated post-transplant regimen, associated with multiple side effects [3–5].

While successful transplantation may afford a patient another 5 to 20 years of life [6], with the uncertain and tenuous transplant process, it is paramount to shift the focus from quantity to quality of life.

What Is Palliative Care?

The World Health Organization defines palliative care as "an approach that improves the quality of life of patients and their families facing the problems associated with life-threatening illness through the prevention and relief of suffering by means of early identification and impeccable assessment and treatment of pain and other problems, physical, psychosocial and spiritual." [7]

Palliative care is medical care provided by an interdisciplinary team including medicine, psychiatry, nursing, social work, chaplaincy, counseling, nursing assistants, and other health professionals, focused on the relief of suffering and support for the best possible QOL for patients facing serious life-threatening illness and their families. Palliative care expands the focus from traditional disease-model medical treatments to include the goals of enhancing QOL, optimizing functioning, and helping with decision-making including decisions regarding end-of-life care [8]. Palliative care includes:

1. The structure and process of care.
2. Physical aspects of care.
3. Psychological and psychiatric aspects of care.
4. Social aspects of care.
5. Spiritual, religious, and existential aspects of care.
6. Cultural aspects of care.
7. Care of the imminently dying patient.
8. Ethical and legal aspects of care.

These core domains of care are used to provide individualized patient- and family-centered care where each patient's and their family's needs are assessed, documented, and addressed individually. Such assessment includes documentation of the disease status, diagnoses, and prognosis, patients' and families' understanding of the disease and prognosis, and patient and family expectations, including goals for care and for living. The palliative care team

A. Piotrowski (✉) · S. Imamura
Department of Psychiatry, Kaiser Permanente, San Jose, CA, USA
e-mail: anna.piotrowski@kp.org

© Springer International Publishing AG, part of Springer Nature 2019
Y. Sher, J. R. Maldonado (eds.), *Psychosocial Care of End-Stage Organ Disease and Transplant Patients*,
https://doi.org/10.1007/978-3-319-94914-7_47

facilitates the documentation of patients' wishes for care along the healthcare continuum via completion of documents such as an advanced care directive or a Physicians Orders for Life-Sustaining Treatment (POLST) [8, 9].

An advanced care directive is a legal document that is completed at any point during the patients' disease process that (1) designates a surrogate decision-maker if a patient becomes unable to make decisions about their own medical care and (2) provides general treatment guidance or instructions in making healthcare decisions (e.g., when to continue, withhold, or withdraw care at the end of life). A POLST is not a legal document and does not designate a surrogate decision-maker. Instead, a POLST is completed when patients are nearing the end of life and are expected to die within a year, and it functions as "portable medical order for specific medical treatments the patient would want tonight" [9] and orders medical personnel to provide specific treatment in an emergency. A POLST contains three major elements including if the patient wishes to receive cardiopulmonary resuscitation if they are nonresponsive, have no pulse, and are not breathing, what type of treatment they wish to receive in an emergency when they have a pulse and are breathing, and if they wish to receive artificial nutrition [9]. After documenting patients' wishes regarding their goals of care, the palliative care team ensures that patients' goals and choices are understood, respected, and implemented within the limits of state and federal law including implementation of do not resuscitate (DNR) orders which instruct medical providers to not provide cardiopulmonary resuscitation if a patient becomes unresponsive, stops breathing, and has no pulse [8, 9].

Aside from assessment, documentation, and implementation of patients' goals for treatment, palliative care can manage symptoms such as pain, shortness of breath, fatigue, nausea, weakness, anorexia, insomnia, anxiety, depression, confusion, and constipation, as well as other symptoms and side effects of the disease process and its treatment. The palliative care team is able to assess and communicate the signs of impending death and care for patients during the dying process and provide grief and bereavement assistance to the patients' families and treatment team [8].

Palliative Care and the Transplant Process

Molmenti and Dunn describe patients eligible for transplants as highly vulnerable physically, socioeconomically, psychologically, and spiritually from the consequences of end-stage organ failure. Their and their families' wishes may evolve over time due to the progression of the underlying disease which changes the goals of care. Once transplanted, patients' and their families' expectations for complete recovery may be incongruent with the nature of their disease, post-transplant complications, age, comorbid medical illness, and previous functional status [10]. The involvement of palliative care in the transplant process has been documented to improve advance care planning and goals of care discussions, increase do not resuscitate (DNR) rates, and decrease length of stay in the hospital, without increasing the rate of mortality. They also decrease the rate and severity of symptoms such as nausea, insomnia, pain, tiredness, constipation, depression, anxiety, anorexia, and dyspnea [1].

The integration of palliative care into the transplant process has been found to be highly effective in supporting patients throughout their disease process [11]. Yet, many misconceptions about palliative care act as barriers to referral [12]. Ouimet Perrin describes key barriers to include the misconception by medical providers, patients, and their families that palliative care is solely appropriate for patients near death and is separate from standard care. Therefore, involvement of palliative care can be seen as undermining the goal of saving the patient's life. Furthermore, the unpredictable disease trajectory of organ failure [1, 13] makes it difficult for clinicians to decide when is the best time to involve palliative care. Santivasi et al. describe the concept of a "therapeutic inertia" where the adherence to a preconceived course of treatment even in the face of new medical problems or risks can prevent the consideration of non-transplant-directed care [14, 15].

The integration of palliative care intro transplant clinics has been discussed in numerous articles and has been increasing over the years. Wentlandt et al. describe the integration of palliative care clinic into the organ transplantation service within the University Health Network's Multi-Organ Transplant Program in Toronto, Canada [13]. They report that since 2011, over 250 patients have been referred to the palliative care clinic. After initial consultation, patients' Edmonton Symptom Distress Score, an assessment of symptom distress in the palliative care setting, improved for pain, tiredness, drowsiness, sleep, cough, depression, and anxiety. Each unique solid organ transplantation program (i.e., heart, lung, kidney, liver, gut) as well as hematopoietic cell transplantation can have their own unique issues, question, and symptom burdens. It is important to address the unique aspects of palliative care in these patient populations separately.

Palliative Care and Heart Failure

Improvements in cardiovascular treatment have led to an increase in those living with heart failure, which is expected to rise to nearly 8 million people by 2030 [16]. With advances in diagnosis and therapy, patients with heart failure have access to a variety of treatments including (1) medical therapy, (2) electrical therapy, (3) surgery, and (4) combination therapy. For many patients, as their disease progresses, medical therapy is no longer enough, and evaluation for placement of ventricular support devices and heart transplantation becomes an option [17].

In 2017, there were 3244 heart transplants in the United States. Despite this number, there are currently 3956 patients who are currently registered and waiting for a heart transplant with the median waiting time between 70 and 535 days [18]. Due to prolonged waiting times for a heart transplant, patients may experience emotional strain as well as physical decompensation marked by shortness of breath, nausea, dizziness, and edema. At times these symptoms may be intractable [19]. These symptoms interfere with the ability to work or complete daily activities and cause significant psychological distress for both patients and their families [20]. Worsening anxiety, anorexia, and sleep disturbance may not only be immediate issues for the patient but also detrimental to their long-term health and jeopardize their transplant status [19]. Patients who receive heart transplant and are discharged from the hospital have decreased 5-year survival of 76.2–79.2%, compared to the general population [18]. This is of course superior to medical therapy alone with 1-year survival of only 25% [20].

Thus, opportunities for palliative care team to offer their services are ample throughout the continuum of end-stage heart disease. Ideally, the utilization of palliative care should be started at the time of diagnosis when a patient's health is not in crisis and there exists ample opportunity to discuss diagnoses, symptoms, prognosis, treatment options, treatment preferences, and healthcare values. This integration of palliative care into the initial visits with the patient and their family can provide support to the patient and their family during their disease process. The palliative care providers have the ability to assist the heart failure team with treatment of changing physical and emotional symptoms and discussions of changes in goals of care which may occur during the disease trajectory [19].

Schwarz et al. describe a pilot study of palliative care consultation in patients with advanced heart failure referred for cardiac transplantation. In this study, 20 patients received a palliative care consultation with resulting decreased use of opioids, increased clarity about treatment plans, and realignment of goals of care. Of these patients, 30% completed advanced care directives. In addition, both patients and their cardiologists reported that the palliative care consult provided either moderate or significant positive impact on the patient care [4]. Another study demonstrated that integration of palliative care into heart failure treatment increased patients' QOL, improved their symptom burden, and increased advanced care planning [21].

Post-transplant, while patient's QOL improves and caregiver burden decreases, physical symptoms, such as pain, may continue. In addition, patients might experience an increase in emotional and psychosocial-spiritual burden with up to 69% of patients endorsing such symptoms after transplant [20]. Overall, early and continual involvement of palliative care throughout the disease and transplant process can help not only delineate and clarify evolving goals of care but provide treatment of distressing symptoms, improve QOL, and support patients and their families throughout the disease process.

Palliative Care and Ventricular Assist Devices

In recent years, ventricular assist devices (VADs) have been used not only as a bridge to transplants but also as a destination therapy when a patient is not eligible or does not wish to receive a heart transplant [2, 22]. As a result, nearly 150,000 to 250,000 patients annually are eligible for a destination VAD therapy, although the current 1-year mortality rate for destination (DT) left ventricular assist devices (LVAD) is around 20% and the average survival only slightly exceeds 2 years after implantation [22]. As such, the therapy itself may be considered aggressive palliation as the risk of complications remains very high and includes rehospitalization, infection, stroke, device malfunction due to clotting, and progressive right heart failure [22].

Some of the psychosocial problems common among LVAD patients are different from transplant patients. The caregiving for patients with an LVAD is more burdensome than care of heart transplant candidates or recipients and has been found to be comparable to patients receiving mechanical ventilation at home [16]. In 2013, the Joint Commission mandated that all accredited DT-LVAD programs must have a palliative care specialist as part of the treatment team, and this is also consistent with the 2014 recommendations by the Centers for Medicare and Medicaid Services [22]. Integration of the palliative care team at the time of the initial discussion and implantation decision-making can facilitate understanding and documentation of patient's goals, preferences, and values, including completion of associated documents such as advanced care directives ideally done prior to device implantation. Palliative care can also increase in-home support as symptom burden and complications progress [16]. Longitudinal care and involvement by the palliative care team from implantation of the DT-LVAD can help continually assess the patients' and their families' evolving goals of care and facilitate transitions in goals of care, including device deactivation and end-of-life care [22].

Palliative Care and End-Stage Lung Disease

For patients with end-stage lung disease, lung transplant may be the therapy of choice that can improve both survival and QOL [23]. Unfortunately, lung transplantation includes many risks including drug toxicities, infections, and rejection [24]. Survival post-lung transplant remains low with 1-year and 5-year survival of 87–89.1% and 52.2–55.4%, respectively [18]. In addition, improvement in lung transplant recipients' QOL may not be fully evident until 1 year after transplant [2]. Long-term concerns include bronchiolitis obliterans, a progressive, insidious, and often fatal lung alloreaction, which affects 49% and 75% of patients 1 year and 5 years post-transplant, respectively, determining the trajectory and outcomes post-lung transplant and significantly affecting patients' QOL [5]. Thus, lung transplantation may be seen not as a curative therapy but more as a continuation along the spectrum of chronic disease which makes early palliative care interventions desirable and necessary. In addition, both the American Thoracic Society and American College of Chest Physicians support the involvement of palliative care in the care of patients with advanced lung disease [25].

Despite the recommendations for integration of palliative care, few patients get referred to palliative care services after lung transplantation. In a survey of transplant pulmonologists and palliative care clinicians from the major US lung transplant programs with at least 15 lung transplant annual volume, 18 centers out of 27 contacted responded [26]. The survey indicated that on average, less than five patients per year were referred to the palliative care services from each center. Of note, 94% of palliative care referrals were made late in the disease trajectory, with average length of survival being less than 30 days after such referrals. Despite lung transplant clinicians endorsing palliative care in assistance with not only end-of-life discussions but also in providing family support, pain and symptom management, psychological support, and planning of care, 45% of lung transplant recipients still died in the intensive care unit (ICU) [26].

Co-management by palliative care of end-stage lung disease patients, both pre- and post-transplant, has demonstrated a decrease in symptom burden as well as an increase in goals of care discussions. Freeman et al. described that in a co-managed palliative care and lung transplant clinic, patients experienced an improvement in their sleep and cough and a trend toward improvement in pain. Discussion of advance care directives occurred 74% of the time. All patients who were started on opioids pre-transplant for dyspnea and cough by the palliative care service discontinued opioids post-transplant, demonstrating effective management of dyspnea by the palliative care team [27]. Rosenberger et al. suggested that by incorporating both palliative and restorative care as integral parts in a patient's overall treatment, clinicians may better address patients' distressing symptoms, prepare patients for pre- and post-transplant challenges, and address their changing needs throughout the disease trajectory [5].

Palliative Care in Cystic Fibrosis and Lung Transplant

Patients with cystic fibrosis (CF) are unique in that they live with the possibility that they may die young [28]. Improvement in medical care has increased the median survival time in a patient with CF to 47 years of age in 2016 [29]. As a result, among patients with CF, studies show that palliative care is often deferred in lieu of aggressive medical treatments that aim to sustain patients until transplantation [5], although most patients die prior to receiving a transplant [28]. Therefore, patients with CF are more likely to die in ICU without having ever discussed their goals of care [5]. Chapman et al. have demonstrated that due to the unique nature of being diagnosed and living with CF, these patients were comfortable when questions of dying were raised early by medical staff, despite the reluctance of staff to discuss goals of care, deterioration, death, and dying [28]. In addition to questions about death and dying, patients with CF are living longer lives with significant symptom burden. In a palliative care survey completed by patients with CF receiving medical care in a major academic institution, 24% of patients reported chronic pain and nearly one-half of these patients reported that pain interfered with general activity, enjoyment of life, and ability to exercise. Only 31% of patients complaining of chronic pain had a treatment plan for pain. Unsurprisingly, patients reporting worse physical symptoms also had worsening lung function. In addition, 43% of patients reported that they frequently think about the impact of CF on their lives and 33% of patients reported that now or earlier was the ideal time to discuss end-of-life care. Despite the fact that 95% of patients reported that they felt comfortable talking to their CF team about end-of-life care, only 25% had completed a healthcare proxy form, a living will, or other written instructions [30]. The disparity between the high amount of symptom burden and actual treatment of patients' symptoms and discussion about their end-of-life care goals highlights an ample opportunity to improve care for patients living with CF. In addition, the disparity between patients' reported comfort and eagerness for such discussions as compared to providers' discomfort and hesitancy demonstrates the need for increasing providers' education and support regarding such discussions. The integration of palliative and active care throughout the life of a patient with CF would allow the patient, their family, and the team to better adapt to the progression of the disease and to improve QOL in physical, psychological, and spiritual domains across the continuum of the illness experience [28].

Palliative Care and End–Stage Renal Disease

There are four treatment modalities established for the management of end-stage kidney disease: hemodialysis, peritoneal dialysis, transplant, and conservative care defined as management of end-stage renal disease (ESRD) without dialysis [31, 32].

In 2017, there was a total of 18,489 kidney transplant nationwide, with adults over the age of 65 representing the third largest age group receiving a kidney transplant with 3666 transplants [18]. While a kidney transplant greatly reduces morbidity and mortality from ESRD compared to patients on the waiting list, larger benefits were seen for patients who were 20 to 39 years old [33]. Patients over the age of 70 did not achieve equal survival benefit compared to those on the waitlist, until 2 months after transplant. Yet these patients are a growing segment of the population with ESRD. Chen et al. describe that this population has a 5-year mortality rate of 60% post-kidney transplantation [34]. In patients continuing dialysis, the annual mortality rate is between 20 and 25%, and the majority of these patients die in acute care facilities without accessing palliative care services [35].

All patients with ESRD report high symptom burden independent of whether there are receiving dialysis or are transplant patients, and studies have shown that many patients have comparable symptom burden to those of patients with advanced cancer [36]. Despite the high symptom burden and high mortality rate, especially for patients ineligible for transplant, few patients have knowledge regarding their disease trajectory and palliative and hospice care services. In a survey of 584 patients with stage 4 and 5 chronic kidney disease who presented to dialysis, transplantation, or pre-dialysis clinics, only 17.9% felt their health would deteriorate in the next 12 months. Despite 60.7% of dialysis patients regretting their decisions to start dialysis, 83.4% did not know about palliative care. Among these surveyed patients, 65.6% reported being comfortable discussing end-of-life care with their nephrology staff, but only 38.2% had completed an advanced directive [32]. These studies demonstrated the need for integration of palliative care services into the renal clinics to address patients' symptoms, to provide support in decision-making around questions of conservative care versus further treatments such dialysis and transplant, and to complete advanced care planning.

Post-transplant patients may continue to have a significant symptom burden. Afshar et al. described a cross-sectional symptom survey of patients in the United Kingdom who had received a renal transplant 1 year prior to completion of the survey. Of the 110 patients surveyed, seven symptoms affected at least one third of the population examined. These included weakness (55%), difficulty sleeping (45%), dyspnea (42%), anxiety (36%), drowsiness (35%), dissatisfaction with body image (35%), and weight gain (33%) [37].

The Renal Palliative Care Initiative at Baystate Medical Center in collaboration with area dialysis and hospice centers describes an integrated palliative care service which included symptom assessment and management protocols, advance care planning, hospice referral, and bereavement services for all patients with ESRD. They have demonstrated an increase in advanced care directives completion from 6% to 32% [38]. Thus, given the previously described roles of palliative care to address ongoing symptoms pre- and post-transplant, discuss goals of care, and support patients throughout their disease process, the integration of palliative care into renal clinics can allow for better management of symptom burden and delivery of patient- and family-driven care.

Palliative Care and End-Stage Liver Disease

More people are affected by liver disease every year due to increased alcohol consumption, viral hepatitis, and obesity. Twenty percent of patients listed for liver transplant will die before a donor becomes available, and many patients living with cirrhosis are not eligible for transplant. End-stage liver disease (ESLD) represents a major cause of mortality and morbidity with 38,000 patients dying annually and is the seventh leading cause of death in the United States [39]. In terms of QOL, patients with ESLD have a significant symptom burden, suffer many complications, and require management of a complicated medication and nutrition regimen [40]. The complexity of symptom management is particularly highlighted in end-of-life care when patients may experience an average of 14 physical symptoms in the last month of care [41, 42]. In addition, some patients describe significant distress waiting for a liver transplant including difficulty coping, loss of trust in medical personal, and uncertainties about their future [43].

Typically goals of care and prognosis discussions in ESLD occur too late and may not include the patient themselves. As described by Low et al. at a tertiary treatment center in North London, United Kingdom, 77% of the time, the prognosis was discussed with family members, and 53% of such discussions occurred at or less than 34 days before the patient's death. In most cases, the medical team and not the patient or their family members had completed DNR orders. Most patients died in the hospital and were referred to palliative care 5 days before death [41]. This study demonstrated that although patients were clearly in poor health, there were limited discussions to address their QOL, goals of care, and prognosis and that referral to palliative care was done too late in the disease process. Low et al. reported that the liver clinicians engaged in "reactive treatment at the expense of palliative care" and that palliative care was only discussed at the initiation of the patient and not the team [41].

Unfortunately, this is not uncommon as it has frequently been reported that only 0.97–7.1% of patients with ESLD and 11% of patients removed from liver transplant lists received palliative care despite their uncontrolled symptoms [30, 41, 44, 45].

Several reasons for late referral to palliative care in patients with ESLD have been described. One of these is the unpredictable trajectory of liver disease, where patients may have frequent admissions and decompensations but may remain stable in between these exacerbations and only develop symptoms of ESLD abruptly. In addition, physicians' desire for active treatment may be secondary to their own perceptions of patient's expectations, their misunderstanding of palliative care, poor continuity of care, and perceived lack of skill and confidence when discussing prognosis and palliative care with patients and their caregivers. Despite this, early palliative care referral is associated with better QOL and can decrease both patient's affective and physical symptoms.

Waiting for liver transplant and receiving palliative care does not need to be a mutually exclusive process. Rossaro et al. describe a case of a 50-year-old man with ESLD secondary to hepatitis C who successfully received both palliative care services and was listed for a liver transplant [40]. While integration of palliative care into the transplant program was met with patient and family barriers and physician reluctance, this new integrated model improved QOL and prepared the patient for end of life in case of not receiving a liver in time. Rossaro proposes that patients too sick for a liver transplant should be immediately referred to palliative care. Patients with an increasing Model for End-stage Liver Disease (MELD) score, signaling worsening liver disease and increasing symptomatology, should be referred concurrently to palliative care and liver transplant and thus be supported and prepared for any eventual outcome. This was also demonstrated in a study at the University of California in Davis where patients were jointly co-managed by hospice and hepatology and showed improvement in their MELD scores [43].

A study published by Baumann et al. [46] demonstrated that an intervention via incorporation of a longitudinal, multidisciplinary early palliative care into the pre-transplant evaluation at Albert Einstein Medical Center in Philadelphia improved moderate to severe symptoms such as pruritus, appetite, and fatigue in 50% of patients. Other improvements that were noted but were not statistically significant included pain, myalgias, sexual dysfunction, sleep disturbance, and dyspnea. In addition, depression symptoms improved in 27.8% [46]. Moreover, 55.6% of patients established new healthcare power of attorneys and 17% completed advanced directives [46]. Other studies have also demonstrated that a palliative intervention for liver transplant patients can

improve DNR status clarification from 52% to 81% [44]. Therefore, these studies demonstrate that palliative care interventions in liver transplantation provide improved patient QOL, decreased disease symptomatology, improved education and goals of care discussions, decrease in ICU length of stays, and improved communication and family satisfaction without impacting patient mortality [43].

Palliative Care and Intestinal Transplant

It is estimated that two to three persons per million per year experience intestinal failure (IF), and 15% of them become candidates for intestinal transplant (ITx) [47]. Unique challenges in ITx include the large number of bacteria in the gut increasing the risk for post-transplantation infection and the large number of white cells in the bowel providing a strong stimulus for rejection. Due to these risks, ITx remains the rarest of organ transplants.

For the majority of patients with IF, total parenteral nutrition (TPN) is the preferred treatment as patients can be managed on home TPN for many years, and presently, long-term survival on TPN is superior to intestinal transplant for short bowel syndrome. In the first 1–2 years, the data varies on TPN's superiority to ITx. While earlier studies showed promising short-term (1-year) patient survival after isolated intestinal transplantation of 88–92%, which is similar to survival on TPN, later studies reported more discouraging statistics of 77% 1-year survival [48–50]. Long-term survival after ITx is consistently found to be lower compared to TPN over the same time frame. The International Intestinal Transplant Registry in 1997 reported that a 5-year patient survival is only 50% after ITx, compared with 60%–80% 5-year survival on TPN [51]. A review article by DeLegge in 2007 reported a 5-year patient survival similarly at 49% [50]. Due to improved survival on TPN compared to intestinal transplant, ITx is not currently indicated for patients dependent on TPN who are not experiencing complications.

For those experiencing complications on long-term TPN, intestinal transplant can be a life-saving procedure and is the only long-term solution. Additionally, ITx does provide a marked improvement in QOL with most patients consuming all their calories orally or via tube feedings and the majority returning to school and work. TPN is time-consuming, taking 10–16 h and up to 24 h to administer with the need for attachment to an intravenous pump. Not surprisingly, long-term TPN affects one's ability to work and maintain usual activities [52].

Due to its comparative infrequency to other organ transplants, studies looking at palliative care interventions and needs specific to the intestinal transplant patient are lacking. The challenges faced by ITx candidates and recipients overlap with the broader challenges of transplant patients magnified by the unique challenges of the gut. Pre-transplant, ITx candidates have the highest mortality for those awaiting transplantation. The US Scientific Registry of Transplant Recipient Data reported mortality rates of 16% per year. Adults aged 35–65 awaiting small bowel and liver transplantation have a mortality rate three to six times that of patients awaiting liver transplantation alone [53].

Additionally, there is not the same degree of conflict between QOL and maintaining optimal physical condition in patients awaiting ITx as compared to patients waiting for another solid organ transplant (SOT). TPN management, associated with such QOL concerns as complexity of catheter care and duration of administration, is critical in optimizing physical strength and resiliency for survival and recuperation from transplant surgery. This is in marked contrast to symptoms like air hunger seen in lung transplant candidates where palliative sedation with opioids can reduce this highly distressing symptom but also decrease level of activity or may even not be compatible with transplant listing. Due to these issues, referral to palliative care is a realistic and needed consult starting with the initial ITx evaluation.

Post-transplant, ITx patients need more intense immunosuppressive protocols than other SOT patients due to large size of the graft and the strong evoked immune response. Thus, opportunistic infections and neoplastic diseases are seen more commonly in ITx recipients compared to other SOT. Graft versus host disease (GVHD) is also more common in ITx than in other SOT due to the large size of the transplanted tissue creating a strong stimulus for an immune response [54]. The heavy immunosuppressant burden needed to prevent GVHD in turn leads to sepsis, the leading cause of death following intestinal transplant. Acute rejection is seen in 50–75% of patients, and chronic rejection occurs in up to 10–15% of recipients [47, 55]. With longer survival, post-transplant lymphoproliferative disease (PTLD) becomes a risk from prolonged immunosuppression and is a leading cause of death long-term in intestinal transplant recipients [56]. Thus, while quality of post-transplant life is markedly high with approximately 80% of surviving patients fully independent of TPN [48] and with a high rate of reduction in narcotic needs, transplant recipients still must deal with a chronic disease process with heavy immunosuppression therapy, multiple complications, and hospitalizations and a gradual deterioration in health over time. With all these challenges, palliative care can provide an invaluable service for both the pre- and post-ITx patients in understanding their illness trajectory, clarification of the uncertainty around the relapsing and remitting course of the disease process, and assisting patients and families with planning around an intervention with low long-term survival rates [47, 48, 50, 56–58].

Palliative Care in Hematopoietic Cell Transplantation

Hematopoietic cell transplantation (HCT) is a potentially life-saving and curative intervention with high recovery rates. Bush et al. found that 1–4 years after HCT, 73% to 81% of survivors rated their overall QOL as good to excellent. By 2 years after transplantation, 71% of survivors reported that they had recovered from their transplantation, up from 41% at 6 months and 66% at 1 year [59]. At the same time, HCT still carries significant risk for acute complications and late effects including GVHD, organ toxicity, osteoporosis, infections, cataracts, secondary cancers, and infertility. In the case of hematological malignancies, patients also experience the side effects from high doses of chemotherapy including nausea, fatigue, mouth sores, extreme weakness, diarrhea, or constipation. HCT procedure requires patients to spend several weeks in the hospital to help protect against increased susceptibility to infections, possible need for blood transfusions, and monitoring/treatment for possible complications. Even after hospital discharge, the recovery process can take several more months before the individual is able to engage fully in life activities prior to the transplant. Additionally, despite the advancements in treating hematological malignancies, the threat of relapsed disease, progression of symptoms, and eventual mortality remain. For all these factors, the involvement of palliative care both pre- and post-HCT and ongoing and active evaluations of one's QOL are a vital part of management in patients undergoing HCT.

While one of the barriers in consulting and benefitting from palliative care has been its equation with end-of-life and hospice care, the concurrent involvement of palliative care with active treatment shows improved outcomes, including decreased symptom burden during hospitalization and increased mood and overall QOL [60]. A randomized control trial in 160 enrolled patients by El-Jawahri et al. had palliative care provide guidelines for addressing nausea, pain, diarrhea, constipation, fatigue, insomnia, anxiety, and depression as well as meeting with the patient for at least four visits during the course of their hospitalization with two of the visits in the first 2 weeks of care. Palliative care involvement was associated with less decline in overall QOL and some improvements in depression and anxiety. Caregivers of patients who had been followed by palliative care reported better coping, improvement in administrative and financial QOL, and fewer depressive symptoms [61].

Currently palliative care services are elicited less frequently in HCT and patients with hematological malignancies as compared to SOT and other oncologies [66]. Howell demonstrated that patients with hematological malignancies were far less likely to receive care from palliative or hospice services compared to other cancers [62]. For the United States specifically, the proportion of patients with all cancers receiving input from palliative care team is 59% versus 21% in specifically hematological cancers. Similarly, a US retrospective study by Cheng et al. showed that 11% of hematological patients accessed palliative care compared to 89% of patient with solid tumors [63].

The causes for the lower rates of palliative care involvement in hematological malignancies vary considerably and reflect the heterogeneity in the indications for HCT. Factors like the belief that symptom burden in hemato-oncological patient is less than other oncological patients have not stood up in studies with hematological patients who experienced similar levels of pain and more drowsiness and delirium than other oncological patients [64]. The chronic trajectory of the illness with intermittent acuity creates strong bonds over a long duration of care with the hematology team. This may lead the patient and family to look to the hematology care team for both active treatment and palliative care needs and may reduce the hematology teams' readiness to involve another specialty, particularly if referral to palliative care may signal too starkly the transition to terminal care. Alternatively, once advanced disease is identified, the rapid mortality of the condition compared to solid tumors may prevent enough time to involve the palliative care team. Fadul et al. determined time from palliative care referral to death in hematological patients was 13 days as compared to 46 days in patients with solid tumors [64]. Given this rapid mortality of hematological malignancies, earlier involvement of palliative care can ease the transition from active treatment to end-of-life care, provide education on clinical indicators of the dying process, and help patients and families better recognize imminent death risk. Hematological patients are also more likely to die in the hospital setting which can be an added strain for patients and their families. End-of-life care in the home environment can be comparatively more complex as terminal patients may require frequent transfusions. However, these challenges highlight the utility of palliative care involvement. Interventions such as transfusions can be performed in prearranged home visits rather than defaulting to day units. For those who have been mostly cared in the acute hospital but wish to pass at home, early involvement with palliative care can provide a much-needed familiarity and connection.

Given that the transition point between life-prolonging care and palliative phases of the disease can be difficult to predict or define, the focus on palliative care as distinct from end-of-life and hospice care in HCT patients is imperative.

Conclusions

Early palliative care involvement in the transplant evaluation and treatment process provides numerous advantages to patients, families, and care teams. In the transplant process, palliative care teams can reduce symptom burden,

improve caregiver support, offer education, clarify goals of care, and provide clear healthcare directives for loved ones and the care team. Even more importantly, early palliative care involvement has demonstrated a survival advantage of 2.7 months for individuals with similar level of disease burden [65].

In contrast to common misperceptions among medical personnel, studies repeatedly have shown that patients welcome honest and early discussions around mortality and disease prognosis. Given the high morbidity and mortality for organ and bone marrow transplant, the discussion of end-of-life care is a realistic and needed part of the care plan and often comes too late in the disease process. When the goals of care change, palliative care can assist in the transition from active to comfort care while maximizing quality of life in the process. Studies have found no disadvantage or harm with involvement of palliative care [39], although limitations like cost remain a potential barrier, as the cost-effectiveness for palliative care involvement has not been adequately explored. However, palliative care services are available at most major institutions where transplants are offered, making the barriers for early involvement of palliative care low compared to the strong benefits this service provides. The support for early and continuous involvement of palliative care throughout the transplant process is strong from many providers and continues to grow.

References

1. Wentlandt K, Weiss A, O'Connor E, Kaya E. Palliative and end of life care in solid organ transplantation. Am J Transplant. 2017;17(12):3008–19.
2. Crone CC, Marcangelo MJ, Shuster JJL. An approach to the patient with organ failure: transplantation and end-of-life treatment decisions. Med Clin N Am. 2010;94:1241–54.
3. Pinter J, Hanson CS, Chapman JR, Wong G, Craig JC, Schell JO, et al. Perspectives of older kidney transplant recipients on kidney transplantation. Clin J Am Soc Nephrol. 2017;12(3):443–53.
4. Schwarz ER, Baraghoush A, Morrissey RP, Shah AB, Shinde AM, Phan A, et al. Pilot study of palliative care consultation in patients with advanced heart failure referred for cardiac transplantation. J Palliat Med. 2012;15(1):12–5.
5. Rosenberger EM, Dew MA, DiMartini AF, DeVito Dabbs AJ, Yusen RD. Psychosocial issues facing lung transplant candidates, recipients and family caregivers. Thorac Surg Clin. 2012;22:517–29.
6. Wright L, Pape D, Ross K, Campbell M, Bowman K. Approaching end-of-life care in organ transplantation: the impact of transplant patients' death and dying. Prog Transplant. 2007;17(1):57–61.
7. Organization WH. WHO Definition of Palliative Care, updated 2018. Available from: http://www.who.int/cancer/palliative/definition/en/.
8. National Consensus Project for Quality Palliative Care: Clinical Practice Guidelines for quality palliative care, executive summary. J Palliat Med. 2004;7(5):611.
9. Force NPPT. National POLST Paradigm 2018 [Available from: http://polst.org/professionals-page/?pro=1.

10. Molmenti EP, Dunn GP. Transplantation and palliative care: the convergence of two seemingly opposite realities. Surg Clin N Am. 2005;85:373–82.

11. Edlin M. Imitation-worthy palliative care programs: five successful initiatives. Manag Healthc Exec. 2017;27(6):8–11.

12. Johnson C. LIVING WITH DIGNITY: a palliative approach to care at the end of life. ANMJ. 2017;25(6):30–3.

13. Wentlandt K, Dall'Osto A, Freeman N, Le LW, Kaya E, Ross H, et al. The transplant palliative care clinic: an early palliative care model for patients in a transplant program. Clin Transpl. 2016;30(12):1591–6.

14. Santivasi WL, Strand JJ, Mueller PS, Beckman TJ. The organ transplant imperative. Mayo Clin Proc. 2017;92(6):940–6.

15. Ouimet Perrin K, Kazanowski M. End-of-life care. Overcoming barriers to palliative care consultation. Crit Care Nurse. 2015;35(5):44–52.

16. Warraich HJ, Hernandez AF, Allen LA. The present and future: how medicine has changed the end of life for patients with cardiovascular disease. J Am Coll Cardiol. 2017;70:1276–89.

17. Kavalieratos D, Gelfman LP, Tycon LE, Riegel B, Bekelman DB, Ikejiani DZ, et al. Palliative Care in Heart Failure: rationale, evidence, and future priorities. J Am Coll Cardiol. 2017;70(15):1919–30.

18. http://optn.transplant.hrsa.gov. Organ Procurement and Transplantation Network. [This work was supported in part by Health Resources and Services Administration contract 234–2005-37011C. The content is the responsibility of the authors alone and does not necessarily reflect the views or policies of the Department of Health and Human Services, nor does mention of trade names, commercial products, or organizations imply endorsement by the U.S. Government.:[.

19. Bramstedt KA. Hoping for a miracle: supporting patients in transplantation and cardiac assist programs. Curr Opin Support Palliat Care. 2008;2(4):252–5.

20. Bayoumi E, Sheikh F, Groninger H. Palliative care in cardiac transplantation: an evolving model. Heart Fail Rev. 2017;22(5):605–10.

21. Sidebottom AC, Jorgenson A, Richards H, Kirven J, Sillah A. Inpatient palliative care for patients with acute heart failure: outcomes from a randomized trial. J Palliat Med. 2015;18(2):134–42.

22. Wordingham SE, McIlvennan CK, Fendler TJ, Behnken AL, Dunlay SM, Kirkpatrick JN, et al. Curbside rounds: state of the art in palliative care: palliative care clinicians caring for patients before and after continuous flow-left ventricular assist device. J Pain Symptom Manag. 2017;54:601–8.

23. Colman R, Singer LG, Barua R, Downar J. Characteristics, interventions, and outcomes of lung transplant recipients co-managed with palliative care. J Palliat Med. 2015;18(3):266–9.

24. McCurry KR, Budev MM. Lung transplant: candidates for referral and the waiting list. Cleve Clin J Med. 2017;84(12 Suppl 3):54–8.

25. Lanken PN, Terry PB, Delisser HM, Fahy BF, Hansen-Flaschen J, Heffner JE, et al. An official American Thoracic Society clinical policy statement: palliative care for patients with respiratory diseases and critical illnesses. Am J Respir Crit Care Med. 2008;177(8):912–27.

26. Song M-K, De Vito DA, Studer SM, Arnold RM. Palliative care referrals after lung transplantation in major transplant centers in the United States. Crit Care Med. 2009;37(4):1288–92.

27. Freeman N, Le LW, Singer LG, Colman R, Zimmermann C, Wentlandt K. Research correspondence: impact of a transplant palliative care clinic on symptoms for patients awaiting lung transplantation. J Heart Lung Transplant. 2016;35:1037–9.

28. Chapman E, Landy A, Lyon A, Haworth C, Bilton D. End of life care for adult cystic fibrosis patients: facilitating a good enough death. J Cyst Fibros. 2005;4:249–57.

29. Foundation CF. Annual data report. Bethesda: Cystic Fibrosis Foundation; 2016.

30. Chen E, Killeen KM, Peterson SJ, Saulitis AK, Balk RA. Evaluation of pain, Dyspnea, and goals of care among adults with cystic fibrosis: a comprehensive palliative care survey. Am J Hosp Palliat Care. 2017;34(4):347–52.

31. Conservative care of the patient with end-stage renal disease.pdf.

32. Alston H, Burns A. Conservative care of the patient with end-stage renal disease. Clin Med (Lond). 2015;15(6):567–70.

33. Wolfe RA, Ashby VB, Milford EL, Ojo AO, Ettenger RE, Agodoa LY, et al. Comparison of mortality in all patients on dialysis, patients on dialysis awaiting transplantation, and recipients of a first cadaveric transplant. N Engl J Med. 1999;341(23):1725–30.

34. Chen LX, Josephson MA, Hedeker D, Campbell KH, Stankus N, Saunders MR. A clinical prediction score to guide referral of elderly Dialysis patients for kidney transplant evaluation. Kidney Int Rep. 2017;2(4):645–53.

35. Davison SN. End-of-life care preferences and needs: perceptions of patients with chronic kidney disease. Clin J Am Soc Nephrol. 2010;5(2):195–204.

36. Berman N, Christianer K, Roberts J, Feldman R, Reid MC, Shengelia R, et al. Disparities in symptom burden and renal transplant eligibility: a pilot study. J Palliat Med. 2013;16(11):1459–65.

37. Afshar M, Rebollo-Mesa I, Murphy E, Murtagh FEM, Mamode N. Original article: symptom burden and associated factors in renal transplant patients in the U.K. J Pain Symptom Manag. 2012;44:229–38.

38. Cohen LM, Germain MJ, Poppel DM. Practical considerations in Dialysis withdrawal: "to have that option is a blessing". JAMA. 2003;289(16):2113.

39. Kelly SG, Campbell TC, Hillman L, Said A, Lucey MR, Agarwal PD. The utilization of palliative Care Services in Patients with cirrhosis who have been denied liver transplantation: a single Center retrospective review. Ann Hepatol. 2017;16(3):395–401.

40. Rossaro L, Troppmann C, McVicar JP, Sturges M, Fisher K, Meyers FJ. A strategy for the simultaneous provision of pre-operative palliative care for patients awaiting liver transplantation. Transpl Int. 2004;17(8):473.

41. Low J, Davis S, Vickerstaff V, Greenslade L, Hopkins K, Langford A, et al. Advanced chronic liver disease in the last year of life: a mixed methods study to understand how care in a specialist liver unit could be improved. BMJ Open. 2017;7(8):e016887.

42. Hansen L, Lyons KS, Dieckmann NF, Chang MF, Hiatt S, Solanki E, et al. Background and design of the symptom burden in end-stage liver disease patient-caregiver dyad study. Res Nurs Health. 2017;40(5):398–413.

43. Potosek J, Curry M, Buss M, Chittenden E. Integration of palliative care in end-stage liver disease and liver transplantation. J Palliat Med. 2014;17(11):1271–7.

44. Poonja Z, Brisebois A, van Zanten SV, Tandon P, Meeberg G, Karvellas CJ. Original article: patients with cirrhosis and denied liver transplants rarely receive adequate palliative care or appropriate management. Clin Gastroenterol Hepatol. 2014;12:692–8.

45. Rush B, Walley KR, Celi LA, Rajoriya N, Brahmania M. Palliative care access for hospitalized patients with end-stage liver disease across the United States. Hepatology. 2017;66(5):1585–91.

46. Baumann AJ, Wheeler DS, James M, Turner R, Siegel A, Navarro VJ. Brief quality improvement report: benefit of early palliative care intervention in end-stage liver disease patients awaiting liver transplantation. J Pain Symptom Manag. 2015;50:882-6.e2.

47. Gürkan A. Advances in small bowel transplantation. Turk J Sur. 2017;33(3):135.

48. Sudan DL, Kaufman SS, Shaw BW Jr, Fox IJ, McCashland TM, Schafer DF, et al. Isolated intestinal transplantation for intestinal failure. Am J Gastroenterol. 2000;95(6):1506–15.

49. Fishbein TM, Kaufman SS, Florman SS, Gondolesi GE, Schiano T, Kim-Schluger L, et al. Isolated intestinal transplantation: proof of clinical efficacy. Transplantation. 2003;76(4):636–40.

50. DeLegge M, Alsolaiman MM, Barbour E, Bassas S, Siddiqi MF, Moore NM. Short bowel syndrome: parenteral nutrition versus intestinal transplantation. Where are we today? Dig Dis Sci. 2007;52(4):876–92.

51. Grant D. Intestinal transplantation: 1997 report of the international registry. Transplantation. 1999;67(7):1061–4.

52. Winkler MF. Quality of life in adult home parenteral nutrition patients. JPEN. 2005;29(3):162.

53. Furukawa H, Manez R, Kusne S, Abu-Elmagd K, Green M, Reyes G, et al. Cytomegalovirus disease in intestinal transplantation. Transplant Proc. 1995;27(1):1357–8.

54. Sudan D. Cost and quality of life after intestinal transplantation. Gastroenterology. 2006;130(2 Suppl 1):S158–62.

55. Lauro A, Oltean M, Marino IR. Chronic rejection after intestinal transplant: where are we in order to avert it? Dig Dis Sci. 2018;63(3):551–62.

56. Harper SJF, Jamieson NV. Transplantation: intestinal and multivisceral transplantation. Surgery (Oxford). 2017;35:391–6.

57. Fryer J, Pellar S, Ormond D, Koffron A, Abecassis M. Mortality in candidates waiting for combined liver-intestine transplants exceeds that for other candidates waiting for liver transplants. Liver Transpl. 2003;9(7):748–53.

58. National Consensus Project for Quality Palliative Care. Clinical practice guidelines for quality palliative care, executive summary. J Palliat Med. 2004;7(5):611–27.

59. Bush NE, Donaldson GW, Haberman MH, Dacanay R, Sullivan KM. Conditional and unconditional estimation of multidimensional quality of life after hematopoietic stem cell transplantation: a longitudinal follow-up of 415 patients. Biol Blood Marrow Transplant. 2000;6(5A):576–91.

60. El-Jawahri A, LeBlanc T, VanDusen H, Traeger L, Greer JA, Pirl WF, et al. Effect of inpatient palliative care on quality of life 2 weeks after hematopoietic stem cell transplantation: a randomized clinical trial. JAMA. 2016;316(20):2094–103.

61. DeFor TE, Burns LJ, Gold E-MA, Weisdorf DJ. A randomized trial of the effect of a walking regimen on the functional status of 100 adult allogeneic donor hematopoietic cell transplant patients. Biol Blood Marrow Transplant. 2007;13(8):948–55.

62. Howell DA, Shellens R, Roman E, Garry AC, Patmore R, Howard MR. Haematological malignancy: are patients appropriately referred for specialist palliative and hospice care? A systematic review and meta-analysis of published data. Palliat Med. 2011;25(6):630–41.

63. Cheng W-W, Willey J, Palmer JL, Zhang T, Bruera E. Interval between palliative care referral and death among patients treated at a comprehensive cancer center. J Palliat Med. 2005;8(5):1025–32.

64. Fadul NA, El Osta B, Dalal S, Poulter VA, Bruera E. Comparison of symptom burden among patients referred to palliative care with hematologic malignancies versus those with solid tumors. J Palliat Med. 2008;11(3):422–7.

65. Temel JS, Greer JA, Muzikansky A, Gallagher ER, Admane S, Jackson VA, et al. Early palliative Care for Patients with metastatic non–small-cell lung Cancer. N Engl J Med. 2010;363(8):733–42.

Ethical Considerations in Transplant Patients

48

Nuriel Moghavem and David Magnus

Introduction

As of April 2018, there are nearly 120,000 Americans waiting for a transplant, without which they might die. The process of getting organs to those Americans involves the procurement of high-quality organs from donors, selection and listing of patients in need of organs, and allocation of organs to those who have been listed. This requires a speedy process: organ quality is maximized when the time an organ spends between a donor and a recipient is minimized. In the case of living organ donors, clinicians must weigh in the tangible risk to the donor versus the potential benefits to recipients. Therefore, behind the selection process, there is a complex set of ethical considerations, which must be seriously considered.

Organ transplantation remains one of the most challenging issues in bioethics because it touches on so many already difficult subjects: end-of-life care, rationing, euthanasia, surrogate decision-making, justice, financial conflicts of interest, and the definition of death itself.

To understand the current model of organ donation in the United States (US), one must wrestle with each of these ethical considerations and understand both the consensus view and its problems. Only then can a provider be sure that they are honoring organ donors, optimizing the recipients, and allocating the organs in a just way.

N. Moghavem
Department of Neurology and Neurological Sciences, Stanford University School of Medicine, Stanford, CA, USA

D. Magnus (✉)
Center of Biomedical Ethics, Stanford University School of Medicine, Stanford, CA, USA
e-mail: dmagnus@stanford.edu

Section 1: Procurement

Dead Donor Rule

Among the key philosophical tenets of transplant ethics is *the dead donor rule*. According to this rule, individuals must be declared dead before any vital organs are removed for transplantation. By this principle, it is permissible to donate a single kidney or a part of liver, for instance, because the removal of the organ does not cause death.

Some bioethicists and clinicians have suggested abandoning the dead donor rule, allowing patients in specific circumstances to die as a result of organ procurement [1]. Doing so would be a special case of active euthanasia, whereby a physician intentionally causes the death of a gravely ill patient with the patient's consent. This is in contrast to assisted dying, whereby a consenting patient with a grave illness causes their own death aided by a prescription by their physician. The active involvement of the physician to accelerate the dying process in euthanasia has proven to be an ethical hurdle in the United States, particularly for physicians. While countries such as the Netherlands, Canada, Belgium, and Colombia permit active euthanasia, in the United States, euthanasia is still considered a crime, and only certain states have permitted assisted dying. Indeed, euthanasia continues to lack public support in the United States, even as support for assisted dying has increased.

Though there are some bioethicists who disagree, a majority believe that the active process of withdrawing life-sustaining treatment is not considered morally equivalent to the active process of euthanasia. The dominant legal view is that once life-sustaining treatment – such as a ventilator – is discontinued, the patient continues on the trajectory they would have otherwise followed without it, which is often a natural death. At this point, patients may become donors.

Many argue that the dead donor rule is necessary to preserve public trust in the medical system and that allowing death by organ procurement may introduce incentives to

© Springer International Publishing AG, part of Springer Nature 2019
Y. Sher, J. R. Maldonado (eds.), *Psychosocial Care of End-Stage Organ Disease and Transplant Patients*,
https://doi.org/10.1007/978-3-319-94914-7_48

obtain viable organs from vulnerable patients [2]; critics point out that this already has illegally occurred in some instances, even with the dead donor rule in place. Critics of the dead donor rule predominantly rely on utilitarian arguments. They point out that abandoning the rule would increase the donor pool by allowing donation in cases where the patient does not meet death criteria but does not have prognosis for meaningful life [3–6]. In addition, they reject the deontological objection to euthanasia, arguing that the potential value of the organs and the wishes of the patient override the imperative not to actively cause the death of another person.

Those who argue for the abandonment of the dead donor rule also point to another tenet of end-of-life ethics: the doctrine of double effect. Many patients at the end of life experience tremendous pain, air hunger, or other discomfort. Patients may require increasing doses of pain medications, even if those doses are likely to hasten death. If medicines are given with the *intention* to treat symptoms, not the *intention* of causing death, death can be considered a side effect of a palliative treatment and, therefore, a foreseeable but unintended consequence of pain relief. Those who want to abandon the dead donor rule see the well-established doctrine of double effect as a fiction that makes euthanasia de facto permissible. Abandoning the dead donor rule is a logical next step [7] for these individuals.

Defining Death

The centrality of the dead donor rule to the availability of viable organs for transplant means it is important for clinicians and for society to clearly define death. New technologies for prolonging life complicate this discussion: historically, death was a unitary phenomenon. The advent of ventilators, ventricular assist devices, dialysis, feeding tubes, and other such technologies has allowed for the support of life despite the loss of a critical organ. In this way, a permanent loss of function can be masked.

In particular, life-sustaining treatments can mask irreversible loss of brain function as a result of stroke, trauma, or other devastating neurological injury. In 1968, an ad hoc committee at Harvard Medical School created a definition for brain death: a series of examination-based criteria that could determine whether patients were in an "irreversible" coma [8]. Despite having a heartbeat and pulmonary or some other bodily function supported by technology, these patients could be considered dead if they had no demonstrable brain activity. Brain death as a new criterion for death would allow the withdrawal of respiratory and other support in brain-dead patients and, in consenting families, or patients who have provided first person consent, would provide a source of high-quality organs for society.

However, the ad hoc committee identified an incongruence with contemporary US case law regarding the definition of death, which was then understood to mean the end of circulatory function. The incongruence was solved in 1981, when The President's Commission for the Study of Ethical Problems in Medicine and Biomedical and Behavioral Research published *Defining Death*, including a recommendation that "a statute is needed to provide a clear and socially-accepted basis for making determinations of death." [9]. This became the Uniform Determination of Death Act (UDDA), which was quickly adopted by all 50 states (45 by statute, 5 by case law).

The UDDA states, "An individual who has sustained either (1) irreversible cessation of circulatory and respiratory functions, or (2) irreversible cessation of all functions of the entire brain, including the brain stem, is dead. A determination of death must be made in accordance with accepted medical standards." Some states did include caveats, for instance, New Jersey allows religious objection to override determination of death. California allows a "reasonably brief period of accommodation" between brain death determination and withdrawal of life-sustaining treatment for family or next-of-kin to gather.

Each of the two definitions of death codified in the UDDA has faced criticisms and complexities of their own which will be discussed in-depth below.

Donation after Cardiac Death

In line with the definition of cardiac death in the UDDA, donation after cardiac death (DCD) refers to a procedure, whereby organs are surgically procured following pronouncement of death due to irreversible cessation of circulatory and respiratory functions.

The typical patient who becomes a DCD donor is one who is severely ill and on life-sustaining treatment, usually in the intensive care unit. In this setting, the removal of life-sustaining treatment, declaration of death, and initiation of organ procurement can happen quickly to preserve organ quality. Organs may not be transplantable in a donor who died at home overnight, for instance, because a prolonged lack of blood flow has led to extensive cell death within the organ.

Most DCD policies allow the family to be present until the patient's "final moments" and occasionally allow a clear wish to be communicated by the patient to be a donor. However, several elements of the DCD process should be highlighted, as they are ethically complex and potential areas for conflict. Here, those elements will be presented in the order they may arise in the DCD process.

Decision to Withdraw Life–Sustaining Treatment
Organs available for transplant are deeply valuable not only to potential recipients but also to the providers who take care

of those recipients and perform the difficult transplantation procedure. It is obviously wrong for a provider or hospital to coerce a family into withdrawing life-sustaining treatment in order to facilitate DCD. For that reason, it is incredibly important that no provider be seen as encouraging a patient or her family into withdrawing life-sustaining treatment explicitly because organ donation may be a benefit. While that benefit is clear, the possibility that such an encouragement could be seen as coercive is very real.

The decision to withdraw life-sustaining treatment must be made entirely independent of the decision to donate organs, unless the patient or their family first bring up the possibility of organ donation on their own. In cases when neither the patient nor their surrogate raises the possibility of DCD, providers must not breach the topic or initiate a discussion on the cessation of life-sustaining treatment for the purpose of facilitating the donation process.

Evaluation of Patient as Potential DCD Donor

Once a family has decided upon removing life-sustaining treatment, it is appropriate for providers to evaluate the patient as a potential DCD donor. Importantly, those caring for the potential donor may not be the same providers for a potential recipient, as this would introduce significant conflicts of interest regarding their duties to both subjects. Medical facilities typically have predefined medical criteria for donors, which usually require that donors are deemed likely to die within a reasonably short period after cessation of life-sustaining treatment. Ideally, an ethics consultation would be incorporated into the process at this time.

Organ Procurement Organization (OPO) Obtains Informed Consent

Once providers have deemed a patient to be an appropriate candidate medically and there are no conflicts of interest (e.g., concern that asking about donation could have a negative impact on care of the patient), an OPO gets involved. An OPO is a nonprofit organization that performs donor and recipient management and streamlines the surgical processes to ensure maximum efficiency while standards are followed. The rule is that the OPO, not the potential donor's provider, will approach the patient and their family and gauge their level of interest in organ donation. They are responsible for discussing the entire procurement process with surrogates, in particular, what efforts will be made before procurement to preserve and optimize organs. Ideally, they will also discuss what happens if the patient does not die as anticipated, within 1–2 h of the removal of life-sustaining treatment.

Life-Sustaining Treatment Is Withdrawn

Once the family has agreed to donate their loved one's organs and an appropriate recipient is located, the DCD donor is taken to the operating room. It is possible, at this point, to administer pharmacological agents to the donor, designed to aid in the viability and preservation of organs after they are procured. This is part of the potential ethical issue, as these medications are expected to provide benefits to the recipient but provide no meaningful benefit to the donor. Some ethicists criticize such a practice as it represents an invasive intervention on the still-living future donor. A provider's primary fiduciary duty is to care for their patient. If the patient is also a donor, there is the potential for a conflict between this duty and the ancillary duty to act in such a way as to maximize organ recovery.

It is not clearly unethical to provide non-beneficial treatment, particularly if there are extenuating circumstances, such as this one. From a utilitarian perspective, the administration of pre-recovery medications to improve procured organ quality, probably, has a net societal benefit. If a provider wishes to administer interventions of this kind, an informed consent must be obtained from the donor's family, detailing the potential benefits to the donated organs and any expected side effects, if any, to the donor.

Usually, the family of the donor says their final goodbyes and is asked to leave the operating room between the withdrawal of life-sustaining treatment and final declaration of death.

Determination of Death

On the surface, determination of circulatory death seems like it should be one of the simpler elements of the DCD process. In reality, it is one of the most contentious aspects of the process.

The UDDA defines circulatory death as the "irreversible cessation of circulatory and respiratory functions." The source of greatest debate surrounds how to define "irreversible." Does irreversible mean "impossible to reverse" or "unlikely to reverse" or when surrogates or providers have "chosen not to reverse"? Bernat has referred to the latter situation as "permanent cessation" of circulatory and respiratory functions, rather than "irreversible" loss [10]. Is the former sufficient to meet the legal and ethical requirements of the dead donor rule? Bernat has argued that it is a "perfect" surrogate for "irreversible cessation," but is this justified? How long does one wait to be sure that cessation is "permanent" or "irreversible"?

Human hearts have the capacity to spontaneously regain function after they have stopped beating for a few minutes, a process known as autoresuscitation or, more poetically, the Lazarus phenomenon [11]. While the literature on this process is scant, and its occurrence may be associated with cardiopulmonary resuscitation (CPR), which is not performed on organ donors, there are documented cases in adults of continuous electrocardiogram (EKG) registering a return of electrical heart activity up to 7 min after its initial cessation. There are also case reports of autoresuscitation in children, up to 25 min after loss of pulse, though these did not benefit from confirmatory EKG monitoring and were associated with CPR [12].

In practice, most transplant centers have adopted a safe "wait time" between the end of heart activity and the initiation of organ procurement to minimize any possibility of autoresuscitation, typically between 2 and 5 min (with the Institute of Medicine recommending 5 min). At that time, the likelihood of the heart regaining pulse is very low, and death is declared.

Two protocols in the last decade have caused controversy for pushing the limits on DCD. The first is a protocol pioneered at the University of Michigan which utilizes an extracorporeal membrane oxygenation (ECMO) machine to oxygenate, warm, and circulate blood through abdominal organs after declaration of circulatory death. Under this protocol, blood flow is blocked above the diaphragm by means of a balloon catheter, and tissue in the heart and brain continues to wither from ischemia, while organs like the kidneys and liver are continuously perfused. This protocol meets all standards of both brain and circulatory death while maintaining excellent tissue quality in abdominal organs bound for transplantation but raises two key ethical questions. The first is alluded to in the previous section regarding interventions performed on the donor prior to the withdrawal of life-sustaining treatment: the ECMO protocol requires the placement of arterial catheters in the donor prior to death, an invasive procedure, which provides no benefit to the patient. If the ECMO protocol is to be followed, family members will need to understand this aspect and consent to it in an informed manner. The second, which remains unresolved, is whether a protocol that restarts circulation and vital function of half the body constitutes a true irreversible cessation of circulatory function.

The second protocol was developed by pediatric heart transplant surgeons in Denver in 2008. Under their protocol, they transplanted one pediatric heart after 3 min of heart function cessation and two hearts after 75 s [13]. This protocol was controversial for two reasons. The first, mentioned briefly above, was whether a heart can ethically be transplanted after DCD; it stands to reason that a heart capable of functioning in a recipient may not fit a certain definition of "irreversible" cessation of function in the donor [14]. Supporters of this protocol would argue that a decision by the parents not to reverse any cessation of function is equivalent to irreversibility of function in the donor (autoresuscitation notwithstanding). Opponents would say that performing a heart transplant from a DCD patient is a suspension of the dead donor rule, since the donated heart has proven itself to have reversible loss of function, and therefore the donor was not dead. However, the focus of the rule is on the donor's irreversible loss of circulation, which could be compatible with circulation being restarted by the same heart in a different individual.

The second controversy is the 75-s waiting time utilized by the transplant team, well under the 2–5-min minimum recommendation from a number of different clinical and

ethical societies and institutes. The transplant team argued that autoresuscitation has never been definitively proven after 60 s in a child, so 75 s was a prudential wait time. Opponents argued that the data on autoresuscitation are thin that unverified case reports exist of longer times before resumption of heart function, and therefore, more extensive study is required to safely declare death before 2 min [15]. If the period of waiting was not long enough, the patient was not dead at the time of procurement.

The declaration of death of the donor in DCD, especially given technological advances, is indeed one of the most complicated points in the process from an ethical standpoint.

The Organ Procurement Process

At this point, the surgical team, typically an outside transplant team responsible for the recipient's care, will begin the procurement process. To ensure no conflict of interest, the surgical team performing procurement has no role in either the care of the donor before their death or in the declaration of death itself. In most cases, the surgical team is not allowed into the operating room at all until the declaration of death. In one controversial case, described in closer detail in our section on "Conflicting Ethical Obligations in the Care of an Organ Donor," a transplant surgeon was accused of administering medications to a donor who was taking longer than expected to pass away in order to hasten his death [16].

Donation after Brain Death

As previously discussed, the dead donor rule stipulates that a donor must be dead before their organs can be harvested and that death can be declared by one of two avenues under the UDDA: cardiac death and brain death. Brain death is defined as the "irreversible cessation of all functions of the entire brain, including the brain stem."

Candidates for donation after brain death (DBD) have usually experienced a devastating neurological injury such as a ruptured aneurysm, suffocation, or trauma from a motor vehicle accident or a gunshot wound. Organs procured from brain-dead patients are often of higher quality than those coming from DCD patients. Because donors who have suffered brain death usually still have a heartbeat and are often under continuous ventilation in the hospital, their organs have not experienced anoxic injury. Moreover, since death is determined without any wait time, those organs can remain perfused until the very moment they leave the donor's body.

Brain death can often be difficult to understand, both for providers and for families. The patients appear warm, relaxed, and their hearts beat independently – for many, these are signs of life. For this reason, many of the controversies in DBD deal with the very definition of brain death, rather than the process of obtaining organs (as in DCD).

Defining Brain Death

The definition of death in the UDDA, as discussed previously, stemmed from the findings of the Harvard ad hoc committee on irreversible coma.

Today, brain death is determined through the brain death examination, which has a well-accepted protocol established by the American Academy of Neurology [17]. A simplified description of the steps is as follows:

1. Diagnose coma by showing that the patient is nonverbal and has no eye or motor response to noxious stimuli.
2. Establish a known irreversible cause for coma.
3. Correct conditions, which may adversely influence the brain death evaluation, such as hypothermia, hypotension, and metabolic derangements. Stop all medications that may similarly affect the brain death examination such as sedatives, paralytics, and anticonvulsants.
4. Demonstrate absence of brain stem reflexes, such as pupillary, oculocephalic, oculovestibular, corneal, and gag reflexes, as well as primitive reflexes, such as rooting or sucking.
5. Perform apnea testing by oxygenating the patient to 100% and then turning off the ventilator: If no respirations are seen and the blood concentration of CO_2 increases, patient is brain dead.
6. If no respirations are observed, but the patient is unable to do an apnea test or arterial CO_2 does not drop, perform an electroencephalogram (EEG) or radionuclide cerebral blood flow test.

Chief Criticisms of Brain Death Determination Method

The primary criticism of brain death is that it is a socially constructed legal fiction, much like legal blindness, for the permissibility of organ transplantation under the dead donor rule [18, 19]. Just as we legally define blindness as 20/200 or worse, rather than total absence of sight, so too brain death is a fiction.

Early elucidation of the concept of brain death focused on the brain's centrality in integrating functions required for life: in the absence of brain activity, that integration falls apart, which is incompatible with life. The position espoused in the original 1981 account of brain death argued that death is a unitary phenomenon with two criteria. Both loss of circulatory and respiratory functions and loss of brain function lead to the loss of the organism as a unified whole. However, critics point out that patients who have been determined to be dead by neurologic criteria continue to show a range of continued complex, integrated biological functions: they can regulate body temperature, secrete hormones, heal cuts, children can grow, and gestating mothers can continue to carry their pregnancies. These critics argue that it is false to claim that these bodies cease to function as integrated wholes.

Furthermore, because temperature and hormonal function often continue undisturbed, there is evidence that the hypothalamus, a deep brain structure, retains some activity. If this is the case, can it be said that there is "cessation of all functions of the entire brain," as the UDDA stipulates? In practice, the AAN requirements evaluate the loss of the function of the brain stem and the cerebral cortex. Hypothalamic functioning is not evaluated (and would be practically impossible to do in a reliable and time effective way).

In response to these observations, the President's Council on Bioethics issued a report in 2008, which reframed the discussion: it is not the integrative function of the brain, which is important, but whether the individual is "no longer able to carry out the fundamental work of a living organism. Such a patient has lost – and lost irreversibly – a fundamental openness to the surrounding environment as well as the capacity and drive to act on this environment on his or her own behalf" [20].

That council report has also been criticized by those who point out that the definition put forward by the President's Council is perhaps too broad and would include those in vegetative states, for instance.

Therefore, there is great disagreement on whether there is a biological basis for the idea of brain death. What almost all bioethicists agree on, however, is that the patient who is brain dead has ceased to exist as the person they once were. What even more agree on is the idea that brain death serves an overall social good, in that it permits transplantation of high-quality organs [10, 21, 22].

In that vein, the dominant ethical opinion at this time is that there is insufficient evidence or public interest in changing the definition of brain death. While there are disagreements about its philosophical underpinnings, there is no clear reason to change the legal definition of brain death, be it a "legal fiction" or not. A less realist approach argues that the perspective of both the defenders and critics of brain death err in believing that "death" names a natural kind [23]. An alternative to this perspective is to recognize (as Ron Green has argued regarding the beginning of life) that biological occurrences are processes rather than events [24].

Thus, the decisions need to be made to determine moral and legal status (i.e., when is someone a person with both ethical and constitutional rights) as well as to clarify the metaphysical issue (i.e., when did your existence start and when does it end). Just as there is no biological event that one can point to that clearly determines when personhood starts, there is no point where we are required to say that the person's life has ended. Dying is a process. As some organ system fails, others will follow. At some point, every cell will die and rigor mortis will set in.

The legal line between life and death needs to be drawn at some point, and the line as currently drawn is well supported. There are good practical grounds for drawing the line where it is currently. The clinical criteria are clear, relatively easy to follow, and can be applied in a timely way. Moreover, to date, when applied correctly, there have been no false positives (no brain-dead patients have recovered). These individuals have irreversibly lost all that made them who they were.

In contrast, while one could argue that permanently vegetative patients have suffered similar loss of identity, a permanent vegetative state is harder to diagnose accurately, cannot be diagnosed in a timely fashion (e.g., for traumatic brain injury it takes a year to definitely state that the condition is permanent), and will not be a practical way of distinguishing life and death.

In short, we should continue with the criteria that practically seem to work. This does not mean brain death is a "fiction" in any way that matters; only that it is conventionally defined. Our current nosology is clearly conventional rather than real; in parallel, we at times define diseases by sets of signs and symptoms, at other times by their physical causes, and often based in historical notions. Nevertheless, a patient still has the flu. And brain death is still death [23].

Conflicting Ethical Obligations in the Care of an Organ Donor

Care must be taken in organ donation to manage often conflicting or competing ethical obligations. From the standpoint of the physician, the challenge is balancing the absolute responsibility to one's patient while pulled by the opportunity to save the life of another through organ donation.

Physicians do not have an obligation to extend the life of a patient indefinitely. They may recommend the cessation of life-sustaining treatment if it is assessed to be futile or perhaps against a patient's wishes, but that recommendation and those assessments can be colored by the opportunity for organ donation. Several steps are taken to mitigate these competing obligations, including the inclusion of an OPO as a third-party entity that discusses donation with donors, selects recipients, and organizes the transplantation process. In addition, donation is never discussed until after the decision is made to withdraw life-sustaining treatment, or a patient is declare dead; in this way, a physician will never feel compelled to recommend withdrawal of care, since the family's perspective on donation will not be known.

There are also conflicting obligations created by the procurement process itself and the inclusion of multiple care teams. The case of Ruben Navarro, a developmentally disabled 25-year-old, and transplant surgeon Dr. Hootan C. Roozrokh in 2008 illustrates these competing obligations [25]. Mr. Navarro's family had agreed to donate his organs after cardiac death, and life-sustaining treatments were ceased. The hospital essentially treated this case the way they would have treated a brain-dead patient. They withdrew life support and sent the patient to the OR for procurement. However, the patient was still alive. The hospital seems to have stopped managing the patient, just as they would for a brain-dead patient, and thus they turned over care to the surgeons who were brought in to do the procurement. However, since Mr. Navarro did not pass away quickly, and the hospital was not managing the patient, Dr. Roozrokh, the procuring surgeon (who should have no role in interacting with the patient until after the patient had expired), stepped in and began managing the still living patient. In the end, he did not die quickly enough for procurement to move forward, and the patient was sent back to the floor where he passed away many hours later. Dr. Roozrokh should clearly never have been involved in caring for the patient while he was alive. He was accused though ultimately found not guilty of administering intravenous medications (including Betadine, an antiseptic) to hasten Mr. Navarro's death [26]. But it is understandable how confusing DCD can be for both the treatment teams and the procurement teams, since their roles are so radically different for DCD versus brain death procurements (which are much more common).

Opt–In Versus Presumed Consent Donation Models

One of the most publicly debated elements of transplant ethics, especially with regard to procurement, is the opt-in vs. presumed consent models of identifying a potential organ donor. In an opt-in system, much like the United States has today, an individual has affirmatively stated during life that they would like to be an organ donor in order to become one. In a presumed consent model, such as in Spain, an individual is automatically considered a donor, unless during life, they stated that they would not want to be one.

Advocates for an opt-in system argue that it preserves individual decision-making and protects marginalized communities, which may not have access to opt-out mechanisms in a presumed consent model. In addition, even in an opt-in system, families of the deceased have substantial decision-making ability over donation, including, in some states, the ability to reverse the organ donation decision of their deceased family member. Moreover, there is still much opportunity to raise the rate of organ donation through improved education and community engagement.

Opponents of an opt-in system, who advocate for a presumed consent model, argue that it affords a sure mechanism to raise the organ donation rate, which provides massive benefits to the public. They also argue that a presumed consent model accurately reflects positive public sentiment for organ donation and would, therefore, allow donation from an individual who may have wanted to become a donor but never expressly articulated the sentiment to friends or family.

In a controversial case in Ohio, in July 2013, the parents of Elijah Smith objected to having his organs procured, though he has provided a first-person authorization through the DMV. The organ procurement organization prevailed in litigation, but this has led some to question the validity of the consent process involved in first-person authorization [27]. The full range of risks and complications are not typically disclosed, and some have argued that the information provided by UNOS is actually misleading [28, 29].

There is some evidence that communities using presumed consent have, on average, higher rates of organ donation than those which use an opt-in, explicit consent model [30, 31]. However, it is not known if that is simply a reflection of existing pro-donation attitudes and conditions locally which predispose to both donation and the development of opt-out policies. In other words, it is not clear that changing from an opt-in system to one of presumed consent causes a significant change in the donation rate.

Section 2: Listing

While many of the controversies in organ transplantation occur at the level of the donor and the procurement of their organ, there are additional complexities at the recipient level. The overall shortage of every transplantable organ necessitates waiting lists, and the question of who is eligible for a place on a waiting list (or who may circumvent such a list) becomes a difficult one. The question of how such lists are organized will be discussed in the third section of this chapter on organ allocation.

In general, either recipients get their organs from a known individual (i.e., directed donation) or they get their organ from a stranger (i.e., altruistic donation). Directed donation circumvents the transplant list, while those receiving a deceased donor organ or an altruistic living donor must wait until one becomes available. We will first discuss directed donation, including its many manifestations and opportunities for abuse, before discussing listing controversies.

Directed Donation: Opportunities for Abuse

In directed donation, an individual who needs an organ can identify a relative, a friend, or a known community member willing to donate their organ; that organ is then procured in short order from the willing donor and transplanted into the recipient. The key requirements in directed donation, beyond normal medical and evolving psychosocial criteria, are that (a) the recipient is able to identify a donor, (b) the donor freely agrees to donation to the recipient, and (c) there are no medical or psychosocial contraindications to proceed with transplantation.

The ability to name a recipient has become very easy with the advent of the Internet, which has ushered in an age of previously unknown social connectivity. Organizations like the now-defunct LifeSharers connected donors and recipients online; while they were frankly unknown to each other on a personal level, donor and recipient did know each other's names, and were therefore able to circumvent a waiting list and perform a directed donation.

There have also been rare cases of racially driven attempts at directed donation. In 1990, Thomas Simons of Tampa, Florida, a Klu Klux Klan sympathizer, was shot and killed by a black teenager. His family chose to make his organs available for transplant, but only to white recipients, and the OPO complied with those wishes [32]. In 1999, a British citizen made the same request in England, and the National Health Service complied with the request [33]. Notably, in neither of these cases was the donor able to name a recipient – they simply stipulated what race they must be.

Somewhat related are several faith-based virtual networks that connect organ donors and recipients of the same religion for the purposes of facilitating directed donation. One such organization is the Brooklyn-based Renewal, which connects Jews for the purpose of providing names and connections to allow for directed donation [34].

In these cases, a long waiting list is circumvented when a compatriot of some form, whether it be someone truly known to a recipient or merely someone of the same religious or racial background, is willing to narrow the potential field of recipients. While a brother donating an organ to his sister raises no red flags, the Klu Klux Klan case is clearly more problematic. In the case of renewal, it is likely that their activities identify donors who may not otherwise have considered donating a kidney at all and, therefore, lead to an overall increase in the available organ pool. However, where should the line be drawn? This is an area of active debate, but, for now, the only limitation on an otherwise acceptable live donor remains that a donor be able to name their recipient.

Solicitation

Closely related to the establishment of virtual networks for connecting donors and recipients is the issue of recipients actively searching for donors. Should individuals in need of an organ and wanting to circumvent the waiting list be able to advertise to the public in search of a directed donor? Should celebrities?

There are several examples of this occurring, perhaps the most famous of which is of Todd Krampitz of Houston, TX. Mr. Krampitz was fairly low on the organ transplant list. However, after his family leased two billboards on busy

Houston roads advertising his need for a liver, an anonymous donor emerged after just a week. Mr. Krampitz received his new liver and died 8 months later [35]. The actual cause of death is not known.

The highest-profile case of organ donation solicitation by a celebrity comes from Ottawa, Canada, where the billionaire hockey team owner of the Ottawa Senators, Eugene Melnyk, issued a public call for an organ donor at a press conference after going into liver failure. An anonymous fan donated his organ, stating that all he wanted was "to help Mr. Melnyk return to good health, to enjoy his family and friends, and most importantly to bring the Stanley Cup home to the Ottawa Senators." The transplant appears to have been successful [36].

While it is easy to understand why a patient who will die without transplant might make a public plea for an organ donor, several ethical issues are raised by the practice. While free speech laws in the United States mean that such advertisements cannot be banned, more widespread use of organ transplant solicitation could give wealthier or more famous patients an advantage in obtaining organs. This would lead to a bias in distribution of organs and an inequality of access to organs.

In addition, the transplant list is thought to be fair, optimizing recipients for the urgency of their need and their ability to do well with a new organ and making the best use of the scare resource. Circumventing the list allows for patients like Mr. Krampitz, who was likely known to have a poor expected outcome after transplant, to get a liver which may have otherwise gone to a recipient that would have lived longer with it.

Organ Donation Markets

The existence of an organ transplant list is a function of the deficit of available organs. One policy proposal that would likely eliminate a waiting list for kidneys is an organ donation market. Many have argued that financially compensating live donors would be a powerful inducement to transplant and would greatly boost the number of available organs. It would be an efficient and market-based solution to the dire need for more kidneys, though it would have some serious ethical hazards.

Only one country currently has a market for kidneys: Iran. There, an Iranian may be paid to donate a kidney to another Iranian (transplant tourism is forbidden), and typical rates run between $2000 and $4000 [30, 37]. Iran was able to eliminate its kidney waiting list within 10 years with this model, though it is important to note that, unlike the United States, healthcare is government-run in Iran.

There are some concerns about establishing an organ transplant market in the United States, most having to do with the concept of justice and equity. The current model of

organ donation does not allow financial compensation, and the financial standing of the potential recipient is not directly considered (though it may be an indirect factor, given a largely income-based insurance model, which may discriminate against the very poor, and the opportunity for listing in multiple states that advantages the very wealthy, both discussed in greater detail later).

An organ donation market would greatly benefit those able to purchase a new kidney and would likely then harm those unable to afford it, creating a significant imbalance in the system and funneling available organs to those who can "buy" them while depleting available organs to the general list. Moreover, there are ethical concerns regarding the social justice effects of such policy change, creating a significant drive on impoverished Americans now having an incentive to donate organs in order to pay off debts or make some money for short-term purposes, without much concern about the long-term health effects of such decision. For example, in Iran, 58% of donors reported negative health outcomes after donation and 65% reported problems finding employment after donation [38]. In India, where a robust black market for kidneys exists, 96% agree to donate to pay off debts, but 79% later say they would not recommend that someone else do the same, perhaps indicating a high level of regret. Most Indians surveyed also had worse economic status after donation than prior to it [39, 40].

Listing at Multiple OPOs

In addition to controversies over directed donation, in which individuals seek to circumvent the waiting list in order to get an organ sooner, several ethical issues exist for those who remain waiting on an organ transplant list.

Perhaps the most well-known is the practice of a potential recipient listing at multiple transplant centers. While listing at multiple transplant centers in the same region would confer no advantage, listing at transplant centers across the country could offer a significant advantage, especially in areas with shorter wait lists. This practice clearly offers an advantage to those with significant financial means, as there are significant economic implications on the need to travel and stay at each of the transplant centers where a given recipient wants to be listed at. In addition, there is the issue that one must be able to rapidly travel to the other state when an organ becomes available, which requires either access to a private plane or the funds to acquire a last minute, rather expensive plane ticket.

Perhaps the most well-known case of multiple listing relates to former Apple CEO and Founder Steve Jobs, who chose to list in his home state of California (6-year average wait for a liver) and in Tennessee (3-month average wait). He was able to take a jet from Northern California to Tennessee when a liver became available and was successfully transplanted [41].

While multiple listing is relatively rare (e.g., around 5% of potential recipients are listed at multiple transplant centers), it raises the question of whether it gives those with financial means an unfair advantage. A more impoverished resident of California would not have the means to get to Tennessee in time for an organ and would, therefore have to stay on a 6-year waiting list, where they may not survive.

Listing of Cognitively Impaired Patients

The current transplant system seeks to enhance equity, by giving all people an equal shot at getting an organ, and efficiency, by optimizing the number of years that can be expected to be gained by transplant in the right person. However, the current system does not consider the post-transplant quality of life or productivity of a recipient or whether they can be expected to appreciate those additional years.

Among adults with cognitive impairment, the chief concern with transplantation involves their ability to adhere to the complex, post-transplant regimen (e.g., immunosuppressant agents, diet, lifestyle adjustments): can adults who are developmentally delayed or suffer from other cognitive impairments (e.g., dementia, anoxic brain injury, traumatic brain injury) be relied upon to take their immunosuppressive medications and appear at follow-up visits with their physicians? Among adults, existing data suggests outcomes for kidney transplantation are comparable to outcomes for non-delayed patients, but less is known for other organs [42].

There is more data with regard to children, and the debate is more pronounced. There have been several cases of cognitively impaired individuals, mostly children, being denied organs. With good social support and involved parents, adherence is less of an issue with children, and the data show equivalent survival outcomes compared to cognitively intact children [43–46]. The chief ethical question with younger transplant recipients is whether there is value in giving a life-extending therapy. Such a question is difficult to answer, as it seems like a judgment about the value of the life of the recipient. However, some recipients may have such severe cognitive deficits that they cannot be reasonably expected to appreciate the extension of life, although some argue the extension of their lives may positively influence the well-being of their parents and siblings. There is great heterogeneity in whether transplant centers use developmental delay as a contraindication to transplant [47]. This raises two distinct ethical issues. First, if similar patients will be listed at some programs and not others, there is significant concern about justice. In addition, the discrepancy between outcomes and listing practice (especially for mild to moderately cognitively impaired patients) makes it difficult to come to any

conclusions at this time, except acknowledgment that there is prejudice and bias in listing decisions in some programs.

Adherence Determinations, Financial Standing, and the Psychosocial Evaluation

In determining whether someone is an acceptable candidate for transplantation, several subjective decisions are made about their candidacy, in addition to more objective measures of their current health status and expected prognosis. Those subjective decisions are largely grouped into two categories: financial standing and psychosocial evaluations, which include adherence determinations.

Adherence determinations, mentioned previously with relation to cognitively impaired patients, attempt to determine whether a transplant recipient is likely to take good care of their new organ. Based on a patient's history, the listing team determines their confidence level that the recipient will take immunosuppressive medications, abstain from alcohol or other drugs, adhere to lifestyle changes, and regularly return for follow-up appointments and laboratory testing.

Ultimately, organs are a precious, limited resource, and this element of the listing process is meant to ensure that recipients will treasure that resource; it is important to maximize how far a scarce organ may help a patient, and an adherent patient may gain more years of utility out of a donated organ than a nonadherent one. In addition, nonadherence will likely translate in a significant larger cost to society in the management of complications and rejection reactions, not counting on the potential benefits never materialized have the transplant been given to a patient who took good care of the organ.

Financial standing, which includes the patient's insurance status, may indicate one's ability to care for the organ they have been given. In the United States, Medicare only pays for 1 year of immunosuppressive therapy. Medicaid policy varies by state but sometimes does not provide long-term coverage for immunosuppressive medications. In these cases, if a patient cannot be expected to pay for immunosuppressive medications a year or two after transplant, they would be likely to go into organ rejection.

In addition, as a part of psychosocial evaluations, the presence and functionality of support network are determined, with the understanding that more support will make transplant more successful. There is data suggesting that the absence of a reliable support system is the single most powerful psychosocial predictor of transplant success [48, 49] and conversely, the lack of social support being a reliable predictor of treatment nonadherence [49–56].

Transplantation is a long, difficult process involving a major surgical procedure, months of recovery, and years of follow-up needed to ensure success. It is nearly impossible to fully recover from transplantation, if socially isolated and without a dedicated psychosocial support system. In addition, some degree of financial resources are also needed to maintain health insurance, afford immunosuppressive medications, and get to appointments on time.

However, as these elements of the listing decision may be subjective in nature and their weight varies among various transplant centers, they may be prone to many human biases – many of them against the poor, immigrants, and other historically marginalized communities. There is sometimes insufficient empirical data to support the adherence determinations or psychosocial evaluations, and there are arguments that transplant recipients should also receive social services to enhance their ability to do well after transplantation. Debates about the appropriateness of many characteristics used as criteria by some programs are ongoing and include alcohol use, marijuana use, psychiatric illness, criminal history, and immigration status. Efforts to create a more objective approach to the evaluation of these factors offer the potential to reduce discriminatory or biased practices [49].

Transplant Tourism

Due to the increased demand for organs in the United States, the practice of transplant tourism (e.g., traveling to another country with the intent of acquiring a paid transplant there) has risen despite some key ethical and medical concerns [57]. Other nations have far more lax standards for both organ procurement (including the ability to buy an organ) and surgical excellence.

China has become a consistent destination for transplant tourists, with a larger supply of available organs including those from executed criminals. While this practice raises concerns from a medical standpoint (e.g., criminals are at higher risk of carrying communicable diseases such as hepatitis or HIV), there are also obvious moral issues with procuring organs from an incarcerated population. In other countries, like Pakistan, a black market for organs raises issues discussed previously in the section on organ markets, including predation on the impoverished local population.

However, what of patients who travel abroad to have their transplants in order to bypass our lengthy transplant list but return to the United States for their continuing care? Is a physician complicit in unethical organ transplant tourism by providing care for these patients? If a patient, once at home, goes into organ rejection and needs another organ immediately, should they be able to jump to the top of the US list? These questions are difficult to answer, and different transplant centers have developed different approaches to these patients [58–61]. Of note, the Organ Procurement and Transplantation Network (OPTN)/United Network for Organ Sharing (UNOS) Board of Directors, at its annual 2006 meeting, approved a resolution affirming, "the OPTN and UNOS are strongly opposed to practices in which patients in need of transplantation travel abroad to purchase an organ in exploitive situations" [62].

Section 3: Allocation

Beyond the complexity of who belongs on the organ transplant list and how the list itself can be circumvented is the method of distributing organs to the patients who wait, often for years, on the transplant list. The existing method seeks to balance several different ethical principles, while remaining appropriate for the local environment, all in an effort to optimize equity and efficiency.

Justice

Ultimately, the desire to allocate organs equitably has its roots in the concept of justice; however, different philosophical schools of thought have difference in their conceptions of justice.

A more utilitarian perspective would seek to maximize the utility across society that might be provided by a single organ: such a perspective would dictate that the patient who would obtain the most benefit from a given organ should be given the organ. Such a patient would be younger, given an excellent prognosis with transplant, and – in the purest utilitarian approach – expect to contribute maximally to society.

A Rawlsian perspective seeks to promote fairness and equality of opportunity among those on a transplant list in allocation decisions. One conception of fairness might be to prioritize the sickest members on the list and prioritize them for transplant, even if they may have lower odds of success than someone more stable. In addition to medical urgency, important factors would also include likelihood of finding another organ in the future, waiting list time, and first transplant versus repeat transplant status.

These two schools of thought, in addition to an understanding of respect for persons, are harmonized to make up the backbone of the Organ Procurement and Transplantation Network's Ethical Principles in the Allocation of Human Organs [63, 64].

Geography

While ensuring justice is a key tenet of organ allocation decisions, allocation decisions often involve difficult and sometimes controversial tradeoffs. Patients living in a metropolis, a smaller city, or in a rural environment might all be subject to different impact depending on the role that geography plays in listing decisions.

Urban settings often have far more recipients waiting for organs than donors available for donation. Consider the case of San Francisco, which is populous – and thus, has many waiting recipients – but has relatively few events of brain death compared to New Orleans, given its lower rates of stroke and trauma (defined as motor vehicle accident, assault, gunshot, and head trauma) [65]. In California, only 30% of patients get a liver within a year of being on the transplant list; in Louisiana, over 50% do [63, 64]. In addition, the highest acuity patients awaiting transplant are often in urban settings at higher-resource medical centers, making the illness of urban patients overall more severe as well. This inequality could be mitigated by broader sharing of organs across larger geographic areas.

However, for some organs, the amount of time between organ procurement and transplantation is incredibly critical; in more rural environments, then, proximity to the transplant center can be an important factor in determining which member of the transplant list is best suited for an available organ or even has access at all. If organs were shared across larger geographic areas, it would almost certainly result in the loss of smaller transplant programs in more rural areas.

Ethical arguments about whether the current role that geography plays in allocation continue.

Conclusions

The process of obtaining organs from willing donors and developing a method of allocating them to recipients fairly is ethically complex and touches on some of our society's most controversial debates. Ethical debates continue over issues related to the procurement of organs, selection and listing of candidates, and finally allocation. As tens of thousands of critically ill patients wait for organs, the scarcity will continue to create challenges for our conceptions of justice.

References

1. Miller FG. Heart donation without the dead donor rule. Ann Thorac Surg. 2014;97(4):1133–4.
2. Bernat JL. Life or death for the dead-donor rule? N Engl J Med. 2013;369(14):1289–91.
3. Sade RM. Consequences of the dead donor rule. Ann Thorac Surg. 2014;97(4):1131–2.
4. Sade RM, Boan A. The paradox of the dead donor rule: increasing death on the waiting list. Am J Bioeth. 2014;14(8):21–3.
5. Truog R. The price of our illusions and myths about the dead donor rule. J Med Ethics. 2016;42(5):318–9.
6. Truog RD, Miller FG. The dead donor rule and organ transplantation. N Engl J Med. 2008;359(7):674–5.
7. Veatch RM. Killing by organ procurement: brain-based death and legal fictions. J Med Philos. 2015;40(3):289–311.
8. A definition of irreversible coma. Report of the Ad Hoc Committee of the Harvard Medical School to examine the definition of brain death. JAMA. 1968;205(6):337–40.
9. President's Commission for the Study of Ethical Problems in Medicine and Biomedical and Behavioral Research. Defining Death: A Report on the Medical, Legal and Ethical Issues in the Determination of Death. Washington, DC, 1981.
10. Bernat JL. Whither brain death? Am J Bioeth. 2014;14(8):3–8.
11. Sahni V. The Lazarus phenomenon. JRSM Open. 2016;7(8):2054270416653523.
12. Hornby K, Hornby L, Shemie SD. A systematic review of autoresuscitation after cardiac arrest. Crit Care Med. 2010;38(5):1246–53.
13. Boucek MM, Mashburn C, Dunn SM, Frizell R, Edwards L, Pietra B, et al. Pediatric heart transplantation after declaration of cardiocirculatory death. N Engl J Med. 2008;359(7):709–14.
14. Veatch RM. Donating hearts after cardiac death--reversing the irreversible. N Engl J Med. 2008;359(7):672–3.
15. Bernat JL. The boundaries of organ donation after circulatory death. N Engl J Med. 2008;359(7):669–71.
16. Sanford J. When are you dead? Resurgent form of organ transplantation raises a new question. Stanford Medicine. 2011:29–33.
17. Wijdicks EF, Varelas PN, Gronseth GS, Greer DM. American Academy of N. Evidence-based guideline update: determining brain death in adults: report of the quality standards Subcommittee of the American Academy of neurology. Neurology. 2010;74(23):1911–8.
18. Nair-Collins M. Death, brain death, and the limits of science: why the whole-brain concept of death is a flawed public policy. J Law Med Ethics. 2010;38(3):667–83.
19. Truog RD, Miller FG. Changing the conversation about brain death. Am J Bioeth. 2014;14(8):9–14.
20. The President's Council on Bioethics. Controversies in the determination of death. Washington, DC, 2008.
21. Bernat JL. The whole-brain concept of death remains optimum public policy. J Law Med Ethics. 2006;34(1):35–43. 3
22. Robertson J. Should we scrap the dead donor rule? Am J Bioeth. 2014;14(8):52–3.
23. Magnus DC, Wilfond BS, Caplan AL. Accepting brain death. N Engl J Med. 2014;370(10):891–4.
24. Green RM. Stem cell research: a target article collection: part III--determining moral status. Am J Bioeth. 2002;2(1):20–30.
25. McKinley J. Transplant surgeon charged in patient's death. The New York Times, 2008 .
26. McKinley J. Doctor cleared of harming man to obtain organs. The New York Times, 2008.
27. McCleskey C. Legal Battle In Ohio Over Organ Donation Highlights Controversy Over Defining Death: Global Bioethics Initiative; 2013, updated July 23, 2013. Available from: http://globalbioethics.org/gbi_old/news-articles-and-public-addresses/news/legal-battle-in-ohio-over-organ-donation-highlights-controversy-over-defining-death/
28. Nair-Collins M. Brain death, paternalism, and the language of "death". Kennedy Inst Ethics J. 2013;23(1):53–104.
29. Iltis AS. Organ donation, brain death and the family: valid informed consent. J Law Med Ethics. 2015;43(2):369–82.
30. Abadie A, Gay S. The impact of presumed consent legislation on cadaveric organ donation: a cross-country study. J Health Econ. 2006;25(4):599–620.
31. Rithalia A, McDaid C, Suekarran S, Myers L, Sowden A. Impact of presumed consent for organ donation on donation rates: a systematic review. BMJ. 2009;338:a3162.
32. Kleindienst L. Lawmakers try to end bias by organ donors. Orlando Sentinel, 1994.
33. Boseley S, Brindle D, Dodd V. NHS took organs donated for whites only. The Guardian, 1999.
34. Renewal. What We Do 2017, updated 2008. Available from: www.life-renewal.org/whatwedo

35. Hopper L. Man who advertised on billboards for liver dies. Houston Chronicle, 2005.
36. Hune-Brown N. Are we entering the age of crowdsourced organ donations? The Guardian, 2015.
37. The Economist. Psst, wanna buy a kidney? The Economist, 2006.
38. Ghods AJ, Savaj S. Iranian model of paid and regulated living-unrelated kidney donation. Clin J Am Soc Nephrol. 2006;1(6):1136–45.
39. Shimazono Y. The state of the international organ trade: a provisional picture based on integration of available information. Bull World Health Organ. 2007;85(12):955–62.
40. Goyal M, Mehta RL, Schneiderman LJ, Sehgal AR. Economic and health consequences of selling a kidney in India. JAMA. 2002;288(13):1589–93.
41. Isaacson W. Steve Jobs. New York: Simon & Schuster; 2011. xxi, 630 p., 8 leaves of plates p.
42. Halpern SD, Goldberg D. Allocating organs to cognitively impaired patients. N Engl J Med. 2017;376(4):299–301.
43. Wightman A, Bartlett HL, Zhao Q, Smith JM. Prevalence and outcomes of heart transplantation in children with intellectual disability. Pediatr Transplant. 2017;21(2)
44. Wightman A, Hsu E, Zhao Q, Smith J. Prevalence and outcomes of liver transplantation in children with intellectual disability. J Pediatr Gastroenterol Nutr. 2016;62(6):808–12.
45. Wightman A, Young B, Bradford M, Dick A, Healey P, McDonald R, et al. Prevalence and outcomes of renal transplantation in children with intellectual disability. Pediatr Transplant. 2014;18(7): 714–9.
46. Martens MA, Jones L, Reiss S. Organ transplantation, organ donation and mental retardation. Pediatr Transplant. 2006;10(6): 658–64.
47. Richards CT, Crawley LM, Magnus D. Use of neurodevelopmental delay in pediatric solid organ transplant listing decisions: inconsistencies in standards across major pediatric transplant centers. Pediatr Transplant. 2009;13(7):843–50.
48. Dew MA, Goycoolea JM, Stukas AA, Switzer GE, Simmons RG, Roth LH, et al. Temporal profiles of physical health in family members of heart transplant recipients: predictors of health change during caregiving. Health Psychol. 1998;17(2):138–51.
49. Maldonado JR, Dubois HC, David EE, Sher Y, Lolak S, Dyal J, et al. The Stanford integrated psychosocial assessment for transplantation (SIPAT): a new tool for the psychosocial evaluation of pre-transplant candidates. Psychosomatics. 2012;53(2):123–32.
50. Christensen AJ, Turner CW, Slaughter JR, Holman JM Jr. Perceived family support as a moderator psychological Well-being in end-stage renal disease. J Behav Med. 1989;12(3):249–65.
51. Debray Q, Plaisant O. Pulmonary transplantation. Psychological aspects. The medical context and indications. Ann Med Psychol. 1990;148(1):105–7. discussion 8–9
52. Feinstein S, Keich R, Becker-Cohen R, Rinat C, Schwartz SB, Frishberg Y. Is noncompliance among adolescent renal transplant recipients inevitable? Pediatrics. 2005;115(4):969–73.
53. Molassiotis A, van den Akker OB, Boughton BJ. Perceived social support, family environment and psychosocial recovery in bone marrow transplant long-term survivors. Soc Sci Med. 1997;44(3):317–25.
54. Schlebusch L, Pillay BJ, Louw J. Depression and self-report disclosure after live related donor and cadaver renal transplants. S Afr Med J= Suid-Afrikaanse tydskrif vir geneeskunde. 1989;75(10): 490–3.
55. Surman OS, Purtilo R. Reevaluation of organ transplantation criteria. Allocation of scarce resources to borderline candidates. Psychosomatics. 1992;33(2):202–12.
56. Teichman BJ, Burker EJ, Weiner M, Egan TM. Factors associated with adherence to treatment regimens after lung transplantation. Prog Transplant. 2000;10(2):113–21.
57. International Summit on Transplant T, Organ T. The declaration of Istanbul on organ trafficking and transplant tourism. Clin J Am Soc Nephrol 2008;3(5):1227–1231.
58. Participants in the International Summit on Transplant T, Organ Trafficking Convened by the Transplantation S, International Society of Nephrology in Istanbul TAM. The Declaration of Istanbul on organ trafficking and transplant tourism. Transplantation 2008;86(8):1013–1018.
59. Danovitch GM, Chapman J, Capron AM, Levin A, Abbud-Filho M, Al Mousawi M, et al. Organ trafficking and transplant tourism: the role of global professional ethical standards-the 2008 declaration of Istanbul. Transplantation. 2013;95(11):1306–12.
60. Cohen IG. Transplant tourism: the ethics and regulation of international markets for organs. J Law Med Ethics. 2013;41(1):269–85.
61. Schiano TD, Rhodes R. Transplant tourism. Curr Opin Organ Transplant. 2010;15(2):245–8.
62. OPTN. OPTN/UNOS Board opposes transplant tourism: U.S. Department of Health & Human Services; 2006. Available from: https://optn.transplant.hrsa.gov/news/board-opposes-transplant-tourism/
63. OPTN. OPTN/UNOS Ethics Committee: Ethical Principles to be Considered in the Allocation of Human Organs: HRSA; 2010, updated June 22, 2010. Available from: http://optn.transplant.hrsa.gov/resources/bioethics.asp?index=5
64. OPTN/UNOS. OPTN/UNOS Ethics Committee General Considerations in Assessment for Transplant Candidacy: HRSA; 2010. Available from: http://optn.transplant.hrsa.gov/resources/bioethics.asp?index=5
65. Sheehy E, O'Connor KJ, Luskin RS, Howard RJ, Cornell D, Finn J, et al. Investigating geographic variation in mortality in the context of organ donation. Am J Transplant. 2012;12(6):1598–602.

Cultural Aspects of Transplantation

Cultural Aspects of Transplantation

49

Sheila Lahijani and Renee Garcia

Introduction

Cultural influences are widespread in medicine and directly impact a patient's healthcare experience starting from initiation of healthcare to determining access to end-of-life care. The most common definition of culture involves a "shared set of (implicit and explicit) values, ideas, concepts, and rules of behavior that allow a social group to function and perpetuate itself" [1]. Culture also can be framed as the dynamic and evolving socially constructed reality that exists in the minds of its social group members. Their shared culture allows members to communicate, work effectively together, and understand motives of behavior. Culture shapes one's perspective on life and death, his/her experiences, and relationships. It is then not surprising that a patient's cultural beliefs would impact his/her perceptions of diagnosis, medical recommendations, and the procurement/transplantation of organs.

The field of transplantation medicine has progressed drastically in the last 20 years, especially with the advent of immunosuppressant medications. Organ transplantation is no longer just confined to the Western world, but it is now a more globally offered procedure. Regional culture has been shown to impact transplantation when diagnosing end-stage organ failure, performing pre-transplant evaluation, waiting lists, transplantation surgery, and post-transplant recovery. The goals of this chapter are to review some of the cultural aspects surrounding perceptions of death, procurement of organs, and impact on post-transplant care and adherence. Additionally, the cultural implications of race and ethnicity, religion, and gender are also reviewed. Finally, the adaptation of screening measures or instruments to specific cultures or languages will be discussed.

S. Lahijani (✉) · R. Garcia
Department of Psychiatry and Behavioral Sciences, Stanford University School of Medicine, Stanford, CA, USA
e-mail: lahijani@stanford.edu

Eastern Versus Western Beliefs on Death Determinations and Perceptions

The transplantation process from cadaveric donors cannot begin until death has occurred in the designated donor. This very early step, as necessary and straightforward as it may seem, is one of the most controversial steps in the transplantation process. Most of the controversy circulates around when "death" occurs and how it is defined – brain, or brainstem death (DBD), or death after cardiac death (DCD) [see Chap. 48 for more details] – and the procurement of cadaveric organs. The labeling of "death" carries with it many emotional, social, legal, and medical ramifications [2]. Medical implications include discontinuation of resuscitative efforts and interventions and, ultimately, organ procurement. Given the finality, it is essential that there is an agreement and understanding as to when exactly death has occurred. Is it a process? Or does death occur at some defined moment when chance of meaningful recovery has passed? Determining when death has occurred not only takes into account a strong medical knowledge base but also requires a social consensus and communal acceptance [2]. It is these latter principles that are most influenced by an individual's cultural perspective.

Historically, a person was determined to be dead when his/her breathing and heart irreversibly came to a stop. With advances in medicine, our ability to prolong life has substantially improved, especially with the development of mechanical ventilation, vasoactive medications to prevent cardiovascular collapse, and/or extracorporeal membrane oxygenation (ECMO) to oxygenate blood [3]. However, there does come a point where additional medical or surgical interventions are futile with no chance of meaningful neurological recovery. The amount of neurologic recovery that is deemed acceptable most certainly varies from person to person. There have been some landmark publications that have attempted to define death in terms other than just cardiopulmonary arrest. The concept of brain death evolved during the twentieth century with the Harvard Criteria in 1968, Uniform Determination of Death Act in 1981, and ultimately in 1995 with the American Academy of Neurology (AAN) publishing their practice parameters to conduct a brain death determination [3] (see Chap. 48 for additional details).

Attitudes about end-of-life decisions and death are deeply rooted in a society's culture and undoubtedly influence perspectives toward brain death and subsequent organ procurement. If these cultural differences are not recognized, family members may not view that patient as truly deceased or perhaps perceive that life-sustaining support has been withdrawn prematurely with the sole purpose of procuring their organs [4]. Knowledge of the specific details of every cultural belief as it relates to perspective on death and dying is not feasible given sheer number of different cultures globally. However, being aware of key cultural beliefs or themes at play in transplantation medicine allows providers to be more sensitive to an individual's specific cultural beliefs, which can facilitate the mutual respect, communication, and understanding that are essential components to the delivery of quality and culturally sensitive care [4].

Many publications have approached conceptualizing "cultural" influences on perception of death by globally categorizing into the Western and Eastern worlds [2, 3, 5, 6]. These two belief systems have different philosophical and religious influences which have developed in parallel and independent of each other. While not universal, ideas in Table 49.1 can help guide providers to anticipate potential aspects of the transplantation process that will be of most concern to patients and family members.

Table 49.1 Western and Eastern World Philosophical and Religious Principles Impacting Perception of Brain Death

Cultural belief	East	West
Body-soul/spirit relationship	Life is composed of an integration of the body, soul/spirit, and nature	Distinct separation of the body and soul
Location of the soul/spirit	Distributed throughout the entire body	Soul or conscious mind dwells in the brain
Determination of death	Ambiguous transition that can take hours	Clear boundary when death occurs
Timing of death	Acceptance of a natural death	Attempts to control mode and timing of death
Priority of values	Interpersonal relationships with a family-centered approach	Autonomous decision making
Perspectives on life	It is to be awed and is mysterious	It is to be controlled, planned for, and explained by physical laws

Adapted from Ref. [2]

The West

The Western world's philosophical underpinning originates from individuals like Socrates, Descartes, and Plato [2]. Socrates was one of the first to propose the idea of the soul being and existing separate from the body [7]. Plato adds to that principle by describing the soul as a "pure spiritual existence" that is imprisoned by the body temporarily [6]. Descartes reinforced this separation by identifying the soul or the ability to think as the source of one's personhood and the body as an "organic machine" for the soul [6]. This focus on the brain, or neuro-essentialism, devalues the physical body and places the brain as the seat of rational thought [8]. Hence, the presence of irreversible brain damage and the loss of one's higher cognitive functions to believe, to make decisions, and to feel and interact with the world indicates that death has occurred [9, 10]. Perspective studies in Europe found that the majority consider life without cognitive capacity as not worth living. Americans may believe that death has already occurred in those who are comatose or in persistent vegetative state [11, 12]. The body without a conscious mind is no longer a person [6].

Additionally, the Western world during its industrial period heralded the doctrines of pragmatism and utilitarianism, which factor into the acceptance of death by brain death as it provides "great instrumental value," or that one's death can still contribute to society [13]. Lock et al. proposed that the DBD criteria in the Harvard Report were the result of the pragmatic philosophy evidenced by the reduction of futile medical care and to facilitate organ procurement [14, 15]. Lock also highlighted that the modern Western world is obsessed with planning and controlling one's life and death; the acceptance of DBD is another manifestation of this propensity by controlling the time and manner of death [14, 15].

The Western world's perspective on death is also influenced by religious beliefs and leaders. Christianity, Judaism, and Islam have all been known to use the term "physiological decapitation" to describe brain death [16]. Orthodox Jews are the exception in that they hold fast to their belief that the soul resides in the heart [16]. The Pope Pius XII made official statement in 1957 affirming that the ultimate authority to set criteria for death are physicians and even specifically advocated against prolonging life in "hopeless situations" where additional medical interventions or treatments are futile [2]. DBD was officially accepted by Chief Rabbinical Councils of Israel and America and the council of Islamic Jurisprudence in 1986, thus further reinforcing the wide acceptance of DBD in the Western world [2].

The East

The Eastern world does not recognize the dichotomy between the body and soul as the Western world does [2]. In fact, the concept is completely foreign to many Asian countries and societies. There are many differing philosophical and religious perspectives within the Eastern world, including Shintoism, Taoism, Confucianism, and Buddhism, but there is the main commonality that one's personhood is not solely found in the brain and is distributed throughout the body [2, 17, 18].

Shintoism is the native religion of Japan and views the body as a whole to be the resting place for the soul and human life to be intimately connected with nature and the surrounding environment [5]. One Shintoism custom involves attempting to call the soul back to the physical body, waiting for period of time to be sure that the soul will not return to the body, and accounts for delaying the death determination as long as possible [5, 19]. Family maintains attachments to the body until the funeral ritual has been completed when the soul of the deceased is thought to be launched onto a new journey [19, 20]. Japan has somewhat honored this tradition legally. In fact, the first transplant in Japan from a brain-dead donor was performed in 1968 and was met with a legal and societal backlash, with the surgeon prosecuted and transplantations from a cadaveric donors coming to an end for some time. The Act on Organ Transplantation regulating donation from brain-dead persons came into effect in 1997, which allowed organ procurement only if the brain-dead person provided consent for organ donation in the event of brain death. The 2010 revision allowed family to provide consent for organ procurement even if the brain-dead person's wishes were not clear in an attempt to increase transplantation [5]. However, the ratio of transplantations performed with organs from living donors versus from deceased donors is strikingly high in Japan, reflecting the societal struggle with the definition of death and obtaining the organs from the deceased. In 2013, there were 14.23 living organ transplants performed per million people in Japan as compared to 0.66 dead organ transplants (as compared to 18.83 versus 25.99 in the United States, 8.59 versus 35.12 in Spain, and 36.54 versus 8.55 in South Korea) [21].

Chinese cultures are influenced by Taoism and Confucian traditions and beliefs. Like Shintoism, Taoism, which is the native religion of Chinese culture, recognizes that humans, both body and soul, are intricately associated with the surrounding environment; Taoism advocates following the laws of nature [2, 18]. Taoists believe that the body is the soul's resting place after death, and the body must be preserved without any form of mutilation to ensure immortality [5, 20]. Confucianism has been considered both a religion and a philosophy for the Chinese people and even has influences into Korea, Japan, and Vietnam [22–24]. Confucians believe that one's body is a gift from their parents/ancestors; thus it is not allowed to be mutilated or damaged in any way [5, 20]. Death is not instantaneous but considered to be a gradual process with disintegration of both spiritual and physical existences, and there are associated rituals to sending off their loved ones. Additionally, after death, the deceased person's spirit lingers near the body protecting it and is able to retaliate against anyone who desecrates his/her body [20]. A Confucian scholar stated "when a person is about to die, heat leaves his body, which indicates the spirit is gone," emphasizing the importance of body heat as an indication of life [18]. However, allowing for the dissipation of body heat is not compatible with viable organ procurement. Any mutilation or disruption to the body's wholeness is considered the premier violation of the "filial piety" or the virtue of respect for one's parents, elders, and ancestors [25].

Buddhism is another widespread religion in Asia which originated in Ancient India with a basis in the teachings of Buddha. Buddhists believe that they will be reborn again after death [20]. The concept of the Eighth Consciousness represents one's personhood or collective identity that is distributed throughout the body, not exclusive to any one bodily location, including the brain [26]. Therefore, a person's consciousness may still be present within the body even in the absence of brain activity and opposing the brain death principle [26]. Buddhists believe the spirit leaves the body immediately but may linger in an in-between state near the body. In this case, it is important that the body is treated with respect so that the spirit can continue its journey in the state of happiness. Additionally, Buddhism has not endorsed a consensus regarding organ donation leaving the decision to the individual conscience [20, 26]. Although it also must be noted that acts of compassion are highly valued in the Buddhist religion and the gift of the body, via organ donation, can be viewed as karmic advantage [6].

Beliefs about the importance of the physical body in Eastern religions are pervasive. The brain is not considered to be the dominant organ, but is only a portion of what constitutes one's personhood. It is these key beliefs that are considered to be contributing to the rejection, or resistance, of brain death in Eastern societies. Eastern religions have not released a clear opinion with regard to acceptance or denial of DBD [2]. Clinicians can provide reassurance to potential donor's family members by recognizing the impact these beliefs can have on an individual's perception of brain death and willingness to donate, and by reinforcing that rigorous efforts have been made to continue both physical and social life of the donor before their death [18].

Religion in Transplantation

Religious concerns may factor into many decisions about organ donation and transplantation. While differences in infrastructures and laws may account for variations between countries, religious beliefs may be attributable for low deceased donation rates among some groups and populations

Table 49.2 Components of various religions related to organ transplantation

Religion	Organ transplantation issues
Islam	Body is sacred, not to be violated Controversial definitions of brain stem death Traditional burial within 24 hours of death Saving a life is highly valued, and "necessity overrides the prohibition" Different decisions by religious scholars
Christianity	An act of altruism Individual decisions
Judaism	Prohibitions concerning cadavers Avoiding any unnecessary interference with the body (e.g., prohibition of autopsy) Saving a life is of fundamental value and represents "mitzvah" (religious ruling) Burial customs
Hinduism	Altruism, selflessness Physical body not crucial to reincarnation
Sikhism	Physical body not crucial to rebirth Doing good actions
Shintoism	Interfering with a corpse may be bad luck and disrupt the relationship between dead person and the bereaved Modern laws may allow transplantation
Buddhism	Generosity and selfless giving Spiritual consciousness within the body
Confucianism	Traditional principles exclude organ donation Modern scholars have different views
Taoism	Organ donation may be attempt to change the natural process of life Modern scholars may approve organ donation
Jehovah's witness	Restrictions on plasma exchange, blood transfusion Transplantation is allowed as long as there is no blood transfusion Contemporary guidance may view it as individual choice
Scientology	No formal indication concerning organ donation and transplantation Physical body is believed to be a transitory and restricting part of existence; accordingly, no medical practice is forbidden Scientologists are allowed to make their own decisions about organ donation The clinical definition of brain death is accepted and the church considers donation as a very valuable act

Adapted from [27]

[27]. See Table 49.2 for particular religious beliefs that might guide organ donation.

Additionally, when transplantation occurs, the role of religion can be viewed in the context of coping. In a longitudinal study of heart transplant patients, patients with strong beliefs who participated in religious activities had better physical and emotional welfare, fewer health concerns, and better adherence at the final 1 year assessment after transplant [28]. Thus, there may be an opportunity to maximize quality of life in transplant recipients with incorporation of faith, when appropriate, among psychosocial interventions.

Organ Procurement

Most would agree that there is an overall knowledge gap when it comes to the process of organ procurement even among healthcare workers. This deficit can lead to one inserting the opinions of misinformed others, use of false assumptions, or even refusal to donate. Perception studies in the West show that both European and American populations equate brain death or death of the conscious mind to the "real death." Eastern societies have many cultural beliefs that, if honored in the truest sense, would not yield any viable donated organs. Most of these beliefs all circulate around the importance of the physical body remaining whole and undamaged. Any real or perceived injury to the physical body can impede the ability of the spirit to transition upon death, have an enjoyable life in the underworld, and to reincarnate into the next life [20].

These cultural factors can be negotiated to salvage viability of donated organs, with appropriate sensitivity. Buddhists believe that death can take up to several hours once the person appears clinically deceased. Family members of Buddhist faith might like additional time with their loved one who has been declared dead, before they will allow organ procurement [6]. The specific timing of organ procurement can be negotiated with families to determine how much time is required, to honor their cultural beliefs or practices, prior to organ procurement [29]. Time requests must be weighed against maintaining the viability of the organs, often requiring continuation of supportive care to maintain blood flow and oxygenation to vital organs. Even if a family is unwilling to donate, it should be explored with family whether it is a result of resistance to one vital organ or donation as a whole (i.e., heart perceived by some as the locus of life). An educational discussion should be conducted to review the range of donations possible, including skin, pancreas, or corneas [6].

Race and Ethnicity

Race and ethnicity are two other important areas of consideration in medicine in general and particularly in transplant care. They may serve as surrogates for other differences, such as perceptions about donation and transplantation, or highlight disparities in medical care received among different groups. For example, racial-ethnic minorities in the United States with end-stage renal disease (ESRD) have been less likely to receive live donor kidney transplantation (LDKT) than their white counterparts. This may be partly due to reported difficulties in identifying live donors for ESRD patients from minority communities. In one US study, the willingness to donate live kidneys varied by race-ethnicity and recipient relationship to the potential donor. Differences in willingness to donate live kidneys were related to socioeconomic factors, medical trust, and concerns about the impact of live donation upon burial or cremation after death [30].

Distinguishing between "differences" and "disparities" is important. Whereas differences are defined as consistent and measurable variations in health outcomes, disparities are unnecessary, avoidable, unfair, and unjust differences. Reducing disparities stems from avoidable, involuntary, and differential risk. Understanding the continuum from a chronic illness, such as chronic kidney disease, to graft survival post-transplantation can increase points of intervention and address barriers [31].

Racial disparities in kidney transplantation have been documented in several steps of the process, including referral, evaluation, and wait listing. Racial disparities exist in the transplant process, and the rate of kidney transplantation in African-Americans has been observed to be 59% lower than whites. Lack of patient education about kidney disease and the kidney transplant process may be one explanation observed. In a retrospective study of education program's impact on the completion of transplant outcomes, the racial disparities were attenuated after the educational intervention [32]. In a systematic review of barriers to renal transplant in African-Americans, both patient-related barriers (personal and cultural beliefs, preferences about transplantation, lower socioeconomic status, lower level of education) and healthcare-related barriers (referral delays, inadequate transplant work-up, HLA-related and physician-related barriers) were identified. Personal and cultural beliefs and preferences of African-Americans were identified across studies. These included religious objections to transplant, better overall health and energy during dialysis, and less negative effects of kidney disease with lesser preference for renal transplantation [33].

Barriers to LKDT consist of the following factors: (1) recipient and donor attitudes, beliefs, and clinical characteristics; (2) healthcare provider knowledge, attitudes and behaviors; (3) population awareness; and (4) disease burden. Among recipient and live donor characteristics, low health literacy may be associated with suboptimal transplant self-care and lower levels of kidney function among LDKT recipients. Lower health literacy rates are reported among Hispanic, African-American, and American Indian/Alaska Native adults. Additionally, perceptions that healthcare providers have of their patients may lead to lower rates of transplant referrals and evaluations and higher rates of incomplete evaluations among minority potential recipients as compared to whites. In addressing these issues, many interventions have been proposed and initiated, including educational programs, social network engagement, financial counseling, and improving cultural competency among healthcare providers [34].

In a retrospective cohort study of US national transplant registry data over 25 years, significant center-level variabilities in graft outcome disparities for African-American kidney recipients were noted. It was concluded that in addition to focusing on patient-related factors, it is important to consider system-related factors to mitigate racial disparities; these refer to variabilities in healthcare systems and how there may be segregation of care. Of further consideration is minimizing acute rejection differences due to biologic and immunologic variations, reducing prolonged hospitalizations, increasing living donation, and using calcineurin inhibitor-based regimens in African-Americans (as opposed to not using them or using them ineffectively) may help improve disparities in transplant outcomes [35]. Of note, a recent multicenter longitudinal cohort study of 602 patients undergoing initial evaluation for kidney transplantation at 4 National VA centers found no significant racial disparities in the time from beginning of transplant evaluation to acceptance for kidney transplant. Authors suggested that specific characteristics of the VA healthcare system or veterans may play a role in mitigating disparities. These characteristics of a healthcare model include free of charge care to qualifying individuals, thus removing differences in insurance and income; support to transplant candidates including travel and lodging to attend the transplant center, again balancing out the financial disparities; and standardized referral and evaluation process throughout the VA system [36].

The US lung transplant registry data has demonstrated variability in adult waitlist mortality by race/ethnicity. For patients being listed for lung transplant, the lung allocation score (LAS) was created and is based on medical urgency and benefit. The introduction of LAS initially resolved differences in waitlist outcomes between African-American and white candidates. However, recent reports have demonstrated significant variation in unadjusted waitlist mortality by race/ethnicity. A recent study assessed the impact of race/ethnicity on transplant access or risk/adjusted mortality among waitlisted candidates. It was concluded that among advanced lung disease patients who are listed for lung transplant, there is no adjusted difference in waitlist mortality by race/ethnicity. However, unadjusted mortality and adjusted waitlist transplant access were worse in nonwhite candidates. This may be partly attributable to greater illness severity and disparities in the management of advanced lung disease patients before transplant listing [37].

Variations in the diagnosis and treatment of chronic liver disease in racial-ethnic minorities may impact access to the liver transplants. Studies indicated a 2.5 times lower response to hepatitis C (HCV) antiviral therapy in African-Americans than whites. There is a demonstrated lower incidence of hepatocellular carcinoma in whites than in African-Americans, Asians, Native Americans, and Alaskan Natives. In the liver transplantation process, many studies report race/ethnicity factors affecting access to liver transplant centers for evaluation, access to the liver transplant waitlist, and from the waitlist to transplant. These may represent the cumulative effect of structural, process, socioeconomic, cultural, and biological barriers that may arise at many stages. Data on racial-ethnicity differences in post-transplant outcomes are inconsistent. They may also be related to biological factors or differences in immunosuppression pharmacokinetics and adherence [38].

These differences may apply also to outcomes in patients listed for and undergoing heart transplant. Hispanic-Latino patients experience an increased risk of death on the waiting list, and African-American heart transplant recipients experience an increased risk of rejection and death post-transplant. By contrast, Asian heart transplant recipients experience a lower risk of rejection and death compared to whites and other minorities. While it is important to address health inequities both prior to and after transplant for minorities, other areas of consideration include gene expression profiling and the use of pharmacogenetics data to customize immunosuppressive regimens [39].

For patients undergoing allogeneic hematopoietic cell transplantation (HCT), biological factors also may contribute to differences in outcomes by race. Studies have demonstrated worse overall survival in African-American patients as compared to Caucasian, Hispanic, and Asian/Pacific Islanders. This association was independent of socioeconomic status. For patients undergoing autologous HCT, studies have demonstrated overall survival in African-American patients to be similar to that of Caucasian patients. More research is indicated to understand the biological, social, cultural, medical, and financial components of race that may influence disparities in donor availability, access to HCT, and outcomes of HCT [40].

Gender

Gender-related differences exist in solid organ transplantation. The relationship between sex hormones and immunological processes has been documented extensively. In females, cell-mediated immunity and natural killer cell activity diminish during pregnancy; there is an increased release of interleukin 1 in menopause. Estrogen may be an immunosuppressant or immunostimulant. Androgens can also affect immune function. Given these variabilities, certain forms of liver and kidney disease are more common in either men or women and may be subject to hormonal fluctuation. Thus, not only may there be unique challenges in pregnancy and menopause, donor and recipient gender may affect graft and patient survival after transplantation. There is also the possibility of gender bias in organ donation and transplantation [41].

In a cross-sectional study evaluating the motives and decision making of potential living liver donors, there were few differences between men and women. Women demonstrated a greater likelihood of being concerned about the impact of the donation on their families and social obliga-

tions, which may relate to their caregiving responsibilities. Women were more likely than men to endorse religion as a reason for donation [42]. A review of gender-specific distributions of living donor liver transplantation demonstrated that more men than women were both donors and recipients. There were noted regional differences; however, in the United States and Europe, the gender distribution was more balanced. Overall there was a paucity of literature on gender in living donors, and further investigation is needed [43].

Special Considerations

Transgender Populations

Over the last several years, standards of care and principles of care for the health of transgender individuals have been published [44, 45]. These guidelines are important given the inconsistencies that may take place with respect to name, gender identity, demographic information, and healthcare records. Cultural sensitivity is of utmost importance in optimizing communication between providers and patients [46].

Transgender individuals may experience specific challenges during the transplant evaluation, the perioperative phase, and the postoperative period. The literature on liver transplantation in transgender individuals is scarce; there is an indication of increased risk of hepatic cirrhosis and hepatocellular carcinoma [47]. There is also a paucity of data regarding early access of care for transgender individuals with chronic kidney disease. Major considerations in the transplant process of transgender individuals include (1) the health and medical history, (2) the surgical history, (3) the physical examination, (4) insurance coverage, (5) the psychological evaluation, (6) the social work evaluation, (7) postsurgical issues, and (8) privacy issues [48]. Addressing both the medical care and those aspects of care specific to the transgender individual are important in providing comprehensive care.

Adaptation of Tools

The increasing use of instruments in multinational studies has resulted in studies evaluating the adaptability of transplant assessment tools as well as the translation of tools into other languages. Specific examples include the Transplant Evaluation Rating Scale (TERS), Psychosocial Assessment of Candidates for Transplantation (PACT) scale, and the Stanford Integrated Psychosocial Assessment for Transplantation (SIPAT). While language is an obvious form of interpretation of a tool, there are a number of other factors that are very important when considering the use of these measures, including reliability, validity, feasibility, and generalizability. Consideration of differences in reported by patients, variations in psychometric properties, diversity knowledge of disease, and adherence norms can all impact the adaptation of tools in different cultures.

Economics of Transplantation

Organ transplantation is a costly procedure but can prolong life and improve its quality. Comorbidities, complications, and immunosuppressant treatment can help determine the cost effectiveness of organ transplant. The economics of organ transplantation considers organ shortage and organ allocation. Two main benefit measures of interest in the economic evaluation of transplant are survival and health-related quality of life. Interrelated aspects of the economics of organ transplantation consist of the following and serve as points of potential intervention: (1) determinants of end-stage organ disease, (2) health benefit measurements, (3) demand of organ transplantation, (4) offer of organs and of organ transplantation, (5) economic evaluation, (6) equilibrium analysis, (7) macro assessment, and (8) planning, budgeting, and monitoring. Economic models can be useful tools analyzing costs and create policies to improve the accessibility to organ transplantation to disparate populations [49].

Conclusions

The role of culture in transplantation extends from the time of the initial clinical diagnosis of disease throughout the period of post-transplant recovery. Perceptions of disease and death, including the procurement of organs, can impact illness and the transplant experience. Cultural implications of race and ethnicity, religion, and gender are evident in the literature and can impact both healthcare policy and healthcare delivery. Culture on a larger scale can influence health system outcomes and public health measures. Additionally, the economics and costs associated with transplant procedures can impact clinical decision making. Consideration of these factors is important in approaching a patient who is being considered for organ transplantation to ensure that the most comprehensive and effective care is offered.

References

1. Hudelson PM. Culture and quality: an anthropological perspective. Int J Qual Health Care. 2004;16:345–6.
2. Yang Q, Miller G. East-West differences in perception of brain death. J Bioeth Inq. 2014;12:211–25.
3. Silva IRFD, Frontera JA. Worldwide barriers to organ donation. JAMA Neurol. 2015;72:112.
4. Forsythe JL, Oniscu GC. An overview of transplantation in culturally diverse regions. Ann Acad Med Singap. 2009;38:365–9.
5. Siemionow MZ, Rampazzo A, Gharb BB. Addressing religious and cultural differences in views on transplantation, including composite tissue allotransplantation. Ann Plast Surg. 2011;66:410–5.
6. Bowman KW, Richard SA. Culture, brain death, and transplantation. Prog Transplant. 2003;13:211–7.
7. Devettere RJ. Neocortical death and human death. Law Med Health Care. 1990;18:96–104.
8. Ohnuki-Tierney E. Brain death and organ transplantation: cultural bases of medical technology. Curr Anthropol. 2014;35:233–54.
9. Arbour R, AlGhamdi HMS. Islam, brain death, and transplantation: culture, faith, and jurisprudence. AACN Adv Crit Care. 2012;23:381–94.
10. Grodin MA. Religious exemptions: brain death and Jewish law. J Church State. 1994;36:357–72.
11. Demertzi A, Ledoux D, Bruno M-A, Vanhaudenhuyse A, Gosseries O, Soddu A, et al. Attitudes towards end-of-life issues in disorders of consciousness: a European survey. J Neurol. 2011;258:1058–65.
12. Siminoff LA, Burant C, Youngner SJ. Death and organ procurement: public beliefs and attitudes. Kennedy Inst Ethics J. 2004;14:217–34.
13. Fins JJ. Across the divide: religious objections to brain death. J Relig Health. 1995;34:33–40.
14. Lock M. Displacing suffering: the reconstruction of death in North America and Japan. Daedalus. 1996;125:207–44.
15. Lock M. Twice dead: organ transplants and the reinvention of death. University of California Press. 2002.
16. Bernat JL. The concept and practice of brain death. Progress in Brain Research The Boundaries of Consciousness: Neurobiology and Neuropathology. 2005:369–379.
17. Kasai K. The religious attitude of Japanese. Research Reports of Chuubu University. 2009;10:35–43.
18. Liao Z. Overview of the view on life and death in Chinese culture. Qinghai Soc Sci. 2005;5:69–72.
19. Hardacre H. Response of Buddhism and Shintō to the issue of brain death and organ transplant. Camb Q Healthc Ethics. 1994;3:585.
20. Different cultural beliefs at time of death [Internet]. Customs and religious protocols. [cited 2018]. Available from: http://www.amemorytree.co.nz/customs.php
21. Okita T, Hsu E, Aizawa K, Nakada H, Toya W, Matsui K. Quantitative survey of laypersons attitudes toward organ transplantation in Japan. Transplant Proc. 2018;50:3–9.
22. Weiming T. Confucianism [Internet]. Encyclopædia Britannica. Encyclopædia Britannica, inc.; 2017 [cited 2018Feb26]. Available from: https://www.britannica.com/topic/Confucianism
23. Jones DG, Nie J-B. Does Confucianism allow for body donation? Anatomical Sciences Education. 2018.
24. McQuay JE. Cross-cultural customs and beliefs related to health crises. Crit Care Nurs Clin North Am. 1995;7
25. Tang Y, Li JH, Wu YX. Status quo and cause analysis and its ethical issues of organ transplantation in China. China J Mod Med. 2008;18:1142–5.
26. Keown D. Buddhism, brain death, and organ transplantation. J Buddhist Ethics. 2010;17:2–34.
27. Oliver M, Woywodt A, Ahmed A, Saif I. Organ donation, transplantation and religion. Nephrol Dial Transplant. 2011 Feb;26(2):437–44.
28. Harris RC, Dew MA, Lee A, Amaya M, Buches L, Reetz D, et al. The role of religion in heart-transplant recipients' long-term health and well-being. J Relig Health. 1995 Mar 1;34(1):17–32.
29. Patterson GM. The path not taken: social and cultural barriers to thoracic transplantation. Clin Chest Med. 2006;27:503–9.
30. Purnell TS, Powe NR, Troll MU, Wang NY, Haywood C, LaVeist TA, et al. Measuring and explaining racial and ethnic differences

in willingness to donate live kidneys in the United States. Clin Transpl. 2013 Sep 1;27(5):673–83.

31. Ladin K, Rodrigue JR, Hanto DW. Framing disparities along the continuum of care from chronic kidney disease to transplantation: barriers and interventions. Am J Transplant. 2009 Apr 1;9(4):669–74.

32. Patzer RE, Perryman JP, Pastan S, Amaral S, Gazmararian JA, Klein M, et al. Impact of a patient education program on disparities in kidney transplant evaluation. Clin J Am Soc Nephrol. 2012 Apr 1;7(4):648–55.

33. Navaneethan SD, Singh S. A systematic review of barriers in access to renal transplantation among African Americans in the United States. Clin Transpl. 2006 Nov 1;20(6):769–75.

34. Purnell TS, Hall YN, Boulware LE. Understanding and overcoming barriers to living kidney donation among racial and ethnic minorities in the United States. Adv Chronic Kidney Dis. 2012 Jul 1;19(4):244–51.

35. Freeman MA, Pleis JR, Bornemann KR, Croswell E, Dew MA, Chang CC, et al. Has the department of veterans affairs found a way to avoid racial disparities in the evaluation process for kidney transplantation? Transplantation. 2017 Jun 1;101(6):1191–9.

36. Taber D, Gebregziabher M, Egede L, Baliga P. Transplant Center Variability in Disparities for African-American Kidney Transplant Recipients. Ann Transplant. 2018 Feb 16;23:119–28.

37. Mooney JJ, Hedlin H, Mohabir P, Bhattacharya J, Dhillon GS. Racial and ethnic disparities in lung transplant listing and waitlist outcomes. J Heart Lung Transplant. 2017 Sep 30.

38. Mathur AK, Sonnenday CJ, Merion RM. Race and ethnicity in access to and outcomes of liver transplantation: a critical literature review. Am J Transplant. 2009 Dec 1;9(12):2662–8.

39. Morris AA, Kransdorf EP, Coleman BL, Colvin M. Racial and ethnic disparities in outcomes after heart transplantation: a systematic review of contributing factors and future directions to close the outcomes gap. J Heart Lung Transplant. 2016 Aug 1;35(8):953–61.

40. Majhail NS, Nayyar S, Santibañez MB, Murphy EA, Denzen EM. Racial disparities in hematopoietic cell transplantation in the United States. Bone Marrow Transplant. 2012 Nov;47(11):1385.

41. Safer JD. Transgender medical research, provider education, and patient access are overdue. Endocr Pract. 2013 Jul 1;19(4):575–6.

42. DiMartini A, Cruz RJ Jr, Dew MA, Fitzgerald MG, Chiappetta L, Myaskovsky L, et al. Motives and decision making of potential living liver donors: comparisons between gender, relationships and ambivalence. Am J Transplant. 2012 Jan 1;12(1):136–51.

43. Hermann HC, Klapp BF, Danzer G, Papachristou C. Gender-specific differences associated with living donor liver transplantation: a review study. Liver Transpl. 2010 Mar 1;16(3):375–86.

44. Ettner R, Monstrey S, Coleman E, editors. Principles of transgender medicine and surgery. Routledge; 2016 May 20.

45. Coleman E, Bockting W, Botzer M, Cohen-Kettenis P, DeCuypere G, Feldman J, et al. Standards of care for the health of transsexual, transgender, and gender-nonconforming people, version 7. Int J Transgend. 2012 Aug 1;13(4):165–232.

46. Gardner IH, Safer JD. Progress on the road to better medical care for transgender patients. Curr Opin Endocrinol Diabetes Obes. 2013 Dec 1;20(6):553–8.

47. Martin KA, Bostwick JM, Vargas HE. Liver transplant case report: transgenderism and liver transplantation. Int J Transgend. 2011 Oct 1;13(1):45–9.

48. Hoch DA, Bulman M, McMahon DW. Cultural sensitivity and challenges in Management of the Transgender Patient with ESRD in transplantation. Prog Transplant. 2016 Mar;26(1):13–20.

49. Machnicki G, Seriai L, Schnitzler MA. Economics of transplantation: a review of the literature. Transplant Rev. 2006 Apr 1;20(2):61–75.

Patient Perspectives

50

Eirik Gumeny, Gerardine Hernandez, Tyson Hughes, and Yelizaveta Sher

When I reflected back on Eirik Gumeny's piece in the *New York Times* section of "Modern Love" [1], I realized that this textbook would not be complete without the voices of individuals who have actually gone through the process of organ transplantation. Mr. Gumeny vividly describes the emotional toll of waiting for a lung transplant, with devouring anxiety and much uncertainty. He recounts the profound effect it had on him and his main support person, his wife. "No one tells you that the physical scars are the easy ones."

While the scientific literature informs us about our clinical decision-making in a cognitive way, real patient stories remind us of the depth of individual's emotions and experiences. They tell us frankly what works and what doesn't; they show us our blind spots as healthcare providers; they teach us in ways no book or article can. While the scientific journals tell us about statistics, numbers, and confidence intervals, our patients remind us why we do what we do, and how we can do it better.

When our patients share with us their experiences, they allow us an opportunity to be helpful to them and to others who will be walking their this path after them. Their journeys are unique, but some themes repeat themselves. Nothing is as powerful as hearing directly from these individuals. From them we learn that despite being surrounded by people, you are alone when facing death. We learn of the extreme psychological strain that accompanies the unraveling of the physical body. From their intensive care unit narratives, we hear stories of being left behind with people coming and going, of not having control and being dependent on others, of medical providers not always acknowledging or showing the acknowledgement of the whole personhood obscured by the attached tubes and machines. Their stories contain themes of incredible pressure of having received the gift of life and feeling an obligation to feel happy and grateful, while struggling with sadness, anxiety, and grief; themes of ongoing discovery and coping with the new post-transplant person and integrating this new version with an old version of self; themes of letting go of the old version of self and discovering what the new version is able to conquer; themes of fear; themes of loss; themes of hope; and themes of love.

Each patient's story is an invaluable gift to us. Below are some of these precious gifts.

Eirik Gumeny

In the last few months before my double lung transplant, my lung function deteriorated to 12 percent. I was barely able to move across my tiny apartment, barely able to get from the bed to the couch, needing 10 liters of oxygen at all times. I was on a large number of medications and therapies for my worsening cystic fibrosis, including frequent intravenous antibiotic treatments. I had a G-tube inserted to keep from wasting away.

As difficult as all that was, however, the sickness and surgeries ended up being the easy parts of getting a transplant. The toll the process took on my mental health was something altogether more difficult.

The physical ailments at least made sense; they were expected and understood. If I got an infection, I was prescribed antibiotics. If I was losing weight, supplemental nutrition was added. There was a cause and effect that made the response to symptoms obvious. Moreover, the physical difficulties were where the medical team excelled – those were the problems they were trained to diagnose and correct.

The significance of the psychological baggage that goes along with a transplant, however, seemed to be less obvious and more mysterious to them.

ОЛ

E. Gumeny · G. Hernandez · T. Hughes
Stanford University Medical Center, Stanford, CA, USA

Y. Sher (✉)
Department of Psychiatry and Behavioral Sciences, Stanford University School of Medicine, Stanford, CA, USA
e-mail: ysher@stanford.edu

© Springer International Publishing AG, part of Springer Nature 2019
Y. Sher, J. R. Maldonado (eds.), *Psychosocial Care of End-Stage Organ Disease and Transplant Patients*,
https://doi.org/10.1007/978-3-319-94914-7_50

Anxiety and depression were anticipated and treated with pills. Guilt, fear, and frustration were shrugged off. I felt that as long as I wasn't suicidal, everything was fine. The bulk of the team's efforts were on keeping me alive, and anything beyond that was a "quality of life" issue – and, understandably, not their top priority.

The burden of sorting out my emotional health was on me. Obviously, this was not an easy task.

For one, it was incredibly difficult for me to even know that I needed psychological help. I was sicker than I had ever been during the run-up to the transplant, my body failing me left and right. I was on new and stronger medications, with new and stronger side effects. I was taking a number of psychoactive medications, including dronabinol, sertraline, and mirtazapine daily, as well as lorazepam as needed – and I needed it often. Beyond simply not trusting my own body, I was continually in a haze, making it difficult to sort out specific problems that might need addressing.

Similarly, physical and mental health often collided, and separating the two became increasingly troublesome. As frail as I was at the time, every little stressor – financial problems, insurance issues, even a television show that hit too close to home – had significant and noticeable impacts on my ability to breathe and function. I was expending so much effort just to be, that any slight change rippled outward, like a pebble dropped in a pond. And while that might have been only a small splash to a healthy person, it hit me like a tidal wave.

I suffered from tremendous panic attacks while awaiting transplant, at one point even falling to the ground and calling for an ambulance in the 2 minutes it took for my wife to pull the car around. In those moments I was fundamentally unable to tell if I was in some kind of respiratory distress or simply succumbing to anxiety. As sick as I was, the issue could easily have been either one – and was often both. I would get short of breath and then panic, or vice versa, one problem feeding into the other until discerning a difference was impossible.

There was, in fact, one thing I could be completely certain of during this time: fear. Not necessarily the fear of the surgery, or of dying – though both were certainly present – but a real, tangible fear that if I got too sick or a test came back with the wrong results, I might lose my place on the transplant list. That if I said the wrong thing or felt the wrong way, I might be kicked out of the hospital. In that cloudy, muddled time, fear, unfortunately, was one of the few emotions I could be sure of.

In hindsight, I'm less sure how justified that feeling was, but, at the time, there was a genuine and constant concern about being perceived as somehow non-compliant by the clinic staff and having to face the ramifications. I was worried that expressing that fear, or any anxiety or doubt, might itself come across as a lack of support and enthusiasm for

transplant, might bring my intentions into question. Compliance is scripture in pre-transplant clinics, and – waiting for a miracle as I was – I didn't want to be seen as anything less than completely reverent and obedient.

Survival, after all, is the predominant concern pre-transplant, for all parties involved. When the patient is coughing up blood, the focus is understandably on stopping the bleeding, not making sure the patient isn't scared. And for the patient himself, in the thick of things, there's no time to sort through what's going on in his head – it's a constant, muffled scream, and he learns to live with it.

As a result, no matter what was going on, or what I was feeling, I convinced myself I was okay, because that was the only way I was going to make it through the process. There were bouts of guilt, terror, worry, but I hid them, ignored them – unconsciously – because it seemed that getting past them was more important than acknowledging and addressing them. With the threat of death ever-present, taking the time to sort myself out felt like a luxury I didn't have. I chalked everything up to "the transplant" and moved on, assuming it would all simply go away after the surgery.

Which it did, almost immediately. Which is what makes all of this so challenging to accurately discuss.

Obviously, ignoring my problems and concerns was not the most emotionally healthy tactic and may even have contributed to the survivor's guilt and occasional depression I still struggle with today, 3.5 years out. More directly, not addressing the psychological issues I was struggling with made an already stressful situation that much more stressful and painful. But then, what alternative did I have? More importantly, what alternative should I have had?

While I readily admit that I, personally, may not have been receptive to or capable of fully utilizing the mental health resources available to me, I do wish that I, and other patients going through the various transplant stages, had early access to additional integrated assistance with facing the psychological pressures of transplantation. The acknowledgment and anticipation by the medical team of the emotional difficulties created by the transplant, along with their already expert addressing of the physical challenges, would certainly help to ease the weight of those emotional difficulties.

Similarly, early access to mental health assistance during – or, ideally, before – the earliest pre-transplant stages, before the paralyzing anxiety and panic set in, would go a long way toward allowing the patient to be more emotionally ready and more receptive to the mental health resources on hand when needed. Cystic fibrosis, or whatever other underlying disease is affecting the patient, takes a psychological toll of its own. A patient already in the habit of healthily addressing his or her emotions and fears would certainly be more receptive and willing to utilize available mental health resources and may not even be as in need of them.

I know that I was not able to sufficiently articulate my emotional concerns until well after the transplant, when I was removed from the maelstrom of the experience, with a therapist completely separate from the clinic and transplantation. Had that occurred before the transplant, I'd like to think that I'd have been in a better place to address the psychological issues confronting me. Addressing the enormity of the impact that transplantation has on a patient's mental health early, before the process begins in earnest, could be a way to alleviate that impact later on.

In the end, there's no getting around the fact that lung transplantation is a traumatic experience, both physically and mentally. Having early and readily available access to more understanding of the latter would significantly help to ease that psychological burden.

Geri Hernandez

In the summer of 2010, I caught a bad cold which seemed to never go away. At the time, I was working as an Interior Designer, remodeling entire house projects, and I started to notice that I was gasping for air walking up the stairs.

I spent the next 4 years going to doctor after doctor to determine the source of my illness. My congestion was strangling me from the inside. If only I could cough up this phlegm I thought, but it wouldn't go away.

As time went by, it became more and more difficult to breathe. I would often have difficulty catching my breath. How many times had I grabbed a stranger's hand, "Hold me, please, stay with me, please don't leave me alone!" in the parking lot, in the dressing room, at the store. Not being able to breathe filled my mind with anxiety and stress. I had to plan every move… How many steps is it to the parking lot from my car? Can I make it to the store? Where is the exit in case I need to run outside? Will I be able to make it to the toilet? It left me with a lot of anxiety about breathing. People often thought I was having panic attacks. In reality, not breathing was causing me anxiety and stress. All I wanted to do was to breathe. It's a natural act that we take for granted, until it's taken from us.

Eventually it became impossible to continue working. I had to stop my business and sell my house. I could no longer walk very far without gasping for air. As my illness progressed, strangers often would stare at me when I coughed uncontrollably. Once a lady told me to go home because she didn't want to catch what I had. Another time a man at the movie theater asked me to leave because my cough was bothering him. So eventually I did stay away from people, ashamed that I coughed too much.

Those years were the loneliest and most depressing periods of my life. I felt so isolated. I could no longer participate in family activities and stopped going to family parties. My

friends stopped inviting me because they knew I was sick. I could no longer go dancing because I could barely walk. I felt very alone, scared about my health, and betrayed by my own body. I could see the old, outgoing, joyful, fun-loving Geri slowly slipping away. The girl with the warm smile and infectious laugh was gone. Laughing would cause me to cough uncontrollably. So who needed to laugh, I just wanted to breathe.

Diagnosis

In the summer of 2014, I ended up in the emergency room. The doctor told me I wasn't going home until they had determined what was wrong with me. And I knew that without a diagnosis, I wasn't going to make it much longer.

After a 3-week stay in the hospital, the doctors confirmed I had pulmonary fibrosis with barely any good lung left. I was placed on oxygen therapy 24/7. At first, it was difficult to accept the fact that I had to be 100% reliant on oxygen. I was always an independent person and I didn't want to be reliant on this machine. However, I could no longer breathe on my own. The doctor reminded me that I would feel better if I used the oxygen. At first I felt ashamed and embarrassed to have to drag around that big cart and tank. It was an outward reminder to me and the world that I was sick, that I wasn't strong, that my body had defeated me. And it made me angry and frustrated. But slowly I adjusted to the tank and cart. And eventually I saw the tank and oxygen as my friend not my foe. I started to feel better, and I concentrated on getting outside. That Halloween I even made a costume for "Tankie" and we both went as Minions.

Welcome to the Family: Stanford

My new pulmonologist told me that I would never recover from the pulmonary fibrosis and that eventually it would end my life. He estimated I had about 3 years with my own lungs. However, he felt I was a good candidate for a lung transplant. My heart sank that day when I heard the words "lung transplant." A rush of emotions entered my mind. I was terrified. I understood first-hand about transplants since my sibling had had two kidney transplants, but I never thought I would need a transplant. I had to keep walking forward. I had already left behind so much stress, pain, tears, and torture. I thought to myself, I've already walked close to death. I knew what that was like, and I am still alive. My only choice was to keep walking through this low valley and go to Stanford.

Right before Christmas of 2014, I received my transplant evaluation packet from Stanford. I was scheduled for 5 days of tests that took about 8 hours each day. It's a testament of your endurance and emotions to make it through the myriad of tests to evaluate your health. When you are going through the evaluation process, you want to be hopeful that the procedure will save your life. But what new transplant patients don't realize is that this is still a new frontier. There are consequences and risks involved in this procedure. The education meeting tells you briefly the facts of a transplant. It focuses on the fact that the surgery is a treatment, and not a cure, and highlights some of the possible complications and shortcomings that you might endure.

Waiting Game

I was accepted into the transplant program in December 2016. I thought of this time as a training period. I would often play that old Rocky song in my head every time I went walking the track. I exercised every day and tried to eat well to be physically ready for the procedure. But in the back of my mind, I could hear a small voice reminding me the clock was ticking, I had an estimated 3 years left with my old lungs. As that thought entered my mind, fear and sadness filled my heart. I wasn't ready to die. God had already been with me through the worst part. I had already come close to death, and I was still alive! "Si se puede," I can do it, I could hear my late father say to me.

I had seen firsthand the success of a transplant from my older sibling, and that gave me hope about my own transplant. However, I had also experienced my sibling's reaction to the medication. I was only a child when my sibling had the first transplant, and the experience had caused me some traumatic stress that was surfacing now. I was frightened I might react the same way to the medication. I didn't want to lose the old Geri.

When I shared my fears with my transplant program, I was referred to the transplant psychiatrist. The psychiatrist was very helpful in working out my fears about the medication and the transplant. The doctor was able to help me better understand and work through my thoughts and fears and to help me learn how to stay in the moment and not predict the future. I realized that my journey is not someone else's, but my own. In retrospect, I wish this referral was initiated at the very start of my transplant journey.

It's only a treatment

On Saturday, June 4, 2016, at 1:45 AM in the morning, I received the call that it was my turn. I had waited about a year and half for my transplant. I asked them twice if they were really calling for me. I felt so nervous and anxious that my life was about to change. I would no longer have my own lungs. I would be out on a limb without a safety net. I could never come back from this. I fell to my knees and prayed to

God to protect me and be with me during the surgery. I called my sister, "Wake up, it's my turn."

We arrived at the emergency department 90 minutes later and checked in. After some preliminary vital checks, a doctor entered the room and told me he was going to pick up my lungs. It was a surreal experience. On one hand, you are so thankful and grateful for the new lungs, but on the other hand, you are mourning the loss of your old lungs. It's a very scary moment to realize there is no going back from this operation.

When I woke up, I felt this rush of air entering into my lungs. I felt like I couldn't control my breathing and that I wasn't in sync with my lungs. Eventually my body adjusted to the new lungs and my breathing leveled. As I opened my eyes for the first time, I asked my sister if I was alive and if I made it. The room seemed to be flashing and changing colors. The nurse told me I was hallucinating. I had no idea that this would happen after surgery and neither did my family. It took about 3 days for the hallucinations to subside and I started to be more like myself. It was a very scary and confusing time for me. I felt comforted knowing that my psychiatrist came to visit me each day at the hospital and gave me the emotional support I needed. She understood my fears and worries about the operation and about the medication. She knew me emotionally.

The odd thing after the surgery was that I felt like I still needed my oxygen, even though I could see my oxygen level was 99%. Yet my mind felt like I still needed it. How strange is it that the one thing I didn't want was now something I felt I couldn't be without. I had become emotionally dependent upon the oxygen, and now I had to be weaned from it.

I felt so good when I left the hospital 11 days later. I was so grateful and thankful I had made it through the surgery and that I was doing so well. However, 3 weeks later, I ended up back in the hospital with a MRSA infection on my incision. The doctors had to cut out more of my chest tissue which left this large noticeable cavity on my chest. It was a disappointing setback. My chest required a wound vacuum for 6 months and I had a PICC line inserted into my arm for antibiotics.

One of the positive aspects of having a chronic condition is realizing how many family and friends step forward and rally around you. I never would have made it through the 4 years of being sick without a diagnosis without my family. After the transplant, my sister and the rest of my family had to come forward and helped me recover. Also, many friends, even new friends, stepped up to volunteer to take me to the countless appointments. No patient can make it through the transplant process without a village of people to help them recover.

I think one of the misconceptions people have about lung transplants is that you have the surgery and then you are cured. In reality, the surgery is a major therapy that tremendously improves your quality of life, but after all it is a treatment that requires constant ongoing monitoring, medication, and even further treatments. The pulmonary fibrosis journey is not over. After surgery you are monitored very closely, and many treatments are required to keep you on track. I felt unprepared for the physical obstacles that happened after the surgery. The doctors are used to handling the numerous types of complications that happen, but the patient is experiencing the problem for the first time and often feels overwhelmed by the setbacks.

I often felt anxious going for my checkups, wondering what else they will find wrong with me. Those initial visits back to the hospital were filled with a lot of anxiousness, worry, and resentment. Of course I was grateful to be breathing on my own, but a part of me still felt resentment that I had to go back to the doctors so many times. I was still trying to accept my new situation and my long-term commitments.

As time went by, and I slowly worked through each obstacle with the help of my psychiatrist, I began to realize that this was really a new phase of my pulmonary fibrosis journey. My job now was to help monitor my progress and to take the best care of myself so I could be as successful as possible. And in time, I realized that the doctors, the nurses, the hospital, and even the medications were not the bad guys, but the good ones who were just as interested in me being successful. What I finally concluded was that these people really did care what happened to me, and that they really were my new family. Just like a family, they were going to be with me through thick and thin, good times and bad ones.

I think the most important lesson I have learned from this experience is that we have to live in the moment. Today I am doing well and I feel great. I'm trying to take it day by day. I'm staying positive and always grateful. And even if I have a future problem, I am confident my new family of doctors and staff will help me through it. Holding my hand through the low valleys of this journey. I'm so thankful for all the people that have helped me live another day. I appreciate the family who donated their loved one's lungs to me. I will try to respect that person by living my life well, and I will try to give back to others who need help. My future is uncertain… like everyone's. However, I still am hopeful about my future. This journey has made me realize that in a way I am one of the lucky ones. I've experienced firsthand how fragile the human body can be, and I have also seen how resilient and strong our bodies and minds are. I am so grateful and amazed each time I just breathe.

Tyson Hughes

My name is Tyson Hughes and I am a heart transplant patient. I use the word patient because I will always be one. Some choose to use the word recipient, but I prefer patient. I'm 4 years post-heart transplant and except for a few hiccups, I am generally doing alright. Most of my days consist of two major medicine interruptions, but these interruptions generally allow me to go about living my life like most other people. Of course, some days are better than others, while others are … not so much. I'm learning to ride the roller coaster that my new life has become, but I also understand that I'll always be learning new, and maybe not so exciting, ways of coping.

Prior to being a transplant patient, I was a 13-year veteran police officer. I loved my job, my co-workers, my friends and family, and my life in general. I was extremely active, both at work and on my own time. I loved to exercise and could pretty much run as far and as fast as I wanted to. I walked full-length golf courses regularly and could play ten games of aggressive racquetball consecutively. I worked as hard as I played and really loved life. As a police officer, I was also extremely active. Immediately after briefing, I would often jog to my patrol car, pull out of the police station, and stay in the field until the end of my shift. I spent most of my time looking for criminal activity, and that really gave me joy in the job. I loved being the barrier between "good" and "bad."

One of my many duties as a police officer was to respond to calls relating to mental health concerns. I handled everything from mental health evaluations, welfare checks, threats of suicide, displays of violence, and sadly, even suicides. All of these I lumped into a category of what I considered to be "just" mental health responses. After responding, taking care of my duties, and writing my report, I would never give it another thought, since I knew there would just be more of the same issues tomorrow.

I didn't truly understand mental health issues … until I became a patient. In fact, even for the first couple of years after I became ill and received the transplant, I didn't comprehend that I was now "having issues." Almost every afternoon, I would start getting these unexplainable episodes. I would tremble, pace around my home anxiously, become nauseous and nervous, then paranoia would set in. I was sure I was going to die, if not today, then surely tomorrow. I didn't like or understand these feelings and was always amazed and thankful that somehow, I survived until the next day. It was the strangest feeling not to have control over my mind, especially given how much trauma my physical body had already endured and overcome. Needless to say, I was confused.

How could it possibly be that a strong police officer such as myself, with many years of experience dealing with psychologically related tragedies, was experiencing, yet not recognizing, the symptoms of what I was going through. At minimum, I had anxiety and I probably experienced full-blown depression when I was at my worst. Initially, I received assistance from a therapist, who unfortunately, did not have specific experience with transplant patients. Although my time with her was valuable, it was clear to me that I wasn't really gaining any tools needed to deal with my daily issues. Consequently, I turned to and sought assistance from the

Stanford Hospital post-transplant team that was established to help me specifically. I came away with the name of a woman who previously worked with the solid organ transplant team at Stanford Hospital but left to start her private practice in nearby Menlo Park. This highly skilled therapist, a Licensed Clinical Social Worker by training, was exactly what I needed. She had previously worked at Stanford Hospital with the exact people who were caring for my physical needs. She had a great working relationship with the transplant psychiatrist at Stanford Hospital. The psychiatrist would be the overseer of my psychological needs. She evaluated me and worked with her team and I to determine the proper medication and dosage amounts for my particular needs. My transplant therapist and I met weekly to talk about and help me normalize the craziness my life had become. After my first few meetings with these two wonderful medical professionals, I had already seen a marked improvement in my mental health. It was clear I was partnered with the appropriate team to care for my mental health needs. They will forever be an integral part of my care team.

Going into the transplant process, I was worried about the surgery and about the good possibility of infection. I knew I needed to commit to following the long list of rules established by the post-transplant team: wash my hands, keep my hospital room and home as tidy and as germ-free as possible, remind friends to avoid me when they were ill, watch my sodium intake, take my 50+ pills a day as prescribed (that's another whole chapter), wear that truly awful, ugly mask to protect me from others who might be ill (did I mention that it was pink???), exercise at the recommended pace (this was very hard for me to scale back given my prior fitness level), attend all of my appointments, adjust my medications as suggested, take my blood pressure and weigh myself daily, stay indoors, and avoid dust. I did all of these things, and more. I worked hard, then I worked harder, and then I pushed myself just a little further. But ... I forgot one thing.

I forgot that although my physical body had taken the brunt of the trauma during the surgeries and throughout the recovery process, my mind had been neglected. My mind had been dealt a huge blow and was traumatized by all of the events, both pre- and post-transplant. I was no longer the same psychologically. My mind was forever changed by the physical transition my body went through. I had forgotten to tend to some very important and critical pieces in my recovery challenge, my brain, my mind, and my mental stability. I had had years of experience identifying, communicating with, and assisting people with mental health-related issues, yet I couldn't even identify that I needed help myself.

I've not been shy about sharing my experiences with other transplant patients or those going through other medical scenarios. I've urged others toward mental health counseling and openly shared my delicate experiences. I had overlooked my need for mental health assistance, but I am glad to report that I'm back on track. I will forever be a patient, but my lifelong mental wellness has significantly improved, allowing me to be a more normal person.

Thank you to all that have helped me through these events!

Further Recommended Reading

Amy Silverstein, *Sick Girl,* Grove Press, New York, Reprint edition (October 1, 2008)

Amy Silverstein, *My Glory Was I Had Such Friends*, New York, NY, Harper Wave (June 27, 2017)

Charity Tilleman-Dick, *The Encore: A Memoir in Three Acts*, New York, NY, Atria Books (October 3, 2017)

Mary Gohlke with Max Jennings, *I'll take Tomorrow: The Story of a Courageous Woman Who Dared to Subject Herself to a Medical Experiment-The First Successful Heart-Lung Transplant*, New York, NY, M Evans & Co (April 1, 1985)

Elizabeth Scarboro, *My Foreign Cities: A Memoir*, New York, NY, Liveright; 1 edition (January 27, 2014)

Isabel Stenzel Byrnes and Anabel Stenzel, *The Power of Two: A Twin Triumph over Cystic Fibrosis*, Columbia, Missouri, University of Missouri Press; Updated, Expanded ed. edition (October 5, 2007)

Reference

1. Gumeny E. When love isn't as simple as standing by your man. The New York Times. 2016.

Index

A

Abatacept, 165
Abdominal trauma, 325
Absolute uterine factor infertility (AUFI), 377, 378
Acamprosate, 131, 151, 464
Accelerated acute rejection, 338
Acceptance and commitment therapy (ACT), 476
Acetylcholinesterase inhibitors (ACHIs), 82, 99, 210
Acute cellular rejection (ACR), 115, 171, 187, 231, 262, 282, 338
Acute kidney injury (AKI), 63, 74, 103, 174, 262, 280, 283
Acute lymphoblastic leukemia (ALL), 389, 391–393
Acute myelogenous leukemia (AML), 391
Acute rejection, 3, 24, 105, 112, 170, 182, 199, 229, 232, 279, 313, 338, 355, 366, 523, 543
Acute respiratory distress syndrome (ARDS), 267, 268
Adenovirus, 421, 427
Adult motility disorders, 302
Adult-to-Adult Living Donor Liver Transplantation Cohort Study (A2ALL), 53, 56
Advanced heart failure
 definition, 196
 diagnosis, 196
 heart transplantation, 195
Adverse effects of marijuana, 39
Airway anastomotic complications, 281
Albuminuria, 63, 64
Alcoholic liver disease (ALD), 24, 33, 127, 139, 147, 171, 182, 184, 188
 causes, 147
 definition, 139
 effects of recidivism after LT, 35
 factors associated with LT failure, 24
 impact on overall health, 182
 sucess rate of ALD vs. other reasons for LT, 33
Alcohol-mediated oncogenesis, 36
Alcohol use, 18, 33, 36, 54, 56, 61, 121, 124, 139, 147, 150, 183, 262, 294, 493, 494
Alcohol use disorders (AUDs), 139, 140, 147, 150, 151, 175, 185, 493
 causes, 147
 definition, 139
 diagnosis, 493
 effects of recidivism after LT, 35
 epidemiology, 493
 factors associated with LT failure, 24
 HCT, in, 404
 impact on overall health, 182
 liver transplant, in, 183
 lung transplant, in, 262
 6-month rule, 33, 143, 494–495, 499, 501
 success rate of ALD vs other reasons for LT, 33
Alcohol Use Disorders Identification Test (AUDIT), 129, 183, 262
Alcohol Use Disorders Identification Test-Consumption (AUDIT-C), 183

Alemtuzumab, 165, 282, 312, 338, 418, 421, 457
Allogeneic hematopoietic stem cell transplantation (allo-HCT), 37
Allograft microbiota, 316
Allosensitization, 199
Allotransplantation, 103
Alpha-1 antitrypsin (A1AT), 247, 248
Amantadine, 97, 99, 446, 456
Ambivalence, 27, 51, 53, 54, 150, 477, 485
American College of Cardiology, 196, 203
American College of Surgeons (ACS), 10, 162, 405
American Medical Association (AMA), 10, 11, 160
Amiodarone
 delirium, 211
 toxicity, 199
 use, 216
Amitriptyline, 98, 153, 207, 259, 326, 444, 455, 460
Amlodipine, 174
Anemia, 165
Antibody-mediated rejection (AMR), 114, 231, 282, 338
Anti-CD25 monoclonal antibodies, 106
Anticoagulation, 113, 171, 221, 269
Antidepressants agent
 monoamine oxidase inhibitors (MAOIs), 460
 selective serotonin reuptake inhibitors (SSRIs), 458
 serotonin norepinephrine reuptake inhibitors (SNRIs), 459
 stimulants, 461
 tricyclic antidepressants (TCAs), 460
 other antidepressants, 459
Antiepileptic drugs (AEDs), 173, 445, 463–464
Antilymphocyte globulin (ALG), 162, 165, 338
Antimetabolites, 230
Antithymocyte globulin (ATG), 106, 112, 115, 172, 232, 282, 312, 338, 418, 421, 457
Anxiety, 3, 4, 18, 30, 53, 54, 75, 79, 95, 401–403
 in CKD, 79–84, 94–97, 120, 127, 130
 in COPD
  epidemiology and risk factor, 256
  pathophysiological mechanisms, 256
  treatment, 257
 in cystic fibrosis
  epidemiology and risk factors, 257
  treatment, 260
 in heart disease, 205, 207–211, 217, 237–240
 kidney transplant recipients, 121
 in liver disease, 148, 151
 liver transplantation, 181, 182
 in lung disease, 255
 post-lung transplantation, 293
 pulmonary hypertension, 4, 142, 198, 241, 247, 250, 255, 260, 267, 273, 281

© Springer International Publishing AG, part of Springer Nature 2019
Y. Sher, J. R. Maldonado (eds.), *Psychosocial Care of End-Stage Organ Disease and Transplant Patients*,
https://doi.org/10.1007/978-3-319-94914-7

Aortohepatic conduit, 171
Aplastic anemia (AA), 397, 398, 464
Apolipoprotein (APO-L1) L1 gene variants, 64
Arteriopathic rejection, 173
Artificial ventilation, 163
Ascites, 140
Asymmetric dimethylarginine (ADMA), 74
ATG, *see* Antithymocyte globulin
ATP-binding cassette (ABC) transporters, 454
Atrial dysrhythmias, 284
AUFI, *see* Absolute uterine factor infertility
Autologous HCT, 387, 393, 395, 421, 430, 544
Autotransplantation, 103
Azathioprine, 105, 112, 161, 162, 173, 175, 225, 230, 274, 332, 379, 457

B
B-ALL, 392
Barbiturates, 40, 113, 499
Basal cell carcinoma (BCC), 116
Basal metabolic rate (BMR), 331
Basiliximab, 106, 112, 165, 172, 173, 230, 457
Beck Anxiety Inventory (BAI), 78, 79, 370
Beck Depression Inventory (BDI), 27, 73, 76–79, 83, 94, 129, 182,
         199, 205, 207, 209, 261, 322, 325, 345, 359, 360, 370
Belatacept, 107, 165, 173, 457
Benzodiazepines, 40, 74, 95, 98, 153, 209, 240, 257, 270, 290, 293,
         403, 408, 454, 456, 461, 463, 465, 499
Bicaval technique, 170, 227, 228
Biliary tract abnormalities (BTA), 171
Biloma/sterile collection of bile, 172
Bipolar disorder, 97, 121, 182, 237, 240, 256, 445, 463
Bisphosphonates, 174, 284, 303, 429
BK virus, 115, 280
Blood and marrow transplantation (BMT), *see* Hematopoietic cell
         transplantation (HCT)
Bone mineral density (BMD), 428
Brain-derived neurotropic factor (BDNF), 74, 441
Brainstem death (DBD), 539
Brief Symptom Inventory-anxiety subscale, 208
Bronchial anastomosis, 273
Bronchial stenosis, 282
Bronchiolitis obliterans syndrome (BOS), 276, 280, 282, 292, 427
Buprenorphine, 151, 326, 465, 497
Bupropion, 97, 98, 131, 151, 206, 208, 257, 408, 444, 460

C
Calcineurin inhibitors (CNIs), 106–108, 113, 173, 230, 283, 291, 339,
         340, 344, 356, 379, 423, 456, 462
California Verbal Learning Test–Second Edition (CVLTII), 80
Canadian Cardiac Randomized Evaluation of Antidepressant and
         Psychotherapy Efficacy (CREATE), 206
Cannabinoid, 40, 74, 151, 185, 497
Cannabis, 38–40, 74, 151–152, 184, 496–497
Carbohydrate-deficient transferrin, 184
Carbon dioxide hyperventilation model, 256
Cardiac allograft, 231
    acute cellular rejection, 37, 231
    assessment of Immunologic Status, 199
    contraindications to Heart Transplantation, 200
    indications for heart transplantation, 197
    quality of life, 229
    re-innervation, 229
    rejection, 231
    survival rates, 229

        tobacco, 37
        transplantation (*see* Heart Transplantation)
        treatment, 232
Cardiac allograft vasculopathy (CAV)
    diagnosis, 232–233
    malignancy, 231
    morphologic features, 232
    mortality, 229
    prevention, 233
    prognosis, 233
    risk factors, 231
    treatment, 230, 233
Cardiac Arrhythmia Suppression Trial, 215
Cardiac denervation, 229, 232
Cardiac failure, 267, 268
Cardiac replacement therapy, 220, 221
Cardiac resynchronization therapy (CRT), 216
Cardiogenic shock, 197, 219, 268
Cardiac transplantation, *see* Heart transplantation
Cardiopulmonary exercise physiology test (CPX), 198
Cardiovascular disease (CVD), 63, 68, 69, 81, 114, 185, 205, 209,
         217, 428, 445, 476, 494, 498
Caspofungin (echinocandin), 176, 419
Ceftriaxone, 141
Center for Epidemiologic Studies Depression Scale (CES-D), 79, 129,
         258, 322, 370, 405
Center for International Blood and Marrow Transplant Research
         (CIBMTR), 387, 414
Centers for Medicare and Medicaid Services (CMS), 12, 32, 50, 304,
         307, 483, 519
Child-Pugh classification/class, 143
Child–Turcotte–Pugh score, 164
Chronic allograft rejection, 173
Chronic ductopenic rejection, 173
Chronic GVHD (cGHVHD), 415, 424, 425, 443
Chronic kidney disease (CKD), 63, 73–79, 82, 284
    anemia, 80, 81, 97, 106
    cardiovascular disease, 63, 68, 81, 114
    classification and prognosis, 64
    complications, 65
    definition, 63
    dialysis, 91
    epidemiology, 64
    etiologies, 64, 65
    pharmacokinetics in, 83, 98
    psychiatric disorders in, 75–82, 94, 96
    referral for transplant evaluation, 66
Chronic liver disease (CLD), 139, 142
    ALD (*see* Alcoholic liver disease (ALD))
    HBV (*see* Hepatitis B virus (HBV))
    HCV (*see* Hepatitis C virus (HCV))
    neurocognitive and neuropsychiatric manifestations
        cognitive impairment, 149
        hepatic encephalopathy, 141, 149
        porphyrias, 150
        Wilson's disease, 149, 150
    NAFLD, 148, 149
    psychotherapeutic issues, 153, 154
Chronic lung allograft dysfunction (CLAD), 268, 280, 282, 292
Chronic obstructive pulmonary disease (COPD), 247–248, 251,
         255–258, 261–263, 294, 475, 498
    BODE score, 247
    clinical factors, 247, 249
    psychiatric conditions
        anxiety, 256
        cognitive disorders, 256–257

depression, 256
severe mental illness, 256
smoking, 255
tobacco use, 255
etiology, 255
ISHLT consensus guidelines, 248
long-term survival outcomes, 247
lung volume reduction surgery, 248
pathophysiological mechanisms, 256
posttransplant survival data, 248
progression, 247
Chronic rejection, 108, 162, 173, 187, 231, 233, 279, 282, 313, 315, 338, 341, 355, 523
Chronic ulcerative colitis, 175
Chylothorax, 281
Cirrhosis
epidemiology of, 139, 140
natural history of, 140
portal hypertension complications
ascites, 140
hepatic encephalopathy, 141–142
HCC, 142
hepatocellular carcinoma, 142
hepatorenal syndrome, 140, 141
pulmonary vascular complications, 142
variceal bleeding, 141
Clinician-Administered PTSD Scale (CAPS-1), 359
Clostridium difficile (C. difficile), 175, 280, 284, 418, 419
Cocaine, 38, 74, 78, 81, 150, 197, 200
Cognitive behavioral therapy (CBT), 83, 95, 149, 151, 153–154, 206, 209–210, 258, 261, 322, 405, 442, 476
anxiety, 209
depression, 206
heart failure, 207
Cognitive behavioral therapy for insomnia (CBT-I), 96, 405
Cognitive Depression Index (CDI), 94
Cognitive disorders, 90, 345
COPD, 256–258
in heart transplant, 240
in HCT, 417
ILD, 258
in lung transplant, 262
mental disorder, 262–263
in pancreatic transplant, 345
pulmonary hypertension, 260
Cognitive impairment, 3, 29, 39, 76–80, 82, 84, 94, 96, 97, 122, 149, 186, 196, 210, 240, 256, 260, 291, 339, 402, 443, 445, 455, 458, 472, 494, 499, 507, 535
Coma depasse, 163
Continuous renal replacement therapy (CRRT), 91
Conventional Ventilatory Support Versus Extracorporeal Membrane Oxygenation for Severe Adult Respiratory Failure (CESAR), 267
Coronary artery disease (CAD), 24, 25, 28, 30, 205–208, 215, 225, 284
Coronary heart disease (CHD), 206–209
Corticosteroids, 105
face transplantation, 355
heart transplantation, 230
Hematopoietic Cell Transplantation, 401, 408, 424, 455
liver transplantation, 172, 187, 338
lung transplantation, 274, 280, 296
renal transplantation, 69
uterine transplantation, 378
CRT, *see* Cardiac resynchronization therapy
Cyclophosphamide, 105

Cyclosporine, 4, 10, 11, 40, 105, 163, 165, 173, 456, 458
calcineurin inhibitor, 105, 456
donor-specific transfusion, 106
efficacy and safety, 106
heart transplantation, 226, 230, 239, 240
hematopoietic cell transplantation, 413–415
liver transplantation, 163–165, 173–174
lung transplantation, 273, 283, 290
muromonab-CD3, 106, 175, 282
renal transplantation, 105–107, 112, 226
uterine transplantation, 379
visceral transplantation, 307
Cystic fibrosis (CF), 176, 247, 249, 255, 258, 259, 284, 291, 337, 520, 547
Cytochrome P450 (CYP 450) enzyme system, 40, 131, 152, 250, 446, 454
Cytolysis, 160, 457
Cytomegalovirus (CMV), 67, 115–116, 173, 176, 274–276, 280, 283, 285, 314, 339, 355, 356, 360, 414–415, 418, 420, 424, 426
antiviral prophylaxis and prevention, 275
oral acyclovir/ganciclovir, 274, 275
valganciclovir prophylaxis, 275

D
Daclizumab, 106, 230, 314
Death after cardiac death (DCD), 67, 112, 164, 172, 275–276, 528–530, 532, 539
Decision-making capacity, 97, 99, 408
Deep venous thrombosis (DVTs), 280
Default mode network (DMN), 32
Delayed airway stenosis, 274
Delayed graft function (DGF), 68, 112, 114, 123, 187, 455
Delirium, 3, 4, 7, 149, 150, 173, 210, 237–240, 242, 263, 270, 289–293, 296, 404, 408, 439, 441–446, 455–458, 461–463, 472–473, 524
Delis-Kaplan Executive Function System (D-KEFS), 80
Demoralization, 81, 211, 403
De novo diabetic nephropathy, 108
De novo malignancy, 337, 339
Depression, 3, 4, 18, 21, 23–31, 53, 402, 403, 499, 511, 518, 522
calcineurin Inhibitors, 456
chronic kidney disease, 74–79, 81–84, 93–99
chronic liver disease, 147, 149, 152
drug interactions, 292
end-stage lung disease, 255–262
face transplantation, 354, 357–361
heart failure, 200, 205–211, 217
heart transplantation, 237–242
hematopoietic cell transplantation, 402–406, 439–446
limb transplantation, 369–370
liver transplantation, 181–182, 186, 188
lung transplantation, 289, 292–296
pharmacotherapy (*see* Antidepressants)
polyclonal and monoclonal antibodies, 457
psychotherapy, 471, 475–477, 484–485
renal transplantation, 120–121, 123, 127, 129–131
uterine transplantation, 380
visceral transplantation, 317, 321–326, 337, 339, 344–346
Diabetes mellitus (DM), 32, 75, 82, 108, 115, 173, 174, 200, 230, 249, 280, 283, 321–323, 334, 337
Diagnosis and Statistical Manual (DSM), 6, 78, 96, 184, 261, 290, 359, 367, 370, 401, 405, 440

Dialysis, 5, 49, 55, 57, 63–70
  discontinuation, 97
  frequency, 92
  modalities, 92
  mortality rate, 64, 68, 96, 97
  psychiatric disorders
    anxiety, 79, 95
    cognitive impairment, 80, 82, 96, 97
    depression (see Depression)
    sexual dysfunction, 97
    sleep disorders, 80, 82, 95, 96
  psychopharmacology, 83, 97
  QOL, 92
  suicide, 94
Dialysis Outcomes and Practice Patterns Study (DOPPS), 93, 96
Diaphragmatic paralysis, 280
Diastolic HF, 195
Diffuse large B-cell lymphoma (DLBCL), 395
Diffuse large cell lymphoma (DLCL), 395
Disordered eating behavior (DEB), 323
Donation after brain death (DBD), 163, 276, 530
  candidates for, 530
  primary criticism, 531, 532
Donation after cardiac death (DCD), 67, 164, 275, 276, 528
  determination of circulatory death, 529
Donation Cognition Instrument (DCI), 54
Donor advocate team, 50
Donor-specific antibodies (DSAs), 112, 114, 115, 282, 313, 315, 316, 356
Double-lung transplant, 4, 20, 252, 273
Draw-A-Person test, 370
Dronabinol, 152, 185, 548
Dual-energy X-ray absorptiometry (DEXA), 303, 317, 429
Dyslipidemia, 174, 284, 428, 455, 462
Dyspnea, 142, 195, 197, 247, 250, 256–258, 280, 282, 293, 295, 391, 393, 457, 464, 518, 520, 522

E
Edmonton protocol, 343
Electroconvulsive therapy (ECT), 239
Empyema, 281, 284
Endomyocardial biopsy, 226, 231
Endoscopic retrograde cholangiography (ERC), 172
End-stage kidney disease, 103, 105–107, 521
End-stage liver disease (ESLD), 29, 31, 33, 139–144, 147, 159, 163, 174, 186, 199, 248, 303, 308, 458, 460, 506, 521, 522
  anemia, 165
  See also Cirrhosis
End-stage renal disease (ESRD), 63–65, 67, 69, 81–84, 91, 96, 121, 175, 343, 345, 459, 475, 488, 521, 542
Enhancing Recovery in Coronary Heart Disease Patients (ENRICHD) trial, 206
Epoetin, 82, 106
Epstein-Barr virus (EBV), 67, 116, 175, 231, 283, 285, 314, 339, 356, 418, 421
Epworth Sleepiness Scale (ESS), 80, 96
Escitalopram, 82, 131, 206–208, 239, 257, 259, 292, 326, 360, 444, 458
Escitalopram for DEPression in Acute Coronary Syndrome (EsDEPACS) study, 206
Estimated glomerular filtration rate (eGFR), 63, 64, 66, 67, 74, 80, 200
Estimated posttransplant survival (EPTS) scores, 67, 506
Eszopiclone, 96
European platform on ethical, legal, and psychosocial aspects of organ transplantation (ELPAT), 52

European Society for Clinical Nutrition and Metabolism (ESPEN), 331
European Society for Organ Transplantation (ESOT), 49
Evaluation of Donor Informed Consent Tool (EDICT), 54
Everolimus, 107, 113, 173, 230, 233, 240, 379, 457, 506
Expanded criteria donors (ECD), 107, 164
Extracorporeal membrane oxygenation (ECMO), 5, 202, 267–270, 530
  gas exchange, 269
  indications, 267
  management, 269–270
  psychological considerations, 270
Ex vivo lung perfusion (EVLP), 275
Eye transplantation, 357

F
Face transplantation (FT), 353
  assessment and communication strategies, 356
  course and complications after, 355
  facial disfigurement and psychological comorbidity, 354
  indication for, 353
  patient selection and psychiatric evaluation, 357, 358
  pediatric face transplantation, 358
  prevalence of facial disfigurement and, 353
  psychological assessment and outcomes, tools for, 359–361
  psychological tasks, adjusting, 358, 359
Facial Disability Index, 360
Fatigue Severity Scale (FSS), 81
Felodipine, 174
Fertility, 377–382, 407, 417, 429
Financial toxicity, 407
Fingolimod, 107
Fluconazole, 176, 419, 424
Fluoxetine, 82, 95, 97, 98, 153, 207, 208, 239, 259, 408, 444, 456, 458, 463
Focal segmental glomerulosclerosis (FSGS), 64, 116
Follicular lymphoma, 395, 396
Following Rehabilitation, Economics and Everyday-Dialysis Outcome Measurements (FREEDOM) Study, 96
Foscarnet, 176, 420
Frank-Starling principle, 229
Frequent Hemodialysis Network (FHN), 96
Functional Assessment of Chronic Illness Therapy-Fatigue (FACIT-F), 81
Functional connectivity strength (FCS) analysis, 32

G
Gabapentin, 82, 83, 95–99, 240, 257, 293, 408, 445, 456, 463
GAD, see Generalized anxiety disorder
Gastrointestinal ischemia, 274
Gastrointestinal malignancy, 69
Gastroparesis, 280–281, 333–334
Generalized anxiety disorder (GAD), 120, 129, 148, 208, 240, 256, 259, 293, 296, 322, 370, 403, 405, 462, 478, 484
Generalized Anxiety Disorder-7 scale (GAD-7), 129, 208, 240, 256, 259, 405
Glomerular disease, 65, 115, 174
Glomerular filtration rate (GFR), 63, 92, 99, 355
Glomerulonephritis, 65, 74, 108, 116
Glucocorticoids, 112, 113, 115, 283, 455
Glycemic control, 55, 174, 200, 283, 321–323, 344
Graft-versus-host disease (GVHD), 308, 311, 313, 340, 356, 387, 389, 401, 403, 406, 414, 419–430, 439–443, 474, 523
  in HCT, 387, 401, 403, 406, 414, 419–430, 439–443
  in visceral transplant, 308, 340

H

HADS, *see* Hospital Anxiety and Depression Scale
HADS-total score, 75
Haloperidol, 97, 238, 290, 445, 462
Healing of Deacon Justinian, 103
Health Care Financing Administration (HCFA), 11
Health literacy, 55, 116, 122, 186, 379, 484, 543
Health-related quality of life (HRQOL), 83, 92, 95, 148, 169, 175,
      188, 207, 240, 258, 285, 293, 295, 307, 317, 443, 511, 545
Heart disease, 27, 29, 67, 196, 198, 202, 205–211
   anxiety
      benzodiazepines, 209
      collaborative care, 209
      epidemilogy, 208–209
      multiple SSRIs, 209
      treatment, 209
   cognitive impairment
      epidemiology, 210
      treatment, 210
   depression
      epidemiology, 205, 206
      mechanisms, 206
      treatment, 206–208
   ICDs (*see* Implantable cardioverter defibrillators)
   severe mental illness, 209–210
      epidemiology, 209
      treatment, 209
   ventricular assistive devices, 210
Heart failure (HF), 195–202
   ACC/AHA stages, 196
   advanced failure (*see* Advanced heart failure)
   classification, 195
   definition, 195
   etiology, 196
   ICDs (*see* Implantable cardioverter-defibrillators)
   prevalence, 195
   stages of, 196
   symptoms, 195
   treatment options, 197
Heart Failure– A Controlled Trial Investigating Outcomes of Exercise
      Training study, 207
Heart Failure Survival Score (HFSS), 198
Heart transplantation, 10, 37, 195–202
   assessment of immunologic status, 199
   assessment for potential transplantation, 198
   cardiac denervation, 232
   contraindications, 200
   Eisenmenger syndrome, 252
   etiologies, 196
   heart failure survival score, 198
   heart transplant listing, 200
   heart transplant survivorship, 238
   history of, 225–226
   HF-related risk and perioperative risk, 198
   immediate postoperative care, 227
   immunocompatibility, 199
   immunosuppression
      induction therapy, 230
      infection, 230
      maintenance therapy, 230
      malignancy, 231
   indications, 197, 198, 227
   invasive right heart catheterization, 198
   mechanical circulatory support, 217, 221
   post-transplant outcomes, 227, 228
   quality of life, 229
   refractory left ventricular failure, 252
   rejection, 231, 232
   Revised (2017) UNOS heart allocation status, 202
   Seattle heart failure model, 198
   stages, 196
   Stanford pre-heart transplantation algorithm, 201
   treatment options, 197, 217
Hematopoietic cell transplantation (HCT), 387,
      401–450
   allogeneic sibling donors, 414
   anemia, 389, 391–394, 397, 404, 414, 445, 464
   anxiety, 401–408, 439–447
   chemotherapy-based preparative regimens, 414
   conditioning/preparative regimens, 417–418
   cytogenetics and molecular abnormalities, 391
   depression, 402–408, 439–446
   disease specific indications
      acute myelogenous leukemia (AML), 389, 391
      acute lymphoblastic leukemia, 392
      aplastic anemia, 397
      diffuse large B-cell lymphoma, 395
      follicular lymphoma, 395
      Hodgkin lymphoma (HL), 397
      lymphoma, 394–398
      mantle cell lymphoma (MCL), 396
      MDS, 393, 394
      multiple myeloma, 394
   evaluation and diagnosis
      financial burden, 407
      psychosocial needs, 407
      quality of life, 396, 402, 404–406
      screening, 405
      social support, 406, 407
   fatal post-transplant infection, 414
   global development, 388
   GVHD (*see* Graft-versus-Host disease (GVHD))
   HLA groups, 413
   indications, 390
   infectious complications
      adenovirus, 421
      antifungal and fungal species, 419
      antimicrobial resistance, 418
      C. difficile infection, 418, 419
      candidemia, 419
      CMV, 420
      DNA viruses, 418
      exogenous exposure, 418
      fecal microbiota, 422
      fever during neutropenia, 419
      fungal infection, 418
      herpesvirus family, 418
      HHV6, 421
      HSV-1, HSV-2, and VZV, 420
      HTLV-1 and HTLV-2, 419, 420
      individual risk assessment, 418
      mold-active agents, 419
      Nocardia spp., 422
      oral health, 418
      posttransplant vaccination, 422
      pre-transplant tests, 418
      PTLD, 421
      respiratory viruses, 421, 422
      timing, frequency, and severity, 419
   National Marrow Donor Program (NMDP), 414
   nonmalignant hematologic diseases, 415
   neurocognitive impairments, 443

Hematopoietic cell transplantation (HCT) (cont.)
    non-infectious complications/organ injury
        CVD, 428 (see also Graft-versus-host disease (GVHD))
        renal, 422–423
        reproduction/fertility, 429
        thyroid gland dysfunction, 429
        VOD/SOS, 423
    overall survival after, 392, 393
    palliative care, 523, 524
    patient evaluation and preparation, 388, 389
    post-HCT outcomes, 439, 440
    pre-HCT period and hospitalization, 439
    psychiatric symptoms and disorders
        anxiety, 401–403, 441
        delirium, 404, 442–443
        demoralization, 403
        depression, 402, 403, 440–441
        post-traumatic stress disorder (PTSD), 442
        substance use disorders, 407–408
        suicide, 403, 404
    sexuality and fertility, 407
    solid organ transplants, 415
    somatic symptoms, 443
        fatigue, 404, 405
        pain, 404
        sleep disorders, 405, 430
    therapeutic immunomodulatory antibodies, 430
Hemodialysis (HD), 63–66, 68, 75, 81, 83–84, 91–93, 96–97
Hepatic artery thrombosis (HAT), 170–172, 498
Hepatic encephalopathy (HE), 31, 32, 140–142, 149, 171, 186–188
Hepatic vein stenosis, 171
Hepatitis B virus (HBV), 139, 142, 148, 155
Hepatitis C virus (HCV), 112, 139, 142, 148, 150–152, 173, 200, 543
Hepatocellular carcinoma (HCC), 142, 144, 148, 151, 154, 162, 164, 170, 176, 185, 543, 544
Hepatopulmonary syndrome, 142
Hepatorenal syndrome, 140–142, 151, 187
Hernandez, Geri, 549
Herpes simplex 1 and 2 (HSV-1, HSV-2), 285, 356, 418, 420, 424
Herrick, Richard, 3, 49, 104
HF with preserved ejection fraction (HFpEF), 195
HF with reduced ejection fraction (HFrEF), 195
High-Risk Alcoholism Relapse (HRAR) score, 34–35
Hodgkin lymphoma, 397
Hospital Anxiety and Depression Scale (HADS), 73, 75–79, 94, 95, 129–130, 258–259, 370, 402, 405, 475
Human herpesvirus (HHV), 285, 421
Human immunodeficiency virus (HIV), 69, 176, 200, 249, 251, 356, 418, 476, 536
Human leukocyte antigen (HLA), 49, 105–106, 114–115, 199, 282, 388, 413
Human metapneumovirus (hMPV), 421
Human T-cell lymphotropic viruses 1 and 2 (HTLV-1/−2), 418–420
Hyperammonemia, 141, 283
Hyperkalemia, 65, 92, 333, 379, 457, 464
Hypersensitivity pneumonitis, 258
Hyponatremia, 66, 74, 99, 140, 240, 332, 340, 458, 464
Hypoxemic/hypercapnic respiratory failure, 248–250, 267, 281

I

Idiopathic interstitial pneumonia (IIP), 247–248, 250, 251
Idiopathic pulmonary arterial hypertension (IPAH), 247
Idiopathic pulmonary fibrosis (IPF), 250, 258, 275
IF-associated liver disease (IFALD), 303–304, 322, 332

ILD complicating connective tissue diseases (CTD-ILD), 258
Immune-modulatory strategy, 312
Immunosuppression, 9, 28, 49, 67–69, 104–108, 112–116, 119, 128, 143, 162, 165, 170, 173–176, 181, 186, 200, 227, 229–233, 249–250, 273, 283, 307, 312, 314–316, 323, 337–340, 344, 355–358, 365–367, 369–370, 377, 389, 394, 421, 439, 455, 478, 513, 523, 544
Immunosuppressive agents, 170, 172–175, 233, 343, 368
Impact of Event Scale, 360
Implantable cardioverter-defibrillators (ICDs), 210
    Class I recommendation, 216
    clinical trials, 216
    complications, 217
    indications, 215
    SCD (see Sudden cardiac death)
    SICD (see Subcutaneous ICD (SICD))
Independent living donor advocate (ILDA), 50, 55
Indirect calorimetry (IC), 330–331
Inflammatory bowel disease (IBD), 249, 301, 325
Informed consent, 28, 43, 51, 53, 56, 355, 370, 380–382, 506, 508, 529
Initiating Dialysis Early and Late (IDEAL) study, 92
Insomnia, 83, 95, 98, 113, 173, 241, 405, 408, 443, 455–458, 471, 476, 518, 523
    CBT, 83, 96, 98, 241
    RLS, 95–96
Interagency Registry for Mechanically Assisted Circulatory Support (INTERMACS), 218–220
Interpleural communication, 281
Interstitial lung disease (ILD), 199, 248–251, 255, 258, 295, 427
    anxiety, 258
    cognitive disorders, 258
    CTD-ILD, 258
    depression, 258
    hypersensitivity pneumonitis, 258
    idiopathic pulmonary fibrosis, 258
    pulmonary rehabilitation programs, 258
    sarcoidosis, 258
    symptoms, 258
Intestinal adaptation, 304
Intestinal dysmotility, 329
Intestinal failure, 329
    causes, 329
    complications, 329
    definition, 301, 329
    etiologies, 301
        acute volvulus, 302
        adult motility disorders, 302
        Crohn's disease (CD), 302
        intra-abdominal malignancy, 302
        mesenteric ischemia, 301
        re-transplantation, 303
    history, 301
    management, 329
    manifestations, 329
Intestinal failure-associated liver disease (IFALD), 303, 324
Intestinal immunogenicity, 341
Intestinal rehabilitation, 304
Intestinal transplant (ITx), see Visceral allograft
Intravenous immunoglobulin (IVIG), 112, 115
Invasive aspergillosis, 176, 285
Invasive self-care behaviors, 322
Ischemic cardiomyopathy (ICM), 30, 196, 239
Islet transplant alone (ITA), 343
Isolated intestinal transplantation, 308, 337, 522
Itraconazole, 176, 419

K

Kaposi sarcoma, 116, 283
Kidney Disease Improving Global Outcomes (KDIGO)
        group, 63, 65
Kidney Disease Outcomes Quality Initiative (KDOQI) workgroup, 92
Kidney Disease Quality of Life (KDQOL) Short Form version 1.3
        (KDQOL-SF 1.3), 93
Kidney donation, 49, 55, 57, 70
Kidney donor profile index (KDPI), 67, 111, 506
Kidney Donor Risk Index (KDRI), 111
Kidney donors, 49
    laparoscopy, 51
    long-term psychosocial outcomes, 56
    psychosocial evaluation, 51
    Rotterdam Renal Replacement Knowledge-Test, 54
Kidney replacement therapy, 107
Kidney transplantation, 10, 49, 57, 63, 66
    evaluation factors
        age, 67, 68
        cardiovascular disease, 68
        cerebrovascular disease, 68
        frailty, 69
        gastrointestinal malignancy, 69
        hematologic disease, 68
        infection, 69
        malignancy, 68
        obesity, 68
        peripheral vascular disease, 68
        psychosocial evaluation, 69
        surgical evaluation, 69
    indications, 66
    living donation, 70
    medical evaluation, 67
    timing of referral, 66, 67 (see also Renal transplantation)
Kidney transplant (KT) recipients, 28, 37
    psychosocial problems
        clinical intervention for, 131
        mental health problems, 120, 121, 123, 127
        nonadherence to medical regimen, 120, 122–124, 126
        substance use, 121, 122, 124, 127
    psychosocial screening, 128, 132
        mental health problems, 130
        nonadherence to medical regimen, 128, 130
        substances use, 130
    retransplantation rate, 119
Kidney xenotransplantation, 160

L

LAM, see Lymphangioleiomyomatosis
Langerhans cell histiocytosis, 247
Lansky and Karnofsky performance scores, 318
LDAT, see Live Donor Assessment Tool
LDKT, see Living donor kidney transplantation
LDLT, see Living donor liver transplantation
Left ventricular assist device (LVAD), 197, 198, 202, 218–222, 519
Left ventricular (LV) function, 195
Limb transplantation, 365
    bioethical issues, 371
    donor family contact, 371
    evaluation, psychosocial domains, 367
        adherence, 367
        body image issues, 368
        motivation and expectations, 367
        psychological reactions, 368
        social support, 367, 368

financial support, 371
    follow-up care, 369
    history and medical course, 366
    informed consent, 370, 371
    pain related to amputation and phantom limb pain, 368
    psychosocial contraindications, 368
    psychosocial evaluation, tools for
        interview guidelines and qualitative assessment,
            369, 370
        psychometric screening, 369, 370
    risk-benefit ratio, 369
    selection of, 367
    technical/anatomic issues, 370
    tolerate loss of function, ability to, 371
Lithium, 74, 82, 97–98, 153, 183, 240, 445, 456,
    464–465
Live donor
    acute recovery period, 55, 56
    ambivalence, 53
    donor surgery, 55, 56
    ethics of live donation, 56, 57
    evaluation process, 51
    expectations after donation, 53
    ILDA, 55
    informed consent process, 53
    kidney transplant evaluation, 70
    long-term outcomes, 55, 56
    medical and surgical evaluation, 50, 51
    motivation, 52
    psychiatric disorders, 54
    psychosocial assessment tools
        Donation Cognition Instrument, 54
        Evaluation of Donor Informed Consent Tool, 54
        Likert scales, 54
        Live Donor Assessment Tool, 54
        Living Donation Expectancies
            Questionnaire, 54
        Psychosocial Assessment Tool, 54
        Rotterdam Renal Replacement Knowledge-Test, 54
        Stanford Integrated Psychosocial
            Assessment Tool, 55
    psychosocial evaluation, 50, 54
    psychosocial factor, 51, 52
    relationship with recipient, 52
    social support network, 53, 54
    stability in life, 53, 54
    substance use disorders, 54
    unhealthy coping, 54
Live Donor Assessment Tool (LDAT), 54, 55, 379
Living organ donor Psychosocial Assessment Tool (EPAT), 54
    adverse psychosocial outcomes, 17–18
    evidence-based guidelines, 18
    medical listing criteria per end-organ system, 17, 20
    negative medical outcomes, 17
    OPTN/UNOS guidelines, 17
    post-transplant psychosocial outcomes, 19
    pre-transplant assessment tools, 22
    pre-transplant evaluation, 21
    pre-transplant psychosocial vulnerability markers, 19
    Psychosocial Assessment of Candidates for
        Transplantation, 21, 22
    psychosocial consultants, 19
    psychosocial eligibility criteria, 18
    Psychosocial Levels System, 21
    Transplant Evaluation Rating Scale, 21, 22
    transplant recipient selection process, 21

Liver disease
    ALD (*see* Alcoholic liver disease (ALD))
    CLD (*see* Chronic liver disease (CLD))
    common mental health disorders
        AUD (*see* Alcohol use disorder (AUD))
        depression, 150
        marijuana, 151, 152
        opioid use disorders, 151
        pain in cirrhosis, 152
        pharmacotherapy, 152, 153
        tobacco use, 151
Liver donation, 49, 52, 54–56
Liver donors, 49
    anatomy, 51
    EDICT, 54
    long-term psychosocial outcomes, 56
Liver-intestinal allograft, 308, 310
Liver transplantation (LT)
    for ALD, 24, 33, 35
    history, 166
        artificial ventilation, 163
        Atlantic, first human successes, 162
        coma depasse, 163
        donor and recipient operation, 163
        early surgical and immunological barriers, outcomes of, 160
        ESLD, 159
        evaluation process, 143
        first human attempt and moratorium, 161, 162
        governing fair organ allocation, 164
        next generation of strategies, 165, 166
        organ shortage drives surgical innovation, 164, 165
        preclinical successes with, 160, 161
    immediate surgical complications
        hepatic artery thrombosis, 171
        portal vein thrombosis, 171
        primary allograft nonfunction, 171
        small-for-size syndrome, 170
    indications for, 142
        evaluation process, 143, 144
        timing of, 143
    late medical complications
        chronic allograft rejection, 173
        CKD, 174, 175
        de novo malignancies, development of, 175
        diabetes mellitus, 173, 174
        dyslipidemia, 174
        fatigue and quality of life of transplant recipient, 175
        fertility, sexuality and pregnancy, 175
        hypertension, 174
        immunization, 176
        immunosuppressive agents, 173
        obesity, 174
        opportunistic infections, 175, 176
        osteopenia and osteoporosis, 174
        prognosis, 176
        recurrence of primary disease, 176
    late surgical complications
        biliary tract abnormalities, 171, 172
        hepatic vein stenosis, 171
    medical course and recovery from, 170
    timing of liver transplantation, 143
    waiting period, 154
Liver transplantation (LT) recipients
    cognitive recovery post-liver transplantation, 186, 187
    immunization, 176
    mental health and behavioral issues
        depression and anxiety, 181, 182

        psychotic disorders, 182, 183
    methadone maintenance therapy, 185
    pharmacologic considerations, 187, 188
    posttransplant quality of life and employment, 188, 189
    substance use and disorders
        alcohol use, 183, 184
        issues, 181
        marijuana use, 184, 185
        nonalcohol substance use disorders, 185
        tobacco use, 185
    treatment adherence, 185, 186
Living Donation Expectancies Questionnaire (LDEQ), 54
Living donor kidney transplantation (LDKT), 49, 50
Living donor liver transplantation (LDLT), 49, 51, 52, 56, 57, 164–166
L-ornithine-L-aspartate (LOLA), 141
Lung allocation score (LAS), 17, 250, 275, 543
Lung transplantation, 549
    absolute contraindications, 252
    airway complications, 273, 274
    contraindications, 252
    COPD (*see* Chronic obstructive pulmonary disease (COPD))
    cystic fibrosis (*see* Cystic fibrosis (CF))
    cytomegalovirus, 274, 275
    donation after cardiac death, 275, 276
    donor lung preservation solutions, 274
    early surgical history, 273
    ex vivo lung perfusion, 275, 276
    Final Rule, 275
    follow-up care, 285
    idiopathic pulmonary fibrosis (*see* Idiopathic pulmonary fibrosis (IPF))
    immunosuppressant regimens, 274
    indications
        A1AT deficiency, 248
        COPD, 247, 248
        cystic fibrosis, 247, 249
        idiopathic interstitial pneumonia, 247, 250
        idiopathic pulmonary arterial hypertension, 247
        LAM, 249
        non-CF bronchiectasis, 249
        pulmonary hypertension, 250, 251
    lung allocation score, 275
    median survival, 285
    overall prognosis, 285
    pulmonary hypertension (*see* Pulmonary hypertension (PH))
    timely referral, 247
Lung volume reduction surgery (LVRS), 248
Lymphangioleiomyomatosis (LAM), 247, 249
Lymphoma, 68, 116, 175, 231, 283, 343, 356, 389, 394–397, 401, 403, HCT

M
Magnetic resonance cholangiopancreatography (MRCP), 172
Major adverse cardiac events (MACE), 208, 233
Major depressive disorder (MDD), 29, 31, 75, 77–79, 82, 83, 93, 148, 150, 206, 239, 292, 322, 326, 440, 478
Malnutrition, 65–66, 96, 140, 149, 196, 252, 284, 302, 329–330, 425, 429
Mammalian target of rapamycin (mTOR) inhibitors, 106–107, 113, 165, 173–176, 230, 233, 312, 356, 423
Mantle cell lymphoma (MCL), 396, 397
Marijuana, 18, 38–40, 55, 121, 122, 124, 151–152, 184–185, 496–497, 501, 536
    carcinogenic effects, 38
    consideration for listing, 38
    effect of short term use, 39

fungal contaminants, 39
legalization, 40
negative psychosocial effects, 39
pharmacokinetic effects, 40
potency, 39
Marsupialization, 113
post-transplant complications, 184
Mechanical circulatory support (MCS)
advanced care planning, 222
advanced heart failure, 217
adverse events
bleeding complications, 221
infections, 221
neurologic events, 221
pump thrombosis and hemolysis, 222
right ventricular failure, 221
valvular heart disease, 222
end-of-life decision making, 222
Mechanical ventilation support, 269
Mechanistic Target of Rapamycin (mTOR) Inhibitors, 457
Medical Cannabis Organ Transplant Act, 184
Medical decisions to end life (MDEL), 475
Medicare ESRD Program, 63
Memantine, 97, 99, 240
Membranoproliferative glomerulonephritis (MPGN), 65, 74, 116
Mesenteric ischemia, 301–302
Metabolic bone disease, 174, 303, 305, 324, 332
Metabolic complications
acute kidney injury, 283
chronic kidney disease, 284
diabetes mellitus, 283
dyslipidemia, 284
hyperammonemia, 283
osteopenia, 284
osteoporosis, 284
Metabolic syndrome (MetS), 32, 139, 173, 199, 428, 455
Methadone, 151, 465, 497, 499
Methadone maintenance therapy (MMT), 185, 497
Metoprolol, 174, 208, 458
Microchimerism, 166
Microdroplet lymphocytotoxicity test, 105
Mindfulness-based cognitive therapy (MBCT), 258, 323, 476–477
Mindfulness-based stress reduction (MBSR), 83, 127, 153, 239–240, 476, 477, 486
Mineral bone disease (MBD), 66, 70, 98
Mini-International Neuropsychiatric Interview (MINI) score, 83, 261, 360
Mini Mental Status Examination (MMSE), 97
Minnesota Multiphasic Personality Inventory PTSD Scale (MMPI-PTSD), 360
Mirtazapine, 98, 206, 208, 239, 257, 259, 292–293, 326, 408, 444, 459
Mobilized peripheral blood (MPB), 419
Modafinil, 82, 99, 175, 446, 456, 461
Model for End-Stage Liver Disease (MELD) score, 17, 20, 42, 143–144, 164, 182, 188, 357, 506, 522
"Modified" multivisceral transplantation, 308
Monoamine Oxidase Inhibitors (MAOIs), 444, 460
Montreal Cognitive Assessment (MoCA), 80, 97, 263, 291
Mood disorders, *see* Depression
Morbid obesity, 25, 174
Motivational enhancement therapy (MET), 151
Motivational interviewing (MI), 53–54, 126, 131, 150, 183, 186, 294, 477, 479, 500
Mucositis, 402, 404, 417–419, 425, 442
Multicenter Automatic Defibrillator Implantation Trial I (MADIT-I), 216
"Multi-organ" transplantation, 308

Multiple myeloma, 389, 391, 394, 401, 517
Multivisceral allografts, 308
Multivisceral and intestinal (MV/I) transplants, 323
intestinal failure, 324
parenteral nutrition
chronic etiologies, 325
"eating for survival", 324
estimated annual cost, 324
loss of autonomy and dependence, 324
physical complications and risks, 324
physical risks, 324
psychiatric comorbidities, 325
psychiatric evaluation, 324
pre-transplant psychosocial assessment, 324
short bowel syndrome, 324
survival rates, 323
Multivisceral/intestinal post-transplant, 345–347
Multivisceral transplantation (MVTx), 304, 307–308, 310–312, 314, 337
Muromonab-CD3, 106, 282
Mycobacterium tuberculosis, 39, 418
Mycophenolate mofetil, 106, 107, 112, 173–175, 230, 457
Mycophenolic acid, 165, 173, 175, 457
Myeloablative TBI, 417
Myelodysplasia, 390–391, 394
Myelodysplastic syndromes (MDS), 393, 394
Myocardial Infarction and Depression Intervention Trial (MIND-IT), 206

N
Nabilone, 152, 185
National Comprehensive Cancer Network (NCCN), 405, 440, 444, 447
National Conference of Commissioners on Uniform State Laws, 106
National Kidney Foundation (NKF), 54, 106
National Kidney Registry (NKR), 57
National Marrow Donor Program (NMDP), 414
National Organ Transplant Act (NOTA), 9–13, 105, 106, 164
Nicardipine, 174
Nicotine replacement therapy, 131, 151, 257
Nicotine use, 23, 33, 37, 144
N-methyl D-aspartate (NMDA) antagonists, 97, 99, 210
Nonalcoholic fatty liver (NAFL), 148
Nonalcoholic fatty liver disease (NAFLD), 139, 148, 149, 151
Nonalcoholic steatohepatitis (NASH), 36, 139, 147–148, 176
Non-anastomotic strictures, 172
Non-CF bronchiectasis, 249
Non-cutaneous malignancies, 231
Non-directed donors (NDD), 52, 57
Non-HLA-identical donor organs, 225
Nonidentical twin transplantation, 105
Nonischemic cardiomyopathy, 196, 215–216, 227
Norfloxacin, 141
Normothermic ex vivo perfusion technology, 316
Nutrition assessment, 330
Nutrition therapy, 332

O
Obesity, 68, 174
Obstructive sleep apnea (OSA), 241
Octreotide, 141
Opiate use disorder, 326
Opioid maintenance therapy (OMT), 151
Opioid use disorder, 54
Opportunistic infections, 175, 176

Oral Mucositis Daily Questionnaire (OMDQ), 404
Organ Donation and Recovery Improvement Act, 12
Organ procurement, 10–13, 17, 106, 164, 275, 527, 530, 533, 536, 539–542
Organ Procurement and Transplantation Network (OPTN), 10–13, 17–18, 42, 49, 57, 106–107, 275, 338–339, 341, 505–506, 509, 536
Organ procurement organizations (OPOs), 10–13
Organ sale, 52
Organ shortage, 13, 108, 164–166, 545
Organ transplant social work
    caregivers, 487, 488
    CMS mandates, 483
    discharge planning, 485
    documentation, 485
    financial stability, 484, 485
    fundraising, 485
    Internet resources, 487
    peer support, 486
    post-transplant intervention, 486
    psychoeducation, 484
    psychosocial evaluation, 483–484
    therapeutic interventions, 485–486
Orthotopic heart transplantation, 227–228
Osteopenia, 174, 284
Osteoporosis, 113, 174, 230, 252, 280, 284, 303, 334, 429, 523

P
Paced Auditory Serial Addition tests, 345
Palliative care
    CF, 520
    definition, 517
    depression, 518, 522–523
    end-stage lung disease, 520
    ESLD, 521, 522
    ESRD, 521
    HCT, 523, 524
    heart failure, 518–519
    individualized patient- and family-centered care, 517
    interdisciplinary team, 517
    ITx, 522, 523
    patients' disease process, 518
    transplant process, 518
    treatment goals, 518
    VADs, 519
Pancreas transplant
    post-transplant, 343
        fear of hypoglycemia and QOL peri-pancreas transplant, 344
        indications for, 343, 344
        psychiatric comorbidities, sexual dysfunction, and cognitive disorders, 345
        psychological evaluation of, 343
    type 1 diabetes (see Type 1 diabetes (T1D))
Pancreas transplant alone (PTA), 343
Panel reactive antibody (PRA), 112, 114
Parainfluenza viruses (PIV), 421
Parathyroid hormone (PTH), 66
Parenteral nutrition (PN)
    acute post-transplant phase, 333, 334
    adverse effects
        catheter-related bloodstream infections (CRBSI), 303
        IF-Associated Liver Disease (IFALD), 303
        metabolic bone disease, 303
    chronic post-transplant phase, 334
    CRBSI, 303
    electrolyte imbalances, 303
    fluid overload, 303

IFALD, 303
Intestinal Transplant Registry (ITR), 329
    definition, 329
    indications, 329
    intestinal adaptation, 304
    intestinal rehabilitation, 304
    management, 329
    mechanical obstruction, 329
    metabolic bone disease, 303
    MV/I transplants (see MV/I transplants)
    outcomes, 303
    pathophysiological conditions, 329
    Protein–Calorie Malnutrition, 329
    specialized rehabilitation programs, 329
Paroxysmal ventricular arrhythmias, 210
Patient Health Questionnaire-9 (PHQ-9), 93, 129–130, 259–260, 296, 370, 405
Pediatric End-Stage Liver Disease (PELD) systems, 164, 506
Pediatric transplantation
    adherence, 512
    medical evaluation, 505, 506
    medical outcomes, 510
    psychosocial evaluation, 506–508
    psychosocial outcomes, 511
    selection/listing process, 508, 509
    transitioning, 513
    waiting list, 509–510
Pediatric Transplant Rating Instrument (P-TRI), 507
Penile injuries, 381
Penile transplantation, 381–382
    societal acceptance, 382
Peribronchiolar and intraluminal fibrosis process, 427
Periodic limb movement disorder (PLMD), 95
Periodic limb movement syndrome (PLMS), 80
Peritoneal dialysis (PD), 63–64, 73, 80, 91, 93–96, 521
Personality disorders, 30–31, 54, 148, 150, 292, 324, 357, 368, 467, 472, 495
PGD, see Primary graft dysfunction (PGD)
P-glycoprotein (P-gp), 40, 454–457, 459–460, 465, 497
Phantom limb pain, 368
Phosphodiesterase type 5 (PDE5) inhibitors, 241
Phrenic nerve injury, 280, 284
Physicians Orders for Life-Sustaining Treatment (POLST), 518
Piper Fatigue Scale (PFS), 81
Pittsburgh Sleep Quality Index (PSQI), 96
Pleural complications, 281
Pleural effusions, 280, 281
PN-associated liver disease (PNALD), see also IF-associated liver disease (IFALD), 326, 332
Pneumocystis pneumonia (PCP), 340
Pneumothorax, 217, 249–250, 280, 281, 303
Pocket Personal Assistant for Tracking Health (Pocket PATH), 295
Polycystic liver disease, 176
Porphyrias, 150
Portal vein thrombosis (PVT), 171
Portocaval shunt, 161, 170
Portopulmonary hypertension, 142
Posterior reversible encephalopathy syndrome (PRES), 291
Post-lung transplantation
    adherence, 294, 295
    anxiety, 293
    depression, 292
    infectious
        bacterial infections, 284
        fungal infections, 285
        viral infections, 285
    intravenous drug use, 294
    methylphenidate, 294

neuropsychiatric disorders
 cognitive impairment, 291, 292
 delirium, 290
 headaches, 291
 PRES, 291
 seizures, 291
 toxic-metabolic encephalopathy, 291
 tremors, 291
noninfectious (*see* noninfectious complications)
patient qualitative experience, 289–290
pentazocine, 294
PTG (*see* Posttraumatic growth (PTG))
PTSD-T, 293
QOL, 295
smoking, 294
talc (magnesium silicate), 294
tobacco use, 293
Post-transplant lymphoproliferative disorder (PTLD), 116, 175, 231, 283, 311–312, 314, 316, 339–340, 356, 421, 457, 523
Post-transplant primary graft dysfunction (PGD), 267–268, 279–281, 283, 285
Posttraumatic growth (PTG), 295
Post-traumatic stress disorder (PTSD), 24–25, 31, 95, 181–182, 208–210, 217, 237–238, 240–241, 263, 270, 289, 293, 325, 354, 357–360, 368, 370, 382, 441–444, 478
Post-traumatic stress disorder associated with transplantation (PTSD-T), 24–25, 31, 263, 289, 293, 296, 478
Posttraumatic stress symptoms (PTSS), 442
PPSV23 vaccination, 176
Prednisolone, 162
Prednisone, 107, 112, 114, 225, 274, 355–356, 441, 455
Pregabalin, 96
Primary graft dysfunction (PGD), 279, 280
Primary graft non-function (PNF), 112
Primary parenchymal disease, 199
Primary sclerosing cholangitis, 175
Profile of Mood State (POMS), 345
Proliferation signal inhibitors, 230
Protein-calorie malnutrition (PCM), 329, 330
Psychiatric disorders
 cognitive impairment, 240
 *d*elirium, 238
 depression
  manic and hypomanic episodes, 240
  non-pharmacological treatment, 239
  prevalence, 239
  psychopharmacological treatment, 239
 generalized anxiety disorder, 240
 mild neuropsychiatric side effects, 238
 PTSD, 240
 sexual dysfunction, 241
 sleep disorders, 241
Psychiatric medications
 AEDs, 463–464
 antipsychotics, 462
 atypical antipsychotics, 462–463
 benzodiazepines, 461–462
 bupropion, 460
 buspirone, 462
 dexmedetomidine, 465
 haloperidol, 462
 herbal supplements, 460
 lithium, 464
 MAOIs, 460
 mirtazapine, 459
 nefazodone, 460
 SNRIs, 459
 SSRIs, 458, 459

 stimulants, 461
 substance use disorders, 464, 465
 TCAs, 460
 trazodone, 460
 vilazodone, 459
 vortioxetine, 460
Psychiatric risk classification, 21, 26
Psychiatric syndromes, 210–211
Psychodynamic psychotherapy (PDT)
 cancer patients, 472
 countertransference, 473
 medically ill patients, 472
 medical professionals, 473
 patient-doctor relationship, 474
 personality attributes and coping styles, 473
 poor transplant outcomes, 472
 psychological mechanisms, 472
 stress hospitalized patients, 472, 473
Psychoeducational interventions, 84
Psychological distress, 401, 406
Psychological stability, 29–33
Psychometric Hepatic Encephalopathy Score, 187
Psychosocial Assessment of Candidates for Transplantation (PACT), 21, 22, 544
Psychosocial consultants, 4, 5, 9, 19, 23
Psychosocial distress, 406
Psychosocial Levels System (PLS), 21
Pulmonary arterial hypertension (PAH), *see* Pulmonary hypertension
Pulmonary aspergillosis, 39
Pulmonary embolism (PE), 280
Pulmonary fibrosis, 549
Pulmonary hypertension (PH), 4, 250, 251
 epidemiology and risk factors, 260
 mental disorders
  anxiety, 261, 262
  childhood physical/sexual abuse, 263
  cognitive disorders, 262–263
  depression, 261, 262
  overall psychosocial risk, 261
  prior abuse history, 263
  tobacco and alcohol use, 262
 treatment
  anxiety, 260, 261
  depression, 260, 261
Pulmonary vascular disease, 199
Pulmonary vein occlusion, 281

Q

Quality of life (QoL), 75–78, 81–84, 92–97, 99, 148, 150, 154, 175, 181–182, 188–189, 255–262, 289, 292–293, 295, 307, 317, 321–326, 329, 334–335, 344–347, 354–356, 358–361, 366–367, 369, 402–409, 440, 442, 506, 510–511, 517, 519–523
 definition, 443
 dialysis, 92–97
 end-stage lung disease, 255–261
 enteral & parenteral nutrition, 329, 334–335
 ESLD, 148, 150, 154
 face transplantation, 355, 358–361
 Palliative care transplant patients, 517, 519–523
 Pediatric populations, 505–506, 510–511
 post_HCT, 402, 406, 409, 440, 442–443
 post- limb transplantation, 366–367, 369
 post-Liver Transplantation, 175, 181, 182, 188–189
 post-lung transplant, 289, 292–293, 295
 post- visceral transplantation, 307, 317, 325–327, 344–347
 Quality of Life Inventory (QOLI), 346

R

Rejection, 17, 21, 24–25, 28, 37, 40, 68–69, 112–115, 123, 125–126,
130, 170, 173–174, 182, 186–187, 199, 229–233, 239, 241,
262, 279–283, 285, 291, 293, 303, 308, 312–315, 323,
333–334, 337–341, 355–356, 358, 368–370, 379, 381,
455–457, 460, 464
   end-stage lung disease, 262
   ESRD, 68–69, 112–115, 123, 125–126, 130
   influenced by psychosocial factors, 17, 21, 24–25, 28, 37, 40
   post-face transplantation, 355–356, 358
   post-HCT, 455–457, 460, 464
   post-heart transplantation, 199, 229–233, 239, 241
   post-limb transplantation, 368–370
   post-liver transplantation, 170, 173–174, 182, 186–187
   post-lung transplantation, 279–283, 285, 291, 293
   post-uterine transplantation, 379, 381
   post-visceral transplantation, 303, 308, 312–315, 323, 333–334, 337–341
Renal and Lung Living Donors Evaluation (RELIVE) study, 56
Renal replacement therapy (RRT), 63, 73, 91, 99, 283, 455
Renal transplantation
   ceasing dialysis, 112
   complications
      BK virus, 155
      cytomegalovirus, 115–116
      disease recurrence, 116
      Epstein-Barr virus, 116
      nonadherence, 116
      posttransplantation lymphoproliferative disorder, 116
      rejection and graft loss, 114, 115
      skin cancer, 116
      ureteric strictures, 115
      urinary tract infection, 115
   current state and challenges, 107, 108
   donor quality, 111
   early twentieth century, 103
   expanding pharmacopeia and age of generics, 106, 107
   history, 103
   immediate postoperative complications
      bleeding and hemorrhage, 113
      lymphocele, 113
      typical hospital course and discharge, 114
      urologic, 113
      vascular, 113
      wound infection, 113
   immunosuppression, 112
   indications, 63
   non-identical twin transplantation, 105
   post-operative course, 112–113
   post-transplant course, 114
   postwar revival, 103–105
   scheduling transplant, 111
   surgery, 112
Repeatable Battery for the Assessment of Neuropsychological Status
(RBANS), 187, 263
Respiratory syncytial virus (RSV), 280, 282, 421–422
Resting energy expenditure (REE), 331
Restless legs syndrome (RLS), 77, 80–82, 95–96, 98, 463
Restrictive allograft syndrome (RAS), 280, 282
Rifabutin, 173
Rifampin, 173
Right ventricular (RV) failure, 221, 251–252, 281
Rituximab, 112, 115–116, 231–232, 282, 338, 356, 421, 430, 457
Rokitansky syndrome, 377–378
Ropinirole, 82, 96
RorschachTest, 370

Rotigotine, 82, 96
Rotterdam Renal Replacement Knowledge-Test (R3K-T), 54

S

Sarcoidosis, 197, 248, 258
SCD-HeFT trial, 216
Scientific Registry of Transplant Recipients (SRTR), 9, 12, 509
Seattle Heart Failure Model (SHFM), 198, 201
Second-generation antipsychotic medications, 326
Seizures, 291
Selective serotonin reuptake inhibitors (SSRIs)
   anxiety, 95, 209, 240, 257, 259–261, 293
   citalopram, 82, 98, 131, 206–208, 239, 257, 292, 326, 444, 458
   depression, 206, 207, 239, 257, 259–261, 292
   escitalopram, 82, 131, 206, 208, 239, 257, 259, 292, 326, 360, 444, 458
   fluoxetine, 82, 95, 97–98, 153, 207, 239, 259, 408, 444, 456, 458, 463
   fluvoxamine, 131, 208, 456, 459
   medical conditions and co-administration, 206–208, 239, 458
   paroxetine, 95, 98, 207, 239, 257, 408, 444, 457–458
   platelet dysfunction, 458, 463
   QTc prolongation, 207
   sertraline, 458
      Sertraline Against Depression and Heart Disease in Chronic
Heart Failure (SADHART-CHF), 207
      Sertraline Antidepressant Heart Attack Randomized Trial
(SADHART), 206
Serious and persistent mental illness (SPMI), 81
Serotonin Norepinephrine Reuptake Inhibitors (SNRIs), 207, 459
Sertraline, 83, 97
Serum-ascites albumin gradient (SAAG), 140
Severe mental illness
   antipsychotic agents, 209, 210
   development and progression, 209
   epidemiology, 209
   in COPD, 256
Sexual dysfunction, 75–78, 93, 96–98, 210–211, 238, 241, 292, 345, 407, 428, 442–443, 522
Sexual function, 56, 75, 80, 345, 360–361, 379–381, 407, 473
Sexuality, 175, 317, 345, 379, 381, 407
Short bowel syndrome, 301, 324–326, 329
Short gut syndrome (SGS), 308, 510
Sildenafil, 175, 241
Sinusoidal obstruction syndrome, 422–423
SIPAT, *see* Stanford Integrated Psychosocial Assessment for
Transplantation
Sirolimus, 106, 107, 113, 173, 175, 230, 233, 239, 281, 291, 338, 356, 379, 457
6-mercaptopurine (6-MP), 105–106, 161, 457
Skin allotransplantation, 160
Skin cancer, 36, 67–68, 116, 144, 175, 231, 256, 283, 425
Sleep-disordered breathing (SDB), 95–96
Sleep disorders, 77, 80, 82, 95, 96, 98, 241, 326, 405, 430
Sleep disturbances, 76, 80, 92, 210, 339, 405, 430, 443
Small-for-size syndrome (SFSS), 169–170
Smoking
   Alcohol, Smoking and Substance Involvement Screening Test
(ASSIST), 129
   CAD, 68
   cessation, 127, 131, 206, 257, 261, 294, 357, 476, 494, 497
   chronic kidney disease, 498
   cerebrovascular disease, 68
   consequences, 36, 37, 54, 121, 124, 206, 209, 493, 497–498
   contraindication to transplantation, 37, 69, 497–498

COPD, 255–256
decreased survival, 498
marijuana use, 38, 39
mental illness, 150, 255–256
pharmacology, 454, 455, 460–462
post-HCT Transplantation, 418
post-heart transplantation, 28, 31, 37, 238
post-liver transplantation, 37, 151, 185, 498
post-lung transplantation, 37, 185, 250, 255, 261–263, 284, 294, 296
post-renal transplantation, 121
post-visceral transplantation, 303
renal transplant recipients, 498
Social support, 1, 3–4, 18, 21–23, 25, 28–31, 33–34, 41–42, 53–55,
77, 82, 92–93, 116, 122–123, 125, 144, 182–184, 200–201,
206, 220, 237–241, 252, 260–263, 292–293, 295, 308,
315–316, 324, 331, 339, 341, 346, 354, 357, 361, 367–368,
388, 401, 403, 406–407, 409, 439, 441–443, 471–472, 486,
494–496, 499, 506–508, 512–513, 535–536
Solid organ transplant shortage, 19
Solute-linked carrier (SLC) transporters, 454
Somatic symptoms
fatigue, 404, 405
pain, 404
sleep disorders, 405
Spontaneous bacterial peritonitis (SBP), 140, 142, 152
Squamous cell carcinoma (SCC), 116, 356, 425
Stanford Integrated Psychosocial Assessment for Transplantation
(SIPAT), 22–23, 26, 40–42, 55, 211, 379, 544
domain measurement, 23
patient's level of readiness, 26–28
psychological stability and psychopathology, 29–33
social support system, 28–29
Effects of Substance Use, 33–40
influence on other tools, 55
multinational scales, 544
psychometric qualities, 40–42
specific psychosocial variables, inclusion of, 23–26
Stanford Pediatric Psychosocial Optimization Tool (SPPOT), 507
Stanford pre-heart transplantation algorithm, 201
State-Trait Anxiety Inventory (STAI), 261, 360, 370
Stepwise Psychotherapy Intervention for Reducing Risk in Coronary
Artery Disease (SPIRR-CAD) trial, 206
Streptococcal mitis, 419
Structured Clinical Interview for DSM Disorders (SCID), 73, 75–80,
95–96, 370
Subcutaneous ICD (SICD), 215
Subjective global assessment (SGA), 330
Substance use disorder (SUD), 4–5, 23, 33, 38–39, 51, 54, 81, 94–95,
121, 122, 124, 127, 130, 143–144, 150, 183, 185, 200,
293–294, 325, 345, 354, 357, 368, 379, 407, 408, 447, 464,
487, 493–495, 499–500, 511
adherence, effect on, 367, 494
anxiety, 95, 354
candidacy, effect on transplant, 4, 54, 143, 200, 211, 325, 354, 357,
367–368, 379, 401, 404, 407, 495–496, 499–500
donor candidacy, effect on, 51, 54, 150, 153, 380
effect on health, 147, 150
epidemiology, 493
screening tools, 129
prevalence, 81, 493
SIPAT score, influence on, 23, 33, 42
social support system, effect on, 29, 487
suicide, influence on, 94
transplant outcomes, influence on, 4, 18, 23, 29, 33, 38–40, 119,
121, 124, 127–131, 181, 183, 185, 186, 218, 241, 293, 324,
345, 495, 511
treatment, 8, 127, 464

Sudden cardiac death (SCD)
primary prevention, 215, 216
secondary prevention, 215
Suicide, 403, 404
contraindication to transplantation, as, 18, 357
medical conditions increasing suicide risk, 94, 95, 97, 150, 403, 441
predictor of negative transplant outcome, as, 21, 25, 31, 56, 211,
353, 360
Supplemental Security Income (SSI), 485
Syndrome of inappropriate antidiuretic hormone secretion
(SIADH), 66
Synthetic cannabinoids, 74
Systolic HF, 195, 197

T
Tacrolimus, 40, 106–107, 112, 125, 307, 340, 355, 456–457, 477, 497
side effects, 173, 230, 291, 346, 379, 456–457, 462
Talc (magnesium silicate), 294
T-cell cytolytic agents, 230
T-cell-mediated (cellular) rejection (TCMR), 338
Telephone-based cognitive behavioral (T-CBT) intervention, 442
Telephone-based mindfulness-based stress reduction (tMBSR), 83
Terlipressin, 141, 170
Tetrahydrocannabinol (THC), 38
See also Marijuana
Thematic Apperception Test, 370
Thrombotic microangiopathy (TMA), 423
Thymoglobulin, 114, 312, 314, 338, 457
Tobacco smoke exposure, 37
Tobacco use, 36, 37, 54, 56, 121, 124, 129, 151, 296, 408, 498
effect on health, 36, 56
COPD, 255, 257, 263
epidemiology and risk factors, 493
post organ transplantation, 37, 54, 121, 124, 151, 185, 189, 200,
263, 293, 494–495, 497–498
treatment, 257
Tofacitinib, 107
Topiramate, 83–84, 445, 464
Total artificial heart (TAH), 202, 215, 220–222
Total body irradiation (TBI), 105, 404, 414–415, 417, 429, 443
Total parenteral nutrition (TPN), 304, 307–308, 314, 317, 325–326,
341, 346–347, 522–523
Toxic-metabolic encephalopathy, 291
Tracheal anastomosis necrosis, 274
Transfusion effect, 106
Transitional model, 359
Transjugular liver biopsy, 427
Transplant coronary artery disease (TxCAD), 24, 28
Transplant ethics, 527
adherence determinations, 535
conflicting ethical obligations in the care of organ donors, 532
dead donor rule, 527
defining death, 528
directed donation, 533
donation after cardiac death (DCD), 528
decision to withdraw life-sustaining treatment, 528–529
evaluation as potential DCD donor, 529
death determination, 529–530
organ procurement process, 530
provision of consent, 529
withdrawal of life-sustaining treatment, 529
donation after brain death, 530
chief criticisms, 531
defining brain death, 531
financial standing, 535
listing at multiple OPOs, 534

Transplant ethics (*cont.*)
  listing of cognitively impaired patients, 535
  opt-in versus presumed consent, 532
  organ allocation, 536
  organ donation markets, 534
  psychosocial evaluation, 535
  solicitation, 533–534
  transplant tourism, 536
Transplant Evaluation Rating Scale (TERS), 21, 22, 379, 544
Transplant mental health, 4, 211, 344
Transplant psychiatrist, 50, 484, 550, 552
Transvenous devices, 215
Tricyclic antidepressants (TCAs), 98, 207, 239, 257, 325, 444, 459, 460
Trimethoprim-sulfamethoxazole, 176, 424, 425
Triple immunosuppression, 105, 321

U
Umbilical cord blood (UCB), 387, 414, 420
Uniform Determination of Death Act (UDDA), 106, 528, 540
United Network for Organ Sharing (UNOS), 11, 12, 17, 20, 49, 50, 52, 57, 66, 106, 164, 188, 201–202, 226, 228, 248, 295, 505–506, 533, 536
United States Preventative Services Task Force (USPSTF), 68
United States Renal Data System (USRDS), 63
Upper extremity transplantation, 371
Ureteric strictures, 115
Ureteroneocystostomy, 113
Uridine 5′-diphosphate glucuronosyltransferase (UGT), 457
Urinary tract infection (UTI), 115, 175
US transplantation data, 17
Uterine transplantation
  ethical considerations, 380–381
  history of, 377, 378
  indications, 377
  psychosocial assessment, 379
    uterine donors, 380
    uterine recipients, 378–380
  VCA versus solid organ transplantation, 378

V
Vagal nerve injury, 280
Valganciclovir, 176, 275, 339
Varenicline, 131, 151, 257
Varicella zoster virus (VZV), 418, 420
Vascular anastomotic complications, 281
Vascularized composite allotransplantation (VCA), 377
  bioethical considerations, 371
  candidate selection, 366
  differences between VCA and solid organ transplantation, 378
  ethical considerations, 380
  factors driving uterine transplantation process, 378
  history, 366, 377, 381
  indications, 377, 381
  limb transplantation, 365
  medical course, 366
  penile transplantation, 381
  pharmacological risk to fetus, 379

psychosocial assessment
  recipients, 378
  donors, 380
psychosocial considerations, 381
psychosocial contraindications, 368
psychological reactions, 368
psychosocial evaluation, 367–370
risk-benefit considerations, 369
steps to successful outcome, 379
uterine transplantation, 377
Venlafaxine, 98, 153, 208, 444, 457, 459
Veno-occlusive disease, 140, 251, 423
Venous thromboembolism (VTE), 280
Ventricular assist devices (VADs), 197, 218
  adverse events, 221
  indications, 197, 218
  mechanism of action, 218
  types, 218–220
Visceral allograft, 307
  acute post-transplant care, 333
  advanced management strategies, 311
  chronic post-transplant care, 334
  complications, 321
    anxiety, 322
    depression, 321
    diabetic distress, 322
    disordered eating behavior, 323
  contraindications, 308
  evaluation for transplantation, 304
  graft function, 316
  history, 307
  indications, 307
  intestinal rehabilitation, 304
  multivisceral-intestinal transplant, 323
  nomenclature, 307
  PN therapy, 304, 314
  psychiatric evaluation pre-transplantation, 324
  quality of life, 316, 334
  rejection, 313
  surgical techniques, 310
  survival, 316
  therapeutic efficacy, 314
  transition to home, 334
  types of visceral allograft, 307
Visual impairment, 356
Volvulus, 301, 302, 308
Voriconazole (azole), 176, 419, 425
VTE, *see* Venous thromboembolism (VTE)
VZV, *see* Varicella zoster virus (VZV)

W
Wernicke-Korsakoff syndrome, 149
West Haven criteria for hepatic encephalopathy, 141
West Nile virus, 418
Wilson's disease (WD), 140, 142, 149

Z
Zaleplon, 96
Zopiclone, 96